CONTEMPORARY CARDIOLOGY

Christopher P. Cannon, MD
Series Editor

Annemarie M. Armani, MD
Executive Editor

For other titles published in this series, go to
www.springer.com/series/7677

José Marín-García, MD

Heart Failure

Bench to Bedside

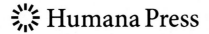 Humana Press

José Marín-García, MD
Director
The Molecular Cardiology and Neuromuscular Institute
Highland Park, NJ
USA
tmci@att.net

ISBN 978-1-60761-146-2   e-ISBN 978-1-60761-147-9
DOI 10.1007/978-1-60761-147-9
Springer New York Dordrecht Heidelberg London

Library of Congress Control Number: 2009943534

Cover illustration: Untitled by Danièle M. Marín

Printed on acid-free paper

Humana Press is a part of Springer Science+Business Media (www.springer.com)

To my wife Danièle, and daughter Mèlanie with love

Preface

Heart Failure (HF), an endemic problem of great magnitude in the world, is essentially the final and common pathway of cardiovascular diseases that result in cardiac systolic and/or diastolic dysfunction. Common underlying disorders in HF include cardiomyopathy, primary or acquired from previous myocardial infarctions, chronic myocardial ischemia, hypertension, diabetes, valvular defects, dysrhythmias, and congenital heart defects. The hallmark of HF is that of relentless clinical progression often manifested as repeated hospitalizations with a significant economic impact to society. Despite considerable clinical and research advances, the morbidity and mortality of HF remain high. Consequently, there is an urgent need to develop new paradigms and to identify novel therapeutic targets for HF.

While invasive and noninvasive procedures such as cardiac catheterization and echocardiography have been for several decades the most important diagnostic tools in children and adults with cardiovascular diseases, presently clinical cardiology is experiencing a period of profound transformation with advances that are changing dramatically our understanding of HF pathophysiology. Upon the completion of the Human Genome Project, new discoveries in molecular and cellular biology have begun to offer significant insights into the basic mechanisms underlying HF, and they are providing clinicians and researchers alike with a large armamentarium of new and largely effective noninvasive diagnostic techniques. With so many new and spectacular developments at hand we believe that this is an appropriate time for a new book on HF that will translate new information from the bench to the bedside. Our goal has been to provide the reader with detailed information of new findings and forthcoming methodologies as well as a critical clinical evaluation of the complex HF syndrome together with available and future therapies. Initially, the clinical phenotypes of HF and known facts concerning its prevalence, relationship to other diseases and incidence in special population defined by age, gender, and ethnicity will be discussed. After that, we will offer the reader clinical terminology employed throughout the book, a primer on gene profiling and bioenergetics of the normal heart and a discussion on molecular, genetic, biochemical, and cellular techniques critical to better understanding HF pathogenesis and pathophysiology. Thenceforth, animal models of HF (one of the most important research tool currently available) will be discussed, including the models of rat coronary artery ligation model, pacing-induced HF, and transgenic animals with either deleted or overexpressed genes. Later, the molecular, genetic, and metabolic variables so far identified in HF, and specific metabolic, signaling pathways, and gene expression patterns that may participate in the causation of HF will be presented. This will be followed by discussions on cardiac remodeling, oxidative stress, and alterations in other organs and systems that are often associated with human HF. Two chapters are specifically dedicated to the pathogenesis and clinical presentation of HF in children together with a comprehensive subsection covering heart transplantation in this age group. This will be followed by another section with two chapters designed to cover basic mechanisms and clinical presentation of HF in the elderly.

Finally in the last four chapters, we will deal with current and forthcoming diagnostic techniques and therapies, including the application of "omics" in HF, pharmaceutical and pharmacogenomic-based individualized medicine, gene and cell-based therapies, and the search for new frontiers.

We have tried to provide the readers of this book with a clear view of current approaches to HF clinical diagnosis and treatment, as well as insightful critiques of original and creative scientific thoughts on postgenomic HF research; however, we are aware of the limitations that a single volume may have to cover in its entirety a subject so complex and extensive as HF.

Nowadays, books dealing with subjects of the complexity and magnitude of HF are often written with the participation of numerous contributors sacrificing at times reading homogeneity. To overcome this potential shortcoming, we purposely decided to limit the number of contributors to only a few hoping that this approach will lend the book a higher sense of homogeneity and clarity.

We hope that new discoveries, innovations, increasing knowledge, and learning will flourish in the future, and hopefully soon there will be no more HF, but until then the work must continue.

> *From the beginning of time,*
> *we are looking for the light,*
> *it is here... it is there.......,*
> *the truth is worth searching.*

José Marín-García, M.D.
Director, The Molecular Cardiology and Neuromuscular Institute,
Highland Park, NJ, USA
tmci@att.net

Contents

Preface.. vii

With Contributions from... xi

Section I   Clinical, Physiology and Genetics Changes in Heart Failure

1   Introduction to Heart Failure 3

2   Cardiac Function in Heart Failure: The Role of Calcium Cycling 15

3   Gene Profiling of the Failing Heart: Epigenetics 23

Section II   Biochemical and Molecular Changes in Heart Failure

4   Bioenergetics and Metabolic Changes in the Failing Heart................. 45

Section III   The Mitochondrial Organelle and the Heart

5   The Multidimensional Role of Mitochondria in Heart Failure 73

Section IV   Experimental Models of Heart Failure

6   Animal Models of Heart Failure................................ 109

Section V   Signaling, Stress and Cellular Changes in Heart Failure

7   Signaling Cascades in Heart Failure: From Cardiomyocytes
     Growth and Survival to Mitochondrial Signaling Pathways 131

8   Cyclic Nucleotides Signaling (Second Messengers)
     and Control of Myocardial Function: Effects of Heart Failure........... 161

9   Calcium Signaling: Receptors, Effectors, and Other
     Signaling Pathways 171

10   Oxidative Stress and Heart Failure... 195

11   Cardiac Remodeling and Cell Death in Heart Failure 213

Section VI   Peripheral Changes and Co-morbid Conditions in Heart Failure

12 **Heart Failure and Changes at the Periphery: Vascular,
    Inflammation, Neurohormonal, and Renal Systems** 235

13 **Comorbidities in Heart Failure** 257

Section VII   Heart Failure in Children

14 **Mechanisms and Clinical Recognition and Management
    of Heart Failure in Infants and Children** 273

15 **Mechanical Circulatory Support and Heart Transplantation
    in Children with Severe Refractory Heart Failure** 297

Section VIII   Aging and the Failing Heart

16 **Basic Mechanisms Mediating Cardiomyopathy
    and Heart Failure in Aging** 315

17 **Heart Failure of Aging: Clinical Considerations** 341

Section IX   Diagnostic Methodology in Heart Failure

18 **Diagnosis of Heart Failure: Evidence-Based Perspective** 353

19 **"Omics" Application in Heart Failure: Novel Diagnostic and Prognostic
    Markers to Understand Pathophysiology and Find New Therapies** 365

Section X   Available and Forthcoming Therapies for Heart Failure

20 **Treatment of Chronic Heart Failure** 379

21 **Gene Therapy in Heart Failure: Forthcoming Therapies** 393

22 **Myocardial Cell-Based Regeneration in Heart Failure** 409

Section XI   Looking to the Future

23 **Future Frontiers in Heart Failure** 431

Glossary 447

Index 459

With Contributions From

Gordon W. Moe, MD
Professor, Department of Medicine
University of Toronto
St. Michael Hospital
Toronto, ON, Canada

Harvey R. Weiss, PhD
Professor, Heart and Brain Circulation Laboratory
Department of Physiology and Biophysics
Robert Wood Johnson Medical School – UMDNJ
Piscataway, NJ, USA

Michael Portman, MD
Professor, Department of Pediatrics
Seattle Children's Hospital and Research Institute
University of Washington
Seattle, WA, USA

Section I
Clinical, Physiology and Genetics Changes in Heart Failure

Chapter 1
Introduction to Heart Failure

Overview

Heart failure (HF) constitutes an important and escalating clinical and public health problem. The overall prevalence of clinically evident HF is around 5–20 cases/1,000 population, but rises to >100 cases/1,000 population in subjects aged >65 years. The overall annual incidence of clinically overt HF in middle-aged men and women is approximately 0.1–0.2%, but with each additional decade of life there is a doubling of the rate. Patients with HF frequently suffer from clinical decompensation requiring hospital admissions. These patients who are admitted and discharged with a diagnosis have a high readmission rate in which these rates appear to be steadily increasing in all industrialized countries, especially among older individuals. In this introductory chapter, contemporary data on the epidemiology, risk factors, as well as the clinical phenotypes of HF will be reviewed.

Introduction

HF is a clinical syndrome that results from any form of cardiac disease that can cause systolic and/or diastolic function or both. HF ensues when the organ is no longer able to generate a cardiac output sufficient to meet the demands of the body without unduly increasing diastolic pressure. As HF may be manifested by symptoms of poor tissue perfusion alone, e.g., fatigue, poor exercise tolerance, confusion or by both symptoms of poor tissue perfusion and congestion of vascular beds, e.g., dyspnea, crackles, pleural effusion, pulmonary edema, distended neck veins, congested liver, peripheral edema, the more general descriptive term HF is preferred over the more restrictive term congestive HF [1].

Prevalence and Incidence

According to the American Heart Association (AHA) 2004 update on heart disease and stroke statistics, 15 million patients are believed to have symptomatic HF worldwide.

In the United States (US), it is estimated that 5 million people have HF and 550,000 new cases are diagnosed each year [2]. In the Framingham study, at the time of entry, 17 of 5,209 persons (3/1,000 cases) screened for HF on the basis of clinical criteria were thought to have HF; all were less that 63 years of age [3]. After 34 years follow up, prevalence rates increased as the cohort matured. The estimated prevalence of HF in the groups aged 50–59, 60–69, 70–79, and >80 years was 8, 23, 49, and 91 cases/1,000 persons, respectively [4]. The National Health and Nutrition Examination Survey (NHANES-1) reported the HF prevalence rate within the US population. Based on self reporting, and using a clinical scoring system, this study screened 14,407 persons of both sexes, aged 25–47 years, between 1971 and 1975, with detailed evaluation of 6,913 subjects and reported a prevalence rate of 20 cases/1,000 [5]. The study of men born in 1913 examined the prevalence of HF in a cohort of 855 Swedish men at ages 50, 54, 57, and 67 years. The prevalence rate of "manifest" HF rose markedly from 21/1,000 at age 50 years to 130/1,000 cases at age 67 years. In Canada, HF affects approximately 490,000 people and accounts for 4,500 deaths each year [6]. Furthermore, there is evidence to indicate that the prevalence of HF is increasing with projected further increases over the next decade (Fig. 1.1) [7]. In the USA, the number of HF incident hospital cases per year is projected to more than double by the year 2025. To keep the current number of incident patients the same as in 1996/97, it is estimated that the incidence of HF would have to decrease by 2.6% per year.

There are less extensive studies that report prevalence but with objective evidence of cardiac dysfunction. A study from Scotland targeted a representative cohort of 2,000 persons aged 25–74 years living north of the River Clyde in Glasgow [8]. Of those selected, 1,640 (83%) underwent a detailed assessment of their cardiovascular status and underwent echocardiography. Left ventricular (LV) systolic dysfunction was defined as a left ventricular ejection fraction (LVEF) <30%. The overall prevalence of LV systolic dysfunction using this criterion was 2.9%. Concurrent symptoms of HF were found in 1.5% of the cohort, while the remaining 1.4% was asymptomatic. Prevalence was both greater in men and it increased with age: in men aged 65–74 years it was 6.4%

J. Marín-García, *Heart Failure*, Contemporary Cardiology,
DOI 10.1007/978-1-60761-147-9_1, © Springer Science+Business Media, LLC 2010

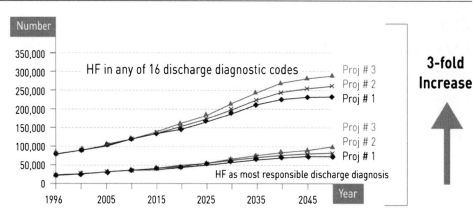

Fig. 1.1 Projected number of incident hospitalizations for heart failure patients, using high, medium and low population growth projections in Canada 1996–2050. It is estimated that the increased longevity of the population alone will result in a doubling of new heart failure (HF) cases by 2025 (Adapted from Johansen et al.[7]. Reproduced with permission of the Can J Cardiol 2003;19(4):430–435)

and in age matched women 4.9%. In a recent study conducted in Minnesota, 21% of the population had mild diastolic dysfunction, 6.6% had moderate diastolic dysfunction, 0.7% had severe diastolic dysfunction, and 5.6% had moderate or severe diastolic dysfunction with normal ejection fraction. The prevalence of any form of systolic dysfunction was 6.0% and moderate or severe systolic dysfunction was 2.0%. HF diagnosis was much more common among those with systolic or diastolic dysfunction than in those with normal ventricular function. Even among those with moderate or severe diastolic or systolic dysfunction, less than 50% had recognized HF. Mild diastolic dysfunction and moderate or severe diastolic dysfunction were predictive of all-cause mortality [9].

Much less has been reported on the incidence when compared to the prevalence of HF. A list of population studies that reported incidence is shown in Table 1.1. In the developed countries, the crude incidence (unadjusted for age) ranges from 1 to 5 cases/1,000 in the general population whereas the crude prevalence of HF ranges from 3 to 20/100, depends on age groups, in the general population [10]. According to the National Heart Lung and Blood Institute (NHLBI) Cardiovascular Health Study (CHS), the annual rates per 1,000 population of new and recurrent HF events for non-black men were estimated to be 21.5 for ages 65–74, 43.3 for ages 75–84, and 73.1 for age 85 and older. For non-black women in the same age groups, the rates are 11.2, 26.3, and 64.9, respectively. For black men, the rates were 21, 52, and 67, and for black women, the rates were 19, 34, and 48, respectively. The most detailed incidence data were reported in the Framingham heart study [4]. At 34 years follow up, the incidence of HF was 2 new cases/1,000 in persons aged 45–54 years increasing to 40 cases/1,000 in men aged between 85 and 94 years. In another report from the Framingham study, at age 40, the lifetime risk of developing HF for both men and women is 1 in 5 [11]. This lifetime risk doubles for people with blood pressure greater than 160/90 mmHg versus those with blood pressure less than 140/90 mmHg.

A more recent study of incidence was from the Hillingdon district of London with a population of approximately 150,000

Table 1.1 Incidence of heart failure from selected population studies.

Study	Location	Incidence
Remes et al. [75]	Eastern Finland	1–4/1,000 (45–74 years)
Ho et al. [4]	Framingham, USA	2/1,000
Rodeheffer et al. [74]	Rochester, USA	1/1,000 (<75 years)
Cowie et al. [12]	London, UK	1/1,000

[12]. In a 15-month period, 122 patients were referred to a special HF clinic. This represented an annual referral rate of 6.5/1,000 population. Using a broad definition of HF, only 29% of these patients were clearly diagnosed as having suffered HF (annual incidence 1.85/1,000 population).

Risk Factors for the Development of Heart Failure

The etiologic importance of associated risk factors for the development of HF depends on the age of the cohort as well as the criteria used to diagnose the disease. Data from the Framingham study into the natural history of coronary heart disease, commenced in the United States in 1949, provided insight into the modifiable risk factors of HF [13]. When these factors are examined in relation to HF, the population-attributable rate for high blood pressure was the greatest, accounting for 39% of HF in men and 59% in women. Previous myocardial infarction, despite its much lower prevalence in the population (3–10%), was the second commonest contributor to HF in men (34%) and in women (13%). Valvular heart diseases accounted for 7–8% of HF. In the subsequent years of follow up, coronary heart disease become increasingly prevalent as the identified new cases of HF, increasing from 22% in the 1950s to closed to 70% in the 1970s. During the same period, the relative contribution of hypertension and valvular heart disease declined (Fig. 1.2).

Other less common but equally important risk factors for HF are diseases of the heart muscle (cardiomyopathy)

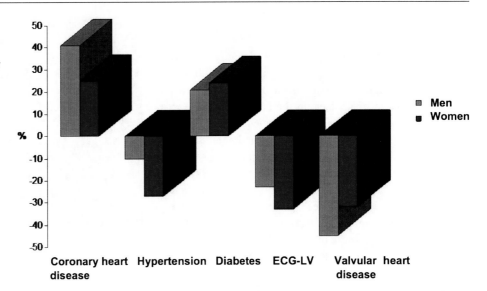

Fig. 1.2 Changes in the etiologic factors in heart failure over time. Changes in causal factors for heart failure in the Framingham heart study during the period 1950–1987

due to alcohol abuse or infections, diabetes, and obesity [14]. Diabetes remains a strong risk factor for the development of HF. Diabetic women with elevated body mass index (BMI) or depressed creatinine clearance are at particularly high risk with annual incidence rates of 7 and 13%, respectively. Among nondiabetic women with no risk factors, the annual incidence rate is only 0.4%. The rate increases with each additional risk factor, and nondiabetic women with three or more risk factors had an annual incidence of 3.4%. Among diabetic participants with no additional risk factors, the annual incidence of HF was 3.0% compared with 8.2% among diabetics with at least three additional risk factors. Diabetics with fasting glucose >300 mg/dL had a threefold adjusted risk of developing heart failure, compared with diabetics with controlled fasting blood sugar levels [15].

Mortality and Morbidity

Patients with HF experience significant mortality and morbidity [2, 7, 8, 16]. Based on the long term follow-up of the Framingham Heart Study reported in the AHA 2006 update, 80% of men and 70% of women under age 65 who have HF die within 8 years. After HF is diagnosed, survival is poorer in men than in women, but fewer than 15% of women survive more than 8–12 years. The 1-year mortality rate is particularly high, with one in five dying after this period. In the original and subsequent Framingham cohort, the probability of someone with a diagnosis of HF dying within 5 years was 62 and 75% in men and 38 and 42% in women, respectively. The Rochester epidemiology project also described the prognosis in 107 patients presenting to associated hospitals with new onset HF in 1981, and 141 patients presenting in 1991. The median follow up in

these cohorts was 1,061 and 1,233 days, respectively. The mean age of the 1981 patients was 75 years, rising to 77 years in 1991. The 1- and 5-year mortality was, respectively, 28 and 66% in the 1981 cohort and 23 and 67% in the 1991 cohort [17, 18]. The NHANES-I initially evaluated 14,407 adults aged 25 and 74 years in the US between 1971 and 1975 [5]. Follow up studies were carried out in 1982–84 and again in 1986, for those aged >55 years and alive during the 1982–84 review. The estimated 10-year mortality in subjects aged 25–74 years with self-reported HF was 42.8% (49.8% in men and 36% in women). Mortality in those aged 65–74 years was 65.4% (71.8 and 59.5% in men and women, respectively). These mortality rates are considerably lower than those observed in Framingham. Patients in NHANES-I were non-institutionalized and their HF was self reported. Follow up was incomplete. NHANES-I was also carried out in a more recent period of time than Framingham when prognosis in HF patients may have improved. Framingham investigators in 1993 looked at patients developing HF in the period 1948–1988 and the Rochester investigators in the period 1981–1991. In both these studies, no temporal change in prognosis was identified.

Hospital admissions for HF constitute an important clinical outcome particularly in more recent clinical trials. Hospital admission rates for several developed countries are shown in Fig. 1.2. Hospitalization for HF is a growing problem globally. In the US, HF continues to be the commonest cause of hospital admission in subjects over the age of 65 years [19]. In the United Kingdom (UK), in the early 1990s, 0.2% of the population was hospitalized for HF per annum and that such admissions accounted for more than 5% of adult general medicine and geriatric hospital admissions, outnumbering those associated with acute coronary syndromes [20]. Hospital admission is frequently prolonged and in many instances followed by readmission within a short time. In Canada, based on 1996/1997 data on 40,958 males and 42,255 females and within the first year, HF patients used an average of 26.9 hospital days and nearly 50% were readmitted to hospital [7]. In the UK, the mean length of stay for a HF related admission in 1990 was 11.4 days in the acute medical wards and 28.5 days in the acute geriatric wards. Within the UK, about one third of patients are readmitted within 12 months of discharge [20]. Hospital admission data for HF in the US are in general very similar [19]. It should be pointed out that these hospital readmission rates are far higher than the other major causes of hospitalization such as stroke and hip fractures. Indeed, in any healthcare delivery system, hospital admissions represent more than one-half of the healthcare expenditure of HF.

There exists some evidence, however, that the overall prognosis of HF may be improving over time. The National Swedish registers on hospital discharges and cause-specific deaths were used to calculate age- and sex-specific trends and sex ratios for HF admissions and deaths [21]. The study included all men and women 45–84 years old hospitalized for the first time for HF in 19 Swedish counties between 1988 and 2000, a mean annual population 2.9 million. A total of 156,919 hospital discharges were included. In 1988, a total of 267 men and 205 women/100,000 inhabitants (age adjusted) were discharged for the first time with a principal diagnosis of HF. After 1993 a yearly decrease was observed, with 237 men and 171 women/100,000 inhabitants discharged during 2000. The 30-day mortality also decreased significantly. The decrease in 1-year mortality was more pronounced in the younger age groups, with a total reduction in mortality of 69% among men and 80% among women aged 45–54 years. The annual decrease was 9% among men and 10% among women aged 45–54 years (95% CI −7 to −12% and −6 to −14% respectively) and 4% among men and 5% among women (95% CI −4 to −5% for both) aged 75–84 years. In spite of this encouraging trend, the 1-year mortality after the first hospitalization for HF is still high. Similarly, a study from Scotland also reported a reduction in 30-day and 1-year case fatality rates among hospitalized patients between 1986 and 1995 [22].

Economic Burden of Heart Failure

Heart failure can incur significant financial burden to societies. The direct and indirect cost of HF in the United States for 2006 is estimated to be $29.6 billion. In 2001, $4.0 billion ($5,912 per discharge) was paid to Medicare beneficiaries for management of HF. In Canada, the annual cost of managing HF patients with NYHA class III/IV symptoms is estimated to be C$1.4–2.3 billion [23]. Figure 1.3 demonstrates that heart failure consumes 1–2% of the total healthcare

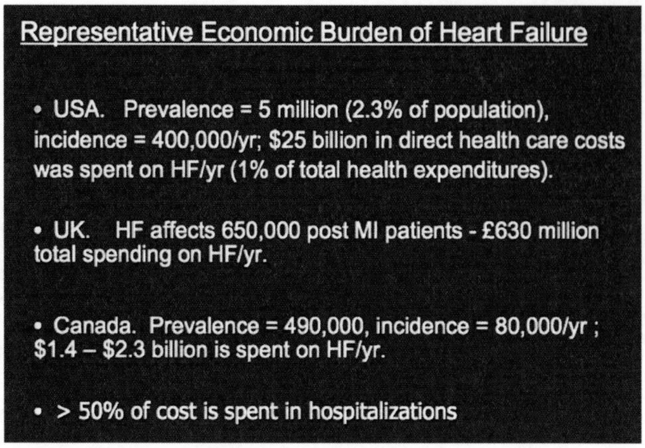

Fig. 1.3 Economic burden of heart failure. Cost of managing heart failure, absolute dollars, and percent of total health care expenditure

expenditure in a number of industrialized countries. Over half of the cost associated with the management of HF is spent on hospital admissions.

Gender, Age, and Ethnicity

Women, the elderly and non-White minorities are typically underrepresented in HF randomized controlled trials [24]. In recent years, however, a great deal of attention has been placed on gender differences, particularly women in cardiovascular disease [25–27]. It is not surprising that the possibility of gender differences in HF has captured some attention. Women with HF have been shown to have a better prognosis than men in both the Framingham cohort [28] as well as in more recent clinical trials [29]. Women also tend to have a higher prevalence of non-ischemic etiologies for HF when compared with men [29]. However, these findings are not entirely uniform. In the population-based Framingham study [3, 4], the prognosis of women was significantly better than men after the onset of symptoms of HF. The median survival time was 1.7 years in men and 3.2 years in women and the 5-year survival rate was 25% in men and 38% in women. In the intervention trials such as the Studies of Left Ventricular Dysfunction (SOLVD) registry, poorer outcome was reported in women than in men at least in the short term [30]. Using the UNC Heart Failure Database at the University of North Carolina, the natural history of patients with HF was studied prospectively to determine whether gender was an independent risk factor for mortality [31]. Follow-up data were available in 99% of patients (mean follow-up period 2.4 years) after study entry, and 201 patients reached the primary study end point of all-cause mortality. By life-table analysis, women were significantly less likely to reach this primary end point than men ($p < 0.001$). A significant association was found between female gender and better survival ($p < 0.001$), which depended on the primary etiology of HF ($p = 0.008$ for the gender–etiology interaction) but not on baseline cardiac function. Women survived longer than men when HF was due to nonischemic causes (men versus women: relative risk [RR] 2.36, 95% confidence interval [CI] 1.59–3.51, $p < 0.001$). In contrast, outcome appeared similar when HF was due to ischemic heart disease (men vs. women: RR 0.85, 95% CI 0.45–1.61, $p = 0.651$). In the Cardiac Insufficiency Bisoprolol Study (CIBIS) II, women ($n = 515$) differed from men ($n = 2,132$) with regard to age, NYHA functional classification, primary cause of HF, and risk factors such as left bundle-branch block [32]. After adjustment for baseline differences, the probability of all-cause mortality was significantly smaller by 36% in women compared with that in men (hazard ratio 0.64, 95% CI 0.47–0.86, $p = 0.003$). Women also had a 39% reduction in cardiovascular deaths (hazard ratio 0.64, 95% CI 0.45–0.91, $p = 0.01$) and a 70% reduction in deaths from pump failure (hazard ratio 0.30, 95% CI 0.13–0.70, $p = 0.005$) compared with men.

The overall quality of care for HF patients has been shown not to differ with gender, although there are also reported gender differences in specific areas in the management and access to care. For example, general practitioners more often treat elderly, female patients with HF than cardiologists [33]. Physicians were also less likely to record findings from the initial physical examination of women [34–36], and women also underwent fewer procedures [20, 36, 37]. Women were less often managed by cardiologists and more seldom referred to a teaching hospital or transferred to other acute-care hospitals than men [20, 34–36, 38]. Compared to women, men had a shorter stay in hospital [20, 36] and lower hospital management costs [36]. There are inconsistent results regarding gender differences with regard to hospital admission. In the SOLVD studies [30], women had a higher annual admission rate than men, whereas Opasich et al. [39] reported no differences between women and men in annual admissions. Readmission rates have been shown to be independent of gender [20, 40] or lower in women [41]. Women with HF tend to be older, suffer from more comorbidities [36], and more likely to be widowed and live alone when the demands due to their illness increase. Women with HF are therefore more likely to need home health aid after hospitalization [42], are more often discharged to skilled nursing facilities and receive more home care post-discharge [34, 36]. It is unclear whether these differences in very specific areas would influence clinical outcomes in the women *versus* men.

As reviewed earlier, HF is the leading cause of hospitalization in the elderly and is therefore the major source of morbidity and mortality in this population. Elderly patients may differ from younger individuals in terms of biologic characteristics and management. Accurate diagnosis of the HF syndrome at older age is complicated by increasing prevalence of atypical symptoms and signs. Exertional dyspnea, orthopnea, lower extremity edema, and impaired exercise tolerance are the cardinal symptoms of HF. However, with increasing age, often accompanied by reduced physical activity, exertional symptoms become less prominent [43]. A prominent feature that distinguishes HF that occurs in the elderly from the younger individuals is the much higher frequency of HF occurring in the absence of systolic dysfunction, i.e., diastolic HF or HF with preserved systolic function [44].

A small number of randomized trials of therapies conducted specifically in the elderly populations, in conjunction with a multitude of data from observational data sets, suggest that most recommendations on HF therapies are applicable to elderly patients. Observational data suggest that ACE inhibitor use in elderly HF patients may preserve cognition, slow functional decline, and reduce hospitalizations and perhaps even mortality, even in patients with relative contraindications such as mild to moderate renal impairment [45]. The β-blocker nebivolol has been studied in over 2,000 patients ≥70 years with clinical evidence of HF, regardless of ejection fraction [46]. After follow up of less than 2 years, a significant benefit for nebivolol was seen with reduction of the combined primary end point of mortality and cardiovascular hospitalization. Elderly patients are vulnerable to adverse drug events (ADE), due to the growing complexity of medication regimens, age-related physiologic changes, and a higher burden of co-morbid illnesses. Cardiovascular medications are frequently associated with ADE in the elderly [47]. Digitalis toxicity can occur at therapeutic serum levels [48]. Falls constitute common clinical presentations of ADE in the elderly, often from postural hypotension. In randomized trials of drug treatment for HF, titration to target doses is less frequently successful in older patients due to higher side effect rates.

Several systematic reviews support the role of HF management programs in elderly HF patient populations [49]. While active involvement of caregivers in patient monitoring and medication adjustment is common to studies showing benefit, the optimal way of providing HF management remains controversial. The precise design of such care delivery systems depends in part upon local resources and infrastructure. Comprehensive geriatric assessment, shown to improve function, prevent hospitalization and institutionalization, reduce the risk of adverse drug reactions, and improve sub-optimal prescribing, may have a role to play in the management of frail elderly patients with HF.

Racial differences in the epidemiology and outcomes of HF have been inferred [50]. However, to gain certainty and insights with such differences would require studies of reasonable sample size that provide simultaneous comparison of two ethnic populations. Because the distribution of ethnic population differs between countries and geographic regions, such comparisons are frequently not feasible. The only racial comparison that is mostly frequently conducted is that between African Americans and the white population in the United States. However, such observations often yielded different results.

Such potential differences in incidence and case fatality of HF in the US were recently examined in the Atherosclerosis Risk in Communities (ARIC) population-based cohort followed from 1987 to 2002 [51]. The age-adjusted incidence rate (per 1,000 person-years) for Caucasian women, 3.4, was significantly less compared with all other groups (Caucasian men, 6.0; African-American women, 8.1; African-American men, 9.1). Age-adjusted HF incidence rates were greater for African-Americans than Caucasians, but adjustment for confounders attenuated the difference. The adjusted African-American-to-Caucasian hazard ratio was 0.86 (95% CI 0.70–1.06) for men, and 0.93 (95% confidence interval, 0.46–1.90) for women during the second half of follow-up. The hazard ratio (HR) for women during the first half of follow-up was 1.79 (95% confidence interval, 1.25–2.55). Thirty-day, 1-year, and 5-year case fatalities following hospitalization for HF were 10.4, 22, and 42.3%, respectively. African-Americans had a greater 5-year case fatality compared with Caucasians ($p<0.05$). HF incidence rates in African-American women were therefore more comparable to those of men than of Caucasian women. The greater HF incidence in African-Americans than in Caucasians was largely explained by African-Americans' greater levels of atherosclerotic risk factors.

The association between race and the natural history of HF has recently been examined in a propensity-matched population of chronic HF from the Digitalis Investigation Group (DIG) trial in which baseline characteristics were balanced between the races [50]. Propensity scores for being nonwhite were calculated for each patient and were used to match 1,018 pairs of white and nonwhite patients. Matched Cox regression analyses were used to estimate associations of race with outcomes during 38 months of median follow-up. All-cause mortality occurred in 34% (rate, 1,180/10,000 person-years) of whites and 33% (rate, 1,130/10,000 person-years) of nonwhite patients (HR when nonwhite patients were compared with whites, 0.95, 95% CI 0.80–1.14; $p=0.593$). All-cause hospitalization occurred in 63% (rate, 3,616/10,000 person-years) of whites and 65% (rate, 3,877/10,000 person-years) of nonwhite patients (HR, 1.03, 95% CI 0.90–1.18; $p=0.701$). Respective hazard ratios (95% CI) for other outcomes were: 0.95 (0.75–1.12) for cardiovascular mortality, 0.82 (0.60–1.11) for HF mortality, 1.05 (0.91–1.22) for cardiovascular hospitalization, and 1.17 (0.98–1.39) for HF hospitalization. Therefore, in a propensity-matched population of HF patients where whites and nonwhites were balanced in all measured baseline characteristics, there appeared to be no racial differences in major

natural history end points. Using the Acute Decompensated Heart Failure National Registry (ADHERE), race-related differences in presentation, treatment, in-patient experiences, and short-term mortality due to acute decompensated HF (ADHF) were analyzed [52]. Demographic and mortality differences in African American and white patients with ADHF entered into the database from its initiation in September 2001 to December 31, 2004. A total of 105,872 episodes of ADHF occurred in white patients and 29,862 occurred in African American patients. African American patients with ADHF were younger than white patients (mean [SD] age, 63.5 [15.4] versus 72.5 [12.5] years) and had lower mean LVEF. The prevalence of hypertension, diabetes mellitus, and obesity was higher in African American patients. African American race was associated with lower in-hospital mortality after adjustment for known predictors (2.1% versus 4.5%; adjusted odds ratio [OR], 0.79; 95% CI 0.72–0.87; $p<0.001$). This association persisted for all age cohorts, was independent of the use of intravenous drugs, and was especially present in African American patients in the nonischemic subgroup (adjusted OR, 0.74; 95% CI 0.57–0.96), but not the ischemic subgroup (adjusted OR, 0.91; 95% CI 0.76–1.09). In this analysis, African American race is therefore associated with lower in-hospital mortality from ADHF compared with white race, despite certain indicators of increased disease severity.

Multiracial Singapore offers an ideal setting to study racial differences in various aspects HF from ethnic groups other than the comparisons of whites and African American that have been explored extensively in the US. In a recent study conducted in Singapore, 668 HF patients, consisting of Chinese (72%), Malays (17.1%), and Indians (10.9%) were prospectively followed up for 24 ± 12 months [53]. Primary outcome measure was the composite endpoint of all-cause mortality or HF readmission. Composite endpoints occurred in 198 (29.6%) patients (133 deaths, 112 HF readmissions). Diabetes mellitus, peripheral vascular disease, and hyperlipidemia were more prevalent in Indians compared to Malays or Chinese (all $p<0.05$). Indians and Malays had higher composite endpoint rates compared to the Chinese ($p=0.01$). Although Indians and Malays had higher HF readmission rates compared to the Chinese ($p<0.01$), a trend towards a higher all-cause mortality rate was seen in Malays ($p=0.12$). Malay race was an independent predictor of the composite endpoint (OR=1.65, 95% CI=1.04–2.63, $p=0.034$), as were age, diabetes mellitus, ischemic cardiomyopathy, β-blocker use, and NYHA class (all $p<0.05$). Therefore, in the multiracial Singapore heart failure population, Indians and Malays had a worse outcome compared to the Chinese, due to higher heart failure readmission rates in Indians and higher mortality and HF readmission rates in Malays. While the worse outcome in Indians may be due to the greater prevalence of diabetes mellitus and atherosclerotic vascular disease, the cause of the poorer prognosis in Malays remains unclear.

There also appear to be very subtle racial differences in terms of quality of care and access to healthcare in heart failure. In the recently published Organized Program to Initiate Lifesaving Treatment in Hospitalized Patients with Heart Failure (OPTIMIZE-HF) registry, data on quality of care measures and outcomes were analyzed for 8,608 African-American patients compared with 38,501 non-African-American patients [54]. African Americans were significantly younger and more likely to receive evidence-based medications but less likely to receive discharge instructions and smoking cessation counseling. In multivariable analyses, African-American race was an independent predictor of lower in-hospital mortality (odds ratio 0.71; 95% confidence interval 0.57–0.87; $p < 0.001$) but similar hospital length of stay. After multivariable adjustment, post-discharge outcomes were similar for American-American and non-African-American patients, but African-American race was associated with higher ACE inhibitor prescription and LV assessment; no other HF quality indicators were influenced by race. In the context of a performance-improvement program as in OPTIMIZE-HF, African Americans with HF received similar or better treatment with evidence-based medications, less discharge counseling, had better in-hospital survival, and similar adjusted risk of follow-up death/repeat hospital stay. In another longitudinal comparative study from eight participant sites in the US, propensity scores were used to adjust for sociodemographic and clinical differences among the ethnic/racial groups [55]. Health-related quality of life was measured using the Minnesota Living with Heart Failure Questionnaire. Significant racial effects were demonstrated, with more favorable Minnesota Living with Heart Failure Questionnaire total scores post-baseline for Hispanic patients compared with both black and white patients, after adjusting for baseline scores, age, gender, education, severity of illness, and care setting (acute vs. chronic), and estimating the treatment effect (intervention vs. usual care). The models based on the physical and emotional subscale scores were similar, with post hoc comparisons indicating more positive outcomes for Hispanic patients than non-Hispanic white patients. To assess the impact of race on healthcare utilization and outcomes in veterans with HF, 4,901 black and 17,093 white veterans hospitalized for HF in 153 Veterans Health Administration (VA) hospital evaluated retrospectively. [56]. The risk-adjusted odds ratios (OR) for 30-day and 2-year mortality in black versus white patients were 0.70 (95% CI 0.60–0.82) and 0.84 (95% CI 0.78–0.91), respectively. In the year following discharge, blacks had the same rate of readmissions as whites. Blacks had a lower rate of medical outpatient clinic visits and a higher rate of urgent care/emergency room visits than whites, although these differences were small. In a system where there is equal access to healthcare, the racial gap in patterns of healthcare utilization is relatively small.

Clinical Phenotypes of Heart Failure

Systolic vs. Diastolic Heart Failure

Systolic and isolated diastolic failure, the latter also known as HF with preserved systolic function, are two phenotypes of HF commonly encountered in clinical practice. Traditionally, HF has been attributed to systolic dysfunction of the left ventricle (LV) and until recently, resources have been invested mostly to understanding the pathophysiology and treatment of systolic HF. As a result, clinicians who manage patients with systolic HF can rely on practice guidelines that are supported by strong evidence from large-scale clinical trials. Over the past decade, there has been a steady rise in the prevalence of HF in those with a preserved systolic function (PSF), related in part to increasing recognition of this condition [57]. In general, patients with HF with PSF can be defined as those with symptomatic HF that occur in the setting of a measured left ventricular ejection fraction ≥40–45% [58, 59]. Thus, the bedside and radiographic findings of the two phenotypes are almost indistinguishable although the epidemiology differs between the two phenotypes. HF with PSF has not been studied as extensively as HF with systolic dysfunction and there is relatively little information on pathophysiology and therefore little evidence-based recommendation to guide the clinicians. This clinical phenotype is frequently equated with diastolic HF [60]. However, not every patient with HF and PSF necessarily has demonstrable diastolic dysfunction, such as that demonstrated on echocardiography, while subjects with objective evidence of diastolic dysfunction, do not necessarily have symptoms [61].

Recent data indicate that 30–55% of patients with HF have PSF [17, 62, 63]. In a large population based study, 8% of persons older than 65 years were found to have HF, and 55% of the patients with HF were noted to have normal LVEF [63]. The same study also found patients with HF and PSF to be twice as likely to have diabetes mellitus as asymptomatic control subjects. In addition, patients with this form of HF are more likely to be older and female and more likely to have a history of hypertension [17, 63, 64].

Similar reductions in quality of life, as measured on standard HF indices, have been noted for patients with the two clinical phenotypes [65]. Patients with either phenotype have significantly decreased peak exercise performance compared with healthy control subjects. Exercise performance, as measured by lactate levels, is also markedly decreased in both when compared with healthy control subjects [65]. Furthermore, for patients hospitalized with HF, readmission rates for patients with an ejection fraction greater than 50% were similar to those with ejection fraction less than 50% [58]. As HF with PSF causes at least as many hospitalization, this condition is also responsible for roughly the same healthcare expenditures as systolic HF [57, 66].

Patients with HF and PSF have similar or lower mortality compared to patients with systolic HF. The Veterans Administration Cooperative Study, an intervention multi-center trial, found that patients with HF and PSF had an annual mortality of 8%; whereas those with a reduced ejection fraction had a 19% annual mortality [67]. Results from the United Kingdom Heart Failure Evaluation and Assessment of Risk Trial (UK-HEART) study reported a 5-year mortality of 25.2% for HF with PSF versus 41.5% for those with reduced systolic function [68]. Analysis of Framingham data also demonstrated a significant difference in mortality between the two phenotypes, annual mortality for PSF of 8.7% versus 3.0% for age-matched control subjects, and for systolic HF 18.9% versus 4.1% for age-matched control subjects [62]. By contrast, a study of newly diagnosed HF in Olmsted County found no difference in mortality between those with preserved and impaired ejection fraction [17].

Acute Heart Failure Syndromes

Although acute HF, often manifested by an acute onset of dyspnea, is likely one of the oldest described clinical syndromes, it was not until recently that this syndrome has received attention from clinicians and researchers. Acute HF syndromes (AHFS) have recently been defined as HF with a relatively rapid onset of signs and symptoms, often resulting in hospitalization or unplanned office or emergency room visits [69]. With only a handful of randomized trials over the past 5 years investigating new treatments of acute decompensated HF, the field has recently received increasing attention.

The Heart Failure Society of America distinguishes patients with AHFS to three categories [70]:

1. The majority of patients hospitalized with acute HF has evidence of hypertension on admission and frequently has preserved systolic function.
2. Most hospitalized patients have volume overload and congestive symptoms.
3. Only a minority have severely impaired systolic function, reduced blood pressure, and symptoms reflective of low cardiac output and poor tissue perfusion.

The European Society of Cardiology also classified acute heart HF patients in six categories (Table 1.2), which is based on newer concepts of AHFS, and which may carry prognostic information [71]. For example, hypertensive acute pulmonary edema likely has a lower mortality rate

Table 1.2 Classification of acute heart failure syndrome based on clinical presentation and pathophysiology [71]

1. Acute decompensated heart failure (do novo or as decompensated from chronic heart failure) with signs and symptoms of acute heart failure, which are mild and do not fulfill criteria of cardiogenic shock, pulmonary edema, or hypertensive crisis
2. Hypertensive acute heart failure: signs and symptoms of acute heart failure are accompanied by high blood pressure and relatively preserved left ventricular function and chest radiograph compatible with pulmonary edema
3. Pulmonary edema (verified by chest X-ray) accompanied by severe respiratory distress, with crackles over the lung and orthopnea, with oxygen saturation usually less than 90% on room air prior to treatment
4. Cardiogenic shock: Cardiogenic shock is defined as evidence of poor tissue perfusion induced by heart failure after correction of preload. Cardiogenic shock is usually characterized by reduced blood pressure (systolic blood pressure <90 mmHg or a drop of mean arterial pressure >30 mmHg) with a pulse rate >60 beats/min with or without evidence of organ congestion
5. High output failure is characterized by high cardiac output, usually with high heart rate, with warm peripheries, pulmonary congestion, and sometimes with low blood pressure as in septic shock
6. Right heart failure is characterized by low output syndrome with increased jugular venous pressure, increased liver size, and hypotension

Table 1.3 Physical findings in patients with phenotype of acute heart failure symptoms

• Prior history of heart failure
• Dyspnea on exertion, orthopnea, or paroxysmal nocturnal dyspnea
• Fatigue
• Increasing edema, weight, or abdominal girth
Physical examination
• Elevated jugular venous pressure
• Peripheral edema or ascites
• Rales, hypoxia or tachypnea
• Tachycardia, arrhythmia
• Diffuse point of maximal intensity
• Ventricular filling gallop (S3)
• Atrial gallop (S4)
• Cool extremities above the hands and feet
• Poor urine output

than decompensated HF with low blood pressure [72]. The rapid diagnosis of acute decompensated HF is necessary to initiate appropriate treatment. Failure to do so increases the need for mechanical ventilatory support, delays hospital discharge, and inflates treatment costs. Unfortunately, the signs and symptoms of acute heart failure often overlap with those of other common medical conditions, particularly chronic obstructive pulmonary disease. In addition, because of the heterogeneous nature of acute decompensated HF, no single finding is perfect for diagnosis, and instead, a broad array of signs and symptoms are associated with the condition (Table 1.3) [73]. Evidence of meaningful outcome benefits with current therapies for acute decompensated HF is often lacking.

Summary

- Heart Failure (HF) is an important clinical and public health problem world wide.
- The overall prevalence of clinically identified HF is estimated to be 3–20 cases/1,000 population, but rises to >100 cases/1,000 population in those aged >65 years.
- Although reported incidence rates are higher in men than women, greater longevity in women balances overall prevalence rates on a sex specific basis.
- The overall annual incidence of clinically overt HF in middle aged men and women is approximately 0.1–0.2%. In each additional decade of life, there is an approximate doubling of this rate and the incidence of HF in those aged >85 years is about 2–3%.
- Annual hospital admission rates for heart failure range from 10 to 40 admissions/10,000 population and increased to >75 admissions/10,000 population in those aged >65 years.
- HF admission rates are increasing in all industrialized countries, especially among older individuals.
- Gender and racial differences in specific parameters related to the natural history and management of HF have been reported. However, there are no systematic differences in any of these parameters with significant variations in observations between studies.

Primer of Terminology

Prevalence. Prevalence is a statistical concept referring to the number of cases of a disease. The prevalence of HF is therefore the proportion of individuals in a population having HF at a given time.

Incidence. Incidence is the number of newly diagnosed cases of HF during a specific period of time. The incidence is distinct from the prevalence, which refers to the number of cases alive on a certain date.

Diastolic heart failure or heart failure with preserved systolic function. HF with PSF can be defined as those cases with symptomatic HF that occur in the setting of a measured left ventricular ejection fraction ≥40–45%.

Acute heart failure. Acute HF or acute heart failure syndromes (AHFS) are HF with a relatively rapid onset of signs and symptoms, often resulting in hospitalization or unplanned office or emergency room visits.

References

1. (2006) Executive summary: HFSA 2006 Comprehensive Heart Failure Practice Guideline. J Card Fail 12:10–38
2. Thom T, Haase N, Rosamond W et al (2006) Heart disease and stroke statistics – 2006 update: a report from the American Heart Association Statistics Committee and Stroke Statistics Subcommittee. Circulation 113:e85–e151
3. McKee PA, Castelli WP, McNamara PM, Kannel WB (1971) The natural history of congestive heart failure: the Framingham study. N Engl J Med 285:1441–1446
4. Ho KK, Pinsky JL, Kannel WB, Levy D (1993) The epidemiology of heart failure: the Framingham Study. J Am Coll Cardiol 22:6A–13A
5. Schocken DD, Arrieta MI, Leaverton PE, Ross EA (1992) Prevalence and mortality rate of congestive heart failure in the United States. J Am Coll Cardiol 20:301–306
6. Heart and Stroke Foundation of Canada (2002) Hospital Morbidity Database 2000/2001
7. Johansen H, Strauss B, Arnold JM, Moe G, Liu P (2003) On the rise: the current and projected future burden of congestive heart failure hospitalization in Canada. Can J Cardiol 19:430–435
8. McDonagh TA, Morrison CE, Lawrence A et al (1997) Symptomatic and asymptomatic left-ventricular systolic dysfunction in an urban population. Lancet 350:829–833
9. Redfield MM, Jacobsen SJ, Burnett JC Jr, Mahoney DW, Bailey KR, Rodeheffer RJ (2003) Burden of systolic and diastolic ventricular dysfunction in the community: appreciating the scope of the heart failure epidemic. JAMA 289:194–202
10. McMurray JJ, Stewart S (2000) Epidemiology, aetiology, and prognosis of heart failure. Heart 83:596–602
11. Lloyd-Jones DM, Larson MG, Leip EP et al (2002) Lifetime risk for developing congestive heart failure: the Framingham Heart Study. Circulation 106:3068–3072
12. Cowie MR, Wood DA, Coats AJ et al (1999) Incidence and aetiology of heart failure; a population-based study. Eur Heart J 20: 421–428
13. Kannel WB, Belanger AJ (1991) Epidemiology of heart failure. Am Heart J 121:951–957
14. Cohn JN (1998) Preventing congestive heart failure. Am Fam Physician 57:1901–1904
15. Bibbins-Domingo K, Lin F, Vittinghoff E et al (2004) Predictors of heart failure among women with coronary disease. Circulation 110:1424–1430
16. Arnold JM, Howlett JG, Dorian P et al (2007) Canadian Cardiovascular Society Consensus Conference recommendations on heart failure update 2007: prevention, management during intercurrent illness or acute decompensation, and use of biomarkers. Can J Cardiol 23:21–45
17. Senni M, Tribouilloy CM, Rodeheffer RJ et al (1998) Congestive heart failure in the community: a study of all incident cases in Olmsted County, Minnesota, in 1991. Circulation 98:2282–2289
18. Senni M, Tribouilloy CM, Rodeheffer RJ et al (1999) Congestive heart failure in the community: trends in incidence and survival in a 10-year period. Arch Intern Med 159:29–34
19. Haldeman GA, Croft JB, Giles WH, Rashidee A (1999) Hospitalization of patients with heart failure: National Hospital Discharge Survey, 1985 to 1995. Am Heart J 137:352–360
20. McMurray J, McDonagh T, Morrison CE, Dargie HJ (1993) Trends in hospitalization for heart failure in Scotland 1980–1990. Eur Heart J 14:1158–1162
21. Schaufelberger M, Swedberg K, Koster M, Rosen M, Rosengren A (2004) Decreasing one-year mortality and hospitalization rates for heart failure in Sweden; Data from the Swedish Hospital Discharge Registry 1988 to 2000. Eur Heart J 25:300–307
22. MacIntyre K, Capewell S, Stewart S et al (2000) Evidence of improving prognosis in heart failure: trends in case fatality in 66 547 patients hospitalized between 1986 and 1995. Circulation 102:1126–1131
23. Bentkover JD, Stewart EJ, Ignaszewski A, Lepage S, Liu P, Cooper J (2003) New technologies and potential cost savings related to

morbidity and mortality reduction in Class III/IV heart failure patients in Canada. Int J Cardiol 88:33–41

24. Heiat A, Gross CP, Krumholz HM (2002) Representation of the elderly, women, and minorities in heart failure clinical trials. Arch Intern Med 162:1682–1688

25. Chou AF, Scholle SH, Weisman CS, Bierman AS, Correa-de-Araujo R, Mosca L (2007) Gender disparities in the quality of cardiovascular disease care in private managed care plans. Womens Health Issues 17:120–130

26. Oliveira CC, Cardoso CR, Rodrigues LH et al (2009) Gender impact on in-hospital outcomes after percutaneous coronary intervention. Int J Cardiol 133:106–109

27. Ordovas JM (2007) Gender, a significant factor in the cross talk between genes, environment, and health. Gend Med 4 Suppl B:S111–S122.

28. Levy D, Larson MG, Vasan RS, Benjamin EJ, Murabito JM (2000) Temporal trends in mortality following the onset of heart failure in subjects from the Framingham Heart Study (abstract). Circulation 102, II412.

29. Frazier CG, Alexander KP, Newby LK et al (2007) Associations of gender and etiology with outcomes in heart failure with systolic dysfunction: a pooled analysis of 5 randomized control trials. J Am Coll Cardiol 49:1450–1458

30. Bourassa MG, Gurne O, Bangdiwala SI et al (1993) Natural history and patterns of current practice in heart failure. The Studies of Left Ventricular Dysfunction (SOLVD) Investigators. J Am Coll Cardiol 22:14A–19A

31. Adams KF Jr, Dunlap SH, Sueta CA et al (1996) Relation between gender, etiology and survival in patients with symptomatic heart failure. J Am Coll Cardiol 28:1781–1788

32. Simon T, Mary-Krause M, Funck-Brentano C, Jaillon P (2001) Sex differences in the prognosis of congestive heart failure: results from the Cardiac Insufficiency Bisoprolol Study (CIBIS II). Circulation 103:375–380

33. Rutten FH, Grobbee DE, Hoes AW (2003) Differences between general practitioners and cardiologists in diagnosis and management of heart failure: a survey in every-day practice. Eur J Heart Fail 5:337–344

34. Ayanian JZ, Weissman JS, Chasan-Taber S, Epstein AM (1999) Quality of care by race and gender for congestive heart failure and pneumonia. Med Care 37:1260–1269

35. Clarke KW, Gray D, Hampton JR (1994) Evidence of inadequate investigation and treatment of patients with heart failure. Br Heart J 71:584–587

36. Philbin EF, DiSalvo TG (1998) Influence of race and gender on care process, resource use, and hospital-based outcomes in congestive heart failure. Am J Cardiol 82:76–81

37. Doughty R, Yee T, Sharpe N, MacMahon S (1995) Hospital admissions and deaths due to congestive heart failure in New Zealand, 1988–91. N Z Med J 108:473–475

38. Taubert G, Bergmeier C, Andresen H, Senges J, Potratz J (2001) Clinical profile and management of heart failure: rural community hospital vs. metropolitan heart center. Eur J Heart Fail 3:611–617

39. Opasich C, Tavazzi L, Lucci D et al (2000) Comparison of one-year outcome in women versus men with chronic congestive heart failure. Am J Cardiol 86:353–357

40. Burns RB, McCarthy EP, Moskowitz MA, Ash A, Kane RL, Finch M (1997) Outcomes for older men and women with congestive heart failure. J Am Geriatr Soc 45:276–280

41. Krumholz HM, Parent EM, Tu N et al (1997) Readmission after hospitalization for congestive heart failure among Medicare beneficiaries. Arch Intern Med 157:99–104

42. Chin MH, Goldman L (1998) Gender differences in 1-year survival and quality of life among patients admitted with congestive heart failure. Med Care 36:1033–1046

43. Tresch DD (2000) Clinical manifestations, diagnostic assessment, and etiology of heart failure in elderly patients. Clin Geriatr Med 16:445–456

44. Vasan RS, Larson MG, Benjamin EJ, Evans JC, Reiss CK, Levy D (1999) Congestive heart failure in subjects with normal versus reduced left ventricular ejection fraction: prevalence and mortality in a population-based cohort. J Am Coll Cardiol 33:1948–1955

45. Ahmed A, Kiefe CI, Allman RM, Sims RV, DeLong JF (2002) Survival benefits of angiotensin-converting enzyme inhibitors in older heart failure patients with perceived contraindications. J Am Geriatr Soc 50:1659–1666

46. Flather MD, Shibata MC, Coats AJ et al (2005) Randomized trial to determine the effect of nebivolol on mortality and cardiovascular hospital admission in elderly patients with heart failure (SENIORS). Eur Heart J 26:215–225

47. Gurwitz JH, Field TS, Harrold LR et al (2003) Incidence and preventability of adverse drug events among older persons in the ambulatory setting. JAMA 289:1107–1116

48. Miura T, Kojima R, Sugiura Y, Mizutani M, Takatsu F, Suzuki Y (2000) Effect of aging on the incidence of digoxin toxicity. Ann Pharmacother 34:427–432

49. Gonseth J, Guallar-Castillon P, Banegas JR, Rodriguez-Artalejo F (2004) The effectiveness of disease management programmes in reducing hospital re-admission in older patients with heart failure: a systematic review and meta-analysis of published reports. Eur Heart J 25:1570–1595

50. Gambassi G, Agha SA, Sui X et al (2008) Race and the natural history of chronic heart failure: a propensity-matched study. J Card Fail 14:373–378

51. Loehr LR, Rosamond WD, Chang PP, Folsom AR, Chambless LE (2008) Heart failure incidence and survival (from the Atherosclerosis Risk in Communities study). Am J Cardiol 101:1016–1022

52. Kamath SA, Drazner MH, Wynne J, Fonarow GC, Yancy CW (2008) Characteristics and outcomes in African American patients with decompensated heart failure. Arch Intern Med 168:1152–1158

53. Lee R, Chan SP, Chan YH, Wong J, Lau D, Ng K (2008) Impact of race on morbidity and mortality in patients with congestive heart failure: a study of the multiracial population in Singapore. Int J Cardiol 134:422–5

54. Yancy CW, Abraham WT, Albert NM et al (2008) Quality of care of and outcomes for African Americans hospitalized with heart failure: findings from the OPTIMIZE-HF (Organized Program to Initiate Lifesaving Treatment in Hospitalized Patients With Heart Failure) registry. J Am Coll Cardiol 51:1675–1684

55. Riegel B, Moser DK, Rayens MK et al (2008) Ethnic differences in quality of life in persons with heart failure. J Card Fail 14:41–47

56. Deswal A, Petersen NJ, Souchek J, Ashton CM, Wray NP (2004) Impact of race on health care utilization and outcomes in veterans with congestive heart failure. J Am Coll Cardiol 43:778–784

57. Owan TE, Hodge DO, Herges RM, Jacobsen SJ, Roger VL, Redfield MM (2006) Trends in prevalence and outcome of heart failure with preserved ejection fraction. N Engl J Med 355:251–259

58. Philbin EF, Rocco TA Jr, Lindenmuth NW, Ulrich K, Jenkins PL (2000) Systolic versus diastolic heart failure in community practice: clinical features, outcomes, and the use of angiotensin-converting enzyme inhibitors. Am J Med 109:605–613

59. Smith GL, Masoudi FA, Vaccarino V, Radford MJ, Krumholz HM (2003) Outcomes in heart failure patients with preserved ejection fraction: mortality, readmission, and functional decline. J Am Coll Cardiol 41:1510–1518

60. Lester SJ, Tajik AJ, Nishimura RA, Oh JK, Khandheria BK, Seward JB (2008) Unlocking the mysteries of diastolic function: deciphering the Rosetta Stone 10 years later. J Am Coll Cardiol 51:679–689

61. Haney S, Sur D, Xu Z (2005) Diastolic heart failure: a review and primary care perspective. J Am Board Fam Pract 18:189–198

62. Vasan RS, Larson MG, Benjamin EJ, Evans JC, Reiss CK, Levy D (1999) Congestive heart failure in subjects with normal versus

reduced left ventricular ejection fraction: prevalence and mortality in a population-based cohort. J Am Coll Cardiol 3:1948–1955

63. Kitzman DW, Gardin JM, Gottdiener JS et al (2001) Importance of heart failure with preserved systolic function in patients > or = 65 years of age. CHS Research Group. Cardiovascular Health Study. Am J Cardiol 87:413–419

64. Devereux RB, Roman MJ, Liu JE et al (2000) Congestive heart failure despite normal left ventricular systolic function in a population-based sample: the Strong Heart Study. Am J Cardiol 86:1090–1096

65. Kitzman DW, Little WC, Brubaker PH et al (2002) Pathophysiological characterization of isolated diastolic heart failure in comparison to systolic heart failure. JAMA 288:2144–2150

66. Liao L, Jollis JG, Anstrom KJ et al (2006) Costs for heart failure with normal vs reduced ejection fraction. Arch Intern Med 166:112–118

67. Cohn JN, Johnson G (1990) Heart failure with normal ejection fraction. The V-HeFT Study. Veterans Administration Cooperative Study Group. Circulation 81:III48–III53

68. MacCarthy PA, Kearney MT, Nolan J et al (2003) Prognosis in heart failure with preserved left ventricular systolic function: prospective cohort study. BMJ 327:78–79

69. Gheorghiade M, Mebazaa A (2005) Introduction to acute heart failure syndromes. Am J Cardiol 96:1G–4G

70. Heart Failure Society of America (2006) Evaluation and management of patients with acute decompensated heart failure. J Card Fail 12:e86–e103

71. Nieminen MS, Bohm M, Cowie MR et al (2005) Executive summary of the guidelines on the diagnosis and treatment of acute heart failure: the Task Force on Acute Heart Failure of the European Society of Cardiology. Eur Heart J 26:384–416

72. Zannad F, Adamopoulos C, Mebazaa A, Gheorghiade M (2006) The challenge of acute decompensated heart failure. Heart Fail Rev 11:135–139

73. Badgett RG, Lucey CR, Mulrow CD (1997) Can the clinical examination diagnose left-sided heart failure in adults? JAMA 277: 1712–1719

74. Rodeheffer RJ, Jacobsen SJ, Gersh BJ et al (1993) The incidence and prevalence of congestive heart failure in Rochester, Minnesota. Mayo Clin Proc 68:1143–1150

75. Remes J, Reunanen A, Aromaa A, Pyörälä K (1992) Incidence of heart failure in eastern Finland: a population-based surveillance study. Eur Heart J 13:588–593

Chapter 2
Cardiac Function in Heart Failure: The Role of Calcium Cycling

Overview

During the cardiac action potential, it is the rise in the level of cytoplasmic calcium as well as the sensitivity of several calcium-sensitive proteins to that released calcium that determines the force of myocardial contraction. Both calcium entry and sensitivity are significantly reduced in heart failure. In this chapter, we discuss how calcium primarily enters the cell through the L-type calcium channel in the plasma membrane. This triggers a large release of calcium primarily through channels (ryanodine receptors) in the sarcoplasmic reticulum. Calcium then binds to several proteins that activate the interaction of actin and myosin in the myofilaments. Finally, this calcium is removed from the cytoplasm back into the sarcoplasmic reticulum and out of the cell through the plasma membrane by several active energy-dependent processes. This calcium removal process is also altered during the development of heart failure. In this chapter, these changes are discussed along with the potential new treatments for heart failure involving changes in calcium entry, exit, and sensitivity.

Introduction

It is the loss of the heart's ability to adequately pump sufficient blood that is the characteristic finding in heart failure. A normal heart can increase its pumping ability to a great extent. Myocardial contractility is primarily controlled by calcium cycling into and out of the cytoplasm of cardiac myocytes as well as calcium sensitivity of various proteins in cardiac myocytes. Calcium initially enters the cell through channels in the plasma membrane, although the major path for calcium entry into the cell cytoplasm is from the sarcoplasmic reticulum. Calcium release channels in the sarcoplasmic reticulum are activated by calcium entry from the plasma membrane. The released cytoplasmic calcium interacts with calcium-sensitive proteins to control the force and rate of contraction. Calcium is then removed from the cytoplasm by several energetic processes, which pump it back into the sarcoplasmic reticulum and

out through the plasma membrane. This calcium cycling of the normal heart is illustrated in Fig. 2.1. Calcium can also enter the mitochondria. All of these processes are altered during the transition to heart failure (HF) [1, 2]. This leads to a loss of contractile reserve. In this chapter, we will first discuss the calcium entry into the cytoplasm both from outside the cell and from the sarcoplasmic reticulum and how this entry is altered in HF. Thereafter calcium sensitivity will be addressed, as well as changes in calcium stores in the sarcoplasmic reticulum. We will also discuss calcium removal and how this parameter is altered in HF. Finally, we will analyze changes in the calcium transients that occur in HF. Some of the changes in calcium cycling that occur in heart failure are presented in Fig. 2.1. It has been proposed that calcium cycling defects may be the final common pathway in the progression to HF [3]. Treatment strategies have been proposed to address the issue of increasing the ability of calcium to ameliorate function in the failing heart [4–7].

Calcium Entry Through the Plasma Membrane

Calcium enters the cardiac myocyte cytoplasm from the extracellular space mainly through L-type Ca^{2+} channels. These channels are one of the main systems in the heart for Ca^{2+} uptake regulation [8, 9]. Their structure has been comprehensively studied and consists of heterotetrameric polypeptide complexes [10, 11]. There are also several accessory subunits of this channel. The L-type Ca^{2+} channels are responsible for the activation of sarcoplasmic reticulum calcium release channels (RyR2) and are controllers of the force of muscle contraction generation in the heart. Thus, the activity of the heart depends on L-type Ca^{2+} channels [8, 12]. The L-type Ca^{2+} channels and the RyR2 receptors are closely linked in the T-tubules of cardiac myocytes [13], and there appears to be a physical connection between these two channels [12]. Phosphorylation of the L-type Ca^{2+} channel-forming subunits by different kinases is one of the most important ways to change the activity of L-type Ca^{2+} channel

J. Marín-García, *Heart Failure*, Contemporary Cardiology,
DOI 10.1007/978-1-60761-147-9_2, © Springer Science+Business Media, LLC 2010

Fig. 2.1 (**a**) Calcium entry and exit from a normal cardiac myocyte. Calcium (■) enters from outside through L-type calcium channels (Ica, L). This triggers Ca²⁺ release from the ryanodine receptors (RyR) in the sarcoplasmic reticulum, called calcium-induced calcium release (CICR). Calcium then activates the myofilaments by binding to troponin C. Calcium is removed from the cytoplasm to the outside of the cell by a sodium–calcium exchanger, which requires an active Na⁺/K⁺ ATPase. There is also a plasma membrane Ca²⁺ ATPase. Calcium is pumped back into the sarcoplasmic reticulum by a Ca²⁺ ATPase (SERCA) that is controlled by a phospholamban. (**b**) Calcium entry and exit from a failing cardiac myocyte. There is reduced calcium entry through the L-type calcium channels and RyR. This is shown by reduced numbers but may also involve reduced activity. Sodium–calcium exchanger activity may increase, but SERCA function is reduced. There is also more diastolic calcium in the cytoplasm

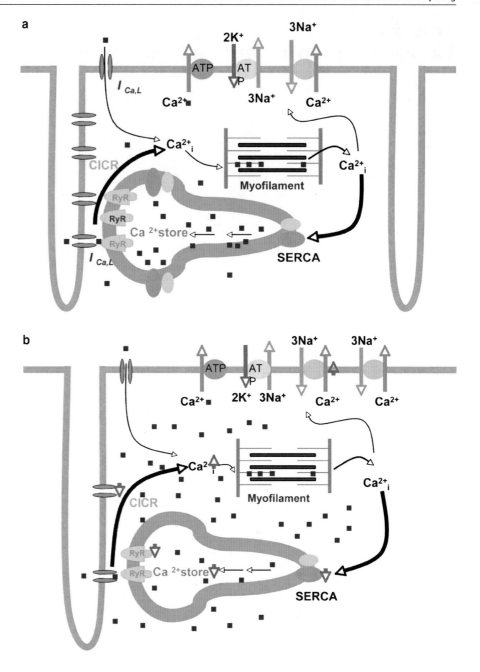

(see Chap. 8). Phosphorylation can either increase or decrease channel activity. Additionally, the activity of L-type Ca²⁺ channels depends on Ca²⁺ concentration in cytoplasm. Other calcium channels may play a minor role in calcium entry into the cardiac myocytes [14]. The Ca²⁺ current entering the cardiac cells through the L-type Ca²⁺ channel facilitate contraction. This entry process is regulated by phosphorylation of L-type Ca²⁺ channels and intracellular Ca²⁺ concentration. Disturbances in cellular Ca²⁺ transport and regulation of L-type Ca²⁺ channels are directly related to HF.

Calcium entry into cardiac myocytes is significantly affected by the development of HF. Some of the changes asso-

ciated with HF are related to changes in the phosphorylation state of the L-type Ca²⁺ channels [4]. In mice, overexpression of L-type Ca²⁺ channels leads to HF [15]. The structure of these channels changes during HF, and their remodeling may prove useful in the treatment of the failing heart [10].

It is not clear whether there are changes in total channel density during the development of HF [11]. Some studies have suggested that there may be reduced expression of these calcium channels in the failing heart [6], in which the coupling between the L-type calcium channels and the calcium release channels of the sarcoplasmic reticulum is also reduced [16]. Although, calcium entry into the cell is reduced in HF, activation of calcium channels has not proved to be useful in the treatment of HF, in which other calcium entry channels may also play a role [14].

Calcium Release from the Sarcoplasmic Reticulum

During the cardiac action potential, Ca^{2+} influx across the cell membrane via L-type Ca^{2+} channels triggers the release of more Ca^{2+} from the sarcoplasmic reticulum, primarily by activating ryanodine receptors (RyR2) in the adjacent sarcoplasmic reticulum membrane [12, 13]. L-type Ca^{2+} channels are located predominantly in the T-tubules, in close proximity to RyR2 channels at the dyad: the junctional region where Ca^{2+} influx from the surface channels triggers sarcoplasmic reticulum Ca^{2+} release [9, 13]. The geometry of this region is of critical importance for proper myocardial function [17]. RyR2 function is regulated by several accessory proteins [18]. Calcium induced calcium release is one of the major controllers of myocardial function [19]. Most of the rise in cytoplasmic calcium that occurs during the cardiac action potential is related to calcium released from the sarcoplasmic reticulum by the RyR2.

Local release of calcium from the RyR2 channels leads to calcium sparks [20] and the rise of intracellular Ca^{2+} activates the contractile proteins. The systolic Ca^{2+} transient is the spatial and temporal sum of such local calcium releases (calcium sparks). The fraction of the total sarcoplasmic reticulum Ca^{2+} content that is released during any given action potential depends on the sarcoplasmic reticulum Ca^{2+} content, the various accessory proteins and the size of the Ca^{2+} trigger [18, 19, 21].

The calcium release channels in the sarcoplasmic reticulum become dysfunctional during the development of HF [5, 19, 22, 23], in which there is evidence for a significant change in the phosphorylation state of these RyR2 channels [4, 12, 24]. However, expression levels of the RyR2 channels may not change significantly [25]. Furthermore, there are slowed calcium transients related to activation of this channel [22, 23].

The structural relationship between the RyR2 channels and the L-type calcium channels is significantly altered with the development of HF [16], in which the physical coupling between these channels is reduced. Moreover, RyR2 channels become leaky during HF [24, 26], although whether this increased leakiness of the RyR2 channels is a cause or an effect of the failing heart is not clear. Fixing this leakiness may prove to be a good therapeutic strategy in the treatment of HF [24]; and this is supported by recent observations suggesting that in HF, RyR2 channels may be useful therapeutic targets [18, 27]. Interestingly, several mutations of the RyR2 channel that affect channel activity have been associated

with the development of human heart failure [22]. These changes in RyR2 and L-type calcium channels lead to reduced calcium transients in failing hearts.

While RyR2 Ca^{2+} release channels have received significant attention, the role of a second pathway for internal Ca^{2+}-release has largely been ignored. The cellular role for inositol 1,4,5-trisphosphate receptors (IP$_3$R) has remained elusive. However, there is great and growing interest in cardiac IP$_3$ signaling due to the known importance of several IP$_3$-inducing agonists (e.g., endothelin, angiotensin II, and norepinephrine) in both hypertrophy and HF [28]. While agonist-induced IP$_3$-dependent Ca^{2+} release is readily observed in most tissues, the role of IP$_3$Rs in cardiac tissue is less clear. The role played by IP$_3$Rs has yet to be convincingly demonstrated in the normal heart. However, there are suggestions that it may lead to amplification of Ca^{2+} signals from the RyR2 or be independently activated through several diverse pathways that lead to the generation of IP$_3$ [29]. This second calcium release channel in the sarcoplasmic reticulum may play a role in normal excitation–contraction coupling. There are also suggestions that the importance of IP$_3$Rs can change significantly during normal aging [30]. This implies that these other calcium release channels may have an increased importance during the development of HF.

Calcium Sensitivity

Myocardial contraction is initiated when Ca^{2+} binds to a specific site on cardiac troponin C [31]. This 12-residue EF-hand loop contains six residues that coordinate Ca^{2+} binding and six residues that do not appear to influence Ca^{2+} binding directly [32]. Structural changes in troponin C affect its calcium sensitivity [32]. Ca^{2+} binding affinity controls contractile force and changes in many types of diseases. Troponin C is part of a troponin complex that together with tropomyosin affects the interaction between actin and myosin leading to the development of myocardial contraction [33, 34]. The interaction between troponin C and calcium is the critical final step of calcium induced control of myocardial contractility. Stretch also affects calcium sensitivity and force development [35]. This is part of the explanation for the Frank–Starling mechanism [36], which may be affected by stretch activated calcium channels. In addition to troponin C, there are several other calcium binding proteins that affect myocardial contractility [37], including calpains and calcium dependent protein kinases [38–41]. These various calcium binding proteins regulate the force of myocardial contraction in the normal heart.

Mutations in troponin C have been associated with the development of HF [34], and changes in calcium sensitivity of troponin may be a potentially useful treatment for HF [42, 43]. As the heart progresses into failure significant reductions in calcium sensitivity occur [33, 44]. Furthermore, decreased phosphorylation level of troponin C occurs in HF [45], and this may be contributory to the decreased contractile function observed in the failing heart [33]. Agents that stabilize troponin C may prove useful.

Several reports have claimed that the increased sensitivity of troponin to calcium observed in the failing heart is due to changes in phosphorylation of troponin I [46]. Several mutations in troponin isoforms have been associated with HF [34]. The ability of the heart to respond to wall stress is also depressed [3]. Other myocardial calcium-binding proteins may also be useful targets for gene therapy in HF [37, 41].

Sarcoplasmic Reticulum Calcium Stores

The major site of internal cellular calcium storage is the sarcoplasmic reticulum (SR). The amount of calcium released by the RyR2 receptors depends, in part, on the amount of calcium in the SR [21]. The calcium content of the SR depends on the balance between calcium uptake by the sarcoplasmic reticulum Ca^{2+}-ATPase (SERCA) and efflux of calcium through RyR2 channels [47]. Calsequestrin is by far the most abundant Ca^{2+}-binding protein in the SR of cardiac muscle [48]. There is a physical link between calsequestrin and RyR2, which allows some control of calcium release during the action potential. This link controls the release of calcium through the RyR2 [49]. Calsequestrin is not the only binding calcium protein in the SR, since calsequestrin null mice are viable suggesting that other protein can also regulate calcium storage in the SR [50]. Other calcium binding proteins including sarcalumenin, calumenin, etc. [51, 52], may also play an important role in calcium storage in the SR.

There are significant alterations in the calsequestrin and SR calcium loads in HF [5]. This may contribute to the increased diastolic calcium levels observed in cardiac myocytes during diastole in HF [49]. Furthermore, calsequestrin loss may also contribute to the development of cardiac hypertrophy [50]. Other calcium binding proteins in the SR may also be affected in the failing heart [51]. Initially, the SR calcium stores may be increased during the early stages of heart failure [53]. However, calcium levels significantly decrease in the SR as the degree of heart failure progresses [37]. Some of these changes are related to increased leakiness from the SR [24, 26]. It is possible that improving calcium storage or its control in the SR may prove a useful target for the treatment of HF.

Calcium Removal

The Na^{+}/Ca^{2+} exchanger is the major plasma membrane transport protein that can cause calcium to exit from the cardiac myocyte [54]. The direction and amplitude of the Na^{+}/Ca^{2+} exchanger current depend on the membrane potential and on the internal and external Na^{+} and Ca^{2+} levels. The Na^{+}/Ca^{2+} exchanger is the main pathway for Ca^{2+} extrusion from ventricular myocytes [54]. This exchanger is regulated by a variety of accessory proteins such as phospholemman [55, 56]. However, the full extent of its control is controversial [57].

Protein phosphorylation is a major regulator of the Na^{+}/Ca^{2+} exchanger [57]. Under some circumstances, the Na^{+}/Ca^{2+} exchanger can operate in the reverse mode and allow calcium entry into the cardiac cell. This exchanger depends in large measure on the activity of the Na^{+}/K^{+} ATPase, which keeps the internal sodium levels low. A plasma membrane calcium ATPase can also aid in the removal of cytoplasmic calcium to the outside [58]. During each heart beat, Ca^{2+} balance is preserved by Ca^{2+} entry via L-type Ca^{2+} channels and Ca^{2+} exit predominantly via the Na^{+}/Ca^{2+} exchanger.

The importance of the Na^{+}/Ca^{2+} exchanger in controlling myocardial contractility actually increases during HF [59]. This suggests downregulation of other important calcium handling proteins in the failing heart. Blockade of the Na^{+}/Ca^{2+} exchanger has been suggested as a possible beneficial therapeutic intervention in heart failure [60]. Classic ways of increasing inotropic activity in failing hearts primarily rely on activation of Na^{+}/Ca^{2+} exchanger by blocking the Na^{+}/K^{+} ATPase in the plasma membrane. Cardiac glycosides such as digitalis and a variety of agents have been used to block Na^{+}/K^{+} ATPase and increase calcium retention in the cytoplasm of failing myocytes [7, 61], which increases the inotropic capacity of the failing cardiac myocytes.

Much of the calcium in the cytoplasm at the end of a cardiac action potential is returned to the SR. The cardiac isoform of the SR calcium ATPase (SERCA2a) is a calcium ion pump powered by ATP hydrolysis [62]. SERCA2a transfers Ca^{2+} from the cytosol of the cardiac myocyte to the lumen of the SR during muscle relaxation. This transporter has a key role in cardiac myocyte calcium regulation [9].

Phospholamban acts as a major control of SERCA [63]. Phospholamban reduces the activity of SERCA, thus reducing calcium reentry into the SR [64]. When phospholamban becomes phosphorylated, inhibition of SERCA2a is reduced. A number of kinases can phosphorylate phospholamban [65–67], that speeds the re-uptake of calcium into the sarcoplasmic reticulum. There are also calcium binding proteins within the SR that help regulate SERCA activity [51, 52, 63]. In addition, there is a calcium ATPase in the plasma membrane that can also remove calcium during normal myocardial functioning although this is a relatively minor pathway for calcium removal from the cytoplasm [1, 5, 6, 58].

The expression of SERCA2a is significantly decreased in HF, which leads to abnormal Ca^{2+} handling and a deficient contractile state [6, 25, 62]. This also leads to reduced calcium removal from the cytoplasm. Following numerous studies in isolated cardiac myocytes and small and large animal models, a clinical trial is underway to restore SERCA2a expression in HF patients by use of adeno-associated virus type 1. Beyond its role in contractile abnormalities in HF, SERCA2a overexpression has beneficial effects in a host of other cardiovascular diseases, and is considered an important target for gene therapy in HF [37, 68].

It is clear that changes in SERCA2a and phospholamban play an important role in the development of HF [5], and preventing the action of phospholamban on SERCA2a may play a beneficial role [69]. Since changes in phospholamban and SERCA2a lead to prolonged calcium transients in failing cardiac myocytes [6, 62, 70], treatment to improve the actions of phospholamban and SERCA2a are currently the major focus of treatment strategies to improve calcium handling during HF.

Changes in Calcium Transients

Calcium transients are involved in regulating electrical signaling and contraction in the heart [1]. The calcium transient that occurs during the action potential in a cardiac myocyte is regulated via ion currents and exchangers, the regulation of other channels or exchangers, and the action potential shape. This is critical for excitation–contraction coupling. When the heart begins to fail, there are alterations in this calcium transient due to the changes discussed above. Since baseline cytosolic diastolic calcium levels are elevated, this may contribute to cardiac diastolic dysfunction [71], that may be partially related to calcium leak from the SR [26].

The rise of the calcium transient is also slowed and diminished in HF. This is related to changes in the L-type calcium channel and the RyR2 channels in the SR [4–6, 19, 22]. The fall in the calcium transient is also slowed in the failing heart. This change is related to reduced calcium removal primarily back into the SR through changes in phospholamban and SERCA2a [6, 62, 70]. Restoring the calcium transient toward its normal functioning may provide several useful targets for the development of novel therapy in the treatment of heart failure.

Conclusions

Ca^{2+} cycling defects in HF are characterized by reduced calcium entry, impaired sarcoplasmic Ca^{2+} release and an associated Ca^{2+} leak, reduced SR Ca^{2+} reuptake, and reduced Ca^{2+} transients. Molecular targeting approaches to correct these abnormalities hold promise as a new therapeutic modality in

the advanced end-stage heart failure patient. These patients have reduced calcium transients and impaired cardiac contractility. Further progress in understanding of Ca^{2+} cycling defects with relevant application in the clinical setting would be useful [72].

Despite remarkable pharmacological advances in the treatment of patients with HF, the rate of development of new therapies, particularly for patients with moderate to severe HF, appears to have slowed. A number of very promising targets have been suggested involving the Ca^{2+} cycling pathway, for selective manipulation using gene transfer approaches. This may provide new treatment approaches for patients with HF.

Summary

- Calcium enters cardiac myocytes primarily through L-type calcium channels.
- Calcium entry is reduced in heart failure.
- Calcium entry triggers activation of ryanodine receptors to release calcium from the sarcoplasmic reticulum.
- Ryanodine receptors release less calcium, more slowly and become leaky during heart failure. Changes in IP$_3$ receptors may also play a role in heart failure.
- Calcium binds to calcium sensitive proteins, primarily troponin C, to cause myofilament activation.
- Calcium sensitivity is depressed in heart failure.
- A large amount of calcium is stored in the sarcoplasmic reticulum and this storage is reduced in heart failure.
- The Na$^+$/Ca^{2+} exchanger is the major mechanism to remove calcium from the cytoplasm to the outside of the cell. It requires an active Na$^+$/K$^+$ ATPase for its functioning. There is also a plasma membrane Ca^{2+} ATPase.
- The Na$^+$/Ca^{2+} exchanger may become more prominent in heart failure.
- Calcium is pumped back into the sarcoplasmic reticulum by a Ca^{2+} ATPase (SERCA2a). This ATPase is primarily controlled by phospholamban.
- SERCA2a activity is reduced in heart failure.
- In heart failure, the diastolic cytoplasmic level is higher and the calcium transients are reduced and slowed.
- Improvements in calcium cycling or sensitivity may prove useful targets for the treatment of heart failure.

References

1. Bers DM (2008) Calcium cycling and signaling in cardiac myocytes. Annu Rev Physiol 70:23–49
2. Francis GS (2001) Pathophysiology of chronic heart failure. Am J Med 110 Suppl 7A:37S–46S

3. Hoshijima M, Knoll R, Pashmforoush M, Chien KR (2006) Reversal of calcium cycling defects in advanced heart failure toward molecular therapy. J Am Coll Cardiol 48:A15–A23

4. Ikeda Y, Hoshijima M, Chien KR (2008) Toward biologically targeted therapy of calcium cycling defects in heart failure. Physiology (Bethesda) 23:6–16

5. Kranias EG, Bers DM (2007) Calcium and cardiomyopathies. Subcell Biochem 45:523–537

6. Kaye DM, Hoshijima M, Chien KR (2008) Reversing advanced heart failure by targeting Ca2+ cycling. Annu Rev Med 59:13–28

7. Degoma EM, Vagelos RH, Fowler MB, Ashley EA (2006) Emerging therapies for the management of decompensated heart failure: from bench to bedside. J Am Coll Cardiol 48:2397–2409

8. Treinys R, Jurevicius J (2008) L-type Ca2+ channels in the heart: structure and regulation. Medicina (Kaunas) 44:491–499

9. Dibb KM, Graham HK, Venetucci LA, Eisner DA, Trafford AW (2007) Analysis of cellular calcium fluxes in cardiac muscle to understand calcium homeostasis in the heart. Cell Calcium 42:503–512

10. Pitt GS, Dun W, Boyden PA (2006) Remodeled cardiac calcium channels. J Mol Cell Cardiol 41:373–388

11. Bodi I, Mikala G, Koch SE, Akhter SA, Schwartz A (2005) The L-type calcium channel in the heart: the beat goes on. J Clin Invest 115:3306–3317

12. Petrovic MM, Vales K, Putnikovic B, Djulejic V, Mitrovic DM (2008) Ryanodine receptors, voltage-gated calcium channels and their relationship with protein kinase A in the myocardium. Physiol Res 57:141–149

13. Orchard C, Brette F (2008) t-Tubules and sarcoplasmic reticulum function in cardiac ventricular myocytes. Cardiovasc Res 77:237–244

14. Horiba M, Muto T, Ueda N et al (2008) T-type Ca2+ channel blockers prevent cardiac cell hypertrophy through an inhibition of calcineurin-NFAT3 activation as well as L-type Ca2+ channel blockers. Life Sci 82:554–560

15. Wang S, Ziman B, Bodi I et al (2009) Dilated cardiomyopathy with increased SR Ca2+ loading preceded by a hypercontractile state and diastolic failure in the alpha(1C)TG mouse. PLoS One 4:e4133

16. Bito V, Heinzel FR, Biesmans L, Antoons G, Sipido KR (2008) Crosstalk between L-type Ca2+ channels and the sarcoplasmic reticulum: alterations during cardiac remodelling. Cardiovasc Res 77:315–324

17. Tanskanen AJ, Greenstein JL, Chen A, Sun SX, Winslow RL (2007) Protein geometry and placement in the cardiac dyad influence macroscopic properties of calcium-induced calcium release. Biophys J 92:3379–3396

18. Phrommintikul A, Chattipakorn N (2006) Roles of cardiac ryanodine receptor in heart failure and sudden cardiac death. Int J Cardiol 112:142–152

19. Gyorke S, Terentyev D (2008) Modulation of ryanodine receptor by luminal calcium and accessory proteins in health and cardiac disease. Cardiovasc Res 77:245–255

20. Guatimosim S, Dilly K, Santana LF, Saleet Jafri M, Sobie EA, Lederer WJ (2002) Local Ca(2+) signaling and EC coupling in heart: Ca(2+) sparks and the regulation of the [Ca(2+)](i) transient. J Mol Cell Cardiol 34:941–950

21. Laver DR (2007) Ca2+ stores regulate ryanodine receptor Ca2+ release channels via luminal and cytosolic Ca2+ sites. Clin Exp Pharmacol Physiol 34:889–896

22. Yano M, Yamamoto T, Ikemoto N, Matsuzaki M (2005) Abnormal ryanodine receptor function in heart failure. Pharmacol Ther 107:377–391

23. Durham WJ, Wehrens XH, Sood S, Hamilton SL (2007) Diseases associated with altered ryanodine receptor activity. Subcell Biochem 45:273–321

24. Neef S, Maier LS (2007) Remodeling of excitation-contraction coupling in the heart: inhibition of sarcoplasmic reticulum Ca(2+) leak as a novel therapeutic approach. Curr Heart Fail Rep 4:11–17

25. Daniels MC, Naya T, Rundell VL, de Tombe PP (2007) Development of contractile dysfunction in rat heart failure: hierarchy of cellular events. Am J Physiol Regul Integr Comp Physiol 293:R284–R292

26. George CH (2008) Sarcoplasmic reticulum Ca2+ leak in heart failure: mere observation or functional relevance? Cardiovasc Res 77:302–314

27. Yamamoto T, Yano M, Xu X et al (2008) Identification of target domains of the cardiac ryanodine receptor to correct channel disorder in failing hearts. Circulation 117:762–772

28. Hund TJ, Ziman AP, Lederer WJ, Mohler PJ (2008) The cardiac IP3 receptor: uncovering the role of "the other" calcium-release channel. J Mol Cell Cardiol 45:159–161

29. Hirose M, Stuyvers B, Dun W, Ter Keurs H, Boyden PA (2008) Wide long lasting perinuclear Ca2+ release events generated by an interaction between ryanodine and IP3 receptors in canine Purkinje cells. J Mol Cell Cardiol 45:176–184

30. Kaplan P, Jurkovicova D, Babusikova E et al (2007) Effect of aging on the expression of intracellular Ca(2+) transport proteins in a rat heart. Mol Cell Biochem 301:219–226

31. Sun YB, Lou F, Irving M (2009) Calcium- and myosin-dependent changes in troponin structure during activation of heart muscle. J Physiol 587:155–163

32. Reece KL, Moss RL (2008) Intramolecular interactions in the N-domain of cardiac troponin C are important determinants of calcium sensitivity of force development. Biochemistry 47:5139–5146

33. Kobayashi T, Jin L, de Tombe PP (2008) Cardiac thin filament regulation. Pflugers Arch 457:37–46

34. Dong WJ, Xing J, Ouyang Y, An J, Cheung HC (2008) Structural kinetics of cardiac troponin C mutants linked to familial hypertrophic and dilated cardiomyopathy in troponin complexes. J Biol Chem 283:3424–3432

35. Shiels HA, White E (2008) The Frank-Starling mechanism in vertebrate cardiac myocytes. J Exp Biol 211:2005–2013

36. Hanft LM, Korte FS, McDonald KS (2008) Cardiac function and modulation of sarcomeric function by length. Cardiovasc Res 77:627–636

37. Vinge LE, Raake PW, Koch WJ (2008) Gene therapy in heart failure. Circ Res 102:1458–1470

38. Letavernier E, Perez J, Bellocq A et al (2008) Targeting the calpain/calpastatin system as a new strategy to prevent cardiovascular remodeling in angiotensin II-induced hypertension. Circ Res 102:720–728

39. Metrich M, Lucas A, Gastineau M et al (2008) Epac mediates beta-adrenergic receptor-induced cardiomyocyte hypertrophy. Circ Res 102:959–965

40. Sucharov CC (2007) Beta-adrenergic pathways in human heart failure. Expert Rev Cardiovasc Ther 5:119–124

41. Heidrich FM, Ehrlich BE (2009) Calcium, calpains, and cardiac hypertrophy: a new link. Circ Res 104:e19–e20

42. Kota B, Prasad AS, Economides C, Singh BN (2008) Levosimendan and calcium sensitization of the contractile proteins in cardiac muscle: impact on heart failure. J Cardiovasc Pharmacol Ther 13:269–278

43. Endoh M (2008) Cardiac Ca2+ signaling and Ca2+ sensitizers. Circ J 72:1915–1925

44. Hamdani N, Kooij V, van Dijk S et al (2008) Sarcomeric dysfunction in heart failure. Cardiovasc Res 77:649–658

45. El-Armouche A, Pohlmann L, Schlossarek S et al (2007) Decreased phosphorylation levels of cardiac myosin-binding protein-C in human and experimental heart failure. J Mol Cell Cardiol 43:223–229

46. Day SM, Westfall MV, Metzger JM (2007) Tuning cardiac performance in ischemic heart disease and failure by modulating myofilament function. J Mol Med 85:911–921

47. Diaz ME, Graham HK, O'Neill SC, Trafford AW, Eisner DA (2005) The control of sarcoplasmic reticulum Ca content in cardiac muscle. Cell Calcium 38:391–396

48. Beard NA, Laver DR, Dulhunty AF (2004) Calsequestrin and the calcium release channel of skeletal and cardiac muscle. Prog Biophys Mol Biol 85:33–69

49. Terentyev D, Kubalova Z, Valle G et al (2008) Modulation of SR Ca release by luminal Ca and calsequestrin in cardiac myocytes: effects of CASQ2 mutations linked to sudden cardiac death. Biophys J 95:2037–2048

50. Song L, Alcalai R, Arad M et al (2007) Calsequestrin 2 (CASQ2) mutations increase expression of calreticulin and ryanodine receptors, causing catecholaminergic polymorphic ventricular tachycardia. J Clin Invest 117:1814–1823

51. Shimura M, Minamisawa S, Takeshima H et al (2008) Sarcalumenin alleviates stress-induced cardiac dysfunction by improving Ca2+ handling of the sarcoplasmic reticulum. Cardiovasc Res 77:362–370

52. Sahoo SK (2008) Kim do H. Calumenin interacts with SERCA2 in rat cardiac sarcoplasmic reticulum. Mol Cells 26:265–269

53. Mork HK, Sjaastad I, Sande JB, Periasamy M, Sejersted OM, Louch WE (2007) Increased cardiomyocyte function and Ca2+ transients in mice during early congestive heart failure. J Mol Cell Cardiol 43:177–186

54. Sher AA, Noble PJ, Hinch R, Gavaghan DJ, Noble D (2008) The role of the Na+/Ca2+ exchangers in Ca2+ dynamics in ventricular myocytes. Prog Biophys Mol Biol 96:377–398

55. Zhang XQ, Ahlers BA, Tucker AL et al (2006) Phospholemman inhibition of the cardiac Na+/Ca2+ exchanger. Role of phosphorylation. J Biol Chem 281:7784–7792

56. Bell JR, Kennington E, Fuller W et al (2008) Characterization of the phospholemman knockout mouse heart: depressed left ventricular function with increased Na-K-ATPase activity. Am J Physiol Heart Circ Physiol 294:H613–H621

57. Zhang YH, Hancox JC (2009) Regulation of cardiac Na+-Ca2+ exchanger activity by protein kinase phosphorylation – still a paradox? Cell Calcium 45:1–10

58. Oceandy D, Stanley PJ, Cartwright EJ, Neyses L (2007) The regulatory function of plasma-membrane Ca(2+)-ATPase (PMCA) in the heart. Biochem Soc Trans 35:927–930

59. Diedrichs H, Frank K, Schneider CA et al (2007) Increased functional importance of the Na, Ca-exchanger in contracting failing human myocardium but unchanged activity in isolated vesicles. Int Heart J 48:755–766

60. Ozdemir S, Bito V, Holemans P et al (2008) Pharmacological inhibition of Na/Ca exchange results in increased cellular Ca2+ load attributable to the predominance of forward mode block. Circ Res 102:1398–1405

61. Schoner W, Scheiner-Bobis G (2007) Endogenous and exogenous cardiac glycosides and their mechanisms of action. Am J Cardiovasc Drugs 7:173–189

62. Kawase Y, Hajjar RJ (2008) The cardiac sarcoplasmic/endoplasmic reticulum calcium ATPase: a potent target for cardiovascular diseases. Nat Clin Pract Cardiovasc Med 5:554–565

63. Bhupathy P, Babu GJ, Periasamy M (2007) Sarcolipin and phospholamban as regulators of cardiac sarcoplasmic reticulum Ca2+ ATPase. J Mol Cell Cardiol 42:903–911

64. Froehlich JP, Mahaney JE, Keceli G et al (2008) Phospholamban thiols play a central role in activation of the cardiac muscle sarcoplasmic reticulum calcium pump by nitroxyl. Biochemistry 47:13150–13152

65. Brittsan AG, Ginsburg KS, Chu G et al (2003) Chronic SR Ca2+-ATPase inhibition causes adaptive changes in cellular Ca2+ transport. Circ Res 92:769–776

66. Zhang Q, Scholz PM, Pilzak A, Su J, Weiss HR (2007) Role of phospholamban in cyclic GMP mediated signaling in cardiac myocytes. Cell Physiol Biochem 20:157–166

67. Vittone L, Mundina-Weilenmann C, Mattiazzi A (2008) Phospholamban phosphorylation by CaMKII under pathophysiological conditions. Front Biosci 13:5988–6005

68. Hajjar RJ, Zsebo K, Deckelbaum L et al (2008) Design of a phase 1/2 trial of intracoronary administration of AAV1/SERCA2a in patients with heart failure. J Card Fail 14:355–367

69. Tsuji T, Del Monte F, Yoshikawa Y et al (2009) Rescue of Ca2+ overload-induced left ventricular dysfunction by targeted ablation of phospholamban. Am J Physiol Heart Circ Physiol 296:H310–H317

70. Kawase Y, Ly HQ, Prunier F et al (2008) Reversal of cardiac dysfunction after long-term expression of SERCA2a by gene transfer in a pre-clinical model of heart failure. J Am Coll Cardiol 51:1112–1119

71. Periasamy M, Janssen PM (2008) Molecular basis of diastolic dysfunction. Heart Fail Clin 4:13–21

72. Roderick HL, Higazi DR, Smyrnias I, Fearnley C, Harzheim D, Bootman MD (2007) Calcium in the heart: when it's good, it's very very good, but when it's bad, it's horrid. Biochem Soc Trans 35:957–961

Chapter 3
Gene Profiling of the Failing Heart: Epigenetics

Overview

In spite of continuing intensive basic and clinical research and new diagnostic modalities and treatment of cardiovascular diseases available, heart failure (HF) remains a severe health problem of dramatic proportions. Nevertheless, in the current era of post-genomics medicine, the development of novel molecular and cellular technologies have awaken a sense of optimism that we will finally be able to unravel the mechanisms of a number of multigenic diseases, in particular, the complex spider-web like HF. These exciting technologies are paving the way to simultaneously assess the expression of tens of thousands of gene transcripts in a single experiment, providing a resolution and precision of phenotypic characterization not previously possible. Within the heart, many examples of genetic and protein changes correlated with functional alterations have been noted both during normal development and during the development of HF from a variety of causes.

While the expectations with genomics (i.e., the association of molecular and cell biology with genetics and computational science) remain high, the progress achieved so far in the clinical diagnosis, prognosis and treatment of HF has been rather limited. True, new diagnostic markers (e.g., BNP) are becoming available, but it seems that progress will be only realized overtime with increasing use of animal models to identify critical genetic loci involved in HF, which may provide important data concerning both gene targeting and therapeutic modulation of HF.

Further investigative efforts in preclinical studies using global and specific gene profiling will be informative regarding the identification of specific genes, which may allow the development of new biomarkers able to assess progression of HF. With the integrated use of genetic technologies (gene profiling, pharmacogenomics, etc.) and clinical medicine it is expected to find effective, individually-tailored, approaches for the treatment of HF. So far, genetic and biochemical studies have shown that epigenetic changes play an important role in the pathophysiology of cardiac hypertrophy and HF, with dysregulation in histone acetylation directly linked to impaired cardiomyocytes contractility.

In this chapter, the molecular basis of HF, with focus on gene function and expression, epigenetics, and metabolic and calcium cycling will be discussed.

Introduction

An endemic problem associated with increasing morbidity and mortality, the HF syndromes include a dynamic and progressive deterioration of myocardial function resulting in inadequate cardiac output to meet the metabolic needs of the body. HF usually involves the loss of viable myocytes by apoptosis, a marked alteration in myocardial bioenergetics, and reprogramming of gene expression. Myocardial remodeling, mediated by both hypertrophy and apoptosis of cardiomyocytes, and stimulated by a number of mechanical and chemical stimuli and signaling factors, cytokines, oxidative stress, NO, endothelin and peptide growth factors (e.g., TNF-α), continues to increase as a result of progressive myocardial dysfunction. These stimuli activate a series of biomechanical stress-dependent signaling cascades involving cardiomyocyte sensors, leading to altered signal transduction pathways and resulting in the activation of transcriptional factors, co-activators, and co-repressors which will orchestrate myocardial gene expression.

Genomics of HF is a rather complex field still under development. Cardiac gene expression is transcriptionally regulated and its activation is dependent on a number of transcription factors together with their DNA regulatory enhancer/promoter sequences. This complexity of gene expression is underlined by the fact that each cardiac gene is under the direction of a number of enhancers, which regulate the spectrum of cardiac gene expression patterns. Undoubtedly, increasing research efforts in this field are desirable because, in spite of considerable clinical advances, the morbidity and mortality of HF remain high; thus, new paradigms and novel diagnostic and therapeutic targets for HF need to be developed.

The Profiling of Gene Expression in HF

Many molecular pathways are responsible for the transduction of hemodynamic and neurohormonal stimuli into changes in gene regulation and expression in HF [1]. The emergence of microarray technology in the early 1990s has paved the way to simultaneously assess the expression of tens of thousands of gene transcripts in a single experiment, providing a resolution and precision of phenotypic characterization not previously possible [2, 3]. Gene expression fingerprints could be good indicators of the etiology of HF. The diverse etiologies and multiple consequences of HF make it attractive to analyze gene array technology especially where HF is idiopathic in nature. For example, in 2002 of 6,606 genes on the GeneChip, Tan et al. [4] using oligonucleotide microarrays reported that 103 genes in ten functional groups were differentially expressed between failing and non-failing hearts with end-stage dilated cardiomyopathy (DCM). Furthermore, using a dendrogram (*used in computational biology to illustrate the clustering of genes, it is a tree diagram often used to show the arrangement of the clusters produced by a clustering algorithm*) the authors identified a gene expression fingerprint of failing and non-failing hearts, which allowed them to distinguish two failing hearts with different etiologies (familial and alcoholic cardiomyopathy, respectively) with different expression patterns. The K means clustering also showed two potentially novel pathways associated with upregulation of atrial natriuretic peptide (ANP) and brain natriuretic peptide (BNP), and with increased expression of extracellular matrix proteins. Preliminary data have suggested that establishing a molecular gene-profiling portrait may help in clinical decision as it relates to the urgency of intervention. Furthermore, expression profiling using a cDNA microarray containing cardiac-relevant genes has been recently conducted in 15 failing and two non-failing hearts [5]. Patients were classified according to expression profile based on differentially expressed genes. Three patient subgroups were identified ("1," "2," and "3" in the patient classification tree), each with a specific molecular portrait. These patient sub-groups did not coincide with a clinical classification based on etiology. However, when the patients were annotated according to their United Network for Organ Sharing Status [6], there appeared to be an association with the molecular patient classification. All patients with Status 1A (i.e., the highest medical urgency status) clustered together in sub-group 2. This sub-group was characterized by a relatively low expression level of sarcomeric genes (e.g., titin) and metabolic genes (e.g., NADH dehydrogenase) and a relatively high expression level of natriuretic peptides. While the clinical relevance of this study remains to be established, it opens up the intriguing possibility that the etiology of human HF can be pinpointed by their molecular portrait.

At present, microarray studies are mainly used in gene discovery and molecular signature analysis. The first application identifies differentially expressed genes characteristics of different disease states through which novel pathways and therapeutic targets can be identified. Using this application, many microarray evaluations in HF have made comparisons between failing and non-failing hearts [5, 7], between DCM and HCM [8] as well as before and after the placement of left ventricle-assisted devices (LVAD) [9]. This approach of gene discovery has also provided new insights into more rare diseases such as giant cell myocarditis [10]. Taken together, these studies have the potential of providing insights into novel genetic pathways and therapeutic targets for common and uncommon conditions associated with HF.

The second application originated from the fact that the state of the transcriptome in a given disease tissue may contain a highly accurate representation of key biologic phenomena. Transcriptome (i.e., a set of all messenger RNA molecules or "transcripts"), is the term used to characterize the total set of transcripts, or a specific subset of transcripts present in the cell. In contrast to the genome, which is approximately fixed in a given cell line (without mutations), the transcriptome can vary with the environmental conditions. Since it contains all mRNA transcripts in the cell, the transcriptome represents every gene being actively expressed at any point in time, except for mRNA degradation events such as transcriptional attenuation. Transcriptomics (also called Expression Profiling) examine the expression level of mRNAs in a cell, employing high-throughput techniques based on DNA microarray technology.

Patterns of gene expression or molecular signatures have the potential to also identify biomarkers useful for diagnostic, prognostic, and therapeutic purposes. With this approach, the goal is to use molecular signature analysis to identify a pattern of gene expression that is associated with a clinical parameter such as etiology, prognosis, or response to treatment, providing a diagnostic or prognostic precision otherwise not possible with standard clinical information. The basic principle of molecular signature analysis is as follow. First, samples are divided into groups based on a clinically relevant parameter such as disease etiology, prognosis, or response to therapy. Then, a molecular signature is created by choosing genes whose expression is associated with the parameter in question, by weighting the genes based on their individual predictive strengths [11, 12]. For example, using prediction analysis of microarrays, Kittleson et al. [13] have identified a gene expression profile that differentiates the two major forms of cardiomyopathy, ischemic and nonischemic, a classification commonly employed in clinical practice and clinical trials.

The potential of transcriptomic biomarkers to predict prognosis in patients with new-onset HF has been recently evaluated by Heidecker et al. [14]. Among a total of 350 endomyocardial biopsy samples, 180 were identified as cases of idiopathic DCM. Patients with phenotypic extremes in survival were selected: good prognosis (event-free survival for at least 5 years; $n = 25$) and poor prognosis (events (death, requirement for LVAD, or cardiac transplant) within the first 2 years of presentation with HF symptoms; $n = 18$). They dissected the data with significance analysis of microarrays and prediction analysis of microarrays. Good versus poor prognosis was identified in 46 overexpressed genes, of which 45 genes were selected by prediction analysis of microarrays for prediction of prognosis in a train set ($n = 29$), with subsequent validation in test sets ($n = 14$ each). The biomarker performed with 74% sensitivity (95% CI 69–79%) and 90% specificity (95% CI 87–93%) after 50 random partitions. Taken together, these findings showed that a transcriptomic signature, generated from a single endomyocardial biopsy, could serve as a novel prognostic biomarker in HF. In addition, these findings may have the potential to identify novel therapeutic targets for HF and cardiomyopathy.

The proteome, represent the entire complement of proteins expressed by a genome, cell, tissue, or organism. It is generally accepted that post-translational and translational processes play key role in determining the cellular proteome [15, 16]. Techniques commonly used in proteomic-based analysis include a combination of 2-D gel electrophoresis (2-DE), mass spectrometry, and autoradiography map changes in myocardial protein expression. An example of the application of these techniques was illustrated by a recent report of an analysis of 27 proteins in the right ventricle (RV) and 21 proteins in the LV in load-induced, and catecholamine-induced RV and LV hypertrophy, respectively [17]. This study represents a potentially novel pathway (BRAP2/BRCA1) that is involved in myocardial hypertrophy. Increased afterload-induced hypertrophy leads to striking changes in energy metabolism with down-regulation of pyruvate dehydrogenase (subunit βE1), isocitrate dehydrogenase, succinyl coenzyme A ligase, NADH dehydrogenase, ubiquinol–cytochrome c reductase, and propionyl coenzyme A carboxylase. These changes go in parallel with alterations of the thin filament proteome (troponin T, tropomyosin), probably associated with Ca^{2+} sensitization of the myofilaments. By contrast, neurohumoral stimulation of the LV increases the abundance of proteins relevant for energy metabolism. Therefore, these techniques allow for an in-depth analysis of global proteome alterations in a controlled animal model of pressure overload-induced myocardial hypertrophy.

Global and Specific Analysis of Gene Expression

During normal cardiac development and during the development of numerous cardiac pathologies, frequent examples of genetic and protein changes correlated with functional altera-

tions have been noted [18]. The association with pathology or cardiac hypertrophy of α-myosin heavy chain (MHC) expression in the ventricles of small rodents, whose normal MHC complement consists largely of α-MHC, has been thoroughly investigated [19]. Similarly, different congenital heart diseases (CHD) are associated with certain shifts in the motor proteins [20]. Expression levels of 6,000–15,000 genes have been compared in the failing and non-failing hearts. In general, up- or down-regulation of different effectors/modulators has been documented in several experimental models, sometimes with conflicting results [21–23]. Remodeling at the transcriptional and translational level is represented by the up-regulation of elongation factors and ribosomal proteins. Most studies also showed increased expression of genes encoding stress protein. For example, in the spontaneously hypertensive rats (SHR), during the transition from LV hypertrophy to frank HF, cardiac α-MHC mRNA was reduced, whereas β-MHC, α-cardiac actin, and myosin light chain-2 mRNAs were not significantly altered. ANP and B-type (brain) natriuretic peptide (BNP) mRNA were significantly increased [23]. Potentials and limitations of the above studies, nevertheless important observations, include occasional high and variable level of ANP and BNP gene expression in the "non-failing hearts" utilized as controls [24], as well as a lack of proof that the new or mutated protein(s) expressed were responsible for the phenotype.

Susceptibility/Modifier Genes/RNAi in HF

An important element in the outcome of a multifactorial disease such as HF is the presence of susceptibility and modifier genes. While susceptibility genes are genes involved in the pathogenesis of the disease, modifier genes are genes that may modulate the severity of HF once it has developed. The modifier genes are not the primary cause of HF, although they can influence the severity of the phenotype following the initiation of the syndrome.

The identification of modifier genes, which will markedly improve the elucidation of genetic risk factors, has been assisted by large-scale genome-wide approaches to identify polymorphic variants correlated with disease severity. Single nucleotide polymorphism-association studies have identified several candidate modifier genes for various cardiac disorders. A number of specific genetic polymorphisms have been found in association with myocardial infarction, coronary artery disease (CAD), and DCM as shown in Table 3.1.

With the increased cataloging of single nucleotide polymorphisms either alone or within a larger chromosomal region (haplotypes) in available shared databases, these modifier loci can be evaluated for their effects in predisposing to specific cardiac defects and severity of HF, and may impact on the choice of diagnostic and treatment options.

Table 3.1 Genes with polymorphic variants contributing to cardiovascular disease

Gene affected (loci)	Normal function	Associated cardiac phenotype	Drug effected
ATP-cassette binding protein (ABC or MDR)	Lipid transport	Coronary artery disease	Digoxin
Angiotensin converting enzyme (ACE)	Renin–angiotensin regulator	Coronary artery disease	Angiotensin converting enzyme inhibitors
β-adrenergic receptor (ADR β-2)	Neurohormone receptor	Congestive heart failure	β-2 adrenergic agonists
Apolipoprotein E (APOE)	Lipid transport	Coronary artery disease	Statin
Cholesterol ester transport protein (CETP)	Lipid transport	Coronary artery disease	Statin
minK related protein (KCNE2/MiRP1)	Potassium channel	Antibiotic-induced cardiac dysrhythmia	Clarithromycin
Plasminogen-activator inhibitor type 1 (PAI-1)	Intravascular fibrinolysis	Myocardial infarction	Nd
Stromelysin-1 (MMP-3)	Matrix metalloproteinase	Myocardial infarction, Angina	Nd
Thrombospondin (TSP-1)	Angiogenesis inhibitor	Premature coronary artery disease	Nd
Nuclear transcription factor (NFATC4)	Transcription factor	Cardiac hypertrophy	Nd
Interleukin-6 (IL-6)	Inflammatory mediator	Myocardial infarction	Nd
Endothelin receptor A (ETA)	Vaso-regulator	Idiopathic DCM	Nd

Nd not determined

By utilizing a genome-wide analysis of cardiovascular disorders, a larger net can be cast for detecting associated disease-related mutations. Recent methodological advances have made it possible to simultaneously assess the entire profile of expressed genes in affected myocardium requiring only very limited amount of biopsied tissue. Foremost among these methods is gene expression profiling using DNA microarrays. Microarrays are artificially-constructed DNA grids in which each element of the grid acts as a probe for a specific RNA. Gene expression by microarray analysis has proved to be a useful tool in establishing pathophysiological features of a disease by comprehensive evaluation of which genes are increased and which are decreased in expression, and can be applied in both diagnosis and in the evaluation of patients' response to therapy.

The association of defective genes with cardiac disorders uncovered by genomic analysis needs to be followed by proteomic analysis (for further discussion on proteomics see Chap. 19) to establish the function and pathophysiological role played by the mutant protein and to reveal interacting modulators. Once the implicated genes and their gene-products have been fully identified, sequence and subsequent bioinformatic analysis can be employed to identify common structural and functional motifs and homologies with known proteins. The potentially significant functional interaction of proteins (which can be an important determinant of the cardiac phenotype) can be further determined by yeast two-hybrid analysis.

Based on genetic association studies (i.e., searching the genome for single nucleotide polymorphisms or SNPs in a population or in a family to find genetic variations associated with a trait or disease) between the severity of the phenotype and sequence variations of selected genes, several polymorphisms in the β1 and β2 adrenergic receptors and angiotensin converting enzyme (ACE) gene have been correlated with HF prognosis in several individuals. Komajda and Charron

[25] have noted that because of the small size of the populations, available studies cannot be considered as definitive because of their lack of replication and ethnic stratification. In addition, their statistical power is rather limited since parameters other than genetic background largely contribute to the phenotypic variability (etiology, treatment, and environment). This low statistical power prevents the analysis of gene–gene and gene–environment interactions, which are likely to play a major role in this multifactorial syndrome that is HF. Moreover, the selection of candidate genes is limited by our incomplete knowledge of the pathophysiology of HF, and consequently, new approaches are needed to improve the identification of modifier and susceptibility genes involved in HF. These new approaches may include the use of genomic-wide screening and the use of transgenic animal models; however, the application of genomic-wide screening to multifactorial diseases in human populations with complex inheritance is difficult. On the other hand, transgenic animal models of HF overexpressing the gene(s) of interest seem a better alternative to study since their phenotype may not be affected by environmental factors, thus variability in the phenotype may be due to differences in the genetic background. In this regard, Le Corvoisier et al. [26] have reported the use of genomic mapping to screen for modifier genes in HF, and found that the prognosis in transgenic mice with HF induced by overexpressing calsequestrin (CSQ), was linked to 2 Quantitative Trait Loci (QTL) localized on chromosome 2 and 3. However, genome mapping in an experimental mouse model of HF has important limitations [25]. For example, the modifier loci identified may not be specific to the animal specific HF induced by CSQ overexpression, implying that studies in other models of HF are warranted. Furthermore, the modifier loci may also be specific to the particular mouse strain, and more importantly, even after the identification of the responsible genes in the mouse, model translation of these discoveries to the multifactorial human

HF syndrome may be not justified since the pathophysiology and the pathways affected may be different between mouse and man.

RNA interference (RNAi) is a molecule that inhibits gene expression at the stage of translation or by hindering the transcription of specific genes. Previously known as post transcriptional gene silencing and transgene silencing, these methods also described the RNAi phenomenon. Recently, using a gene knock-out approach Gupta et al. [27] have shown that inhibition of the nuclear factor (NF-κB), using direct gene delivery of sh-p65 RNA, results in regression of cardiac hypertrophy. Since activation of the NF-κB signaling pathway may be associated with the development of cardiac hypertrophy progressing to HF, these investigators have employed the transgenic Myo-Tg mouse, which develops hypertrophy and HF as a result of overexpression of myotrophin in the heart, associated with an elevated level of NF-κB activity. Furthermore, using this mouse model and a NF-κB-targeted gene array, the components of NF-κB signaling cascade and the NF-κB-linked genes that are expressed during the progression to cardiac hypertrophy and HF were determined. In addition, the effects of inhibition of NF-κB signaling events, using a gene knockdown approach such as RNAi through delivery of a short hairpin RNA against NF-κB p65 using a lentiviral vector (L-sh-p65), were explored. Following the direct delivery of a short hairpin RNA into the hearts of 10-week-old Myo-Tg mice, a significant regression of cardiac hypertrophy, associated with a significant reduction in NF-κB activation and atrial natriuretic factor expression occurred. These novel findings suggest that inhibition of NF-κB using direct gene delivery of sh-p65 RNA results in regression of cardiac hypertrophy and this could be used as a therapeutic target in the prevention of HF. Parenthetically, it has been demonstrated that the human failing heart, explanted at the time of heart transplantation, exhibits marked nuclear translocation of NF-κB in cardiac myocytes when compared to control hearts [28]. NF-κB as well as AP-1 have been found to be significantly activated in chronic HF due to ischemic or DCM. This suggests that NF-κB and AP-1 have significant involvement in the cardiac remodeling process.

MicroRNAs and HF

MicroRNAs (miRNAs) are fundamental post-transcriptionally regulators of gene expression in eukaryotic cells and they represent a new paradigm for cardiac gene regulation. Targeting a high number of a variety of mRNA, these small, non-coding RNAs have the potential to modulate genes that are participant in metabolic and/or signaling pathways. Interestingly, they can also act in reverse, turning on and off mRNA translation. Recently, these novel

genes have been found to be required for normal heart development and function, and also they are expressed in heart disease. A number of specific miRNAs have shown distinct roles in the development of the heart, during cardiac remodeling, in the modulation of cardiac hypertrophy and cardiac conduction system.

It is important to understand that whereas both miRNA and small interfering RNA (siRNA) are used for gene inactivation, endogenous miRNA-induced silencing complexes (miRISC) inhibit translation by binding imperfectly matched sequences in the 3′ UTR of target mRNA. On the other hand, siRNA-programmed RISC (siRISC) is a synthetic or exogenous dsRNA that silences gene expression by cleaving a perfectly complementary target mRNA (see section "Epigenetics and HF"). Thus, miRNAs function as guide molecules in diverse gene silencing pathways modulating gene function and are characterized functionally as part of ribonucleoprotein (RNP) complexes, also referred as miRNPs or miRNA-induced silencing complexes (miRISCs). Although analysis of in vivo and cell-free extracts has shed some light on the miRNA-mediated repression, the mechanistic details are not still fully understood [29].

Even though initially miRNAs were reported to be transcribed by RNA polymerase II (Pol II), and that the primary miRNA transcripts (pri-miRNAs) contain cap structures as well as poly(A) tails, which are the unique properties of class II gene transcripts [30], the view of miRNA origins and the transcriptional machinery driving their expression has been modified. After genomic analysis of miRNAs in the human chromosome 19 miRNA cluster (C19MC), Borchert et al. [31] have found that these molecules are interspersed among Alu repeats. Since Alu transcription occurs through RNA Pol III recruitment, and the Alu elements upstream of C19MC miRNAs retain sequences important for Pol III activity, the authors tested the promoter requirements of C19MC miRNAs. Using chromatin immunoprecipitation and cell-free transcription assays they concluded that Pol III, but not Pol II, is associated with miRNA genomic sequence and sufficient for transcription. Thus, originally transcribed as long RNA precursors denominated primary RNA, the formation of premature miRNA requires to be trimmed by the nuclear encoded RNA polymerase III Drosha. Later on, to become a mature miRNA, this molecule is further trimmed by Dicer in the cytoplasm, an endonuclease that cleaves double-stranded RNA and that is required for miRNA biogenesis [32]. According to Viswanathan et al. [33], mature miRNAs to be produced from primary miRNA requires sequential cleavages by the Microprocessor (Fig. 3.1), which is comprised by a double-stranded RNA binding protein DGCR8 besides Drosha and the Dicer enzyme complexes.

Interestingly, post-translational control of miRNA expression occurs in a tissue-specific manner [34, 35], and is developmentally regulated [36–38]. Some miRNAs are highly expressed in human [39] and mouse embryonic cells, mouse

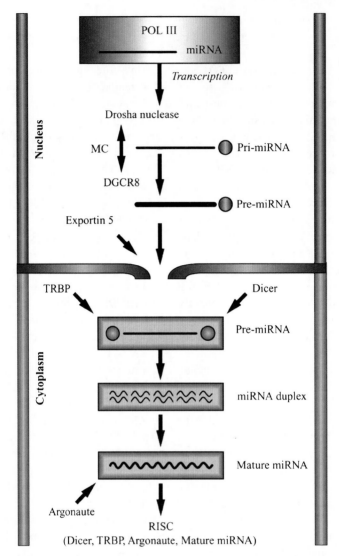

Fig. 3.1 Pathway for miRNA biogenesis. MicroRNAs (miRNA) are single-stranded RNA molecules of about 21–23 nucleotides in length, which regulate gene expression. The genes that encode miRNAs are transcribed from DNA but not translated into protein (non-coding RNA). They are processed from primary transcripts known as pri-miRNA to short stem-loop structures called pre-miRNA and finally to functional miRNA. Mature miRNA molecules are partially complementary to one or more messenger RNA (mRNA) molecules, and their main function is to downregulate gene expression. Analysis of miRNAs in the human chromosome 19 miRNA cluster (C19MC), by Borchert et al. showed that Pol III, but not Pol II, is associated with miRNA genomic sequence and sufficient for transcription (see text) [31]. The initial transcript is called primary microRNA (pri-miRNA) whose 5′ and 3′ ends are cleaved by the Drosha nuclease, which needs a dedicated double-stranded RNA binding protein to convert the long nuclear primary microRNA transcripts into shorter pre-microRNA stem-loops, the cytoplasmic precursors from which mature microRNAs are ultimately excised. Drosha nuclease is complexed with the RNA-binding protein DGCR8 forming the Microprocessor complex (MC). The cleavage product is called the pre-microRNA (pre-miRNA), a product of about 60–70 nt. The resulting pre-miRNA, bound by Exportin-5, is translocated across the nuclear pore into the cytoplasm. In the cytoplasm, the pre-miRNA is bound and cleaved by the Dicer ribonuclease in complex with the RNA-binding protein (TAR binding-protein (TRBP)). The product becomes an imperfectly double-stranded miRNA of about 21–23 nucleotides. At this stage, the miRNA has two strands: the passenger strand, which will be removed and degraded, and the guide strand, which will be retained and guides the RISC to target mRNAs. The Argonaute protein is already bound to the Dicer:miRNA complex or subsequently binds the complex. The resulting single-stranded miRNA (the guide strand) remains in a complex containing Argonaute, Dicer, TRBP, and other proteins termed as the RNA-induced Silencing Complex (RISC)

embryonic carcinoma as well as in human primary tumors although their mature types were not detectable [37].

The discovery of miRNAs has completely changed the understanding of selective silencing of a gene product in vivo. It is estimated that approximately 1% of predicted genes in animals encode these small regulatory molecules, which consist of about 20–25 noncoding nucleotides that regulate gene expression post-transcriptionally, by hybridization to messenger RNAs (mRNAs) with subsequent mRNA degradation or translational inhibition of the targeted transcripts [40].

Thomas et al. reported that as miRNAs regulate the translation of target mRNAs, the up- or downregulation of a particular miRNA from its "normal" state can cause the miRNA to act as either a tumor suppressor or an activator [41]. The upregulation of a particular miRNA is likely to lead to a decrease in its targeted protein levels, while downregulation should lead to an increase. Since multiple miRNAs can regulate one transcript, the correlation of levels of a particular miRNA with its protein targets is rather complicated.

A significant fraction of human genes are regulated by microRNAs, which play essential roles in critical processes such as cellular proliferation, development, differentiation, and apoptosis [40, 42–45]; therefore, a search for the role of microRNAs in cardiovascular diseases, and in particular in HF is actively being pursued.

As our understanding of the role of the molecular elements lying in miRNA regulation advances, many RNA-based targets will probably begin to show from these powerful translational regulators. Expectations are that this new research field will significantly contribute to decipher gene expression regulation in cardiovascular diseases, and in particular in myocardial hypertrophy regulation and HF. Interestingly, Thum et al., using microarray and miRNA stem loop RT-PCR techniques, have evaluated miRNA profiles and the cardiac mRNA transcriptome in the LV from end-stage HF individuals, and compared to healthy subjects and fetal human heart [46]. Marked changes were found in the miRNAs expression in HF patients, and these changes appear to closely mimic the miRNAs expression pattern observed in fetal cardiac tissue. Employing bioinformatic analysis a strong agreement was noted between regulated mRNA expression in HF and the presence of miRNA binding sites in the respective 3′ untranslated regions. Messenger RNAs upregulated in the failing heart contained preferentially binding sites for downregulated miRNAs and vice versa. Furthermore, transfection of cardiomyocytes with a set of fetal miRNAs induced cellular hypertrophy as well as changes in gene expression comparable to the failing heart. Hopefully, local or systemic application of precursor or inhibitory miRNA molecules effecting heart miRNAs may be beneficial by modulating heart gene networks; and targeting miRNAs may become a new therapeutic form for the prevention and treatment of HF.

Cardiac miRNAs may play a major role in the regulation of genes expression during heart development, cardiac function, and electrical conductance. Furthermore, vasculoproliferative conditions such as angiogenesis and neointimal lesion formation have been found associated to miRNAs.

The roles of Dicer and miRNAs in mammalian skeletal muscle development have been studied by O'Rourke et al. [47]. They found that during embryogenesis Dicer activity was essential for normal muscle development since Dicer muscle mutants have reduced muscle miRNAs, and die perinatally while displaying decreased skeletal muscle mass accompanied by abnormal myofiber morphology. Also, Dicer mutant muscles showed increased apoptosis and Cre-mediated loss of Dicer in Myod-converted myoblasts, resulting in increased cell death. Thus, Dicer RNase III endonuclease has an essential role in skeletal muscle development and implies that miRNAs are vital components for embryonic myogenesis.

The importance of miRNAs in development and cardiac homeostasis is also supported by the recent findings of Chen et al. [48] that cardiac-specific knockout of Dicer, leads to rapidly progressive DCM, HF, and postnatal lethality. Dicer mutant mice exhibit abnormal expression of cardiac contractile proteins and marked sarcomere disarray. In addition, these mutant mice showed decreased heart rates and fractional shortening. Consistent with the role of Dicer in animal hearts, Dicer expression was also decreased in end-stage human DCM and in failing hearts. On the other hand, significant increase of Dicer expression was observed in the failing hearts after insertion of LVADs. Taken together, these findings support the notion that the Dicer gene has a role of paramount significance in cardiac contractility and not only miRNAs play a critical role in normal cardiac function but also in the development of cardiac pathology. Myogenic miRNAs, encoded by bicistronic transcripts or nestled within intron of myosin genes, have been shown to modulate muscle function in a number of cardiovascular conditions such as hypertrophy, CHD, HF, cardiac dysrhythmias, and muscle dystrophy. This plurality of roles makes miRNAs very desirable targets to develop new therapeutic strategies.

To determine whether miRNAs have a role in cardiac development and/or homeostasis, Wang et al. searched for miRNAs that were expressed in the mouse cardiovascular system, and were conserved across species ranging from flies to humans. On the basis of their in silico data and information from previous observations, a particular miRNA subgroup, the miR-1 subfamily appears to be cardiac-enriched [49, 50]. This subfamily consists of two closely related miRNAs encoded by distinct genes that share near complete identity and are designated miR-1-1 and miR-1-2 (see Table 3.1). Northern blot analysis of both miR-1 genes demonstrated that they are 21 base pairs (bp) in length and were expressed specifically in the heart and skeletal muscle of adult mice. Of special interest is that miR-1-1 and miR-1-2 are specifically expressed in cardiac and skeletal muscle precursor cells, and miR-1 genes seem to be direct transcriptional targets of muscle differentiation regulators, including serum response factor, MyoD, and Mef2. It is worth noting that excess of miR-1 in the developing heart leads to a decreased pool of proliferating ventricular cardiomyocytes. Using a new algorithm for microRNA target identification that incorporates features of RNA structure and target accessibility, these investigators [49, 50] showed that Hand2, a transcription factor that promotes ventricular cardiomyocyte expansion, is a target of miR-1 and that miR-1 genes titrate the effects of critical cardiac regulatory proteins to control the balance between differentiation and proliferation during cardiogenesis. A pair of muscle-specific miRNAs miR 206/133b (Table 3.1) has been reported by Chen et al. [51]. miRNA-1 (miR-1) and miRNA-133 (miR-133), clustered on the same chromosomal loci, were transcribed together in a tissue-specific manner during development, and miR-1 promotes myogenesis by targeting histone deacetylase 4 (HDAC4), a transcriptional repressor of muscle gene expression. On the other hand, miR-133 enhances myoblast proliferation by repressing serum response factor (SRF). These findings suggest that two mature miRNAs, derived from the same miRNA polycistron and transcribed together, can carry out distinct biological functions and that miRNAs participate in transcriptional circuits that control skeletal muscle gene expression and embryonic development. Liu et al. [52] have shown how MEF2 transcription factor directly activates transcription of a bicistronic primary transcript encoding miR-1-2 and 133a-1, via an intragenic muscle-specific enhancer located between the miR-1-2 and 133a-1 coding regions. This MEF2-dependent enhancer is activated in the linear heart tube during mouse embryogenesis and thereafter controls transcription throughout the atrial and ventricular chambers of the heart. MEF2 together with MyoD also regulates the miR-1-2/-133a-1 intragenic enhancer in the somite myotomes and in all skeletal muscle fibers during embryogenesis and adulthood. A similar muscle-specific intragenic enhancer controls transcription of the miR-1-1/-133a-2 locus. Taken together, these findings reveal a commonality of regulatory elements associated with the miR-1/-133 genes and underscore the central role of MEF2 as a regulator of the transcriptional and posttranscriptional pathways that control cardiac and skeletal muscle development.

MiRNAs, by modulating the balance between the antagonistic processes of myoblast growth and differentiation, become essential components of the regulation of muscle development [53], and to find out whether disease-associated miRNAs are contributory to the disease process and if so, whether therapeutic modulation might affect the severity and/or progression of the disease may be of great significance. Assigning a specific miRNA to a specific target represent a great challenge; although, finding the potential targets of miRNA may provide not only new insights into the mechanism of disease but may also allow the discovery of novel therapies.

That miRNAs miR-1 and miR-133 are preferentially expressed in the heart and skeletal muscle, and have opposing effects in cardiomyocytes apoptosis have been reported by Xu et al. [54]. Single target sites for miR-1 in the 3′-untranslated regions of the HSP60 and HSP70 genes, and multiple putative target sites for miR-133 throughout the sequence of

the caspase-9 gene were detected. miR-1 reduced the levels of HSP60 and HSP70 proteins without changing their transcript levels, whereas miR-133 did not affect HSP60 and HSP70 expression at all. On the other hand, miR-133 repressed caspase-9 expression at both the protein and mRNA levels. Thus, increased miR-1 and/or decreased miR-133 levels favor apoptosis and decreased miR-1 and/or miR-133 levels favor survival. These investigators have also noted that overexpression of miR-1 occur in patients with CAD, and when miR-1 was overexpressed either in normal or infarcted rat hearts it intensified dysrhythmogenesis [55]. In contrast, elimination of miR-1 by an antisense inhibitor in infarcted rat hearts ameliorated the dysrhythmias. miR-1 overexpression slowed conduction and depolarized the cytoplasmic membrane by post-transcriptionally repressing KCNJ2 (encodes the K+ channel subunit Kir2.1) and GJA1 (encodes connexin 43), and likely this accounts, at least in part, for its dysrhythmogenic potential. Therefore, miR-1 may have an important pathophysiological role in the heart, and is a potential target for dysrhythmias.

Notwithstanding the current explosion of information regarding miRNAs, its use in diagnosis and therapeutic modulation of individual miRNAs or miRNA clusters in cardiovascular diseases need further investigation, since it is likely that therapies that specifically regulate cardiovascular miRNAs, either mimicking or antagonizing miRNAs actions [56], might normalize dysfunctional gene networks and may constitute a new paradigm in the prevention/treatment of cardiovascular diseases, including HF.

MiRNA expression-profiling studies demonstrate that expression levels of specific miRNAs change in diseased human hearts, pointing to their involvement in cardiomyopathies and HF [46]. Identification of the targets of specific miRNAs is necessary to understand the correct molecular mechanisms underlying their function.

As observed by Callis and Wang [57], most animal miRNAs are partially complementary to their target sites, which thwart simple homology searches to identify target sequences. In response, several bioinformatic-prediction algorithms that weigh various criteria, including sequence conservation and thermal stability have been developed and they have shown to be an indispensable guide for advancing miRNA research [58–60]. On the other hand, these *in silico* predictions require experimental testing and, to date, only a handful of miRNA targets with roles in the heart have been validated in biological systems (see Table 3.1).

Previous profiling studies in human samples show that changes in miRNA expression also occur in the failing human hearts, including the up-regulation of miRNAs that are normally expressed in the developing heart [46, 51]. According to van Rooij et al. [61] continued miR-195 overproduction led to DCM and HF in young mice, although the mechanisms underlying miR-195 function have not been clearly defined since no target genes have been yet identified. MiR-214 is also up-regulated during hypertrophy, although transgenic mice over-expressing miR-214 did not cause an abnormal heart phenotype. Unlike miR-195 and miR-214, miR-1 and miR-133 are down-regulated during hypertrophy [61–64], and miR-208 is expressed specifically in the heart and has been deleted from the mouse genome [65]. Interestingly, miR-208 null animals were viable and appeared normal without evidence of gross developmental defects. On the other hand, the miR-208 null animals showed at 2 months of age mild reduction in contractility and progressive cardiac dysfunction.

It is apparent that the genetic pathways controlling cardiac hypertrophy share a common component that is regulated by miR-208. The thyroid hormone receptor-associated protein 1 (Thrap1), a co-factor of the thyroid hormone nuclear receptor that can influence transcription positively and negatively has been considered such a component [57]. While the exact nature of miR-21 function remains unclear, inhibition of miR-21 using antisense oligonucleotides suppresses agonist-induced hypertrophic growth in primary cardiomyocytes [66]. In contrast, inhibition of miR-21 using locked nucleic acid-modified miR-21 antisense oligonucleotides stimulated hypertrophic growth in vitro. Moreover, introduction of functional miR-21 or

miR-18b into cardiomyocytes represses myocyte hypertrophy [67]. These findings suggests that miRNAs, and in particular miR-1, miR-21, miR-133, miR-195 and miR-208, are novel players in animal models of cardiac hypertrophy (Table 3.2).

Identification of specific targets for miRNAs involved in the hypertrophic response might provide insights on the molecular mechanisms underlying cardiac hypertrophy/ remodeling. Notably, since changes in miRNA expression occur in cardiac diseases, the molecules could be used not only as biomarkers for clinical diagnosis but also, because of their small size, their in vivo delivery becomes a feasible therapy. On the other hand, recent observations suggested that miR-1 and miR-133a expression are decreased during skeletal muscle hypertrophy. McCarthy and Esser have studied the expression level of the muscle-specific miRNAs in the soleus and plantaris muscles, and also whether their expression in the plantaris was altered in response to functional overload [68]. From a group of miRNAs examined only miR-206 was differentially expressed between soleus and plantaris muscles. This was confirmed by a sevenfold higher expression in the soleus for both the primary miRNA (pri-miR) and mature miR. After functional overload, transcript levels for both pri-miR-1-2 and pri-miR-133a-2 increased by approximately twofold,

Table 3.2 Validated Heart/Muscle-Specific MicroRNAs

microRNA	Expression pattern	Functions	Target sites	Refs
miR-1	Heart, skeletal muscle	Inhibition of hypertrophy, cell proliferation	RasGAP, Cdk9	[63]
		Control of cardiac conductance	Hand2	[69]
		Myogenesis	Irx5, KCND2	[70]
		Cardiogenesis	HDAC4	[51]
		Pro-apoptotic	Notch ligand, Delta	[71]
		Dysrhythmias when overexpressed in CAD	3′ untranslated regions of HSP60 and HSP70	[54]
			KCNJ2 (Kir2.1), GJA1(connexin 43)	[57]
miR-133	Heart, skeletal muscle	Inhibition of cardiac hypertrophy	RhoA, Cdc-42	[62]
		Promotion of proliferation	WHSC2	[51]
		Control of cardiac conductance	SRF	[72]
		Anti-apoptotic	HERG	[54]
			Caspase-9	
miR-206	Skeletal muscle	Myogenesis	Cx43, Fst11, Utrn	[73]
			PolA1	[74]
				[75]
miR-208	Heart	β-MHC expression	THRAP1	[65]
		Stress-dependent cardiac remodeling		
miR-21	Heart (also in spleen, small intestine, colon)	Inhibition of cardiac hypertrophy	Fas & TGF-β receptor (?)	[65]
		Tumor suppressor genes	PTEN, TPM1	[66]
				[76]
				[77]

RasGAP Ras GTPase activating protein; *Cdk9* cyclin-dependent kinase 9; *Hand2* heart and neural crest derivatives expressed transcript 2; *Irx5* Iroquois homeobox protein 5; *KCND2* potassium voltage-gated channel; *HDAC4* histone deacetylase 4; *HSP60* heat shock protein 60; *KCNJ2* potassium inwardly-rectifying channel, subfamily J, member 2; *GJA1* gap junction protein α1; *RhoA* Ras homolog gene family, member A; *Cdc-42* cell division cycle 42; *WHSC2* Wolf–Hirschhorn syndrome candidate gene 2; *SRF* serum response factor; *HERG* human ether-a-go-go related gene; *Cx43* Connexin 43; *Fst11* Follistatin-like 1; *Utrn* utrophin (*Homo sapiens*); *PolA1* polymerase (DNA directed) α1; *TGF* tumor necrosis factor; *PTEN* phosphatase and tensin homolog gene; *TPM1* tropomyosin 1 (*Homo sapiens*)

whereas pri-miR-206 levels were elevated 18.3-fold. In contrast, the expression of miR-1 and miR-133a were downregulated by approximately 50% following overload. This difference between pri-miR and miR expression following overload could not be explained by a change in the expression of components of the miRNA biogenesis pathway, since Drosha and Exportin-5 transcript levels were significantly increased (by 50%) in response to functional overload, whereas Dicer expression was unchanged. These findings suggest that miRNAs may have a role in the adaptation to functional overload in skeletal muscle, but if this also occurs in the heart is not known.

Finally, since single miRNAs appear to have multiple mRNA targets, with some of those miRNA regulatory targets seemingly working in concert to control a common pathway and/or biological function, miRNAs potentially may become efficient tools for targeting a particular disease pathway or process [57]. That miRNAs involvement occurs in cardiac diseases has been confirmed by the dysregulated expression of miRNAs and Dicer, a miRNA pathway component in HF; however, further research is needed in order to understand how the integration of miRNAs into the genetic networks occurs in cardiac pathology, and importantly in order to develop miRNAs as potential novel therapeutic targets.

Epigenetics and HF

Gene expression is significantly affected in the failing heart and knowing which genes are affected may be very helpful in the understanding of the pathophysiology of HF. An important part in the regulation of gene expression is play by epigenetics, thru histone modification. Epigenetics is thought of as changes in gene expression that are stable between cell divisions, and sometimes between generations, through modification of chromosomal components, but do not involve changes in the underlying DNA sequence of the organism. Central to eukaryotic biology, epigenetics is better demonstrated in the process of cellular differentiation, which allows cells to stably maintain different characteristics despite containing the same genomic material. Such epigenetic modifications include methylation of genomic DNA as well as acetylation, phosphorylation, ubiquitination, and SUMOylation of core histone proteins.

Genetic and biochemical studies have shown that epigenetic changes play an important role in the pathophysiology of cardiac hypertrophy and HF, with dysregulation in histone acetylation shown to be directly linked to impaired cardiomyocytes contractility. In this section we will describe some general concepts and the available information on the role of epigenetic modifications with a survey of the current status and prospects for epigenetic (also on gene therapy in a later chapter) in human with cardiac pathology/HF.

Histone/Chromatin Modifications; Epigenetic Control of Gene Expression

The amino termini of histones contain a diversity of posttranslational modifications. The most prominent are acetylation and methylation of lysine residues in the highly conserved N termini of histones H3 and H4. Increased acetylation invariably correlates with up-regulation of transcriptional activity whereas decreased acetylation correlates with transcriptional repressed states (the heterochromatic state is associated with hypoacetylation of histones). Interestingly, the inactivation of genes in heterochromatin contrasts with euchromatin that is characterized by genes with robust gene expression and activation (Fig. 3.2a).

The regulation of heterochromatin assembly is also mediated by modifying enzymes that act directly on histones or by factors that bind them [78], as depicted in Fig. 3.2b. The status of histone acetylation, at a given promoter, is determined by the balanced action of histone acetyltransferases (HATs) and histone deacetylases (HDACs). This includes the NAD-dependent HDAC (SIR2), a key mediator of heterochromatin assembly and gene silencing. Also, there is ample evidence for the role of repetitive DNA elements and noncoding RNAs in the regional targeting (and propagation) of heterochromatin complexes. For instance, siRNAs are involved in post-transcriptional gene silencing and in initiating heterochromatin complexes at repetitive DNA. Moreover, centromeric repeat sequences produce small double-stranded RNAs (dsRNA) that are sufficient to recruit heterochromatin [79]. Small RNAs are involved in dosage compensation and genomic imprinting [80] and dsRNAs complementary to promoter regions can cause gene silencing mediated via DNA methylation [81].

It is worth noting that although the process is mediated by naturally-occurring double-stranded RNA molecules, it can also be induced by adding chemically-synthesized siRNAs that will silence specific cardiomyocytes genes by altering the RNA sequence to match the corresponding gene sequence. This approach may have therapeutic potential in HF patients (see Chap. 21) since it provides a new way of targeting known disease-causing genes, including those for which small-molecule drugs have not been found.

Histone Acetylation/Chromatin Remodeling Plays a Critical Role in the Triggering/ Progression of Cardiac Hypertrophy

Among the best-characterized control points for gene regulation in hypertrophic myocardium is histone acetylation [82]. Together with other histone modifications, the change in chromatin structure and remodeling is a prerequisite for

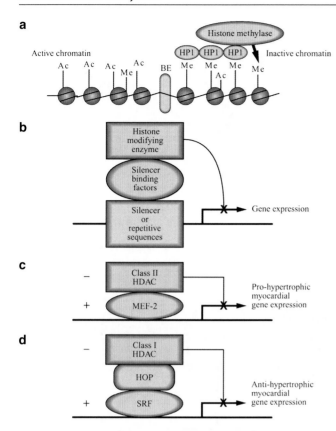

Fig. 3.2 Epigenetic chromatin histone modifications and gene expression. (**a**) Representation of transcriptionally active (euchromatin) and silenced chromatin (heterochromatin) with acetylated (Ac) and methylated (ME) histone N-termini. HP1 is a transcription-inhibiting protein recruited by methylated histone residues. BE is a boundary element, which separates areas of active and inactive chromatin. (**b**) Model of the formation of heterochromatic gene silencing. (**c**) Chromatin modification can block cardiac hypertrophy. A pro-hypertrophic transcriptional program mediated by the binding of myocyte enhancing factor-2 (MEF-2) is repressed with the recruitment and functional modification of chromatin by specific histone deacetylases (class II HDAC). (**d**) Other settings of chromatin can promote cardiac hypertrophy. An anti-hypertrophic transcriptional program mediated by the binding of SRF (serum response factor) is repressed by the binding of the HOP protein and the recruitment of class I HDAC, promoting hypertrophic growth response

access of transcription factors to their target DNA. The essential role of a HAT protein in cardiac muscle was first proven by deletion of the coactivator p300, which perturbed heart development and cell proliferation [83]. Class II HDACs can act as signal-responsive repressors of cardiac hypertrophy, inhibiting gene expression that is dependent on myocyte enhancer factor-2 [84]. Furthermore, overexpression of the transcriptional corepressor homeodomain-only protein (HOP) causes cardiac hypertrophy by the recruitment of a class I HDAC. In addition, the activity of different HDACs can act, in some contexts, as repressors of cardiac hypertrophy by inhibiting the gene expression of pro-hypertrophic genes (Fig. 3.2c) and in other contexts (e.g., recruitment by HOP)

by inhibiting the expression of a novel growth-suppressing anti-hypertrophic transcriptional pathway (Fig. 3.2d) HDAC activity effectively contributes to cardiac hypertrophy [85, 86].

Other Regulators of Chromatin Remodeling Have Been Recently Identified Which May Be Operative in the Heart

In a genome-wide search for cardiogenic genes, the simjang gene, which encodes a protein component of the chromatin remodeling complex recruited by methyl-CpG-DNA binding proteins was found, suggesting that epigenetic information may be crucially involved in early cardiac development [87].

Can these data be used for therapeutic purposes? At first glance, the large scale and global nature of the transcriptional suppression engendered by this type of chromatin modification/remodeling might be difficult to apply to modulating specific pathways without compromising the gene expression, that is essential for cardiac function; however, the possibility that this modification could be finely targeted by the appropriate administration of specific small RNAs and/or repeated elements, opens the door for the directed use of global transcriptional inactivation reagents in the treatment of cardiovascular diseases in general, and specifically in HF.

DNA Modification-Methylation

DNA methylation is a key epigenetic mechanism implicated in genomic imprinting, gene regulation, chromatin structure, genome stability and disease, and is the focus of a human epigenome project [88].

It is well established that a major mechanism for down-regulation of gene expression involves the methylation of a cytosine and guanosine rich area in the promoter region of genes termed the CpG island (see Fig. 3.3). This promoter associated CpG methylation has been associated with the permanent inactivation of gene transcription [89]. This process has also been shown to be involved in the inactivation of the X chromosome in which promoter methylation is critical in maintaining the silenced state, and where demethylation results in renewed gene expression [90]. Promoter methylation is also involved in genomic imprinting in which the silenced state of the affected allele is determined by methylation of the promoter regions for numerous imprinted genes, and demethylation results in bi-allelic gene expression [91].

Until now, there has been limited systematic study addressing the relationship of DNA methylation to the expression of cardiac genes either during myocardial development, normal physiological transition or during cardiac disease.

Fig. 3.3 Model of the epigenetic role of DNA methylation in mediating gene expression, DNA damage, and stability

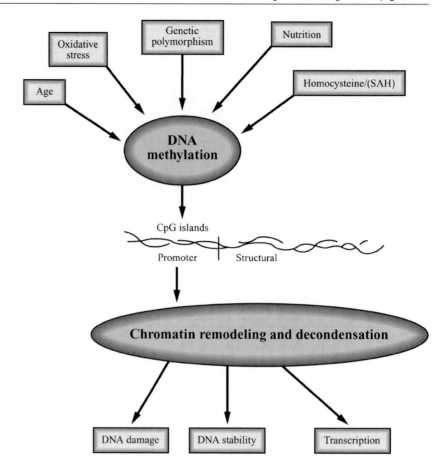

Several observations have shown that the stability and expression of the cardiac troponin gene associated with normal cardiac function and cardiac pathology is affected by cytosine methylation [92]. Also, it has been demonstrated that the expression of genes known to be essential in maintaining homeostatic cardiac physiology can be modulated by targeted DNA methylation, e.g., the KVLQT1 gene involved in cardiac membrane transport is subject to regulation by DNA methylation which alters its expression [93, 94]. Interestingly, defects in this gene are associated with long QT syndrome, cardiac dysrhythmias and sudden cardiac death. Moreover, the mtTFA gene associated with mitochondrial biogenesis, is also regulated by DNA methylation [95].

The promoter of human mtTFA contains 67 CpG dinucleotides particularly evident at its NRF1 binding site. In vitro methylation of NRF-1 site by HhaI methylase abolished the mtTFA promoter activity up to 90%, implying that the CpG methylation of NRF-1 site inactivate mtTFA promoter-driven transcriptional activity. The significance of a normal functioning mtTFA has been recently demonstrated in transgenic mice which developed DCM by harboring a deleted mtTFA allele. Moreover, it has been reported that methylation of the estrogen receptor gene was prevalent, with a non-uniform distribution, in human cardiovascular

tissues including right atrium, saphenous veins and proximal aorta [96]. Furthermore, elevated levels of DNA methylation have been found to be age and not gender-dependent, and were more prevalent in patients with CAD as compared to normal tissues. Interestingly, high levels of homocysteine correlated with decreased levels of DNA methylation (or increased hypomethylation).

Hyperhomocysteinemia has been implicated in several cardiovascular pathologies including its participation in the pathogenesis of occlusive CAD [97]. The mechanism of the relationship between DNA methylation and homocysteine levels has already been defined [98]. Chronic elevation in homocysteine levels results in parallel increases in intracellular S-adenosylhomocysteine (SAH) with the consequent inhibition of DNA methyl-transferases [99]. Hence, elevated levels of DNA hypomethylation is associated with increased levels of homocysteine. Increased SAH-mediated DNA hypomethylation and associated alterations in gene expression and chromatin structure may prove informative in understanding the pathogenesis of diseases related to homocysteinemia including cardiac pathologies.

A linkage of SAH-mediated DNA hypomethylation with increased oxidative damage to DNA has been proposed [98]. This suggests that DNA hypomethylation increases DNA's vulnerability and sensitivity to free radical damage. Parenthetically, it has been well documented that DNA hypomethylation is associated with elevated levels of hyper-acetylated and decondensed chromatin, due to decreased binding of methyl-sensitive proteins such as methyl CpG binding protein and histone deacetylase. This is supported by the promotion of chromatin decondensation by hypomethy-lating agents such as SAH and 5-azacytidine. A more open DNA conformation associated with hypomethylated chro-matin would constitute an easier target for endonuclease digestion and increased DNA strand breaks.

In summary, genomic methylation appears to function as a final step in the modulation of gene transcription but its role in the profiling of gene expression in HF remains unknown. Therefore, the potential therapeutic application of these findings in HF is unclear at this time. While DNA methylation-mediated regulation is generally "broad-brush" or global (similar to that described above with altered chro-matin in relation to heterochromatic gene expression), site-specificity might be directed by the introduction of CpG islands into non-coding regions of introduced genetic con-structs in the cardiovascular system.

Transcriptional Coactivator p300 and Cardiac Hypertrophy

The transcriptional coactivator p300 is a ubiquitous nuclear phosphoprotein and transcriptional cofactor with intrinsic acetyltransferase activity. It controls the expression of numerous genes in cell-type and signal-specific manner, and plays a pivotal role in cellular proliferation, apoptosis, and embryogenesis [100]. By catalyzing acetylation of histones and transcription factors, p300 plays a significant role in epi-genetic regulation. Abnormal p300 function is associated with deregulated target gene expression, and is implicated in cardiac hypertrophy, inflammation, cancer, and genetic dis-orders. Recently, Wei et al. [101] have assessed in vivo the quantitative control of adaptive cardiac hypertrophy by acetyltransferase p300 and its effect in the development of HF. In this study, pressure overload induced by transverse aortic coarctation, postnatal physiological growth, and human HF were associated with large increases in p300. With minimal transgenic overexpression of p300 (1.5- to 3.5-fold) striking myocyte and cardiac hypertrophy were detected, and both mortality and cardiac mass were directly related to p300 protein dosage. Heterozygous loss of a single p300 allele reduced pressure overload-induced hypertrophy by approximately 50% and rescued the hypertrophic pheno-type of p300 overexpressers. Furthermore, increased expres-sion of p300 did not have effect on total histone deacetylase activity but was associated with proportional increases in

p300 acetyltransferase activity and acetylation of the p300 substrates histone 3 and GATA-4. The doubling of p300 lev-els was associated with the de novo acetylation of myocyte enhancer factor-2 (MEF2). Consistent with this, genes spe-cifically upregulated in p300 transgenic hearts were highly enriched for MEF2 binding sites. Taken together, these find-ings suggest that small increments in p300 are necessary and sufficient to drive myocardial hypertrophy, possibly through acetylation of MEF2 and upstream of signals promoting phosphorylation or nuclear export of histone deacetylases. Induction of myocardial p300 content appears to be a pri-mary rate-limiting event in the response to hemodynamic loading in vivo and p300 availability drives and constrains adaptive myocardial growth. Thus, specific reduction of p300 content or activity may diminish stress-induced hyper-trophy and prevent the development of HF.

Energy Metabolism Profiling

There is increasing evidence that metabolic abnormalities may contribute to the development and progression of myo-cardial disease. Data obtained from animal models have sug-gested a "metabolic switch" from fatty acid to glucose oxidation during evolving HF; however, whether the same pathologic process is operative in human HF [5, 102] awaits further confirmation.

Gathered observations have shown up-regulation of genes involved in OXPHOS that might reflect a decrease in activity of mitochondrial respiratory pathways during developing HF [8, 24, 103]; although genes involved in FAO did not show consistent up- or down-regulation, highlighting the difficulty of reproducing findings from animal models to humans. When assessing only end-stage HF there appears to be a trend towards down-regulation of glycolysis, in apparent contradiction with the hypothesis that a switch from fatty acid to glucose oxidation occurs in the failing heart, but rather favoring a decreased use of glucose as an energy sub-strate [104, 105]. None of the transcriptional regulators of cardiac mitochondrial biogenesis and respiratory function have been found to be deregulated. This may be related to the fact that most studies lacked an experimental design that would allow the detection of relatively small expression changes [105].

The peroxisome proliferator-activated receptor (PPAR) family of nuclear receptor transcription factors can regulate cardiac metabolism at the gene expression level. According to Madrazo and Kelly [106], the three PPAR family members (α, β/δ and γ) are unique to serve as transducers of develop-mental, physiological, and dietary cues that influence cardiac fatty acid and glucose metabolism. Murine PPAR loss- and gain-of-function models have provided insights on the roles of these receptors in regulating myocardial metabolic pathways and have defined key links to disease states, including the hypertensive and diabetic heart. Nevertheless, further research is needed before we can translate these findings to human HF.

Further proof that changes in energy metabolism contribute to HF comes from observations in patients and experimental models of cardiomyopathy/HF, in which cardiac dysfunction is associated with alterations in a number of key pathways including energy metabolism, cell survival, cytokine signaling, calcium handling, adrenergic receptor signaling, cytoskeletal and contractile proteins, extracellular matrix, and endothelial and microvascular functions. Some of these alterations appear to be reversible and regulated by left ventricular assisted devices (LVAD) treatment. LVAD by lowering cardiac pressure and volume overload in the myocardium, followed by decreased ventricular wall tension, reduced cardiomyocyte hypertrophy, improved coronary perfusion, and decreased chronic ischemia. Improvement in coronary blood flow and myocardial perfusion as well as decreased ventricular wall tension may affect the molecular pathways involved in the development of chronic HF [107]. While traditionally considered as a bridge to transplantation, LVAD is now considered by themselves a definitive form of therapy, since it may reverse at least some of the changes in the above signaling pathways with the potential for myocardial recovery through reverse remodeling, a potential that is further enhanced by combination with pharmacologic therapy. Furthermore, thru LVAD we are beginning to distinguish changes associated with recovery from those of mechanical unloading alone, opening the door to potential predictors and novel therapeutic targets capable of repairing the myocardial damage [108]. Nevertheless, further research to confirm these findings is warranted.

Intracellular Calcium Cycling Profiling

Observations on the molecular basis of HF have emphasized the existence of a variety of potentially important new therapeutic targets, and among them important components of the cardiomyocyte calcium-handling pathway exhibit distinctive alterations in HF. Studies from Kaye et al. [109] on the effect of restoration these changes in experimental models of HF, whether in genetically engineered mouse models or by myocardial gene transfer, support the concept that calcium-handling pathway is a potential target for clinical intervention.

HF is characterized by abnormal sarcoplasmic reticulum (SR) function, with markedly decreased myocyte contractility and development of dysrhythmias. Evidence has shown that intracellular Ca^{2+} cycling is a key regulator of contraction in the human heart. During membrane depolarization

Ca^{2+} enters the cardiomyocyte through the L-type Ca^{2+} channel (as discussed in Chap. 2). In this section, it suffices to say that the influx of Ca^{2+} into the cell triggers Ca^{2+} release from the SR through the ryanodine receptor. This then triggers muscle contraction through the actin–myosin complex. Subsequently, relaxation is initiated by Ca^{2+} reuptake in the SR by Ca^{2+}ATPase-2 (SERCA2). Although not all studies have yielded consistent results, altered functional properties of the L-type Ca^{2+} channel, the ryanodine receptor, ATPase-2 and related regulatory proteins have been linked to human HF [110]; changes in calcium cycling factors are thought to contribute to the reduced velocity of contraction present in the failing heart [111]. On the other hand, it has recently been pointed out that although there is evidence for the existence of an abnormal ryanodine receptor (RyR2)-mediated Ca^{2+} leak in HF, it is not known if this is the cause or rather it is the consequence of the disease [112]. Thus, the SR Ca^{2+} leak may be an important contributor in the development of dysrhythmias in HF but it may not be the direct cause of the abnormal myocyte contractility, rather the secondary effect of abnormal metabolism and energy utilization.

Gene profiling studies in human have consistently revealed a pattern of down-regulation of SERCA2 expression in the failing heart [24, 113, 114]. This is concordant with the results at both the mRNA and protein levels [114]. This down-regulation could be related to decreased SR Ca^{2+} content, found in cardiomyocytes from failing hearts. In most gene profiling studies in human failing hearts, the negative regulator of Ca^{2+}ATPase-2 – phospholamban – was not differentially expressed between failing and non-failing states. The only exception was the study by Grzeskowiak et al. [115] who found that phospholamban was up-regulated in the failing heart. These data corroborate the proposed mechanism that HF is associated with a decreased Ca^{2+}ATPase-2/phospholamban ratio and therefore decreased Ca^{2+}ATPase-2. Phospholamban will only inhibit Ca^{2+}ATPase-2 activity when it is hypophosphorylated. The dephosphorylation of phospholamban is accomplished by type 1 phosphatase, which is inhibited by the protein phosphatase inhibitor PPP1R1A. In one transcriptomal study, this inhibitor was down-regulated in the failing hearts [4], suggesting activation of phospholamban. Moreover, down-regulation of PPP1R1A may also increase the dephosphorylation of other Ca^{2+} cycling proteins, such as the L-type Ca^{2+} channel and the ryanodine receptor [116].

In general, protein dephosphorylation is associated with impaired cardiac function, and increased type 1 phosphatase levels and activity have been found in human HF [117]. Furthermore, ablation of PPP1R1A in murine hearts is associated with impaired β-adrenergic contractile responses [118]. Other protein phosphatase inhibitors such as PPP1R14C [119], PPP1R12A, [117] and PPP1R15A were found up-regulated in failing hearts [119]. Nevertheless, it remains unclear whether the encoded proteins play a role in the regulation of intracellular Ca^{2+} cycling proteins. The fact that in the transcriptomal studies of HF relatively few proteins involved in intracellular Ca^{2+} cycling were differentially expressed indicated that either disturbed Ca^{2+} cycling is mostly regulated at the protein level, or that it is regulated by expression changes so small that were below the detection threshold.

The Genetics of Human HF

Although the genesis of most forms of adult HF does not appear to be primarily genetic, HF, like other forms of adult heart disease, can be precipitated by an underlying genetic condition that results in the expression of a causative protein from birth, with inherited DCM and adult HCMs being particularly salient examples [120]. There exists substantial cross-talk between genetic and acquired processes in both adult and CHD. Environmental factors can profoundly disturb normal cardiac development, and it is increasingly apparent that common genetic variations can act as important modifiers of acquired adult heart disease, influencing susceptibility or progression, and determining the response to therapy. The development of cardiac hypertrophy and subsequent HF are accompanied by the reprogramming of cardiac gene expression and the activation of "fetal" cardiac genes that encode proteins involved in contraction, calcium handling, and metabolism (Fig. 3.4). Molecular pathways that participate in the control of cardiac hypertro-

phy program include: natriuretic peptides, the adrenergic system, adhesion and cytoskeletal proteins, IL-6 cytokine family, MEK-ERK1/2 signaling, histone acetylation, calcium-mediated modulation, and the recent discovery that microRNAs play a role in controlling cardiac hypertrophy [121]. This transcriptional reprogramming is related to a loss of cardiac function, while improvement in cardiac function following LVAD is frequently accompanied by normalization of cardiac gene expression [122, 123].

From the perspective of the etiology of HF, the greatest insight has been gained from the discovery that HCM and DCM can result from mutations in genes encoding an astonishingly broad range of cardiac proteins. The vast spectrum of causative mutations and new insights into their mechanisms of action has been extensively reviewed [120]. To date, hundreds of mutations that cause HCM have been discovered, with varying phenotypes resulting from missense mutations in a given protein. An intriguing handful of mutations can promote aggressive clinical courses. Determining the way in which human myosin heavy chain mutations alter force-generation in single-molecule motility studies is a triumph of the reductionist approach. In contrast, it is unclear how hyperdynamic properties at this level of organization "trickle up" to myofiber disarray, sporadic cell death, and reactive fibrosis; this illustrates a gap in the present understanding of pathogenesis, as opposed to etiology. From one point of view, many hereditary cardiomyopathies may differ little from acquired cardiac disorders; the instigating signal is known in both cases, whether it is a mutation, long-standing hypertension, or past ischemic injury, yet the mechanisms of

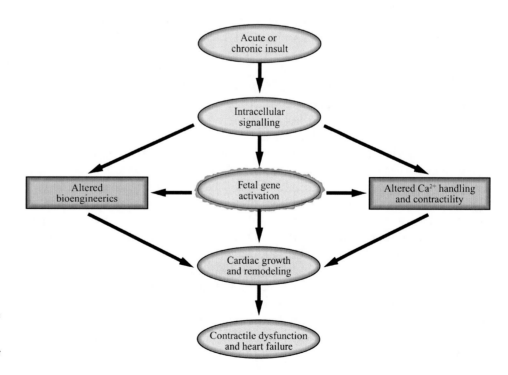

Fig. 3.4 Flow-chart showing the role of fetal gene activation in cardiac remodeling, pathologic hypertrophy, and progression to HF

disease progression are still cryptic. Because genetic defects alter cells in highly precise and defined ways, it is reasonable to hope that dissecting their effector pathways might prove simpler than dissecting those of other forms of heart disease. Human mutations are an experiment of nature through which extraordinary details of cardiac proteins' structure and function have come to be unmasked – not only for the sarcomeric and cytoskeletal proteins that are most familiar in hereditary heart disease, but also for genetic defects in energy-generating mechanisms, calcium-cycling mechanisms, and transcriptional control, some of which were discussed earlier.

Recent progress in genomic applications has led to a better understanding of the relationship between genetic background and HF. A considerable component of the variability in HF outcome is due to modifier genes, i.e., genes that are not involved in the genesis of a disease but which modify the severity of the phenotypic expression once the disease has developed [124]. The strategy most commonly used to identify modifier genes, the candidate strategy, is based on association studies correlating the severity of the phenotype of the disease (morbidity and/or mortality) and the sequence variation(s) of selected candidate gene(s). Single nucleotide polymorphisms (SNPs) are the most common among these genetic variations, and are widely used in association studies. This strategy has showed that, for example, several polymorphisms of the β-1 and β-2 adrenergic receptors genes and the angiotensin-converting enzyme gene are correlated to prognosis in HF patients. For example, a polymorphism at the nucleotide position 145 leads to a missense mutation of amino-acid residue 49 of the β-1 adrenergic receptor (β1-AR) and replacement of a serine (Ser-49) by a glycine (Gly-49). The consequence of this Ser49Gly polymorphism on the risk to develop HF and the time course of the disease has been examined in a study of 184 patients and 77 healthy controls [124]. The allele frequency of the Gly49 variant was 0.13 in controls and 0.18 in patients. At the time of the 5-year follow-up, 62% of the patients with the wild type gene and 39% of the patients with the Ser49Gly variant had died or had experienced hospitalization. Patients without the mutation had significantly poorer survival compared to those with the mutation.

Genome mapping has been employed for the identification of HF modifier genes [125], and also has been used with success to identify genes involved in the development of both monogenic and multifactorial diseases. Furthermore, it has been shown that the prognosis of mice with HF, induced through overexpressing calsequestrin, is linked to two Quantitative Trait Loci (QTL) localized on chromosome 2 and 3 [126]. Using the two strategies in combination, candidate gene and genome mapping, it may be possible in the near future identification of an increasing number of modifier genes, which may provide a more rational approach to detect patients at risk for disease, as well as their response to therapy.

Conclusion

HF, the final common pathway of a plurality of cardiovascular disorders, results from impairment of myocardial systolic and/or diastolic function. Since the publication of the human genome, there have been many changes in the field of genetic research, and has provided investigators with a vast new array of potential therapeutic genes to test in animal models in vivo. The emergence of microarray technology has paved the way to simultaneously assess the expression of tens of thousands of gene transcripts in a single experiment, providing a resolution and precision of phenotypic characterization not previously possible. Within the heart, many examples of genetic and protein changes correlated with functional alterations have been noted both during normal development and during the development of HF from diverse etiologies. Detailed profiling has been performed on structural changes, as well as functional alterations including energy metabolism and intracellular calcium handling as mentioned earlier.

With the discovery of miRNAs, there is now a need to further re-evaluate the mechanisms and pathophysiology of cardiovascular diseases. These small molecules appear to be tissue specific and have been found in the heart. Interestingly, many miRNAs have been found to be dysregulated in human HF and they are actively involved in cardiac growth and development, electrical conduction, and cardiac pumping function [127].

Although established genetic tools are sufficient for uncovering the underlying causes for monogenic diseases, the genetic basis underlying the pathogenesis of complex, polygenic diseases such as HF remain mostly unknown. At present, it is likely that the combined use of novel genetic research with emerging epigenetic tools will be the method of choice to explore the molecular causes that underlie the pathophysiology of HF. Moreover, understanding how small molecules (nutrients and chemicals) interact with the epigenome may allow us to design a new generation of epigenetic drugs for complex diseases such as cancer and Metabolic Syndrome [64]. Similarly, besides advances in the understanding of genetic mechanisms, understanding the effect of epigenetic in cardiac disease-related gene deregulation is also providing new insights. Knowledge about the genetic and molecular changes occurring in the human failing heart has begun to have clinical applications as diagnostic and prognostic markers, as well as in the development of new therapies for those conditions associated with HF.

The potential for HDAC inhibitors in HF therapy has been outlined by McKinney and Olson [128]. HDAC inhibitors thru curbing cardiac hypertrophy and normalization of gene expression may modify the current therapy of HF. We agree that improvement in our understanding of the fundamental processes that control stress-response pathways and cardiac gene expression, together with novel high throughput screening of molecular modifiers of cellular function, novel transcriptional therapies will be developed to further the treatment of HF.

Finally, increasing research in genomics with data coming from multiple fields, ranging from cancer research, neurobiology, and chemical sciences, will facilitate progress in understanding the pathophysiology and clinical management of HF. Novel insights into the genetic background of HF and the cardiovascular consequences of abnormal gene function and expression may ultimately impact on the development of targeted therapeutic strategies and disease management replacing less effective treatment modalities directed solely at rectifying structural cardiac defects and temporal improvement of function in the failing heart.

Summary

- HF is the final common pathway of cardiovascular disorders resulting from impairment of myocardial systolic and/or diastolic function.
- Global and specific gene profiling in preclinical studies has proved informative about the involvement of specific genes and the development of useful biomarkers in the progression of HF.
- Gene profiling studies have shown distinctive profiles of gene expression in association with different types of cardiomyopathy leading to HF (e.g., ischemic, DCM, or HCM).
- Early clinical studies suggest that the integrated use of genetic technologies (gene profiling, pharmacogenomics) with clinical medicine may enable a highly effective individually-tailored approach to treating Cardiomyopathy/HF.
- Modifier *loci* and SNPs have been identified to impact HF progression.
- The combined use of novel genetic research with emerging epigenetic tools will be the method of choice to explore the molecular causes that underlie the pathophysiology of HF.
- With the discovery of miRNAs, there is a need to further re-evaluate the mechanisms and pathophysiology of cardiovascular diseases.
- HDAC inhibitors thru curbing cardiac hypertrophy and normalization of gene expression may modify the current therapy of HF.
- Gene therapies and cell transplantation studies have just begun to be employed in clinical studies of HF with modest but encouraging preliminary results.
- Research in genomics with novel findings arriving from multiple fields, ranging from cancer research to neurobiology and chemical sciences, may facilitate progress in understanding the pathophysiology and clinical management of HF.

References

1. Mann DL (1999) Mechanisms and models in heart failure: a combinatorial approach. Circulation 100:999–1008
2. Kittleson MM, Hare JM (2005) Molecular signature analysis: using the myocardial transcriptome as a biomarker in cardiovascular disease. Trends Cardiovasc Med 15:130–138
3. Sanoudou D, Vafiadaki E, Arvanitis DA, Kranias E, Kontrogianni-Konstantopoulos A (2005) Array lessons from the heart: focus on the genome and transcriptome of cardiomyopathies. Physiol Genomics 21:131–143
4. Tan FL, Moravec CS, Li J, Apperson-Hansen C, McCarthy PM, Young JB, Bond M (2002) The gene expression fingerprint of human heart failure. Proc Natl Acad Sci USA 99:11387–11392
5. Steenman M, Lamirault G, Le Meur N, Le Cunff M, Escande D, Leger JJ (2005) Distinct molecular portraits of human failing hearts identified by dedicated cDNA microarrays. Eur J Heart Fail 7:157–165
6. Renlund DG, Taylor DO, Kfoury AG, Shaddy RS (1999) rules: historical background and implications for transplantation management. United Network for Organ Sharing. J Heart Lung Transplant 18:1065–1070
7. Kaab S, Barth AS, Margerie D et al (2004) Global gene expression in human myocardium-oligonucleotide microarray analysis of regional diversity and transcriptional regulation in heart failure. J Mol Med 82:308–316
8. Hwang JJ, Allen PD, Tseng GC, Lam CW, Fananapazir L, Dzau VJ, Liew CC (2002) Microarray gene expression profiles in dilated and hypertrophic cardiomyopathic end-stage heart failure. Physiol Genomics 10:31–44
9. Hall JL, Grindle S, Han X et al (2004) Genomic profiling of the human heart before and after mechanical support with a ventricular assist device reveals alterations in vascular signaling networks. Physiol Genomics 17:283–291
10. Kittleson MM, Minhas KM, Irizarry RA et al (2005) Gene expression in giant cell myocarditis: altered expression of immune response genes. Int J Cardiol 102:333–340
11. Carey VJ, Gentry J, Whalen E, Gentleman R (2005) Network structures and algorithms in Bioconductor. Bioinformatics 21:135–136
12. Simon R, Radmacher MD, Dobbin K, McShane LM (2003) Pitfalls in the use of DNA microarray data for diagnostic and prognostic classification. J Natl Cancer Inst 95:14–18
13. Kittleson MM, Ye SQ, Irizarry RA et al (2004) Identification of a gene expression profile that differentiates between ischemic and nonischemic cardiomyopathy. Circulation 110:3444–3451
14. Heidecker B, Kasper EK, Wittstein IS et al (2008) Transcriptomic biomarkers for individual risk assessment in new-onset heart failure. Circulation 118:238–246
15. Song Q, Schmidt AG, Hahn HS et al (2003) Rescue of cardiomyocyte dysfunction by phospholamban ablation does not prevent ventricular failure in genetic hypertrophy. J Clin Invest 111:859–867
16. Wilkie GS, Dickson KS, Gray NK (2003) Regulation of mRNA translation by 5′- and 3′-UTR-binding factors. Trends Biochem Sci 28:182–188
17. Schott P, Singer SS, Kogler H et al (2005) Pressure overload and neurohumoral activation differentially affect the myocardial proteome. Proteomics 5:1372–1381
18. Figueredo VM, Camacho SA (1995) Basic mechanisms of myocardial dysfunction: cellular pathophysiology of heart failure. Curr Opin Cardiol 10:246–252
19. Barany M (1967) ATPase activity of myosin correlated with speed of muscle shortening. J Gen Physiol 50:197–218
20. Morano M, Zacharzowski U, Maier M, Lange PE, Alexi-Meskishvili V, Haase H, Morano I (1996) Regulation of human heart contractility by essential myosin light chain isoforms. J Clin Invest 98:467–473

21. Braz JC, Bueno OF, Liang Q et al (2003) Targeted inhibition of p38 MAPK promotes hypertrophic cardiomyopathy through upregulation of calcineurin-NFAT signaling. J Clin Invest 111:1475–1486

22. Dorn GW, Molkentin JD (2004) Manipulating cardiac contractility in heart failure: data from mice and men. Circulation 109:150–158

23. Boluyt MO, O'Neill L, Meredith AL et al (1994) Alterations in cardiac gene expression during the transition from stable hypertrophy to heart failure. Marked upregulation of genes encoding extracellular matrix components. Circ Res 75:23–32

24. Yung CK, Halperin VL, Tomaselli GF, Winslow RL (2004) Gene expression profiles in end-stage human idiopathic dilated cardiomyopathy: altered expression of apoptotic and cytoskeletal genes. Genomics 83:281–297

25. Komajda M, Charron P (2004) A new approach for the identification of modifier genes in heart failure. Pharmacogenomics J 4:221–223

26. Le Corvoisier P, Park HY, Carlson KM, Marchuk DA, Rockman HA (2003) Multiple quantitative trait loci modify the heart failure phenotype in murine cardiomyopathy. Hum Mol Genet 12:3097–3107

27. Gupta S, Young D, Maitra RK et al (2008) Prevention of cardiac hypertrophy and heart failure by silencing of NF-kappaB. J Mol Biol 375:637–649

28. Frantz S, Fraccarollo D, Wagner H et al (2003) Sustained activation of nuclear factor kappa B and activator protein 1 in chronic heart failure. Cardiovasc Res 57:749–756

29. Filipowicz W, Bhattacharyya SN, Sonenberg N (2008) Mechanisms of post-transcriptional regulation by microRNAs: are the answers in sight? Nat Rev Genet 9:102–114

30. Lee Y, Kim M, Han J, Yeom KH, Lee S, Baek SH, Kim VN (2004) MicroRNA genes are transcribed by RNA polymerase II. EMBO J 23:4051–4060

31. Borchert GM, Lanier W, Davidson BL (2006) RNA polymerase III transcribes human microRNAs. Nat Struct Mol Biol 13:1097–1101

32. Wang Z, Luo X, Lu Y, Yang B (2008) miRNAs at the heart of the matter. J Mol Med 86:771–783

33. Viswanathan SR, Daley GQ, Gregory RI (2008) Selective blockade of microRNA processing by Lin28. Science 320:97–100

34. Smirnova L, Gräfe A, Seiler A, Schumacher S, Nitsch R, Wulczyn FG (2005) Regulation of miRNA expression during neural cell specification. Eur J Neurosci 21:1469–1477

35. Obernosterer G, Leuschner PJ, Alenius M, Martinez J (2006) Post-transcriptional regulation of microRNA expression. RNA 12:1161–1167

36. Mineno J, Okamoto S, Ando T et al (2006) The expression profile of microRNAs in mouse embryos. Nucleic Acids Res 34:1765–1771

37. Thomson JM, Newman M, Parker JS, Morin-Kensicki EM, Wright T, Hammond SM (2006) Extensive post-transcriptional regulation of microRNAs and its implications for cancer. Genes Dev 20:2202–2207

38. Wulczyn FG, Smirnova L, Rybak A et al (2007) Post-transcriptional regulation of the let-7 microRNA during neural cell specification. FASEB J 21:415–426

39. Suh MR, Lee Y, Kim JY et al (2004) Human embryonic stem cells express a unique set of microRNAs. Dev Biol 270:488–498

40. Karp X, Ambros V (2005) Developmental biology. Encountering microRNAs in cell fate signaling. Science 310:1288–1289

41. Thomas JR, Hergenrother PJ (2008) Targeting RNA with small molecules. Chem Rev 108:1171–1224

42. Rajewsky N, Socci ND (2004) Computational identification of microRNA targets. Dev Biol 267:529–535

43. Cheng AM, Byrom MW, Shelton J, Ford LP (2005) Antisense inhibition of human miRNAs and indications for an involvement of miRNA in cell growth and apoptosis. Nucleic Acids Res 33:1290–1297

44. Chen CZ, Li L, Lodish HF, Bartel DP (2004) MicroRNAs modulate hematopoietic lineage differentiation. Science 303:83–86

45. Xu P, Guo M, Hay BA (2004) MicroRNAs and the regulation of cell death. Trends Genet 20:617–624

46. Thum T, Galuppo P, Wolf C et al (2007) MicroRNAs in the human heart: a clue to fetal gene reprogramming in heart failure. Circulation 116:258–267

47. O'Rourke JR, Georges SA, Seay HR et al (2007) Essential role for Dicer during skeletal muscle development. Dev Biol 311:359

48. Chen JF, Murchison EP, Tang R et al (2008) Targeted deletion of Dicer in the heart leads to dilated cardiomyopathy and heart failure. Proc Natl Acad Sci USA 105:2111–2116

49. Wang Z, Wang DZ, Hockemeyer D, McAnally J, Nordheim A, Olson EN (2004) Myocardin and ternary complex factors compete for SRF to control smooth muscle gene expression. Nature 428: 185–189

50. Wang DZ, Olson EN (2004) Control of smooth muscle development by the. myocardin family of transcriptional coactivators. Curr Opin Genet Dev 14:558–566

51. Chen JF, Mandel EM, Thomson JM et al (2006) The role of microRNA-1 and microRNA-133 in skeletal muscle proliferation and differentiation. Nat Genet 38:228–233

52. Liu N, Williams AH, Kim Y et al (2007) An intragenic MEF2-dependent enhancer directs muscle-specific expression of microRNAs 1 and 133. Proc Natl Acad Sci USA 104: 20844–20849

53. van Rooij E, Liu N, Olson EN (2008) MicroRNAs flex their muscles. Trends Genet 24:159–166

54. Xu C, Lu Y, Pan Z et al (2007) The muscle-specific microRNAs miR-1 and miR-133 produce opposing effects on apoptosis by targeting HSP60, HSP70 and caspase-9 in cardiomyocytes. J Cell Sci 120:3045–3052

55. Yang B, Lin H, Xiao J et al (2007) The muscle-specific microRNA miR-1 regulates cardiac arrhythmogenic potential by targeting GJA1 and KCNJ2. Nat Med 13:486–491

56. Scalbert E, Bril A (2008) Implication of microRNAs in the cardiovascular system. Curr Opin Pharmacol 8:181–188

57. Callis TE, Wang DZ (2008) Taking microRNAs to heart. Trends Mol Med 14:254–260

58. Lewis BP, Burge CB, Bartel DP (2005) Conserved seed pairing, often flanked by adenosines, indicates that thousands of human genes are microRNA targets. Cell 120:15–20

59. Krek A, Grün D, Poy MN et al (2005) Combinatorial microRNA target predictions. Nat Genet 37:495–500

60. Griffiths-Jones S, Saini HK, van Dongen S, Enright AJ (2008) miR-Base: tools for microRNA genomics. Nucleic Acids Res 36: D154–D158

61. van Rooij E, Sutherland LB, Liu N et al (2006) A signature pattern of stress-responsive microRNAs that can evoke cardiac hypertrophy and heart failure. Proc Natl Acad Sci USA 103: 18255–18260

62. Carè A, Catalucci D, Felicetti F et al (2007) MicroRNA-133 controls cardiac hypertrophy. Nat Med 13:613–618

63. Sayed D, Hong C, Chen IY, Lypowy J, Abdellatif M (2007) MicroRNAs play an essential role in the development of cardiac hypertrophy. Circ Res 100:416–424

64. Liu L, Li Y, Tollefsbol TO (2008) Gene-environment interactions and epigenetic basis of human diseases. Curr Issues Mol Biol 10:25–36

65. van Rooij E, Sutherland LB, Qi X, Richardson JA, Hill J, Olson EN (2007) Control of stress-dependent cardiac growth and gene expression by a microRNA. Science 316:575–579

66. Cheng Y, Ji R, Yue J et al (2007) MicroRNAs are aberrantly expressed in hypertrophic heart: do they play a role in cardiac hypertrophy? Am J Pathol 170:1831–1840

67. Tatsuguchi M, Seok HY, Callis TE et al (2007) Expression of microRNAs is dynamically regulated during cardiomyocyte hypertrophy. J Mol Cell Cardiol 42:1137–1141

68. McCarthy JJ, Esser KA (2007) MicroRNA-1 and microRNA-133a expression are decreased during skeletal muscle hypertrophy. J Appl Physiol 102:306–313

69. Zhao Y, Samal E, Srivastava D (2005) Serum response factor regulates a muscle-specific microRNA that targets Hand2 during cardiogenesis. Nature 436:214–220

70. Zhao Y, Ransom JF, Li A et al (2007) Dysregulation of cardiogenesis, cardiac conduction, and cell cycle in mice lacking miRNA-1–2. Cell 129:303–317

71. Kwon C, Han Z, Olson EN, Srivastava D (2005) MicroRNA1 influences cardiac differentiation in Drosophila and regulates Notch signaling. Proc Natl Acad Sci USA 102:18986–18991

72. Xiao J, Luo X, Lin H et al (2007) MicroRNA miR-133 represses HERG K+ channel expression contributing to QT prolongation in diabetic hearts. J Biol Chem 282:12363–12367

73. Anderson C, Catoe H, Werner R (2006) MIR-206 regulates connexin 43 expression during skeletal muscle development. Nucleic Acids Res 34:5863–5871

74. Rosenberg MI, Georges SA, Asawachaicharn A, Analau E, Tapscott SJ (2006) MyoD inhibits Fstl1 and Utrn expression by inducing transcription of miR-206. J Cell Biol 175:77–85

75. Kim HK, Lee YS, Sivaprasad U, Malhotra A, Dutta A (2006) Muscle specific microRNA miR-206 promotes muscle differentiation. J Cell Biol 174:677–687

76. Zhu S, Si ML, Wu H, Mo YY (2007) MicroRNA-21 targets the tumor suppressor gene tropomyosin 1 (TPM1). J Biol Chem 282:14328–14336

77. Meng F, Henson R, Wehbe-Janek H, Ghoshal K, Jacob ST, Patel T (2007) MicroRNA-21 regulates expression of the PTEN tumor suppressor gene in human hepatocellular cancer. Gastroenterology 133:647

78. Grewal SI, Moazed D (2003) Heterochromatin and epigenetic control of gene expression. Science 301:798–802

79. Reinhart BJ, Bartel DP (2002) Small RNAs correspond to centromeric heterochrtomatin repeats. Science 297:1831

80. Volpe TA, Kidner C, Hall IM, Teng G, Grewal SI, Martienssen RA (2002) Regulation of heterochromatin silencing and histone H3 lysine-9 methylation by RNAi. Science 297:1833–1837

81. Mette MF, Aufsatz W, van der Winder J, Matzke MA, Matzke AJM (2000) Transcriptional silencing and promoter methylation triggered by double-stranded RNA. EMBO J 19:5194–5201

82. Metzger JM (2002) HDAC lightens a heavy heart. Nat Med 8:1078–1079

83. Gusterson RJ, Jazrawi E, Adcock IM, Latchman DS (2003) The transcriptional co-activators CREB-binding protein (CBP) and p300 play a critical role in cardiac hypertrophy that is dependent on their histone acetyltransferase activity. J Biol Chem 278:6838–6847

84. Zhang CL, McKinsey TA, Chang S, Antos CL, Hill JA, Olson EN (2002) Class II histone deacetylases act as signal-responsive repressors of cardiac hypertrophy. Cell 110:479–488

85. Hamamori Y, Schneider MD (2003) HATs off to Hop: recruitment of a class I histone deacetylase incriminates a novel transcriptional pathway that opposes cardiac hypertrophy. J Clin Invest 112:824–826

86. Kook H, Lepore JJ, Gitler AD et al (2003) Cardiac hypertrophy and histone deacetylase-dependent transcriptional repression mediated by the atypical homeodomain protein Hop. J Clin Invest 112:863–871

87. Kim YO, Park SJ, Balaban RS, Nirenberg M, Kim Y (2004) A functional genomic screen for cardiogenic genes using RNA interference in developing Drosophila embryos. Proc Natl Acad Sci USA 101:159–164

88. Novik KL, Nimmrich I, Genc B, Maier S, Piepenbrock C, Olek A, Beck S (2002) Epigenomics: genome-wide study of methylation phenomena. Curr Issues Mol Biol 4:111–289

89. Bird AP (1986) CpG rich islands and the function of DNA methylation. Nature 321:209–213

90. Beggs AH, Migeon BR (1989) Chromatin loop structure of the human X chromosome: relevance to X inactivation and CpG clusters. Mol Cell Biol 9:2322–2331

91. Ferguson-Smith AC, Sasaki H, Cattanach BM, Surani MA (1993) Parental-origin-specific epigenetic modification of the mouse H19 gene. Nature 362:751–755

92. D'Cruz LG, Baboonian C, Phillimore HE et al (2000) Cytosine methylation confers instability on the cardiac troponin T gene in hypertrophic cardiomyopathy. J Med Genet 37:E18

93. Smilinich NJ, Day CD, Fitzpatrick GV et al (1999) A maternally methylated CpG island in KvLQT1 is associated with an antisense paternal transcript and loss of imprinting in Beckwith-Wiedemann syndrome. Proc Natl Acad Sci USA 196:8064–8069

94. Cerrato F, Vernucci M, Pedone PV et al (2002) The 5′ end of the KCNQ1OT1 gene is hypomethylated in the Beckwith-Wiedemann syndrome. Hum Genet 111:105–107

95. Choi YS, Kim S, Pak YK (2001) Mitochondrial transcription factor A (mtTFA) and diabetes. Diabetes Res Clin Pract 54:S3–S9

96. Post WS, Goldschmidt-Clermont PJ, Wilhide CC et al (1999) Methylation of the estrogen receptor gene is associated with aging and atherosclerosis in the cardiovascular system. Cardiovasc Res 43:985–991

97. Chen P, Poddar R, Tipa EV, Jacobsen DW (1999) Homocysteine metabolism in cardiovascular cells and tissues: implications for hyperhomocysteinemia and cardiovascular disease. Adv Enzyme Regul 39:93–109

98. James SJ, Melnyk S, Pogribna M, Pogribny IP, Caudill MA (2002) Elevation in S-adenosylhomocysteine and DNA hypomethylation: potential epigenetic mechanism for homocysteine-related pathology. J Nutr 132:2361S–2366S

99. Cox R, Prescott C, Irving CC (1977) The effect of S adenosylhomocysteine on the DNA methylation in isolated rat liver nuclei. Biochim Biophys Acta 474:493–499

100. Ghosh AK, Varga J (2007) transcriptional coactivator and acetyltransferase p300 in fibroblast biology and fibrosis. J Cell Physiol 213:663–667

101. Wei JQ, Shehadeh LA, Mitrani JM, Pessanha M, Slepak TI, Webster KA, Bishopric NH (2008) Quantitative control of adaptive cardiac hypertrophy by acetyltransferase p300. Circulation 118:934–946

102. Huss JM, Kelly DP (2005) Mitochondrial energy metabolism in heart failure: a question of balance. J Clin Invest 115:547–555

103. Yang J, Moravec CS, Sussman MA et al (2000) Decreased SLIM1 expression and increased gelsolin expression in failing human hearts measured by high-density oligonucleotide arrays. Circulation 102:3046–3052

104. Paolisso G, Gambardella A, Galzerano D et al (1994) Total-body and myocardial substrate oxidation in congestive heart failure. Metabolism 43:174–179

105. Steenman M, Lamirault G, Le MN, Leger JJ (2005) Gene expression profiling in human cardiovascular disease. Clin Chem Lab Med 43:696–701

106. Madrazo JA, Kelly DP (2008) The PPAR trio: regulators of myocardial energy metabolism in health and disease. J Mol Cell Cardiol 44:968–975

107. Wohlschlaeger J, Schmitz KJ, Schmid C et al (2005) Reverse remodeling following insertion of left ventricular assist devices (LVAD): a review of the morphological and molecular changes. Cardiovasc Res 68:376–386

108. Soppa GK, Barton PJ, Terracciano CM, Yacoub MH (2008) Left ventricular assist device-induced molecular changes in the failing myocardium. Curr Opin Cardiol 23:206–218

109. Kaye DM, Hoshijima M, Chien KR (2008) Reversing advanced heart failure by targeting Ca2+ cycling. Annu Rev Med 59:13–28

110. Hasenfuss G (1998) Alterations of calcium-regulatory proteins in heart failure. Cardiovasc Res 37:279–289

111. Yano M, Ikeda Y, Matsuzaki M (2005) Altered intracellular Ca2+ handling in heart failure. J Clin Invest 115:556–564

112. George CH (2008) Sarcoplasmic reticulum Ca2+ leak in heart failure: mere observation or functional relevance? Cardiovasc Res 77:302–314

113. Nadal-Ginard B, Kajstura J, Leri A, Anversa P (2003) Myocyte death, growth, and regeneration in cardiac hypertrophy and failure. Circ Res 92:139–150

114. Barrans JD, Allen PD, Stamatiou D, Dzau VJ, Liew CC (2002) Global gene expression profiling of end-stage dilated cardiomyopathy using a human cardiovascular-based cDNA microarray. Am J Pathol 160:2035–2043

115. Grzeskowiak R, Witt H, Drungowski M et al (2003) Expression profiling of human idiopathic dilated cardiomyopathy. Cardiovasc Res 59:400–411

116. Rapundalo ST (1998) Cardiac protein phosphorylation: functional and pathophysiological correlates. Cardiovasc Res 38: 559–588

117. Neumann J, Eschenhagen T, Jones LR, Linck B, Schmitz W, Scholz H, Zimmermann N (1997) Increased expression of cardiac phosphatases in patients with end-stage heart failure. J Mol Cell Cardiol 29:265–272

118. Carr AN, Schmidt AG, Suzuki Y et al (2002) Type 1 phosphatase, a negative regulator of cardiac function. Mol Cell Biol 22: 4124–4135

119. Peterson JT, Hallak H, Johnson L et al (2001) Matrix metalloproteinase inhibition attenuates left ventricular remodeling and dysfunction in a rat model of progressive heart failure. Circulation 103:2303–2309

120. Morita H, Seidman J, Seidman CE (2005) Genetic causes of human heart failure. J Clin Invest 115:518–526

121. Barry SP, Davidson SM, Townsend PA (2008) Molecular regulation of cardiac hypertrophy. Int J Biochem Cell Biol 40:2023–2039

122. Blaxall BC, Tschannen-Moran BM, Milano CA, Koch WJ (2003) Differential gene expression and genomic patient stratification following left ventricular assist device support. J Am Coll Cardiol 41:1096–1106

123. Abraham WT, Gilbert EM, Lowes BD et al (2002) Coordinate changes in Myosin heavy chain isoform gene expression are selectively associated with alterations in dilated cardiomyopathy phenotype. Mol Med 8:750–760

124. Le CP, Park HY, Rockman HA (2003) Modifier genes and heart failure. Minerva Cardioangiol 51:107–120

125. Borjesson M, Magnusson Y, Hjalmarson A, Andersson B (2000) A novel polymorphism in the gene coding for the beta(1)-adrenergic receptor associated with survival in patients with heart failure. Eur Heart J 21:1853–1858

126. Wheeler FC, Fernandez L, Carlson KM, Wolf MJ, Rockman HA, Marchuk DA (2005) QTL mapping in a mouse model of cardiomyopathy reveals an ancestral modifier allele affecting heart function and survival. Mamm Genome 16:414–423

127. van Rooij E, Olson EN (2007) MicroRNAs put their signatures on the heart. Physiol Genomics 31:365–366

128. McKinsey TA, Olson EN (2005) Toward transcriptional therapies for the failing heart: chemical screens to modulate genes. J Clin Invest 115:538–546

Section II
Biochemical and Molecular Changes in Heart Failure

Chapter 4
Bioenergetics and Metabolic Changes in the Failing Heart

Overview

In the failing heart, there are changes in energy substrate metabolism whose etiology and effects are poorly understood. These changes may contribute to deterioration in cardiac contractility as well as to increasing left ventricular remodeling that are the landmarks of the failing heart. Early in HF, the myocardial substrate selection is relatively normal; however, with further HF progression, there is a down-regulation of fatty acid oxidation (FAO), increased glycolysis and glucose oxidation, decreased mitochondrial respiratory chain activity, and abnormal mitochondrial OXPHOS.

Since the literature is abundant on the subject of acquired and inherited lipid disorders in the development of coronary artery disease and stroke (e.g., cholesterol, the apolipoproteins and HDL/LDL), we have decided to omit these subjects. In this chapter, we deal with the metabolic changes that occur in progressive HF, particularly on the mechanisms that regulate metabolic genes expression and metabolic signaling pathways, the effects of these metabolic changes on cardiac performance; the effect of abnormal myocardial substrate metabolism on HF progression, and finally on the effect of therapeutic use of cardiac substrate metabolism in HF.

Introduction

Dysregulation of energy generating pathways occurs in a number of cardiac diseases, including HF. In HF following cardiac hypertrophy, there is a major switch in myocardial bioenergetic substrate used–from fatty acid to glucose. A key component and marker of the switch is the coordinated down-regulation of FAO enzymes and mRNA levels (>40%) in the human left ventricle with a concomitant increase in glucose uptake and oxidation [1]. This switch is thought to represent a reversal to a fetal energy substrate preference pattern of glucose oxidation in the heart. During the development of cardiac hypertrophy, a fetal metabolic gene program is initiated via the complicity of transcription factors that bind to regulatory elements, reducing gene expression

of FAO enzymes (e.g., MCAD and CPT-I β) and is often accompanied by increased expression of ANF, BNP, and β-MHC. Although the molecular mechanisms mediating this down-regulation are not entirely understood, the participation of several nuclear receptors, intermediate metabolites, and transcription factors (e.g., SP1 and PPAR) has been implicated in the programmatic change in myocardial gene expression [2].

The regulation of FAO, the main and critical source of ATP in the healthy heart, occurs at multiple levels, including a strong gene transcriptional component, with members of the peroxisome proliferator-activated receptor (PPAR) family of transcription factors functioning as primary regulators of the FAO enzymes gene expression. Since PPARs are ligand-activated by endogenous lipids and synthetic small molecules, they become attractive targets for pharmaceutical intervention [3]. Furthermore, abnormalities in glucose and fatty acid metabolism associated with diabetes and Metabolic syndrome (MetSyn), chronic diseases increasingly prevalent in the urbanized world, also have an associated spectrum of cardiovascular abnormalities ranging from hypertension to cardiomyopathy and HF. In this chapter, a discussion on the molecular, genetic and cellular basis of abnormal cardiac metabolism, including fatty acid, lipid, and glucose metabolic defects, that can lead to HF is presented.

Bioenergetics of Fatty Acid and Glucose Oxidation

The mitochondrial fatty acid β oxidation pathway contains four reaction steps including acyl-CoA dehydrogenases (short-chain, SCAD, medium-chain, MCAD, long-chain, LCAD and very long chain, VLCAD), short-chain enoyl-CoA hydratase, β-hydroxyacyl CoA dehydrogenase, and β-ketoacyl CoA thiolase as shown in Fig. 4.1. Using long-chain fatty acids as substrates, the latter three steps are performed by a highly organized single enzymatic complex known as the mitochondrial trifunctional protein (MTP) associated with the mitochondrial inner membrane.

J. Marín-García, *Heart Failure*, Contemporary Cardiology,
DOI 10.1007/978-1-60761-147-9_4, © Springer Science+Business Media, LLC 2010

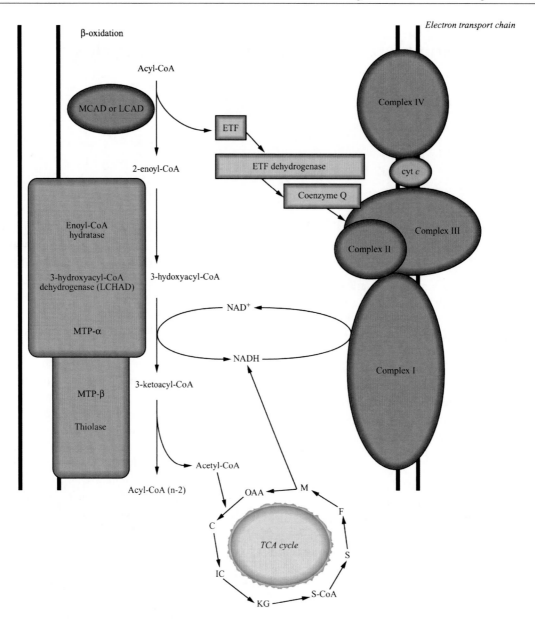

Fig. 4.1 The intersection of mitochondrial bioenergetic pathways: Fatty acid β-oxidation, OXPHOS, and TCA cycle. *ETF* electron transfer flavoprotein; *cytc* cytochrome c; *MTP* mitochondrial trifunctional protein; *MCAD* medium-chain acyl-CoA dehydrogenase; *LCAD* long-chain acyl-CoA dehydrogenase; *LCHAD* long-chain 3-hydroxylacyl-CoA dehydrogenase; *OAA* oxaloacetate; *M* malate; *C* citrate; *F* fumarate; *IC* isocitrate; *KG* ketoglutarate; *S* succinate; *S-CoA* succinyl CoA

Several studies have demonstrated that an entirely different set of enzymes responsible for the β-oxidation of medium and short-chain fatty acids is present in the mitochondrial matrix [4, 5].

The process of FAO is termed β-oxidation since it occurs through the sequential removal of 2-carbon units by oxidation at the β-carbon position of the fatty acyl-CoA molecule. Each round of β-oxidation produces NADH, FADH$_2$, and acetyl-CoA. The acetyl-CoA, the end product of each round of β-oxidation, enters the TCA cycle, where it is further oxidized to CO$_2$ with the concomitant generation of NADH, FADH$_2$, and ATP. The NADH and FADH$_2$ generated during the fat oxidation and acetyl-CoA oxidation in the TCA cycle will subsequently enter the respiratory pathway for the production of ATP. Consequently, the oxidation of fatty acids yields more energy per carbon atom than does the oxidation of carbohydrates. However, while fatty acids produce more ATP during complete aerobic oxidation than glucose, this occurs at the expense of a higher rate of oxygen consumption; thus, the supply of oxygen should be an important determinant of myocardial fuel utilization. As we will see later, a normal balance in the myocardial utilization of these substrates is critical since disruption of this balance can comprise a primary defect resulting in cardiac disease.

Carbohydrate substrates for myocardial glycolytic oxidation are provided by exogenous glucose (obtained by transport) and internal glycogen stores. Upon entry into the cytosol, glucose is rapidly phosphorylated by hexokinase to glucose 6 phosphate and either catabolized by subsequent cytosolic glycolysis or converted into glycogen. The glycolytic pathway produces ATP (two molecules/every glucose molecule oxidized), NADH, and pyruvate, which can either be converted into NAD and cytosolic lactate (often secreted) or transported into the mitochondria for further oxidation by the TCA cycle and oxidative phosphorylation (OXPHOS). The myocardium only generates significant lactate levels as a net producer under conditions of accelerated glycolysis and impaired pyruvate oxidation, which occurs in ischemia and often in diabetes [6]. The oxidative metabolism of pyruvate, once transported to the mitochondria (via a monocarboxylate carrier [7]) generates acetyl-CoA for fueling the TCA cycle and is often termed glucose oxidation.

The regulation of cardiac glycolysis occurs at several steps. Glucose phosphorylation by hexokinase comprises the first regulatory step that commits glucose to further metabolism. Two different isozymes of hexokinase are present in the heart, hexokinases I and II (HKI and HKII), with HKI predominant in the fetal and newborn heart, and the insulin-regulated HKII prevalent in the adult heart [8].

The first regulatory site that commits glucose to the glycolytic pathway occurs at the level of phosphofructokinase (PFK1), catalyzing the phosphorylation of fructose 6-phosphate to fructose 1,6-bisphosphate. The PFK1-mediated conversion of fructose 6-phosphate into fructose 1,6-bisphosphate is a rate-limiting step of glycolysis. Negative allosteric effectors include ATP, citrate, and protons [9], whereas positive effectors consist of AMP and fructose 2,6-bisphosphate, the main activator of PFK-1 in normoxic heart that stimulates glycolysis [10, 11]. Levels of this later effector increases when the glycolytic flux is stimulated and decreases when the heart oxidizes competing substrates [11]. Fructose 1,6-bisphosphate generated by PFK-1 also stimulates pyruvate kinase, which catalyzes the transformation of phosphoenolpyruvate into pyruvate, indicating a further role of PFK-1 in synchronizing several glycolytic reactions, allowing an acceleration of the glycolytic pathway without glycolytic intermediate accumulation [12].

The pyruvate dehydrogenase complex (PDC), an allosteric enzyme that transforms pyruvate into acetyl-CoA by a process called oxidative decarboxylation, is a key determinant in the rate of glucose oxidation. This large multiprotein complex located in the mitochondrial matrix includes 132 subunits (30 E1 dimers, 60 E2 monomers, and 6 E3 dimers) with a variety of coenzymes including thiamine pyrophosphate, lipoamide, CoA, FAD, and NAD and also contains three catalytic subunits responsible for different enzymatic reactions. The PDC complex is highly regulated by its substrates and products and by the activation/inactivation of its catalytic components (i.e., E1, E2, and E3) by their dephosphorylation/phosphorylation. Phosphorylation of PDC by the associated enzyme pyruvate dehydrogenase kinase (PDK) inactivates the PDC whereas pyruvate dehydrogenase phosphatase (stimulated primarily by Ca^{2+}) dephosphorylates and reactivates the enzyme. Both the PDC-activating phosphatase and PDC-deactivating kinase have several cardiac-specific isoforms subject to regulation by diverse developmental, dietary, and hormonal stimuli [13, 14]. The PDK-1 isoform is up-regulated in the adult when compared to the neonatal heart, and is primarily involved in regulating glucose oxidation through the inhibitory phosphorylation of PDC. Expression of the cardiac PDH kinase 4 isoform is responsive to changes in myocardial lipid supply; its up-regulation in the postnatal heart contributes to the perinatal developmental switch to fatty acids as the primary myocardial energy source. This myocardial kinase isoform is also up-regulated in response to thyroid hormone and high-fat diet. Starvation and diabetes decrease myocardial PDC levels by both activating PDK gene expression and by the inactivation of myocardial PDH phosphatase (PDHP) activity, affected largely by promoting a reduced expression of the PDHP2 gene [15].

In addition to its regulation by reversible phosphorylation, PDC is regulated through negative feedback by acetyl-CoA and NADH, end-products of both the PDC reaction and mitochondrial FAO. Acetyl-CoA and NADH accumulation (produced primarily by FAO) also activate PDK, which phosphorylates and inhibits PDC, thereby decreasing glucose oxidation. In addition, increased pyruvate supply can inhibit PDK, thereby stimulating PDC, a process that may occur in isolated hearts perfused with insulin.

When circulating glucose and insulin levels are high, as occurs in the postprandial state, glucose is a primary contributor to cardiac energy metabolism [16], and during the fasting state free fatty acids become the dominant fuel. With increased FAO and the mitochondrial production of acetyl-CoA, NADH and citrate, cytosolic glycolysis and glucose oxidation are inhibited through inactivation of the PDC and phosphofructokinase activities. During oxygen deprivation and anoxia, the inhibition of glucose utilization is removed, and glycolysis is accelerated. A significant increase in carbohydrate oxidation also occurs in the adult heart in response to an acute increase in cardiac work. Since increase in glucose uptake is delayed in this cardiac response, the increase in glucose oxidation is initiated by rapid glycogen breakdown [17].

Glycogen turnover has been proposed as a control site for myocardial glucose metabolism. The myocardial glycogen pool in the adult heart is relatively small occupying only about 2% of the cell volume and is more abundant in the fetal and newborn cardiomyocyte comprising 30% of the cell volume and has a relatively rapid turnover [18]. Unlike liver and skeletal muscle, heart muscle increases its glycogen content with fasting, consistent with the premise that fatty acids, the predominant fuel for the heart during fasting, inhibit glycolysis more than glucose uptake, thereby rerouting glucose toward glycogen synthesis [19]. Myocardial glycogen levels are also increased by insulin, from the concerted stimulation of both glucose transport and glycogen synthase activity [20]. At the other end of the spectrum, glycogen is rapidly broken down when glycogen phosphorylase, the main regulator of glycogenolysis, is stimulated by adrenergic agonist (e.g., epinephrine) or glucagons [21]. It is activated by phosphorylation, either by cAMP-dependent protein kinase or by Ca^{2+}-activated phosphorylase kinase [22]. Glycogen breakdown is also rapidly stimulated during sudden increases of heart work, decreased tissue content of ATP, and increased levels of inorganic phosphate accompanying ischemia or intense physical activities [23, 24].

The role of AMP Kinase (AMPK), a key sensor and mediator in cellular energy metabolism, in glycogen turnover was identified upon the discovery that mutations in the γ-2 regulatory subunit (PRKAγ-2) of the AMPK enzyme, eliciting a constitutively active AMPK, resulted in increased myocardial glycogen, hypertrophic cardiomyopathy (HCM), and preexcitation syndrome (Wolff–Parkinson–White) [25]. However, the relationship between glycogen storage diseases and the development of cardiomyopathy and preexcitation syndrome remains unclear. In contrast, acute AMPK activation leads to increased glycogenolysis. Isolated working hearts perfused with 5-aminoimidazole-4-carboxamide 1-β-D-ribofuranoside (AICAR), an adenosine analog and cell-permeable activator of AMPK, caused an allosteric activation of glycogen phosphorylase responsible for glycogenolysis [26]. Moreover, AMPK contains a putative glycogen-binding site in its β subunit and has been found to be associated with specific subcellular structures containing both glycogen and glycogen phosphorylase [27].

Fatty Acid and Glucose Metabolism in the Normal Cardiomyocyte

Fatty acids play an integral role in determining the structural and functional nature of the cardiomyocyte plasma and mitochondrial membranes. Their role on the fluidity and stability of membrane structure markedly impacts on membrane functions such as the transport of ions and substrates, and on the electrophysiology that is intrinsic to cardiac function and cardiac excitability. Besides the structural and functional roles played within the cardiac membranes, fatty acids and associated lipids are also regulatory molecules that participate in cell signaling, as second messengers in transduction, as effectors in apoptosis and in response to oxidative and ischemic damage.

Glucose metabolism, which provides the bulk of ATP during prenatal growth, contributes significantly to the ATP production in the adult heart (up to 30% of myocardial ATP can be generated by glucose oxidation). In myocardial ischemia and hypertrophy, profound changes in both glucose and fatty acid metabolism occur, with glucose metabolism taking on increasing importance.

Fatty Acids Transport into the Cardiomyocyte

The entry of fatty acids into the myocardial cell, while not fully understood, is thought to be mediated by several proteins including fatty acid binding proteins (FABP) and a myocardial-specific integral membrane transporter (fatty acid translocase or FAT). The nonenzymatic FABP also serves as a facilitator of intracellular transport of relatively insoluble long-chain fatty acids to sites of metabolic utilization (e.g., mitochondria). In mammals, the FABP content in skeletal and cardiac muscle is related to the FAO capacity of the tissue [28]. Interestingly, human FABP has been reported to be a sensitive early marker for acute myocardial infarction, being more sensitive than troponin I [29, 30].

Prior to transport into the mitochondria, fatty acids must be activated in the cytoplasm. The net result of this activation process is the consumption of ATP, and requires CoA-SH. Activation is catalyzed by fatty acyl-CoA synthetases (at least three different acyl-CoA synthetase enzymes have been described whose specificities depend on fatty acid chain length) associated with either the endoplasmic reticulum or the mitochondrial outer membrane.

For the β-oxidation pathway to function, the fatty acyl-CoA has to be transported across the inner mitochondrial membrane. Long-chain fatty acyl-CoA molecules cannot pass directly across the inner mitochondrial membrane and need to be transported as carnitine esters, whereas short-chain and medium-chain fatty acids can be easily transported without the assistance of carnitine.

The transport of long-chain fatty acyl-CoA into the mitochondria, depicted in Fig. 4.2, is accomplished via an acyl-carnitine intermediate, which itself is generated by the action of carnitine palmitoyltransferase I (CPT-I), an enzyme residing in the inner face of the outer mitochondrial membrane. The resulting acyl-carnitine molecule is subsequently transported into the mitochondria by the carnitine translocase, a transmembrane protein residing in the inner membrane, which delivers acyl-carnitine in exchange for free carnitine from the mitochondrial matrix. Carnitine palmitoyltransferase II (CPT-II) located within the inner mitochondrial membrane catalyzes the regeneration of the fatty acyl-CoA molecule, with the acyl group transferred back to CoA from carnitine. Once inside the mitochon-

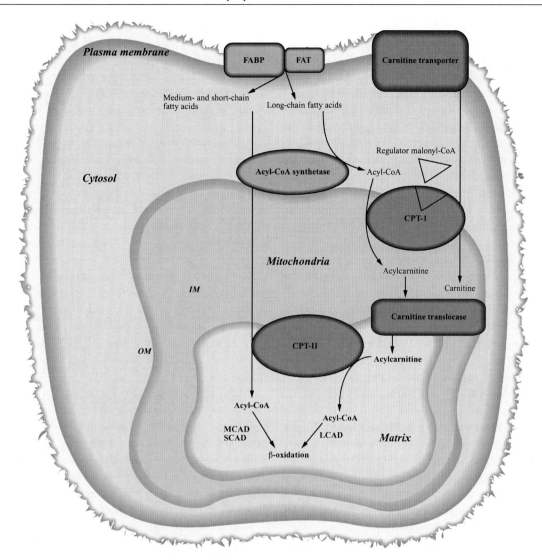

Fig. 4.2 Mitochondrial fatty acid import and oxidation. Fatty acid and carnitine after entry into the cardiomyocyte are transported into the mitochondria for oxidation. *FABP* fatty acid binding protein; *FAT* fatty acid translocase; *CPT-I* carnitine palmitoyltransferase I; *CPT-II* carnitine palmitoyltransferase II; *MCAD* medium-chain acyl-CoA dehydrogenase; *SCAD* short-chain acyl-CoA dehydrogenase; *LCAD* long-chain acyl-CoA dehydrogenase

drion, the fatty acid-CoA is a substrate for the β-oxidation machinery.

A critical regulatory event in the uptake of fatty acids into myocardial mitochondria involves changes in the levels of the metabolite malonyl-CoA that functions as a potent allosteric inhibitor of CPT-I. Malonyl-CoA is synthesized by the enzyme acetyl-CoA carboxylase (ACC) from cytoplasmic acetyl-CoA. Levels of malonyl-CoA are altered by changed levels of the acetyl-CoA or by modulation of the ACC activity. Levels of the cytoplasmic acetyl-CoA increase either as a function of decreased TCA cycle activity reflecting lowered metabolic demand or as a result of increased pyruvate dehydrogenase activity. Therefore, malonyl-CoA production linked to modified metabolic demand or utilization of carbohydrate resources can in turn impact on either the down or up-regulation of fatty acid import into mitochondria and myocardial FAO. ACC activity is allosterically regulated by citrate and by kinase-mediated phosphorylation.

Glucose Transport into the Cardiomyocyte

As in all other cells, the entry of glucose into cardiac myocytes is dependent on the transmembrane glucose gradient and is facilitated by members of the glucose transport (GLUT) family of facilitative glucose transporters [31]. The GLUT-1 transporter, which is localized in the plasma membrane under basal conditions, is considered to be the primary mediator of basal glucose uptake in the heart [32]. Its myocardial expression is steadily increased within hours of ischemia or the induction of hypertrophy. The most abundant glucose transporter in the heart is the insulin-responsive GLUT-4 transporter. Insulin mediates the translocation of GLUT-4 to the plasma membrane from a pool of intracellular vesicles and represents a critical control point, by which the net flux of glucose is regulated. A number of physiological stimuli including hypoxia, ischemia, and cardiac overload can induce this translocation, thereby increasing glucose uptake and glycolytic metabolism [34]. Other stimuli including catecholamines, calcium, and exercise induce stimulation of GLUT-4 translocation and enhance glucose uptake by cardiac tissues and myocytes that are insulin-independent [34–36].

Studies with mice containing muscle-specific deletions in the insulin receptor gene revealed that normal expression of muscle insulin receptors is not needed for the exercise-mediated increase in glucose uptake and glycogen synthase activity in vivo [37]. Furthermore, GLUT-4 translocation to the plasma membrane can also be stimulated by activation of AMPK activity, which occurs during exercise [33]. Studies with transgenic mice containing an inactive form of AMPK have shown normal GLUT-4 levels and glucose uptake, but no increase in glucose uptake, glycolysis or FAO during ischemia [33]. Taken together, these findings have led to the conclusion that AMPK is involved in mediating glucose uptake and glycolysis during ischemia presumably as a protective adaptation. Gathered observations have also demonstrated that changes in myocardial AMPK activity in exercise-trained rats (which increased in proportion to exercise intensity) were associated with physiological AMPK effects (e.g., GLUT-4 translocation to the myocardial sarcolemma) and are consistent with AMPK as a key mediator in the cardiac response to exercise, as previously demonstrated with skeletal muscle [38].

Defects in the ability of insulin to regulate GLUT-4 translocation may be contributory (as one of many effects of insulin) to the development of insulin resistance and noninsulin-dependent type 2 diabetes. Mice heterozygous for a null GLUT-4 allele display reduced muscle glucose uptake, insulin-resistance, and diabetes [39]. On the other hand, mice homozygous for a null GLUT-4 were growth-retarded and exhibited decreased longevity associated with cardiac hypertrophy, although displayed little effect on muscle glucose uptake in either fasted or fed state, but GLUT-4 deleted animals had postprandial hyperinsulinemia suggesting possible insulin resistance. Targeting muscle-specific GLUT-4 revealed a profound reduction in basal glucose transport and near-absence of stimulation by insulin or contraction demonstrating severe insulin resistance and glucose intolerance from an early age [40].

In a model of type 2 diabetes utilizing the Goto-Kakizaki (GK) rat, insulin-stimulated glucose uptake was 50% lower in GK rat hearts when compared with their Wistar controls with marked GLUT-4 protein depletion [41]. Moreover, these animals exhibited significant decreases in levels of the myocardial insulin receptor substrate-1 (IRS-1), as well as reduced IRS-1 association with PI3K, all key upstream events in the insulin signaling pathway. While this study also revealed decreased levels of the myocardial insulin receptor in GK rats, other studies have found conflicting findings about its role in muscle insulin resistance [42]. Interestingly, while most transgenic studies addressing the complicity of insulin signaling pathway on the development of insulin resistance have utilized targeting of muscle-specific components such as GLUT-4 and the insulin receptor, data on the myocardial-specific inactivation of these critical genes are limited. In transgenic mice containing a Cre/LoxP generated construct of GLUT-4 directed to the heart, reduction of the GLUT-4 to a level as low as 15% of the wild type levels was sufficient to allow normal levels of insulin-stimulated glucose uptake, which was markedly reduced with further reduction of GLUT-4 levels. If GLUT-4 levels were reduced to 5% of the wild type, cardiac hypertrophy resulted [43].

Marked down-regulation of myocardial GLUT transporters, limiting both glucose uptake and oxidation and contributing to the heart's inability to generate much needed ATP, has been reported in HF patients [44]. Also, GLUT-4 transcripts have been found to be markedly down-regulated in the human failing heart [45]. Furthermore, in diabetic cardiomyopathy, reduced glucose utilization resulted in an almost exclusive utilization of fatty acids as the myocardial energy source [46, 47]. It is worth noting that data on increased myocardial insulin resistance, accompanying advanced DCM, limiting both glucose uptake and oxidation, may provide critical targets for therapeutic intervention [48, 49]. This myocardial insulin resistance may further impair myocardial glucose uptake and lead to a state of energy depletion.

Experimental and preliminary clinical observations suggest that in patients with chronic HF metabolic modulators that enhance myocardial glucose oxidation may improve cardiac function. Significantly, acute free fatty acid (FFA) deprivation can be harmful [50]. Thus, optimization of myocardial energy metabolism might be an important approach in the treatment of HF. Furthermore, insulin sensitivity and insulin secretion were found to be impaired in chronic HF patients in whom biomarkers of HF and atherosclerotic disease (e.g., NT-proBNP, MR-proADM, CT-proET-1, and MR-proANP) correlated with glucose metabolism [51].

Insulin resistance, characterized by lower myocardial insulin-sensitive glucose uptake and a reduced GLUT-4 protein level, was found in patients with severe cardiac hypertrophy in the absence of hypertension, diabetes, and CAD [52, 53]. Interestingly, myocardial insulin independent glucose uptake (and basal glucose uptake) as well as glycolytic metabolism are enhanced in patients with hypertension and in experimental animals with cardiac hypertrophy, the latter in striking contrast to insulin-stimulated glucose uptake that is depressed in these animals, and suggests that hearts subjected to pressure-overload appear to be resistant to the metabolic effects of insulin [54, 55]. This may have important therapeutic consequences in the setting of individuals with hypertension/hypertrophy, in whom treatment with glucose–potassium–insulin aimed at altering myocardial glucose utilization may be less effective [56]. The expression of myocardial GLUT-4, although at low levels, is present throughout embryonic development, while GLUT-1 is highly expressed in the prenatal heart [57].

At birth, the expression of genes that control myocardial glucose transport and oxidation is down-regulated. In the adult heart, GLUT-4 becomes the main glucose transporter, although GLUT-1 is expressed at a considerable level. Regulation of myocardial glucose transporter levels is primarily exerted transcriptionally [58]. Data collected from several studies suggest that in the failing heart a fetal metabolic gene profile is established largely by down-regulation of adult gene transcripts of metabolic proteins (e.g., GLUT-4) rather than by up-regulation of fetal genes (e.g., GLUT-1) [59]. Similar findings of reactivation of a fetal metabolic program involving the down-regulation of adult but not fetal isoforms as well as a reexpression of growth factors and proto-oncogenes, has been reported in both the hypertrophied heart and after mechanical unloading of the heart [60–62]. Reactivation of these fetal genes includes a pivotal metabolic switch from fat to glucose oxidation, which though initially adaptive, ultimately results in a loss of insulin sensitivity and hence, a loss of metabolic flexibility. This loss of flexibility then becomes an early feature of metabolic dysregulation in the failing heart, which also exhibits all the features of insulin resistance [59].

Cellular Location of FAO and Glucose Oxidation

Both peroxisomes and mitochondria have multiple enzymes involved in fatty acid β-oxidation. The peroxisomal enzymes include palmitoyl-CoA oxidase, L-functional protein and 3-ketoacyl oxidase that are all inducible enzymes acting on straight chain substrates; in addition, peroxisomes contain branched chain acyl-CoA oxidase, D-functional protein and sterol-carrier protein X, which are noninducible and primarily use branched chain substrates. The inducible enzymes increase in response to the peroxisomal proliferating activating receptor (PPAR) resulting in increased peroxisomal biogenesis (see below).

It is important to note that while specific deficiencies in the mitochondrial-located enzymes involved in fatty acid β-oxidation may result in cardiomyopathy and HF; defects in the peroxisomal fatty acid β-oxidation enzymes primarily result in neurological defects including seizures, hypotonia and psychomotor retardation. Interestingly, cardiac abnormalities have been rarely described in peroxisomal deficiencies. This is also true of diseases involving general peroxisomal biogenesis abnormalities such as Zellweger syndrome and neonatal adrenoleukodystrophy, where there is little or no cardiac involvement. There is evidence (discussed below) showing a pivotal role of the PPAR regulation in both mitochondrial FAO and mitochondrial biogenesis, not only in normal cardiac growth and development but also in HF. This suggests an important inter-relationship between the two cellular compartments and further underscores the mitochondrial compartment as a critical effector of cardiac homeostasis. The commonality of biogenesis and potential feedback between these two cellular organelles needs further elucidation in both normal growth and development and in cardiac disease (both fatty acid and mitochondrial OXPHOS disorders).

After entering the plasma membrane, glucose is oxidized by the glycolytic enzymes located primarily in the cytosol but often in association with specific organelles. Glyceraldehyde 3-phosphate dehydrogenase and pyruvate kinase bind to sarcolemmal and sarcoplasmic reticulum membranes. *In silico* (i.e., performed on computer or via computer simulation) studies that simulate the glycolytic burst associated with the onset of ischemia in vivo have suggested the presence of compartmentation of glycolytic function to a defined cytosolic subdomain [63]. Similarly, several observations support the organization of the TCA enzymes within the mitochondrial matrix as constituting a supercomplex or metabolon, providing a kinetic advantage in concentrating intermediates and channeling substrates within the supercomplex [64]. In addition, an association of glycolytic enzymes with mitochondria has been detected [65]. Both the first enzyme in the glycolytic pathway (i.e., hexokinase) and the primary enzyme in glucose oxidation (i.e., PDC) are associated with the mitochondria. Hexokinase binds at the outer membrane to peripheral protein complexes such as the PT pore, while PDC (which determines the fate of the glycolytic product pyruvate) is entirely located within the mitochondrial matrix.

As previously noted, in HF, there is a major switch in myocardial bioenergetic substrate used, from fatty acid to glucose; however, the time course and the role that this metabolic switch plays in the progression of the HF syndrome have not been clearly determined. A key component and marker of the switch is the co-ordinate down-regulation of fatty acid β-oxidation enzymes and mRNA levels (>40%) in the human left ventricle [1]. This switch is thought to represent a reversal to a fetal energy substrate preference pattern in the heart. During the development of cardiac hypertrophy, a fetal metabolic gene program is initiated via the complicity of transcription factors which bind to regulatory elements reducing FAO gene expression (e.g., MCAD and CPT-I b). Although the molecular mechanism(s) mediating this down-regulation is not fully understood, the participation of several nuclear receptors, intermediate metabolites, and transcription factors (e.g., SP1 (human transcription factor involved in gene expression in the early development of an organism) and PPAR) have been implicated in this programmatic change in gene expression (see further discussion in the molecular section below) [2].

According to Lehman and Kelly [66], the transcriptional control mechanisms governing FAO enzyme gene expression in the cardiac myocyte have defined a central role for the fatty acid-activated nuclear receptor PPAR-α. Cardiac FAO enzyme gene expression was shown to be coordinately downregulated in murine models of ventricular pressure overload, consistent with the energy substrate switch away from fatty acid utilization in the hypertrophied heart. Nuclear protein levels of PPAR-α decline in the ventricle in response to pressure overload, while several Sp and nuclear receptor transcription factors are induced to fetal levels, consistent with their binding to DNA as transcriptional repressors of rate-limiting FAO enzyme genes with hypertrophy.

Secondary Effects on Mitochondrial Fatty Acid β-Oxidation: Relationship to Mitochondrial Respiration and OXPHOS

As pointed out in Chap. 6, utilization of fatty acids as an energy source requires the functional operation of the mitochondrial electron transport chain (ETC) and OXPHOS;

the NADH and $FADH_2$ feed into the ETC at complex I and electrons are transferred from acyl-CoA dehydrogenases, via the electron-transfer flavoprotein (ETF), and ETF dehydrogenase and ubiquinone (or coenzyme Q) to complex III as shown in Fig. 4.1. Individuals with deficiencies in the ETF pathway display impaired FAO and abnormal intramitochondrial accumulation of fatty acids and glutaric acid and may develop a fatal cardiomyopathy. Similarly, patients with defects in respiratory complexes (e.g., complex I and IV) will frequently develop cardiomyopathy and HF, largely as a result of impaired energy production [67]. However, the extent of the effects on the cardiac fatty acid β-oxidation and on lipid accumulation in patients with defined respiratory activity defects and with defective coenzyme Q levels has not yet been fully established.

Fatty Acid Metabolism Defects Associated with Cardiomyopathy/Heart Failure

With the exception of defects in the MTP that affect long-chain L-3 hydroxylacyl-CoA activity and are associated with DCM [68], most of the disturbances in fatty acid metabolism are found in patients with hypertrophic cardiomyopathy (HCM), and many of the reported mutations in fatty acid β-oxidation pathway result in HCM rather than dilated DCM [69, 70]. Inherited disorders of fatty acid metabolism that can result in cardiomyopathy and/or HF with their characterized genetic loci are presented in Table 4.1.

Barth syndrome, an X-linked disorder characterized by a triad of DCM, neutropenia and increased levels of 3-methylglucaconic aciduria with onset often occurring in infancy frequently present with dysrhythmias and HF. The protein tafazzin (encoded by the G4.5 gene) is mutated and responsible for Barth syndrome with associated car-

Table 4.1 Inherited fatty acid metabolism defects

Specific fatty acid defect	Affected Loci	Human chromosome location	References
CPT-II	CPT2	1p32	[71]
Barth syndrome	G4.5/TAZ	Xq28	[72]
SCADD	SCADD (ACADS)	12q22-qter	[73]
MTP (also called TFP) (includes LCHAD)	MTP-α (HADHA)	2p24.1–23.3	[74]
	MTP-β (HADHB)	2p23	[75]
VLCAD	ACADVL	17p13	[76, 77]
CPT-I	CPT1	22qter	[78]
Carnitine transport	OCTN2 (SLC22A4)	5q31	[79]
Carnitine translocase	CACT (SLC25A20)	3p21.31	[80, 81, 83]
MCAD	MCAD	1p31	[82]
ETFA	ETFα subunit	15q25–q26	[83]
FAT/CD36	CD36	7q11.2.	[84]
PGC-1α variant	PGC-1	4p15.1	[85]
PPAR-α variant	PPAR-α	22q12.2–13.1	[86]

SCADD short-chain acyl-CoA dehydrogenase deficiency; *ETFA* electron transfer flavoprotein α

diomyopathy [72, 87]. While the biochemical function of the tafazzin protein has not yet been determined, structural analysis suggests that tafazzin belongs to a family of acyltransferases involved in phospholipid synthesis [88]. Levels of cardiolipin have been found markedly reduced in cultured fibroblasts from patients with the G4.5 mutation, likely making this the first report of a human disorder with a defect in cardiolipin metabolism [89], and it may prove to be useful to assess the cardiac levels of cardiolipin in patients with Barth syndrome.

Defects in mitochondrial acyl-CoA dehydrogenase are also inborn errors associated with cardiomyopathy and HF [90]. Generally, defects in the oxidation of long-chain fatty acids are more likely to cause cardiomyopathy than defects in medium-chain or short-chain fatty acids. Specific defects in enzymes involved in long-chain and very long fatty acid chains have been identified [91–93], and the genetic defects will be further analyzed in the molecular section below. While severe cardiomyopathy is unusual in patients with MCAD deficiency, sudden death in children is a common outcome although its pathogenetic mechanism is presently unknown. Furthermore, cardiomyopathy can be part of the clinical phenotype of SCAD deficiency [94].

Carnitine deficiency has been frequently associated with severe cardiomyopathy/HF. Mutations in proteins that participate in carnitine transport and metabolism may cause DCM as a recessive trait [71, 95]. One of the loci affected in carnitine-associated cardiac involvement includes the plasma-membrane localized carrier, which transports carnitine into the cell, and its deficiency has been described as primary carnitine deficiency [96]. This transport deficiency is due to specific defects in the gene (OCTN2) encoding the plasma membrane localized organic cation/carnitine transporter [79]. Defects in a second locus, the mitochondrial membrane localized carnitine translocase also lead to carnitine deficiency resulting in cardiomyopathy and HF [97].

Although not found associated with cardiomyopathy/HF, evidence suggests that CPT-I deficiency might result in cardiac involvement [98]. In contrast, there is a general consensus that deficiency in CPT-II, (specifically infantile CPT-II deficiency), an autosomal recessive disorder, is associated with cardiac damage and sudden death [99].

Fatty Acids and Glucose Metabolism Defects in Cardiac Remodeling and Apoptosis

Since it will be further discussed in later chapters, here suffice to say that apoptosis (programmed cell death) plays a prominent role in the myocyte loss that occurs in human HF [100, 101]. In addition, it plays a major role in the extensive cardiac remodeling that encompasses the transition from cardiac

hypertrophy to HF (in models such as the spontaneously hypertensive rat) [102].

Mitochondrial membrane permeabilization is a critical early step of apoptosis preceding the caspase cascade. This permeabilization is accompanied by an early dissipation of the mitochondrial transmembrane potential [103]. Opening the mitochondrial permeability transition (PT) pore is accompanied by the depolarization of the mitochondrial membrane. A component of the inner membrane that is associated with the mitochondrial pore as well as with cytochrome c is the phospholipid cardiolipin. Cardiolipin also mediates the targeting of the pro-apoptotic protein tBid to mitochondria implicating cardiolipin in the pathway for cytochrome c release [104]. Also, carnitine plays a role in membrane permeability and proton conductance, as well as in the functioning of cytochrome c oxidase.

During ischemia, oxidation of the saturated fatty acid palmitate is associated with diminished myocyte function [105]. Saturated long-chain fatty acid substrates such as palmitate (but not mono-unsaturated fatty acids) readily induce apoptosis in rat neonatal cardiomyocytes [106, 107].

As an early feature of palmitate-induced cardiomyocyte apoptosis, palmitate diminishes the content of the mitochondrial cardiolipin by causing a marked reduction of cardiolipin synthesis. Decreased levels of cardiolipin synthesis and cytochrome c release have been reported to be, although temporally, directly correlated. This suggests that cardiolipin modulates the association of cytochrome c with the mitochondrial inner membrane [108]. Palmitate also decreases the oxidative metabolism of fatty acids and causes increase in the intracellular second messenger ceramide [105], paralleling a decrease in complex III activity. The decrease in fatty acid metabolism (e.g., CPT-I activity declines) and complex III activities and ceramide accumulation have been shown to be downstream events occurring well after cytochrome c release (and changes in the PT pore) [107–109].

Glucose and glucose uptake can play an important role in modulating myocardial apoptosis. Glucose uptake in cardiomyocytes reduces hypoxia-induced apoptosis [110]. Overexpression of GLUT-1, to promote increased glucose uptake, also blocked the progression of apoptosis in hypoxia-treated cardiomyocytes [111]. The protective antiapoptotic role of glucose is further supported by studies in which glucose deprivation promoted myocardial apoptosis. Insulin administration attenuates cardiac I/R-induced apoptosis via activation of the Akt-mediated cell-survival signaling [112, 113]. In contrast to normal myocardial glucose uptake and signaling, which promote cell survival pathways, there is evidence that defective glucose uptake and hyperglycemia, as found in diabetic cardiomyopathy, can lead to increased myocardial apoptosis. Hyperglycemia induces myocyte apoptosis, cytochrome c release, and high levels of ROS in cardiomyocytes in culture as well as in a mouse model of diabetes produced by streptozocin treatment [114].

Molecular Players and Events in Fatty Acid-Related Cardiomyopathy/HF

Genes and Modulation of Gene Expression

MCAD

MCAD deficiency is autosomally recessive and associated with sudden death. Over 90% of cases of MCAD deficiency are associated with a homozygous mutation at bp 985 (A985G). This mutation directs a glutamate replacement of lysine at residue 304 in the mature MCAD subunit causing impairment of tetramer assembly and increased protein instability [115]. MCAD deficiency is the most frequent inborn metabolic disorder in populations of NW European origin [116].

At the gene level, three of the seven reported non A985G mutations found in MCAD deficiency localize to exon 11. At the protein level, the mutant residues cluster in helix H of the MCAD protein and are proposed to have their primary effect on the correct folding and assembly of the tetrameric MCAD enzyme structure. The amino acid residues affected are: M301T, S311R, and K304E [117].

VLCAD

Pediatric cardiomyopathy is the most common clinical phenotype of VLCAD deficiency. A severe form of infantile cardiomyopathy is found in over 67% of cases, often resulting in sudden death [118]. VLCAD deficiency is characterized by a marked reduction of VLCAD mRNA and decreased levels and/or absence of VLCAD enzyme activity. Mutation analysis of the VLCAD gene revealed a large number of different mutant loci (21 in 19 patients) with few repeated mutations [119]. Distinguishing between truly pathogenic mutations and polymorphic variations remains to be done.

CPT-II

The infantile form of CPT-II deficiency has frequent cardiac involvement and is associated with specific CPT-II mutations. This is in contrast to the adult form of CPT-II deficiency which does not present with cardiac involvement.

The infantile CPT-II deficiency has been associated with several mutations including a homozygous mutation at A2399C causing a Tyr → Ser substitution at residue 628. This mutation produces a marked decrease in CPT-II activity in patient fibroblasts [120]. Another mutation has been reported at C1992T predicting an Arg → Cys substitution at residue 631 which is associated with drastic reduction of CPT-II catalytic activity [121].

MTP

MTP, an enzyme of β-oxidation of long-chain fatty acids, is a multienzyme complex composed of four molecules of the α-subunit (encoded by HADHA) which contains both the enoyl-CoA hydratase and 3-hydroxyacyl-CoA dehydrogenase domains, and four molecules of the β-subunit (encoded by HADHB) containing the 3-ketoacyl-CoA thiolase domain. MTP deficiency is classified into two different biochemical phenotypes: (1) both α and β subunits are present and only the 3-hydroxyacyl-CoA dehydrogenase (LCHAD) activity is affected; (2) the absence of both subunits, and the complete lack of all three enzymatic activities of MTP. Although there is some overlap between the clinical features found in each molecular/biochemical phenotype, patients with neonatal cardiomyopathy have the second biochemical phenotype only. The most common mutation associated with MTP deficiency (G1528C) is associated with the first phenotype and not with the second. Mutations have been localized to the 5′ donor splicing site of the α subunit gene which can result in the entire loss of an exon in the mRNA (exon 3) [68], and are associated with the second phenotype. Both DNA and enzymatic testing can be performed in fetal screening of this often devastating disease [122].

PPAR

Although a discussion on PPAR is outlined in Chap.5, here it suffices to say that PPAR activity is dependent on the presence of a variety of activating ligands (e.g., prostaglandins, eicosanoids, long- chain unsaturated fatty acids, etc.) and interacting proteins (i.e., coactivators and corepressors). Activated PPAR-ligand complex binds to a DNA response element in the promoter region of specific genes activating transcription [123]. Cardiac metabolic gene expression is activated by PPAR-α regulation during postnatal development, during short-term starvation, and in response to exercise training. One marker of PPAR activation is up-regulated MCAD expression. Conversely, pressure-overload hypertrophy results in the deactivation of PPAR-α with lower fatty acid oxidation expression, abnormal cardiac lipid homoeostasis and reduced energy production [124]. The negative regulation of PPAR-α is mediated at several levels with PPAR gene expression being reduced in mice during ventricular overload. In addition, PPAR activity is altered at the posttranscriptional level via the extracellular signal-regulated MAP kinase pathway. Ventricular overload therefore results in hypertrophied myocytes with intracellular fat accumulation (in response to oleate loading). Notwithstanding, the PPAR role in the activation of fetal gene program occurring during hypertrophy and HF has not yet been fully delineated.

There is also evidence that the PPAR interacting coactivators affect gene regulation by modulation of the chromatin structure surrounding the DNA (by changing the extent of acetylation of histone residues). PPAR plays also a pivotal role in mediating the effect of hypoxia on mitochondrial FAO in cardiac myocytes resulting in diminished CPT-I β mRNA levels. This is accomplished via PPAR transcriptional regulation (due to reduced binding of PPAR-α) and its obligate partner, retinoid X receptor α (RXR-α) to a DNA response element residing within the CPT-I β promoter [125]. Immunoblot analysis has shown that during hypoxia, nuclear and cytoplasmic levels of RXR-α are reduced, whereas there is no change in PPAR levels.

PGC-1

A detailed discussion on mitochondria and peroxisome proliferator-activated receptor gamma coactivator-1 (PGC-1) has been presented in Chap. 6. Here, we will only note that expression of PGC-1 in cardiac myocytes induces nuclear and mitochondrial gene expression involved in multiple mitochondrial energy-transduction production pathways, increased mitochondrial number, and increased respiration. Cardiac-specific overexpression of PGC-1 in transgenic mice resulted in uncontrolled mitochondrial proliferation in cardiac myocytes leading to loss of sarcomeric structure, DCM and HF. These results identify PGC-1 as a critical regulatory molecule in controlling mitochondrial number and function in response to energy demands [126]. Moreover, it has also been implicated in both the increased expression of mitochondrial transcription factor A (mTFA), which is involved in the control of both mitochondrial DNA transcription and replication, and levels of the NRF-1 and NFR-2 transcription factors (Fig. 4.3) that mediate the expression of a number of nuclear genes involved in mitochondrial OXPHOS including, subunits of cytochrome c oxidase and ATP synthase [127].

Effects of Abnormal Fatty Acid and Glucose Metabolism on Cardiac Structure/Function

Undoubtedly, the main sources for energy production in the heart are glucose and long-chain fatty acid (LCFA), but the mechanism for LCFA uptake is not completely understood.

Recently, the regulation of sarcolemmal glucose and fatty acid transporters in cardiac disease were addressed by Schwenk et al. [128]. It was pointed out that proteins with high-affinity binding sites to LCFA, referred to as LCFA transporters, are responsible for the majority of LCFA uptake and, similar to the and GLUT-1 and GLUT-4, the LCFA transporters CD36 and fatty acid-binding protein (FABP (pm or plasma membrane fraction)) can be recruited from an intracellular storage compartment to the sarcolemma to increase the rate of substrate uptake. Furthermore, permanent relocation of LCFA transporters, from intracellular stores to the sarcolemma is accompanied by accumulation of lipids and lipid metabolites in the heart. Thus, impaired insulin signaling and glucose utilization may lead to decreased cardiac contractility. These observations underline the particular role and interplay of substrate carriers for glucose and LCFA in modulating cardiac metabolism, and the development of HF.

In a progressive way, the hypertrophied and failing heart becomes increasingly dependent on glucose as energy substrate. However, it is unlikely that increased anaerobic glycolysis can compensate in ATP production for the decline in FAO that occurs in the failing heart, together with diminished levels of high-energy phosphates, characterized by a decreased phosphocreatine (PCr): ATP ratio (resulting from declining PCr content), diminished creatine kinase activity, and mitochondrial OXPHOS dysfunction. Moreover, despite the rise in glycolysis, the rate of mitochondrial-localized pyruvate oxidation does not keep up with the increased pyruvate levels [129]. This has led to the conclusion that the failing heart is energetically severely compromised [130].

Use of Cellular and Animal Models to Study Metabolic Defects

Studies using the isolated cardiomyocyte have been particularly useful in the study of rapid and transient signal transduction events occurring in the metabolic signaling pathways in response to specific defined stimuli. An important limitation with such studies is that most metabolic stressors and insults endured by the heart are less well defined and often feature a broad range of effects including neuroendocrine, intercellular signaling involving several cell types and circulatory/hemodynamic effects extending well beyond oxygen availability. Therefore, hypoxic simulations of ischemia or electrical stimulation studies with isolated cardiomyocytes can be useful in delineating a subset of the signaling pathways and molecules involved in the in vivo response.

Research in animal models of HF, and in particular the use of transgenic mouse models, has been extremely helpful in our understanding of the initiation, severity, and progression of

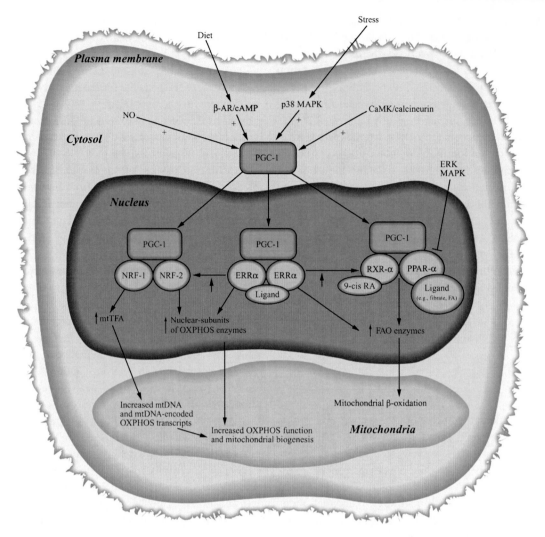

Fig. 4.3 PGC-1 and its metabolic pathway. PGC-1 transduces cell signals associated with physiologic stimuli to regulate cardiac metabolic genes. Numerous signaling pathways downstream of physiologic stimuli, like fasting and exercise, activate the PGC-1 cascade either by increasing PGC-1 expression or activity. PGC-1, in turn, coactivates transcriptional partners, including nuclear respiratory factor-1 and 2 (NRF-1 and 2), estrogen-related receptor (ERR) and PPAR-α, resulting in downstream activation of mitochondrial biogenesis and FAO pathways, respectively

metabolic abnormalities to cardiac phenotypes. Using isotopic tracers, Lei et al. directly measured the progression of substrate oxidation/metabolic changes in different HF stages [131].

These alterations were within normal range in early and middle stages of HF, but changed from FAO to glucose oxidation in the more severe, late stages. When compared to normal control animals, in the canine model of mild pacing-induced HF, no differences in myocardial glucose, lactate or fatty acid metabolism were detected, probably because down-regulation of FAO occurs only in advanced, severe HF [132]. On the other hand, observations from the rat infarct/HF model have suggested that down-regulation of the mRNA for FAO enzymes may occur as early as at 8 weeks [133, 134], and after perfusion, the isolated hearts showed marked increase in glucose oxidation without changes in palmitate

oxidation [133]. Therefore, it is apparent that in the early stages of HF, there are increases in glucose metabolism but not decreases in exogenous fatty acid metabolism. While the mechanisms responsible for the down-regulation of FAO pathway in severe, late HF are not completely understood, several investigators have pointed out that the decreased expression of PPAR-α and/or RXR-α may play a critical role in the myocardial substrate changes observed under these conditions [135–137] .

While decreased PPAR-α protein levels have been found in the failing human heart [136], in dogs with severe pacing-induced HF myocardial protein levels of RXR-α (but not PPAR-α) were decreased [137]. Nevertheless, the fact that differences in HF etiology and animal species can explain the observed differences in myocardial PPAR-α and RXR-α protein expression, if the down-regulation of PPAR-α and/or RXR-α and FAO enzymes happened early or in late HF cannot be definitely established.

The recent availability of transgenic mouse models to assess cardiac metabolism has been also extremely helpful in furthering our understanding of the correlation of diverse cardiac phenotypes to specific abnormalities, in both fatty acid and glucose metabolism [138]. While some of these studies have employed global knock-out of specific genes of interest, the use of cardiac-specific gene disruption generally achieved by the Cre/loxP technology has proved to be useful in preventing embryonic or fetal lethality that may result from global gene ablation, as well as in allowing the distinction of primarily cardiac-specific events from systemic events occurring secondary to altered gene expression in other tissues. Moreover, the addition of inducible elements to the gene of interest allows the manipulation of gene expression within specific developmental or environmental conditions.

In addition to selected mouse models of metabolic genes described in Chap. 7, other affecting metabolic pathways and cardiac phenotypes are presented in Table 4.2. Both global

and cardiac-specific disruption of GLUT-4 in transgenic mice result in marked cardiac hypertrophy [39, 139]. Insulin-mediated glucose uptake is abolished in mice with the cardiac-specific GLUT-4 disruption, and display a compensatory-like increase in GLUT-1 and basal glucose uptake; moreover, decreased FAO suggests a switch from fatty acid to glucose metabolism. Eventually, both models show marked cardiac dysfunction.

Interestingly, male heterozygous GLUT-4$^{+/-}$ knock-out mice become diabetic and hypertensive with features of diabetic cardiomyopathy [140]. These mice exhibit decreased GLUT-4 expression in adipose tissue and skeletal muscle leading to increased serum glucose and insulin, reduced muscle glucose uptake, hypertension, and diabetic histopathology in the heart and liver, similar to humans with noninsulin-dependent diabetes.

Mice lacking PPAR-α have a cardiac phenotype of increased myocyte lipid accumulation [155], and mice lacking MTP-α and -β subunits alleles show necrosis and acute degradation of the cardiac myocytes. These mice also accumulate long-chain fatty acid metabolites, have low birth

Table 4.2 Cardiac phenotype resulting from altered metabolic genes in transgenic mice

Protein (gene)	Alteration	Myocardial phenotype	References
Fatty acid transport protein 1 (FATP1)	Cardiac-specific overexpression	Lipotoxic CM	[141]
Insulin-sensitive glucose transporter (Glut-4)	Null	Cardiac hypertrophy; ↓ FAO	[142]
Long-chain acyl-CoA synthetase (ACS)	Cardiac-specific overexpression	Lipotoxic CM, hypertrophy, TG accumulation	[141]
Peroxisome proliferator-activated receptor-α (PPAR-α)	Cardiac-specific overexpression	↑ FAO; ↓ glucose uptake and oxidation	[143]
Peroxisome proliferator-activated receptor-δ (PPAR-δ)	Cardiac-specific deletion	Lipotoxic CM with ↓ FAO	[144]
Leptin (Lep)	Null	↑ FAO, FA uptake, TG + lipid accumulation; ↑ diastolic dysfunction	[145]
Very-long-chain acyl-coenzyme A dehydrogenase (VLCAD)	Null	Lipid accumulation, CM, mitochondrial proliferation, facilitated PVT induction	[146]
Mitochondrial transcription factor A (Tfam)	Cardiac-specific deletion	↓ MtDNA, ETC and ATP; ↓ FAO + ↑ glycolytic expression	[147]
Lipoprotein lipase (LpL)	Cardiac-specific deletion	↑ TG; ↓ FAO and ↑ Glut expression + glucose uptake	[148]
Fatty acid translocase (FAT/CD36)	Null	↓ Cardiac FA uptake +TG; DCM	[149]
Fatty acid translocase (FAT/CD36)	Overexpression	↑ FAO; ↓ plasma TG + FA; no cardiac pathology; ↑ glucose	[150]
Insulin receptor (Insr)	Cardiac-specific deletion	↓ FAO; ↓ GLUT-1 + basal glucose uptake; ↑ GLUT-4, insulin-glucose uptake + oxidation; smaller heart	[151]
Heart-type fatty acid binding protein (H-FABP)	Null	↓ Free LCFA uptake; ↑ Glucose usage; hypertrophy	[152]
Mitochondrial trifunctional protein (Mtpa)	Null	Accumulate LCFA metabolites; growth retardation, neonatal hypoglycemia + SD	[153]
Peroxisome proliferator-activated receptor γ coactivator-1 (PGC-α)	Null	↓ ETC + ATP; lower work output in response to chemical or electrical stimulation	[154]
Peroxisome proliferator-activated receptor γ coactivator-1 (PGC-α)	Cardiac-specific overexpression	Mitochondrial proliferation, loss of sarcomeric structure and DCM in adults	[126]

Lipotoxic CM cardiac hypertrophy; cardiac dysfunction, progressive myocardial lipid accumulation, and congestive HF with reduced survival; *PVT* polymorphic ventricular tachycardia; *FA* fatty acid: *SD* sudden death; *DCM* dilated cardiomyopathy; *ETC* electron transport chain; *TG* triglyceride

weight, and develop neonatal hypoglycemia with sudden death between 6 and 36 h after birth [153]. In Table 4.3, known PPAR-α regulated genes in cardiac metabolism are presented.

In mice knockouts of PPAR-α, there is reduced myocardial expression of genes involved in fatty acid uptake (CD36/FAT, FATP, FACS-1), mitochondrial transport (CPT I, CPT II), β-oxidation (MCAD, VLCAD, SCAD, SCHAD, MTP) as well as myocardial LCFA uptake and oxidation rates [171, 172]. While unstressed hearts are relatively normal in these knockout strains, a fasting stress, which in wild-type mice induces cardiac FAO enzyme gene expression, promotes hypoglycemia and hepatic and cardiac triglyceride accumulation. In contrast, transgenic mice containing cardiac-specific PPAR-α overexpression, display activated myocardial gene expression for fatty acid utilization including fatty acid uptake and FAO, whereas glucose utilization is reciprocally decreased [161, 173].

Reduced glucose utilization is due to the aforementioned inhibitory effects of acetyl-CoA and NADH (increased during high rates of FAO) on PDC activity as well as on direct gene down-regulation of the glucose transporter, GLUT-4, and the glycolytic enzyme phosphofructokinase, and up-regulation of PDK4 (which decreases glucose oxidation through PDH inhibition) in hearts with increased PPAR levels. These results suggest that PPAR-α provides a critical link in circuits involved in myocardial fatty acid and glucose utilization.

Recently, abnormalities in carbohydrate metabolism and its regulation have been studied in PPAR-α null mouse hearts by Gélinas et al. [174]. When compared with control C57BL/6 mice, isolated working hearts from PPAR-α null mice exhibited abnormal capacity to withstand a rise in preload. At the metabolic level, besides the shift from FA (fivefold down) to CHO at both preloads, PPAR-α null hearts also showed a greater contribution from exogenous lactate and glucose and/or glycogen (twofold up) to endogenous

pyruvate formation, whereas that of exogenous pyruvate remained unchanged and with only marginal alterations in citric acid cycle-related parameters. Lactate production rate was the only measured parameter that was affected differently by preloads in control and PPAR-α null mouse hearts, suggesting a restricted reserve for the latter hearts to enhance glycolysis when the energy demand is increased. Abnormalities in the expression of some glycolysis-related genes suggested the potential mechanisms involved in this defective CHO metabolism. These highlight the importance of metabolic defects in CHO metabolism associated with FA oxidation defects, which may result in HF under stress conditions even in the fed state.

Transgenic mice null for the MTP-α allele lack both MTP-α and -β subunits and display necrosis and acute degradation of the cardiac myocytes. They also accumulate LCFA metabolites, have low birth weight, and develop neonatal hypoglycemia, with sudden death occurring between 6 and 36 h after birth [153].

PGC-1α overexpression in the myocardium can display strikingly developmental-specific differences. While constitutive cardiac-specific overexpression of PGC-1α proved to be lethal resulting in the early development of DCM, marked fibrosis and the accumulation of high numbers of large mitochondria [126], inducible cardiac-specific PGC-1α over expression (driven by a tetracycline-responsive promoter) was useful in examining developmental stage-specific responses [175]. For instance, in the neonatal myocardium, PGC-1α overexpression leads to increased cardiac mitochondrial size and number, concurrent with the increased gene expression associated with mitochondrial biogenesis and with no overt effect on neonatal cardiac function. However, in the adult mouse, PGC-1α overexpression resulted in a moderate increase in mitochondrial number, many organelles containing striking abnormalities in structure (e.g., vacuoles, inclusions), and within 2 weeks, development of cardiomyopathy featuring increased ventricular mass, wall thinning, and chamber dilation. Cessation of PGC-1α expression reverses the cardiac phenotype over time.

To further test the hypothesis that a disturbance in myocardial fatty acid uptake and utilization leads to the accumulation of cardiotoxic lipid species and to establish a mouse model of metabolic cardiomyopathy, transgenic mouse lines that overexpress long-chain acyl-CoA synthetase in the heart have been generated. These mice showed cardiac-restricted expression of the transgene and marked cardiac myocyte triglyceride accumulation, similar to that found in mice with disrupted PPAR-α. Lipid accumulation was associated with initial cardiac hypertrophy, followed by the development of left-ventricular dysfunction and premature death [141].

Lipotoxic cardiomyopathy (LCM) is a significant entity associated with alterations in cellular lipid metabolism. It

Table 4.3 PPAR-α regulated genes in cardiac metabolism

Function	Gene product	References
Fatty acid uptake/ esterification	LPL	[156]
	CD36/FAT, FABP	[157]
	FATP1, FACS-1	[158]
Glucose oxidation	PDK4	[159, 160]
	GLUT-4	[161]
Mitochondrial and peroxisomal β-oxidation	MCAD	[123]
	LCAD, VLCAD	[157]
	M-CPT I (CPT-Iβ)	[162, 163]
	Bifunctional enzyme	[164, 165]
	ACO	[166, 167]
	MCD	[168]
Uncoupling proteins	UCP3	[169, 170]
	UCP2	[161, 170]

can occur as a result of lipid accumulation stemming from defective fat oxidation with leptin deficiency [176], increased oxidation and increased expression of fatty acid transporters due to PPAR overexpression [161], and accumulation of more fatty acids due to expression of long-chain fatty acyl-CoA synthase [141]. In addition, mouse hearts with targeted overexpression of anchored lipoprotein lipase (LpL), the primary enzyme responsible for conversion of lipoprotein triglyceride (TG) into free fatty acids, also develop LCM because of increased myocardial lipid uptake and accumulation [177, 178]. Increased lipid uptake in LpL-overexpressed strains is also associated with the increased expression of genes mediating FAO (e.g., ACO, CPT-I), "heart failure" markers such as atrial natriuretic factor (ANF), brain natriuretic factor (BNP), myosin, apoptosis markers (e.g., caspase-3, cytcochrome c release), a decrease in glucose transporters (GLUT-1, GLUT-4), and AMPK expression [178].

Lipotoxicity and lipid accumulation may also be, at least partly, responsible for the development of myocardial dysfunction in strains with type 2 diabetes and diabetic cardiomyopathy, as well as with FAO defects. The myocardial lipid accumulation that occurs with high fat diets in the PPAR-α null strains has been temporally correlated with cardiac contractile dysfunction and both can be reversed by diet change. Notably, among patients with nonischemic HF, a significant subset (approximately 30%) exhibited intramyocardial lipid accumulation associated with an up-regulation of PPAR-α-regulated genes, as well as MHC-β, and TNF-α. Similarly, intramyocardial lipid and triglyceride overload in the hearts of Zucker diabetic fatty (ZDF) rats was found to be associated with contractile dysfunction and similar changes in gene expression as found in failing human hearts with lipid overload [179]. An extract derived from Salacia oblonga root (SOE), an antidiabetic and antiobesity medicine, improves hyperlipidemia in ZDF rats and possesses PPAR-α activating properties. Chronic oral SOE administration in ZDF rats reduces myocardial triglyceride and fatty acid content and suppressed cardiac overexpression of fatty acid transporter protein-1 mRNA and protein, suggesting inhibition of increased cardiac fatty acid uptake as the basis for decreased cardiac fatty acid levels [180]. SOE treatment also inhibited the overexpression in ZDF rat heart of PPAR-α mRNA and protein and CPT-1, acyl-CoA oxidase, and AMPK mRNAs thereby down-regulating myocardial FAO. This suggests that SOE ameliorates excess of cardiac lipid accumulation and increased cardiac FAO in diabetes and obesity primarily by reducing cardiac fatty acid uptake, and thereby modulating cardiac PPAR-α-mediated FAO gene transcription.

In most cases, both the precise cellular mechanism of cardiac remodeling and the molecular identity of the lipotoxic stimulus remain to be determined, although lipotoxicity has frequently been postulated to result from excess lipid oxidation [181], or from the accumulation of a toxic lipid intermediate [182]. Cellular studies have shown that palmitate, but not oleate, leads to apoptosis [183], but it remains to be determined whether this saturated fatty acid, its metabolic product, or cellular processes affected by palmitate lead to cellular dysfunction or death.

The role of RXR-α in HF has been examined in the transgenic mouse as well. RXR-α null mutant mice display ocular and cardiac malformations and liver developmental delay and die from HF in early embryo life. A large percentage (over 50%) of the downstream target genes, identified by subtractive hybridization, encode proteins involved in fatty acid metabolism and electron transport, suggesting energy deficiency in the null RXR-α embryos. ATP content and MCAD mRNA were significantly lower in RXR-α mutant hearts when compared to wild-type mice. These findings suggest that defects in intermediary metabolism may be a causative factor in the RXR-α$^{-/-}$ phenotype, an embryonic form of DCM [184].

Our understanding of the role that mitochondrial gene expression and function play in defining cardiac metabolism has also been greatly enhanced by transgenic studies. The previously discussed studies with PGC-1 overexpression suggest that increased mitochondrial function and biogenesis may be fine in the neonatal heart but may result in cardiomyopathy in the adult. Disturbing mitochondrial bioenergetic function by creating null mutations in ANT1 can also lead to mitochondrial proliferation with dysfunctional mitochondria and cardiomyopathy [185]. Similarly, null mutations in mtTFA in the mouse cause progressive cardiac dysfunction with depleted mtDNA and an associated decline in OXPHOS ATP production [186]. An early feature in the progression of this cardiac mitochondrial dysfunction is the activation of a fetal metabolic gene-expression program characterized by the decreased expression of FAO genes and increased expression of glycolytic genes [147]. The switch in the programming of cardiac metabolism was followed by increased myocardial mitochondrial biogenesis, which could not compensate in ATP production but rather contributes to the progression of HF, probably in a way similar to the PCG-1α overexpression in the adult heart.

Are the Metabolic Changes Occurring in Heart Failure Tissue-Specific?

A number of changes occur in skeletal muscle during HF, including histological and electromyographic evidence of generalized myopathy and exercise intolerance. Evaluation of skeletal muscle metabolism by the noninvasive methodology of phosphorus nuclear magnetic resonance spectroscopy in patients with HF revealed abnormal levels of phosphocreatine and inorganic phosphate following moderate physical activities [187, 188]. Furthermore, patients with desmin and β-MHC mutations known to cause HCM and HF have defined changes in skeletal muscle fibers. Patients with specific β-MHC mutations may develop abnormal mitochondrial number and function in skeletal muscle as well as type I fiber abnormalities and atrophy [189] .

Congestive HF is often accompanied by skeletal myopathy with a shift from slow aerobic fatigue-resistant fibers to fast anaerobic ones. Many of the cardiac cellular changes as well as the mitochondrial abnormalities often detected in HF appear to be present in skeletal muscle. Alterations in energy metabolism including decreased mitochondrial ATP production as well as defective transfer of energy through the phosphotransfer kinases occur in both cardiac and skeletal muscles and suggest a generalized metabolic myopathy in HF [190]. While more evidence confirming these findings is needed, at least evaluation of skeletal muscle mitochondrial function can be informative in the overall diagnostic and prognostic evaluation of patients with HF. Determining what other parts of the HF signaling pathway are truly cardiac specific and which might be also operative in skeletal muscle awaits further studies. Such studies might shed light about the relationship between signaling pathways and mitochondrial bioenergetics in HF patients.

Diagnostics and Metabolic Therapies

Diagnostic Advances

Before treatment is undertaken, it is critical that the information concerning the site of defect within the fatty acid/carnitine metabolic pathway be evaluated. At the biochemical level, the diagnostic evaluation of fatty acid and glucose metabolic defects and determination of carnitine levels are easily performed. Rapid and correct diagnosis (including newborn screening using a noninvasive, highly sensitive methodology profiling specific metabolic intermediates e.g., acylcarnitines, and carnitines via tandem mass spectrometry, on blood spot collected on a Guthrie card) is particularly critical since dramatic recovery from or prevention of dysrhythmias and HF have been demonstrated in a number of these disorders (e.g., VLCAD deficiency) [191, 192]. In the last few years, the development of noninvasive techniques to evaluate intermediates has greatly progressed, including the use of nuclear magnetic resonance (NMR) spectroscopy to assess glucose transport, glycogen levels, and cellular levels of triglyceride content (in skeletal muscle) [193–195]. These methods may allow noninvasive evaluation of specific lipid levels, of accumulated "toxic" metabolites and of insulin resistance. Although the use of genetic analysis is also available, the presence of nonrepeating mutations makes this analysis rather problematic.

Therapies

Avoidance of fasting is an important step in the treatment of disorders of mitochondrial long-chain FAO, as well as the use of low fat diet with restriction of LCFA intake, frequent carbohydrate rich feeding, and the replacement of normal dietary fat by medium-chain triglyceride. The activation of PPAR-α using lipid-lowering fibrates may also be an effective supplement in some cases of FAO deficiency [196]. PPAR-α and PPAR-β/δ are transcriptional regulators that play an important role in myocardial energy and lipid homeostasis, and both PPAR subtypes, likely with overlapping functions, are necessary in order to maintain the myocardial lipid and energy homeostasis [197], thus defining the roles of each PPAR subtype might provide new targets to treat heart diseases, including HF.

Knowledge of the precise site of the biochemical or molecular defect is extremely important in regard to the choice of therapeutic modality to be applied. For instance, deficiencies in CPT-II, carnitine acylcarnitine translocase, or MTP can be treated with drugs targeted to enhance glucose use and pyruvate oxidation energy, at the expense of FAO, to prevent the accumulation of long-chain acylcarnitines that can result in cardiac conduction defects and dysrhythmias [198]. In contrast, acute cardiomyopathy associated with VLCAD deficiency, which can be diagnosed by acylcarnitine analysis, can be effectively treated with the aforementioned dietary therapy, including medium-chain triglycerides [199]. The accumulation of LCFA and their side effects can also be effectively reversed by inhibition of CPT-I activity with perhexiline and amiodarone [200]. Perhexiline has also been used to reduce ventricular ectopic beats associated with chronic ischemic injury and chronic HF [201, 202]. As previously discussed, the use of carnitine supplementation in patients with carnitine deficiency may be helpful in the prevention and in the treatment of potentially lethal disorders. In addition, gene and cell-based therapies for some of the fatty acid disturbances of cardiac function and structure, to decrease LCFA intermediates and redirect metabolic programs hold great promise, albeit the collected experience at this time is mainly limited to animals [203]. In a rat model of MetSyn caused by leptin insufficiency and abnormal fat accumulation, it was found that a single central administration of recombinant adeno-associated virus vector containing the gene encoding leptin severely depletes fat and ameliorates the major symptoms of MetSyn for an extended period of time [204].

Metabolic therapies utilizing modulation of myocardial glucose and fatty acid metabolism is recognized as a potential approach in the treatment of the failing and ischemic heart. Treatment of congestive HF patients with carvedilol, a β-adrenoreceptor blocker, results in marked improvement in myocardial energy efficiency and a reduction in myocardial oxygen consumption by shifting myocardial oxidative substrates from fatty acid to glucose [205]. Earlier studies with β-blocker treatment indicated that along with some improvement in both HF and hypertension, some components of the MetSyn (including glycemic control) may be worsened, mainly due to its negative effects on carbohydrate metabolism; therefore, their use in diabetics was restricted [206]. On the other hand, nonselective β-blockers vasodilators, such as carvedilol, do not exhibit the same negative metabolic consequences with glucose utilization seen with the use of earlier generation β-blocker and may be used in patients with CVD and diabetes.

Free fatty acids are a primary source of energy during myocardial ischemia and can also serve to uncouple OXPHOS and increase myocardial O_2 consumption. However, inhibitors of FAO can increase glucose oxidation and may serve to improve cardiac efficiency. It is noteworthy that inhibitors of β-FAO can help prevent the hyperglycemia that occurs in noninsulin-dependent diabetes. Since the inhibition of FAO is effective in controlling some of the abnormalities in diabetes, FAO inhibitors targeting enzymes such as CPT-I may also be useful in the treatment of diabetic cardiomyopathy. FAO inhibition can be achieved using a number of enzymatic inhibitors such as etomoxir, oxfenicine, perhexiline, aminocarnitine, trimetazidine, ranolazine, and dichloroacteic acid (DCA) [207, 208]. In animal models, etomoxir, an inhibitor of CPT-I, reversed changes in myocardial fetal gene expression, preserved cardiac function, and prevented ventricular dilatation [209]. Studies using pacing-induced HF, have shown that CPT-I inhibition mediated by oxfenicine treatment not only attenuates ventricular dilatation but also significantly slows left ventricular remodeling and delays the time to end-stage failure [210]. Clinical studies in HF patients treated with etomoxir revealed improved systolic ventricular function, increased ejection fraction, and decreased pulmonary capillary pressure [211]. Partial inhibition of FAO has also proved to ameliorate many of the hemodynamic abnormalities associated with myocardial ischemia and HF [212]. Treatment with ranolazine mediates a partial inhibition of FAO (it is termed a pFOX inhibitor) as it reduces cellular acetyl-CoA content and activates PDH activity. In dogs in which chronic HF was induced by intracoronary microembolizations, intravenous administration of ranolazine significantly increased LV ejection fraction and systolic function [213]. Clinically, ranolazine has been used to treat both ischemia and angina [214]. This metabolic switch from FAO to glucose oxidation increases ATP production, reduces the rise in lactic acidosis, and improves myocardial function under conditions of reduced myocardial oxygen delivery leading to reduced gluconeogenesis and improved economy of cardiac work. Furthermore, trimetazidine treatment provides cardioprotective affects against myocardial

ischemia, diabetic cardiomyopathy, and exercise-induced angina in numerous clinical and experimental investigations [208, 215]. Particularly significant is the amelioration of cardiac function and exercise performance in diabetic patients with ischemic heart disease [216]. While initially trimetazidine has been considered to be an inhibitor of the activity of the long-chain isoform of the last enzyme involved in mitochondrial fatty acid β-oxidation, 3-ketoacyl coenzyme A thiolase [217], gathered observations have cast doubt on FAO inhibition as being the primary mechanism by which trimetazidine mediates cardiac recovery [218]. Other related cardioprotective effects of trimetazidine, which may contribute to its antiischemic action, are its acceleration of phospholipid synthesis and turnover with significant consequences for α-adrenergic signaling [219], and its inhibition of mitochondrial PT pore opening resulting in the prevention of lethal ischemia-reperfusion injury [220].

Polyunsaturated fatty acids (e.g., N-3 PUFA) or fish oil supplementation appears to reduce mortality and the incidence of sudden death, as well as dysrhythmias, associated with HF [221]. Its effect on mortality and morbidity have been gauged in the GISSI HF project, a large-scale, randomized, double-blind study, and shown to significantly reduce sudden death incidence, particularly in patients with left ventricular systolic dysfunction [222, 223]. A smaller study has also confirmed that N-3 PUFA treatment markedly reduces the incidence of both atrial and ventricular dysrhythmias [224]. Among a large assortment of PUFA-mediated effects on cardiomyocyte membrane lipid organization and function, the incorporation of N-3 PUFA (normally associated with reduced arachidonic acid) induces a reduction of mitochondrial β-FAO and oxygen consumption in the heart. These effects on mitochondrial metabolism are manifested primarily during postischemic reperfusion as improved metabolic and ventricular function. Both aging and ischemia markedly decrease levels of N-3 PUFA and cardiolipin in myocardial membranes, effects that have been correlated to increased mitochondrial Ca^{2+} levels and the effects of Ca^{2+} on mitochondrial enzymatic activities [225].

Conclusion

A major switch in myocardial bioenergetic substrate used from fatty acid to glucose occurs in HF following cardiac hypertrophy. Key component and marker of the switch is the coordinated down-regulation of FAO enzymes and mRNA levels in the human left ventricle, with a concomitant increase in glucose uptake and oxidation. This switch is thought to represent a reversal to a fetal energy substrate preference pattern of glucose oxidation in the heart.

The regulation of FAO, the main and critical source of ATP in the healthy heart, occurs at multiple levels, including a strong gene transcriptional component, with members of the peroxisome proliferator-activated receptor (PPAR) family of transcription factors functioning as primary regulators of the FAO gene expression. Changes in glucose and fatty acid metabolism associated with diabetes and MetSyn also have an associated spectrum of cardiovascular abnormalities ranging from hypertension to cardiomyopathy and HF. Deficits in insulin signaling lead to diminished myocardial glucose uptake and utilization resulting in an increased reliance of the heart on FAO for energy generation. This contributes to an increased accumulation of lipid intermediates, elevated cellular acidosis, decreased cardiac efficiency, and contractile dysfunction [226]. Interestingly, increasing evidence derived from human and animal studies suggests that excess of substrate may lead to HF, and this could be prevented or slowed by maintaining low body fat and high insulin sensitivity and by consuming a diet of low glycemic load that is high in mono- and polyunsaturated fatty acids [227]. Spontaneous hypertensive aging rats in HF receiving standard high-carbohydrate diet or high-fat diet supplemented with high-linoleate safflower oil or lard until death have been studied by Chicco et al. [228], to assess their effects on disease progression and mortality. Both high-fat diets ameliorated cardiac hypertrophy, left ventricular dilatation, and systolic function often seen in rats consuming high-carbohydrate diet. The prosurvival effect of linoleate diet was found to be associated with a greater myocardial content and linoleate-enrichment of cardiolipin, which as noted earlier in this chapter, is deficient in the failing heart. Thus, a high-fat diet may accelerate or attenuate the mortality in severe hypertensive heart disease depending on its fatty acid composition. Even though the mechanism responsible for the divergent effects of the lard and linoleate-enriched diets is not completely clear, it may involve diet-induced changes in the content and/or composition of cardiolipin in the heart.

Hyperglycemia and diabetes affect cardiac mitochondria function directly since mitochondria from a variety of diabetic animal models show diminished respiratory control, as well as increased OS [229, 230]. These changes are reversed with insulin administration. Conversely, the activity of the PPAR-α gene regulatory pathway is increased in the diabetic heart, which relies primarily on FAO for energy production, providing further stimulus for the excessive fatty acid import and oxidation underlying the cardiac remodeling of the diabetic heart. It appears that shifts in metabolic programming (from fatty acid to glucose utilization), using specific metabolic inhibitors and cardioprotective agents may be beneficial in the treatment of both specific metabolic defects and more global defects due to myocardial ischemia, HF, and diabetes.

Summary

- Fatty acid utilization is a critical source of bioenergy for the adult heart. Fatty acid transport into the cardiomyocytes and within the cell is a highly regulated process involving specific transport proteins located in the plasma membrane, fatty acid binding proteins and transporters within the mitochondrial membranes.
- Defects in transport proteins function may result in a number of cardiac defects resulting in deficiencies of FAO, or an accumulation of fatty acid metabolic intermediates, which can promote a lipotoxic cardiomyopathy.
- The use of animal models, particularly transgenic mice, has been highly informative.
- FAO, to provide energy for the downstream TCA and oxidative phosphorylation cycles, is largely localized to the mitochondrial organelle and is also present in the peroxisome. This process is governed by substrate levels, a variety of physiological stimuli and regulators including AMP kinase, several members of the nuclear receptor transcription factor family including the PPARs, and associated coactivators such as PGC-1.
- Regulatory factors are modulated by many physiological stimuli as well as by pathophysiological conditions such as myocardial ischemia, HF, and diabetes.
- Several mutations in genes encoding FAO proteins can lead to cardiomyopathy and cardiac dysrhythmias.
- Glucose transport in the heart is facilitated by the function of specific membrane transporters (GLUT-1 and GLUT-4), regulated by a complex signaling pathway, which includes insulin and its receptor, a variety of kinase transducers, by the fatty acid oxidation process, and by other physiological stimuli. Subsequent glycolytic metabolism and glucose oxidation (mainly in the mitochondria) is also highly regulated by many of the same signals and transducers.
- Alterations in CHO metabolism associated with FA oxidation defects may result in HF under stress conditions, even in the fed state.
- Present therapeutic approaches for these metabolic defects include dietary modification, elimination of stresses (e.g., fasting), and supplementation with carnitine.
- Shifts in metabolic programming (from fatty acid to glucose utilization) using specific metabolic inhibitors and cardioprotective agents have proven beneficial in treating both specific metabolic defects and more global defects due to myocardial ischemia, HF, and diabetes.
- Metabolic therapy utilizing fibrates and agonists of PPAR have also shown promise in redirecting bioenergetic pathways with beneficial cardiovascular effect. Gene and cell-mediated therapy holds promise in treating fatty acid and metabolic storage disorders as well as diabetes and insulin resistance.

- It has been proposed that the excess of substrate may lead to HF, and this could be prevented or slowed by keeping low body fat and high insulin sensitivity, and by following a diet with low glycemic load that is high in mono-and polyunsaturated fatty acids.

References

1. Sack MN, Rader TA, Park S, Bastin J, McCune SA, Kelly DP (1996) Fatty acid oxidation enzyme gene expression is downregulated in the failing heart. Circulation 94:2837–2842
2. Kanda H, Nohara R, Hasegawa K, Kishimoto C, Sasayama S (2000) A nuclear complex containing PPARa/RXR is markedly downregulated in the hypertrophied rat left ventricular myocardium with normal systolic function. Heart Vessels 15:191–196
3. Tian Q, Barger BM (2006) Deranged energy substrate metabolism in the failing heart. Curr Hypertens Rep 8:465–471
4. Liang X, Le W, Zhang D, Schulz H (2001) Impact of the intramitochondrial enzyme organization on fatty acid organization. Biochem Soc Trans 29:279–282
5. Jackson S, Schaefer J, Middleton B, Turnbull DM (1995) Characterization of a novel enzyme of human fatty acid beta-oxidation: a matrix-associated, mitochondrial 2-enoyl CoA hydratase. Biochem Biophys Res Commun 214:247–253
6. Stanley WC, Recchia FA, Lopaschuk GD (2005) Myocardial substrate metabolism in the normal and failing heart. Physiol Rev 85:1093–1129
7. Poole RC, Halestrap AP (1993) Transport of lactate and other monocarboxylates across mammalian plasma membranes. Am J Physiol 264:C761–C782
8. Printz RL, Koch S, Potter LR, O'Doherty RM, Tiesinga JJ, Moritz S, Granner DK (1993) Hexokinase II mRNA and gene structure, regulation by insulin, and evolution. J Biol Chem 268:5209–5219
9. Uyeda K (1979) Phosphofructokinase. Adv Enzymol Relat Areas Mol Biol 48:193–244
10. Hue L, Rider MH (1987) Role of fructose 2, 6-bisphosphate in the control of glycolysis in mammalian tissues. Biochem J 245:313–324
11. Depre C, Rider MH, Veitch K, Hue L (1993) Role of fructose 2, 6-bisphosphate in the control of heart glycolysis. J Biol Chem 268:13274–13279
12. Kiffmeyer WR, Farrar WW (1991) Purification and properties of pig heart pyruvate kinase. J Protein Chem 10:585–591
13. Sugden MC, Langdown ML, Harris RA, Holness MJ (2000) Expression and regulation of pyruvate dehydrogenase kinase isoforms in the developing rat heart and in adulthood: role of thyroid hormone status and lipid supply. Biochem J 352:731–738
14. Denton RM, McCormack JG, Rutter GA, Burnett P, Edgell NJ, Moule SK, Diggle TA (1996) The hormonal regulation of pyruvate dehydrogenase complex. Adv Enzyme Regul 36:183–198
15. Huang B, Wu P, Popov KM, Harris RA (2003) Starvation and diabetes reduce the amount of pyruvate dehydrogenase phosphatase in rat heart and kidney. Diabetes 52:1371–1376
16. Opie LH, Sack MN (2002) Metabolic plasticity and the promotion of cardiac protection in ischemia and ischemic preconditioning. J Mol Cell Cardiol 34:1077–1089
17. Goodwin GW, Taegtmeyer H (2000) Improved energy homeostasis of the heart in the metabolic state of exercise. Am J Physiol Heart Circ Physiol 279:H1490–H1501
18. Shelley HJ (1961) Cardiac glycogen in different species before and after birth. Br Med Bull 17:137–156
19. Schneider CA, Nguyên VTB, Taegtmeyer H (1991) Feeding and fasting determine postischemic glucose utilization in isolated working rat hearts. Am J Physiol 260:H542–H548
20. Moule SK, Denton RM (1997) Multiple pathways involved in the metabolic effects of insulin. Am J Cardiol 80:41A–49A
21. Goodwin GW, Arteaga JR, Taegtmeyer H (1995) Glycogen turnover in the isolated working rat heart. J Biol Chem 270:9234–9240
22. Morgan HE, Parmeggiani A (1964) Regulation of glycogenolysis in muscle, II: control of glycogen phosphorylase reaction in isolated perfused heart. J Biol Chem 239:2435–2439
23. Goodwin G, Ahmad F, Taegtmeyer H (1996) Preferential oxidation of glycogen in isolated working rat heart. J Clin Invest 97:1409–1416
24. Stanley WC, Lopaschuk GD, Hall JL, McCormack JG (1997) Regulation of myocardial carbohydrate metabolism under normal and ischaemic conditions. Potential for pharmacological interventions. Cardiovasc Res 33:243–257
25. Gollob MH (2003) Glycogen storage disease as a unifying mechanism of disease in the PRKAG2 cardiac syndrome. Biochem Soc Trans 31:228–231
26. Longnus SL, Wambolt RB, Parsons HL, Brownsey RW, Allard MF (2003) 5-Aminoimidazole-4-carboxamide 1-beta-D-ribofuranoside (AICAR) stimulates myocardial glycogenolysis by allosteric mechanisms. Am J Physiol Regul Integr Comp Physiol 284:R936–R944
27. Polekhina G, Gupta A, Michell BJ, van Denderen B, Murthy S, Feil SC, Jennings IG, Campbell DJ, Witters LA, Parker MW, Kemp BE, Stapleton D (2003) AMPK beta subunit targets metabolic stress sensing to glycogen. Curr Biol 13:867–871
28. Glatz JF, Storch J (2001) Unraveling the significance of cellular fatty acid binding-protein. Curr Opin Lipidol 12:267–274
29. Liao J, Chan CP, Cheung YC, Lu JH, Luo Y, Cautherley GW, Glatz JF, Renneberg R (2009) Human heart-type fatty acid-binding protein for on-site diagnosis of early acute myocardial infarction. Int J Cardiol 133:420–423
30. McCann CJ, Glover BM, Menown IB, Moore MJ, McEneny J, Owens CG, Smith B, Sharpe PC, Young IS, Adgey JA (2008) Novel biomarkers in early diagnosis of acute myocardial infarction compared with cardiac troponin T. Eur Heart J 29:2843–2850
31. Abel ED (2004) Glucose transport in the heart. Front Biosci 9:201–215
32. Flier JS, Mueckler MM, Usher P, Lodish HF (1987) Elevated levels of glucose transport and transporter messenger RNA are induced by ras or src oncogenes. Science 235:1492–1495
33. Russell RR 3rd, Li J, Coven DL, Pypaert M, Zechner C, Palmeri M, Giordano FJ, Mu J, Birnbaum MJ, Young LH (2004) AMP-activated protein kinase mediates ischemic glucose uptake and prevents postischemic cardiac dysfunction, apoptosis, and injury. J Clin Invest 114:495–503
34. Chou SW, Chiu LL, Cho YM, Ho HY, Ivy JL, Ho CF, Kuo CH (2004) Effect of systemic hypoxia on GLUT4 protein expression in exercised rat heart. Jpn J Physiol 54:357–363
35. Till M, Kolter T, Eckel J (1997) Molecular mechanisms of contraction-induced translocation of GLUT4 in isolated cardiomyocytes. Am J Cardiol 80:85A–89A
36. Rattigan S, Appleby GJ, Clark MG (1991) Insulin-like action of catecholamines and Ca2+ to stimulate glucose transport and GLUT4 translocation in perfused rat heart. Biochim Biophys Acta 1094:217–223
37. Wojtaszewski JF, Higaki Y, Hirshman MF, Michael MD, Dufresne SD, Kahn CR, Goodyear LJ (1999) Exercise modulates postreceptor insulin signaling and glucose transport in muscle-specific insulin receptor knockout mice. J Clin Invest 104:1257–1264
38. Coven DL, Hu X, Cong L, Bergeron R, Shulman GI, Hardie DG, Young LH (2003) Physiological role of AMP-activated protein kinase in the heart: graded activation during exercise. Am J Physiol Endocrinol Metab 285:E629–E636

39. Katz EB, Stenbit AE, Hatton K, DePinho R, Charron MJ (1995) Cardiac and adipose tissue abnormalities but not diabetes in mice deficient in GLUT4. Nature 377:151–155

40. Zisman A, Peroni OD, Abel ED, Michael MD, Mauvais-Jarvis F, Lowell BB, Wojtaszewski JF, Hirshman MF, Virkamaki A, Goodyear LJ, Kahn CR, Kahn BB (2000) Targeted disruption of the glucose transporter 4 selectively in muscle causes insulin resistance and glucose intolerance. Nat Med 6:924–928

41. Desrois M, Sidell RJ, Gauguier D, King LM, Radda GK, Clarke K (2004) Initial steps of insulin signaling and glucose transport are defective in the type 2 diabetic rat heart. Cardiovasc Res 61: 288–296

42. Bruning JC, Michael MD, Winnay JN, Hayashi T, Horsch D, Accili D, Goodyear LJ, Kahn CR (1998) A muscle-specific insulin receptor knockout exhibits features of the metabolic syndrome of NIDDM without altering glucose tolerance. Mol Cell 2:559–569

43. Kaczmarczyk SJ, Andrikopoulos S, Favaloro J, Domenighetti AA, Dunn A, Ernst M, Grail D, Fodero-Tavoletti M, Huggins CE, Delbridge LM, Zajac JD, Proietto J (2003) Threshold effects of glucose transporter-4 (GLUT4) deficiency on cardiac glucose uptake and development of hypertrophy. J Mol Endocrinol 31:449–459

44. Razeghi P, Young ME, Ying J, Depre C, Uray IP, Kolesar J, Shipley GL, Moravec CS, Davies PJ, Frazier OH, Taegtmeyer H (2002) Downregulation of metabolic gene expression in failing human heart before and after mechanical unloading. Cardiology 97:203–209

45. Razeghi P, Young ME, Alcorn JL, Moravec CS, Frazier OH, Taegtmeyer H (2001) Metabolic gene expression in fetal and failing human heart. Circulation 104:2923–2931

46. Razeghi P, Young ME, Cockrill TC, Frazier OH, Taegtmeyer H (2002) Downregulation of myocardial myocyte enhancer factor 2C and myocyte enhancer factor 2C-regulated gene expression in diabetic patients with nonischemic heart failure. Circulation 106:407–411

47. Stanley WC, Lopaschuk GD, McCormack JG (1997) Regulation of energy substrate metabolism in the diabetic heart. Cardiovasc Res 34:25–33

48. Nikolaidis LA, Sturzu A, Stolarski C, Elahi D, Shen YT, Shannon RP (2004) The development of myocardial insulin resistance in conscious dogs with advanced dilated cardiomyopathy. Cardiovasc Res 61:297–306

49. Shah A, Shannon RP (2003) Insulin resistance in dilated cardiomyopathy. Rev Cardiovasc Med 4:S50–S57

50. Tuunanen H, Ukkonen H, Knuuti J (2008) Myocardial fatty acid metabolism and cardiac performance in heart failure. Curr Cardiol Rep 10:142–148

51. Clodi M, Resl M, Stelzeneder D, Pacini G, Tura A, Mörtl D, Struck J, Morgenthaler NG, Bergmann A, Riedl M, Anderwald-Stadler M, Luger A, Pacher R, Hülsmann M (2009) Interactions of glucose metabolism and chronic heart failure. Exp Clin Endocrinol Diabetes 117:99–106

52. Paternostro G, Pagano D, Gnecchi-Ruscone T, Bonser RS, Camici PG (1999) Insulin resistance in patients with cardiac hypertrophy. Cardiovasc Res 42:246–253

53. Nuutila P, Maki M, Laine H, Knuuti MJ, Ruotsalainen U, Luotolahti M, Haaparanta M, Solin O, Jula A, Koivisto VA, Voipio-Pulkki LM, Yki-Jarvinen H (1995) Insulin action on heart and skeletal muscle glucose uptake in essential hypertension. J Clin Invest 96: 1003–1009

54. Paternostro G, Clarke K, Heath J, Seymour AM (1995) Radda GK Decreased GLUT-4 mRNA content and insulin-sensitive deoxyglucose uptake show insulin resistance in the hypertensive rat heart. Cardiovasc Res 30:205–211

55. Nascimben L, Ingwall JS, Lorell BH, Pinz I, Schultz V, Tornheim K, Tian R (2004) Mechanisms for increased glycolysis in the hypertrophied rat heart. Hypertension 44:662–667

56. Brownsey RW, Boone AN, Allard MF (1997) Actions of insulin on the mammalian heart: metabolism, pathology and biochemical mechanisms. Cardiovasc Res 34:3–24

57. Vannucci SJ, Rutherford T, Wilkie MB, Simpson IA (2000) Lauder JM Prenatal expression of the GLUT4 glucose transporter in the mouse. Dev Neurosci 22:274–282

58. Santalucia T, Boheler KR, Brand NJ, Sahye U, Fandos C, Vinals F, Ferre J, Testar X, Palacin M, Zorzano A (1999) Factors involved in GLUT-1 glucose transporter gene transcription in cardiac muscle. J Biol Chem 274:17626–17634

59. Taegtmeyer H, Sharma S, Golfman L, Razeghi P, van Arsdall M (2004) Linking gene expression to function: metabolic flexibility in normal and diseased heart. Ann N Y Acad Sci 1015:1–12

60. Young LH, Coven DL, Russell RR 3rd (2000) Cellular and molecular regulation of cardiac glucose transport. J Nucl Cardiol 7: 267–276

61. Depre C, Shipley GL, Chen W, Han Q, Doenst T, Moore ML, Stepkowski S, Davies PJ, Taegtmeyer H (1998) Unloaded heart in vivo replicates fetal gene expression of cardiac hypertrophy. Nat Med 4:1269–1275

62. Doenst T, Goodwin GW, Cedars AM, Wang M, Stepkowski S, Taegtmeyer H (2001) Load-induced changes in vivo alter substrate fluxes and insulin responsiveness of rat heart in vitro. Metabolism 50: 1083–1090

63. Zhou L, Salem JE, Saidel GM, Stanley WC, Cabrera ME (2005) Mechanistic model of cardiac energy metabolism predicts localization of glycolysis to cytosolic subdomain during ischemia. Am J Physiol Heart Circ Physiol 288:H2400–H2411

64. Srere PA, Sumegi B, Sherry AD (1987) Organizational aspects of the citric acid cycle. Biochem Soc Symp 54:173–178

65. Ishibashi S (1999) Cooperation of membrane proteins and cytosolic proteins in metabolic regulation – involvement of binding of hexokinase to mitochondria in regulation of glucose metabolism and association and complex formation between membrane proteins and cytosolic proteins in regulation of active oxygen production. Yakugaku Zasshi 119:16–34

66. Lehman JJ, Kelly DP (2002) Gene regulatory mechanisms governing energy metabolism during cardiac hypertrophic growth. Heart Fail Rev 7:175–185

67. Marin-Garcia J, Goldenthal MJ, Moe GW (2001) Mitochondrial pathology in cardiac failure. Cardiovasc Res 49:17–26

68. Brackett JC, Sims HF, Rinaldo P et al (1995) Two a-subunit donor splice site mutations cause human trifunctional protein deficiency. J Clin Invest 95:2076–2082

69. Kelly DP, Gordon JI, Alpers R, Strauss AW (1989) The tissue-specific expression and developmental regulation of two nuclear genes encoding rat mitochondrial proteins. Medium chain acyl-CoA dehydrogenase and mitochondrial malate dehydrogenase. J Biol Chem 264:18921–18925

70. Schonberger J, Seidman CE (2001) Many roads lead to a broken heart: the genetics of dilated cardiomyopathy. Am J Hum Genet 69:249–260

71. Roe CR, Ding JH (2001) Mitochondrial fatty acid oxidation disorders. In: Scriver C et al (eds) Metabolic and molecular basis of inherited disease, vol 2. McGraw-Hill, New York, pp 2297–2326

72. D'Adamo P, Fassone L, Gedeon A et al (1997) The X-linked gene G4.5 is responsible for different infantile dilated cardiomyopathies. Am J Hum Genet 61:862–867

73. Jethva R, Bennett MJ, Vockley J (2008) Short-chain acyl-coenzyme A dehydrogenase deficiency. Mol Genet Metab 95:195–200

74. Sims HF, Brackett JC, Powell CK, Treem WR, Hale DE, Bennett MJ, Gibson B, Shapiro S (1995) Strauss AW The molecular basis of pediatric long chain 3-hydroxyacyl-CoA dehydrogenase deficiency associated with maternal acute fatty liver of pregnancy. Proc Natl Acad Sci USA 92:841–845

75. Matern D, Strauss AW, Hillman SL, Mayatepek E, Millington DS, Trefz FK (1999) Diagnosis of mitochondrial trifunctional protein deficiency in a blood spot from the newborn screening card by tandem mass spectrometry and DNA analysis. Pediatr Res 46:45–49

76. Strauss AW, Powell CK, Hale DE et al (1995) Molecular basis of human mitochondrial very-long-chain acyl-CoA dehydrogenase deficiency causing cardiomyopathy and sudden death in childhood. Proc Natl Acad Sci USA 92:10496–10500

77. Mathur A, Sims HF, Gopalakrishnan D et al (1999) Molecular heterogeneity in very-long-chain acyl-CoA dehydrogenase deficiency causing pediatric cardiomyopathy and sudden death. Circulation 99:1337–1343

78. Brivet M, Boutron A, Slama A, Costa C, Thuillier L, Demaugre F, Rabier D, Saudubray JM, Bonnefont JP (1999) Defects in activation and transport of fatty acids. J Inherit Metab Dis 22:428–441

79. Nezu J, Tamai I, Oku A et al (1999) Primary systemic carnitine deficiency is caused by mutations in a gene encoding sodium ion-dependent carnitine transporter. Nat Genet 21:91–94

80. Iacobazzi V, Invernizzi F, Baratta S, Pons R, Chung W, Garavaglia B, Dionisi-Vici C, Ribes A, Parini R, Huertas MD, Roldan S, Lauria G, Palmieri F, Taroni F (2004) Molecular and functional analysis of SLC25A20 mutations causing carnitine-acylcarnitine translocase deficiency. Hum Mutat 24:312–320

81. Iacobazzi V, Pasquali M, Singh R, Matern D, Rinaldo P (2004) Amat di San Filippo C, Palmieri F, Longo N. Response to therapy in carnitine/acylcarnitine translocase (CACT) deficiency due to a novel missense mutation. Am J Med Genet 126:150–155

82. Feillet F, Steinmann G, Vianey-Saban C, de Chillou C, Sadoul N, Lefebvre E, Vidailhet M (2003) Bollaert PE.Adult presentation of MCAD deficiency revealed by coma and severe arrythmias. Intensive Care Med 29:1594–1597

83. Finocchiaro G, Ito M, Ikeda Y, Tanaka K (1988) Molecular cloning and nucleotide sequence of cDNAs encoding the alpha-subunit of human electron transfer flavoprotein. J Biol Chem 263:15773–15780

84. Okamoto F, Tanaka T, Sohmiya K, Kawamura K (1998) CD36 abnormality and impaired myocardial long-chain fatty acid uptake in patients with hypertrophic cardiomyopathy. Jpn Circ J 62:499–504

85. Sookoian S, Garcia SI, Porto PI, Dieuzeide G, Gonzalez CD, Pirola CJ (2005) Peroxisome proliferator-activated receptor gamma and its coactivator-1 alpha may be associated with features of the metabolic syndrome in adolescents. J Mol Endocrinol 35:373–380

86. Doney AS, Fischer B, Lee SP, Morris AD, Leese G, Palmer CN (2005) Association of common variation in the PPARA gene with incident myocardial infarction in individuals with type 2 diabetes: A Go-DARTS study. Nucl Recept 3:4

87. Bione S, D'Adamo P, Maestrini E, Gedeon AK, Bolhuis PA, Toniolo D (1996) A novel X-linked gene, G4.5. is responsible for Barth syndrome. Nat Genet 12:385–389

88. Neuwald AF (1997) Barth syndrome may be due to an acyltransferase deficiency. Curr Biol 7:R465–R466

89. Vreken P, Valianpour F, Nijtmans LG et al (2000) Defective remodeling of cardiolipin and phosphatidylglycerol in Barth syndrome. Biochem Biophys Res Commun 279:378–382

90. Kelly DP, Strauss AW (1994) Inherited cardiomyopathies. N Eng J Med 330:913–919

91. Hale DE, Batshaw ML, Coates PM, Frerman FE, Goodman SI, Singh I, Stanley CA (1985) Long-chain acyl coenzyme A dehydrogenase deficiency: an inherited cause of nonketotic hypoglycemia. Pediatr Res 19:666–671

92. Rocchiccioli F, Wanders RJ, Aubourg P et al (1990) Deficiency of long-chain 3-hydroxyacyl-CoA dehydrogenase: a cause of lethal myopathy and cardiomyopathy in early childhood. Pediatr Res 28:657–662

93. Strauss AW, Powell CK (1995) Hale DE et al Molecular basis of human mitochondrial very-long-chain acyl-CoA dehydrogenase deficiency causing cardiomyopathy and sudden death in childhood. Proc Natl Acad Sci USA 92:10496–10500

94. Tein I, Haslam RH, Rhead WJ, Bennett MJ, Becker LE, Vockley J (1999) Short-chain acyl-CoA dehydrogenase deficiency: a cause of ophthalmoplegia and multicore myopathy. Neurology 52:366–372

95. Engel AG, Angelini C (1973) Carnitine deficiency of human skeletal muscle with associated lipid storage myopathy: a new syndrome. Science 179:899–902

96. Stanley CA, Treem WR, Hale DE, Coates PM (1990) A genetic defect in carnitine transport causing primary carnitine deficiency. Prog Clin Biol Res 321:457–464

97. Roschinger W, Muntau AC, Duran M et al (2000) Carnitine-acylcarnitine translocase deficiency: metabolic consequences of an impaired mitochondrial carnitine cycle. Clin Chim Acta 298:55–68

98. Olpin SE, Allen J, Bonham JR et al (2001) Features of carnitine palmitoyltransferase type I deficiency. J Inherit Metab Dis 24:35–42

99. Demaugre F, Bonnefont JP, Colonna M, Cepanec C, Leroux JP, Saudubray JM (1991) Infantile form of carnitine palmitoyltransferase II deficiency with hepatomuscular symptoms and sudden death. Physiopathological approach to carnitine palmitoyltransferase II deficiencies. J Clin Invest 87:859–864

100. Narula J, Haider N, Virmani R et al (1996) Apoptosis in myocytes in end-stage heart failure. N Engl J Med 335:1182–1189

101. Olivetti G, Abbi R, Quaini F et al (1997) Apoptosis in the failing human heart. N Engl J Med 336:1131–1141

102. Li Z, Bing OH, Long X, Robinson KG, Lakatta EG (1997) Increased cardiomyocyte apoptosis during the transition to heart failure in the spontaneously hypertensive rat. Am J Physiol 272:H2313–H2319

103. Marzo I, Brenner C, Zamzani N et al (1998) The permeability transition pore complex: a target for apoptosis regulation by caspases and Bcl-2 related proteins. J Exp Med 187:1261–1271

104. Lutter M, Fang M, Luo X, Nishijima M, Xie X, Wang X (2000) Cardiolipin provides specificity for targeting of tBid to mitochondria. Nat Cell Biol 2:754–761

105. Hickson-Bick DL, Buja ML, McMillin JB (2000) Palmitate-mediated alterations in the fatty acid metabolism of rat neonatal cardiac myocytes. J Mol Cell Cardiol 32:511–519

106. DeVries JE, Vork MM, Roemen TH et al (1997) Saturated but not mono-unsaturated fatty acids induce apoptotic cell death in neonatal rat ventricular myocytes. J Lipid Res 38:1384–1394

107. Sparagna GC, Hickson-Bick DL, Buja LM, McMillin JB (2001) Fatty acid-induced apoptosis in neonatal cardiomyocytes: redox signaling. Antioxid Redox Signal 3:71–79

108. Ostrander DB, Sparagna GC, Amoscato AA, McMillin JB, Dowhan W (2001) Decreased cardiolipin synthesis corresponds with cytochrome c release in palmitate-induced cardiomyocyte apoptosis. J Biol Chem 276:38061–38067

109. Sparagna GC, Hickson-Bick DL, Buja LM, McMillin JB (2000) A metabolic role for mitochondria in palmitate-induced cardiac myocyte apoptosis. Am J Physiol Heart Circ Physiol 279: H2124– H2132

110. Malhotra R, Brosius FC (1999) Glucose uptake and glycolysis reduce hypoxia-induced apoptosis in cultured neonatal rat cardiac myocytes. J Biol Chem 274:12567–12575

111. Lin Z, Weinberg JM, Malhotra R, Merritt SE, Holzman LB, Brosius FC (2000) GLUT-1 reduces hypoxia-induced apoptosis and JNK pathway activation. Am J Physiol Endocrinol Metab 278:E958–E966

112. Fujio Y, Nguyen T, Wencker D, Kitsis RN, Walsh K (2000) Akt promotes survival of cardiomyocytes in vitro and protects against ischemia-reperfusion injury in mouse heart. Circulation 101:660–667

113. Aikawa R, Nawano M, Gu Y, Katagiri H, Asano T, Zhu W, Nagai R (1000) Komuro I Insulin prevents cardiomyocytes from oxidative stress-induced apoptosis through activation of PI3 kinase/Akt. Circulation 102:2873–2879

114. Cai L, Li W, Wang G, Guo L, Jiang Y, Kang YJ (2002) Hyperglycemia-induced apoptosis in mouse myocardium: mitochondrial cytochrome c-mediated caspase-3 activation pathway. Diabetes 51:1938–1948

115. Kelly DP, Hale DE, Rutledge SL et al (1992) Molecular basis of inherited medium-chain acyl-CoA dehydrogenase deficiency causing sudden child death. J Inherit Metab Dis 15:171–180

116. Tanaka K, Yokota I, Coates PM (1992) Mutations in the medium chain acyl-CoA dehydrogenase (MCAD) gene. Hum Mutat 1:271–279

117. Andresen BS, Jensen TG, Bross P et al (1994) Disease-causing mutations in exon 11 of the medium-chain acyl-CoA dehydrogenase gene. Am J Hum Genet 54:975–988

118. Strauss AW, Powell CK, Hale DE, Anderson MM, Ahuja A, Brackett JC, Sims HF (1995) Molecular basis of human mitochondrial very-long-chain acyl-CoA dehydrogenase deficiency causing cardiomyopathy and sudden death in childhood. Proc Natl Acad Sci USA 92:10496–10500

119. Mathur A, Sims HF, Gopalakrishnan D, Gibson B, Rinaldo P, Vockley J, Hug G, Strauss AW (1999) Molecular heterogeneity in very-long-chain acyl-CoA dehydrogenase deficiency causing pediatric cardiomyopathy and sudden death. Circulation 99:1337–1343

120. Bonnefont JP, Taroni F, Cavadini P et al (1996) Molecular analysis of carnitine palmitoyltransferase II deficiency with hepatocardiomuscular expression. Am J Hum Genet 58:971–978

121. Taroni F, Verderio E, Fiorucci S et al (1992) Molecular characterization of inherited carnitine palmitoyltransferase II deficiency. Proc Natl Acad Sci USA 89:8429–8433

122. Ibdah JA, Zhao Y, Viola J, Gibson B, Bennett MJ, Strauss AW (2001) Molecular prenatal diagnosis in families with fetal mitochondrial trifunctional protein mutations. J Pediatr 138:396–399

123. Gulick T, Cresci S, Caira T, Moore DD, Kelly DP (1994) The peroxisome proliferator activated receptor regulates mitochondrial fatty acid oxidative enzyme gene expression. Proc Natl Acad Sci USA 91:11012–11016

124. Barger PM, Brandt JM, Leone TC, Weinheimer CJ, Kelly DP (2000) Deactivation of peroxisome proliferator-activated receptor-alpha during cardiac hypertrophic growth. J Clin Invest 105:1723–1730

125. Huss JM, Levy FH, Kelly DP (2001) Hypoxia inhibits the peroxisome proliferator-activated receptor alpha/retinoid X receptor gene regulatory pathway in cardiac myocytes: a mechanism for O$_2$-dependent modulation of mitochondrial fatty acid oxidation. J Biol Chem 276:27605–27612

126. Lehman JJ, Barger PM, Kovacs A, Saffitz JE, Medeiros DM, Kelly DP (2000) Peroxisome proliferator-activated receptor gamma coactivator-1 promotes cardiac mitochondrial biogenesis. J Clin Invest 106:847–856

127. Vega RB, Huss JM, Kelly DP (2000) The coactivator PGC-1 cooperates with peroxisome proliferator-activated receptor in transcriptional control of nuclear genes encoding mitochondrial fatty acid oxidation enzymes. Mol Cell Biol 20:1868–1876

128. Schwenk RW, Luiken JJ, Bonen A, Glatz JF (2008) Regulation of sarcolemmal glucose and fatty acid transporters in cardiac disease. Cardiovasc Res 79:249–258

129. Leong HS, Brownsey RW, Kulpa JE, Allard MF (2003) Glycolysis and pyruvate oxidation in cardiac hypertrophy: why so unbalanced? Comp Biochem Physiol A Mol Integr Physiol 135:499–513

130. van Bilsen M, Smeets PJ, Gilde AJ, van der Vusse GJ (2004) Metabolic remodelling of the failing heart: the cardiac burn-out syndrome? Cardiovasc Res 61:218–226

131. Lei B, Lionetti V, Young ME, Chandler MP, D'Agostino C, Kang E, Altarejos M, Matsuo K, Hintze TH, Stanley WC, Recchia FA (2004) Paradoxical downregulation of the glucose oxidation pathway despite enhanced flux in severe heart failure. J Mol Cell Cardiol 36:567–576

132. Chandler MP, Kerner J, Huang H, Vazquez E, Reszko A, Martini WZ, Hoppel CL, Imai M, Rastogi S, Sabbah HN, Stanley WC (2004) Moderate severity heart failure does not involve a downregulation of myocardial fatty acid oxidation. Am J Physiol Heart Circ Physiol 287:H1538–H1543

133. Remondino A, Rosenblatt-Velin N, Montessuit C, Tardy I, Papageorgiou I, Dorsaz PA, Jorge-Costa M, Lerch R (2000) Altered expression of proteins of metabolic regulation during remodeling of the left ventricle after myocardial infarction. J Mol Cell Cardiol 32:2025–2034

134. Rosenblatt-Velin N, Montessuit C, Papageorgiou I, Terrand J, Lerch R (2001) Postinfarction heart failure in rats is associated with upregulation of GLUT-1 and downregulation of genes of fatty acid metabolism. Cardiovasc Res 52:407–416

135. Huss JM, Kelly DP (2004) Nuclear receptor signaling and cardiac energetics. Circ Res 95:568–578

136. Karbowska J, Kochan Z, Smolenski RT (2003) Peroxisome proliferator-activated receptor alpha is downregulated in the failing human heart. Cell Mol Biol Lett 8:49–53

137. Osorio JC, Stanley WC, Linke A, Castellari M, Diep QN, Panchal AR, Hintze TH, Lopaschuk GD, Recchia FA (2002) Impaired myocardial fatty acid oxidation and reduced protein expression of retinoid X receptor-alpha in pacing-induced heart failure. Circulation 106:606–612

138. Hartil K, Charron MJ (2005) Genetic modification of the heart: transgenic modification of cardiac lipid and carbohydrate utilization. J Mol Cell Cardiol 39:581–593

139. Abel ED, Kaulbach HC, Tian R, Hopkins JC, Duffy J, Doetschman T, Minnemann T, Boers ME, Hadro E, Oberste-Berghaus C, Quist W, Lowell BB, Ingwall JS, Kahn BB (1999) Cardiac hypertrophy with preserved contractile function after selective deletion of GLUT4 from the heart. J Clin Invest 104:1703–1714

140. Irrcher I, Adhihetty PJ, Sheehan T, Joseph AM, Hood DA (2003) PPARgamma coactivator-1alpha expression during thyroid hormone- and contractile activity-induced mitochondrial adaptations. Am J Physiol Cell Physiol 284:C1669–C1677

141. Chiu HC, Kovacs A, Ford D, Hsu FF, Garcia R, Herrero P, Saffitz JE, Schaffer JE (2001) A novel mouse model of lipotoxic cardiomyopathy. J Clin Invest 107:813–822

142. Stenbit AE, Katz EB, Chatham JC, Geenen DL, Factor SM, Weiss RG, Tsao TS, Malhotra A, Chacko VP, Ocampo C, Jelicks LA, Charron MJ (2000) Preservation of glucose metabolism in hypertrophic GLUT4-null hearts. Am J Physiol Heart Circ Physiol 279:H313–H318

143. Finck B, Lehman JJ, Leone TC, Welch MJ, Bennett MJ, Kovacs A, Han X, Gross RW, Kozak R, Lopaschuk GD, Kelly DP (2002) The cardiac phenotype induced by PPARalpha overexpression mimics that caused by diabetes mellitus. J Clin Invest 109:121–130

144. Cheng L, Ding G, Qin Q, Huang Y, Lewis W, He N, Evans RM, Schneider MD, Brako FA, Xiao Y, Chen YE, Yang Q (2004) Cardiomyocyte-restricted peroxisome proliferator-activated receptor-delta deletion perturbs myocardial fatty acid oxidation and leads to cardiomyopathy. Nat Med 10:1245–1250

145. Christoffersen C, Bollano E, Lindegaard ML, Bartels ED, Goetze JP, Andersen CB, Nielsen LB (2003) Cardiac lipid accumulation associated with diastolic dysfunction in obese mice. Endocrinology 144:3483–3490

146. Exil VJ, Roberts RL, Sims H, McLaughlin JE, Malkin RA, Gardner CD, Ni G, Rottman JN, Strauss AW (2003) Very-long-chain acyl-coenzyme a dehydrogenase deficiency in mice. Circ Res 93:448–455

147. Hansson A, Hance N, Dufour E, Rantanen A, Hultenby K, Clayton DA, Wibom R, Larsson NG (2004) A switch in metabolism precedes increased mitochondrial biogenesis in respiratory chain-deficient mouse hearts. Proc Natl Acad Sci USA 101:3136–3141

148. Augustus A, Yagyu H, Haemmerle G, Bensadoun A, Vikramadithyan RK, Park SY, Kim JK, Zechner R, Goldberg IJ (2004) Cardiac-specific knock-out of lipoprotein lipase alters plasma lipoprotein triglyceride metabolism and cardiac gene expression. J Biol Chem 279:25050–25057

149. Coburn CT, Hajri T, Ibrahimi A, Abumrad NA (2001) Role of CD36 in membrane transport and utilization of long-chain fatty acids by different tissues. J Mol Neurosci 16:117–121

150. Ibrahimi A, Bonen A, Blinn WD, Hajri T, Li X, Zhong K, Cameron R, Abumrad NA (1999) Muscle-specific overexpression of FAT/CD36 enhances fatty acid oxidation by contracting muscle, reduces plasma triglycerides and fatty acids, and increases plasma glucose and insulin. J Biol Chem 274:26761–26766

151. Belke DD, Betuing S, Tuttle MJ, Graveleau C, Young ME, Pham M, Zhang D, Cooksey RC, McClain DA, Litwin SE, Taegtmeyer H, Severson D, Kahn CR, Abel ED (2002) Insulin signaling coordinately regulates cardiac size, metabolism, and contractile protein isoform expression. J Clin Invest 109:629–639

152. Binas B, Danneberg H, McWhir J, Mullins L, Clark AJ (1999) Requirement for the heart-type fatty acid binding protein in cardiac fatty acid utilization. FASEB J 13:805–812

153. Ibdah JA, Paul H, Zhao Y et al (2001) Lack of mitochondrial trifunctional protein in mice causes neonatal hypoglycemia and sudden death. J Clin Invest 107:1403–1409

154. Arany Z, He H, Lin J, Hoyer K, Handschin C, Toka O, Ahmad F, Matsui T, Chin S, Wu PH, Rybkin II, Shelton JM, Manieri M, Cinti S, Schoen FJ, Bassel-Duby R, Rosenzweig A, Ingwall JS, Spiegelman BM (2005) Transcriptional coactivator PGC-1 alpha controls the energy state and contractile function of cardiac muscle. Cell Metab 1:259–271

155. Djouadi F, Brandt JM, Weinheimer CJ, Leone TC, Gonzalez FJ, Kelly DP (1999) The role of the peroxisome proliferator-activated receptor alpha (PPAR a) in the control of cardiac lipid metabolism. Prostaglandins Leukot Essent Fatty Acids 60:339–343

156. Schoonjans K, Peinado-Onsurbe AM, Heyman RA, Briggs M, Deeb S, Staels B, Auwerx J (1996) PPARalpha and PPARgamma activators direct a distinct tissue-specific transcriptional response via a PPRE in the lipoprotein lipase gene. EMBO J 15:5336–5348

157. van der Lee KAJM, Vork MM, de Vries JE, Willemsen PHM, Glatz JFC, Reneman RS, Van der Vusse GJ, Van Bilsen M (2000) Long-chain fatty acid-induced changes in gene expression in neonatal cardiac myocytes. J Lipid Res 41:41–47

158. Martin G, Schoonjans K, Lefebvre AM, Staels B, Auwerx J (1997) Coordinate regulation of the expression of the fatty acid transport protein and acyl-CoA synthetase genes by PPARalpha and PPARgamma activators. J Biol Chem 272:28210–28217

159. Sugden MC, Bulmer K, Gibbons GF, Holness MJ (2001) Role of peroxisome proliferator-activated receptor-alpha in the mechanism underlying changes in renal pyruvate dehydrogenase kinase isoform 4 protein expression in starvation and after refeeding. Arch Biochem Biophys 395:246–252

160. Wu P, Peters JM, Harris RA (2001) Adaptive increase in pyruvate dehydrogenase kinase 4 during starvation is mediated by peroxisome proliferator-activated receptor alpha. Biochem Biophys Res Commun 287:391–396

161. Finck B, Lehman JJ, Leone TC et al (2002) The cardiac phenotype induced by PPARalpha overexpression mimics that caused by diabetes mellitus. J Clin Invest 109:121–130

162. Brandt JM, Djouadi F, Kelly DP (1998) Fatty acids activate transcription of the muscle carnitine palmitoyltransferase I gene in cardiac myocytes via the peroxisome proliferator-activated receptor alpha. J Biol Chem 273:23786–23792

163. Mascaro C, Acosta E, Ortiz JA, Marrero PF, Hegardt FG, Haro D (1998) Control of human muscle-type carnitine palmitoyltransferase Iβ gene promoters by fatty acid enzyme substrate. J Biol Chem 273:32901–32909

164. Zhang BW, Marcus SL, Sajjadi FG, Alvares K, Reddy JK, Subramani S, Rachubinski RA, Capone JP (1992) Identification of a peroxisome proliferator-responsive element upstream of the gene encoding rat peroxisomal enoyl-CoA hydratase/3-hydroxyacyl-CoA dehydrogenase. Proc Natl Acad Sci USA 85:7541–7545

165. Bardot O, Aldridge TC, Latruffe N, Green S (1993) PPAR-RXR heterodimer activates a peroxisome proliferator response element upstream of the bifunctional enzyme gene. Biochem Biophys Res Commun 19:237–245

166. Osumi T, Wen JK, Hashimoto T (1991) Two cis-acting regulatory sequences in the peroxisome proliferator-responsive enhancer region of the rat acyl-CoA oxidase gene. Biochem Biophys Res Commun 175:866–871

167. Dreyer C, Krey G, Keller H, Givel F, Helftenbein G, Wahli W (1992) Control of the peroxisomal β-oxidation pathway by a novel family of nuclear hormone receptors. Cell 68:879–887

168. Campbell FM, Kozak R, Wagner A et al (2002) A role for PPARalpha in the control of cardiac malonyl-CoA levels: reduced fatty acid oxidation rates and increased glucose oxidation rates in the hearts of mice lacking PPARalpha are associated with higher concentrations of malonyl-CoA and reduced expression of malonyl-CoA decarboxylase. J Biol Chem 277:4098–4103

169. Young ME, Patil S, Ying J et al (2001) Uncoupling protein 3 transcription is regulated by peroxisome proliferator-activated receptor alpha in the adult rodent heart. FASEB J 15:833–845

170. Murray AJ, Panagia M, Hauton D, Gibbons GF, Clarke K (2005) Plasma free fatty acids and peroxisome proliferator-activated receptor alpha in the control of myocardial uncoupling protein levels. Diabetes 54:3496–3502

171. Schreiber SN, Emter R, Hock MB, Knutti D, Cardenas J, Podvinec M, Oakeley EJ, Kralli A (2004) The estrogen-related receptor alpha (ERRalpha) functions in PPARgamma coactivator 1alpha (PGC-1alpha)-induced mitochondrial biogenesis. Proc Natl Acad Sci USA 101:6472–6477

172. Dressel U, Allen TL, Pippal JB, Rohde PR, Lau P, Muscat GE (2003) The peroxisome proliferator-activated receptor beta/delta agonist, GW501516, regulates the expression of genes involved in lipid catabolism and energy uncoupling in skeletal muscle cells. Mol Endocrinol 17:2477–2493

173. Hopkins TA, Sugden MC, Holness MJ, Kozak R, Dyck JRB, Lopaschuk GD (2003) Control of cardiac pyruvate dehydrogenase activity in peroxisome proliferator-activated receptor-alpha transgenic mice. Am J Physiol Heart Circ Physiol 285:H270–H276

174. Gélinas R, Labarthe F, Bouchard B, Mc Duff J, Charron G, Young ME, Des Rosiers C (2008) Alterations in carbohydrate metabolism and its regulation in PPARalpha null mouse hearts. Am J Physiol Heart Circ Physiol 294:H1571–H1580

175. Russell LK, Mansfield CM, Lehman JJ, Kovacs A, Courtois M, Saffitz JE, Medeiros DM, Valencik ML, McDonald JA, Kelly DP (2004) Cardiac-specific induction of the transcriptional coactivator peroxisome proliferator-activated receptor gamma coactivator-1alpha promotes mitochondrial biogenesis and reversible cardiomyopathy in a developmental stage-dependent manner. Circ Res 94:525–533

176. Zhou YT, Grayburn P, Karim A, Shimabukuro M, Higa M, Baetens D, Orci L, Unger RH (2000) Lipotoxic heart disease in obese rats: implications for human obesity. Proc Natl Acad Sci USA 97:1784–1789

177. Yagyu H, Chen G, Yokoyama M, Hirata K, Augustus A, Kako Y, Seo T, Hu Y, Lutz EP, Merkel M, Bensadoun A, Homma S, Goldberg IJ (2003) Lipoprotein lipase (LpL) on the surface of cardiomyocytes increases lipid uptake and produces a cardiomyopathy. J Clin Invest 111:419–426

178. Augustus AS, Kako Y, Yagyu H, Goldberg IJ (2003) Routes of FA delivery to cardiac muscle: modulation of lipoprotein lipolysis alters uptake of TG-derived FA. Am J Physiol Endocrinol Metab 284:E331–E339

179. Sharma S, Adrogue JV, Golfman L, Uray I, Lemm J, Youker K, Noon GP, Frazier OH, Taegtmeyer H (2004) Intramyocardial lipid accumulation in the failing human heart resembles the lipotoxic rat heart. FASEB J 18:1692–1700

180. Huang TH, Yang Q, Harada M, Uberai J, Radford J, Li GQ, Yamahara J, Roufogalis BD, Li Y (2006) Salacia oblonga root improves cardiac lipid metabolism in Zucker diabetic fatty rats: modulation of cardiac PPAR-alpha-mediated transcription of fatty acid metabolic genes. Toxicol Appl Pharmacol 210:78–85

181. Finck BN, Han X, Courtois M, Aimond F, Nerbonne JM, Kovacs A, Gross RW, Kelly DP (2003) A critical role for PPARalpha-mediated lipotoxicity in the pathogenesis of diabetic cardiomyopathy: modulation by dietary fat content. Proc Natl Acad Sci USA 100:1226–1231

182. Pillutla P, Hwang YC, Augustus A, Yokoyama M, Yagyu H, Johnston TP, Kaneko M, Ramasamy R, Goldberg IJ (2005) Perfusion of hearts with triglyceride-rich particles reproduces the metabolic abnormalities in lipotoxic cardiomyopathy. Am J Physiol Endocrinol Metab 288:E1229–E1235

183. Listenberger LL, Ory DS, Schaffer JE (2001) Palmitate-induced apoptosis can occur through a ceramide-independent pathway. J Biol Chem 276:14890–14895

184. Ruiz-Lozano P, Smith SM, Perkins G, Kubalak SW, Boss GR, Sucov HM, Evans RM, Chien KR (1998) Energy deprivation and a deficiency in downstream metabolic target genes during the onset of embryonic heart failure in RXR alpha -/- embryos. Development 125:533–544

185. Graham BH, Waymire KG, Cottrell B, Trounce IA, MacGregor GR, Wallace DC (1997) A mouse model for mitochondrial myopathy and cardiomyopathy resulting from a deficiency in the heart/muscle isoform of the adenine nucleotide translocator. Nat Genet 16:226–234

186. Wang J, Wilhelmsson H, Graff C, Li H, Oldfors A, Rustin P, Bruning JC, Kahn CR, Clayton DA, Barsh GS, Thoren P, Larsson NG (1999) Dilated cardiomyopathy and atrioventricular conduction blocks induced by heart-specific inactivation of mitochondrial DNA gene expression. Nat Genet 21:133–137

187. Wiener DH, Fink LI, Maris J, Jones RA, Chance B, Wilson JR (1986) Abnormal skeletal muscle bioenergetics during exercise in patients with heart failure: role of reduced blood flow. Circulation 73:1127–1136

188. Duboc D, Jehenson P, Tamby JF, Payen JF, Syrota A, Guerin F (1991) Abnormalities of the skeletal muscle in hypertrophic cardio-myopathy: spectroscopy using phosphorus-31 nuclear magnetic reso-nance. Arch Mal Coeur Vaiss 84:185–188

189. Caforio AL, Rossi B, Risaliti R, Siciliano G, Marchetti A, Angelini C, Crea F, Mariani M, Muratorio A (1989) Type 1 fiber abnormalities in skeletal muscle of patients with hypertrophic and dilated cardiomyopathy. J Am Coll Cardiol 14:1464–1473

190. Ventura-Clapier R, Garnier A, Veksler V (2004) Energy metabolism in heart failure. J Physiol 555:1–13

191. Cavedon CT, Bourdoux P, Mertens K, Van Thi HV, Herremans N, de Laet C, Goyens P (2005) Age-related variations in acylcarnitine and free carnitine concentrations measured by tandem mass spectrometry. Clin Chem 51:745–752

192. Delolme F, Vianey-Saban C, Guffon N, Favre-Bonvin J, Guibaud P, Becchi M, Mathieu M, Divry P (1997) Study of plasma acylcarnitines using tandem mass spectrometry. Application to the diagnosis of metabolism hereditary diseases. Arch Pediatr 4:819–826

193. Sinha R, Dufour S, Petersen KF, LeBon V, Enoksson S, Ma YZ, Savoye M, Rothman DL, Shulman GI, Caprio S (2002) Assessment of skeletal muscle triglyceride content by (1)H nuclear magnetic resonance spectroscopy in lean and obese adolescents: relationships to insulin sensitivity, total body fat, and central adiposity. Diabetes 51:1022–1027

194. Laurent D, Hundal RS, Dresner A, Price TB, Vogel SM, Petersen KF, Shulman GI (2000) Mechanism of muscle glycogen autoregulation in humans. Am J Physiol Endocrinol Metab 278:E663–E668

195. Petersen KF, Dufour S, Befroy D, Lehrke M, Hendler RE, Shulman GI (2005) Reversal of nonalcoholic hepatic steatosis, hepatic insulin resistance, and hyperglycemia by moderate weight reduction in patients with type 2 diabetes. Diabetes 54:603–608

196. Olpin SE (2005) Fatty acid oxidation defects as a cause of neuro-myopathic disease in infants and adults. Clin Lab 51:289–306

197. Yang Q, Li Y (2007) Roles of PPARs on regulating myocardial energy and lipid homeostasis. J Mol Med 85:697–706

198. Saudubray JM, Martin D, de Lonlay P et al (1999) Recognition and management of fatty acid oxidation defects: a series of 107 patients. J Inherit Metab Dis 22:488–502

199. Brown-Harrison MC, Nada MA, Sprecher H, Vianey-Saban C, Farquhar J Jr, Gilladoga AC, Roe CR (1996) Very long-chain acyl-CoA dehydrogenase deficiency: successful treatment of acute cardiomyopathy. Biochem Mol Med 58:59–65

200. Kennedy JA, Unger SA, Horowitz JD (1996) Inhibition of carnitine palmitoyltransferase-1 in rat heart and liver by perhexiline and amiodarone. Biochem Pharmacol 52:273–280

201. Myburgh DP, Goldman AP (1978) The anti-arrhythmic efficacy of perhexiline maleate, disopyramide and mexiletine in ventricular ectopic activity. S Afr Med J 54:1053–1055

202. Lee L, Campbell R, Scheuermann-Freestone M, Taylor R, Gunaruwan P, Williams L, Ashrafian H, Horowitz J, Fraser AG, Clarke K, Frenneaux M (2005) Metabolic modulation with perhexiline in chronic heart failure: a randomized, controlled trial of short-term use of a novel treatment. Circulation 112:3280–3288

203. Angdisen J, Moore VD, Cline JM, Payne RM, Ibdah JA (2005) Mitochondrial trifunctional protein defects: molecular basis and novel therapeutic approaches. Curr Drug Targets Immune Endocr Metabol Disord 5:27–40

204. Kalra SP, Kalra PS (2005) Gene-transfer technology: a preventive neurotherapy to curb obesity, ameliorate metabolic syndrome and extend life expectancy. Trends Pharmacol Sci 26:488–495

205. Wallhaus TR, Taylor M, DeGrado TR, Russell DC, Stanko P, Nickles RJ, Stone CK (2001) Myocardial free fatty acid and glucose use after carvedilol treatment in patients with congestive heart failure. Circulation 103:2441–2446

206. Bell DS (2005) Optimizing treatment of diabetes and cardiovascular disease with combined alpha, beta-blockade. Curr Med Res Opin 21:1191–1200

207. Rupp H, Zarain-Herzberg A, Maisch B (2002) The use of partial fatty acid oxidation inhibitors for metabolic therapy of angina pectoris and heart failure. Herz 27:621–636

208. Stanley WC (2002) Partial fatty acid oxidation inhibitors for stable angina. Expert Opin Investig Drugs 11:615–629

209. Zarain-Herzberg A, Rupp H (1999) Transcriptional modulators targeted at fuel metabolism of hypertrophied heart. Am J Cardiol 83:31H–37H

210. Lionetti V, Linke A, Chandler MP, Young ME, Penn MS, Gupte S, d'Agostino C, Hintze TH, Stanley WC, Recchia FA (2005) Carnitine palmitoyl transferase-I inhibition prevents ventricular remodeling and delays decompensation in pacing-induced heart failure. Cardiovasc Res 66:454–461

211. Schmidt-Schweda S, Holubarsch C (2000) First clinical trial with etomoxir in patients with chronic congestive heart failure. Clin Sci 99:27–35

212. Stanley WC (2004) Myocardial energy metabolism during ischemia and the mechanisms of metabolic therapies. J Cardiovasc Pharmacol Ther 9:S31–S45

213. Sabbah HN, Chandler MP, Mishima T, Suzuki G, Chaudhry P, Nass O, Biesiadecki BJ, Blackburn B, Wolff A, Stanley WC (2002) Ranolazine, a partial fatty acid oxidation (pFOX) inhibitor,

improves left ventricular function in dogs with chronic heart failure. J Card Fail 8:416–422

214. Pepine CJ, Wolff AA (1999) A controlled trial with a novel anti-ischemic agent, ranolazine, in chronic stable angina pectoris that is responsive to conventional antianginal agents. Am J Cardiol 84:46–50

215. Fragasso G, Piatti Md PM, Monti L, Palloshi A, Setola E, Puccetti P, Calori G, Lopaschuk GD, Margonato A (2003) Short- and long-term beneficial effects of trimetazidine in patients with diabetes and ischemic cardiomyopathy. Am Heart J 146:E18

216. Stanley WC (2005) Rationale for a metabolic approach in diabetic coronary patients. Coron Artery Dis 16:S11–S15

217. Kantor PF, Lucien A, Kozak R, Lopaschuk GD (2000) The antianginal drug trimetazidine shifts cardiac energy metabolism from fatty acid oxidation to glucose oxidation by inhibiting mitochondrial long-chain 3-ketoacyl coenzyme A thiolase. Circ Res 86:580–588

218. MacInnes A, Fairman DA, Binding P, Rhodes J, Wyatt MJ, Phelan A, Haddock PS, Karran EH (2003) The antianginal agent trimetazidine does not exert its functional benefit via inhibition of mitochondrial long-chain 3-ketoacyl coenzyme A thiolase. Circ Res 93:e26–e32

219. Tabbi-Anneni I, Helies-Toussaint C, Morin D, Bescond-Jacquet A, Lucien A, Grynberg A (2003) Prevention of heart failure in rats by trimetazidine treatment: a consequence of accelerated phospholipid turnover? J Pharmacol Exp Ther 304:1003–1009

220. Argaud L, Gomez L, Gateau-Roesch O, Couture-Lepetit E, Loufouat J, Robert D, Ovize M (2005) Trimetazidine inhibits mitochondrial permeability transition pore opening and prevents lethal ischemia-reperfusion injury. J Mol Cell Cardiol 39:893–899

221. Chung MK (2004) Vitamins, supplements, herbal medicines, and arrhythmias. Cardiol Rev 12:73–84

222. Tavazzi L, Tognoni G, Franzosi MG, Latini R, Maggioni AP, Marchioli R, Nicolosi GL, Porcu M (2004) Rationale and design of the GISSI heart failure trial: a large trial to assess the effects of n-3 polyunsaturated fatty acids and rosuvastatin in symptomatic congestive heart failure. Eur J Heart Fail 6:635–641

223. Macchia A, Levantesi G, Franzosi MG, Geraci E, Maggioni AP, Marfisi R, Nicolosi GL, Schweiger C, Tavazzi L, Tognoni G, Valagussa F, Marchioli R; GISSI-Prevenzione Investigators (2005) Left ventricular systolic dysfunction, total mortality, and sudden death in patients with myocardial infarction treated with n-3 polyunsaturated fatty acids. Eur J Heart Fail 7:904–909

224. Singer P, Wirth M (2004) Can n-3 PUFA reduce cardiac arrhythmias? Results of a clinical trial. Prostaglandins Leukot Essent Fatty Acids 71:153–159

225. Pepe S, Tsuchiya N, Lakatta EG, Hansford RG (1999) PUFA and aging modulate cardiac mitochondrial membrane lipid composition and Ca2+ activation of PDH. Am J Physiol 276:H149–H158

226. Avogaro A, Vigili de Kreutzenberg S, Negut C, Tiengo A, Scognamiglio R (2004) Diabetic cardiomyopathy: a metabolic perspective. Am J Cardiol 93:13A–16A

227. Chess DJ, Stanley WC (2008) Role of diet and fuel overabundance in the development and progression of heart failure. Cardiovasc Res 79:269–278

228. Chicco AJ, Sparagna GC, McCune SA, Johnson CA, Murphy RC, Bolden DA, Rees ML, Gardner RT, Moore RL (2008) Linoleate-rich high-fat diet decreases mortality in hypertensive heart failure rats compared with lard and low-fat diets. Hypertension 52: 549–555

229. Mokhtar N, Lavoie JP, Rousseau-Migneron S, Nadeau A (1993) Physical training reverses defect in mitochondrial energy production in heart of chronically diabetic rats. Diabetes 42:682–687

230. Tomita M, Mukae S, Geshi E, Umetsu K, Nakatani M, Katagiri T (1996) Mitochondrial respiratory impairment in streptozotocin induced diabetic rat heart. Jpn Circ J 60:673–682

Section III
The Mitochondrial Organelle and the Heart

Chapter 5
The Multidimensional Role of Mitochondria in Heart Failure

Overview

Mitochondria are at the center of the pathophysiology of the failing heart and, as shown by both clinical studies and animal models, mitochondrial-based oxidative stress together with myocardial apoptosis and cardiac bioenergetic dysfunction are profoundly implicated in the progression of heart failure (HF). In this chapter, we will review the body of evidence that multiple defects in mitochondria are central and primary to HF development. In addition, novel approaches to therapeutic targeting of mitochondrial bioenergetic, biogenic, and signaling abnormalities that can impact will be discussed.

Introduction

The failing heart encompasses a complex phenotype that includes reduced myocardial contractility, diminished capacity to respond to specific hypoxic and oxidative stresses resulting from myocardial ischemia and diverse neurohormonal stimuli, changes in ion channels and electrophysiological function, increased myocardial fibrosis, cellular and subcellular remodeling with increased myocyte loss, and marked changes in myocardial bioenergetic reserves and substrate utilization. These alterations generally are present both at the tissue and cellular level.

The heart in great part depends for its function on the energy generated by mitochondria, primarily by the β-oxidation of fatty acids, ETC, and OXPHOS but also by maintaining normal signaling pathways and crosstalking between mitochondria and other cellular organelles. Evidence from transgenic animal models supports the concept that defects in mitochondrial energy generation at specific loci or pathways may result in HF and numerous molecular and cellular changes leading to HF are being continuously identified.

Besides the organelle contribution to bioenergetic function, mitochondria are intimately involved in the regulation of intracellular Ca^{2+} flux, cardiomyocyte cell death, remodeling events, ROS generation and antioxidant response, and in furnishing cardioprotective actions in response to physiological and pathological insults. Interestingly, the organelle with its manifold roles in energy production, sensor and transport, ROS generation and signaling, cell death, Ca^{2+} levels and contractility, has often been overlooked (Table 5.1).

A discussion about which mitochondrial changes occur in HF will be presented in this chapter, with emphasis on the organelle role on bioenergetics and biogenesis, ROS and oxidative stress (OS), downstream effects on myocyte function (i.e., contractility and stimuli response), and cell death (i.e., apoptosis and necrosis). Such a discussion requires a larger view of the mitochondria function within the cellular context in the pathogenesis of HF including interaction and cross talk with other organelles. Moreover, we will review current investigative work from experimental animal models, the use of transgenic models, gene profiling analysis, in vitro studies with isolated cardiomyocytes (to identify pathway components in HF), and potential targets for new therapeutic interventions.

Centrality of Mitochondria in Cardiac Bioenergetics

The overall centrality of the mitochondrial organelle in HF with its manifold roles is shown in Fig. 5.1. The role of fuel supply and in particular ATP levels are critical for myocardial contractility and electrophysiology [1–5]. The primary ATP-utilizing reactions in the myocyte involve actomyosin ATPase in the myofibril, the Ca^{2+}-ATPase in the sarcoplasmic reticulum (SERCA), and the Na^+/K^+-ATPase in the sarcolemma. ATP produced by mitochondrial oxidative phosphorylation (OXPHOS) is used preferentially to support myocyte contractile activity [6]. Indeed, mitochondria appear to be clustered at sites of high ATP demand and are organized into highly ordered elongated bundles, regularly spaced between rows of myofilaments and in contact with the sarcoplasmic reticulum (SR). Moreover, structural contacts between the SR and mitochondria have been revealed by electron microscopy, and there is compelling evidence of a coordination between

J. Marín-García, *Heart Failure*, Contemporary Cardiology,
DOI 10.1007/978-1-60761-147-9_5, © Springer Science+Business Media, LLC 2010

these organelles at the level of Ca²⁺ homeostasis and regulation of ATP production [7].

Fatty acids are the primary energy substrate for heart muscle ATP generation by mitochondrial OXPHOS and the respiratory chain, the most important energetic pathway providing over 90% of cardiac energy. The supply of ATP from other sources such as cytosolic glycolytic metabolism is limited in normal cardiac tissue. In addition, mitochondrial-localized fatty acid β-oxidation (FAO) and the oxidation of carbohydrates, through the matrix-localized TCA cycle, generate the majority of intramitochondrial NADH and FADH, which are the direct source of electrons for the electron transport chain (ETC) and also produce a portion of the ATP supply (Fig. 5.2).

Furthermore, the heart maintains stored pools of high-energy phosphates including ATP and phosphocreatine (PCr). The enzyme creatine kinase (CK), which has both mitochondrial and cytosolic isoforms, transfers the phosphoryl group between ATP and PCr at a rate estimated to be ten times greater than the rate of ATP synthesis by OXPHOS [8]. Under conditions that increase ATP demand in excess of ATP supply such as in acute pump failure in ischemia, utilization of PCr via the CK reaction is an important mechanism that maintains steady myocardial ATP levels. Another relevant enzyme-mediated transfer system dedicated to maintaining ATP levels involves adenylate kinase (AK) transferring phosphoryl groups among adenine nucleotides. In addition, the adenine nucleotide translocators (ANT) are a family of inner membrane proteins that exchange mitochondrial ATP for cytosolic ADP,

Table 5.1   Mitochondria changes in heart failure

Defects in the electron transport chain (ETC) and in oxidative phosphorylation (OXPHOS)

Decreased levels of tricarboxylic acid cycle (TCA)

Decreased levels of fatty acid oxidation (FAO)

Increased production of reactive oxygen species (ROS) and oxidative stress (OS)

Increased ROS-mediated damage to DNA, proteins, and lipids

Abnormal membrane potential

Changes in mitochondrial biogenesis and turnover

Abnormal mitochondrial permeability transition

Abnormal mitochondrial energy transfer via the adenine nucleotide translocator (ANT) and mitochondrial creatine kinase

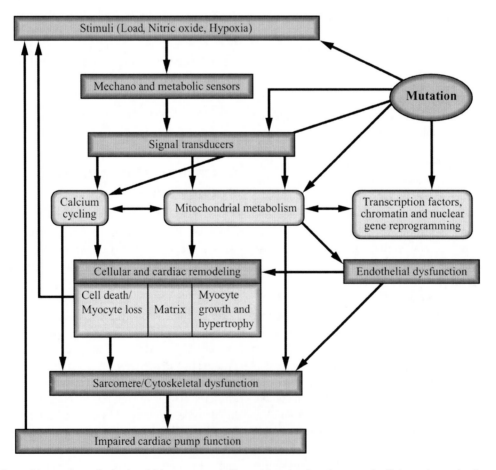

Fig. 5.1   Centrality and interactions of mitochondrial energy metabolism with molecular triggers and cellular pathways leading to heart failure

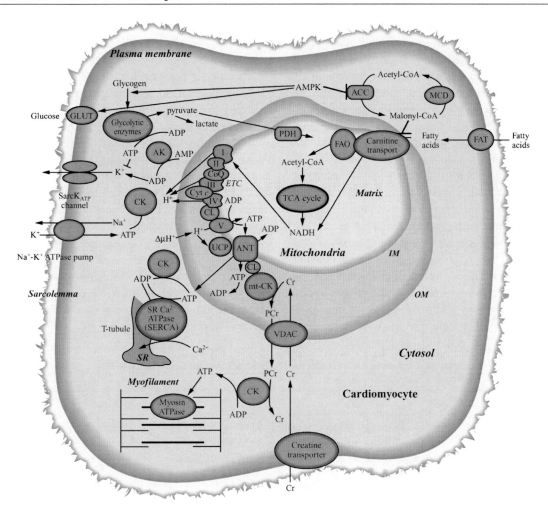

Fig. 5.2 Mitochondrial bioenergetic pathways and their interplay with critical cellular sites of myocardial ATP utilization

providing new ADP to the mitochondria while delivering ATP to the cytoplasm for cellular work.

The concept of an energy-starved or deficient myocardial phenotype has been buttressed by the use of powerful analytical technologies such as nuclear magnetic resonance (NMR) spectroscopy and positron emission tomography (PET) [1–5]. Moreover, this concept has significant clinical implications in the management of patients with HF since pharmacological interventions that reduce metabolic demand, such as ACE inhibitors, angiotensin blockers, and β-blockers improve clinical outcomes, and conversely agents that increase metabolic demand, such as positive inotropic drugs, are less effective in improving outcomes and often increase mortality [2, 3].

Observations from patients in HF have shown reduced activity levels of mitochondrial bioenergetic enzymes including selected respiratory enzymes and mt-CK [9–12]. Moreover, the failing human heart has a 25–30% decline in ATP levels as gauged from observations with human biopsy specimens [13], and by ^{31}P NMR spectroscopy [14]. Data from animal

models of HF have also shown that the loss of ATP associated with a loss in the total adenine nucleotide pool in the failing myocardium is slow and progressive suggesting that a decline in ATP content might only be detectable in severe HF [15].

In animal models of HF, the total pool of cardiac creatine, phosphorylated by CK to form PCr, is reduced by as much as 60% [16, 17] and the magnitude of creatine depletion correlated with the severity of HF in patients [18]. Similarly, PCr levels as measured by ^{31}P NMR and PCr/ATP ratios were significantly lower in subjects with dilated cardiomyopathy (DCM) and HF [19]. Even at moderate workloads, a decrease in PCr/ATP ratio has been consistently reported in the failing human heart and in experimental HF. This is a strong predictor of cardiovascular mortality in patients with DCM (even better than LV ejection fraction) [20]. While PCr levels or PCr/ATP ratios are not specific markers of HF (since they also decline in compensated left ventricular hypertrophy), they are markers of mismatch between ATP supply and ATP demand for utilization. Potential mechanisms responsible for the decline in PCr include reduced number or activity of the creatine transporter [21], and altered CK expression/function [22].

In transgenic mice, targeting of genes associated with mitochondrial bioenergetic function can also lead to cardiomyopathy and HF. For instance, mutational inactivation of the heart/muscle isoform of *Ant1* gene in transgenic mice will result in the development of skeletal myopathy and cardiomyopathy leading to HF [23]. The *Ant1* gene deficient mice exhibit mitochondrial abnormalities including a partial deficit in ADP-stimulated respiration, consistent with impaired translocation of ADP into mitochondria in both skeletal muscle and heart. *Ant1$^{-/-}$* mice also exhibit a progressive cardiac hypertrophic phenotype coincident with the proliferation of mitochondria [24]. This mitochondrial biogenic response may be a compensatory mechanism to correct the energy deficit, but could also be contributory to cardiac remodeling. Interestingly, null mutations in either the mitochondrial or cytosolic creatine kinase gene in mice also lead to increased LV dilation and hypertrophy [25, 26]. Palmieri et al. have reported the

presence of a recessive mutation in the heart/muscle specific-isoform of ANT1 in a patient with HCM and mild myopathy with exercise intolerance and lactic acidosis [27]. This mutation resulted in complete loss of adenine nucleotide transport function and was also associated with increased levels of muscle mitochondrial DNA (mtDNA) deletions.

Clinical evidence indicating that mitochondrial bioenergetic metabolism may be critical and primary in the development of HF has come from the identification in individuals with a variety of cardiomyopathies of specific nuclear gene defects in mitochondrial/metabolic proteins including ANT, respiratory complex enzyme subunits, molecules involved in complex IV assembly, and FAO enzymes (Table 5.2). Specific mtDNA gene defects associated with clinical CM/HF (Table 5.3), often with associated neuropathy, have also been identified in tRNA genes [28], although mutations in structural genes such as ATP6/ATP8 and cyt*b* (mitochondrial genes encoding subunits of complex V and III respectively) can also lead to CM/HF [29–31].

Table 5.2 Specific nuclear gene defects in mitochondrial metabolism leading to cardiomyopathy and HF

Gene loci	Protein function	Cardiac phenotype
Nuclear genes		
PRKAG2	AMP-activated protein kinase (regulatory subunit); energy sensor	HCM
SCO2	Cytochrome c oxidase (COX) assembly	HCM
NDUFV2	Respiratory complex I subunit	HCM
NDUFS2	Respiratory complex I subunit	HCM
ANT	Adenine nucleotide transporter/mtDNA maintenance	HCM
ACADVL	VLCAD activity (FAO)	HCM/DCM
FRDA	Mitochondrial iron import	HCM/FA
COX10	Cytochrome c oxidase (COX) assembly	HCM
SLC22A4	Carnitine transporter (OCTN2)	HCM/DCM
COX15	Cytochrome c oxidase (COX) assembly	HCM
TAZ (G4.5)	Tafazzin (FAO)	DCM/Barth syndrome
MTP/HADHA	Mitochondrial trifunctional protein (FAO)	DCM

FAO fatty acid oxidation; *FA* Friedreich ataxia; *HCM* hypertrophic cardiomyopathy; *DCM* dilated cardiomyopathy

Table 5.3 Specific mitochondrial gene defects leading to clinical cardiomyopathy and HF

Gene loci	Protein function	Cardiac phenotype
MtDNA		
*Leu*3243 (A → G)	Mitochondrial tRNA Biogenesis	DCM
*Leu*3303 (C → T)	Mitochondrial tRNA Biogenesis	Fatal CM
Ile 4300 (A → G)	Mitochondrial tRNA Biogenesis	HCM – adult onset, HF
Ile 4320 (C → T)	Mitochondrial tRNA Biogenesis	Fatal CM
Ile 4269 (A → G)	Mitochondrial tRNA Biogenesis	CM, HF
Lys 8334 (A → G)	Mitochondrial tRNA Biogenesis	HCM, MERRF
Lys 8363 (G → A)	Mitochondrial tRNA Biogenesis	HCM, deafness, LS
Lys 8296 (A → G)	Mitochondrial tRNA Biogenesis	Fatal HCM
Gly 9997 (T → C)	Mitochondrial tRNA Biogenesis	Dysrhythmia, HCM
16S rRNA 3093 (C → G)	Mitochondrial tRNA Biogenesis	MELAS, CM
12S rRNA 1555 (A → G)	Mitochondrial tRNA Biogenesis	CM, HF
Cytb 15498 (G → A) Gly → Asp	Cytochrome *b*, ETC	HiCM
ATPase6 8993 (T → G) Leu → Arg	Mitochondrial ATP synthase, OXPHOS	LS, HCM

HiCM histiocytoid cardiomyopathy; *LS* Leigh syndrome; *HCM* hypertrophic cardiomyopathy; *DCM* dilated cardiomyopathy; *MELAS* mitochondrial myopathy, encephalopathy, lactic acidosis, and stroke

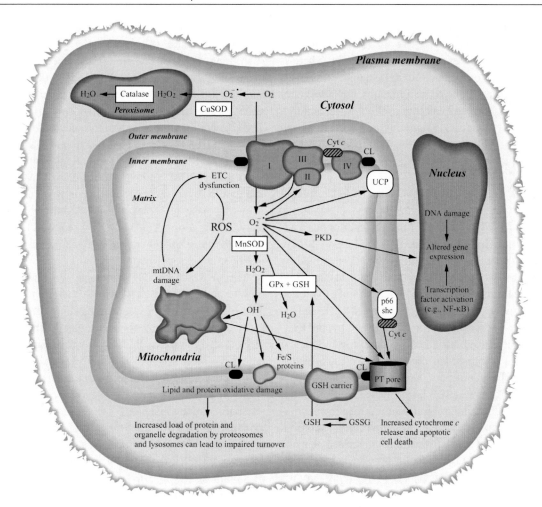

Fig. 5.3 Molecular and subcellular events leading to ROS and oxidative stress. Damage to proteins, lipids, and mtDNA caused by mitochondrial-generated ROS including H_2O_2, superoxide (O_2^{-}), and hydroxyl radicals (OH^-), leads to PT pore opening and apoptotic cell death, mitochondrial enzyme dysfunction, and nuclear DNA damage as well as modulated DNA repair and gene expression in the nucleus. Also shown are antioxidant factors in peroxisomes (catalase), mitochondria (GPx, GSH, and MnSOD), and in the cytosol (CuSOD) that function to scavenge ROS and reduce their impact

Hence, mitochondrial bioenergetic pathways including ETC, OXPHOS, the TCA cycle, and FAO are crucial for the myocardial intracellular ATP-requiring pumps that control sarcomeric contractile functioning, calcium cycling, and membrane ion transport. While there is evidence that suggests that multiple deficits in these pathways likely contribute to the bioenergetic decline in observed human HF, indicative of a programmatic shift in bioenergetic production and utilization, it is unclear when and how this occurs.

Mitochondrial ROS Generation and Antioxidant Response

One attractive hypothesis for mitochondrial contribution to HF relates to its role in ROS production. The generation of a majority of intracellular ROS including superoxide and hydroxyl radicals, and hydrogen peroxide (H_2O_2) is a by-product of normal mitochondrial metabolism and bioenergetic activities (Fig. 5.3). Side reactions of mitochondrial respiratory enzymes (primarily complex I and III) with oxygen directly generate the superoxide anion radical; either excessive or diminished electron flux at these sites can stimulate the auto-oxidation of flavins and quinones (including coenzyme Q) producing superoxide radicals. The superoxide radicals can react with NO to form peroxynitrite, which is a highly reactive and deleterious free radical species or can be converted by superoxide dismutase (SOD) to H_2O_2 that can further react to form highly reactive hydroxyl radicals. The high reactivity of the hydroxyl radical and its extremely short physiological half-life of 10^{-9} s restrict its damage to a small radius from its origin since it is too short-lived to diffuse a considerable distance. Mitochondrial-generated ROS can lead to extensive oxidative damage to macromolecules such as proteins, DNA, and lipids particularly targeting proximal mitochondrial components including mitochondrial respiratory enzymes, matrix enzymes (e.g., aconitase), and membrane phospholipids such as cardiolipin. There is also indication that mitochondrial ROS damage affects a wide spectrum of cardiomyocyte functions including contractility, ion transport, and calcium cycling. Mitochondrial ROS also play a role in cell signaling (e.g., in triggering cardioprotective pathways) and in the transcriptional activation of select nuclear genes eliciting a novel transcriptional programming.

The limited data available from animal models of HF have shown an increase in hydroxyl and superoxide radicals. In murine HF created by ligation of the left anterior descending coronary artery for 4 weeks, Ide et al. [32] found that LV dilatation and decreased contractility were accompanied by significant increases in levels of hydroxyl radicals and lipid peroxides. In addition, the infarcted LV from mice exhibited diminished activity of respiratory complexes I, III, and IV (enzymes each containing subunits encoded by mtDNA) while the mitochondrial enzymes encoded only by nuclear DNA (e.g., citrate synthase and complex II) were unaffected. Ide et al. [33, 34] using electron spin resonance (ESR) spectroscopy to directly assess ROS levels in the canine model of pacing-induced HF, found a significant increase in superoxide anion and hydroxyl radical levels in myocardial submitochondrial fractions. These observations suggested that the elevated myocardial ROS production was secondary to the functional block of electron transport, resulting from a marked decrease in mitochondrial respiratory complex activities (primarily complex I) and also showed a significant positive correlation between myocardial ROS levels and abnormal LV contractility.

Nevertheless, direct measurement of short-lived ROS is extremely difficult and several laboratories have reported increased levels of ROS-mediated damage (e.g., lipid peroxidation, DNA, and protein oxidation) as an indirect index of ROS/OS in several animal models, including pacing-induced HF [35–37]. The left ventricle from paced animals exhibited increased aldehyde levels and marked reductions in the activity of respiratory complex III and V together with increased levels of large-scale mtDNA deletions [37].

While elevated ROS activation in the failing heart has been shown to arise from both mitochondrial and extramitochondrial sources, the role of endogenous antioxidants in ameliorating myocardial OS and the dynamic balance between these counteracting forces should be considered. It is well known that both cytosolic antioxidant enzymes (e.g., catalase, SOD1/CuSOD) and mitochondrial-localized antioxidants including SOD2/MnSOD, thioredoxin, and glutathione peroxidase can reduce ROS levels. Also, thioredoxin and thioredoxin reductase form an enzymatic antioxidant and redox regulatory system implicated in the regeneration of many antioxidant molecules, including

ubiquinone, selenium-containing substances, lipoic acid, and ascorbic acid [38].

Among the most compelling evidence supporting a primary role for mitochondrial ROS and OS in cardiomyopathy and HF are findings with antioxidant genes in transgenic mice. Strains harboring null mutations in either MnSOD or TrxR2 encoding mitochondrial thioredoxin reductase exhibit DCM and HF [39–42]. Li et al. [42] found that mice homozygous for MnSOD deficiency resulted in early neonatal death from severe DCM, and metabolic acidosis. Moreover, these strains displayed severe reduction in myocardial succinate dehydrogenase (complex II) and aconitase (a TCA cycle enzyme) suggesting that MnSOD is required for maintaining the integrity of mitochondrial enzymes susceptible to direct inactivation by superoxide.

Mice in which MnSOD-deficiency was targeted to skeletal muscle and heart (i.e., H/M-$Sod2^{-/-}$ strains) displayed progressive HF with depressed cardiac contractility by 8 weeks, cardiac enlargement by 16 weeks, and death from HF by 22 weeks [42]. Cardiac pathology was associated with specific defects in mitochondrial respiration (i.e., severely reduced respiratory complex II and moderately reduced complex I and III activities) and in myocardial mitochondrial ultrastructure. Immunoblot analyses showed significant expression of the SDHA and SDHB subunits from myocardial complex II H/M-$Sod2^{-/-}$ mice, with moderate suppression of complex Iα 9, Rieske iron–sulfur protein and Core I subunit of complex III, and α and β subunits of complex V. Mitochondrial superoxide production was also significantly higher in these mice as was mitochondrial (but not cytosolic) lipid peroxidation suggesting that oxidative damage was specifically localized in mitochondria. In addition, myocardial ATP production and content were significantly diminished, which may account for the absence of energy-dependent apoptosis in H/M-$Sod2^{-/-}$ mice. This study also offered further evidence that ROS and OS are intimately linked to the progression of cardiomyopathy/HF, since the administration at 8 weeks of age of the antioxidant MnSOD mimetic (MnTBAP) significantly improved cardiac contractility and ameliorated the overall phenotype.

Overexpression of the antioxidant glutathione peroxidase in transgenic mice inhibited the development of LV remodeling and failure after myocardial infarct (MI), and was associated with the attenuation of myocyte hypertrophy, apoptosis, and interstitial fibrosis [43]. Moreover, Schriner et al. have demonstrated that overexpression of catalase (primarily a peroxisomal-localized enzyme) targeted to the mitochondria increased overall mouse longevity, diminished OS and ROS-mediated mitochondrial protein and mtDNA damage, and delayed the onset of aging-mediated cardiac pathology including subendocardial interstitial fibrosis, vacuolization of cytoplasm, variable myofiber size, hypercellularity, collapse of sarcomeres, mineralization, and arteriosclerosis, changes commonly observed in elderly human hearts, and often found in association with congestive HF [44]. Another important finding was that it mattered in which subcellular compartment the over-expressed catalase was localized with little evidence of benefits from nuclear or peroxisomal-localized as compared to striking benefits of mitochondrial-localized catalase activity.

In clinical cases, a clear link between OS/ROS and chronic ventricular dysfunction has only been established in anthracycline-mediated and alcoholic cardiomyopathies. In contrast, it remains unclear whether ROS or OS have a pathophysiologic role in the vast majority of patients with congestive HF or cardiomyopathy due to ischemic, hypertensive, valvular, or idiopathic causes [45]. Superoxide anions as assessed by EPR with an $O_2^{\cdot-}$ spin trap were reported to increase more than twofold in the failing ventricular myocardium from patients with end-stage HF undergoing transplant [46]. Moreover, despite increased MnSOD mRNA levels, a marked decline in mitochondrial-localized MnSOD protein and activity was detected. Both increased ROS levels and decreased antioxidant response would be expected to lead to enhanced OS in the failing heart, which in turn may result in increased transcription of antioxidant enzymes. That excessive ROS/OS in HF may serve as a potent trigger for changes in specific nuclear gene expression, may also underlie the programmatic shift in mitochondrial bioenergetic function previously discussed, as well as acting as a catalyst in myocyte remodeling.

Mitochondrial Role in HF Apoptosis and Necrosis

The overall role that apoptosis play in HF has not been definitively established. Presently, there is only limited morphological evidence that significant cardiomyocyte apoptosis occurs in MI or at any stage of HF. Apoptotic rates are higher after human MI (ranging from 2 to 12%) than in end-stage (NYHA class III–IV) human HF (range 0.1–0.7%) [47, 48]. While the rate of apoptosis is quite low when viewed in absolute terms, when the relatively low rates are viewed in the context of months or years, the actual chronic cell loss attributable to apoptosis (particularly among non-dividing myocytes) could be substantial. Moreover, apoptotic measurements represent only the number of cells undergoing apoptosis at a single point of time and the accurate assessment of true rates and their consequences remain to be established.

The mitochondrial-mediated intrinsic apoptotic pathway features an extensive dialog between the mitochondria, the nucleus, the endoplasmic reticulum (ER), and other subcellular organelles as depicted in Fig. 5.4. The release of several mitochondrial-specific proteins from the intermembrane space including cytochrome c, endonuclease G (EndoG), apoptosis inducing factor (AIF), and Smac are central to the early triggering events in the apoptotic pathway including downstream caspase activation, nuclear DNA fragmentation, and cell death [49]. The release of EndoG and AIF, and their translocation to the nucleus, specifically promote nuclear DNA degradation, even in the absence of caspase activation [50, 51]. The release of both Smac and cytochrome c, which required modification in the mitochondrial organelle to become apoptotically active, are involved in cytosolic caspase activation, i.e., Smac binds and inhibits endogenous cytosolic signaling complexes (e.g., IAPs) that modulate apoptosis, thereby promoting caspase activity. Interestingly, Smac is highly expressed in the heart. In the cytosol, cytochrome c binds Apaf-1 along with dATP and promotes procaspase-9 recruitment into the apoptosome, a multiprotein complex, resulting in caspase activation [52].

The release of these mitochondrial peptides involves the permeabilization of the outer membrane mediated by proapoptotic cytosolic factors Bax, Bak, and tBID. In response to both external pro-death signals largely provided by the extrinsic apoptosis pathway (e.g., ischemia/hypoxia, TNF-α, and Fas ligand) and nuclear signals (e.g., p53), these factors translocate to mitochondria where they bind outer membrane proteins (e.g., VDAC) and can initiate outer membrane channel formation [49].

Protein release from the intermembrane space and cristae, where the majority of cytochrome c is localized, is also associated with opening of the voltage-sensitive PT pore located at the contact sites between inner and outer membranes. Opening of this non-specific pore is responsive to mitochondrial membrane potential ($\Delta\psi M$), mitochondrial ROS and Ca^{2+} overload, pro-oxidant accumulation, and NO [53]. The peptide composition of the PT pore while still controversial is thought to involve several key players in mitochondrial bioenergetic metabolism, including ANT, mt-CK, the outer membrane porin (VDAC), and inner membrane cyclophilin-D. Opening of the PT pore promotes significant changes in mitochondrial structure and metabolism, including increased mitochondrial matrix volume leading to mitochondrial swelling, release of matrix Ca^{2+}, altered cristae, and cessation of ATP production secondary to the uncoupling of ETC and dissipation of $\Delta\psi M$ [54]. Therefore, cytochrome c efflux appears to be coordinated with activation of a mitochondrial remodeling pathway characterized by changes in inner membrane morphology and organization, ensuring complete release of cytochrome c and the onset of mitochondrial dysfunction, which might further contribute to the HF phenotype [55].

Opposing the progression of this apoptotic pathway, antiapoptotic proteins (e.g., Bcl-2), localized to the outer mitochondrial membrane, either directly compete with or impede proapoptotic factor activity, stabilizing mitochondrial

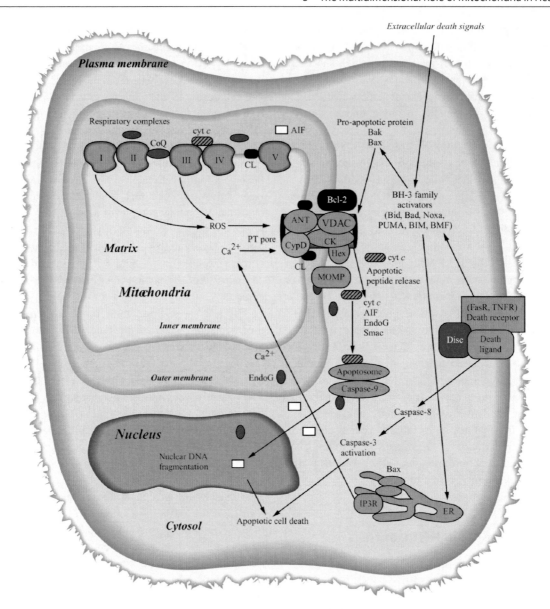

Fig. 5.4 The intrinsic pathway of apoptosis. An array of extracellular and intracellular signals triggers the intrinsic apoptotic pathway, which is regulated by proapoptotic proteins (e.g., Bax, Bid, and Bak) binding to the outer mitochondrial membrane leading to outer-membrane permeabilization and PT pore opening. Elevated levels of mitochondrial Ca^{2+} as well as ETC-generated ROS also promote PT pore opening. This is followed by the release of cytochrome c (Cyt c), *Smac*, EndoG, and AIF from the mitochondria intermembrane space to the cytosol and apoptosome formation (with Cyt c) leading to caspase 9 activation, DNA fragmentation (with nuclear translocation of AIF and EndoG), and inhibition of IAP (by Smac), further stimulating activation of caspases 9 and 3. Bax and Bid-mediated mitochondrial membrane permeabilization and apoptogen release are prevented by antiapoptogenic proteins (e.g., Bcl-2). Also shown are the major proteins comprising the PT pore, including adenine nucleotide translocator (ANT), creatine kinase (CK), cyclophilin D (CyP-D), and porin (VDAC). Intracellular stimuli trigger ER release of Ca^{2+} through both Bax and BH3-protein interactions. Endogenous myocardial factors including apoptosis repressor with caspase recruitment domain (ARC) can target discrete loci impacting mitochondrial-based apoptotic progression

membranes and their channels thereby preventing mitochondrial disruption and inhibiting PT pore opening. The endoplasmic reticulum (ER) has been recognized as an important organelle in the intrinsic pathway. Similar to their roles in transducing upstream signals to the mitochondria, proapoptotic proteins appear to relay upstream death signals to the ER triggering Ca^{2+} release which in turn can rapidly accumulate in mitochondria promoting PT pore opening [49]. In addition to its role in mediating cellular responses to traditional ER stresses, such as misfolded proteins, this organelle appears to be critical in mediating cell death elicited by a subset of stimuli originating outside of the ER, such as OS [56]. Moreover, similar to their roles in transducing upstream signals to the mitochondria, BH3-only proteins appear to relay upstream death signals to the ER [57].

As shown in Fig. 5.4 endogenous myocardial factors including ARC, a master regulator of cardiac death signaling, whose regulation during HF is of great interest, can target discrete loci impacting mitochondrial-based apoptotic progression and preserving mitochondrial function [58]. In addition, prosurvival factors from growth factor signaling pathways (e.g., IGF-1) can inhibit the progression of the apoptotic pathway as well as hypoxia-mediated cardiomyocyte mitochondrial dysfunction albeit their precise mechanism of action is unknown [59].

Recently, it has been suggested that myocardial apoptosis is not a feature of end-stage disease. Akyurek et al. have reported the presence of higher Bax levels in mild HF compared with moderate or severe HF suggesting that cardiomyocytes are more prone to apoptosis in earlier stages of the disease [60]. This susceptibility to apoptosis showed a close correlation with echocardiographic and hemodynamic data indicative that apoptosis may have a role in the transition from mild to end-stage HF.

While myocardial apoptotic induction is frequently associated with abnormal mitochondrial respiratory function, the basis of this relationship remains unclear. Targeting apoptotic factors has been shown to reverse the cardiomyopathy/HF phenotype and associated mitochondrial dysfunction underscoring the interconnected roles of apoptosis and mitochondrial dysfunction in HF. Bcl-2 proteins attenuate p53-mediated apoptosis in cardiomyocytes [61], increase the Ca^{2+} threshold for PT pore opening, decrease mitochondrial Ca^{2+} efflux due to Na^+-dependent Ca^{2+} exchanger in mouse heart mitochondria [62], and inhibit hypoxia-induced apoptosis in isolated adult cardiomyocytes [63]. In desmin-null transgenic mice, which develop cardiomyopathy and HF as well as defective mitochondrial function, there is extensive cardiomyocyte loss in focal areas, and decreased cytochrome c levels in heart mitochondria [64, 65].

Bcl-2 overexpression in these desmin deficient mice dramatically ameliorated the cardiomyopathic phenotype, restored ETC function, and changed the mitochondrial sensitivity to Ca^{2+} exposure [66]. Furthermore, Bcl-2 family proteins are potential regulators of mitochondrial energetics [67]. During ischemia, when mitochondrial ETC and ATP generation are inhibited because of lack of oxygen, the mitochondrial F1F0-ATPase (complex V) runs in reverse and pumps protons out of the matrix while glycolytic ATP is consumed in an attempt to restore $\Delta\psi M$. Bcl-2 has been demonstrated to reduce the rate of ATP consumption during ischemia by inhibiting the F1F0-ATPase. Imahashi et al. have reported that transgenic mice overexpressing Bcl-2 in the heart displayed a decreased rate of ATP decline during ischemia as well as reduced acidification, suggesting that Bcl-2 may provide myocardial protection by inhibiting consumption of glycolysis-generated ATP by the F1F0-ATPase [67].

Another link between apoptosis and mitochondrial respiratory function was established with the demonstration that mice containing a cardiac-specific deletion of AIF developed severe DCM, HF and decreased ETC activities, particularly of complex I [68, 69]. In addition, isolated hearts of AIF-deficient animals developed poor contractile performance in response to ETC-dependent energy substrates, but not in response to glucose consistent with the concept that impaired heart function in AIF-deficient mice results from abnormal ETC function. These results also suggest that AIF similar to cytochrome c serves an essential (albeit largely uncharacterized) role in OXPHOS. With apoptosis, mitochondrial loss of both AIF and cytochrome c impacts ETC and promotes AIF nuclear translocation and DNA degradation, demonstrating another side of nuclear–mitochondrial cross-talk.

Other types of cell death including necrosis are evident in the failing heart at similar (and in some cases greater) numbers [70–72]. In contrast to apoptosis, necrotic cell death is not energy requiring and exhibits characteristic features that include swelling of the cell and its organelles, extensive mitochondrial disruption, blebbing and ultimately irreversible disintegration of the plasma membrane. Necrotic disruption of the plasma membrane leads to release of cellular content into the extracellular space (e.g., release of CK from necrotic myocardial cells), which promotes further inflammatory reaction and subsequent damage or death of neighboring cells. Many of the morphological differences between apoptotic and necrotic processes appear to result from caspase action that is unique to apoptosis, although there is a rather fine line between apoptosis and necrosis that complicates their differentiation. Honda et al. have shown that in the absence of phagocytic cells (to remove damaged apoptotic cells), plasma membrane disruption of apoptotic cells can occur leading to secondary necrosis [73]. Furthermore, shared signaling pathway elements between these different modes of cell death include mitochondrial-based events. For instance, a common event leading to both apoptosis and necrosis is mitochondrial permeabilization and dysfunction (i.e., both involve mitochondrial PT pore opening), although the mechanistic basis of mitochondrial injury appears to vary in different settings [74]. ATP level is a critical factor determining which type of cell death will proceed [75–77]. If ATP levels fall profoundly, plasma membrane permeabilization and cell rupture ensue leading to necrosis. If ATP levels are partially maintained, apoptosis (which requires ATP for its progression) follows PT pore opening. In transgenic mice with enhanced sarcolemmal, L-type Ca^{2+} channel activity with progressive myocyte necrosis that led to pump failure and premature death, necrosis in association with dysregulated Ca^{2+} handling and β-adrenergic receptor signaling and subsequent HF could be prevented by the targeted loss of cyclophilin-D, a regulator of the mitochondrial PT pore [78].

A third type of cell death associated with autophagy has recently been described in HF [72, 79]. In contrast with necrosis, autophagic cell death similar to apoptosis is characterized by the absence of tissue inflammatory response. However, in contrast to apoptosis, which features early collapse of cytoskeletal elements with preservation of organelles until late in the process, autophagic cell death exhibits early degradation of organelles and preservation of cytoskeletal elements until later stages. Also, unlike apoptosis, caspase activation and DNA fragmentation occur very late (if at all) in autophagic cell death [80]. Although the information currently available concerning its signaling pathway and interaction with mitochondria is rather limited, autophagy appears to be triggered by mitochondrial ROS and the role(s) of defective mitochondria in autophagasome biogenesis and in selective cell removal in aging are being actively explored [81].

Mitochondria in Experimental Animal Models of HF

Enzyme Dysfunction

Mitochondrial OXPHOS dysfunction and ROS production have been investigated at least in two experimental animal models of HF, the pacing-induced canine HF, and in rat infarct. A canine model in which rapid ventricular pacing leads to an increase in chamber dimension, wall thinning, elevation in ventricular wall stress, and congestive HF recapitulates many features of human DCM and HF [82], and using proteomic analysis, many of the cardiac proteins altered in the canine model of pacing-induced HF are involved in energy metabolism [83]. That cardiac metabolism plays a role in HF was confirmed by O'Brien et al. observations of significant decrease in ATP-utilizing enzymes including SERCA and myofibrillar Ca^{2+} ATPase activities in dogs that were paced to advanced HF (4 weeks of pacing), whereas in dogs with early HF (1 weeks of pacing), there was a significant decline in activities of the SR Ca^{2+} release channel, mitochondrial ATP synthesis, and creatine kinase [84, 85].

Data obtained from biochemical analysis in paced dogs documented a significant decrease in cardiac respiratory complex III and V activities [37]. Included in this study was a limited temporal course analysis that showed significant reduction in specific ETC enzymes activities in early HF (between 1 and 2 weeks of pacing) [86]. Moreover, this early ETC dysfunction correlated with the appearance of markers of myocyte apoptosis and OS, whose presence has been previously described in paced failing hearts [36, 87]. Using electron spin resonance (ESR) spectroscopy to directly

assess ROS levels in paced dog hearts, Ide et al. demonstrated a significant increase in superoxide anion levels in myocardial submitochondrial fractions; the elevated ROS production was attributed to the functional block of electron transport, resulting from a marked decrease in mitochondrial respiratory complex activities [33]. Furthermore, later studies by Ide et al. [34] using the paced dog HF model and modified ESR analysis showed a significant increase in hydroxyl radical levels, and a significant positive correlation between myocardial ROS levels and increases in LV contractile dysfunction.

While initial studies in paced canine hearts, carried out in our laboratory, revealed mtDNA damage (i.e., large-scale mtDNA deletions detected by PCR), the levels of deletion relative to wild-type mtDNA were very low (less than 1%) and their significance is unclear [37]. Furthermore, using quantitative PCR analysis, no significant changes were noted in the overall mtDNA levels nor was there any significant changes in either mtDNA-encoded complex IV or nuclear DNA-encoded complex II and citrate synthase activities, making a claim for a generalized loss or increase of mitochondrial number, mitochondrial gene expression, or mtDNA in this HF model unlikely. A potential explanation and a testable hypothesis for these findings is that post-transcriptional changes (potentially ROS-induced) of specific enzyme subunits underlie the pacing-induced mitochondrial enzymatic dysfunction, a hypothesis that is being currently investigated. Furthermore, analysis of isolated mitochondria from paced and control animals showed that the respiratory ETC defects (including complex I as well as complex III and V activities) were present in both interfibrillar and subsarcolemmal mitochondrial sub-populations. These findings do not support previous observations of differences in ETC-related mitochondrial fractions.

Similar respiratory dysfunction (relative to enzymes affected) was present in both skeletal muscle and cardiac tissues supporting the view that pacing induced HF involves a generalized metabolic myopathy. The effect that experimental HF has on skeletal muscle metabolic function is consistent with observations of early muscular fatigue and exercise intolerance in patients with HF [88]. Besides myocardial changes, analysis of biopsied skeletal muscle in HF patients showed a 20% reduction in mitochondrial volume (irrespective of age), which correlates with the reduced aerobic capacity observed in these patients [89]. Moreover, these patients displayed decreased oxidative capacity with significantly reduced activities of complex IV [89], succinate dehydrogenase (complex II), and 3-hydroxyacyl CoA dehydrogenase, a mitochondrial enzyme involved in FAO [90]. A role for ROS and increased OS in skeletal muscle metabolic dysfunction in HF has been suggested from observations in several animal models. For instance, increased ROS levels have been found in limb skeletal muscles of HF mice in association with both increased ROS-mediated lipid peroxidation and reduced levels of respiratory complex I and III activities [91], suggesting that ROS-induced damage may in part underlie the skeletal muscle mitochondrial dysfunction. Moreover, endothelial dysfunction occurring secondary to ROS and OS has been suggested to play a contributory role in skeletal muscle dysfunction [92], albeit limited data is thus far available in human HF. We also found that paced dogs have markedly elevated myocardial aldehyde levels, indicative of increased peroxidation (another OS-marker) as shown in Table 5.4.

Myocardial ROS/OS and apoptosis (as gauged by either enzyme immunoassay (ELISA) of cytoplasmic histone-associated DNA fragments or by in situ TUNEL analysis) were further assessed in early HF (1 week pacing) and late HF (3–4 week pacing), and found increasing levels of both over the pacing period (Fig. 5.5). These findings were extended to

include a limited temporal course showing that substantial levels of myocardial dysfunction in specific ETC enzymes were present in early HF at 1–2 weeks of pacing (Fig. 5.6).

Interestingly, the decline in complex III activity continued over the full 4-week time-course of pacing while complex V dysfunction was most pronounced in early pacing and showed no significant further decline by 4 weeks of pacing. This suggests that the biochemical mechanisms involved in the inactivation of these two enzymes during pacing may be different.

Western immunoblot analysis of LV homogenate proteins further corroborated that specific mitochondrial bioenergetic proteins are quantitatively affected in the paced myocardium. On the other hand, no significant differences were detected in paced animals for overall levels of cytochrome c, the COX4 subunit of complex IV and the gamma subunit of complex V or for either of the PT pore components, VDAC/porin or ANT (see Table 5.5). However, significant reductions were found in cytochrome b levels (the mtDNA-encoded subunit of complex III) and in a protein reacting with a mitochondrial ATP synthase monoclonal antibody of the approximate size (52 kDa) of the ATP synthase β subunit. Likely, these peptide deficiencies contribute to the complex III and V activity defects noted in the paced animals. In addition, we found in the paced animals a definitive decline in the mt-CK isoform.

Table 5.4 Levels of oxidative stress as gauged by lipid peroxidation

	Control	Paced
Total aldehyde content	7,047.85±447.9	11,760.63±1,409.6*
Malondialdehydes	1,265.96±121.9	5,804.36±1,306.2*
2 Nonenal	92.76±4.3	145.7±13.6*
4 Hydroxyhexenal	1,332.1±97.2	2,019.51±30.1*

Dura shown correspond to the calculated mean values±SEM
*$p < 0.05$ vs. control

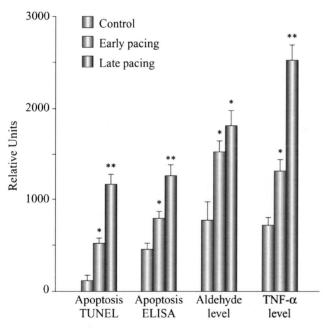

Fig. 5.5 Levels of myocardial apoptosis and oxidative stress in control animals, early and late pacing-induced heart failure. Levels of myocyte apoptosis as determined by in situ TUNEL assay or by enzyme immunoassay (ELISA) for cytoplasmic histone-associated DNA fragments, and myocardial oxidative stress as determined by levels of myocardial aldehydes and the pro-inflammatory cytokine TNF-α were assessed in untreated control, in early HF (1 week paced) and in late (3–4 week paced) animals. *$p = 0.05$ compared to control; **$p < 0.05$ compared to either control or to early paced values

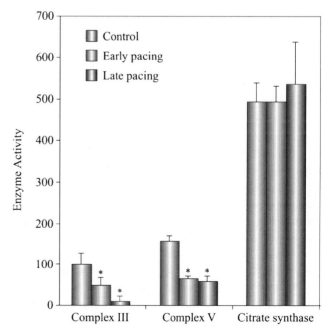

Fig. 5.6 Selected mitochondrial enzyme activities in the course of pacing-induced HF. Activity levels of mitochondrial respiratory complex III and V and citrate synthase (CS) in left ventricle of untreated control, in early HF (1 week paced) and in late HF (3–4 week paced) animals. Data shown in both panels represent mean and SEM values for six animals in each group (unpaced control, early and later pacing) with level of significance ($p < 0.05$) indicated by *

Table 5.5 Peptide levels of specific mitochondrial bioenergetic proteins

Peptide	Function	Control	Paced	Paced/Control	Significance
COX4	ETC/complex IV subunit	135	119	0.88	ns
Cytb (cytochrome b)	ETC/complex III subunit	39	28	0.72	*
V-ATP synthase – γ subunit	OXPHOS/complex V subunit	112	112	1.0	ns
V-ATP synthase – 52 kDa[a]	OXPHOS/complex V subunit	54	41	0.76	*
VDAC/porin	Mitochondrial outer membrane permeability/PT pore protein	115	108	0.94	ns
ANT	Adenine nucleotide transporter/PT pore protein	130	124	0.95	ns
Cytc (cytochrome c)	ETC/apoptogen	125	120	0.96	ns
Mt-CK	Mitochondrial creatine kinase	111	65	0.59	*
PGC-1	Peroxisome proliferator-activated receptor γ coactivator-1α	62	46	0.76	*

ns not significant
[a]Likely ATP synthase β subunit
*$p < 0.05$

Table 5.6 Peptide levels of selected apoptotic and OS proteins

Peptide	Function	Control	Paced	Paced/Control	Significance
Antioxidant					
MnSOD	Mitochondrial-located ROS scavenger	152	174	1.14	ns
Catalase	Peroxisomal-located ROS scavenger	142	147	1.03	ns
Apoptosis					
AIF-65 kDa	Mitochondrial-located uncleaved precursor; apoptogen	65.5	83.2	1.27	*
AIF-57 kDa	Cleaved product; apoptogen	8.8	57.3	6.5	*
Caspase-32 kDa	Protease precursor	90.5	48.5	0.54	*
Caspase-17 kDa	Activated protease cleavage product	5.8	12.5	2.2	*
p21/WAF	Anti-cyclin	3.7	94	25.4	*
p53	Nuclear factor	7.4	50.9	6.9	*

ns not significant
*$p < 0.05$

Previously, markedly reduced transcript levels of ATP synthase β and of mt-CK have been noted in the LV (among the manifold transcript changes) in a profiling analysis of pacing-induced HF in dogs. The findings suggested that orchestrated changes in both nuclear-encoded and mitochondria-encoded enzyme subunit expression are likely an important component of pacing-induced HF [93].

Western immunoblot analysis was carried out to determine levels of antioxidant proteins (as a potential gauge of OS) and of apoptotic markers as well (see Table 5.6). The mitochondrial-located MnSOD showed a modest increase in paced dogs LV (not significant) while catalase levels were unchanged. Among several markers of apoptosis evaluated, the activated form of caspase 3 (17 kDa) showed a substantial 2.2-fold increase in the paced compared to control LV. Levels of p53 (a DNA-damage induced nuclear factor) and of a p53-target (p21/WAF1) were both significantly increased in the paced LV compared to controls of 6.9- and 25.4-fold, respectively.

Transcription of p21/WAF, a potent inhibitor of cyclin-dependent kinase activity required for the progression of cell division from the G1 phase to S phase of mitosis, is known to be induced following DNA damage (oxidative damage), and often has been linked with the accumulation of p53, a tumor suppressor gene. In addition, expression of p21 selectively inhibits a set of genes involved in mitosis, DNA replication and repair, and can trigger growth-arrest in many cell types. This transcription factor has been shown to upregulate genes implicated in age-related diseases including atherosclerosis, Alzheimer's disease, amyloidosis, and arthritis. A number of markers of cell aging are expressed after the transcription of p21. The finding of upregulation in the paced heart further underlines the relationship between HF and the aging process. Moreover, in the LV of paced animals, levels of the mitochondrial-apoptogen AIF was elevated (1.3-fold) and the cleaved 57 kDa form of AIF was significantly increased (6.5-fold). These observations are of interest because they indicate that several apoptotic pathways are active in the failing paced heart.

Data from several laboratories have shown that two major sub-populations of mitochondria are present in skeletal and cardiac muscle. One of these organelle sub-populations is associated with the sarcolemma (i.e., the subsarcolemmal or SSM) and the second population, the interfibrillar mitochondria or IFM, is proximal to the myofilaments. A preferential decline in IFM oxidative function in aged rats has been reported, with concomitant reduction of complex III and complex IV activities [94–96]. Presently, there is limited data concerning the different susceptibility of these mitochondrial sub-populations and its contribution to the overall mitochondrial dysfunction observed in HF, and therefore we undertook their analysis in the pacing dog model left ventricle, left atrial, and in skeletal muscle. Analysis of LV mitochondria revealed that both IFM and SSM showed a pacing-associated decline in complex I, III, and V activities albeit IFM showed a more definitive decline for all three enzymes (Fig. 5.7).

Analysis of LA mitochondria revealed a significant decline in both IFM and SSM of only complex V (somewhat more extensive in IFM). Surprisingly, both subtypes of LA mitochondria had significant increase in complex IV activity in the paced animals. Atrial SSM mitochondria also showed a trend for increased CS and complex I activities, which together with the increases in complex IV may indicate increased mitochondrial proliferation in the atrial compartment (Fig. 5.8).

Interestingly, in our analysis of skeletal muscle, we found a pacing-associated decline in complex I and III activities but limited to SSM mitochondria. On the other hand, a significant decline in complex V activity was detected in both IFM

and SSM (with a higher decline in the IFM fraction) as shown in Fig. 5.9. Taken together, these findings reveal that both discrete defects in bioenergetics and the onset of increased apoptosis are present in pacing-induced CM/HF and operative in the early stages of pacing.

The specificity and reproducibility of these changes suggest that these are not stochastic defects. Both changes were in parallel with elevated ROS/OS levels. The abnormal activity of several mitochondrial enzymes and the increased apoptogenic pathway appear to be underlied, at least in part, by an orchestrated shift in expression (both nuclear and mtDNA) of several respiratory chain subunits (e.g., cyt b, ATP-β), mitochondrial bioenergetic enzymes (e.g., mt-CK), global transcription factor (e.g., PGC-1) and apoptotic proteins (e.g., p53, p21).

Furthermore, these data also suggest that differences in specific mitochondrial subpopulations associated with distinct cardiac compartments may contribute to the observed enzymatic dysfunction observed in HF. Further studies appear to be necessary to unravel the genesis of the orchestration of the inter-communication involved, and identify potential targets for new therapies (Fig. 5.10).

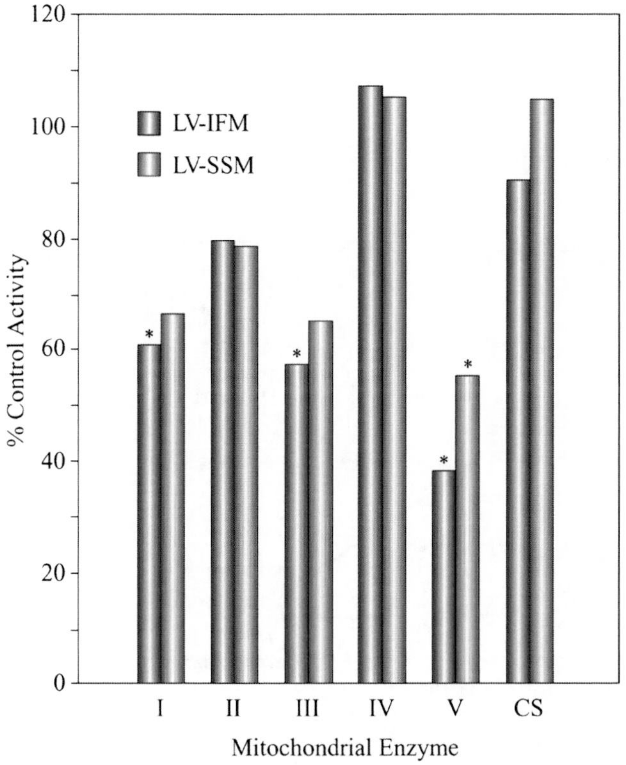

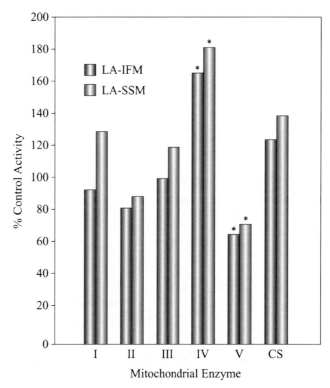

Fig. 5.7 Selected enzymes in different mitochondrial subpopulations in the left ventricle of mongrel dogs with pacing-induced HF. Activity levels of respiratory complex I, II, III, IV, and V and the Krebs cycle enzyme citrate synthase (CS) were assessed in subsarcolemmal (SSM) and interfibrillar (IFM) mitochondria isolated from left ventricle of control ($n = 4$) and 3–4-week ($n = 5$) paced animals. Results shown as expressed as % control value with level of significance ($p < 0.05$)

Fig. 5.8 Selected enzymes in different mitochondrial subpopulations in the left atrium of mongrel dogs with pacing-induced HF. Activity levels of respiratory complex I, II, III, IV, and V and the Krebs cycle enzyme citrate synthase (CS) were assessed in subsarcolemmal (SSM) and interfibrillar (IFM) mitochondria isolated from left atrium of control ($n = 4$) and 3–4-week ($n = 5$) paced animals. Results shown as expressed as % control value with level of significance ($p < 0.05$) indicated by *

Fig. 5.9 Selected enzymes in different mitochondrial subpopulations in skeletal muscle of mongrel dogs with pacing-induced HF. Activity levels of respiratory complex I, II, III, IV, and V and the Krebs cycle enzyme citrate synthase (CS) were assessed in subsarcolemmal (SSM) and interfibrillar (IFM) mitochondria isolated from skeletal muscle of control ($n=4$) and 3–4-week ($n=5$) paced animals. Results shown as expressed as % control value with level of significance ($p<0.05$) indicated by *

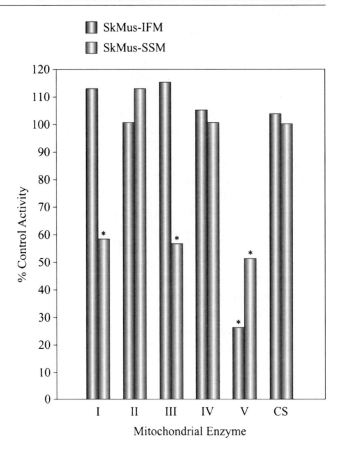

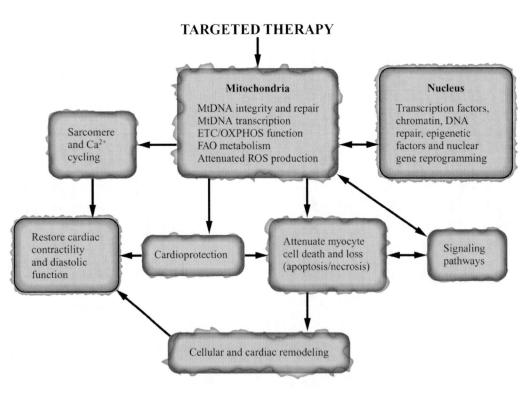

Fig. 5.10 Targeted therapies in HF. This diagram shows the effects of targeting specific organelles/events associated with heart failure (*shaded boxes*) including sarcomeric/calcium cycling, cytosolic signaling pathways, mitochondria, lysosomes, and nuclei. Phenotypic consequences of these therapies including attenuated cell death, increased growth, and increased contractility are shown in the *bottom tier*

In another model of HF, the murine model of myocardial infarct (MI) created by ligation of the left anterior descending coronary artery for 4 weeks, Ide et al. found that LV dilation and contractility dysfunction were accompanied by significant increases in levels of mitochondrial ROS (i.e., hydroxyl radicals) and lipid peroxides [32, 97]. Moreover, infarcted LV from MI mice exhibited diminished enzymatic activity of respiratory complexes I, III, and IV (enzymes each containing subunits encoded by mtDNA) while the mitochondrial enzymes encoded only by nuclear DNA (e.g., citrate synthase and complex II) were unaffected. These investigators also reported a parallel decrease in steady-state levels of several mtDNA-encoded transcripts, including subunits of complexes I, III, and IV as well as 12S and 16S rRNAs and a significant decline in mtDNA copy number. These data are consistent with the concept that membrane lipids, mtDNA, and mitochondrial respiratory enzymes are well-established targets of ROS oxidative damage (see Fig. 5.3), albeit the absence of effect on complex II, a particular common ROS target was unexpected.

Another marker of enhanced OS in the mouse failing heart was increased level of mitochondrial 8-oxo-dGTPase, a DNA repair enzyme which prevents the incorporation of 8-oxo-dGTP into DNA, a significant type of ROS-induced DNA damage which can lead to defects in DNA replication. This HF model illustrates both the development of mitochondrial ROS, a number of its downstream deleterious effects (e.g., enzyme dysfunction, mtDNA damage) as well as an adaptive response (i.e., increased DNA repair activity) to remove that damage.

It is also important to note that while a number of animal studies have shown ROS activation in the failing heart, both arising from mitochondrial and extramitochondrial sources, some observations have suggested that endogenous antioxidants and ROS defense pathways can ameliorate ROS-mediated cardiac abnormalities and the dynamic balance between these counteracting forces should be considered. Both cytosolic antioxidant enzymes (e.g., catalase, SOD1, thioredoxin) and mitochondrial-localized antioxidants including SOD2, thioredoxin, and glutathione peroxidase can reduce ROS levels. Moreover, thioredoxin and thioredoxin reductase form an enzymatic antioxidant and redox regulatory system implicated in the regeneration of many antioxidant molecules, including ubiquinone (Q10), selenium-containing substances, lipoic acid, and ascorbic acid [38]. As we will see later, the relationship of antioxidants with HF has been underlined by several transgenic mouse studies.

While the mechanism by which the antioxidant response signaled in the presence of ROS remains unknown, recent observations suggest that mitochondria can act as an OS sensor and signal to the nucleus to upregulate antioxidant production. Storz et al. have shown that mitochondrial ROS release can activate a signal relay pathway in which the serine/threonine protein kinase D (PKD), acting as a mitochondrial sensor of OS, activates the NF-κB transcription factor leading to induction of SOD2 [98, 99]. PKD has been localized to the mitochondria in cells exposed to both exogenous and mitochondrial ROS, where it is phosphorylated and activated. Upon subsequent dissociation from mitochondria, activated PKD phosphorylates substrates participate in NF-κB activation, although how this is accomplished is not yet known. Experiments in which RNAi-mediated silencing of PKD blunted *SOD2* induction confirm that *SOD2* promoter activation is dependent on PKD. While the role of PKD in HF has not yet been established, the critical involvement of mitochondrial ROS in the signaling and generation of an antioxidant response suggests potential limitations with the use of antioxidants, which target mitochondrial ROS.

Although studies with animal models suggested that ROS and defective ETC play an integral role in the genesis and progression of HF, these findings were correlative, and did not however, establish a direct link between ROS, defective ETC, and either skeletal muscle or cardiac dysfunction. Notwithstanding, these observations did foreshadow recent findings using heart/muscle-specific MnSOD-deficient mice, a transgenic mice in which OS, which selectively impaired mitochondrial respiration, can directly cause HF [39]. Furthermore, ROS may trigger a multiplicity of mechanisms that can lead to HF. For instance, complex IV (affected at both the transcriptional and activity levels in Ide's studies) was not significantly decreased in the MnSOD-deficient mouse. On the other hand, this model exhibited a moderate decline in both complex I and III and particularly, a marked decline in the nuclear DNA-encoded complex II activity (shown to be mediated at the post-transcriptional level). Taken together, this latter study and the aforementioned pacing dog studies do not support the view of ROS-mediated decline in mtDNA copy number and in mitochondrial transcription as the definitive mechanism leading to reduced respiration and cardiac bioenergetic metabolism in HF.

Nuclear–Mitochondrial Communication

Since the majority of the components of mitochondrial bioenergetic, biogenesis, and signaling pathways are encoded by nuclear DNA, regulation of the mitochondrial programmed changes detected in HF largely arise in the nucleus. Even direct damage to mitochondrial-specific molecules such as mtDNA mutations and large-scale mtDNA deletions may arise from defective nuclear gene functions (e.g., DNA polymerase γ, ANT1), leading to cardiomyopathy and/or HF [23, 24, 100]. On the other hand, mitochondria can influence nuclear transcriptional events by virtue of ROS generation and signaling, and numerous observations suggest the presence of significant nuclear–mitochondrial cross talk, which likely will contribute to the failing heart phenotype.

Over the last decade, many nuclear factors have been identified that regulate the biosynthesis of both nuclear-encoded and cytoplasmic-translated mitochondrial proteins (recently estimated to be over 1,500 types), as well as mitochondrial DNA-encoded (and translated) proteins ($n = 13$) as represented in Fig. 5.11. The latter include seven subunits of complex I, one subunit of complex III, three subunits of complex IV, and two for complex V. The nuclear factors include the nuclear respiratory factors-1 and -2 (NRF-1 and -2), the mitochondrial

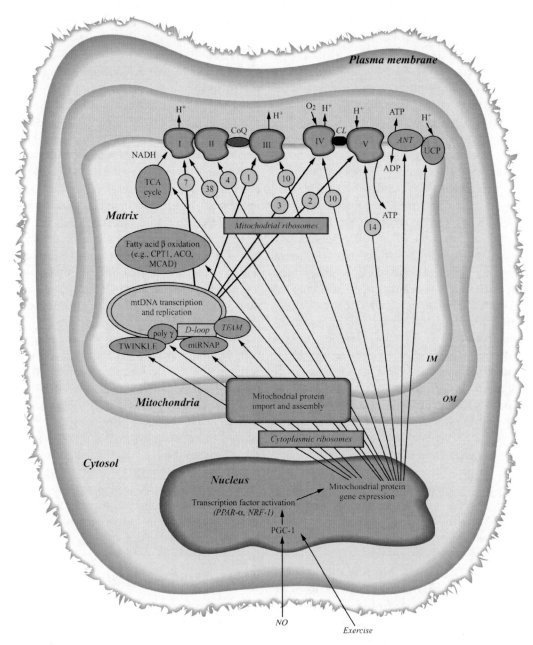

Fig. 5.11 Heart mitochondrial biogenesis and bioenergetic pathways are signal driven. Shown are the major mitochondrial bioenergetic pathways (fatty acid oxidation (FAO)), TCA cycle, and the respiratory complexes (I–V) involved in ETC and OXPHOS; the subunits comprising the majority of mitochondrial proteins including the enzymes of the FAO and TCA cycles, proteins involved in ATP production/distribution, and electron transport coupling (e.g., ANT and UCP). All but 13 proteins involved in respiratory complexes I, III, IV, and V are encoded by nuclear genes translated on cytoplasmic ribosomes and incorporated in the mitochondria by a dedicated mitochondrial import apparatus comprised of inner and outer membrane proteins and molecular chaperones. These genes are under the regulation of specific nuclear transcription factors and co-activators including NRF-1, PGC-1, and PPAR-α that can be modulated by physiological stimuli including thyroid hormone (TH), nitric oxide (NO), electrical stimulation, and exercise. Expression of the mtDNA genes generates 2 rRNA, 22 tRNA, and the 13 proteins encoding respiratory complex subunits (translated on mitochondrial ribosomes) dependent on nuclear-encoded proteins regulating both the transcription and replication of mtDNA (e.g., mitochondrial DNA polymerase (pol γ)), the helicase Twinkle, mtRNA polymerase and TFAM, the latter which is modulated by the nuclear transcription factors (e.g., PGC-1, NRF-1) in response to physiological stimuli

transcription factor A (mtTFA or TFAM), a pivotal factor involved in mtDNA transcription, replication and maintenance, and the nuclear receptor proteins including the peroxisome proliferator-activated receptors (PPAR) [101–103].

Upstream of these factors, is the transcriptional co-activator of peroxisome proliferator activated receptor γ (PPARγ), known as PGC-1, a key regulator of mitochondrial function and mitochondrial biogenesis, which participates in the transduction of physiological stimuli to myocardial energy production. In response to a variety of stimuli, PGC-1 can activate NRF expression and activity which in turn upregulates the expression of nuclear-encoded mitochondrial proteins and of the nuclear-encoded TFAM [104, 105].

In addition to TFAM, other nuclear-encoded proteins play important roles in mtDNA replication, repair, and gene expression. These include the mitochondrial DNA polymerase γ (pol γ), the helicase TWINKLE, the SSB protein, and an additional transcription factor (TFB). As we will discuss later, defects in TWINKLE and pol γ as well as in nuclear regulatory factors can result in HF, implying that some defects in nuclear–mitochondrial cross talk can lead to cardiomyopathy and HF.

Mitochondrial Transcription in HF

The issue and extent of mitochondrial transcriptional changes in different animal models of HF remains largely unsettled. Using a rat model of HF-induced by aortic banding, Garnier et al. reported decreased levels of myocardial oxidative capacity and reduced mitochondrial enzyme activities (i.e., citrate synthase and complex IV), together with a parallel decrease in mRNA levels of complex IV subunits COX I and IV, but no change in overall mtDNA content [105]. Furthermore, in this animal model, marked downregulated expression of nuclear-encoded regulatory factors, including TFAM, NRF2, and PGC1 was detected. Similarly, using a model of rat heart subjected to either 12 or 18 weeks of coronary artery ligation (CAL), Javadov et al., have shown significant downregulation of mitochondrial gene expression and mitochondrial transcription factors induced by postinfarction remodeling [106]. In addition, mRNA level of PGC-1 and its downstream factors, including nuclear respiratory factor 1 and 2, TFAM, and the COX I and COX IV transcripts were also significantly reduced in both 12 and 18 weeks in CAL groups compared with sham-operated hearts.

Transgenic Mice and Mitochondria

Although a comprehensive discussion on transgenic animal models and HF will be presented in Chap. 6, here it suffices to mention that the use of transgenic mice with abnormal

expression of genes involved in bioenergetic metabolism has provided unique insights into the dynamic balance of the mouse heart to maintain energy status and cardiac function, as well as to explore the cause–effect relationships between mitochondrial function and HF. These include either loss-of function mutations (i.e., generation of null alleles or gene "knock-outs") or gain-of-function (e.g., overexpression). A list of transgenic models with heart metabolic changes associated with cardiomyopathy and HF phenotype is shown in Table 5.7.

Loss-of-function model systems using knockouts of a relatively wide spectrum of genes encoding mitochondrial proteins results in severe cardiac dysfunction. These include genes for proteins directly involved in ATP transport including ANT and creatine kinase, antioxidants including MnSOD, TXD, and frataxin (the protein responsible for Friedreich Ataxia), factors involved in cytosolic and mitochondrial fatty acid metabolism such as PPAR, MTP subunits, ACS, OCTN2, VLCAD, FATP1 and LCAD, the energy sensor AMP kinase (PRKAG2), mitochondrial biogenesis factors including TFAM mitochondrial DNA pol γ, and PGC-1. Currently, there is limited information about the impact on the myocardium of knocking-out genes involved directly in OXPHOS, with either nuclear OXPHOS genes or mtDNA structural genes. The generation of the latter represents a formidable technical challenge, which likely will require a novel approach for the creation of a mitochondrial transgenic animal, albeit progress is being made in that direction. In the next section, we will examine selected metabolic components implicated by transgenic studies including ANT1, mitochondrial biogenesis factors, regulatory transcription factors and antioxidants, and their role in the development of HF.

Mitochondrial DNA Integrity and HF in Transgenic Mice

ANT-1, TFAM, and DNA polymerase γ are among the many metabolic related genes for which either deletion or overexpression can promote the development of cardiomyopathy and HF in transgenic mice (shown in Table 5.7). While TFAM and DNA polymerase γ play well-established roles in the maintenance, replication, and expression of mitochondrial DNA (mtDNA), ANT which is pivotally involved in mitochondrial ATP/ADP exchange and transport, as well as a component of the mitochondrial permeability transition (PT) pore, has been reported to have a role in mtDNA maintenance, possibly arising from its participation in the regulation of deoxynucleotide levels [120].

The adenine nucleotide translocators (ANT) are a family of proteins that exchange mitochondrial ATP for cytosolic ADP, providing new ADP substrate to the mitochondria

Table 5.7 Selected transgenic mouse models of metabolic genes involved in CM and HF

Gene (protein)	Genetic alteration	Function	Phenotype	Refs
MTP	Null	FAO; Mitochondrial trifunctional protein	CM, sudden death	[107]
LCAD	Global ablation	FAO; long chain acyl-CoA dehydrogenase	CM, ↑ myocardial lipid and fibrosis	[108]
Frataxin	Cardiac-specific knock-out	Iron metabolism; FRDA	CM, hypertrophy	[109]
TFAM/mtTFA	Cardiac-specific knock-out	Mitochondrial transcription factor A	DCM, AV heart conduction block, HF	[110]
LpL	Cardiac-specific overexpression of GPI-anchored LPL	Lipoprotein lipase	DCM, ↓ FAO	[111]
PRKAG2	Cardiac-specific overexpression of N488I mutation	AMP kinase regulatory subunit	LV hypertrophy, ventricular preexcitation and sinus node dysfunction	[112]
DNA polymerase γ	Cardiac-specific knock-in mutation	Mitochondrial DNA polymerase γ	DCM	[100]
Mito-CK	Null	Mitochondrial creatine kinase	↑ LV dilation and hypertrophy	[25]
Cyto-CK	Null	Cytosolic creatine kinase	↑ LV dilation and hypertrophy	[26]
AIF	Cardiac-specific null	Apoptosis inducing factor	DCM	[69]
TrxR2	Cardiac-specific null	Mitochondrial thioredoxin reductase	Fatal DCM	[41]
MnSOD/SOD2	Null	Mn superoxide dismutase	DCM	[40]
PGC-1α	Cardiac-specific overexpression	Peroxisome proliferator-activated receptor gamma coactivator-1α	Cardiomyopathy and mitochondrial defects only in adult not neonate	[113]
5-HT2B receptor	Cardiac-specific overexpression	Serotonin receptor	HCM with mitochondrial proliferation	[114]
OCTN2	Heterozygous carriers of mutation	Carnitine transporter	Age-associated CM with lipid deposition, hypertrophy	[115]
ANT1	Null	Adenine nucleotide translocator	CM, cardiac hypertrophy with ↑ mitochondrial number	[24]
FATP1	Cardiac-specific overexpression	Fatty acid transport protein 1	Lipotoxic cardiomyopathy	[116]
PPAR-α	Cardiac-specific overexpression	Peroxisome proliferator-activated receptor-α	Diabetic CM with ↑ FAO, ↓ glucose uptake and use, cardiac hypertrophy	[117]
PPAR-δ	Cardiac-specific null	Peroxisome proliferator-activated receptor-δ	HF. Lipotoxic CM with ↑ myocardial lipid, hypertrophy	[118]
ACS	Cardiac-specific overexpression	Long chain acyl-CoA synthetase	Cardiac lipid accumulation and hypertrophy, LV dysfunction and HF	[119]

while delivering ATP to the cytoplasm for cellular work. Mutational inactivation of the mouse *Ant1* gene encoding the heart/muscle isoform of the mitochondrial ANT results in mitochondrial abnormalities including a partial deficit in ADP-stimulated respiration, consistent with impaired translocation of ADP into mitochondria in both skeletal muscle and heart. In addition, *Ant1* gene deficient mice exhibit multiple myocardial mtDNA deletions associated with elevated production of ROS (e.g., H_2O_2) and the development of skeletal myopathy and cardiomyopathy leading to HF [23]. Moreover, *Ant1*-deficient mice displayed an increase in tissue-specific antioxidant defenses (e.g., MnSOD) in skeletal muscle mitochondria but not in heart mitochondria. *Ant1*$^{-/-}$ mice exhibit a progressive cardiac hypertrophic phenotype coincident with the proliferation of mitochondria [24]. It has been suggested that this mitochondrial biogenic response is a compensatory mechanism to correct

the energy deficit, although could also be contributory to cardiac remodeling.

Transgenic mice heterozygous for a null allele of TFAM showed decreased myocardial mtDNA copy number and ETC defects, whereas homozygous TFAM knockout strains exhibited severe mtDNA depletion with decreased OXPHOS function and died in embryonic development [121]. Wang et al. reported that mouse strains containing conditional cardiac and muscle-specific null TFAM alleles developed a mosaic pattern of progressive and severe ETC defects in the postnatal heart, resulting in DCM, atrioventricular conduction block, early HF and death between 2 and 4 weeks [110]. Reduced activities of complex I and IV together with a significant decline in cardiac and skeletal muscle mtDNA levels and gene expression were reported.

Along with the development of severe cardiomyopathy, tissue-specific TFAM knockout mice exhibited increased apoptosis in the in vivo heart consistent with the finding of massive apoptosis in *Tfam* knockout embryos and suggesting that defects in ETC may predispose cells to apoptosis [122]. Global gene profiling analyses in tissue-specific *Tfam* knockout mice revealed a metabolic switch in the early progression of cardiac mitochondrial dysfunction akin to the activation of a fetal gene expression program in which a number of genes, encoding critical enzymes in FAO, showed decreased expression, while several genes encoding glycolytic enzymes showed increased expression [123]. In more advanced disease, the metabolic switch was followed by an increase in mitochondrial biomass or biogenesis, which did not result in increase of overall myocardial mitochondrial ATP production rate. On the basis of these findings, it was inferred that the observed switch in metabolism appeared unlikely to benefit energy homeostasis in the respiratory chain-deficient hearts and may actually promote further cardiac dysfunction.

TFAM overexpression in transgenic mice can ameliorate the mitochondrial dysfunction and HF resulting from myocardial infarction [124]. TFAM overexpression attenuated the decline in mtDNA level and respiratory activities in post-MI hearts, and significantly reduced the LV dilatation and dysfunction accompanied by a decrease in LV remodeling (i.e., decreased myocyte hypertrophy and interstitial fibrosis). The survival of the infarcted animals was affected but not the infarct size.

Cumulative damage to mtDNA, which can result in point mutations, large-scale deletions, or changes in mtDNA copy number has been implicated in the progression of HF. Mice that express a proofreading-deficient mitochondrial DNA polymerase γ targeted to the heart generated cardiac mtDNA mutations (average 2 per mitochondrial genome) and eventually (over several weeks) developed DCM and interstitial fibrosis, often leading to HF [100]. Surprisingly, the mechanism of the pathogenesis in these strains does not appear to involve increased OS levels [125]. Measurements of enzyme function or oxidative defense systems in the transgenic heart fail to detect increased levels of oxidative adducts in DNA or protein, nor signs of increased OS. Furthermore, mitochondrial respiratory function, mitochondrial ultrastructure and number remained normal in these strains although the detection of cytochrome *c* release from mitochondria, a landmark of apoptosis, suggested that the elevated frequency of mtDNA mutations might trigger the initiation of apoptotic cell death. Interestingly, further studies have noted that the activation of myocardial programmed cell death pathway precedes (and may itself trigger) a vigorous prosurvival response including the upregulation of antiapoptotic proteins Bcl-2, Bcl-xl, Bfl1, heat shock protein 27, and X-linked inhibitor of apoptosis protein (XIAP) [126].

PGC-1

The heart appears to function best when it simultaneously oxidizes both carbohydrates and fatty acids as bioenergetic substrates [127]. Under pathologic conditions, the heart relies more on glucose, as seen in cardiac hypertrophy, or may rely almost solely on fatty acids, as observed in cardiac tissue of animal models of diabetes [128]. Furthermore, the failing heart exhibits a decline in overall mitochondrial oxidative catabolism (including FAO), which is most evident in advanced HF while reliance on anaerobic glycolytic pathways tends to be increased [129–131]. Recent observations in an animal model of HF have downplayed the role of myocardial FAO downregulation in early, compensated HF [132]. Thus, initially this switch in metabolic substrate use provides adequate energy to maintain normal cardiac function, and may have an adaptive function by diminishing oxygen consumption. However, over time substrate switch in concert with declining OXPHOS, becomes maladaptive, leading to a state of myocyte energy insufficiency (related to reduced capacity for myocardial mitochondrial ATP production, and depletion in high-energy phosphates), resulting in diastolic HF. As previously noted, alterations in high-energy phosphates (PCr and ATP) have been identified by magnetic resonance spectroscopy both in animal models and human hearts with LV hypertrophy or HF [131, 133], and may be contributory to the pathological remodeling that occurs in end-stage HF.

The programmatic decline in expression of genes involved in mitochondrial oxidative metabolism in the hypertrophied and failing heart has been confirmed by Gene profiling analysis [105, 134–136]. Global nuclear regulators, including the ligand-activated transcription factors such as (PPARs) and the cofactor PGC-1, are important regulatory factors in cardiac mitochondrial metabolism (including FAO) and biogenesis and therefore have been intensively studied in regards to the metabolic switch.

PGC-1 transduces cell signals associated with physiologic stimuli to regulate cardiac metabolic genes (Fig. 5.12). Initially, PGC-1α was identified as a PPAR γ coactivator involved in the regulation of energy metabolic pathways in tissues specialized for thermogenesis (e.g., brown adipose tissue and skeletal muscle) [137]. PGC-1 is selectively expressed in highly oxidative tissues such as heart, skeletal muscle, brown adipose, and liver. Its tissue expression and inducibility in response to a variety of physiological stimuli that increase ATP demand and stimulate mitochondrial oxidation (e.g., exercise, cold exposure and fasting) are intricately linked to its role as a regulator of energy metabolism including myocardial mitochondrial biogenesis and oxidation, hepatic gluconeogenesis, and skeletal muscle glucose uptake [138–140]. *PGC-1α* gene expression is developmentally regulated, with induction in the mouse heart after birth coincident with the perinatal shift from glucose metabolism to FAO; it can also be subsequently induced in response to short-term fasting, conditions known to increase cardiac mitochondrial energy production. Expression of PGC-1α in cardiac myocytes has been found to induce both nuclear and mitochondrial gene expression involved in multiple mitochondrial bioenergetic pathways, with increased mitochondrial biogenesis, respiration, and FAO. Gain-of-function studies utilizing constitutive cardiac-specific overexpression of PGC-1α (MHC-PGC-1) in transgenic mice resulted in uncontrolled mitochondrial proliferation, severe DCM and HF [140]. Regulated overexpression of a tetracycline-inducible PGC-1 construct during the neonatal stages of mouse development led to a dramatic increase in cardiac mitochondrial number and size coincidently with upregulation of genes associated with mitochondrial biogenesis. In contrast, PGC-1α overexpression in the heart of adult mice resulted in a modest increase in mitochondrial number, derangements of mitochondrial ultrastructure, and development of a reversible cardiomyopathy characterized by loss of sarcomeric structure and increased ventricular mass and chamber dilatation [113].

Two independent mouse models of PGC-1α loss-of-function with constitutive inactivation have been developed. In the first, *PGC-1* knock-out mice develop cardiac dysfunction with progressive age; gene profiling analysis of these strains revealed markedly diminished expression of myocardial OXPHOS and FAO genes, associated with reduced mitochondrial enzymatic activities and cardiac myocyte state 3 mitochondrial respiration rates, decreased levels of ATP, and a diminished ability to increase myocardial work output in response to chemical or electrical stimulation [139].

The second PGC-1α$^{-/-}$ mice did not directly display cardiac dysfunction at baseline [140]. However, extensive phenotyping revealed multi-system abnormalities indicative of an abnormal energy metabolic phenotype including blunted postnatal heart growth and slow-twitch skeletal muscle, organs with high mitochondrial energy demands. These PGC-1α$^{-/-}$ mice exhibited decreased mitochondrial number and respiratory capacity in slow-twitch skeletal muscle leading to reduced muscle performance and exercise capacity, and displayed a modest diminution in cardiac function largely related to abnormal control of heart rate. This rate defect was accentuated in response to exercise and β-adrenergic stimulation.

PPAR

Over the last decade, PPARs have been identified as playing a central role in the transcriptional regulation of genes involved in intracellular lipid and energy metabolism including FAO enzymes [128, 136]. Three isoforms of the PPAR

subfamily (α, β, and γ) are enriched in tissues that are dependent on lipid utilization for energy metabolism (e.g., heart, liver, brown adipose tissue as well as in all critical vascular cells) and have been implicated in the rapid mobilization of bioenergetic stores in response to physiological stresses. Each PPAR factor acts in concert with the nuclear retinoid X receptor (RXR) as a heterodimer binding to a consensus DNA response element with the sequence AGGTCA-NAGGTCA (direct repeat with a single nucleotide spacing), contained within the regulatory regions of target genes (see Fig. 5.12).

This is followed by the transcriptional activation and increased gene expression of these target genes, including a constellation of genes encoding enzymes involved in both peroxisome and mitochondrial FAO (e.g., mitochondrial MCAD, CPT-I, and peroxisomal acyl-CoA oxidase). The functional specificity of the PPARs is determined by isoform-specific tissue distribution, specific interaction with activating ligands (e.g., prostaglandins, eicosanoids, leukotriene B4, and long-chain unsaturated fatty acids), and cofactor interactions (i.e., coactivators and corepressors) [130]. While several lines of evidence suggest that all three isoforms modulate cardiac energy metabolism, PPAR-α has been characterized as the central regulator of myocardial mitochondrial fatty acid catabolism, whereas PPAR-γ is thought to be involved in myocardial lipid storage regulation.

While PPAR-α is activated by a number of lipid-derived molecules, the endogenous ligand for PPAR has not yet been precisely determined [141, 142]. Synthetic PPAR ligands including the fibrate class of anti-hyperlipidemic drugs such as ciprofibrate, bezafibrate, fenofibrate, and gemfibrozil are widely used clinically. Interestingly, while some of the synthetic agonists are highly specific for PPAR-α activation, others exhibit dual specificity activating both PPAR-α and PPAR-γ (e.g., glitazars) and some activate all PPARs (e.g., bezafibrate) equally [143].

As with PGC-1, cardiac metabolic gene expression is activated by PPAR-α regulation during post-natal development, during short-term starvation and in response to exercise training [144]. Conversely, pressure-overload hypertrophy results in PPAR-α deactivation leading to lower FAO enzyme expression, abnormal cardiac lipid homeostasis, and reduced energy production [136]. This suggests that PPAR-α may play a contributory role in the energy substrate switch away from fatty acid utilization in the hypertrophied failing heart. Lower nuclear levels of the PPAR-α protein in these tissues have been largely explained to occur as a function of the negative regulation of PPAR-α mediated at the transcriptional level during ventricular overload in mice. In addition, PPAR activity is altered at the post-transcriptional level, by phosphorylation by protein kinases including PKA, PKC, MAPKs, and AMPK [145–148].

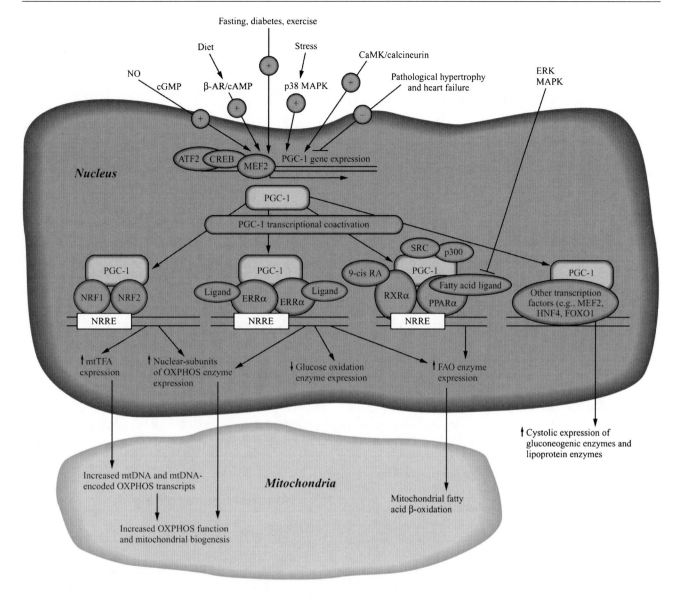

Fig. 5.12 PGC-1 and its metabolic pathway. PGC-1 transduces cell signals associated with physiologic stimuli to regulate cardiac metabolic genes. Numerous signaling pathways downstream of physiologic stimuli, like fasting and exercise, activate the PGC-1 cascade either by increasing PGC-1 expression or activity. PGC-1, in turn, coactivates transcriptional partners, including nuclear respiratory factor-1 and 2 (NRF-1/2), estrogen-related receptor (ERR) and PPAR-α, resulting in downstream activation of mitochondrial biogenesis and FAO pathways, respectively

The cardiac PPAR-α/PGC-1α system is activated in diabetes and has been suggested to contribute to the promotion of diabetic cardiomyopathy. This metabolic shift associated with high level of fatty acid import and oxidation may eventually lead to abnormal mitochondrial and cardiac remodeling. Transgenic mice with cardiac restricted overexpression of PPAR-α (i.e., MHC-PPAR-α mice) exhibit increased expression of genes encoding enzymes involved in multiple steps of mitochondrial FAO with strong reciprocal downregulation of glucose transporter (GLUT-4) and glycolytic enzyme gene expression [149]. Myocardial fatty acid uptake and mitochondrial FAO are markedly increased in MHC-PPAR-α hearts, whereas glucose uptake and oxidation are profoundly diminished in MHC-PPAR-α mice. Echocardiographic assessment identified LV hypertrophy and dysfunction in the MHC-PPAR-α mice in a transgene expression-dependent manner [117, 150, 151].

Defects in Cytosolic Proteins Can Cause HF with Mitochondrial Dysfunction

Even mouse strains containing null genes encoding cytosolic proteins, such as desmin and calcineurin, develop HF associated with significant mitochondrial dysfunction [64, 152–154].

Table 5.8 Mitochondrial proteins effected in Desmin-related HF

Downregulated genes

ATP synthase α chain (complex V)

Creatine kinase, sarcomeric mitochondrial (S-MtCK)

Cytochrome $c1$, heme protein

Core protein 2 of Ubiquinol–cytochrome c reductase (complex III subunit II)

Upregulated genes

Long-chain acyl-CoA synthetase (ACS1)

β-keto-thiolase

Annexin

VDAC/porin

Analysis of desmin-deficient strains revealed a role for desmin-associated cytoskeletal intermediate filaments in myocardial mitochondrial function [155]. Mice lacking desmin exhibited disruption of muscle architecture with numerous mitochondrial abnormalities, including significant organelle clumping, extensive mitochondrial proliferation and number, loss of normal positioning, swelling and degeneration of the mitochondrial matrix as well as compromised respiratory function. These mitochondrial abnormalities occur early and are followed by myocardial degeneration with extensive fibrosis and dystrophic calcification. While the precise mechanism by which desmin affects mitochondrial function is not yet known; proteomic analysis of desmin-null mice found significant changes in protein levels of several respiratory enzymes (see Table 5.8) suggesting altered activity of regulatory factors, underscoring and probably expanding the role of nuclear–cytosol–mitochondrial cross-talk in HF [155]. In calcineurin-null mice, loss of this signaling molecule also results in decreased mitochondrial respiratory subunit protein levels leading to impaired ETC. Furthermore, this was associated with high levels of superoxide production that might contribute to HF development [154].

Clinical Studies

Clinical observations have shown marked cardiac mitochondrial respiratory enzyme dysfunction in HF, albeit there is no consensus on the extent of this dysfunction and the specific enzymes affected. Increased incidence of complex III deficiency in DCM has been reported by some investigators [10, 11], while others have reported increased complex IV deficiency [9]. Scheubel et al. in a study of a series of 43 explanted failing hearts found significantly decreased myocardial complex I activity (30%), while complex III and IV activities were unchanged. Furthermore, no changes were found in heart mtDNA (either integrity or levels) or TFAM levels, nor in mtDNA-encoded transcripts excluding a generalized defect in mitochondrial gene expression or mtDNA damage

as a reason for the cardiac enzyme deficiency noted [156]. This suggests that complex I deficiency likely arose from a post-transcriptional modification of complex I subunits, presumably the result of oxidative injury.

A clear link between OS and chronic ventricular dysfunction has been established only in cases of anthracycline-mediated and alcoholic cardiomyopathies. On the other hand, it is unclear whether ROS or OS have a pathophysiologic role in congestive HF or cardiomyopathy due to ischemic, hypertensive, valvular, or idiopathic etiologies [45]. Since levels of short-lived ROS (i.e., superoxide and hydroxyl radicals) are difficult to directly gauge, increased ROS levels in patients with HF has been difficult to confirm. Recently, superoxide anions as assessed by EPR with an O_2-spin trap have been reported to increase more than twofold in the myocardium of patients with end-stage HF undergoing transplant [157]. Interestingly, despite increased MnSOD mRNA levels, a marked decline in mitochondrial-localized MnSOD protein and activity was detected. Both increased ROS levels and decreased antioxidant response would be expected to lead an enhanced OS in the failing heart, which in turn may result in increased transcription of antioxidant enzymes.

An important caveat raised by these data should be noted. The finding of bioenergetic defects in tissues from patients is essentially correlative evidence and can be interpreted as a consequence of the pathological state.

Mitochondrial Gene Profiling

Observations from animal models have suggested a "metabolic switch" from fatty acid to glucose oxidation during evolving HF. However, there is no consensus that the same pathologic processes are operative in human HF [158, 159]. Upregulation of genes involved in OXPHOS, which might reflect a decrease in activity of mitochondrial respiratory pathways during progressive HF has been reported [160–162]. Whether this reflects a compensatory adaptation to mitochondrial dysfunction or damage similar to that found in studies of mitochondrial cytopathies remains to be seen. No consistent pattern of up- or downregulation of genes involved in FAO has emerged highlighting the difficulty of reproducing findings from animal models to humans. When only considering end-stage HF, there appears to be a trend toward the downregulation of glycolysis contradicting the hypothesis that the failing heart switches from fatty acid to glucose oxidation, but rather favoring a decreased use of glucose as an energy substrate [163]. None of the transcriptional regulators of cardiac mitochondrial biogenesis and respiratory function were found to be deregulated. This may be related to the fact that most studies lacked an experimental design that would allow the detection of relatively small expression changes.

Implication of Metabolic Genes in HF

The significance of adequate bioenergetic function to the heart has been underscored by the discovery of several inherited disorders in which defective components of the metabolic pathways lead to cardiac pathologies, including cardiomyopathy, hypertrophic remodeling, and HF. This provides further evidence that deranged mitochondrial metabolism leads to cardiac dysfunction, rather than being its consequence. Specific metabolic gene mutations have been localized in both nuclear and/or mitochondrial-encoded genes (see Table 5.2).

Mutations in mtDNA resulting in global impairment of mitochondrial respiratory function cause HCM or DCM and cardiac conduction defects (see Table 5.3). Point mutations in mitochondrial tRNA genes have been most often found (such as leucine, lysine, and isoleucine) although mutations in mitochondrial rRNA and structural genes have also been reported to lead to cardiomyopathy and HF. The presentation of these pathogenic mutations is most often heteroplasmic (i.e., mixture of wild-type and mutant alleles), although rarely homoplasmic mutations have also been described. Most of the pathogenic mtDNA mutations have been located in highly conserved nucleotides, and were accompanied by decreased levels of respiratory enzyme activity(s). The cardiac phenotype arising from these mutations may be isolated cardiomyopathy or may be a part of a constellation of primarily neurological findings associated with mitochondrial defects (such as MELAS, MERRF, and Leigh syndrome).

In addition to inherited mtDNA mutations (entirely of maternal origin), acquired and/or sporadic mtDNA mutations have been reported. For instance, sporadic large-scale mtDNA deletions (usually of a discrete single size) have been associated with Kearns–Sayre syndrome (KSS) in which patients may display cardiomyopathy, mitral valve prolapse, and/or cardiac conduction abnormalities [164]. An increase in the abundance of somatic mtDNA deletions in the heart has been documented with increased aging and has also been reported to be increased in patients with cardiomyopathy, presumably arising from increased OS [165–167]. However, the overall levels of deleted genomes (relative to wild type genomes) in these patients is extremely low (often less than 1%) and their significance relative to cardiac phenotype or respiratory deficiency is not evident.

Other mtDNA deletion-associated phenotypes can arise as a result of defects in autosomal nuclear DNA loci (showing either dominant or recessive inheritance patterns) [168, 169]. For instance, progressive external ophthalmoplegia (PEO) with autosomal recessive inheritance results in multiple mtDNA deletions phenotype commonly presenting as a severe cardiomyopathy in infancy [169]. Mutations in several nuclear encoded mitochondrial proteins including ANT1, DNA polymerase γ, and the helicase Twinkle have been reported to lead to PEO with increased tissue-specific mtDNA deletions [170].

Palmieri et al. have reported the presence of a recessive mutation in the heart/muscle specific-isoform of ANT1 in a patient with HCM, mild myopathy with exercise intolerance and lactic acidosis but no ophthalmoplegia. This mutation resulted in a complete loss of adenine nucleotide transport function and was associated with increased multiple deletions of muscle mtDNA [27].

Sporadic cases of cardiomyopathy (primarily infantile) with a severe mtDNA depletion and associated reduction in cardiac and/or skeletal muscle mitochondrial respiratory activities have also been reported, albeit the primary site of defect was not identified in these studies [171, 172]. However, in patients with Alpers syndrome, a developmental mitochondrial DNA syndrome depletion characterized by reduced mitochondrial respiration, including complex IV deficiency and extensive mtDNA depletion may display HCM with skeletal muscle ragged-red fibers [173]. This disorder is primarily attributed to a pronounced mtDNA polymerase γ deficiency [174] with specific lesions in the Pol γ gene and reported to account for over 90% of cases [175]. Therefore, these disorders illustrate the cardiomyopathic phenotype resulting from mutations in nuclear genes compromising the stability of the mitochondrial genome, a significant disruption of the nuclear–mitochondrial communication whose hallmark is the accumulation of mtDNA large-scale deletions and mtDNA depletion in post-mitotic tissues.

Mutations in nuclear genes encoding mitochondrial FAO enzymes may also manifest as cardiomyopathy. Interestingly, cardiomyopathies resulting from inborn errors in mitochondrial FAO enzymes are often provoked by physiological or pathophysiological conditions that increase dependence on FAO for myocardial ATP production, such as prolonged exercise or fasting associated with infectious illness. Inherited FAO disorders caused by mutations in nuclear genes, encoding enzymes in the mitochondrial FAO pathways, may lead to impaired mitochondrial catabolism of fatty acids and may manifest as a cardiomyopathic phenotype leading to HF. Cardiomyopathy in these patients usually appears during childhood and often presents sudden onset HF or ventricular dysrhythmias induced by stress. Mitochondrial dysfunction involving FAO has also been reported in acquired cardiomyopathies. Furthermore, in end-stage HF and in pressure overload hypertrophy, FAO and OXPHOS pathways are impaired [1–3, 26].

Potential Mechanisms and Downstream Effects of Metabolic Damage in HF

Contractile dysfunction and cardiac remodeling in HF can be seen as downstream events occurring as a function of metabolic dysfunction/deficits. Viewed at the cellular level, mitochondria which is at the epicenter of the generation of ATP via OXPHOS,

TCA and FAO cycles and of OS/ROS production also impact the overall Ca^{2+} levels to the proximally located ER/SR and play a pivotal role in the events of cell-death, including the triggering of apoptosis and signaling of necrosis. In this section, we will discuss evidence concerning the involvement of mitochondria in both cardiac contractile dysfunction and in myocyte cell death and assess their significance in HF progression.

Calcium Handing, Homeostasis, and Contractility

Altered Ca^{2+} homeostasis is recognized as a key pathophysiological mechanism in HF, leading to altered contractile function, activation of signaling pathways, and transcriptional activity. As shown in Fig. 5.13, Ca^{2+} homeostasis depends on efficient energy-driven ion pumps, while Ca^{2+} concentration in turn influences energy expenditure through its activation of cellular ATPases and mitochondrial dehydrogenases.

Disturbances in these finely controlled cellular processes make the myocyte enter a vicious cycle of energy mismatch and Ca^{2+} dysregulation that may turn out to be highly detrimental, especially in periods of increased workload. The impairment of contractile function during progressive HF reflects significant cellular changes that include altered expression of membrane and contractile proteins, altered energy metabolism, and impaired excitation–contraction coupling. Interestingly, altered energetics has been proposed to underlie myocardial dysfunction even in HCM, in which sarcomeric/contractile proteins are either deficient in function or expression [176].

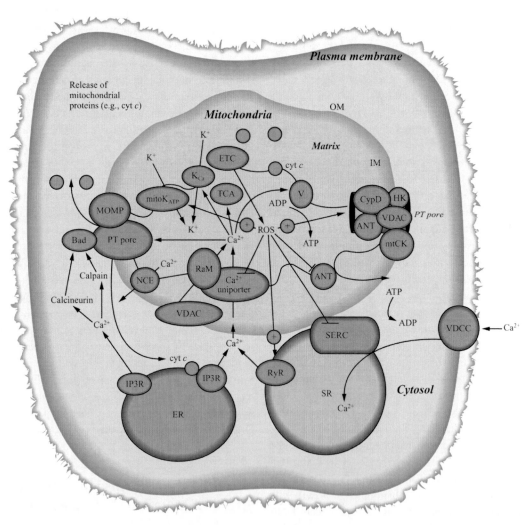

Fig. 5.13 Mitochondrial channels impact calcium and potassium flux in the failing heart. The opening of mitochondrial K^+ channel (mito K_{ATP}) in the inner membrane is normally triggered by ROS, ATP levels, ligands binding to an assortment of membrane receptors, and the involvement of protein kinases (PKC, PI3K). In addition to K^+ influx, matrix volume and the level of ROS are affected by the opening of these channels. Mitochondrial K^+ influx is also mediated by the K_{Ca} channel which is activated by Ca^{2+}. Ca^{2+} enters the mitochondria via an aging-regulated uniporter (with VDAC involvement), and by RaM transporter. Increased mitochondrial Ca^{2+} can activate enzymes of the TCA cycle, ETC, and complex V as well as modulate the opening of the PT pore. Ca^{2+} efflux is primarily managed by the Na^+/Ca^{2+} exchanger (NCE). Ca^{2+} can also enter the mitochondria as can a large number of small metabolites via the PT pore opening

Another important factor by which mitochondria impact contractility is via ROS production. ROS accumulation significantly alters myocardial ion channel flux and membrane ion pump function in part by generalized membrane damage arising from ROS-mediated lipid peroxidation. More specific effects of ROS include targeting the L-type calcium channels on the myocyte sarcolemma and suppressing the Ca^{2+} current [177] and targeting the activity of the sarcoplasmic reticulum Ca^{2+}ATPase(SERCA2), a membrane Ca^{2+} pump involved in cardiac Ca^{2+} handling and a determinant of myocardial contractility [178]. ROS generation can also affect the function of cardiac sodium channels, potassium channels, and ion exchangers, such as the Na^+/Ca^{2+} exchanger [179]. In addition, ROS can decrease the Ca^{2+} sensitivity of the myofilaments via ROS-mediated phosphorylation of contractile proteins such as troponin T [180], which could lead to abnormalities in excitation–contraction coupling. Whether this pathway actually contributes to human HF remains unknown.

It is noteworthy that while contractile dysfunction clearly contributes to HF, there is no direct evidence that depressed contractility has a causative role in its initiation and progression nor in the profound structural remodeling that occurs in the failing heart since substantial cardiac remodeling can occur in HF in the absence of depressed myocyte contractility [181, 182].

Magnitude of Cellular and Molecular Changes Associated with Mitochondria in HF

A number of the aforementioned cellular/molecular changes observed during HF involve mitochondria and bioenergetic production. However, this relationship requires further exploration. It could be argued that mitochondrial dysfunction plays an integral part in the mechanism of cardiac dysfunction, even when other factors are more evident or it may represent a common downstream event in the pathways leading to HF. In most cases of HF, it remains to be established whether the mitochondrial abnormalities associated with other myocardial changes are truly primary or secondary to other abnormalities in myocardium (e.g., hypertrophy, remodeling, etc.) as compared to the less speculative nature of the mitochondrial defects in the cases discussed of primary mitochondrial dysfunction. Cardiac hypertrophic changes have been associated with increased mitochondrial number and size as well as increased mtDNA synthesis [183, 184]. Early studies of rat cardiac hypertrophy found a coordination between complex IV activity, nuclear-encoded mRNA, and mitochondrial rRNA synthesis. Within 24 h after growth stimulus, a specific decrease was found only in mitochondrial mRNA synthesis [176]. Furthermore, thyroid hormone can affect mitochondrial structure and function.

For instance, thyroid hormone treatment causes cardiac hypertrophy similar to aortic stenosis in rats [185]. Both models of cardiac hypertrophy show increases in total tissue RNA accompanying increases in ventricular weight as well as in both cytosolic and mitochondrial ribosomes. Thyroxin can also modulate increases in mitochondrial enzyme activities [186]. It has been suggested that regulation is exerted at the level of transcriptional regulation of nuclear genes encoding mitochondrial proteins (including components of the respiratory pathway). This regulatory effect may occur as a result of many of the nuclear-encoded mitochondrial genes having thyroxin-sensitive promoter elements.

What Events Occurring in HF Are Truly Tissue Specific

The finding of shared events in skeletal muscle and heart during HF has considerable prognostic implication for the clinician. Yet to date, despite (and possibly because) of the immense research effort in this area, the relationship between cardiac and skeletal muscle events in HF at the cellular and molecular levels has not been comprehensively examined. A number of changes occur in skeletal muscle during HF, such as histological and electromyographic evidence of generalized myopathy and exercise intolerance. Evaluation of skeletal muscle metabolism by the non-invasive methodology of phosphorus nuclear magnetic resonance spectroscopy demonstrated altered levels of phosphocreatine and inorganic phosphate in HF patients following moderate exercise [187, 188]. Patients with desmin and β-MHC mutations known to cause HCM and HF have defined changes in skeletal muscle fibers; patients with specific β-MHC mutations may develop abnormal mitochondrial number and function in skeletal muscle, as well as type I fiber abnormalities and atrophy [189–191]. HF is often accompanied by skeletal myopathy with a shift from slow aerobic fatigue-resistant fibers to fast anaerobic ones. Is the fiber atrophy mediated by apoptosis? Evidence of apoptosis as gauged by TUNEL, as well as significantly reduced expression of Bcl-2 has been demonstrated in both skeletal muscle tissues of patients with chronic HF [192], and from rats with experimentally-induced HF [193]. Interestingly, evidence of increased iNOS was also noted in the HF patients.

Structural and functional changes in skeletal muscle mitochondria have also been found in cardiomyopathy/HF [194, 195]. In addition, pathogenic mtDNA mutations (e.g., 3243, 3260, 4269, 8344, 8363, 9997) present in cardiomyopathy with a broad spectrum of myopathies and accompanying respiratory enzyme defects, are present at relatively high levels in skeletal muscle. Furthermore, the use of skeletal muscle biopsies (instead of endomyocardial biopsy) for analysis of respiratory enzyme dysfunction has been recommended in the diagnostic evaluation of mitochondrial-mediated cardiac abnormalities [196]. Furthermore, reduction in specific enzyme activities has been found in both skeletal and cardiac muscle in a group of children with cardiomyopathy [196]. Similarly, pronounced complex IV defects have been found in both cardiac and skeletal muscle of patients with KSS and cardiomyopathy [197]. In some patients, the mitochondrial dysfunction is treatable by supplementation with vitamins, coenzyme Q, and/or carnitine.

While an increasing incidence of cardiac mtDNA deletions in patients with DCM has been reported [166, 198, 199], scarce data are available regarding the tissue-specificity or correlation of the extent of cardiac mtDNA deletions with skeletal muscle deletions in the same patient. In isolated cases of KSS with cardiomyopathy, both skeletal muscle and heart harbored high amount of mtDNA deletion [200]. Also, multiple mtDNA deletions have been detected in skeletal muscle of patients with cardiomyopathy. However, it remained unknown whether deletions were present in cardiac tissue since cardiac biopsies were not available [169]. Similarly, patients with decreased levels of cardiac mtDNA have not been studied with regards to the levels of skeletal muscle mtDNA. Patients with both cardiomyopathy and myopathy have been reported to contain skeletal muscle mtDNA depletion (not investigated in heart) [201]. The pathological effects of AZT on mtDNA levels, respiratory complex activities and on phenotype have been demonstrated in both heart and skeletal muscle from human and animal models [202].

Taken together, many of the cellular cardiac changes as well as mitochondrial abnormalities often found in HF appear to be present in skeletal muscle. While more evidence confirming these findings is warranted, evaluation of skeletal muscle mitochondrial function could be helpful in the overall diagnostic and prognostic evaluation of HF. To determine what other parts of the HF signaling-pathway are truly cardiac specific and which might be also operative in skeletal muscle awaits further studies. Such studies might shed light about the relationship between the signaling pathway(s) and mitochondrial energetics.

Conclusion: The Road Ahead

The critical involvement of mitochondria and mitochondrial pathways in myocardial bioenergetic regulation, in the balance of oxidants and antioxidants, and in the progression of cell-death are critical contributory factors to the cardiac dysfunction and remodeling found in the failing heart. The identification of nuclear and mitochondrial components of these pathways and delineation of their cross-talk has suggested a number of potential targets for the clinical treatment of HF.

Among the novel intervention strategies being developed include the targeting of apoptosis which appears to be reversible, at least in part. Such an approach will have to be finely targeted since apoptotic inhibition or prosurvival pathway stimulation could result in unwanted proliferative growth. A second approach involves the targeting of metabolic remodeling. As pointed out by Neubauer [2], the multiple metabolic loci that can cause HF and cardiac dysfunction if ablated is a testimonial to the fully integrated metabolic machinery that is necessary for normal cardiac function, supporting the concept that chronic HF is multifactorial and begs the question whether perturbation of any metabolic components can lead to HF.

Several observations suggest that increasing the capacity for glucose utilization may delay HF progression; however, it remains unclear whether upregulating FAO will be helpful. Findings from rodent models that this metabolic modulation can be effected by targeting global nuclear receptors/transcriptional regulators (i.e., PPARs and PGC-1) with exogenous agonists or by nutritional interventions (e.g., caloric restriction) may eventually be clinically applied in treating HF. This approach of targeting transcriptional regulation addresses the programmatic shift in mitochondrial bioenergetic function indicated by the broad array of bioenergetic loci affected in HF and by transcriptional profiling studies in both human and animal models [93, 162, 203].

Although the use of transgenic mice with defined mutations to study their impact and relationship to HF has also been very informative, there still remains a gap in information about the physiological, biochemical, and molecular events happening in the normal mouse heart. What is needed is a rigorous standardization of quantitative measurements relevant to mitochondrial bioenergetics, structure, and function in both cardiac and skeletal muscle tissues. This should include an evaluation of the levels of mitochondrial enzyme activities, mtDNA, ATP, ADP and NADH, as well as a comprehensive investigation of mitochondrial changes (including mtDNA deletions) as a function of age. Particular focus should be directed to the activity levels and content of mitochondrial ATP synthase and ANT, given the degree to which they appear affected in HF. Such information should provide the requisite database, to investigate and compare the direct effects of introducing mutant genes in animal model (e.g., mouse) to test for pathogenic mutations that effect both mitochondria and cardiac function. Further refinement will also be needed to overcome the technical hurdle that presently exists in introducing and testing specific mtDNA mutations and their pathogenic effects in a whole animal model, as well as more precise monitoring of cellular and molecular events in the myocardium in a less invasive manner than endomyocardial biopsy.

Furthermore, novel approaches to increase ATP or PCr levels and ATP synthesis in the failing heart are critically needed; while new pharmacological approaches are likely in the more immediate future, down the road, both genetic and cell-mediated therapies (e.g., stem-cells), which have shown promise in preclinical models may be utilized for clinical treatment. Along these lines, strategies aimed at activating mitochondrial responses against OS and targeting the signaling pathways identified in pharmacological and ischemic conditioning (which feature mitochondrial elements) may also offer the potential to provide clinical cardioprotection in the treatment of human HF.

In addition, gene therapy for treatment of mitochondrial cytopathies is under development and promise to be useful in targeting mitochondrial-based disorders. Hopefully, future studies will also allow an understanding of the temporal order of changes in mitochondrial structure and function, as well as their contribution to the pathophysiological events in HF.

Summary

- The failing heart encompasses a complex phenotype that includes reduced myocardial contractility, diminished capacity to respond to specific hypoxic and oxidative stresses resulting from myocardial ischemia and diverse neurohormonal stimuli, changes in ion channels and electrophysiological function, increased myocardial fibrosis, cellular and subcellular remodeling with increased myocyte loss, and marked alterations in myocardial bioenergetic reserves and substrate utilization.
- Mitochondrial bioenergetic metabolism may be critical and primary in the development of HF.
- Mitochondrial defects may underlie several aspects of the HF phenotypes.
- The role of fuel supply, and in particular, ATP levels are critical for myocardial contractility and electrophysiology.
- Fatty acids are the primary energy substrate for heart muscle ATP generation by mitochondrial OXPHOS and the respiratory chain, the most important energetic pathway providing over 90% of cardiac energy.
- Under conditions which increase ATP demand in excess of ATP supply such as in acute pump failure in ischemia, utilization of PCr via the CK reaction is an important mechanism that maintains steady myocardial ATP levels.
- Observations from patients in HF have shown reduced activity levels of mitochondrial bioenergetic enzymes including selected respiratory enzymes and mt-CK.
- Data from animal models of HF have also shown that the loss of ATP associated mitochondrial ROS damage affects a wide spectrum of cardiomyocyte functions including contractility, ion transport, and calcium cycling.
- Loss in the total adenine nucleotide pool in the failing myocardium is slow and progressive suggesting that a decline in ATP content might only be detectable in severe HF.
- Even at moderate workloads, a decrease in PCr/ATP ratio has been consistently reported in the failing human heart and in experimental HF. This is a strong predictor of cardiovascular mortality in patients with DCM (even better than LV ejection fraction).
- Mitochondrial contribution to HF may relate to its role in ROS production.
- Mitochondrial-generated ROS can lead to extensive oxidative damage to macromolecules such as proteins, DNA, and lipids particularly targeting proximal mitochondrial components including mitochondrial respiratory enzymes, matrix enzymes (e.g., aconitase), and membrane phospholipids such as cardiolipin.
- Mitochondrial ROS damage affects a wide spectrum of cardiomyocyte functions including contractility, ion transport, and calcium cycling.
- Among the most compelling evidence supporting a primary role for mitochondrial ROS and OS in cardiomyopathy and HF are findings with antioxidant genes in transgenic mice.
- While elevated ROS activation in the failing heart has been shown to arise from both mitochondrial and extramitochondrial sources, the role of endogenous antioxidants in ameliorating myocardial OS and the dynamic balance between these counteracting forces should be considered.
- Overexpression of the antioxidant glutathione peroxidase in transgenic mice inhibited the development of LV remodeling and failure after myocardial infarct (MI), and was associated with the attenuation of myocyte hypertrophy, apoptosis, and interstitial fibrosis.
- The mitochondrial-mediated intrinsic apoptotic pathway features an extensive dialog between the mitochondria, the nucleus, and other subcellular organelles.
- The release of several mitochondrial-specific proteins from the intermembrane space including cytochrome c, endonuclease G (EndoG), apoptosis inducing factor (AIF), and Smac are central to the early triggering events in the apoptotic pathway including downstream caspase activation, nuclear DNA fragmentation, and cell death.
- Protein release from the intermembrane space and cristae, where the majority of cytochrome c is localized, also is associated with opening of the voltage-sensitive PT pore located at the contact sites between inner and outer membranes.
- While myocardial apoptotic induction is frequently associated with abnormal mitochondrial respiratory function, the basis of this relationship remains unclear.

- Targeting apoptotic factors has been shown to reverse the cardiomyopathy/HF phenotype and associated mitochondrial dysfunction underscoring the interconnected roles of apoptosis and mitochondrial dysfunction in HF.
- In contrast to apoptosis, necrotic cell death is not energy-requiring and exhibits characteristic features that include swelling of the cell and its organelles, extensive mitochondrial disruption, blebbing and ultimately irreversible disintegration of the plasma membrane.
- In contrast with necrosis, autophagic cell death similar to apoptosis is characterized by the absence of tissue inflammatory response.
- A canine model in which rapid ventricular pacing leads to an increase in chamber dimension, wall thinning, elevation in ventricular wall stress, and congestive HF recapitulates many features of human DCM and HF.
- By proteomic analysis, many of the cardiac proteins altered in the canine model of pacing-induced HF are involved in energy metabolism.
- Data obtained from biochemical analysis in paced dogs documented a significant decrease in cardiac respiratory complex III and V activities.
- Similar respiratory dysfunction (relative to enzymes affected) was present in both skeletal muscle and cardiac tissues supporting the view that pacing inducing HF involves a generalized metabolic myopathy.
- Differences in specific mitochondrial subpopulations associated with distinct cardiac compartments may contribute to the observed enzymatic dysfunction observed in HF.
- While initial studies in paced canine hearts revealed mtDNA damage (i.e., large-scale mtDNA deletions detected by PCR), the levels of deletion relative to wild-type mtDNA were very low (less than 1%) and their significance is unclear.
- In another model of HF, the murine model of myocardial infarct (MI) was found that LV dilation and contractility dysfunction were accompanied by significant increases in levels of mitochondrial ROS (i.e., hydroxyl radicals) and lipid peroxides.
- The issue and extent of mitochondrial transcriptional changes in different animal models of HF remains largely unsettled.
- Transgenic mice with abnormal expression of genes involved in bioenergetic metabolism have provided unique insights into the cause–effect relationships between mitochondrial function and HF.
- Since the majority of the components of mitochondrial bioenergetic, biogenesis, and signaling pathways are encoded by nuclear DNA, regulation of the mitochondrial programmed changes detected in HF largely arise in the nucleus.
- Expression of PGC-1α in cardiac myocytes has been found to induce both nuclear and mitochondrial gene expression involved in multiple mitochondrial bioenergetic pathways, with increased mitochondrial biogenesis, respiration, and FAO.
- PGC-1α overexpression in the heart of adult mice resulted in a modest increase in mitochondrial number, derangements of mitochondrial ultrastructure, and development of a reversible cardiomyopathy characterized by loss of sarcomeric structure and increased ventricular mass and chamber dilatation.
- PPAR-α may play a contributory role in the energy substrate switch away from fatty acid utilization in the hypertrophied failing heart.
- Mouse strains containing null genes encoding cytosolic proteins, such as desmin and calcineurin, develop HF associated with significant mitochondrial dysfunction.
- Altered Ca^{2+} homeostasis is recognized as a key pathophysiological mechanism in HF, leading to altered contractile function, activation of signaling pathways and transcriptional activity.
- Ca^{2+} homeostasis depends on efficient energy-driven ion pumps, while Ca^{2+} concentration in turn influences energy expenditure through its activation of cellular ATPases and mitochondrial dehydrogenases.
- Many of the cellular cardiac changes as well as mitochondrial abnormalities often found in HF appear to be present in skeletal muscle.
- Sporadic cases of cardiomyopathy with a severe mtDNA depletion and associated reduction in cardiac and/or skeletal muscle mitochondrial respiratory activities have also been reported.
- The identification of nuclear and mitochondrial components of these pathways and delineation of their cross-talk has suggested a number of potential targets for the clinical treatment of HF.
- Some technical hurdles need to be overcome in the testing of specific mtDNA mutations and their pathogenic effects in whole animal model.

References

1. Ventura-Clapier R, Garnier A, Veksler V (2004) Energy metabolism in heart failure. J Physiol 555:1–13
2. Neubauer S (2007) The failing heart – An engine out of fuel. N Engl J Med 356:1140–1151
3. van Bilsen M, Smeets PJ, Gilde AJ, van der Vusse GJ (2004) Metabolic remodeling of the failing heart: the cardiac burn-out syndrome? Cardiovasc Res 61:218–226
4. Katz AM (2004) Is the failing heart energy depleted? Cardiol Clin 16:633–644
5. Ingwall JS, Weiss RG (2004) Is the failing heart energy starved? On using chemical energy to support cardiac function. Circ Res 95:135–145
6. Weiss JN, Lamp ST (1989) Cardiac ATP-sensitive K+ channels: evidence for preferential regulation by glycolysis. J Gen Physiol 94:911–935

7. Rizzuto R, Pinton P, Carrington W, Fay FS, Fogarty KE, Lifshitz LM, Tuft RA, Pozzan T (1998) Close contacts with the endoplasmic reticulum as determinants of mitochondrial Ca^{2+} responses. Science 280:1763–1766

8. Bittl JA, Ingwall JS (1985) Reaction rates of creatine kinase and ATP synthesis in the isolated rat heart. A ^{31}P NMR magnetization transfer study. J Biol Chem 260:3512–3517

9. Jarreta D, Orus J, Barrientos A, Miro O, Roig E, Heras M, Moraes CT, Cardellach F, Casademont J (2000) Mitochondrial function in heart muscle from patients with idiopathic dilated cardiomyopathy. Cardiovasc Res 45:860–865

10. Marin-Garcia J, Goldenthal MJ, Pierpont ME, Ananthakrishnan R (1995) Impaired mitochondrial function in idiopathic dilated cardiomyopathy: biochemical and molecular analysis. J Card Fail 1:285–291

11. Quigley AF, Kapsa RM, Esmore D, Hale G, Byrne E (2000) Mitochondrial respiratory chain activity in idiopathic dilated cardiomyopathy. J Card Fail 6:47–55

12. Ingwall JS, Atkinson DE, Clarke K, Fetters JK (1990) Energetic correlates of cardiac failure: changes in the creatine kinase system in the failing myocardium. Eur Heart J 11:108–115

13. Starling RC, Hammer DF, Altschuld RA (1998) Human myocardial ATP content and in vivo contractile function. Mol Cell Biochem 180:171–177

14. Beer M, Seyfarth T, Sandstede J, Landschutz W, Lipke C, Kostler H, von Kienlin M, Harre K, Hahn D, Neubauer S (2002) Absolute concentrations of high-energy phosphate metabolites in normal, hypertrophied, and failing human myocardium measured noninvasively with (31)P-SLOOP magnetic resonance spectroscopy. J Am Coll Cardiol 40:1267–1274

15. Shen W, Asai K, Uechi M, Mathier MA, Shannon RP, Vatner SF, Ingwall JS (1999) Progressive loss of myocardial ATP due to a loss of total purines during the development of heart failure in dogs: a compensatory role for the parallel loss of creatine. Circulation 100:2113–2118

16. Tian R, Ingwall JS (1999) The molecular energetics of the failing heart from animal models-small animal models. Heart Fail Rev 4:235–253

17. Zhang J, Bache RJ (1999) The molecular energetics of the failing heart from animal models - large animal models. Heart Fail Rev 4:255–267

18. Nakae I, Mitsunami K, Omura T, Yabe T, Tsutamoto T, Matsuo S, Takahashi M, Morikawa S, Inubushi T, Nakamura Y, Kinoshita M, Horie M (2003) Proton magnetic resonance spectroscopy can detect creatine depletion associated with the progression of heart failure in cardiomyopathy. J Am Coll Cardiol 42:1587–1593

19. Hardy CJ, Weiss RG, Bottomley PA, Gerstenblith G (1991) Altered myocardial high-energy phosphate metabolites in patients with dilated cardiomyopathy. Am Heart J 122:795–801

20. Neubauer S, Horn M, Cramer M, Harre K, Newell JB, Peters W, Pabst T, Ertl G, Hahn D, Ingwall JS, Kochsiek K (1997) Myocardial phosphocreatine-to-ATP ratio is a predictor of mortality in patients with dilated cardiomyopathy. Circulation 96:2190–2196

21. Neubauer S, Remkes H, Spindler M, Horn M, Weismann F, Prestle J, Walzel B, Ertl G, Hasenfuss G, Wallimann T (1999) Down regulation of the Na(+)-creatine co-transporter in failing human myocardium and in experimental heart failure. Circulation 100: 1847–1850

22. Saupe KW, Spindler M, Hopkins JC, Shen W, Ingwall JS (2000) Kinetic, thermodynamic, and developmental consequences of deleting creatine kinase isoenzymes from the heart. Reaction kinetics of the creatine kinase isoenzymes in the intact heart. J Biol Chem 275:19742–19746

23. Esposito LA, Melov S, Panov A, Cottrell BA, Wallace DC (1999) Mitochondrial disease in mouse results in increased oxidative stress. Proc Natl Acad Sci USA 96:4820–4825

24. Graham BH, Waymire KG, Cottrell B, Trounce IA, MacGregor GR, Wallace DC (1997) A mouse model for mitochondrial myopathy and cardiomyopathy resulting from a deficiency in the heart/muscle isoform of the adenine nucleotide translocator. Nat Genet 16:226–234

25. Nahrendorf M, Spindler M, Hu K, Bauer L, Ritter O, Nordbeck P, Quaschning T, Hiller KH, Wallis J, Ertl G, Bauer WR, Neubauer S (2005) Creatine kinase knockout mice show left ventricular hypertrophy and dilatation, but unaltered remodeling post-myocardial infarction. Cardiovasc Res 65:419–427

26. De Sousa E, Veksler V, Minajeva A, Kaasik A, Mateo P, Mayoux E, Hoerter J, Bigard X, Serrurier B, Ventura-Clapier R (1999) Subcellular creatine kinase alterations – Implications in heart failure. Circ Res 85:68–76

27. Palmieri L, Alberio S, Pisano I, Lodi T, Meznaric-Petrusa M, Zidar J, Santoro A, Scarcia P, Fontanesi F, Lamantea E, Ferrero I, Zeviani M (2005) Complete loss-of-function of the heart/muscle-specific adenine nucleotide translocator is associated with mitochondrial myopathy and cardiomyopathy. Hum Mol Genet 14:3079–3088

28. Marín-García J, Goldenthal MJ (2002) Understanding the impact of mitochondrial defects in cardiovascular disease: a review. J Card Fail 8:347–361

29. Andreu AL, Checcarelli N, Iwata S, Shanske S, DiMauro S (2000) A missense mutation in the mitochondrial cytochrome b gene in a revisited case with histiocytoid cardiomyopathy. Pediatr Res 48:311–314

30. Pastores GM, Santorelli FM, Shanske S, Gelb BD, Fyfe B, Wolfe D, Willner JP (1994) Leigh syndrome and hypertrophic cardiomyopathy in an infant with a mitochondrial DNA point mutation (T8993G). Am J Med Genet 50:265–271

31. Jonckheere A, Hogeveen M, Nijtmans L, van den Brand M, Janssen A, Diepstra H, van den Brandt F, van den Heuvel L, Hol F, Hofste T, Kapusta L, Dillmann U, Shamdeen M, Smeitink J, Rodenburg R (2008) A novel mitochondrial ATP8 (MT-ATP8) gene mutation in a patient with apical hypertrophic cardiomyopathy and neuropathy. J Med Genet 45:129–133

32. Ide T, Tsutsui H, Hayashidani S, Kang D, Suematsu N, Nakamura K, Utsumi H, Hamasaki N, Takeshita A (2001) Mitochondrial DNA damage and dysfunction associated with oxidative stress in failing hearts after myocardial infarction. Circ Res 88:529–535

33. Ide T, Tsutsui H, Kinugawa S, Utsumi H, Kang D, Hattori N, Uchida K, Arimura K, Egashira K, Takeshita A (1999) Mitochondrial electron transport complex I is a potential source of oxygen free radicals in the failing myocardium. Circ Res 85:357–363

34. Ide T, Tsutsui H, Kinugawa S, Suematsu N, Hayashidani S, Ichikawa K, Utsumi H, Machida Y, Egashira K, Takeshita A (2000) Direct evidence for increased hydroxyl radicals originating from superoxide in the failing myocardium. Circ Res 86:152–157

35. Giordano FJ (2005) Oxygen, oxidative stress, hypoxia, and heart failure. J Clin Invest 115:500–508

36. Cesselli D, Jakoniuk I, Barlucchi L, Beltrami AP, Hintze TH, Nadal-Ginard B, Kajstura J, Leri A, Anversa P (2001) Oxidative stress–mediated cardiac cell death is a major determinant of ventricular dysfunction and failure in dog dilated cardiomyopathy. Circ Res 89:279–286

37. Marin-Garcia J, Goldenthal MJ, Moe GW (2001) Abnormal cardiac and skeletal muscle mitochondrial function in pacing-induced cardiac failure. Cardiovasc Res 52:103–110

38. Nordberg J, Arner ES (2001) Reactive oxygen species, antioxidants, and the mammalian thioredoxin system. Free Radic Biol Med 31:1287–1312

39. Nojiri H, Shimizu T, Funakoshi M, Yamaguchi O, Zhou H, Kawakami S, Ohta Y, Sami M, Tachibana T, Ishikawa H, Kurosawa H, Kahn RC, Otsu K, Shirasawa T (2006) Oxidative stress causes heart failure with impaired mitochondrial respiration. J Biol Chem 281:33789–33801

40. Huang TT, Carlson EJ, Kozy HM, Mantha S, Goodman SI, Ursell PC, Epstein CJ (2001) Genetic modification of prenatal lethality and dilated cardiomyopathy in Mn superoxide dismutase mutant mice. Free Radic Biol Med 31:1101–1110

41. Conrad M, Jakupoglu C, Moreno SG, Lippl S, Banjac A, Schneider M, Beck H, Hatzopoulos AK, Just U, Sinowatz F, Schmahl W, Chien KR, Wurst W, Bornkamm GW, Brielmeier M (2004) Essential role for mitochondrial thioredoxin reductase in hematopoiesis, heart development, and heart function. Mol Cell Biol 24:9414–9423

42. Li Y, Huang TT, Carlson EJ, Melov S, Ursell PC, Olson JL, Noble LJ, Yoshimura MP, Berger C, Chan PH, Wallace DC, Epstein CJ (1995) Dilated cardiomyopathy and neonatal lethality in mutant mice lacking manganese superoxide dismutase. Nat Genet 11: 376–381

43. Shiomi T, Tsutsui H, Matsusaka H, Murakami K, Hayashidani S, Ikeuchi M, Wen J, Kubota T, Utsumi H, Takeshita A (2004) Overexpression of glutathione peroxidase prevents left ventricular remodeling and failure after myocardial infarction in mice. Circulation 109:544–549

44. Schriner SE, Linford NJ, Martin GM, Treuting P, Ogburn CE, Emond M, Coskun PE, Ladiges W, Wolf N, Van Remmen H, Wallace DC, Rabinovitch PS (2005) Extension of murine life span by overexpression of catalase targeted to mitochondria. Science 308:1909–1911

45. Mak S, Newton GE (2001) The oxidative stress hypothesis of congestive heart failure radical thoughts. Chest 120:2035–2046

46. Sam F, Kerstetter DL, Pimental DR, Mulukutla S, Tabaee A, Bristow MR, Colucci WS, Sawyer DB (2005) Increased reactive oxygen species production and functional alterations in antioxidant enzymes in human failing myocardium. J Card Fail 11:473–480

47. Narula J, Haider N, Virmani R, DiSalvo TG, Kolodgie FD, Hajjar RJ, Schmidt U, Semigran MJ, Dec GW, Khaw BA (1996) Apoptosis in myocytes in end-stage heart failure. N Engl J Med 35: 1182–1189

48. Olivetti G, Abbi R, Quaini F, Kajstura J, Cheng W, Nitahara JA, Quaini E, Di Loreto C, Beltrami CA, Krajewski S, Reed JC, Anversa P (1997) Apoptosis in the failing heart. N Engl J Med 336:1131–1141

49. Danial NN, Korsmeyer SJ (2004) Cell death: critical control points. Cell 116:205–219

50. Li LY, Luo X, Wang X (2001) Endonuclease G is an apoptotic DNase when released from mitochondria. Nature 412:95–99

51. Susin SA, Lorenzo HK, Zamzami N, Marzo I, Snow BE, Brothers GM, Mangion J, Jacotot E, Costantini P, Loeffler M, Larochette N, Goodlett DR, Aebersold R, Siderovski DP, Penninger JM, Kroemer G (1999) Molecular characterization of mitochondrial apoptosis-inducing factor. Nature 397:441–446

52. Liu X, Kim CN, Yang J, Jemmerson R, Wang X (1996) Induction of apoptotic program in cell-free extracts: requirement for dATP and cytochrome c. Cell 86:147–157

53. Kroemer G (2003) Mitochondrial control of apoptosis: an introduction. Biochem Biophys Res Commun 304:433–435

54. Marzo I, Brenner C, Zamzami N, Susin SA, Beutner G, Brdiczka D, Remy R, Xie ZH, Reed JC, Kroemer G (1998) The permeability transition pore complex: a target for apoptosis regulation by caspases and Bcl-2 related proteins. J Exp Med 187:1261–1267

55. Scorrano L, Ashiya M, Buttle K, Weiler S, Oakes S, Mannella CA, Korsmeyer SJ (2002) A distinct pathway remodels mitochondrial cristae and mobilizes cytochrome c during apoptosis. Dev Cell 2:55–67

56. Scorrano L, Oakes SA, Opferman JT, Cheng EH, Sorcinelli MD, Pozzan T, Korsmeyer SJ (2003) BAX and BAK regulation of endoplasmic reticulum Ca2+: a control point for apoptosis. Science 300:135–139

57. Morishima N, Nakanishi K, Tsuchiya K, Shibata T, Seiwa E (2004) Translocation of Bim to the endoplasmic reticulum (ER) mediates ER stress signaling for activation of caspase-12 during ER stress-induced apoptosis. J Biol Chem 279:50375–50381

58. Neuse M, Monticone R, Lundberg MS, Chesley AT, Fleck E, Crow MT (2001) The apoptotic regulatory protein ARC (apoptosis repressor with caspase recruitment domain) prevents oxidant stress-mediated cell death by preserving mitochondrial function. J Biol Chem 276:33915–33922

59. Pi Y, Goldenthal MJ, Marín-García J (2007) Mitochondrial involvement in IGF-1 induced protection of cardiomyocytes against hypoxia/reoxygenation injury. Mol Cell Biochem 301:181–189

60. Akyurek O, Akyurek N, Sayin T, Dincer I, Berkalp B, Akyol G, Ozenci M, Oral D (2001) Association between the severity of heart failure and the susceptibility of myocytes to apoptosis in patients with idiopathic dilated cardiomyopathy. Int J Cardiol 80: 29–36

61. Kirshenbaum LA, de Moissac D (1997) The bcl-2 gene product prevents programmed cell death of ventricular myocytes. Circulation 96:1580–1585

62. Zhu L, Yu Y, Chua BH, Ho YS, Kuo TH (2001) Regulation of sodium-calcium exchange and mitochondrial energetics by Bcl-2 in the heart of transgenic mice. J Mol Cell Cardiol 33:2135–2144

63. Kang PM, Haunstetter A, Aoki H, Usheva A, Izumo S (2000) Morphological and molecular characterization of adult cardiomyocyte apoptosis during hypoxia and reoxygenation. Circ Res 87:118–125

64. Milner DJ, Mavroidis M, Weisleder N, Capetanaki Y (2000) Desmin cytoskeleton linked to muscle mitochondrial distribution and respiratory function. J Cell Biol 150:1283–1298

65. Linden M, Li Z, Paulin D, Gotow T, Leterrier JF (2001) Effects of desmin gene knockout on mice heart mitochondria. J Bioenerg Biomembr 33:333–341

66. Weisleder N, Taffet GE, Capetanaki Y (2004) Bcl-2 overexpression corrects mitochondrial defects and ameliorates inherited desmin null cardiomyopathy. Proc Natl Acad Sci USA 101:769–774

67. Imahashi K, Schneider MD, Steenbergen C, Murphy E (2004) Transgenic expression of Bcl-2 modulates energy metabolism, prevents cytosolic acidification during ischemia, and reduces ischemia/reperfusion injury. Circ Res 95:734–741

68. Vahsen N, Cande C, Briere JJ, Benit P, Joza N, Larochette N, Mastroberardino PG, Pequignot MO, Casares N, Lazar V, Feraud O, Debili N, Wissing S, Engelhardt S, Madeo F, Piacentini M, Penninger JM, Schagger H, Rustin P, Kroemer G (2004) AIF deficiency compromises oxidative phosphorylation. EMBO J 23: 4679–4689

69. Joza N, Oudit GY, Brown D, Benit P, Kassiri Z, Vahsen N, Benoit L, Patel MM, Nowikovsky K, Vassault A, Backx PH, Wada T, Kroemer G, Rustin P, Penninger JM (2005) Muscle-specific loss of apoptosis-inducing factor leads to mitochondrial dysfunction, skeletal muscle atrophy, and dilated cardiomyopathy. Mol Cell Biol 25:10261–10272

70. Kajstura J, Cheng W, Reiss K, Clark WA, Sonnenblick EH, Krajewski S, Reed JC, Olivetti G, Anversa P (1996) Apoptotic and necrotic myocyte cell death are independent contributing variables of infarct size in rats. Lab Invest 74:86–107

71. Rayment NB, Haven AJ, Madden B, Murday A, Trickey R, Shipley MJ, Katz DR (1999) Myocyte loss in chronic heart failure. J Pathol 188:213–219

72. Gill C, Mestril R, Samali A (2002) Losing heart: the role of apoptosis in heart disease – a novel therapeutic target? FASEB J 16: 135–146

73. Honda O, Kuroda M, Joja I, Asaumi J, Takeda Y, Akaki S, Togami I, Kanazawa S, Kawasaki S, Hiraki Y (2000) Assessment of secondary necrosis of Jurkat cells using a new microscopic system and double staining method with annexin V and propidium iodide. Int J Oncol 16:283–288

74. Malhi H, Gores GJ, Lemasters JJ (2006) Apoptosis and necrosis in the liver: a tale of two deaths? Hepatology 43:S31–S44

75. Kim JS, He L, Lemasters JJ (2003) Mitochondrial permeability transition: a common pathway to necrosis and apoptosis. Biochem Biophys Res Commun 304:463–470

76. Lemasters JJ, Nieminen AL, Qian T, Trost LC, Elmore SP, Nishimura Y, Crowe RA, Cascio WE, Bradham CA, Brenner DA, Herman B (1998) The mitochondrial permeability transition in cell death: a common mechanism in necrosis, apoptosis and autophagy. Biochim Biophys Acta 1366:177–196

77. Zamzami N, Hirsch T, Dallaporta B, Petit PX, Kroemer G (1997) Mitochondrial implication in accidental and programmed cell death: apoptosis and necrosis. J Bioenerg Biomembr 29:185–213

78. Nakayama H, Chen X, Baines CP, Klevitsky R, Zhang X, Zhang H, Jaleel N, Chua BH, Hewett TE, Robbins J, Houser SR, Molkentin JD (2007) Ca2+- and mitochondrial-dependent cardiomyocyte necrosis as a primary mediator of heart failure. J Clin Invest 117:2431–2444

79. Knaapen MW, Davies MJ, De Bie M, Haven AJ, Martinet W, Kockx MM (2001) Apoptotic versus autophagic cell death in heart failure. Cardiovasc Res 51:304–312

80. Levine B, Yuan J (2005) Autophagy in cell death: an innocent convict? J Clin Invest 115:2679–2688

81. Scherz-Shouval R, Elazar Z (2007) ROS, mitochondria and the regulation of autophagy. Trends Cell Biol 17:422–427

82. Moe GW, Armstrong PW (1999) Pacing-induced heart failure: a model to study the mechanism of disease progression and novel therapy in heart failure. Cardiovasc Res 42:591–599

83. Heinke MY, Wheeler CH, Yan JX, Amin V, Chang D, Einstein R, Dunn MJ, Dos Remedios CG (1999) Changes in myocardial protein expression in pacing-induced canine heart failure. Electrophoresis 20:2086–2093

84. O'Brien PJ, Ianuzzo CD, Moe GW, Stopps TP, Armstrong PW (1990) Rapid ventricular pacing of dogs to heart failure: biochemical and physiological studies. Can J Physiol Pharmacol 68: 34–39

85. O'Brien PJ, Moe GW, Nowack LM, Grima EA, Armstrong PW (1994) Sarcoplasmic reticulum Ca-release channel and ATP-synthesis activities are early myocardial markers of heart failure produced by rapid ventricular pacing in dogs. Can J Physiol Pharmacol 72:999–1006

86. Ananthakrishnan R, Moe GW, Goldenthal MJ, Marín-García J (2005) Akt signaling pathway in pacing-induced heart failure. Mol Cell Biochem 268:103–110

87. Liu Y, Cigola E, Cheng W, Kajstura J, Olivetti G, Hintze TH, Anversa P (1995) Myocyte nuclear mitotic division and programmed myocyte cell death characterize the cardiac myopathy induced by rapid ventricular pacing in dogs. Lab Invest 73: 771–787

88. Ventura-Clapier R, De Sousa E, Veksler V (2002) Metabolic myopathy in heart failure. News Physiol Sci 17:191–196

89. Drexler H, Riede U, Munzel T, Konig H, Funke E, Just H (1992) Alterations of skeletal muscle in chronic heart failure. Circulation 85:1751–1759

90. Sullivan MJ, Green HJ, Cobb FR (1990) Skeletal muscle biochemistry and histology in ambulatory patients with long-term heart failure. Circulation 81:518–527

91. Tsutsui H, Ide T, Hayashidani S, Suematsu N, Shiomi T, Wen J, Nakamura Ki, Ichikawa K, Utsumi H, Takeshita A (2001) Enhanced generation of reactive oxygen species in the limb skeletal muscles from a murine infarct model of heart failure. Circulation 104: 134–136

92. López Farré A, Casado S (2001) Heart failure, redox alterations, and endothelial dysfunction. Hypertension 38:1400–1405

93. Gao Z, Xu H, DiSilvestre D, Halperin VL, Tunin R, Tian Y, Yu W, Winslow RL, Tomaselli GF (2006) Transcriptomic profiling of the canine tachycardia-induced heart failure model: global comparison to human and murine heart failure. J Mol Cell Cardiol 40:76–86

94. Hoppel CL, Moghaddas S, Lesnefsky EJ (2002) Interfibrillar cardiac mitochondrial comples III defects in the aging rat heart. Biogerontology 3:41–44

95. Fannin SW, Lesnefsky EJ, Slabe TJ, Hassan MO, Hoppel CL (1999) Aging selectively decreases oxidative capacity in rat heart interfibrillar mitochondria. Arch Biochem Biophys 372:399–407

96. Lesnefsky EJ, Gudz TI, Moghaddas S, Migita CT, Ikeda-Saito M, Turkaly PJ et al (2001) Aging decreases electron transport complex III activity in heart interfibrillar mitochondria by alteration of the cytochrome c binding site. J Mol Cell Cardiol 33:37–47

97. Tsutsui H, Ide T, Shiomi T, Kang D, Hayashidani S, Suematsu N, Wen J, Utsumi H, Hamasaki N, Takeshita A (2001) 8-oxo-dGTPase, which prevents oxidative stress-induced DNA damage, increases in the mitochondria from failing hearts. Circulation 104:2883–2885

98. Storz P (2007) Mitochondrial ROS-radical detoxification, mediated by protein kinase D. Trends Cell Biol 17:13–18

99. Storz P, Doppler H, Toker A (2005) Protein kinase D mediates mitochondrion-to-nucleus signaling and detoxification from mitochondrial reactive oxygen species. Mol Cell Biol 25: 8520–8530

100. Zhang D, Mott JL, Farrar P, Ryerse JS, Chang SW, Stevens M, Denniger G, Zassenhaus HP (2003) Mitochondrial DNA mutations activate the mitochondrial apoptotic pathway and cause dilated cardiomyopathy. Cardiovasc Res 57:147–157

101. Scarpulla RC (2002) Nuclear activators and coactivators in mammalian mitochondrial biogenesis. Biochim Biophys Acta 1576:1–14

102. Parisi MA, Clayton DA (1991) Similarity of human mitochondrial transcription factor 1 to high mobility group proteins. Science 252:965–969

103. Scarpulla RC (2008) Transcriptional paradigms in mammalian mitochondrial biogenesis and function. Physiol Rev 88:611–638

104. Wu ZD, Puigserver P, Andersson U, Zhang CY, Adelmant G, Mootha V, Troy A, Cinti S, Lowell B, Scarpulla RC, Spiegelman BM (1999) Mechanisms controlling mitochondrial biogenesis and respiration through the thermogenic coactivator PGC-1. Cell 98:115–124

105. Garnier A, Fortin D, Delomenie C, Momken I, Veksler V, Ventura-Clapier R (2003) Depressed mitochondrial transcription factors and oxidative capacity in rat failing cardiac and skeletal muscles. J Physiol 551:491–501

106. Javadov S, Purdham DM, Zeidan A, Karmazyn M (2006) NHE-1 inhibition improves cardiac mitochondrial function through regulation of mitochondrial biogenesis during postinfarction remodeling. Am J Physiol Heart Circ Physiol 291:H1722–H1730

107. Ibdah JA, Paul H, Zhao Y, Binford S, Salleng K, Cline M, Matern D, Bennett MJ, Rinaldo P, Strauss AW (2001) Lack of mitochondrial trifunctional protein in mice causes neonatal hypoglycemia and sudden death. J Clin Invest 107:1403–1409

108. Kurtz DM, Rinaldo P, Rhead WJ, Tian L, Millington DS, Vockley J, Hamm DA, Brix AE, Lindsey JR, Pinkert CA, O'Brien WE, Wood PA (1998) Targeted disruption of mouse long-chain acyl-CoA dehydrogenase gene reveals crucial roles for fatty acid oxidation. Proc Natl Acad Sci USA 95:15592–15597

109. Puccio H, Simon D, Cossee M, Criqui-Filipe P, Tiziano F, Melki J, Hindelang C, Matyas R, Rustin P, Koenig M (2001) Mouse models for Friedreich ataxia exhibit cardiomyopathy, sensory nerve defect and Fe-S enzyme deficiency followed by intramitochondrial iron deposits. Nat Genet 27:181–186

110. Wang J, Wilhelmsson H, Graff C, Li H, Oldfors A, Rustin P, Bruning JC, Kahn CR, Clayton DA, Barsh GS, Thoren P, Larsson NG (1999) Dilated cardiomyopathy and atrioventricular conduction blocks induced by heart-specific inactivation of mitochondrial DNA gene expression. Nat Genet 21:133–137

111. Yokoyama M, Yagyu H, Hu Y, Seo T, Hirata K, Homma S, Goldberg IJ (2004) Apolipoprotein B production reduces lipotoxic cardiomyopathy: studies in heart-specific lipoprotein lipase transgenic mouse. J Biol Chem 279:4204–4211

112. Arad M, Moskowitz IP, Patel VV, Ahmad F, Perez-Atayde AR, Sawyer DB, Walter M, Li GH, Burgon PG, Maguire CT, Stapleton D, Schmitt JP, Guo XX, Pizard A, Kupershmidt S, Roden DM, Berul CI, Seidman CE, Seidman JG (2003) Transgenic mice overexpressing mutant PRKAG2 define the cause of Wolff-Parkinson-White syndrome in glycogen storage cardiomyopathy. Circulation 107:2850–2856

113. Russell LK, Mansfield CM, Lehman JJ, Kovacs A, Courtois M, Saffitz JE, Medeiros DM, Valencik ML, McDonald JA, Kelly DP (2004) Cardiac-specific induction of the transcriptional coactivator peroxisome proliferator-activated receptor gamma coactivator-1alpha promotes mitochondrial biogenesis and reversible cardiomyopathy in a developmental stage-dependent manner. Circ Res 94:525–533

114. Nebigil CG, Jaffre F, Messaddeq N, Hickel P, Monassier L, Launay JM, Maroteaux L (2003) Overexpression of the serotonin 5-HT2B receptor in heart leads to abnormal mitochondrial function and cardiac hypertrophy. Circulation 107:3223–3229

115. Xiaofei E, Wada Y, Dakeishi M, Hirasawa F, Murata K, Masuda H, Sugiyama T, Nikaido H, Koizumi A (2002) Age-associated cardiomyopathy in heterozygous carrier mice of a pathological mutation of carnitine transporter gene, OCTN2. J Gerontol A Biol Sci Med Sci 57:B270–B278

116. Chiu HC, Kovacs A, Blanton RM, Han X, Courtois M, Weinheimer CJ, Yamada KA, Brunet S, Xu H, Nerbonne JM, Welch MJ, Fettig NM, Sharp TL, Sambandam N, Olson KM, Ory DS, Schaffer JE (2005) Transgenic expression of fatty acid transport protein 1 in the heart causes lipotoxic cardiomyopathy. Circ Res 96:225–233

117. Finck BN, Lehman JJ, Leone TC, Welch MJ, Bennett MJ, Kovacs A, Han X, Gross RW, Kozak R, Lopaschuk GD, Kelly DP (2002) The cardiac phenotype induced by PPARα overexpression mimics that caused by diabetes mellitus. J Clin Invest 109:121–130

118. Cheng L, Ding G, Qin Q, Huang Y, Lewis W, He N, Evans RM, Schneider MD, Brako FA, Xiao Y, Chen YE, Yang Q (2004) Cardiomyocyte-restricted peroxisome proliferator-activated receptor-delta deletion perturbs myocardial fatty acid oxidation and leads to cardiomyopathy. Nat Med 10:1245–1250

119. Chiu HC, Kovacs A, Ford DA, Hsu FF, Garcia R, Herrero P, Saffitz JE, Schaffer JE (2001) A novel mouse model of lipotoxic cardiomyopathy. J Clin Invest 107:813–822

120. Kaukonen J, Juselius JK, Tiranti V, Kyttala A, Zeviani M, Comi GP, Keranen S, Peltonen L, Suomalainen A (2000) Role of adenine nucleotide translocator 1 in mtDNA maintenance. Science 289:782–785

121. Larsson NG, Wang J, Wilhelmsson H, Oldfors A, Rustin P, Lewandoski M, Barsh GS, Clayton DA (1998) Mitochondrial transcription factor A is necessary for mtDNA maintenance and embryogenesis in mice. Nat Genet 18:231–236

122. Wang J, Silva JP, Gustafsson CM, Rustin P, Larsson NG (2001) Increased in vivo apoptosis in cells lacking mitochondrial DNA gene expression. Proc Natl Acad Sci USA 98:4038–4043

123. Hansson A, Hance N, Dufour E, Rantanen A, Hultenby K, Clayton DA, Wibom R, Larsson NG (2004) A switch in metabolism precedes increased mitochondrial biogenesis in respiratory chain-deficient hearts. Proc Natl Acad Sci USA 101:3136–3141

124. Ikeuchi M, Matsusaka H, Kang D, Matsushima S, Ide T, Kubota T, Fujiwara T, Hamasaki N, Takeshita A, Sunagawa K, Tsutsui H (2005) Overexpression of mitochondrial transcription factor a ameliorates mitochondrial deficiencies and cardiac failure after myocardial infarction. Circulation 112:683–690

125. Mott JL, Zhang D, Stevens M, Chang S, Denniger G, Zassenhaus HP (2001) Oxidative stress is not an obligate mediator of disease provoked by mitochondrial DNA mutations. Mutat Res 474:35–45

126. Zhang D, Mott JL, Chang SW, Stevens M, Mikolajczak P, Zassenhaus HP (2005) Mitochondrial DNA mutations activate programmed cell survival in the mouse heart. Am J Physiol Heart Circ Physiol 288:H2476–H2483

127. Taegtmeyer H (2000) Metabolism – The lost child of cardiology. J Am Coll Cardiol 36:1386–1388

128. Huss JM, Kelly DP (2004) Nuclear receptor signaling and cardiac energetics. Circ Res 95:568–578

129. Mettauer B, Zoll J, Garnier A, Ventura-Clapier R (2006) Heart failure: a model of cardiac and skeletal muscle energetic failure. Pflugers Arch 452:653–666

130. Osorio JC, Stanley WC, Linke A, Castellari M, Diep QN, Panchal AR, Hintze TH, Lopaschuk GD, Recchia FA (2002) Impaired myocardial fatty acid oxidation and reduced protein expression of retinoid X receptor-alpha in pacing-induced heart failure. Circulation 106:606–612

131. van Bilsen M (2004) "Energenetics" of heart failure. Ann N Y Acad Sci 1015:238–249

132. Chandler MP, Kerner J, Huang H, Vazquez E, Reszko A, Martini WZ, Hoppel CL, Imai M, Rastogi S, Sabbah HN, Stanley WC (2004) Moderate severity heart failure does not involve a down-regulation of myocardial fatty acid oxidation. Am J Physiol Heart Circ Physiol 287:H1538–H1543

133. Neubauer S, Horn M, Pabst T, Harre K, Stromer H, Bertsch G, Sandstede J, Ertl G, Hahn D, Kochsiek K (1997) Cardiac high-energy phosphate metabolism in patients with aortic valve disease assessed by 31P-magnetic resonance spectroscopy. J Investig Med 45:453–462

134. Razeghi P, Young ME, Alcorn JL, Moravec CS, Frazier OH (2001) Taegtmeyer H Metabolic gene expression in fetal and failing human heart. Circulation 104:2923–2931

135. Sack MN, Rader TA, Park S, Bastin J, McCune SA, Kelly DP (1996) Fatty acid oxidation enzyme gene expression is downregulated in the failing heart. Circulation 94:2837–2842

136. Barger PM, Brandt JM, Leone TC, Weinheimer CJ, Kelly DP (2000) Deactivation of peroxisome proliferator-activated receptor-alpha during cardiac hypertrophic growth. J Clin Invest 105:1723–1730

137. Puigserver P, Wu Z, Park CW, Graves R, Wright M, Spiegelman BM (1998) A cold-inducible coactivator of nuclear receptors linked to adaptive thermogenesis. Cell 92:829–839

138. Lehman JJ, Barger PM, Kovacs A, Saffitz JE, Medeiros D, Kelly DP (2000) PPARgamma coactivator-1 (PGC-1) promotes cardiac mitochondrial biogenesis. J Clin Invest 106:847–856

139. Herzig S, Long F, Jhala US, Hedrick S, Quinn R, Bauer A, Rudolph D, Schutz G, Yoon C, Puigserver P, Spiegelman B, Montminy M (2001) CREB regulates hepatic gluconeogenesis through the coactivator PGC-1. Nature 413:179–183

140. Michael LF, Wu Z, Cheatham RB, Puigserver P, Adelmant G, Lehman JJ, Kelly DP, Spiegelman BM (2001) Restoration of insulin-sensitive glucose transporter (GLUT4) gene expression in muscle cells by the transcriptional coactivator PGC-1. Proc Natl Acad Sci USA 98:3820–3825

141. Arany Z, He H, Lin J, Hoyer K, Handschin C, Toka O, Ahmad F, Matsui T, Chin S, Wu PH, Rybkin II, Shelton JM, Manieri M, Cinti S, Schoen FJ, Bassel-Duby R, Rosenzweig A, Ingwall JS, Spiegelman BM (2005) Transcriptional coactivator PGC-1 alpha controls the energy state and contractile function of cardiac muscle. Cell Metab 1:259–271

142. Leone TC, Lehman JJ, Finck BN, Schaeffer PJ, Wende AR, Boudina S, Courtois M, Wozniak DF, Sambandam N, Bernal-Mizrachi C, Chen Z, Hollosy JO, Medeiros DM, Schmidt RE, Saffitz JE, Abel ED, Semenkovich CF, Kelly DP (2005) PGC-1alpha deficiency causes multi-system energy metabolic derangements: muscle dysfunction, abnormal weight control and hepatic steatosis. PLoS Biol 3:e101

143. Forman BM, Chen J, Evans RM (1997) Hypolipidemic drugs, polyunsaturated fatty acids, and eicosanoids are ligands for peroxisome proliferator-activated receptors alpha and delta. Proc Natl Acad Sci USA 94:4312–4317

144. Devchand PR, Keller H, Peters JM, Vazquez M, Gonzalez FJ, Wahli W (1996) The PPARalpha-leukotriene B4 pathway to inflammation control. Nature 384:39–43

145. Tenenbaum A, Motro M, Fisman EZ (2005) Dual and pan-peroxisome proliferator-activated receptors (PPAR) co-agonism: the bezafibrate lessons. Cardiovasc Diabetol 4:14

146. Lehman JJ, Kelly DP (2002) Gene regulatory mechanisms governing energy metabolism during cardiac hypertrophic growth. Heart Fail Rev 7:175–185

147. Diradourian C, Girard J, Pegorier JP (2005) Phosphorylation of PPARs: from molecular characterization to physiological relevance. Biochimie 87:33–38

148. Bronner M, Hertz R, Bar-Tana J (2004) Kinase-independent transcriptional co-activation of peroxisome proliferator-activated receptor alpha by AMP-activated protein kinase. Biochem J 384: 295–305

149. Blanquart C, Mansouri R, Paumelle R, Fruchart JC, Staels B, Glineur C (2004) The protein kinase C signaling pathway regulates a molecular switch between transactivation and transrepression activity of the peroxisome proliferator-activated receptor alpha. Mol Endocrinol 18:1906–1918

150. Lazennec G, Canaple L, Saugy D, Wahli W (2000) Activation of peroxisome proliferator-activated receptors (PPARs) by their ligands and protein kinase A activators. Mol Endocrinol 14:1962–1975

151. Finck BN, Han X, Courtois M, Aimond F, Nerbonne JM, Kovacs A, Gross RW, Kelly DP (2003) A critical role for PPARalpha-mediated lipotoxicity in the pathogenesis of diabetic cardiomyopathy: modulation by dietary fat content. Proc Natl Acad Sci USA 100:1226–1231

152. Milner DJ, Weitzer G, Tran D, Bradley A, Capetanaki Y (1996) Disruption of muscle architecture and myocardial degeneration in mice lacking desmin. J Cell Biol 134:1255–1270

153. Capetanaki Y (2002) Desmin cytoskeleton: a potential regulator of muscle mitochondrial behavior and function. Trends Cardiovasc Med 12:339–348

154. Sayen MR, Gustafsson AB, Sussman MA, Molkentin JD, Gottlieb RA (2003) Calcineurin transgenic mice have mitochondrial dysfunction and elevated superoxide production. Am J Physiol Cell Physiol 284:C562–C570

155. Fountoulakis M, Soumaka E, Rapti K, Mavroidis M, Tsangaris G, Maris A, Weisleder N, Capetanaki Y (2005) Alterations in the heart mitochondrial proteome in a desmin null heart failure model. J Mol Cell Cardiol 38:461–474

156. Scheubel RJ, Tostlebe M, Simm A, Rohrbach S, Prondzinsky R, Gellerich FN, Silber RE, Holtz J (2002) Dysfunction of mitochondrial respiratory chain complex I in human failing myocardium is not due to disturbed mitochondrial gene expression. J Am Coll Cardiol 40:2174–2181

157. Sam F, Kerstetter DL, Pimental DR, Mulukutla S, Tabaee A, Bristow MR, Colucci WS (2005) Sawyer DB.Increased reactive oxygen species production and functional alterations in antioxidant enzymes in human failing myocardium. J Card Fail 11: 473–480

158. Huss JM, Kelly DP (2005) Mitochondrial energy metabolism in heart failure: a question of balance. J Clin Invest 115:547–555

159. Steenman M, Lamirault G, Le MN, Leger JJ (2005) Gene expression profiling in human cardiovascular disease. Clin Chem Lab Med 43:696–701

160. Yung CK, Halperin VL, Tomaselli GF, Winslow RL (2004) Gene expression profiles in end-stage human idiopathic dilated cardiomyopathy: altered expression of apoptotic and cytoskeletal genes. Genomics 83:281–297

161. Yang J, Moravec CS, Sussman MA, DiPaola NR, Fu D, Hawthorn L, Mitchell CA, Young JB, Francis GS, McCarthy PM, Bond M (2000) Decreased SLIM1 expression and increased gelsolin expression in failing human hearts measured by high-density oligonucleotide arrays. Circulation 102:3046–3052

162. Hwang JJ, Allen PD, Tseng GC, Lam CW, Fananapazir L, Dzau VJ, Liew CC (2002) Microarray gene expression profiles in dilated and hypertrophic cardiomyopathic end-stage heart failure. Physiol Genomics 10:31–44

163. Paolisso G, Gambardella A, Galzerano D, D'Amore A, Rubino P, Verza M, Teasuro P, Varricchio M, D'Onofrio F (1994) Total-body and myocardial substrate oxidation in congestive heart failure. Metabolism 43:174–179

164. Zeviani M, Moraes CT, DiMauro S, Nakase H, Bonilla E, Schon EA, Rowland LP (1988) Deletions of mitochondrial DNA in Kearns-Sayre syndrome. Neurology 38:1339–1346

165. Marin-Garcia J, Goldenthal MJ, Ananthakrishnan R, Pierpont ME, Fricker FJ, Lipshultz SE, Perez-Atayde A (1996) Specific mitochondrial DNA deletions in idiopathic dilated cardiomyopathy. Cardiovasc Res 31:306–313

166. Li YY, Hengstenberg C, Maisch B (1995) Whole mitochondrial genome amplification reveals basal level multiple deletions in mtDNA of patients with dilated cardiomyopathy. Biochem Biophys Res Commun 210:211–218

167. Ozawa T, Tanaka M, Sugiyama S, Hattori K, Ito T, Ohno K, Takahashi A, Sato W, Takada G, Mayumi B, Yamamoto K, Adachi K, Koga Y, Toshima H (1990) Multiple mitochondrial DNA deletions exist in cardiomyocytes of patients with hypertrophic or dilated cardiomyopathy. Biochem Biophys Res Commun 170:830–836

168. Suomalainen A, Kaukonen J, Amati P, Timonen R, Haltia M, Weissenbach J, Zeviani M, Somer H, Peltonen L (1995) An autosomal locus predisposing to deletions of mitochondrial DNA. Nat Genet 9:146–151

169. Bohlega S, Tanji K, Santorelli FM, Hirano M, al-Jishi A, DiMauro S (1996) Multiple mitochondrial DNA deletions associated with autosomal recessive ophthalmoplegia and severe cardiomyopathy. Neurology 46:1329–1334

170. Agostino A, Valletta L, Chinnery PF, Ferrari G, Carrara F, Taylor RW, Schaefer AM, Yurnbull DM, Tiranti V, Zeviani M (2003) Mutations of ANT 1, Twinkle, and POLG1 in sporadic progressive external ophthalmoplegia (PEO). Neurology 60:1354–1356

171. Marin-Garcia J, Ananthakrishnan R, Goldenthal MJ (1998) Hypertrophic cardiomyopathy with mitochondrial DNA depletion and respiratory enzyme defects. Pediatr Cardiol 19:266–268

172. Poulton J, Sewry C, Potter CG, Bougeron T, Chretien D, Wijburg FA, Morten KJ, Brown G (1995) Variation in mitochondrial DNA levels in muscle from normal controls: is depletion of mtDNA in patients with mitochondrial myopathy a distinct clinical syndrome? J Inherit Metab Dis 18:4–20

173. Rasmussen M, Sanengen T, Skullerud K, Kvittingen EA, Skjeldal OH (2000) Evidence that Alpers-Huttenlocher syndrome could be a mitochondrial disease. J Child Neurol 15:473–477

174. Naviaux RK, Nyhan WL, Barshop BA, Poulton J, Markusic D, Karpinski NC, Haas RH (1999) Mitochondrial DNA polymerase gamma deficiency and mtDNA depletion in a child with Alpers' syndrome. Ann Neurol 45:54–58

175. Naviaux RK, Nguyen KV (2004) POLG mutations associated with Alpers' syndrome and mitochondrial DNA depletion. Ann Neurol 55:706–712

176. Ashrafian H, Redwood C, Blair E, Watkins H (2003) Hypertrophic cardiomyopathy: a paradigm for myocardial energy depletion. Trends Genet 19:263–268

177. Guerra L, Cerbai E, Gessi S, Borea PA, Mugelli A (1996) The effect of oxygen free radicals on calcium current and dihydropyridine binding sites in guinea-pig ventricular myocytes. Br J Pharmacol 118:1278–1284

178. Kaplan P, Babusikova E, Lehotsky J, Dobrota D (2003) Free radical-induced protein modification and inhibition of Ca2+-ATPase of cardiac sarcoplasmic reticulum. Mol Cell Biochem 248:41–47

179. Goldhaber JI (1996) Free radicals enhance Na+/Ca2+ exchange in ventricular myocytes. Am J Physiol 271:H823–H833

180. He X, Liu Y, Sharma V, Dirksen RT, Waugh R, Sheu SS, Min W (2003) ASK1 associates with troponin T and induces troponin T phosphorylation and contractile dysfunction in cardiomyocytes. Am J Pathol 163:243–251

181. Houser SR, Margulies KB (2003) Is depressed myocyte contractility centrally involved in heart failure? Circ Res 92:350–358

182. Davies CH, Davia K, Bennett JG, Pepper JR, Poole-Wilson PA, Harding SE (1995) Reduced contraction and altered frequency response of isolated ventricular myocytes from patients with heart failure. Circulation 92:2540–2549

183. Zak R, Rabinowitz M, Rajamanickam C, Merten S, Kwiatkowska-Patzer B (1980) Mitochondrial proliferation in cardiac hypertrophy. Basic Res Cardiol 75:171–178

184. Wiesner RJ, Aschenbrenner V, Ruegg JC, Zak R (1994) Coordination of nuclear and mitochondrial gene expression during the development of cardiac hypertrophy in rats. Am J Physiol 267:C229–C235

185. Goldenthal MJ, Weiss HR, Marin-Garcia J (2004) Bioenergetic remodeling of heart mitochondria by thyroid hormone. Mol Cell Biochem 265:97–106

186. Tanaka T, Morita H, Koide H, Kawamura K, Takatsu T (1985) Biochemical and morphological study of cardiac hypertrophy. Effect of thyroxin on enzyme activities in the rat myocardium. Basic Res Cardiol 80:165–174

187. Wiener DH, Fink LI, Maris J, Jones RA, Chance B, Wilson JR (1986) Abnormal skeletal muscle bioenergetics during exercise in patients with heart failure: role of reduced blood flow. Circulation 73:1127–1136

188. Duboc D, Jehenson P, Tamby JF, Payen JF, Syrota A, Guerin F (1991) Abnormalities of the skeletal muscle in hypertrophic cardiomyopathy. Spectroscopy using phosphorus-31 nuclear magnetic resonance. Arch Mal Coeur Vaiss 84:185–188

189. Caforio AL, Rossi B, Risaliti R et al (1989) Type 1 fiber abnormalities in skeletal muscle of patients with hypertrophic and dilated cardiomyopathy. J Am Coll Cardiol 14:1464–1473

190. Fananapazir L, Dalakas MC, Cyran F, Cohn G, Epstein ND (1993) Missense mutations in the beta-myosin heavy-chain gene cause central core disease in hypertrophic cardiomyopathy. Proc Natl Acad Sci USA 90:3993–3997

191. Thompson CH, Kemp GJ, Taylor DJ et al (1997) Abnormal skeletal muscle bioenergetics in familial hypertrophic cardiomyopathy. Heart 78:177–181

192. Adams V, Jiang H, Yu J et al (1999) Apoptosis in skeletal myocytes of patients with chronic heart failure is associated with exercise intolerance. J Am Coll Cardiol 33:959–965

193. Vescovo G, Zennaro R, Sandri M et al (1998) Apoptosis of skeletal muscle myofibers and interstitial cells in experimental heart failure. J Mol Cell Cardiol 30:2449–2459

194. Issacs H, Muncke G (1975) Idiopathic cardiomyopathy and skeletal muscle abnormality. Am Heart J 90:767–773

195. Hubner G, Grantzow R (1983) Mitochondrial cardiomyopathy with involvement of skeletal muscle. Virchows Arch A Pathol Anat Histopathol 399:115–125

196. Marin-Garcia J, Ananthakrishnan R, Goldenthal MJ, Filiano J, Perez-Atayde A (1999) Mitochondrial dysfunction in skeletal muscle of children with cardiomyopathy. Pediatrics 103:456–459

197. Muller-Hocker J, Johannes A, Droste M, Kadenbach B, Pongratz D, Hubner G (1986) Fatal mitochondrial cardiomyopathy in Kearns–Sayre syndrome with deficiency of cytochrome c oxidase in cardiac and skeletal muscle. An enzyme histochemical-ultra-immunocytochemical-fine structural study in longterm frozen autopsy tissue. Virchows Arch B Cell Pathol Incl Mol Pathol 52:353–367

198. Suomalainen A, Paetau A, Leinonen H, Majander A, Peltonen L, Somer H (1992) Inherited idiopathic dilated cardiomyopathy with multiple deletions of mitochondrial DNA. Lancet 340:1319–1320

199. Marin-Garcia J, Goldenthal MJ, Ananthakrishnan R et al (1996) Specific mitochondrial DNA deletions in idiopathic dilated cardiomyopathy. Cardiovasc Res 31:306–314

200. Anan R, Nakagawa M, Higuchi I, Nakao S, Nomoto K, Tanaka H (1992) Deletion of mitochondrial DNA in the endomyocardial biopsy sample from a patient with Kearns–Sayre syndrome. Eur Heart J 13:1718–1719

201. Poulton J, Sewry C, Potter CG et al (1995) Variation in mitochondrial DNA levels in muscle from normal controls. Is depletion of mtDNA in patients with mitochondrial myopathy a distinct clinical syndrome? J Inherit Metab Dis 18:4–20

202. Lewis W, Dalakas MC (1995) Mitochondrial toxicity of antiviral drugs. Nat Med 1:417–422

203. Razeghi P, Young ME, Alcorn JL, Moravec CS, Frazier OH, Taegtmeyer H (2001) Metabolic gene expression in fetal and failing human heart. Circulation 104:2923–2931

Section IV
Experimental Models of Heart Failure

Chapter 6
Animal Models of Heart Failure

Overview

The great achievements made in our understanding of the pathophysiology and treatment of heart failure (HF) would not have been possible without the use of animal models of HF. Experimental models are often needed to address specific questions not easily answered in patients, but in the case of HF, no single model can reproduce exactly any of the clinical phenotypes of these patients. The species and interventions used to create HF depend not only on the scientific question but also on factors such as ethical and economical considerations, accessibility, and reproducibility of the model. The syndrome of HF may be induced experimentally by pressure loading, volume loading, myocardial infarction, rapid pacing, or by the creation of other disease states within the myocardium. Pressure loading may be especially useful in the study of ventricular hypertrophy, cellular derangements, and vascular changes. Volume loading may be useful when examining the pathogenesis of hormonal and electrolyte disturbances. Models of myocardial infarction or destruction are likely to be most suitable for assessing novel therapy provided that peripheral reflexes are maintained. Experimental cardiomyopathy such as those induced by rapid pacing can provide an important means of identifying pathological subcellular mechanisms. They may also be of use in the evaluation of therapy. Any one model may be useful if it permits study of a single variable in isolation or at a time when information is not obtainable from patients. In this chapter, animal models of HF are discussed with particular focus on similarities between the animal model and the failing human heart regarding myocardial function as well as molecular and subcellular mechanisms.

Introduction

The search for experimental models that would simulate the human clinical syndrome of HF has captured the imagination of several generations of investigators. The heterogeneous etiology and the uncertainty in defining its time of onset conspire to make HF a particularly difficult condition to investigate. A list of animal models that induce a clinical phenotype of HF is shown on Table 6.1; only models that have been used extensively and that address broader issues and concepts in HF are listed. In general, rat models are relatively inexpensive and because of short gestation periods, a large sample size can be produced in a relatively short period. Therefore, rat models have been extensively used to study long-term pharmacological interventions including long-term survival studies [1]. However, there are limitations to the use of rat models related to the differences in myocardial function when compared to the human heart. First, rat myocardium exhibits a very short action potential, which normally lacks a plateau phase. Second, calcium removal from the cytosol is predominated by the activity of the sarcoplasmic reticulum calcium pump whereas Na^+/Ca^{2+}-exchanger activity is less relevant [2]. Third, in normal rat myocardium, myosin heavy-chain isoform predominates and a shift toward the β-myosin isoform occurs with hemodynamic load or hormonal changes [3].

Dog and other large animal models of HF may allow the study of left (LV) function and volumes more accurately than in the rodent models. In particular, they better allow for chronic instrumentation. Furthermore, in dog, like in the human myocardium, the β-myosin heavy-chain isoform predominates and excitation–contraction coupling processes seem to be similar to the human myocardium [4]. The force–frequency relation, as evaluated by E_{max}, the slope of the end-systolic pressure–volume relation, was shown to be positive in autonomically intact awake dogs as well as during autonomic blockade [5]. On the other hand, dog models are costly and require substantial resources with respect to the housing and care.

Pressure and Volume Overload

Volume overload, pressure overload, and the combination of both models have been used to induce HF particularly in the rabbits. Chronic severe aortic regurgitation in rabbits,

Table 6.1 Animal models of heart failure

Species and model	Functional features
Rat	
Coronary ligation	Clinical characteristics similar to human heart failure; survival studies
Aortic banding	Studies of transition from hypertrophy to failure; survival studies
Salt-sensitive hypertension	Studies of transition from hypertrophy to failure
Spontaneous hypertension	Extracellular matrix changes; apoptosis; studies of transition from hypertrophy to failure
SH-HF/Mcc-facp	Altered NOS expression; altered calcium triggered calcium release
Aorto-caval fistula	Left ventricular hypertrophy; moderate LV dysfunction
Toxic cardiomyopathy	Decreased myocardial performance; myocyte loss with chronic ethanol application. Cardiomyopathy following catecholamine infusion or associated with *Diabetes mellitus*
Dog	
Tachycardia	Studies of remodeling and neurohumoral activation; studies on molecular mechanism of subcellular dysfunction; no hypertrophy
Coronary artery ligation	Studies on progression of heart failure; high mortality and dysrhythmias
Direct-current shock	Studies of neurohumoral mechanisms and therapeutic interventions
Volume overload	Aorto-caval fistula
	Mitral regurgitation
Vena caval constriction	Low cardiac output failure
Toxic cardiomyopathy	Left ventricular dysfunction
Genetic	Spontaneous cardiomyopathy in Doberman Pinscher dogs
Pig	
Tachycardia	Comparable with dog model for most aspects
Coronary artery ligation	Congestive heart failure; altered myocardial energetics
Rabbit	
Volume and pressure overload	Myocardial alterations similar to failing human myocardium
Pacing tachycardia	Myocardial alteration similar to failing human myocardium
Toxic cardiomyopathy	Studies of functional consequences of altered ryanodine receptors
Guinea pig	
Aortic banding	Myocardial function and alteration of calcium handling similar to human heart failure
Syrian hamster	
Genetic	Hypertrophy and failure; alterations critically dependent on strain and age
Cat	
Pulmonary artery constriction	Transition from compensated right ventricular hypertrophy to failure
Turkey	
Toxic cardiomyopathy	Alteration of calcium handling and myocardial energetics
Bovine	
Genetic	Similar to human heart failure regarding changes in β-adrenergic system
Sheep	
Pacing tachycardia	Similar to dog and swine model of pacing tachycardia
Aortic constriction	Transition from compensated hypertrophy to left ventricular dysfunction

created by aortic valve perforation with a catheter, produces left ventricular hypertrophy, followed by systolic dysfunction and HF after a period of months [6]. Occurrence of HF is more rapidly achieved when aortic regurgitation is combined with aortic constriction. In the model developed by Ezzaher et al., aortic insufficiency was produced by destroying the aortic valve with a catheter introduced through the carotid artery. After 14 days, aortic constriction was performed just below the diaphragm. HF occurs about 4 weeks after the initial procedure [7, 8].

HF is associated with alterations in the β-adrenoceptors system similar to those in humans [8]. Furthermore, in this

model, there is an inversion of the force–frequency relation and alteration of post-rest potentiation that closely resembles the situation in the human heart [9]. Protein and mRNA levels of Na^+/Ca^{2+}-exchanger were significantly increased in failing compared to nonfailing hearts whereas sarcoplasmic reticulum Ca^{2+}-ATPase was not significantly altered. This may indicate that increased trans-sarcolemmal calcium loss by increased Na^+/Ca^{2+}-exchanger activity may decrease calcium availability to contractile proteins and decrease myocardial function even without direct alteration of sarcoplasmic reticulum function. Because this model closely mimics alterations of myocardial function observed in the end-stage failing human myocardium, this model may be well suited to study alterations in excitation–contraction coupling processes occurring during the transition from compensated hypertrophy to failure.

In dogs, volume overload has also been produced by creation of an arteriovenous fistula or by destruction of the mitral valve [10, 11]. Chronic mitral regurgitation produced in closed-chest dogs by disruption of mitral chordae or leaflets using an arterially placed grasping forceps results in LV hypertrophy and dilatation within 3 months and development of overt HF occurs in this model [10]. Neurohumoral activation including local activation of the renin–angiotensin–aldosterone system (RAAS) was observed, which is associated with depressed myocardial function [12, 13]. The model has been utilized to study the influence of chronic β-adrenoceptor blockade on myocyte and left ventricular function, both of which significantly improved with this treatment [13].

Suprarenal aortic coarctation results in a very short-term reactive hyperreninemia of less than 4 days. Thereafter, the circulating RAAS is no longer activated, but the ventricular angiotensin-converting enzyme (ACE) activity begins to rise. After a period of several weeks, ventricular ACE activity may decrease again to normal values, which may be related to normalization of wall stress with increasing hypertrophy [14]. Numerous studies have been performed using aortic banding in rats to evaluate different aspects of left ventricular hypertrophy. Furthermore, after several months, a subset of animals goes into clinical HF. Chronic experimental aortic constriction imposed by banding of the ascending aorta in weanlings resulted in compensated left ventricular hypertrophy of the adult rats for several weeks. After 20 weeks of aortic banding, two distinct groups could be identified: rats without change in LV systolic pressure development and those with a significant reduction in LV systolic pressure [15]. The latter group exhibited increased LV volumes, reduced ejection fraction, and clinical signs of overt HF [16]. Left ventricular hypertrophy and failure was associated with increased β-myosin heavy chain mRNA and atrial natriuretic factor mRNA. Interestingly, a decrease in SR-Ca^{2+}-ATPase mRNA levels by the polymerase chain reaction (PCR) occurred in left ventricular myocardium from failing animals after 20 weeks of banding but not in nonfailing hypertrophied hearts. From this data, it was suggested that the decrease in SR-Ca^{2+}-ATPase mRNA levels may be a marker of the transition from compensatory hypertrophy to failure in these animals [15]. During compensated hypertrophy, while catecholamine levels are normal, there is activation of the local myocardial renin–angiotensin system, which may be important for the development of myocardial failure. With the development of HF, plasma catecholamine levels can increase [17]. This model therefore appears to be well suited for studying the transition from hypertrophy to failure at the level of the myocardium. Nevertheless, one

should keep in mind that considerable differences in the function of subcellular systems may exist between rat and human myocardium.

Models of Transition of Compensated Cardiac Hypertrophy to Heart Failure

Dahl Salt-Sensitive Rats

An animal model that appears to be well suited for studying the transition from compensated hypertrophy to failure is the Dahl salt-sensitive rat [18, 19]. This strain of rats develops systemic hypertension after receiving a high-salt diet. This results in the development of concentric LV hypertrophy at 8 weeks, followed by marked LV dilatation, and overt clinical HF at 15–20 weeks. Rats with HF die within a short period. This type of HF is associated with reduced myocardial performance as shown in isolated muscle strip preparations [19].

Spontaneous Hypertensive Rats

The spontaneous hypertensive rat (SHR) is a well-established model of genetic hypertension in which cardiac pump function is initially preserved [20]. At 18–24 months, HF develops which includes reduced myocardial performance and increased fibrosis. In this model, although altered calcium cycling has been observed, no decrease in mRNA of the sarcoplasmic reticulum calcium pump was found during the transition from compensated hypertrophy to failure [21, 22]. It was suggested that the transition to failure is associated with significant alterations in the expression of genes encoding extracellular matrix [21]. Furthermore, an increased number of apoptotic myocytes was observed, suggesting that apoptosis might be a mechanism involved in the reduction of myocyte mass that accompanies the transition from stable compensation to HF in the model. Interestingly, the angiotensin-converting enzyme inhibitor captopril was associated with reduction in the exaggerated apoptosis that accompanied the HF syndrome [23].

Spontaneously hypertensive rats which develop failure before 18 months of age have been selectively bred (SH-HF). Development of HF occurs earlier in SH-HF rats, which carry the *facp* (corpulent) gene that encodes a defective leptin receptor (SH-HF/Mcc-facp) [24]. In these animals, renin-plasma activity, ANP, and aldosterone levels progressively increase with age, and renin-plasma activity is independently correlated to cardiac hypertrophy [25]. Interestingly, hearts from the SH-HF rat exhibit a more negative force–frequency relationship than control rats [26].

Gómez et al. have reported that calcium current density, density and function of ryanodine receptors, and sarcoplasmic reticulum calcium uptake are normal. However, they showed that the relationship between calcium current density and the probability of evoking a spark was reduced indicating that calcium influx is less effective at inducing SR calcium release. It was speculated that these changes may be related to spacial remodeling between L-type calcium channels and ryanodine receptors [27]. Of note, Ca^{2+}-dependent NOS activity and expression of endothelial NOS appear to be increased in hypertensive SH-HF rats [28].

Cardiomyopathic Hamster

Cardiomyopathic strains of the Syrian hamster have been widely used as a model for cardiac hypertrophy and transition to HF [29]. This model displays an autosomal recessive mode of inheritance [29, 30]. Cardiac disease proceeds progressively in several histologic and clinical phases during the life of the animal and overt HF develops after 7–10 months. Histologically, necrotic, calcified myocardial lesions are observed initially in the development of the disease. Microvascular spasms and disturbed calcium handling have been suggested to be relevant for the pathophysiology in this model and beneficial effects of verapamil have been observed [31, 32]. The density of L-type calcium channels seems to be increased in younger animals before morphological evidence for the myopathy is present. However, when there is a fully developed myopathy, there seems to be no appreciable difference between control and myopathic hamsters [33, 34]. Kuo et al. have showed decreased gene expression of sarcoplasmic reticulum calcium pump in Syrian hamsters. Interestingly, this alteration in gene expression preceded any noticeable myocyte damage [35]. On the other hand, Whitmer et al. have observed that sarcoplasmic reticulum calcium uptake is decreased in 9-month-old animals exhibiting HF but not in hypertrophic hearts without signs of HF [32].

Enhanced activity of the Na^+/Ca^{2+}-exchanger in failing animals was recently suggested from electrophysiological measurements [36]. Furthermore, time-dependent changes in myosin isoform expression have also been observed [36, 37]. A genetic linkage map localized the cardiomyopathy locus on hamster chromosome 9qa2.1-b1 [38]. Furthermore, it was shown that the cardiomyopathy results from a mutation in the δ-sarcoglycan gene [39]. The advantages of this model are: absence of surgical manipulations, low costs, and the ease with which large numbers of animals can be studied. It is important to state that there are differences among the strains, and in the time course of the pathologic changes, and therefore, the time point at which measurements are performed is critically important in this model.

Coronary Artery Ligation and Microembolization Models

Due to its apparent clinical relevance and the relatively easy technique involved, myocardial infarction in the rat is a widely used small-animal model of HF. Myocardial infarction following coronary artery ligation in Sprague-Dawley rats is a widely used rat model of HF. If the left coronary artery is not completely ligated, HF may still occur as a consequence of chronic myocardial ischemia [40]. Complete occlusion of the left coronary artery results in myocardial infarction of variable sizes with occurrence of overt HF after 3–6 weeks in animals with large infarcts. The impairment of LV function is related to the loss of myocardium. Heart failure is associated with LV dilatation, reduced systolic function, and increased filling pressures [1]. The progression of LV dysfunction and myocardial failure is associated with neurohumoral activation similar to that seen in patients with HF [41, 42]. In particular, it was shown that ACE activity in the LV correlated inversely with LV function and that ACE activity in the kidney was only increased late after the induction of HF [43]. Depressed myocardial function is associated with altered calcium transients [44]. The density of L-type calcium channels, as evaluated by antagonist binding was shown to be decreased in moderate to severe stages of congestive HF [45]. Furthermore, it was shown that after 4, 8, and 16 weeks following coronary artery ligation, $SR-Ca^{2+}$-ATPase mRNA and protein levels decrease continuously with increasing severity of HF. Interestingly, $SR-Ca^{2+}$-ATPase activity was found to be more depressed than expected from the reduction in protein levels [46]. Although alterations in neurohumoral systems as well as in baroreflex control have been well studied in HF, little is known about changes in the central nervous system itself. A recent study assessed hexokinase activity in various brain regions in rats with myocardial infarction and HF [47]. Hexokinase activity appears to be a reliable indicator of metabolic changes in discrete regions of the brain. The animals had increased hexokinase activity in the parvicellular and magnicellular divisions of the paraventricular nucleus of the hypothalamus as well as in the locus caeruleus. These regions contain vasopressin-producing neurons or sympathoexcitatory sites, respectively. Therefore, for the first time in an animal model of chronic HF, this study demonstrated changes in specific brain regions involved in central modulation of volume homeostasis and cardiovascular control, which may contribute to the observed peripheral alterations in HF.

Although a high initial mortality and induction of mild HF in most cases may be a real disadvantage of this model, it seems to be very useful for long-term studies of pharmacological interventions on neurohumoral activation. In rats, if the left coronary artery is not completely ligated but is chronically narrowed by an incompletely tied suture, a non-occlusive stenosis leading to chronic myocardial ischemia and LV dysfunction with decreased contractility and elevated filling pressures is produced [48]. Reductions in blood pressure, cardiac output, and stroke volume suggest forward failure. The hearts of these animals are characterized by LV dilatation and hypertrophy. Myocyte loss, hypertrophy, and hyperplasia all contribute to the changes associated with LV remodeling [40]. Being primarily a model of myocardial ischemia rather than of HF, this preparation appears to be of some relevance to chronic ischemic LV dysfunction.

Coronary artery ligation and microembolization have also been used to produce myocardial infarction and HF in dogs. In closed-chest dogs, approximately up to seven embolization procedures are performed 1–3 weeks apart. Three months after the final microembolization, there are clinical signs of HF, LV dilatation, decreased ejection fraction, and neurohumoral activation similar to that observed in humans [49]. A decreased number of β-adrenoceptors and L-type calcium channels have been observed 3 months after the final embolization procedure [50]. Furthermore, sarcoplasmic reticulum Ca^{2+}-ATPase activity and protein levels were reduced in LV myocardium in the HF animals [51]. With this model, the progression from LV dysfunction to HF and the influence of pharmacological interventions can be studied [52]. The model does have several disadvantages. Because of extensive collateral circulation, there are important differences in the pattern of infarction between the human and the dog. The model is therefore time consuming, technically demanding and expensive, and is associated with high mortality and with a high incidence of dysrhythmias.

Pacing Induced Cardiomyopathy

In 1962, Whipple et al. first reported that atrial pacing at over 330 beats/min can induce physical signs of HF [53]. Although these investigators initially devised the model to reproduce the human condition of tachycardia-induced cardiomyopathy, over the past two decades, the model has increasingly been used to evaluate broader questions related to HF [54–56]. There are several features that make this model particularly suitable for the study of HF. First, the model, at least when used in most laboratories, avoids major surgical trauma, such as thoracotomy and pericardectomy, which may confound the interpretation of physiological data. Second, HF evolves over a period of several weeks, which permits sequential observations [54, 57, 58]. Third, the magnitude of the provoking stimulus can be calibrated by employing a programmable pacemaker. Fourth, rapid pacing produces a well defined

clinical syndrome of biventricular failure with cardiomegaly, hypoperfusion, pulmonary congestion, cachexia and ascites, all of which mimic the human state. Finally, HF induced in this fashion is reversible after cessation of pacing [59, 60]. A comprehensive description of the general aspects of this model, including the various methods of pacing, has been discussed in several reviews [54, 56, 61, 62]. In brief, the most commonly used method is right ventricular pacing in the dog using transvenous endocardial leads. In our institution, we have employed programmable pulse generators and the pacing rate is programmed at 250 beats/min. With this protocol, we have consistently induced severe HF in 3–4 weeks. With daily physical examination and weekly radiographic and echocardiographic assessments, premature mortality was seldom encountered. Other investigators have induced HF in the pig by chronic supraventricular tachycardia using atrial electrodes implanted after thoracotomy [56, 63, 64]. The hemodynamic and neurohormonal changes induced in the pig model are quite similar to those of the canine model that uses endocardial right ventricular pacing. The pacing model has also been modified for use in the sheep and, more recently, in rabbits using epicardial electrodes. It is quite likely that other animal species and pacing protocols will be employed in future. Specific aspects of HF and the contemporary experimental data derived from this model as well as on how these data provide further insights into our understanding of the mechanisms of progression of heart failure are discussed in this section.

Cardiac Remodeling and Dysfunction

In almost all species studied, chronic atrial or ventricular rapid pacing both produce marked dilatation of all cardiac chambers [54, 56, 59, 65]. This profound cardiac chamber dilatation is surprisingly accompanied by little or no cardiac hypertrophy at the whole organ level. Indeed, in both dogs and pigs subjected to pacing, ventricular wall thinning in the absence of increased heart weight appears to be the rule [59, 66, 67]. Interestingly, at 4 weeks following pacing cessation, whereas all hemodynamic and neurohormonal parameters returned to the baseline values, both systolic and diastolic chamber volume remained increased from baseline while heart weight actually increased from the time of HF. It was initially believed that these findings reflected a relative metabolic deficiency induced by rapid pacing. Thus, chronic rapid pacing resulted in severe depletion of myocardial high-energy phosphate [68], potentially impairing the development of hypertrophy. The dramatic recovery of hemodynamic and clinical parameters as well as the development of hypertrophy after cessation of pacing appeared to support this hypothesis. To test this hypothesis, we devised a

7-week protocol of intermittent pacing, consisting of 48 h of rapid pacing alternating with 24 h of resumption of sinus rhythm, reasoning that there would have been intermittent recovery of energy substrate to permit the development of hypertrophy [69]. However, both the continuously paced and intermittently paced dogs failed to develop cardiac hypertrophy. Although the reasons why cardiac hypertrophy at a whole-organ level does not develop in this model remain unclear, these unique features of this model suggest that the insult is sufficiently intense such that these paced animals never enter a stage of compensated LV hypertrophy. Furthermore, the persistent chamber dilatation in spite of hemodynamic recovery at 4 weeks would suggest that structural remodeling is ongoing in spite of cessation of pacing. In contrast to the left ventricle, we first observed a significant increase in left atrial dimension in conjunction with an increase in left and right atrial appendage weights, indicating the development of significant biatrial hypertrophy [70, 71]. The basis for the dissociation between atrial and left ventricular hypertrophy is unclear, given a similar systemic hemodynamic and neurohumoral environment. It could, however, relate in part to the different atrial and ventricular rates and, therefore, high atrial wall stress and the different oxygen requirements of these chambers under the stress of rapid ventricular pacing. The differential wall stress of the left atrium and left ventricle appears to be accompanied by higher increased collagen content in the left atrium but not in the left ventricle of the paced dogs [71].

Our group and others have recently demonstrated that significant atrial remodeling occurs in addition to LV remodeling in the setting of HF [72, 73]. We first characterized the structural basis for atrial remodeling in our canine model of HF induced by right ventricular (RV) pacing [73]. HF is accompanied by atrial interstitial fibrosis with increased heterogeneity in local conduction, a substrate for the development of atrial fibrillation [74]. Atrial myocytes are hypertrophied. In addition, collagen synthesis is increased with a concurrent increase in proteolytic enzyme activity and collagen breakdown suggesting dynamic turnover [73, 74]. To specifically study atrial remodeling and atrial fibrillation in the setting of HF, we have recently validated a canine simultaneous atrioventricular pacing (SAVP) model [75, 76]. The pacemakers were programmed to capture both chambers simultaneously (AV delay 0-ms) at 220 beats/min with 1.0-ms pulses at three times threshold current. The SAVP dogs display clinical signs and echocardiographic changes of HF. Compared to controls and RV pacing, SAVP induced more profound atrial chamber dilatation and dysfunction with slightly less LV dysfunction (Table 6.2). Importantly, SAVP exacerbated the vulnerability to induced atrial fibrillation when compared to normal controls and RV pacing (Table 6.3). These abnormalities were accompanied by structural changes including denser fibrosis and more intense activation of matrix

Table 6.2 Comparison of echocardiographic parameters of LA and LV remodeling and dysfunction, expressed as percent change from baseline induced by chronic rapid right ventricular pacing (RVP) versus those by simultaneous atrioventricular pacing (SAVP) [76]

	RVP ($n = 8$)	SAVP ($n = 14$)
LA diastolic area	77±41%	62±35%
LA systolic area	64±38%	88±48%
LAFAS	−26±30%	−61±17%*
LV diastolic area	156±53%	43±17%
LV systolic area	58±27%	92±50%
LVFAS	−55±10%	−36±18%*

Data are mean ± SD. *LA* left atrium; *LV* left ventricle; *FAS* area fractional shortening
*$P < 0.05$ versus RVP

Table 6.3 Comparison of the vulnerability to atrial fibrillation in heart failure induced by RVP and SAVP [76]

	CTRL ($n = 5$)	RVP ($n = 5$)	SAVP ($n = 14$)
AF inducibility			
AERP induced-AF (%)	0	0	50
Percent of burst attempts leading to AF > 1 min	1.0±1.7	8.2±4.1	20±14*,†
AF maintenance			
AF duration, median and interquartile range (s)	0	710 (160–1,180)	1,600 (1,195–2,400)†
Percent of dogs with AF duration >10 min	0	40	83*,†

CTRL control dogs without pacing; *AERP* atrial effective refractory period
*$P < 0.05$ versus normal dogs
†$P < 0.05$ versus RVP dogs

metalloproteinase-9 (MMP-9) compared to RV pacing [76]. The profound electrophysiological and structural changes enabled us to explore the effects of intervention using MMP inhibition [77] as well as the effects of Omega-3 polyunsaturated fatty acids (PUFA) [78]. SAVP dogs treated with the MMP inhibitor had less atrial fibrillation inducibility than SAVP dogs treated with the vehicle. The treated dogs also had significantly smaller increases in atrial myocyte cross sectional area, collagen area fraction, and MMP-9 activity relative to the controls than in the vehicle treated dogs. There were no significant differences in the changes in chamber dimension and function in the left atrium. PUFA-treated paced dogs had less atrial fibrillation inducibility than untreated dogs. Histochemical analyses using picrosirius red staining of atrial appendages revealed smaller collagen area fraction in the treated dogs.

Fluid Retention and Edema

Pulmonary congestion and edema formation are two hallmarks of the syndrome of HF. The mechanisms for fluid retention in HF are multiple and include the development in the kidney of Starling forces, such as increased venous capillary pressure and decreased oncotic pressure, as well as the effects of local and systemic neurohormonal activation [79]. In our experience, chronic RV pacing in dogs at 250 beats/min for more than 3 weeks invariably produces severe radiographic pulmonary congestion [57, 60]. Peripheral edema occurs and is often manifested as ascites [57]. Significant increases in body weight may or may not occur, which probably reflect the net balance between accumulation of edema fluid and loss of lean body mass. In an earlier study, we made detailed comparisons of the sequential changes of plasma neurohormonal parameters during evolving pacing-induced HF to gain insights into the role of neurohormonal activation on fluid retention. Atrial natriuretic peptide (ANP) was activated early during the course of evolving HF, suggesting that this vasodilator, natriuretic neurohormone played an important role in early HF [79, 80]. It acts to prevent fluid retention at this early stage when the other neurohormones, such as norepinephrine, renin, and aldosterone, were not significantly increased. At the time of severe HF, hyponatremia developed, possibly related in part to the intense activation of the renin–angiotensin system, which is apparent at this advanced stage. Others have reported that the glomerular filtration rate, renal blood flow, and urinary Na excretion all decreased significantly. Increased natriuretic peptides likely play a homeostatic role. Intrarenal administration of the inhibitor of the natriuretic peptide receptor antagonist HS-142-1 to dogs with acute HF induced by rapid pacing resulted in reduced urinary cGMP and Na excretion accompanied by a reduced glomerular filtration rate [81]. We have demonstrated that in spite of increased circulating levels of ANP and BNP, the release of these peptides to an acute, further increase of atrial pressures, and the natriuretic responses to exogenous administration of ANP and BNP are both attenuated at HF [82, 83]. These probably constitute additional mechanisms contributing to the fluid retention.

In order to evaluate whether the response to hypertonic saline challenge can predict the propensity for fluid retention in HF, we classified normal dogs according to whether they drank more or less water than required to dilute the saline challenge to isotonicity [84]. These dogs were then paced for 1 or 3 weeks. At HF, the fluid retention score was higher in dogs that drank more after the saline challenge at baseline. There was a direct correlation between water intake following saline challenge at baseline and subsequent fluid retention. There was also an inverse correlation between the ability to concentrate urine at baseline and the degree of fluid retention at HF. These data suggest that the ability to regulate a salt load may be a useful predictor of the propensity for fluid retention in HF.

Neurohormonal and Cytokine Activation

Modulation of the neurohormonal system represents the most important treatment modality that has been developed in the management of patients with HF. The original neurohormone hypothesis states that prolonged neurohormone activation not only explains the clinical, hemodynamic, and metabolic perturbations but also contributes to disease progression in HF [85]. The model of pacing-induced cardiomyopathy was ideal for the studies of the pathophysiologic role of neurohormonal activation in HF because of its ability to produce intense stimulation of almost every neurohormonal system and cytokines including the endothelin system [79, 83, 86].

The pronounced alterations in the sympathetic nervous system, the RAAS, and the natriuretic peptides in this model have been comprehensively described in previous reviews [17, 54, 56, 61]. Among these parameters, endothelin-1 (ET-1) is one of the most potent vasoconstrictor peptides with diverse biological properties, which have recently been implicated in the pathogenesis of HF [54, 87, 88]. In dogs with pacing-induced HF, plasma ET-1 levels are consistently elevated [86, 89]. To elucidate some of the mechanisms for the increased circulating ET-1 level, we studied pulmonary clearance of ET-1 in dogs with pacing-induced HF [86]. Compared to baseline, the capacity of the lung to clear ET-1, as measured by the permeability-surface product, was markedly reduced at HF. This was accompanied by a reduced binding affinity of the type B endothelin receptors in the lungs. Our findings suggest that reduced pulmonary clearance of ET-1 likely contributes to the increased circulating ET-1 levels observed in this model. Using a ribonuclease protection assay, we have also demonstrated markedly increased mRNA expression of preproET-1 in the LV and the lungs of paced dogs [90]. The increased cardiac expression of ET-1 raises the possibility that ET-1 may play an important paracrine role in HF. Furthermore, the increased pulmonary expression strongly supports the hypothesis that increased ET-1 mediates the pulmonary hypertension in HF. The availability of specific antagonists of the endothelin receptors has allowed the examination of the functional role of the activation of the endothelin system in HF with the potential of establishing a novel therapy. We examined the effects of a 3-week oral administration of the specific type A endothelin receptor (ET_A) antagonist LU 135252 on hemodynamic and neurohormonal parameters in dogs with pacing-induced HF [91]. Administration of LU

135252 was associated with attenuation of the markedly increased LV end diastolic and pulmonary artery pressures observed in the placebo-treated dogs, and the rise in systemic and pulmonary vascular resistance observed in the placebo-treated dogs was prevented. The beneficial hemodynamic effects were obtained with no adverse effects on neurohormonal parameters such as norepinephrine and ANP. In a rabbit model of pacing-induced HF, administration of another ET_A antagonist was accompanied by restoration of function of the isolated myocytes [92]. Therefore, data derived from the canine and rabbit pacing-induced HF models suggest that an activated endothelin system may mediate the pulmonary and systemic vasoconstriction and impairment of myocyte function observed in HF.

There is now evidence in support of a pathological role of the proinflammatory cytokines such as tumor necrosis factor-α (TNF-α) in the pathogenesis of HF [93]. Several studies have reported in patients with advanced HF elevated circulating levels of TNF-α and its soluble receptors (sTNF-R1 and sTNF-R2) [94, 95]. In the canine pacing-induced HF model, we have reported serial changes of plasma TNF-α levels during evolving HF [54]. As early as 1 week after the onset of pacing, there was a trend of the plasma TNF-α levels increasing from baseline. At 3 weeks of pacing, the plasma TNF-α level was markedly elevated. Immunohistochemical studies of the LV tissue demonstrated intense staining of TNF-α, which was not observed in the control normal dogs. Furthermore, there were very few inflammatory cells in the paced dogs. The spleen stained only mildly positive. Our findings therefore suggest that, in the canine model of pacing-induced HF, there is a marked activation of the proinflammatory cytokine TNF-α. Furthermore, the heart is one source of production of cytokines in HF and this activation may occur in the absence of any major concurrent immune activation.

We recently tested the hypothesis that administration of a TNF-α blocking protein would prevent the induction of MMPs and alter the course of myocardial remodeling in developing LV failure. Adult dogs were randomly assigned to the following groups: (1) chronic pacing, (2) chronic pacing with concomitant administration of a TNF-α blocking protein using a soluble p75 TNF receptor fusion protein (TNFR:Fc); administered at 0.5 mg/kg twice a week subcutaneously, and (3) normal controls [96]. LV end-diastolic volume increased in control with chronic pacing and was reduced with TNF-α blockade. MMP zymographic levels (92 kDa, pixels) increased in control with chronic pacing and was normalized by TNF block (Fig. 6.1). Myocardial MMP-9 and MMP-13 levels assessed by immunoblot increased with pacing relative to controls and was normalized by TNF-α blockade. These results suggest that TNF-α contributes to the myocardial remodeling process in evolving HF through the local induction of specific MMPs.

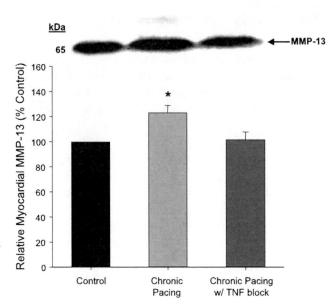

Fig. 6.1 Effect of cytokine blockade on matrix metalloproteinase abundance in heart failure. Immunoblotting for matrix metalloproteinase (MMP)-9 revealed an increase in the chronic pacing group that returned to normal in the TNF-blocking protein group. The emergence of a higher molecular weight band for MMP-9 in the chronic pacing-only group likely reflects increased abundance of a proform of MMP-9 (Reprinted from Bradham et al. [96]. With kind permission from the American Physiological Society)

Another mechanism by which the cytokines exert an adverse effect on the failing heart may be through an increased expression of inducible nitric oxide synthase (iNOS) [97]. In vitro studies in myocytes [98] and in vivo studies in animals [99] have demonstrated that NO decreases myocardial contractility and attenuates the contractile response to β-adrenergic stimulation. We have demonstrated that, in the canine model of pacing-induced HF, the inotropic response to β-adrenergic stimulus is attenuated [100]. It is therefore conceivable that enhanced myocardial NO may mediate in part the β-adrenergic hyporesponsiveness in HF in this model. To test the hypothesis, one study examined the effects of NOS inhibitor on contractile function in myocytes isolated from dogs with pacing-induced cardiomyopathy [101]. Total myocardial NOS activity, as measured by the conversion of arginine to citrulline, was significantly increased in dogs with HF compared to the normal controls. Contractile function of the myocyte was assessed by sarcomere shortening velocity. The addition of N-nitro-L-arginine methyl ester (L-NAME), an inhibitor of NOS, alone had no effects on basal sarcomere shortening velocity in the normal or HF dogs. However, L-NAME augmented the inotropic response to isoproterenol in HF dogs but not in the controls. These findings were interpreted to indicate that increased myocardial NOS activity contributes to an autocrine alteration in myocardial function in HF. We recently examined NOS activities as well as the protein expression of Ca^{2+}-dependent NOS, e.g., endothelial NOS (eNOS), and inducible Ca^{2+}-independent NOS in the LA and LV of the paced dogs [102]. Ca^{2+}-dependent NOS activity was increased in the left atrium but not in the left ventricle of the paced dogs. Likewise, protein expression of eNOS was increased only in the left atrium. On the other hand, inducible Ca^{2+}-independent NOS activity was not detectable in either the left atrium or left ventricle. These data suggest that there is differential regulation of NOS activities between the left atrium and left ventricle. One wonders whether the increased expression of eNOS in the left atrium may serve as a compensatory mechanism to counteract the atrial hypertrophy. In another study that also used the canine model [103], vascular rings from the coronary arteries of the paced dogs had a greater endothelium-dependent relaxation to BHT920, an $\alpha2$-adrenergic agonist compared to controls. However, the relaxation caused by BHT920 in the paced dogs was attenuated by NG monomethyl-L-arginine (L-NMMA), indicating that increased NOS in the coronary arteries enhances endothelium-dependent relaxation in the coronary arteries in the paced dogs. Notwithstanding differences in observations between different studies, the data obtained from the pacing model, on balance, suggest that increased NO may play a "protective role" by down-regulating the inotropic response of the heart to β-adrenergic stimulation, thereby counteracting hypertrophy while preserving coronary blood flow.

Transgenic Models

The recent development of techniques to alter specifically the expression of genes greatly improved our understanding of the pathophysiology of HF. Moreover, several genetic models of HF by addition or deletion of genes in mice have been developed. Several of these models have also provided interesting data about the genes involved in HF, as well as providing significant information regarding their phenotypic expression in the elderly.

Mutations in Sarcomeric and Intermediate Filament Proteins

The effects of specific mutations on sarcomere and cytoskeletal structure and function, as well as on overall cardiac structure and function in vivo have been examined in genetically engineered mouse models. A large number of transgenic studies have provided a wealth of information in the identification of new genetic targets, the confirmation of pathogenic mutations described in clinical studies, and in some cases elucidation of the role of these specific pathogenic mutations,

and resultant proteins in the progression of cardiac hypertrophy, fibrosis and onset of cardiomyopathy, either hypertrophic or dilated. Several specific alterations in genes involved in cytoskeletal and sarcomeric function, which generate cardiomyopathy and frequently induces HF in transgenic mice, are presented in Table 6.4.

The age-specific phenotypic expression of specific sarcomeric protein mutations was compared between heterozygous mice bearing a cardiac MHC missense mutation ($\alpha MHC^{403/+}$) and mice bearing a cardiac MyBP-C mutation (MyBP-$C^{t/+}$) [104]. While both mutant strains exhibited progressive LV hypertrophy, by 30 weeks of age $\alpha MHC^{403/+}$ mice showed considerably more LV hypertrophy than MyBP-$C^{t/+}$ mice. Moreover, increased expression of molecular markers of cardiac hypertrophy was observed in hearts from 50 week-old $\alpha MHC^{403/+}$ mice while MyBP-$C^{t/+}$ mice did not show expression of these markers until the mice were >125 weeks old. Electrophysiological assessment also indicated that MyBP-$C^{t/+}$ mice were not as likely to have inducible ventricular tachycardia as $\alpha MHC^{403/+}$ mice, and significant cardiac dysfunction was noted in $\alpha MHC^{403/+}$ mice before the development of LV hypertrophy whereas the cardiac function of MyBP-$C^{t/+}$ mice was not impaired even after the development of cardiac hypertrophy. Although it is not yet clear as to the extent to which these murine models mimic their human counterparts of familial HCM, both the use of electrophysiological and cardiac function studies may enable better risk stratification in older patients. Other studies with the R403Q mutation in cardiac αMHC murine model of familial HCM showed gender-specific differences with age [105]. Interestingly, cardiac hypertrophy was significantly increased with age in female animals while male hearts exhibited severe dilation by 8 months of age, in the absence of increased mass.

In addition to mutations in the sarcomere and cytoskeleton which mediate cardiomyopathy, we have previously noted that mutations in the intermediate filament lamin proteins of the nuclear lamina (lamin A/C) underlying the inner nuclear membrane are associated with clinical DCM with conduction defects. A mouse line that might recapitulate this clinical phenotype was constructed using homologous recombination and expressed the LMNA-N195K lamin A variant analogous to the asparagine-to-lysine substitution at amino acid 195, which causes DCM in humans [106]. Several phenotypes observed in the LMNA-N195K/N195K mice were consistent with DCM including heart chamber dilation, increased heart weight, interstitial fibrosis, upregulation of a fetal gene expression profile, and progressive conduction defects albeit neither apoptosis in the ventricular myocardium nor ventricular myocyte hypertrophy was detected. Also, similar to the human disorder, an age-dependent phenotypic progression was observed in the transgenic mouse. Despite a minor growth defect, LMNA-N195K/N195K mice appeared healthy,

Table 6.4 Selected mouse models of cardiomyopathy and heart failure – sarcomeric and structural genes

Gene (protein)	Genetic alteration	Function	Phenotype
α-MHC	S532P + F764LR 403 Q	Myosin heavy chain	DCM
			HCM
cMyBP-C	Cardiac-specific KO; truncated C-terminus	Cardiac myosin binding protein C	HCM
cTnT	R92 Q, I79N	Cardiac troponin T	HCM
MLP	Null	Muscle LIM protein	DCM
SGCD	Null	Delta-sarcoglycan	DCM, necrosis
Lamin A/C (LMNA)	Null; L85R + N195K	Nuclear membrane protein	DCM
TIMP-3	Null	Matrix metalloproteinases (MMP) inhibitor	DCM, hypertrophy
ABCA5	Null	Lysosomal ABC transporter	DCM
Desmin	Null	Cytoskeletal protein	DCM, fibrosis
Plakoglobin	Plakoglobin +/−	Desmosomal protein	ARVCM
SERCA2a	Gene-replacement with SERCA2b (>Ca^{2+} affinity)	SR Ca^{2+} transport ATPase, calcium cycling	HCM
N-cadherin (Cdh2)	Cardiac-specific null or overexpression	Cell adhesion molecule in intercalated disc	DCM
Tmod	Cardiac-specific overexpression	Tropomodulin	DCM
Calsarcin	Null	Sarcomeric Z-disc protein	Accelerated CM in response to pathological biomechanical stress
RLC	Cardiac-specific expression of E22K-RLC mutation	Myosin regulatory light-chain	Inter-ventricular septal hypertrophy and enlarged papillary muscles with no filament disarray

with no diminished activity levels or behavioral defects, and were difficult to distinguish from littermates until just before their demise, which generally followed an acute period of deterioration. This tended to occur between 11 and 14 weeks of age, with most mutant homozygous animals dying in that period (average, 12 weeks), none surviving past 16 weeks. Similarly, although impulse propagation initially appeared normal, the conduction system showed a deficit with increasing age. Interestingly, the LMNA-N195K/N195K mice live twice as longer as LMNA null mice and show earlier mortality (3 months) compared to another LMNA mutant model (H222P) (4–9 months) despite the fact that all three LMNA-deficient murine strains have similar cardiovascular phenotypes (i.e., conduction defects, lack of hypertrophy, dilation of heart chambers, and nuclear shape defects) and the LMNA-N195K/N195K strain does not exhibit the multiple tissue pathologies of the LMNA null mice nor the muscular dystrophy seen with the LMNA mutant model (H222P) [107, 108].

Mutations and Signal Transduction Pathways

It is well-known that diverse neurohormonal signals acting through a series of interwoven signal transduction pathways contribute to pathological cardiac hypertrophy and HF. Many such agonists act on the myocardium through cell surface receptors coupled with G-proteins to mobilize intracellular Ca^{2+}, with consequent activation of downstream kinases and the Ca^{2+}- and calmodulin-dependent phosphatase calcineurin. In addition, MAPK signaling pathways are interconnected at multiple levels with intracellular Ca^{2+}, with consequent activation of downstream kinases and the Ca^{2+}-dependent kinases and calcineurin [109]. β-adrenergic agonists also influence cardiac growth and function through the generation of cAMP, which activates protein kinase A (PKA) and other downstream effectors [110]. These signaling pathways target a variety of substrates in the cardiomyocyte, including components of the contractile apparatus, intracellular Ca^{2+}, with consequent activation of downstream kinases, the Ca^{2+} channels, and their regulatory proteins.

Mutations in proteins involved in a number of signal transduction pathways in the heart have also been found to lead to cardiomyopathy and HF in transgenic mice. A list of several identified gene mutations in cardiac signaling proteins, which can lead to cardiomyopathy and their phenotypic effects, is presented in Table 6.5. The functions of genes involved cover an extremely wide spectrum ranging from kinases e.g., p38 MAPK, DMPK, PKA, the receptor tyrosine kinase ErbB2, integrin-linked kinase, ILK, growth factors e.g., FGF-2, receptors e.g., angiotensin II type 2 receptor (AT2R), bradykinin B$_2$ receptor, α-adrenergic receptor 1B (α-AR 1B), β$_1$-adrenergic receptors e.g., β$_2$-AR, β$_1$-AR; transcription factors e.g., CREB, CHF1/HEY2, G-proteins (Gsα), caveolins e.g., CAV1, CAV3, calcium regulatory factors e.g., calcineurin, and splicing factors e.g., CELF, SC35.

Interestingly, transgenic mice with cardiac-specific overexpression of the stimulatory GTP-binding protein Gsα

Table 6.5 Selected mouse models of cardiomyopathy and heart failure – signaling genes

Gene (protein)	Genetic alteration	Function	Phenotype
CAV-1	Homozygous null	Caveolin signaling proteins	HCM, DCM
CAV-3	Null, P 104 L	Caveolin signaling proteins	HCM
DMPK	Overexpression	Protein kinase	HCM, fibrosis
p38 MAPK	Cardiac-specific dominant-negative	Mitogen-activated protein kinase	HCM
AGT	Null	Angiotensinogen-deficient	DCM
FGF-2	Null	Fibroblast growth factor	DCM
BK B2 receptor	Null	Bradykinin B2 signaling	DCM
AT2R	Cardiac-targeted overexpression	Angiotensin II type 2 receptor	DCM
CHF1 (Hey2)	Null	HLH transcription factor	DCM
Ena-VASP	Cardiac-specific dominant-negative	Vasodilator-stimulated phosphoprotein	DCM, hypertrophy
CELF	Cardiac-specific dominant-negative	RNA binding proteins involved in alternative splicing	DCM, hypertrophy
ABCA5	Null	Lysosomal ABC transporter	DCM
α-AR 1B	Cardiac-specific overexpressiom	Alpha-adrenergic receptor 1B	DCM
β2-AR	Overexpression	Beta2-adrenergic receptor	DCM, HF
β1-AR	Overexpression	Beta1-adrenergic receptor	DCM, HF
PKA	Cardiac-specific constitutive expression-catalytic subunit	Protein kinase A	DCM
SC35	Cardiac-specific null	Trans-acting splicing factor	DCM
ErbB2 (Her2)	Cardiac-specific conditional mutant allele	Receptor tyrosine kinase	DCM
Calcineurin	Cardiac-specific expression of constitutively active gene	Calcium signaling regulator	HCM/HF
CREB	Cardiac-specific dominant negative	Transcription factor	DCM
ILK	Cardiac-specific KO	Integrin-linked kinase	DCM, HF
iNOS	Cardiac-specific overexpression	Inducible nitric oxide synthase	Cardiac fibrosis, hypertrophy, dilatation and sudden death
Gs α	Cardiac-specific overexpression	Stimulatory G-protein	Hypertrophy, fibrosis; DCM in older mice

subunit exhibit increased cardiac contractility in response to β-adrenergic receptor stimulation. However, with aging, these mice develop a cardiomyopathy, which involves induction of apoptosis of cardiac myocytes [111].

Overexpression of the G-protein Gαq or constitutively active components of its signaling pathway have been shown in transgenic studies to lead to increased cardiac mass, cardiomyocyte hypertrophy, contractile dysfunction, and ventricular remodeling. These studies also demonstrated that massive cardiomegaly and extensive ventricular dilation were limited to animals with much elevated levels of Gαq and that a relatively modest overexpression of Gαq produced features of compensated LV hypertrophy with more extensive LV dilation, and HF only arising as a consequence of hemodynamic overload or neurohormonal stress (e.g., occurs with pregnancy) [112]. Mende et al., in transgenic mouse line containing a constitutively active Gαq allele (Gαq52), found that a cardiomyopathic phenotype including increased ventricular mass and dilation was present by 10 weeks of age [113]. Moreover, undetectable levels of the constitutively activated transgene product were found at 10 weeks suggesting that persistent expression of the transgene was not required for the progression of the cardiomyopathic phenotype. Another transgenic mouse line containing an epitope-tagged Gαq 44 allele expressed a lower level of transgene product, and ultimately displayed the same DCM phenotype with severely impaired left ventricular systolic function (assessed by M-mode and 2D echocardiography), but with a much delayed disease onset [114]. At 12–14 months, over 60% of mice with Gαq 44 still had normal cardiac function and ventricular weight/body weight ratio but manifested increased phospholipase C (PLC) levels compared to either wild-type mice or mice with the Gαq52 allele. This suggests that different Gαq alleles (in the same genetic background) can exert markedly different age-dependent phenotypes including disease onset; that PLC activation is not correlated with Gαq-determined phenotype, and that environmental modifiers may be involved in the age-dependent phenotypic expression.

Cytokine signaling and inflammation are well recognized for their involvement in the pathogenesis of HF. Several important components of these signaling pathways are the IL-6 family of cytokines, the extracellular gp130 receptor, and the signal transducer and activator of transcription 3 (STAT3) activated through gp130 – all of which have integral roles in cardiac myocyte survival and hypertrophy. Mice containing a cardiomyocyte-restricted deletion of STAT3 are significantly more susceptible to cardiac injury after doxorubicin treatment than age-matched controls [115]. Moreover, suggestive of a potential role of STAT3 in protecting against inflammation-induced heart damage, STAT3-deficient mice treated with lipopolysaccharide (LPS) displayed significantly more apoptosis than their wild-type counterparts. Also cardiomyocytes with STAT3 deleted secreted significantly more tumor necrosis factor (TNF) in response to LPS, and cardiomyocyte-restricted STAT3-deficient mice exhibited a dramatic increase in cardiac fibrosis in aged mice. While no overt signs of HF were present in young STAT3-deficient mice, heart dysfunction develops with advancing age. Therefore, these studies reveal a crucial role for STAT3 in mediating cardiomyocyte resistance to inflammation and other acute injury and in the pathogenesis of age-related HF.

Metabolic Defects

It is well-recognized that the adult heart is strongly reliant on fatty acids as its key fuel supply and a number of studies have shown that a variety of pathological conditions (e.g., cardiac hypertrophy) can shift the utilization of metabolic substrates [116, 117]. It has been proposed that initially this switch in metabolic substrate provides adequate energy to maintain normal cardiac function, however, over time diastolic dysfunction and HF may occur in association with depletion in high-energy phosphates. Importantly, the functioning of mitochondrial bioenergetic pathways (e.g., TCA cycle, FAO pathway, and the ETC/OXPHOS) provides most of the cellular ATP necessary for contractile and electrophysiological function. Results from both animal and human studies have confirmed that a variety of cardiomyopathic disorders and HF can be an important consequence of compromised mitochondrial bioenergetic function [116–119].

The creation of transgenic mice with altered expression of genes involved in carbohydrate, lipid, and mitochondrial metabolism has provided unique insights into the fine balance within the mouse heart to maintain energy status and cardiac function as well as to explore the cause–effect relationships between mitochondrial function and myocardial disease. A list of transgenic models of metabolic modification in the heart that are associated with cardiac dysfunction and/or HF phenotype is shown in Table 6.6.

Loss-of-function model studies, which disrupt mitochondrial metabolism, can exhibit specific cardiac phenotypes. Mouse models demonstrating a causal relationship between a mitochondrial energetic defect and cardiomyopathy include the Ant1 null and the TFAM null mice [120, 121]. The affected proteins are critically involved in mitochondrial bioenergetics, the adenine-nucleotide-translocator (ANT) protein, involved in mitochondrial nucleotide transport, and the mitochondrial

transcription factor (TFAM/mtTFA) that plays a variety of roles in mtDNA function (e.g., gene transcription, mtDNA replication, and maintenance) as well as in mitochondrial biogenesis. In addition, null mutation of mitochondrial creatine kinase can lead to LV dilation and hypertrophy [122].

Transgenic models of specific defects in the mitochondrial fatty acid oxidation (FAO) pathways have also been established. Two distinct mouse models with genetic deletion of the second step in the mitochondrial FAO pathway, a fatty acid chain-length-specific dehydrogenase enzyme (VLCAD and LCAD), display a cardiomyopathic phenotype [123, 124]. Furthermore, mice null for the PPAR-δ gene also exhibit diminished myocardial fat catabolic capacity and mild cardiomyopathic phenotype that accompanies aging [125]. A null mutation in the mitochondrial trifunctional protein (MTP) encoding a multifunctional enzyme in the β oxidation of fatty acids also results in cardiomyopathy and can lead to increased incidence of sudden death [126].

Several studies have shown that loss-of-function of critical mitochondrial antioxidant proteins can lead to cardiac dysfunction and cardiomyopathy. Strains harboring null mutations in either the Mn superoxide dismutase (MnSOD) or in TrxR2 encoding the mitochondrial thioredoxin reductase exhibit DCM [127, 128]. Mouse strains with a null mutation in frataxin (FRDA), a mitochondrial protein thought to be involved in regulating iron accumulation and flux and a regulator of oxidative stress (OS), also develop cardiac hypertrophy and cardiomyopathy [128, 129]. These strains appear to reliably recapitulate Friedreich ataxia, a human disorder with both neuropathic (e.g., ataxia) and cardiac involvement (e.g., HCM) caused by alterations in the gene for frataxin (most often trinucleotide repeats).

In addition to transgenic models with loss-of-function, studies utilizing "gain of function"/overexpression of a transgene have provided insights into the relation between mitochondrial dysfunction and cardiac dysfunction, particularly in cardiomyopathy associated with diabetes. Transgenic mice with cardiac-restricted overexpression of PPAR-α (the MHC-PPAR-α mice) exhibit increased expression of genes encoding enzymes involved in multiple steps of mitochondrial FAO with strong reciprocal down-regulation of glucose transporter (GLUT4) and glycolytic enzyme gene expression [130]. This activation of FAO via the elevation of the cardiac PPAR-α/PGC-1α mimics events occurring in the diabetic heart in which this metabolic shift is associated with high level of fatty acid import and oxidation can eventually lead to pathological mitochondrial and cardiac remodeling typical of diabetic cardiomyopathy. Echocardiographic assessment identified LV hypertrophy and dysfunction in the MHC-PPAR-α mice, in a transgene expression-dependent manner.

In these mouse models, overexpression of several genes with roles in metabolic regulation can also lead to cardiomyopathy and HF. These include overexpression of genes involved in

Table 6.6 Selected mouse models of metabolic genes involved in cardiomyopathy and heart failure

Gene (protein)	Genetic alteration	Function	Phenotype
MTP	Null	FAO; Mitochondrial trifunctional protein	CM; sudden death
LCAD	Global ablation	FAO; long chain acyl-CoA dehydrogenase	CM, ↑ myocardial lipid + fibrosis
Frataxin	Cardiac-specific KO	Iron metabolism; FRDA	CM, hypertrophy
TFAM/MtTFA	Cardiac-specific KO	Mitochondrial transcription factor A	DCM, AV heart conduction block
LpL	Cardiac-specific LPL with a GPI anchor	Lipoprotein lipase	DCM; ↓ FAO
PRKAG2	Cardiac-specific overexpression of N488I mutation	AMP kinase regulatory subunit	LV hypertrophy, ventricular preexcitation + sinus node dysfunction
Polymerase γ	Cardiac-specific knock-in mutation	Mitochondrial DNA polymerase	DCM
Mito-CK	Null	Mitochondrial creatine kinase	Increased LV dilation and hypertrophy
AIF	Cardiac-specific null	Apoptosis inducing factor	DCM
TrxR2	Cardiac-specific null	Mitochondrial thioredoxin reductase	Fatal DCM
MnSOD/SOD2	Null	Mn superoxide dismutase	DCM
PGC-1α	Cardiac-specific inducible overexpression	Peroxisome proliferator-activated receptor gamma coactivator-1α	Cardiomyopathy and mitochondrial defects only in adult not neonate
5-HT2B receptor	Cardiac-specific overexpression	Serotonin receptor	HCM with mitochondrial proliferation
OCTN2	Heterozygous carriers of mutation	Carnitine transporter	Age-associated CM with lipid deposition, hypertrophy
ANT1	Null	Adenine nucleotide translocator	CM, cardiac hypertrophy with ↑ mitochondria
FATP1	Cardiac-specific overexpression	Fatty acid transport protein 1	Lipotoxic cardiomyopathy
PPAR-α	Cardiac-specific overexpression	Peroxisome proliferator-activated receptor-α	Diabetic CM with ↑ FAO, ↓ glucose uptake + use, cardiac hypertrophy
PPAR-δ	Cardiac-specific null	Peroxisome proliferator-activated receptor-δ	Lipotoxic CM with ↑ myocardial lipid, dysfunction, hypertrophy, HF
ACS	Cardiac-specific overexpression	Long chain acyl-CoA synthetase	Cardiac lipid accumulation + hypertrophy, LV dysfunction and HF

fatty acid transport and utilization (e.g., ACS, FATP1) [130, 131] and of genes acting as global transcription regulators of metabolic regulation (PGC1) [132]. The latter gene is of particular relevance with respect to aging since it appears to show little overall affect on the heart when overexpressed in neonates, while overexpression in adult mice leads to extensive mitochondrial defects and cardiomyopathy.

Antioxidants and Reactive Oxygen Species

The age-mediated accumulation of ROS and their potent damaging effects on cellular macromolecules (particularly mitochondrial) and their function is particularly evident in aging cardiomyocytes and appears also to be involved in aging of the vasculature. Accumulative data have shown that mitochondrial defects resulting in the accumulation of OS can lead to cardiomyopathy and HF [133]. Associated with the cardiomyopathy resulting from murine knock-out of MnSOD, thioredoxin and TFAM genes are increased levels of mtDNA damage and OS. While in some cases global overexpression of antioxidants have not proven to be able to reverse the OS and aging-mediated dysfunction in the heart, recent studies have demonstrated that cardiac targeted-overexpression

of the antioxidant catalase can successfully ameliorate aging-mediated cardiac dysfunction. Schriner et al. have noted that overexpression of catalase targeted to the mitochondria increased overall mouse longevity, diminished OS, reduced mitochondrial protein and mtDNA damage, and delayed the onset of aging-mediated cardiac pathology [134]. Similarly, diminished levels of protein carbonyls, advanced glycation end-products (AGE) and of age-induced mechanical defects in myocyte contractility, and increased lifespan have been observed by Ren et al. in mice with cardiac-specific catalase overexpression [135]. Furthermore, catalase overexpression exerted attenuation of aging-induced contractile defect and cardiomyocyte relaxation dysfunction in part by improving intracellular Ca^{2+} cycling, and mainly by restoring the expression levels of the Na^+/Ca^{2+} exchanger (NCX) and the Kv1.2 K^+ channel [136].

Other Genetic Animal Models

In addition to the wealth of molecular information concerning age-mediated cardiomyopathy and HF which has emerged from mouse transgenic models, studies with genetic models highlighting the involvement of specific genes in cardiomyopathic and HF pathways have also been provided by other animal models including rat, rabbit, hamster, and even the fly Drosophila [137]. Studies with aging spontaneously hypersensitive rat (SHR) strains and with a rat strain prone to heart failure (SHHF), have contributed greatly to our understanding of signaling pathways involved in HF including generalized activation of the RAA, endothelin, and ANP systems [138, 139]. For instance, left ventricular homogenates from SHHF rats showed marked increases in Ca^{2+}-dependent NOS activity with age, accompanied by enhanced expression of endothelial NOS (eNOS), a change not seen in SHR or wild type rats [28]. In addition, the SHR strains are a useful model to study the transition from stable, compensated hypertrophy to decompensated HF in the context of aging, and have allowed the identification of programmatic changes in myocardial gene expression including increased expression of genes encoding elements of the ECM associated with this transition [140]. Moreover, pharmacological treatments that prevent matrix gene expression in the SHR heart have been shown to improve myocardial function and survival, albeit with limited success in reversing myocardial dysfunction [138].

Similarly, studies in cardiomyopathic-prone strains of hamsters have shown to mimic many of the changes occurring in otherwise healthy aged mammalian hearts [141]. These strains also exhibit age-associated changes in the ECM. Several hamster strains including CHF147 present a progressive DCM due to a large deletion of the δ-sarcoglycan gene leading to HF [39, 142]. These strains have been useful in both elucidating the changes leading to cardiomyopathy and HF and in testing strategies for reversing the cardiac dysfunction. In addition to its hereditary origin, in these strains HF can be aggravated by treatment with catecholamines and ameliorated by the administration of β-antagonists, both in genetic cardiomyopathic hamsters and in humans. Furthermore, in the CHF147 hamster, short-term treatment with recombinant human IGF-1 (without significant increases in IGF-1 serum levels) slowed down the progression of DCM, and significantly increased survival [143]. In addition, δ-sarcoglycan (δ-SG)-null cardiomyopathic hamsters fed from weaning to death with an α-lipoic acid (ALA)-enriched diet had a significant increase in viability with marked preservation of myocardium structure and function, and attenuation of myocardial fibrosis. At the cellular level, ALA treatment resulted in increased eicosapentaenoic/arachidonic acid ratio with preserved plasmalemma and mitochondrial membrane integrity, maintenance of proper cell/extracellular matrix contacts and signaling, normal gene expression profile (in terms of MHC isoforms, ANP, and TGF-β1) and limited development of fibrotic areas within the ALA-fed cardiomyopathic hearts [144]. In the TO-2 strain of hamsters with DCM, gene therapy by intramural delivery into the cardiac apex and left ventricle of a δ-SG gene, in a recombinant AAV vector, resulted in amelioration of the morphological and physiological cardiac abnormalities [145].

New Genetic Models

As research progresses in this field, new animal models of cardiomyopathy and genes mutations are being reported. Recently, Leatherbury et al. [146] have developed a mouse model of X-linked cardiac hypertrophy. This model exhibited neonatal lethality associated with severe fetal cardiac hypertrophy, with a number of adult mice dying suddenly with HCM. Histopathology analysis showed increased ventricular wall thickness, increased cardiomyocyte size, and mild myofiber disarray. Ultrastructural analysis by electron microscopy revealed mitochondria hyperproliferation and dilated sarcoplasmic reticulum. While genome scanning using microsatellite DNA markers mapped the mutation to the X chromosome, DNA sequencing showed no mutation in the coding regions of several candidate genes on the X chromosome, including several known to be associated with HCM. Likely, this mouse line may harbor a mutation in a novel gene causing X-linked cardiomyopathy. Also, Tsoutsman et al. have recently reported a double-mutant murine model of familial HCM (FHCM) [147]. This model has a TnI-203/MHC-403 double-mutant mice that develop into a severe cardiac phenotype characterized by HF and early death. By age 16–18 days, TnI-203/MHC-403 mice rapidly developed severe DCM and HF, with inducibility of ventricular dysrhythmias that led to death by 21 days. Downregulation of mRNA levels of key regulators of Ca^{2+} homeostasis in TnI-203/MHC-403 mice was observed. In addition, the TnI-203/MHC-403 mice showed increased levels of phosphorylated STAT3, which corresponded with the onset of disease suggesting a possible cardioprotective response. Thus, the presence of two disease-causing mutations may predispose individuals to a greater risk of developing severe HF than that caused by a single gene mutation. Furthermore, supporting the concept that a common mechanism may be involved in LV hypertrophy and LV dilatation, Kaneda et al. [148] have found that a novel β-myosin heavy chain gene mutation, p.Met531Arg, identified in isolated LV non-compaction in humans, resulted in the progression from LV hypertrophy to LV dilation in a mouse model.

Conclusions

The progress made in our understanding of the pathophysiology and treatment of HF would not have been possible without a number of animal models of HF and hypertrophy, each one having unique advantages as well as disadvantages. The common advantage is the availability of adequate healthy controls and the absence of confounding factors such as marked differences in age, concomitant pathologies, and pharmacological treatments. When starting a research project, investigators should always choose the model most suitable to address their specific aims, since significant differences always exist between human and experimentally-induced pathology. In this chapter, we have highlighted the critical importance that experimental animal models of HF assume for the difficult process of translation of basic scientific knowledge from bench to bedside.

Summary

- There are many animal models of heart failure and hypertrophy, each one having unique advantages as well as disadvantages.
- The species and interventions used to create heart failure depend on the scientific question as well as on factors such as ethical and economical considerations, accessibility, and reproducibility of the model.
- Besides basic ethical and philosophical questions, the use of animal models of heart failure and hypertrophy needs careful consideration because of at least two reasons: the disease may be associated with discomfort and pain to the animal and results from animal studies are not readily transferable to the situation in patients with heart failure.
- Rat models are relative inexpensive to utilize and because of short gestation periods, a large sample size can be produced in a short period of time. Rats are very robust animals: in an anesthetized rat, it is possible to exteriorize the heart via a small thoracic incision, occlude a coronary artery, reposition the heart in the thoracic cavity, repair the incision in a few minutes, and obtain a rapid recovery within hours. Therefore, rat models are extensively used to study long-term pharmacological interventions including long-term survival studies. However, there are limitations to the use of rat models regarding differences in myocardial function when compared to the human heart.
- Dog and other large animal models of heart failure may allow the study of left ventricular function and volumes more accurately than rodent models. They better allow for chronic instrumentation. Furthermore, in dog, many changes, such as the β-myosin heavy-chain isoform predominates and excitation–contraction coupling processes seem to be similar to the human myocardium. On the other hand, dog models are costly and require substantial resources with respect to housing and care.
- Rabbit models are less expensive than dog models. In addition, non-failing rabbit myocardium exhibits interesting similarities to the human heart. This model may be particularly suited to study functional consequences of altered ryanodine receptor expression.
- Cardiomyopathic strains of the Syrian hamster have been widely used as a model for cardiac hypertrophy and heart failure. The advantages of this model are (1) absence of surgical manipulations, (2) low costs, and (3) the ease with which large numbers of animals can be studied.
- At present, transgenic animal models of hypertrophy and heart failure are critically important for understanding the molecular alterations underlying the development of the disease. Addition or deletion of genes in transgenic mice together with miniaturized physiological techniques to evaluate the resulting cardiac phenotypes may allow the identification of genes that are causative for heart failure and evaluation of the molecular mechanisms responsible for the development and progression of the disease.

References

1. Pfeffer MA, Pfeffer JM, Fishbein MC, Fletcher PJ, Spadaro J, Kloner RA, Braunwald E (1979) Myocardial infarct size and ventricular function in rats. Circ Res 44:503–512
2. Hasenfuss G (1998) Animal models of human cardiovascular disease, heart failure and hypertrophy. Cardiovasc Res 39:60–76
3. Swynghedauw B (1986) Developmental and functional adaptation of contractile proteins in cardiac and skeletal muscles. Physiol Rev 66:710–771
4. Schwartz K, Lecarpentier Y, Martin JL, Lompre AM, Mercadier JJ, Swynghedauw B (1981) Myosin isoenzymic distribution correlates with speed of myocardial contraction. J Mol Cell Cardiol 13:1071–1075
5. Freeman GL, Little WC, O'Rourke RA (1987) Influence of heart rate on left ventricular performance in conscious dogs. Circ Res 61:455–464
6. Magid NM, Opio G, Wallerson DC, Young MS, Borer JS (1994) Heart failure due to chronic experimental aortic regurgitation. Am J Physiol 267:H556–H562
7. Ezzaher A, el Houda BN, Su JB, Hittinger L, Crozatier B (1991) Increased negative inotropic effect of calcium-channel blockers in hypertrophied and failing rabbit heart. J Pharmacol Exp Ther 257:466–471
8. Gilson N, el Houda BN, Corsin A, Crozatier B (1990) Left ventricular function and beta-adrenoceptors in rabbit failing heart. Am J Physiol 258:H634–H641
9. Ezzaher A, el Houda BN, Crozatier B (1992) Force-frequency relations and response to ryanodine in failing rabbit hearts. Am J Physiol 263:H1710–H1715
10. Kleaveland JP, Kussmaul WG, Vinciguerra T, Diters R, Carabello BA (1988) Volume overload hypertrophy in a closed-chest model of mitral regurgitation. Am J Physiol 254:H1034–H1041
11. McCullagh WH, Covell JW, Ross J Jr (1972) Left ventricular dilatation and diastolic compliance changes during chronic volume overloading. Circulation 45:943–951
12. Nagatsu M, Zile MR, Tsutsui H, Schmid PG, DeFreyte G, Cooper G, Carabello BA (1994) Native beta-adrenergic support for left ventricular dysfunction in experimental mitral regurgitation normalizes indexes of pump and contractile function. Circulation 89:818–826

13. Tsutsui H, Spinale FG, Nagatsu M, Schmid PG, Ishihara K, DeFreyte G, Cooper G, Carabello BA (1994) Effects of chronic beta-adrenergic blockade on the left ventricular and cardiocyte abnormalities of chronic canine mitral regurgitation. J Clin Invest 93:2639–2648

14. Holtz J, Studer R, Reinecke H, Just H, Drexler H (1992) Modulation of myocardial sarcoplasmic reticulum Ca(++)-ATPase in cardiac hypertrophy by angiotensin converting enzyme? Basic Res Cardiol 87:191–204

15. Feldman AM, Weinberg EO, Ray PE, Lorell BH (1993) Selective changes in cardiac gene expression during compensated hypertrophy and the transition to cardiac decompensation in rats with chronic aortic banding. Circ Res 73:184–192

16. Weinberg EO, Schoen FJ, George D, Kagaya Y, Douglas PS, Litwin SE, Schunkert H, Benedict CR, Lorell BH (1994) Angiotensin-converting enzyme inhibition prolongs survival and modifies the transition to heart failure in rats with pressure overload hypertrophy due to ascending aortic stenosis. Circulation 90:1410–1422

17. Elsner D, Riegger GA (1995) Characteristics and clinical relevance of animal models of heart failure. Curr Opin Cardiol 10:253–259

18. LK Dahl, Heine M, Tassinari L (1962) Role of genetic factors in susceptibility to experimental hypertension due to chronic excess salt ingestion. Nature 194:480–482

19. Inoko M, Kihara Y, Morii I, Fujiwara H, Sasayama S (1994) Transition from compensatory hypertrophy to dilated, failing left ventricles in Dahl salt-sensitive rats. Am J Physiol 267:H2471–H2482

20. Okamoto K, Aoki K (1963) Development of a strain of spontaneously hypertensive rats. Jpn Circ J 27:282–293

21. Bing OH, Brooks WW, Conrad CH, Sen S, Perreault CL, Morgan JP (1991) Intracellular calcium transients in myocardium from spontaneously hypertensive rats during the transition to heart failure. Circ Res 68:1390–1400

22. Boluyt MO, O'Neill L, Meredith AL, Bing OH, Brooks WW, Conrad CH, Crow MT, Lakatta EG (1994) Alterations in cardiac gene expression during the transition from stable hypertrophy to heart failure. Marked upregulation of genes encoding extracellular matrix components. Circ Res 75:23–32

23. Li Z, Bing OH, Long X, Robinson KG, Lakatta EG (1997) Increased cardiomyocyte apoptosis during the transition to heart failure in the spontaneously hypertensive rat. Am J Physiol 272: H2313–H2319

24. Chua SC Jr, Chung WK, Wu-Peng XS, Zhang Y, Liu SM, Tartaglia L, Leibel RL (1996) Phenotypes of mouse diabetes and rat fatty due to mutations in the OB (leptin) receptor. Science 271:994–996

25. Holycross BJ, Summers BM, Dunn RB, McCune SA (1997) Plasma renin activity in heart failure-prone SHHF/Mcc-facp rats. Am J Physiol 273:H228–H233

26. Narayan P, McCune SA, Robitaille PM, Hohl CM, Altschuld RA (1995) Mechanical alternans and the force-frequency relationship in failing rat hearts. J Mol Cell Cardiol 27:523–530

27. Gomez AM, Valdivia HH, Cheng H, Lederer MR, Santana LF, Cannell MB, McCune SA, Altschuld RA, Lederer WJ (1997) Defective excitation-contraction coupling in experimental cardiac hypertrophy and heart failure. Science 276:800–806

28. Khadour FH, Kao RH, Park S, Armstrong PW, Holycross BJ, Schulz R (1997) Age-dependent augmentation of cardiac endothelial NOS in a genetic rat model of heart failure. Am J Physiol 273:H1223–H1230

29. Bajusz E (1969) Hereditary cardiomyopathy: a new disease model. Am Heart J 77:686–696

30. Forman R, Parmley WW, Sonnenblick EH (1972) Myocardial contractility in relation to hypertrophy and failure in myopathic Syrian hamsters. J Mol Cell Cardiol 4:203–211

31. Jasmin G, Proschek L (1982) Hereditary polymyopathy and cardiomyopathy in the Syrian hamster. I. Progression of heart and skeletal muscle lesions in the UM-X7.1 line. Muscle Nerve 5:20–25

32. Whitmer JT, Kumar P, Solaro RJ (1988) Calcium transport properties of cardiac sarcoplasmic reticulum from cardiomyopathic Syrian hamsters (BIO 53.58 and 14.6): evidence for a quantitative defect in dilated myopathic hearts not evident in hypertrophic hearts 2. Circ Res 62:81–85

33. Finkel MS, Marks ES, Patterson RE, Speir EH, Steadman KA, Keiser HR (1987) Correlation of changes in cardiac calcium channels with hemodynamics in Syrian hamster cardiomyopathy and heart failure. Life Sci 41:153–159

34. Wagner JA, Reynolds IJ, Weisman HF, Dudeck P, Weisfeldt ML, Snyder SH (1986) Calcium antagonist receptors in cardiomyopathic hamster: selective increases in heart, muscle, brain. Science 232:515–518

35. Kuo TH, Tsang W, Wang KK, Carlock L (1992) Simultaneous reduction of the sarcolemmal and SR calcium ATPase activities and gene expression in cardiomyopathic hamster. Biochim Biophys Acta 1138:343–349

36. Hatem SN, Sham JS, Morad M (1994) Enhanced Na(+)-Ca2+ exchange activity in cardiomyopathic Syrian hamster. Circ Res 74:253–261

37. Malhotra A, Karell M, Scheuer J (1985) Multiple cardiac contractile protein abnormalities in myopathic Syrian hamsters (BIO 53:58). J Mol Cell Cardiol 17:95–107

38. Okazaki Y, Okuizumi H, Ohsumi T, Nomura O, Takada S, Kamiya M, Sasaki N, Matsuda Y, Nishimura M, Tagaya O, Muramatsu M, Hayashizaki Y (1996) A genetic linkage map of the Syrian hamster and localization of cardiomyopathy locus on chromosome 9qa2.1-b1 using RLGS spot-mapping. Nat Genet 13:87–90

39. Nigro V, Okazaki Y, Belsito A, Piluso G, Matsuda Y, Politano L, Nigro G, Ventura C, Abbondanza C, Molinari AM, Acampora D, Nishimura M, Hayashizaki Y, Puca GA (1997) Identification of the Syrian hamster cardiomyopathy gene. Hum Mol Genet 6:601–607

40. Kajstura J, Zhang X, Reiss K, Szoke E, Li P, Lagrasta C, Cheng W, Darzynkiewicz Z, Olivetti G, Anversa P (1994) Myocyte cellular hyperplasia and myocyte cellular hypertrophy contribute to chronic ventricular remodeling in coronary artery narrowing-induced cardiomyopathy in rats. Circ Res 74:383–400

41. Teerlink JR, Loffler BM, Hess P, Maire JP, Clozel M, Clozel JP (1994) Role of endothelin in the maintenance of blood pressure in conscious rats with chronic heart failure. Acute effects of the endothelin receptor antagonist Ro 47-0203 (bosentan). Circulation 90:2510–2518

42. van Veldhuisen DJ, van Gilst WH, de Smet BJ, de Graeff PA, Scholtens E, Buikema H, Girbes AR, Wesseling H, Lie KI (1994) Neurohumoral and hemodynamic effects of ibopamine in a rat model of chronic myocardial infarction and heart failure. Cardiovasc Drugs Ther 8:245–250

43. Pinto YM, de Smet BG, van Gilst WH, Scholtens E, Monnink S, de Graeff PA, Wesseling H (1993) Selective and time related activation of the cardiac renin-angiotensin system after experimental heart failure: relation to ventricular function and morphology. Cardiovasc Res 27:1933–1938

44. Litwin SE, Morgan JP (1992) Captopril enhances intracellular calcium handling and beta-adrenergic responsiveness of myocardium from rats with postinfarction failure. Circ Res 71:797–807

45. Gopalakrishnan M, Triggle DJ, Rutledge A, Kwon YW, Bauer JA, Fung HL (1991) Regulation of K+ and Ca2+ channels in experimental cardiac failure. Am J Physiol 261:H1979–H1987

46. Zarain-Herzberg A, Afzal N, Elimban V, Dhalla NS (1996) Decreased expression of cardiac sarcoplasmic reticulum Ca(2+)-pump ATPase in congestive heart failure due to myocardial infarction. Mol Cell Biochem 163–164:285–290

47. Patel KP, Zhang PL, Krukoff TL (1993) Alterations in brain hexokinase activity associated with heart failure in rats. Am J Physiol 265:R923–R928

48. Anversa P, Zhang X, Li P, Capasso JM (1992) Chronic coronary artery constriction leads to moderate myocyte loss and left ventricular dysfunction and failure in rats. J Clin Invest 89:618–629

49. Sabbah HN, Stein PD, Kono T, Gheorghiade M, Levine TB, Jafri S, Hawkins ET, Goldstein S (1991) A canine model of chronic heart failure produced by multiple sequential coronary microembolizations. Am J Physiol 260:H1379–H1384

50. Gengo PJ, Sabbah HN, Steffen RP, Sharpe JK, Kono T, Stein PD, Goldstein S (1992) Myocardial beta adrenoceptor and voltage sensitive calcium channel changes in a canine model of chronic heart failure. J Mol Cell Cardiol 24:1361–1369

51. Gupta RC, Shimoyama H, Tanimura M, Nair R, Lesch M, Sabbah HN (1997) SR Ca(2+)-ATPase activity and expression in ventricular myocardium of dogs with heart failure. Am J Physiol 273:H12–H18

52. Sabbah HN, Shimoyama H, Kono T, Gupta RC, Sharov VG, Scicli G, Levine TB, Goldstein S (1994) Effects of long-term monotherapy with enalapril, metoprolol, and digoxin on the progression of left ventricular dysfunction and dilation in dogs with reduced ejection fraction. Circulation 89:2852–2859

53. Whipple GH, Sheffield LT, Woodman EG, Theophilis C, Friedman S (1962) Reversible congestive heart failure due to chronic rapid stimulation of the normal heart. Proc N Engl Cardiovasc Soc 20:39–40

54. Moe GW, Armstrong P (1999) Pacing-induced heart failure: a model to study the mechanism of disease progression and novel therapy in heart failure. Cardiovasc Res 42:591–599

55. Recchia FA, Lionetti V (2007) Animal models of dilated cardiomyopathy for translational research. Vet Res Commun 31:35–41

56. Shinbane JS, Wood MA, Jensen DN, Ellenbogen KA, Fitzpatrick AP, Scheinman MM (1997) Tachycardia-induced cardiomyopathy: a review of animal models and clinical studies. J Am Coll Cardiol 29:709–715

57. Armstrong PW, Stopps TP, Ford SE, De Bold AJ (1986) Rapid ventricular pacing in the dog: pathophysiologic studies of heart failure. Circulation 74:1075–1084

58. Riegger AJ, Liebau G (1982) The renin-angiotensin-aldosterone system, antidiuretic hormone and sympathetic nerve activity in an experimental model of congestive heart failure in the dog. Clin Sci (Lond) 62:465–469

59. Howard RJ, Moe GW, Armstrong PW (1991) Sequential echocardiographic-Doppler assessment of left ventricular remodelling and mitral regurgitation during evolving experimental heart failure. Cardiovasc Res 25:468–474

60. Moe GW, Stopps TP, Howard RJ, Armstrong PW (1988) Early recovery from heart failure: insights into the pathogenesis of experimental chronic pacing-induced heart failure. J Lab Clin Med 112:426–432

61. Armstrong PW, Howard RJ, Moe GW (1989) Clinical lessons learned from experimental heart failure. Int J Cardiol 24:133–136

62. Smith HJ, Nuttall A (1985) Experimental models of heart failure. Cardiovasc Res 19:181–186

63. Spinale FG, Coker ML, Thomas CV, Walker JD, Mukherjee R, Hebbar L (1998) Time-dependent changes in matrix metalloproteinase activity and expression during the progression of congestive heart failure: relation to ventricular and myocyte function. Circ Res 82:482–495

64. Spinale FG, Gunasinghe H, Sprunger PD, Baskin JM, Bradham WC (2002) Extracellular degradative pathways in myocardial remodeling and progression to heart failure. J Card Fail 8:S332–S338

65. Morgan DE, Tomlinson CW, Qayumi AK, Toleikis PM, McConville B, Jamieson WR (1989) Evaluation of ventricular contractility indexes in the dog with left ventricular dysfunction induced by rapid atrial pacing. J Am Coll Cardiol 14:489–495

66. Shannon RP, Komamura K, Stambler BS, Bigaud M, Manders WT, Vatner SF (1991) Alterations in myocardial contractility in conscious dogs with dilated cardiomyopathy. Am J Physiol 260:H1903–H1911

67. Tanaka R, Spinale FG, Crawford FA, Zile MR (1992) Effect of chronic supraventricular tachycardia on left ventricular function and structure in newborn pigs. J Am Coll Cardiol 20:1650–1660

68. Moe GW, Montgomery C, Howard RJ, Grima EA, Armstrong PW (1993) Left ventricular myocardial blood flow, metabolism, and effects of treatment with enalapril: further insights into the mechanisms of canine experimental pacing-induced heart failure. J Lab Clin Med 121:294–301

69. Moe GW, Howard RJ, Grima EA, Armstrong PW (1995) How does intermittent pacing modify the response to rapid ventricular pacing in experimental heart failure? J Card Fail 1:223–228

70. Moe GW, Grima EA, Howard RJ, Armstrong PW (1996) Biatrial appendage hypertrophy but not ventricular hypertrophy: a unique feature of canine pacing-induced heart failure. J Card Fail 2:127–132

71. O'Brien DW, Fu Y, Parker HR, Chan SY, Idikio H, Scott PG, Jugdutt BI (2000) Differential morphometric and ultrastructural remodelling in the left atrium and left ventricle in rapid ventricular pacing-induced heart failure. Can J Cardiol 16:1411–1419

72. Boixel C, Fontaine V, Rucker-Martin C, Milliez P, Louedec L, Michel JB, Jacob MP, Hatem SN (2003) Fibrosis of the left atria during progression of heart failure is associated with increased matrix metalloproteinases in the rat. J Am Coll Cardiol 42:336–344

73. Khan A, Moe GW, Nili N, Rezaei E, Eskandarian M, Butany J, Strauss BH (2004) The cardiac atria are chambers of active remodeling and dynamic collagen turnover during evolving heart failure. J Am Coll Cardiol 43:68–76

74. Li D, Fareh S, Leung TK, Nattel S (1999) Promotion of atrial fibrillation by heart failure in dogs: atrial remodeling of a different sort. Circulation 100:87–95

75. Laurent G, Moe GW, Hu X, Pui-Sze SP, Ramadeen A, Leong-Poi H, Doumanovskaia L, Konig A, Trogadis J, Courtman D, Strauss BH, Dorian P (2008) Simultaneous right atrioventricular pacing: a novel model to study atrial remodeling and fibrillation in the setting of heart failure. J Card Fail 14:254–262

76. Laurent G, Moe G, Hu X, Leong-Poi H, Connelly KA, So PP, Ramadeen A, Doumanovskaia L, Konig A, Trogadis J, Courtman D, Strauss B, Dorian P (2008) Experimental studies of atrial fibrillation: a comparison of two pacing models. Am J Physiol Heart Circ Physiol 294:H1206–H1215

77. Moe GW, Laurent G, Doumanovskaia L, Konig A, Hu X, Dorian P (2008) Matrix metalloproteinase inhibition attenuates atrial remodeling and vulnerability to atrial fibrillation in a canine model of heart failure. J Card Fail 14:768–776

78. Laurent G, Moe G, Hu X, Holub B, Leong-Poi H, Trogadis J, Connelly K, Courtman D, Strauss BH, Dorian P (2008) Long chain n-3 polyunsaturated fatty acids reduce atrial vulnerability in a novel canine pacing model. Cardiovasc Res 77:89–97

79. Moe GW, Stopps TP, Angus C, Forster C, De Bold AJ, Armstrong PW (1989) Alterations in serum sodium in relation to atrial natriuretic factor and other neuroendocrine variables in experimental pacing-induced heart failure. J Am Coll Cardiol 13:173–179

80. Moe GW, Grima EA, Wong NL, Howard RJ, Armstrong PW (1996) Plasma and cardiac tissue atrial and brain natriuretic peptides in experimental heart failure. J Am Coll Cardiol 27:720–727

81. Stevens TL, Rasmussen TE, Wei CM, Kinoshita M, Matsuda Y, Burnett JC Jr (1996) Renal role of the endogenous natriuretic peptide system in acute congestive heart failure. J Card Fail 2:119–125

82. Moe GW, Forster C, De Bold AJ, Armstrong PW (1990) Pharmacokinetics, hemodynamic, renal, and neurohormonal effects of atrial natriuretic factor in experimental heart failure. Clin Invest Med 13:111–118

83. Moe GW, Grima EA, Wong NL, Howard RJ, Armstrong PW (1993) Dual natriuretic peptide system in experimental heart failure. J Am Coll Cardiol 22:891–898

84. Fu Y, O'Brien DW, Chan SY, Kaufman S, Moe GW, Armstrong PW (1997) Does a hypertonic saline load predict fluid retention in pacing induced heart failure? Cardiovasc Res 33:172–180

85. Packer M (1992) The neurohormonal hypothesis: a theory to explain the mechanism of disease progression in heart failure. J Am Coll Cardiol 20:248–254

86. Dupuis J, Moe GW, Cernacek P (1998) Reduced pulmonary metabolism of endothelin-1 in canine tachycardia-induced heart failure. Cardiovasc Res 39:609–616

87. Colucci WS (1996) Myocardial endothelin. Does it play a role in myocardial failure? Circulation 93:1069–1072

88. Yanagisawa M, Kurihara H, Kimura S, Tomobe Y, Kobayashi M, Mitsui Y, Yazaki Y, Goto K, Masaki T (1988) A novel potent vasoconstrictor peptide produced by vascular endothelial cells. Nature 332:411–415

89. Margulies KB, Hildebrand FL Jr, Lerman A, Perrella MA, Burnett JC Jr (1990) Increased endothelin in experimental heart failure. Circulation 82:2226–2230

90. Huntington K, Picard P, Moe G, Stewart DJ, Albernaz A, Monge JC (1998) Increased cardiac and pulmonary endothelin-1 mRNA expression in canine pacing-induced heart failure. J Cardiovasc Pharmacol 31:S424–S426

91. Moe GW, Albernaz A, Naik GO, Kirchengast M, Stewart DJ (1998) Beneficial effects of long-term selective endothelin type A receptor blockade in canine experimental heart failure. Cardiovasc Res 39:571–579

92. Spinale FG, Walker JD, Mukherjee R, Iannini JP, Keever AT, Gallagher KP (1997) Concomitant endothelin receptor subtype-A blockade during the progression of pacing-induced congestive heart failure in rabbits. Beneficial effects on left ventricular and myocyte function. Circulation 95:1918–1929

93. Mann DL, Young JB (1994) Basic mechanisms in congestive heart failure. Recognizing the role of proinflammatory cytokines. Chest 105:897–904

94. Ferrari R, Bachetti T, Confortini R, Opasich C, Febo O, Corti A, Cassani G, Visioli O (1995) Tumor necrosis factor soluble receptors in patients with various degrees of congestive heart failure. Circulation 92:1479–1486

95. Torre-Amione G, Kapadia S, Lee J, Durand JB, Bies RD, Young JB, Mann DL (1996) Tumor necrosis factor-alpha and tumor necrosis factor receptors in the failing human heart. Circulation 93:704–711

96. Bradham WS, Moe G, Wendt KA, Scott AA, Konig A, Romanova M, Naik G, Spinale FG (2002) TNF-alpha and myocardial matrix metalloproteinases in heart failure: relationship to LV remodeling. Am J Physiol Heart Circ Physiol 282:H1288–H1295

97. Finkel M, Finkel ER, Harris AI (1978) Von Recklinghausen's disease with involvement of the colon: an endoscopic view. Mt Sinai J Med 45:387–389

98. Brady AJ, Warren JB, Poole-Wilson PA, Williams TJ, Harding SE (1993) Nitric oxide attenuates cardiac myocyte contraction. Am J Physiol 265:H176–H182

99. Hare JM, Colucci WS (1995) Role of nitric oxide in the regulation of myocardial function. Prog Cardiovasc Dis 38:155–166

100. Spinale FG, Tempel GE, Mukherjee R, Eble DM, Brown R, Vacchiano CA, Zile MR (1994) Cellular and molecular alterations in the beta adrenergic system with cardiomyopathy induced by tachycardia. Cardiovasc Res 28:1243–1250

101. Yamamoto S, Tsutsui H, Tagawa H, Saito K, Takahashi M, Tada H, Yamamoto M, Katoh M, Egashira K, Takeshita A (1997) Role of myocyte nitric oxide in beta-adrenergic hyporesponsiveness in heart failure. Circulation 95:1111–1114

102. Khadour FH, O'Brien DW, Fu Y, Armstrong PW, Schulz R (1998) Endothelial nitric oxide synthase increases in left atria of dogs with pacing-induced heart failure. Am J Physiol 275:H1971–H1978

103. O'Murchu B, Miller VM, Perrella MA, Burnett JC Jr (1994) Increased production of nitric oxide in coronary arteries during congestive heart failure. J Clin Invest 93:165–171

104. McConnell BK, Fatkin D, Semsarian C, Jones KA, Georgakopoulos D, Maguire CT, Healey MJ, Mudd JO, Moskowitz IP, Conner DA, Giewat M, Wakimoto H, Berul CI, Schoen FJ, Kass DA, Seidman CE, Seidman JG (2001) Comparison of two murine models of familial hypertrophic cardiomyopathy. Circ Res 88:383–389

105. Vikstrom KL, Factor SM, Leinwand LA (1996) Mice expressing mutant myosin heavy chains are a model for familial hypertrophic cardiomyopathy. Mol Med 2:556–567

106. Mounkes LC, Kozlov SV, Rottman JN, Stewart CL (2005) Expression of an LMNA-N195K variant of A-type lamins results in cardiac conduction defects and death in mice. Hum Mol Genet 14:2167–2180

107. Arimura T, Helbling-Leclerc A, Massart C, Varnous S, Niel F, Lacene E, Fromes Y, Toussaint M, Mura AM, Keller DI, Amthor H, Isnard R, Malissen M, Schwartz K, Bonne G (2005) Mouse model carrying H222P-Lmna mutation develops muscular dystrophy and dilated cardiomyopathy similar to human striated muscle laminopathies. Hum Mol Genet 14:155–169

108. Nikolova V, Leimena C, McMahon AC, Tan JC, Chandar S, Jogia D, Kesteven SH, Michalicek J, Otway R, Verheyen F, Rainer S, Stewart CL, Martin D, Feneley MP, Fatkin D (2004) Defects in nuclear structure and function promote dilated cardiomyopathy in lamin A/C-deficient mice. J Clin Invest 113:357–369

109. Sugden PH, Clerk A (1998) "Stress-responsive" mitogen-activated protein kinases (c-Jun N-terminal kinases and p38 mitogen-activated protein kinases) in the myocardium. Circ Res 83:345–352

110. Rockman HA, Koch WJ, Lefkowitz RJ (2002) Seven-transmembrane-spanning receptors and heart function. Nature 415:206–212

111. Geng YJ, Ishikawa Y, Vatner DE, Wagner TE, Bishop SP, Vatner SF, Homcy CJ (1999) Apoptosis of cardiac myocytes in Gsalpha transgenic mice. Circ Res 84:34–42

112. Adams JW, Sakata Y, Davis MG, Sah VP, Wang Y, Liggett SB, Chien KR, Brown JH, Dorn GW (1998) Enhanced Galphaq signaling: a common pathway mediates cardiac hypertrophy and apoptotic heart failure. Proc Natl Acad Sci USA 95:10140–10145

113. Mende U, Kagen A, Cohen A, Aramburu J, Schoen FJ, Neer EJ (1998) Transient cardiac expression of constitutively active Galphaq leads to hypertrophy and dilated cardiomyopathy by calcineurin-dependent and independent pathways. Proc Natl Acad Sci USA 95:13893–13898

114. Mende U, Semsarian C, Martins DC, Kagen A, Duffy C, Schoen FJ, Neer EJ (2001) Dilated cardiomyopathy in two transgenic mouse lines expressing activated G protein alpha(q): lack of correlation between phospholipase C activation and the phenotype. J Mol Cell Cardiol 33:1477–1491

115. Jacoby JJ, Kalinowski A, Liu MG, Zhang SS, Gao Q, Chai GX, Ji L, Iwamoto Y, Li E, Schneider M, Russell KS, Fu XY (2003) Cardiomyocyte-restricted knockout of STAT3 results in higher sensitivity to inflammation, cardiac fibrosis, and heart failure with advanced age. Proc Natl Acad Sci USA 100:12929–12934

116. Russell LK, Finck BN, Kelly DP (2005) Mouse models of mitochondrial dysfunction and heart failure. J Mol Cell Cardiol 38:81–91

117. Carvajal K, Moreno-Sanchez R (2003) Heart metabolic disturbances in cardiovascular diseases. Arch Med Res 34:89–99

118. Kelly DP, Strauss AW (1994) Inherited cardiomyopathies. N Engl J Med 330:913–919

119. Smeitink J, van den HL, DiMauro S (2001) The genetics and pathology of oxidative phosphorylation. Nat Rev Genet 2: 342–352

120. Graham BH, Waymire KG, Cottrell B, Trounce IA, MacGregor GR, Wallace DC (1997) A mouse model for mitochondrial myopathy and cardiomyopathy resulting from a deficiency in the heart/muscle isoform of the adenine nucleotide translocator. Nat Genet 16:226–234

121. Wang J, Wilhelmsson H, Graff C, Li H, Oldfors A, Rustin P, Bruning JC, Kahn CR, Clayton DA, Barsh GS, Thoren P, Larsson NG (1999) Dilated cardiomyopathy and atrioventricular conduction blocks induced by heart-specific inactivation of mitochondrial DNA gene expression. Nat Genet 21:133–137

122. Nahrendorf M, Spindler M, Hu K, Bauer L, Ritter O, Nordbeck P, Quaschning T, Hiller KH, Wallis J, Ertl G, Bauer WR, Neubauer S (2005) Creatine kinase knockout mice show left ventricular hypertrophy and dilatation, but unaltered remodeling post-myocardial infarction. Cardiovasc Res 65:419–427

123. Exil VJ, Gardner CD, Rottman JN, Sims H, Bartelds B, Khuchua Z, Sindhal R, Ni G, Strauss AW (2006) Abnormal mitochondrial bioenergetics and heart rate dysfunction in mice lacking very-long-chain acyl-CoA dehydrogenase. Am J Physiol Heart Circ Physiol 290:H1289–H1297

124. Kurtz DM, Rinaldo P, Rhead WJ, Tian L, Millington DS, Vockley J, Hamm DA, Brix AE, Lindsey JR, Pinkert CA, O'Brien WE, Wood PA (1998) Targeted disruption of mouse long-chain acyl-CoA dehydrogenase gene reveals crucial roles for fatty acid oxidation. Proc Natl Acad Sci USA 95:15592–15597

125. Cheng L, Ding G, Qin Q, Huang Y, Lewis W, He N, Evans RM, Schneider MD, Brako FA, Xiao Y, Chen YE, Yang Q (2004) Cardiomyocyte-restricted peroxisome proliferator-activated receptor-delta deletion perturbs myocardial fatty acid oxidation and leads to cardiomyopathy. Nat Med 10:1245–1250

126. Ibdah JA, Paul H, Zhao Y, Binford S, Salleng K, Cline M, Matern D, Bennett MJ, Rinaldo P, Strauss AW (2001) Lack of mitochondrial trifunctional protein in mice causes neonatal hypoglycemia and sudden death. J Clin Invest 107:1403–1409

127. Conrad M, Jakupoglu C, Moreno SG, Lippl S, Banjac A, Schneider M, Beck H, Hatzopoulos AK, Just U, Sinowatz F, Schmahl W, Chien KR, Wurst W, Bornkamm GW, Brielmeier M (2004) Essential role for mitochondrial thioredoxin reductase in hematopoiesis, heart development, and heart function. Mol Cell Biol 24:9414–9423

128. Huang TT, Carlson EJ, Kozy HM, Mantha S, Goodman SI, Ursell PC, Epstein CJ (2001) Genetic modification of prenatal lethality and dilated cardiomyopathy in Mn superoxide dismutase mutant mice. Free Radic Biol Med 31:1101–1110

129. Puccio H, Simon D, Cossee M, Criqui-Filipe P, Tiziano F, Melki J, Hindelang C, Matyas R, Rustin P, Koenig M (2001) Mouse models for Friedreich ataxia exhibit cardiomyopathy, sensory nerve defect and Fe-S enzyme deficiency followed by intramitochondrial iron deposits. Nat Genet 27:181–186

130. Finck BN, Lehman JJ, Leone TC, Welch MJ, Bennett MJ, Kovacs A, Han X, Gross RW, Kozak R, Lopaschuk GD, Kelly DP (2002) The cardiac phenotype induced by PPARalpha overexpression mimics that caused by diabetes mellitus. J Clin Invest 109:121–130

131. Chiu HC, Kovacs A, Ford DA, Hsu FF, Garcia R, Herrero P, Saffitz JE, Schaffer JE (2001) A novel mouse model of lipotoxic cardiomyopathy. J Clin Invest 107:813–822

132. Russell LK, Mansfield CM, Lehman JJ, Kovacs A, Courtois M, Saffitz JE, Medeiros DM, Valencik ML, McDonald JA, Kelly DP (2004) Cardiac-specific induction of the transcriptional coactivator peroxisome proliferator-activated receptor gamma coactivator-1alpha promotes mitochondrial biogenesis and reversible cardiomyopathy in a developmental stage-dependent manner. Circ Res 94:525–533

133. Marin-Garcia J, Pi Y, Goldenthal MJ (2006) Mitochondrial-nuclear cross-talk in the aging and failing heart. Cardiovasc Drugs Ther 20:477–491

134. Schriner SE, Linford NJ, Martin GM, Treuting P, Ogburn CE, Emond M, Coskun PE, Ladiges W, Wolf N, Van RH, Wallace DC, Rabinovitch PS (2005) Extension of murine life span by overexpression of catalase targeted to mitochondria. Science 308:1909–1911

135. Wu S, Li Q, Du M, Li SY, Ren J (2007) Cardiac-specific overexpression of catalase prolongs lifespan and attenuates ageing-induced cardiomyocyte contractile dysfunction and protein damage. Clin Exp Pharmacol Physiol 34:81–87

136. Ren J, Li Q, Wu S, Li SY, Babcock SA (2007) Cardiac overexpression of antioxidant catalase attenuates aging-induced cardiomyocyte relaxation dysfunction. Mech Ageing Dev 128:276–285

137. Ocorr K, Akasaka T, Bodmer R (2007) Age-related cardiac disease model of Drosophila. Mech Ageing Dev 128:112–116

138. Bing OH, Conrad CH, Boluyt MO, Robinson KG, Brooks WW (2002) Studies of prevention, treatment and mechanisms of heart failure in the aging spontaneously hypertensive rat. Heart Fail Rev 7:71–88

139. Heyen JR, Blasi ER, Nikula K, Rocha R, Daust HA, Frierdich G, Van Vleet JF, De CP, McMahon EG, Rudolph AE (2002) Structural, functional, and molecular characterization of the SHHF model of heart failure. Am J Physiol Heart Circ Physiol 283:H1775–H1784

140. Boluyt MO, Bing OH (2000) Matrix gene expression and decompensated heart failure: the aged SHR model. Cardiovasc Res 46:239–249

141. Minieri M, Fiaccavento R, Carosella L, Peruzzi G, Di NP (1999) The cardiomyopathic hamster as model of early myocardial aging. Mol Cell Biochem 198:1–6

142. Sakamoto A, Ono K, Abe M, Jasmin G, Eki T, Murakami Y, Masaki T, Toyo-oka T, Hanaoka F (1997) Both hypertrophic and dilated cardiomyopathies are caused by mutation of the same gene, delta-sarcoglycan, in hamster: an animal model of disrupted dystrophin-associated glycoprotein complex. Proc Natl Acad Sci USA 94:13873–13878

143. Serose A, Salmon A, Fiszman MY, Fromes Y (2006) Short-term treatment using insulin like growth factor-1 (IGF-1) improves life expectancy of the delta-sarcoglycan deficient hamster. J Gene Med 8:1048–1055

144. Fiaccavento R, Carotenuto F, Minieri M, Masuelli L, Vecchini A, Bei R, Modesti A, Binaglia L, Fusco A, Bertoli A, Forte G, Carosella L, Di Nardo P (2006) Alpha-linolenic acid-enriched diet prevents myocardial damage and expands longevity in cardiomyopathic hamsters. Am J Pathol 169:1913–1924

145. Toyo-oka T, Kawada T, Xi H, Nakazawa M, Masui F, Hemmi C, Nakata J, Tezuka A, Iwasawa K, Urabe M, Monahan J, Ozawa K (2002) Gene therapy prevents disruption of dystrophin-related proteins in a model of hereditary dilated cardiomyopathy in hamsters. Heart Lung Circ 11:174–181

146. Leatherbury L, Yu Q, Chatterjee B, Walker DL, Yu Z, Tian X, Lo CW (2008) A novel mouse model of X-linked cardiac hypertrophy. Am J Physiol Heart Circ Physiol 294:H2701–H2711

147. Tsoutsman T, Kelly M, Ng DC, Tan JE, Tu E, Lam L, Bogoyevitch MA, Seidman CE, Seidman JG, Semsarian C (2008) Severe heart failure and early mortality in a double-mutation mouse model of familial hypertrophic cardiomyopathy. Circulation 117:1820–1831

148. Kaneda T, Naruse C, Kawashima A, Fujino N, Oshima T, Namura M, Nunoda S, Mori S, Konno T, Ino H, Yamagishi M, Asano M (2008) A novel beta-myosin heavy chain gene mutation, p. Met531Arg, identified in isolated left ventricular non-compaction in humans, results in left ventricular hypertrophy that progresses to dilation in a mouse model. Clin Sci (Lond) 114:431–440

Section V
Signaling, Stress and Cellular Changes in Heart Failure

Chapter 7
Signaling Cascades in Heart Failure: From Cardiomyocytes Growth and Survival to Mitochondrial Signaling Pathways

Overview

Over the last decade, signal transduction pathways have been identified in normal cardiovascular growth processes, metabolic homeostasis, and during the development of the myocardium and vasculature. Alterations in discrete components of these signaling pathways are contributory factors in the pathogenesis and progression of a broad spectrum of cardiovascular disorders, dysrhythmias, atherosclerosis, hypertension, diabetes, and metabolic syndrome, and in the cardiovascular dysfunction associated with aging, as well as heart failure (HF).

Introduction

Cardiovascular signaling has come to light as a by-product of intensive research on the mechanisms of cardiac hypertrophy, cell death, and myocardial remodeling. The targeting and localization of signaling factors and enzymes to discrete subcellular compartments or substrates are important regulatory mechanisms that ensure specific signaling events in response to local stimuli. These systems should be examined both, from a sub-cellular/organellar and functional standpoint under physiological and pathophysiological conditions. It is worth noting that cardiovascular signaling encompasses built-in specificity, reversibility, and a redundancy of its components, which while making their analysis a very complex undertaking, provides the cardiac cells with a great plasticity to respond to insult, as well as to growth stimuli.

In this and next two chapters, we will discuss cell signaling in HF with an emphasis on myocardial signaling as well as signaling pathways that are involved in vascular cells.

Signaling in Physiological Cardiovascular Growth

It is well established that cardiac myocytes rapidly proliferate in the embryo but exit the cell cycle irreversibly shortly after birth, with the predominant form of growth shifting from hyperplastic to hypertrophic. Extensive research has focused on identifying the mitogenic stimuli and signaling pathways that mediate these distinct growth processes in isolated cells, and in vivo hearts. The molecular mechanisms underlying the proliferative growth of embryonic myocardium and adult cardiac myocyte hypertrophy in vivo remain largely undetermined, although considerable progress has recently been made using postgenomic analysis. This includes studies involving the manipulation of the murine genome in concert with mutational analysis of these signaling and growth control pathways in vivo, and in cardiomyocytes grown in vitro including the use of gene transfer/knock-out. For instance, cell cycle control can be mediated by p38 MAP kinase activity, which regulates the expression of genes required for mitosis in cardiomyocytes including cyclin A and cyclin B. Cardiac-specific p38MAPK knock-out mice show a 92% increase in neonatal cardiomyocyte mitosis. Furthermore, inhibition of p38 MAPK promotes cytokinesis in adult cardiomyocytes [1].

Evidence has been gathered that cyclin D1, a cell-cycle regulator involved in promoting the G_1-to-S phase progression via phosphorylation of the retinoblastoma (Rb) protein, is localized in the nucleus of fetal cardiomyocytes but is primarily cytoplasmic in neonatal and adult cardiomyocytes (concomitant with Rb underphosphorylation). Ectopic expression of a variant of cyclin D1 equipped with nuclear localization signals dramatically promote neonatal cardiomyocyte proliferation and Rb phosphorylation [2]. Growth factors such as FGF-2 significantly promote neonatal cardiac myocyte proliferation [3], and overexpression of the FGF-2 receptor (FGF-R1) in neonatal rat cardiomyocytes results in marked proliferation [4]. Cardiotrophin (CT-1) an interleukin 6-related cytokine, has been shown to promote both the survival and proliferation of cultured neonatal cardiac myocytes [5]. This likely is mediated by the PI3K/Akt pathway since CT-1 phosphorylates and activates Akt [6]. These diverse approaches have confirmed the importance of suspected pathways, and implicated unexpected pathways leading to new paradigms for the control of cardiac growth as well. Furthermore, in the regulation of cardiomyocyte growth and/or proliferation, there are several signal transductions acting as redundant mechanisms converging on one or several serine/threonine kinases. Several G-protein-coupled receptors (GPCRs) such as α-AR, β-AR, angiotensin II, and endothelin-1 are able to activate these signaling cascades, and induce changes in cell growth and proliferation. A general scheme involves the following: Signals received at the plasma membrane receptors are transmitted via GPCR/G-proteins second messengers to a wide-spectrum of protein kinases, and phosphatases, which are in turn activated. These activated protein modifiers may lead to the activation and/or deactivation of specific transcription factors, which modulate specific gene expression affecting a broad spectrum of cellular events, or they can directly target proteins involved in metabolic pathways, ion transport, Ca^{2+} regulation, and handling influencing contractility and excitability, as well as the pathways of cardiomyocyte apoptosis and/or survival. Also, transcriptional networks implicated in mitochondrial biogenesis and function [7], include PPARγ coactivator-1 (PGC-1), the ensemble of downstream nuclear receptor partners (e.g., PPARs and estrogen-related receptors (see Chap. 5), converging molecular signals such as Ca^{2+} (see below in this chapter), NO, MAPKs, β-adrenergic mechanisms, cAMP (see Chap. 8), and signal transduction pathways (e.g., ERKs).

Prosurvival Pathways

Protein kinase B or Akt and PI3K

The PI3K/Akt pathway is a key regulator of four intersecting biological processes: cell growth and survival, cell-cycle progression, and metabolism. In the heart, Akt contributes to both pathological and physiological cardiac growth, myocyte survival, and contractile function [8].

Akt

Akt or protein kinase B (PKB) represents a family of serine and threonine kinases, which include Akt1, Akt2, and Akt3 encoded by three distinct genetic loci with extensive homology (approximately 80%) [9]. There are considerable differences in both the expression and function of the Akt isoforms with

only Akt1 and Akt2 being highly expressed in the heart. All three Akt isoforms contain a kinase domain (with structural homology to PKA and PKC), which contains the primary site (Thr^{308}) of phosphorylation by PDK-1. Although Thr^{308} phosphorylation partially activates Akt, subsequent phosphorylation of Akt at a C-terminal site, Ser^{473} is required for its full activation; under some conditions, this phosphorylation may be produced by PDK-1, another kinase (PDK-2) or by autophosphorylation.

Akt1 knock-out mice weigh approximately 20% less than wild-type littermates, and have a proportional reduction in the size of all somatic tissues including the heart. In contrast, Akt2 knock-out mice have only a modest reduction in organ size. Thus, data from the available Akt knock-out models support a critical role specifically for Akt1 in the normal growth of the heart. On the other hand, Akt1/Akt2 double-knock-out mice suffer marked growth deficiency, and striking defect in cell proliferation. Interestingly, activation of Akt in these transgenic models induced cardiac hypertrophy primarily by increasing the size of cardiomyocytes [10]. Furthermore, Akt expression confers protection from ischemia-induced cell death and cardiac dysfunction.

Akt in Pacing-induced HF

In the canine model of pacing-induced chronic HF, Rhada et al. have studied the potential role of the Akt pathway in signaling the metabolic transitions central to progression to HF [11]. Myocardial Akt levels were found elevated in early HF (after 1–2 weeks of pacing) accompanied by increased severity of oxidative stress (OS), the cytokine tumor necrosis factor-α (TNF-α) and free fatty acid accumulation, reduced activity levels of mitochondrial respiratory complex III and complex V, and apoptosis initiation. In severe HF (3–4 weeks of pacing), there was significant increase in myocardial apoptosis, with pronounced decline in myocardial Akt kinase activity. At this later stage, there were no further changes in free fatty acid accumulation, complex V activity or in OS indicating that these changes primarily occurred in the earlier stage of evolving HF. In contrast, during severe HF, both the reduction in complex III activity and increase in TNF-α level became more pronounced.

A major and novel finding of this study was the identification of both myocardial Akt kinase activation and the role of specific Akt phosphorylation as significant signaling events occurring in early HF. While its upstream regulators are not yet known, both OS and TNF-α levels, which also increased in early HF, could play a contributory role in the activation of Akt [12]. One potential downstream target of the Akt pathway is the shift in myocardial substrate utilization, including FAO. The role of ventricular pacing in down-regulating FAO has been previously documented [13, 14]. In the canine model of pacing-induced HF, there is reduced gene expression of mitochondrial FAO enzymes (e.g., MCAD, CPT1), and marked reduction in FFA consumption that preceded increasing glucose utilization [13]. By 2 weeks of pacing, when Akt kinase activity is at its peak (and concurrent with high levels of Akt phosphorylation at residue Ser^{473}), higher levels of FFA accumulate in the heart, and are not utilized for energy by β-oxidation. These findings support the view that the failing heart reverts to a fetal mode of glucose oxidation, characterized by reduced FFA consumption and increased utilization of glucose [15]; this is potentially advantageous for the failing heart, which needs less oxygen to produce ATP from glucose, when compared to FFA. Down-regulation of RXR-α, a global transcription regulator of genes encoding mitochondrial FAO enzymes also occurs in pacing-induced severe HF [14]. Similarly, activation of myocardial Akt kinase promotes down-regulation of specific transcriptional regulators involved in FAO gene expression [16]. Notwithstanding, the precise mechanisms by which Akt kinase exerts its regulatory effects on myocardial FAO metabolism, including the delineation of both upstream and downstream events within the Akt signaling pathway remain to be elucidated. While Akt kinase has not been previously implicated in modulating specific mitochondrial OXPHOS/ETC enzyme activities, such a role would also be consistent with the overall down-regulation of myocardial FAO and could contribute to the overall myocardial shift to glycolytic metabolism. Of related interest, is the finding that Akt activation can directly down-regulate the activity of cardiac AMPK, an energy sensor that acts as a modulator of glucose uptake and FAO [17].

Another novel finding in this study [11] was the demonstration that enzymatic dysfunction in mitochondrial complex III and V is an early event in pacing, occurring well before significant clinical signs of HF are evident (usually by 3–4 weeks of pacing). The onset of mitochondrial enzymatic dysfunction was accompanied by both increased levels of OS and TNF-α levels in the early paced group. Whether the observed OS is in fact generated from the mitochondrial enzyme defects (particularly in complex III, see Chap. 10) remains to be determined, although this is an attractive hypothesis that requires further testing. Indeed, further studies directed at elucidating these events at days 1–7 of pacing may shed light on the precise role and generation of OS in this model.

Akt, Oxidative Stress and Apoptosis

The increased in OS noted in early HF, in association with both stimulated Akt kinase activation and apoptotic initiation, is also consistent with the concept that OS promotes both of these pathways [18]. Dogs with severe HF exhibit both increased in TNF-α level and a more severe complex III

deficiency; this correlation may be significant since TNF-α has been found to promote complex III deficiency in isolated cardiomyocytes, presumably acting through the ceramide signaling pathway [19]. It is noteworthy that with increasing pacing time, myocardial Akt kinase activity is significantly reduced. This coincides with both the development of clinical signs of HF as well as with further increase in myocardial apoptosis, as measured by TUNEL or cell death ELISA.

It has long been recognized that Akt acts as an antiapoptotic factor important in cardiomyocyte survival, and one way it can modulate apoptotic progression is by phosphorylation of pro-apoptotic peptide factors (e.g., BAD) [20]. Conversely, apoptosis can trigger or stimulate factors capable of de-phosphorylating signaling stimulators such as Akt [21, 22]. Also, caspase induction stimulates specific phosphatase activities which can target Akt [21]. Changes in calcium flux (also a pivotal feature of myocardial apoptosis) can also induce specific phosphatase activities thereby down-regulating Akt activity and signaling, and further promoting apoptosis [22]. Moreover, end-stage HF can stimulate the increase in expression and activities of multiple myocardial phosphatases [23]. The reduction of myocardial Akt activity observed by Rhada et al. with increased duration of pacing [11] was consistent with other reports showing a decline in phosphorylated Akt in dogs with severe DCM, paced for 4.5–5 weeks [24]. This study also demonstrated a marked decline in myocardial ATP levels in late HF in the paced dogs, likely a consequence of the documented severe complex III and V dysfunction and further underscores the value of characterizing early events in HF.

Akt kinase is activated by phosphorylation at Thr^{308} and within its C-terminus at Ser^{473}. Akt activation promotes cell survival by inhibiting apoptosis [25], has a crucial role in stimulating glucose uptake by regulating glycogen synthase kinase, modulates gene expression of FAO enzymes, and intracellular calcium regulating proteins [26]. In addition to stimulation by OS and TNF-α, myocardial Akt activity can also be modulated by long chain fatty acids such as palmitate and by calcium-induced phosphatases [27, 28]. Thus, Akt may play a crucial role in the dynamics and signaling of substrate regulation during pacing-induced HF. Taken together, these findings provide the first demonstration that the Akt signaling pathway is a contributory element in the early signaling events leading to the progression of pacing-induced HF, accompanying a shift in substrate utilization from fatty acid to glucose utilization. In early HF, increased Akt activity and Akt phosphorylation correlated with elevated levels of OS and TNF-α, FFA accumulation, the initial onset of myocardial apoptosis and reduced activity levels of specific mitochondrial respiratory enzymes (i.e., complex III and complex V) as noted above. During severe HF, there is a significant increase in myocardial apoptosis, with a pronounced decline in myocardial Akt kinase activity and no further change in the levels of FFA, complex V activity, or in OS, indicating that these changes occurred primarily during early pacing-induced HF. In contrast, both reduced complex III activity and elevated myocardial TNF-α level become more pronounced during late HF.

Akt and Mammalian Target of Rapamycin

Akt is positioned at a signaling cascade branch point [29]. One branch leads to mammalian target of rapamycin (mTOR) and the activation of the protein synthetic machinery, which is essential for all forms of hypertrophy (Fig. 7.1).

It has been reported that insulin rapidly activates the 70-kDa ribosomal S6 kinase (p70S6k), and this effect is inhibited both by rapamycin and by inhibitors of PI3K [32]. Peptide growth factors (e.g., GH, IGF) are primary activators

of mTOR in mammalian cells, and activate mTOR primarily via Akt. Interestingly, downstream activation of p70S6k is mediated by a signaling pathway involving mTOR, a molecule that responds to the nutritional status and amino acid availability, and is centrally involved in cell growth and proliferation. Moreover, one downstream target of mTOR signaling is the 4E binding protein (4E-BP), a translational repressor that directly regulates the activity of the eIF4 translational initiation factor. In addition, activated mTOR is able to phosphorylate p70S6k, which can inactivate eEF2 kinase (regulating translational elongation), as well as phosphorylate the 40S ribosomal protein S6. In several cell types, activation of the TSC1–TSC2 complex (Tuberous sclerosis gene) negatively regulates p70S6k; it also inhibits mTOR signaling, reducing cell growth (and insulin signaling), and is inhibited by Akt-dependent phosphorylation [33, 34]. The TSC complex mediates its effect on mTOR signaling by

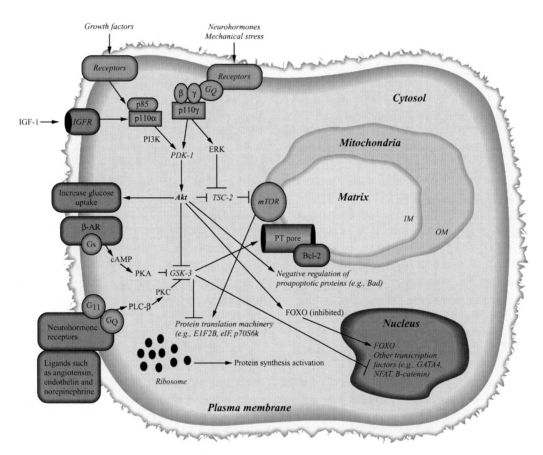

Fig. 7.1 Akt signaling. Akt is positioned at a signaling cascade branch point. One branch leads to mammalian target of rapamycin (mTOR) and the activation of the protein synthetic machinery, which is essential for all forms of hypertrophy. Downstream effects of Akt kinase activity include changes in myocardial bioenergetic substrates, effected by increasing glucose uptake, and by down-regulating FAO metabolism via direct effect on transcription regulators (e.g., PPAR-α and RXR-α). It may also impact mitochondrial OXPHOS activities, which decline in parallel with increased Akt activity. Both mTOR and Akt modulate cytoplasmic protein synthesis by activation of

translation initiation factor (IF), and of ribosomal proteins. Also shown are peptide growth factors (GH, IGF) and other downstream targets of mTOR. FOXO sustained activation in cardiomyocytes leads to increased Akt phosphorylation and kinase activity. As depicted, upstream of FOXO, the activity of Akt itself is governed by several protein kinases and phosphatases including phosphorylation at Thr[308] within its catalytic domain by 3-phosphoinositide-dependent protein kinase-1 (PDK1) and by phosphorylation at Ser[473] within a C-terminal hydrophobic motif by mammalian target of rapamycin (mTOR) [30, 31] targeting Rheb, which is a small Ras-homologous GTPase implicated with mTOR in the activation of p70S6k [35, 36]. However, the identification and the contribution of the TSC complex and Rheb to the signaling events occurring in cardiomyocyte growth, and cardiac hypertrophy remain to be determined.

Akt and Glycogen Synthase Kinase

A second branch of the signaling cascade leads to glycogen synthase kinase-3 (GSK-3), which also regulates the general protein translational machinery, as well as specific transcription factors implicated in both normal and pathologic cardiac growth. GSK-3β, which was among the first negative regulators of cardiac hypertrophy to be identified, blocks cardiomyocyte hypertrophy in response to endothelin (ET-1), isoproteronol, and Fas signaling [37–39]. In addition, GSK-3β has been found to be a negative regulator of both normal and pathologic stress-induced growth (e.g., pressure overload) [39]. GSK-3β plays a key inhibitory role in both insulin signaling, and in the Wnt signaling pathway, which has been implicated in early cardiomyocyte differentiation as well as in myocardial hypertrophic growth responses. In unstimulated cells, GSK-3β phosphorylates the N-terminal domain of β-catenin, thereby targeting it for ubiquitylation (protein modification by the covalent attachment of one or more ubiquitin monomers, is implicated in a number of metabolic pathways and nonproteolytic cellular functions) and proteasomal degradation. GSK-3β is constitutively active unlike most kinases; it is turned "off" by cell stimulation by growth factors and hypertrophic agonists. GSK-3β negatively regulates most of its substrates, including the protein translation initiation factor eIF2B [40], as well as transcription factors implicated in cardiac growth, including c-Myc, GATA-4, and β-catenin [40, 41]. In addition, GSK-3β is a counter-regulator of calcineurin/NFAT signaling phosphorylating NFAT N-terminal residues, which are dephosphorylated by calcineurin, preventing nuclear translocation of the NFATs [38]. Moreover, Akt phosphorylates GSK-3β at serine-9 inhibiting its activity.

Inhibition of GSK-3β releases a number of transcription factors from tonic inhibition and also releases eIF2B allowing translational activation. Transgenic mice overexpressing GSK-3β in the heart exhibit significantly defective postnatal cardiomyocyte growth, as well as markedly abnormal cardiac contractile function related to down-regulation of SERCA expression (resulting in abnormal calcium handling), and severe diastolic dysfunction with progressive HF [42]. In addition, it has been suggested that a family of dimeric phophoserine-binding molecules, the 14-3-3 proteins (which are implicated in cell-cycle control and the stress response), participate in the regulation of GSK-3β phosphorylation [43].

It is noteworthy that the activation of protein translation affected by both of these signaling branches can also be regulated by stress-activated mechanisms, which are independent of Akt. For instance, AMP-activated protein kinase (AMPK), a key regulator of cellular energy homeostasis, is involved in modulating the activity of mTOR, and can affect the translational response in cardiac hypertrophy [44]. Moreover, hypoxia can rapidly and reversibly trigger mTOR hypo-phosphorylation, and mediate changes in its effectors such as 4E-BP1 and p70S6K, independent of Akt or AMPK signaling [45]. Also, the TSC complex can be phosphorylated and inactivated by stress-mediated stimuli, and the ERK pathway independent of Akt signaling. The Akt-independent mechanism of activation of mTOR may be particularly relevant to pathological stress-induced growth.

Inactivation of GSK-3β by S9 phosphorylation may also occur independent of the PI3K/Akt pathway, and this includes involvement of growth factors such as EGF and PDGF which stimulate the GSK-3β-inactivating kinase p90 RSK through MAP kinases, activators of cAMP-activated PKA, and PKC activators. Moreover, exposure of cells to Wnt protein ligands leads to inactivation of GSK-3β by an undefined mechanism [46].

Cardiac Akt Activation

The stimuli that result in Akt activation in the heart are shown in Table 7.1. Upon activation, myocardial Akt can phosphorylate a number of downstream targets, including cardioprotective factors involved in glucose and mitochondrial metabolism, apoptosis and regulators of protein synthesis, as discussed below. The regulation of Akt is also achieved by its dephosphorylation effected by the protein phosphatase PP2A. Inhibitors of PP2A activity, including okadaic acid, increase Akt activity, while ceramide, which is involved in enhanced apoptotic signaling, stimulates PP2A. In the heart, Akt signaling has a pronounced antiapoptotic effect, significantly increases cardiomyocyte growth, and enhance

Table 7.1 Stimuli activating myocardial Akt

Stimuli	References
Insulin	[47, 48]
IGF-1	[49, 50]
Cardiotrophin-1	[51]
LIF	[52]
β-AR agonists	[10]
Angiotensin-II	[53]
Endothelin-1	[54]
Acetylcholine	[55]
Adrenomedullin	[56]
Pressure overload	[57]
Ischemia (hypoxia)	[58]

function. Apoptotic progression of hypoxic cardiomyocytes is abrogated with IGF-1 treatment, which activates PI3K and Akt [49]. Overexpression of constitutively active transgenes, either PI3K or Akt, in cultured hypoxic cardiomyocytes reduces apoptosis. Moreover, after transient ischemia in vivo, gene transfer of constitutively active Akt to the heart resulted in reduced apoptosis and infarct size [50]. Several mechanisms and/or effectors by which the PI3K/Akt pathway stems apoptosis have been identified, and it appears likely that these effectors might be enhanced when applied in combination. These include the phosphorylation and inactivation of the proapoptotic protein Bad, NF-κB activation, enhanced NO release and eNOS activation, changes in the mitochondrial membrane pores and membrane potential suppressing apoptotic progression, as well as cytochrome c release induced by several proapoptotic proteins. Gathered observations have also shown that Akt's effect on apoptosis and cell survival is mediated by its phosphorylation of the forkhead transcription factor FOXO3 that in turn reduces the transcription of specific proapoptotic molecules [51].

PI3K

Both PI3K and Akt can modulate cardiomyocyte growth with significant effects on both cell and organ size. Transgenic mice with cardiac-specific overexpression of either the constitutively active or dominant-negative alleles of PI3K exhibited an increase or decrease in cardiomyocyte size, respectively [51]. The constitutive activation of PI3K led to an adaptive hypertrophy, and did not change into a maladaptive hypertrophy, consistent with a critical role for the PI3K/PDK-1/Akt pathway in regulating normal cardiac growth. Interestingly, none of the transgenic models in which PI3K or Akt activation were associated with cardiac enlargement demonstrated increased cardiomyocyte proliferation in contrast to findings in transgenic mice with cardiac specific expression of IGF-1. This suggests that PI3K activation is not sufficient to induce cardiomyocyte proliferation, which likely involves the coordination of other signaling pathways downstream of IGF-1, and upstream of PI3K.

The PI3K/Akt pathway promotes cell survival in several ways. By intervening in the mitochondrial apoptosis cascade at events before cytochrome c release and caspase activation, Akt activation inhibits changes in the inner mitochondrial membrane potential that occur in apoptosis (suppressing apoptotic progression and cytochrome c release induced by several proapoptotic proteins). While Akt also contributes to the phosphorylation and inactivation of the proapoptotic protein Bad, it remains unclear whether Bad phosphorylation is the mechanism by which Akt ensures cell survival and mitochondrial integrity since other mitochondrial targets of Akt remain to be identified. PI3K/Akt signaling promotes

glucose uptake, growth, and survival of cardiomyocytes and has been implicated in heart growth [59]. Growth factors are known to effect cardiomyocyte growth (e.g., IGF-1) signal through the PI3K/Akt pathway [60]. Microarray analysis of cardiomyocytes have demonstrated that treatment with IGF-1 results in the differential expression of genes involved in cellular signaling and mitochondrial function, and confirmed that this IGF-1-mediated gene regulation required the activation of ERK and PI3K [16].

Transgenic mice with cardiac specific expression of activated Akt exhibit up-regulation of IGF-binding protein (consistent with its growth signaling/antiapoptotic role) and down-regulation of both PGC-1 and PPARα (activators of mitochondrial FAO and mitochondrial biogenesis), presumably shifting cardiomyocytes towards glycolytic metabolism. Deprivation of nutrients (e.g., specific amino acids), glucose and serum growth factors, which can lead to cardiomyocyte apoptosis [61] has been found to signal via the mitochondrial associated mTOR protein [62]. Moreover, both the Akt pathway and the downstream mTOR proteins impact cardiomyocyte survival and cell size largely through promoting cytoplasmic protein synthesis mediated by the activation of translational initiation factors and ribosomal proteins. Also, Akt can provide cardioprotection against ischemic injury induced by exposure of cardiomyocytes to diverse treatments including cardiotrophin-1, acetylcholine, adenosine, and bradykinin mediated preconditioning. The precise target of Akt action in cardioprotection remains undetermined since Akt has not been associated directly with mitoK$_{ATP}$ channels. Several studies have suggested that cardioprotective signaling is mediated in part by blocking PT pore opening (functioning as an end-effector) regulated by modulation of GSK-3β activity arising from either of several convergent signaling pathways including ROS-activated PKC or by receptor tyrosine kinases (RTKs) triggering Akt and mTOR/p70s6k pathways (shown in Fig. 7.1) [63].

Insulin-Like Growth Factor-1: Activator of Akt Signaling

Insulin-like growth factor-1 (IGF-1), a 70 amino acid polypeptide, is one of the most potent natural activators of the Akt signaling pathway, a stimulator of cell growth and multiplication and a potent inhibitor of programmed cell death. Because of its ability to improve flow-metabolism coupling, IGF-1 could indeed represent a new cardiovascular disease treatment option for many cardiac disorders such as ischemic heart disease and heart failure [64].

IGF-1 binds to at least two cell surface receptors: the IGF-1 receptor (IGFR) (see Fig. 7.1), and the insulin receptor. The IGF-1 receptor binds IGF-1 at significantly higher affinity than IGF-1 is bound to the insulin receptor; as the insulin receptor, the IGFR is a tyrosine kinase, an enzyme that mediates signaling by transferring a phosphate group from ATP to a tyrosine residue in a protein. IGF-1 activates the insulin receptor at approximately 0.1× the potency of insulin. Part of this signaling may be via IGFR/insulin receptor heterodimers.

Several lines of evidence indicate that IGF-1 has a protective effect on ischemia/reperfusion (I/R) injury in a variety of tissues including the heart. IGF-1 has been shown to ameliorate I/R-induced acute renal failure [65], recover neurons from severe cerebral hypoxic–ischemic injury [66], improve cardiac function and reduce structural damage during I/R [50, 67–72], and prevent apoptosis and promote survival of cardiomyocytes [50, 71–74]. Davani et al. observed that the histological and functional cardiac improvements generated by IGF-1 treatment in an ex vivo model of myocardial I/R injury were accompanied by the maintenance of the ratio of mitochondrial to nuclear DNA in the mouse heart after I/R [68]. Using cultured neonatal rat cardiomyocytes, Lai et al. found that IGF-1 can prevent the loss of the mitochondrial electrochemical gradient and membrane depolarization resulting from doxorubicin-induction and demonstrated that IGF-1 signaling to the organelle involved the PI3 kinase-Akt pathway [75].

Observations in animal models of myocardial I/R revealed that the administration of IGF-1 can provide substantial cardioprotective effect. IGF-1 signaling can trigger multiple signal cascade pathways in cardiomyocytes [50, 71–76], and the activation of the PI3K-Akt pathway and/or ERK 1/2 kinase cascade by IGF-1 can initiate efficient anti-cell death mechanisms, and show evidence of mitochondrial involvement. For instance, systemic IGF-1 treatment in rat up-regulates Bcl-Xl expression but down-regulates pro-apoptotic Bax protein in heart mitochondria, as well as significantly reduces PTP opening and cytochrome c release in response to I/R injury [71]. In addition, overexpression of Bcl-Xl affects mitochondrial membrane potential, matrix swelling, and prevents cell death induced by OXPHOS inhibitors [77]. These findings suggest that IGF-1 may regulate mitochondrial function and in turn protect myocytes against a lethal stimulus like hypoxia/reoxygenation (HR).

IGF-1 has been reported to decrease Ca^{2+}-stimulated mitochondrial cytochrome c release and inhibit Ca^{2+}-sensitive mitochondrial swelling [71], suggesting that IGF-1 signaling can modulate PTP in the heart. Juhaszova et al. found that GSK-3, a potential downstream target of the IGF-signaling pathway can regulate the opening of mitochondrial PTP in cardiomyocytes [78].

Also, IGF-1 can prevent mitochondrial DNA damage following postischemic reperfusion injury [68], and promote increased mitochondrial ATP synthesis in rat heart myocytes [71]. These salutary actions of IGF-1 would enable mitochondria to be more resistant to insult stress and protect cardiac muscle against OS. The highly-targeted application of IGF-1 by somatic gene transfer may provide cardioprotection against transient ischemia and ischemic HF, offering potential strategic advantages over the systemic delivery of the IGF-I peptide [79]. Nonetheless, the mechanisms by which IGF-1 prevents myocardial ischemia-reperfusion injury are not fully understood.

Pi et al. [80] have addressed whether mitochondrial bioenergetic pathways are involved in the cardioprotective effects of IGF-1. Using single cardiomyocytes from adult rats incubated in the absence or presence of IGF-1 for 60 min and subjected to 60 min hypoxia followed by 30 min reoxygenation at 37°C (HR), mitochondrial function was evaluated by assessment of enzyme activities of oxidative phosphorylation and Krebs cycle pathways. HR caused significant inhibition of mitochondrial respiratory complex IV and V activities and of the Krebs cycle enzyme citrate synthase, whereas pretreatment with IGF-1 maintained enzyme activities in myocytes at or near control levels. Mitochondrial membrane potential, evaluated with JC-1 staining, was significantly higher in IGF-1 + HR-treated myocytes than in HR alone, with levels similar to those found in normal control cardiomyocytes.

As shown in Figs. 7.2 and 7.3, red fluorescence intensity, in particular, the ratio of red to green fluorescence was significantly decreased in HR-treated cardiomyocytes when compared to control, suggesting that HR caused the loss of mitochondrial electrochemical gradient in cultured adult cardiomyocytes. On the other hand, in cardiomyocytes pretreated with IGF-1, the ratio of red to green fluorescence after HR was significantly higher when compared to HR alone indicating that IGF-1 prevented the collapse of the mitochondrial electrochemical gradient. These data suggest that rapid IGF-1 signaling is able to effectively maintain or to promote full recovery of $\Delta\Psi_m$ in cardiomyocytes undergoing HR stress. In addition, IGF-1 reduced both HR-induced lactate dehydrogenase (LDH) release and malondialdehyde production (an indicator of lipid peroxidation) in cardiomyocytes. These results indicate that IGF-1 protects cardiomyocytes from HR injury via stabilizing mitochondria and reducing reactive oxidative (ROS) damage.

Welch et al. [81] have tested the hypothesis that IGF-1, can positively affect HF progression in a tropomodulin (Tmod)-overexpressing transgenic mouse model of DCM. In an attempt to counteract the remodeling and dysfunction leading to DCM, the Tmod-overexpressing transgenic (TOT) mice line was crossbred with homozygous transgenic mice overexpressing IGF-1 in cardiac myocytes to create Tmod-IGF-1-overexpressing mice. The beneficial effects of IGF-1 were apparent by multiple indices of cardiac structure and function, including normalization of heart mass, anatomy, hemodynamics, and apoptosis. IGF-1 expression also acted as a proliferative stimulus as evidenced by calculated increases in myocyte number as well as expression of Ki67, a nuclear marker of cellular replication. Cellular analyses showed that

Control   **HR**   **IGF-1+HR**

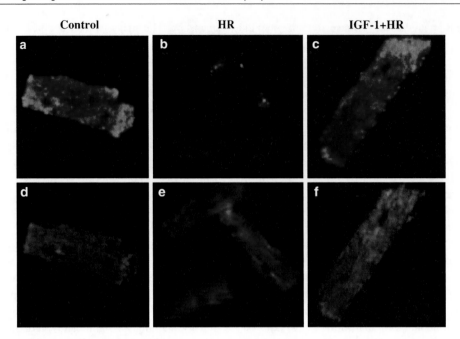

Fig. 7.2 Representative fluorescence microscopic images of JC-1 staining in myocytes. IGF-1 (100 nM) was added to the culture medium 1 h prior and during HR. **a–f** show the changes in mitochondrial fluorescence intensity in myocytes with or without HR stress. **a–c** show cells with *red filter*; **d–f** with *green filter* (Reprinted from Pi et al. [80]. With kind permission from Springer)

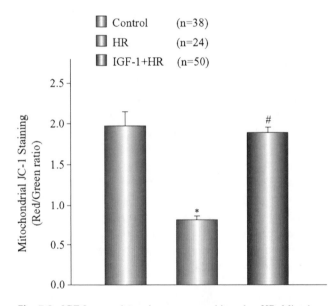

Fig. 7.3 IGF-I rescued $\Delta\psi_m$ in myocytes subjected to HR. Mitochondrial membrane depolarization was characterized by the reduction of red/green ratio. Data derived from four independent experiments are shown. *n* number of cells determined; *$p < 0.0001$ vs. control. #$p < 0.0001$ vs. HR (Adapted from Pi et al. [80]. With kind permission from Springer)

IGF-1 inhibited characteristic cardiomyocyte elongation in dilated hearts and restored calcium dynamics, comparable to that observed in normal cells. This study provided significant information about (1) the ability of IGF-1 to inhibit progression of cardiomyopathic disease in a defined model system and suggest that HF may benefit from early interventional IGF-1 treatment; (2) the cellular mechanisms that lead to heart remodeling, thus contributing to the existing controversy regarding the roles of cardiomyocyte apoptosis and regeneration in the pathogenesis of HF.

Other Growth and Pro-survival Pathways

SIR/Sirtuins

Using the genetically tractable model organism baker's yeast, *Saccharomyces cerevisiae*, primary genetic determinants of replicative life span in yeast were initially identified from genetic screens of starvation-resistant strains for long-lived mutants. Among these mutants, there were members of the SIR (silent information regulator) gene family [82]. Subsequent studies revealed that loss-of-function of SIR2 (whose homolog in mammals is known as SIRT1, SIR2L1 or Sir2α) significantly shortened yeast life span, whereas increased SIR2 gene dosage extended it [83]. An SIR2 orthologue subsequently detected in *C. elegans* was similarly shown to extend life span with increased dosage [84].

Interestingly, SIR2 had been previously identified as a mediator of gene silencing of the mating type loci in yeast [85]. In yeast, transcriptional silencing occurs at a number of chromosomal loci including telomeres, the two mating-type loci (HML and HMR), and rDNA locus RDN1.

The establishment of inactive heterochromatin at telomeres, mating-type loci, and at the rDNA requires a complex including SIR2. Overexpression of SIR2 increases the extent of silencing at both telomeres and rDNA, suggesting that SIR2 is a limiting component of the silencing apparatus. Evidence strongly suggests that SIR2 mediates its effect on yeast aging primarily through its generation of heterochromatin at the rDNA, and suppression of both the recombination between rDNA repeats, and the formation of extra-chromosomal circulars forms of rDNA (ERCs) [86].

SIR2's action as an NAD$^+$-dependent histone deacetylase (HDAC) mediates chromatin remodeling effect, and has rendered it the founding member of a large family of NAD-dependent histone deacetylases termed the sirtuins. The sirtuin proteins are conserved from prokaryotes to eukaryotes, and include seven human sirtuin isoforms. The NAD$^+$ dependence of SIR2 may permit the regulation of its activity through changes in the availability of this cosubstrate, allowing the enzyme to sense the bioenergetic and redox states of the cell and set the life span accordingly. Moreover, SIR2 activity can be increased by genetic and physiological interventions that decrease the levels of NADH, a competitive inhibitor of SIR2 [87].

In Fig. 7.4, a number of targets of SIRT1/SIRT2 are shown. Overexpression of Sir2α protects cardiac myocytes from apoptosis in response to serum starvation and significantly increase the size of cardiac myocytes. Moreover, endogenous Sir2α plays an essential role in mediating cell survival, whereas Sir2α overexpression protects myocytes from apoptosis and causes modest hypertrophy.

Sir2α expression has been found increased in hearts from dogs with HF induced by rapid pacing superimposed on stable, severe hypertrophy. An increase in Sir2α expression during HF suggests that Sir2α may play a cardioprotective role in pathologic hearts in vivo [88]. In HF, reduced Sir2α deacetylase activity and NAD$^+$ depletion mediate poly(ADP-ribose) polymerase-1 (PARP)-dependent cardiac myocyte cell death. Pillai et al. [89] reported that in both failing hearts and cultured cardiac myocytes, the increased activity of PARP was associated with depletion of cellular NAD$^+$ levels and reduced Sir2α deacetylase activity. Myocyte cell death induced by PARP activation was prevented by repletion of cellular NAD$^+$ levels either by adding NAD$^+$ directly to the culture medium or by overexpressing NAD$^+$ biosynthetic enzymes. The beneficial effect of NAD$^+$ repletion was seen, however, only when Sir2α was intact. Knocking down Sir2α levels by small interfering RNA eliminated this benefit, indicating that Sir2α is a downstream target of NAD$^+$ replenishment leading to cell protection. NAD$^+$ repletion also prevented loss of the transcriptional regulatory activity of the Sir2α catalytic core domain resulting from PARP activation. Furthermore, PARP activation and the concomitant reduction of Sir2α activity in failing hearts regulate the post-translational acetylation of p53. Thus, in stressed cardiac myocytes, depletion of cellular NAD$^+$ levels forms a link between PARP activation and reduced Sir2α deacetylase activity, contributing to myocyte cell death during HF.

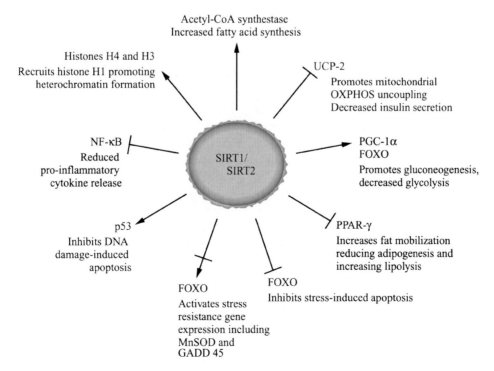

Fig. 7.4 Targets of SIRT1/SIR2

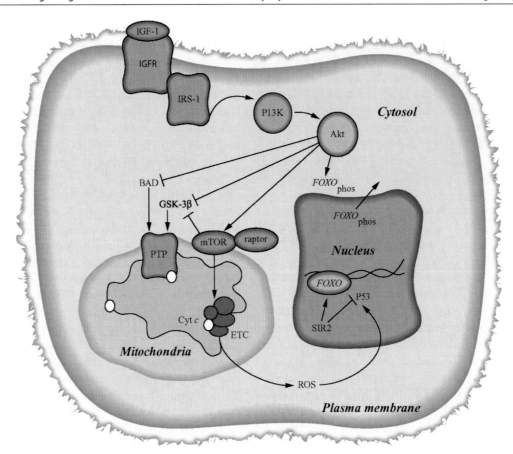

Fig. 7.5 Interacting signaling pathways, including IGF-1, mTOR and SIR2. Shown is the IGF-1 ligand binding to its cell surface receptor associated with insulin receptor substrate-1 (IRS-1). Downstream of the receptor, the signal is transmitted to the kinases (P13K and subsequently Akt). The activated Akt inhibits the translocation of the proapoptotic BAD to the mitochondria, stemming mitochondrial PT pore (mPTP) and inhibiting apoptosis; similarly, it attenuates glycogen synthase kinase-3β (GSK-3β) activity-reducing mPTP. Akt also activates mTOR signaling part of the mitochondrial retrograde pathway. Akt phosphorylates FOXO, inactivating it, increasing its translocation from the nucleus to the cytosol, reducing its DNA binding and stemming its positive effect on longevity. In contrast, the sirtuin (SIR2) activates FOXO transcriptional activity by reversing its acetylation. Similarly, SIR2 inactivates p53 by deacetylation and attenuates its apoptotic program

A critical target of the SIR2 deacetylase activity is the FOXO forkhead transcription factors (Fig. 7.5), shifting FOXO dependent responses away from cell death and toward cell survival contributing to enhanced longevity. In addition to the demonstration by genetic analysis in *C. elegans* that SIR2 acts upstream of DAF-16 in the insulin-like signaling pathway [84], several studies have shown that SIRT1, the mammalian homologue of SIR2, deacetylates FOXO factors (e.g., FOXO 1,3 and/or 4) and modulates their transactivation function [90–92]. The effect on FOXO function leads to the attenuation of FOXO-induced apoptosis and potentiation of FOXO3's ability to induce resistance to OS. Other recently identified SIRT1-regulated transcription factors of considerable significance in cardiovascular signaling pathways include PPAR-γ, PGC-1α, NF-κB, p53, p300, and the cell-cycle and apoptosis regulator E2F1 [93–96].

Caloric restriction (CR) appears to extend the life span in a number of animal models, and it had shown to improve cardiac remodeling and diastolic dysfunction in the Dahl salt-sensitive rat model of decompensated pressure-overload hypertrophy [97]. Although the mechanisms underlying CR in HF and extension of life span remain unclear, a direct connection between SIR2 activation and CR has been found in studies with Drosophila [98]. Increase in Drosophila Sir2 (dSir2) extends the fly life span, whereas a decrease in dSir2 blocks the life span-extending effect of CR. Studies have suggested that the mammalian Sir2 orthologue, SIRT1, is required for the induction of at least a phenotypic component of the complex physiological and behavior patterns associated with CR in mice [99]. Moreover, SIRT1 activates a critical tissue-specific component of CR in mammals; i.e., fat mobilization in white adipocytes [100]. Upon food withdrawal, SIRT1 protein binds to and represses PPAR-γ transcriptional activation downregulating genes mediating fat storage. In SIRT1[+/−] mice, mobilization of fatty acids from white adipocytes upon fasting is compromised. In 3T3-L1 adipocytes, overexpression of SIRT1 attenuates adipogenesis, and RNAi-mediated silencing of SIRT1 expression enhances it.

In addition, upregulation of SIRT1 in differentiated fat cells triggers lipolysis and loss of fat. The involvement of SIRT1 in fat reduction is likely a contributory factor in extending life span. Furthermore, assessment of long-term CR effects in mice using microarray gene expression techniques showed changes in expression consistent with decreased cardiac remodeling and improvement in contractility and energy production via FAO [101].

TOR

Target of rapamycin (TOR) is an integrator of nutrient and growth factor signals and also a coordinator of cell growth and cell cycle progression. The mammalian TOR (mTOR) is a component of the insulin–phosphoinositide 3-kinase pathway, which is known to play a critical role in the determination of cell, organ, and body size. Several components (mTOR and raptor) (Fig. 7.5) of another nutrient sensing pathway have been implicated in both life span extension in several model organisms, and as part of the CR pathway in yeast [102]. TOR gene encodes a protein kinase that mediates a highly conserved signaling pathway that couples amino acid availability to ribosomal S6 protein kinase activation, translation initiation, and cell growth. In addition, TOR responds to changes in growth factors, amino acids, oxygen tension, and energy status. Also, overexpression of upstream regulators such as tuberous sclerosis complex genes 1 and 2 (dTsc1, dTsc2), which inhibit TOR expression, or dominant-negative forms of dTOR or dS6K all cause life span extension, dependent on the nutritional status [103].

Similar to findings with the insulin/IGF-1 pathway, modulation of TOR signaling expression in fat tissues is sufficient for life span extension, and disruption in TOR signaling, as a result of either mutation or targeted pharmacological intervention (e.g., rapamycin treatment), resulted in enhanced chronological life span in yeast (i.e., the time cells in a stationary phase culture remain viable), a potential model for aging of postmitotic tissues in mammals [104]. Decreased TOR activity also resulted in increased accumulation of storage carbohydrates and enhanced stress resistance. Furthermore, removal of either asparagine or glutamate from the media significantly increased stationary phase survival suggesting that TOR plays a role in starvation-induced stress and CR modulation of life span. In addition, TOR modulates replicative life span in yeast in response to nutrients and modulates CR, but CR failed to increase life span in TOR mutants [102].

Another critical aspect of TOR action is its effect on stress response and signaling of mitochondrial dysfunction. The mTOR is mainly localized in the mitochondrial outer membrane (see Fig. 7.5), although a cytosolic form has also been reported [105]. mTOR along with accessory proteins such as raptor form a stress-sensing module consisting

of mitochondria and mitochondrial outer membrane-associated mTOR, integrate diverse stress signals, including nutrients, cAMP levels, and osmotic stress with cellular responses such as transcription, translation, and autophagy. Mitochondrial bioenergetic function and membrane potential serve as a regulatory intermediate on TOR activity [106, 107]. Moreover, raptor (regulatory associated protein of mTOR) binds to p70S6k and 4E-BP1 and is essential for TOR signaling in vivo, and it appears to serve as an mTOR scaffold protein; binding to mTOR substrates is required for effective mTOR-catalyzed phosphorylation in vivo [108].

Interestingly, mTOR pathway plays a significant role in determining both resting oxygen consumption and oxidative capacity [109]. This conclusion was mainly inferred from the correlation of mTOR/raptor complex formation with overall mitochondrial activity. Following treatment with the mTOR inhibitor rapamycin, disruption of this complex lowered membrane potential, oxygen consumption, and ATP synthetic capacity. Furthermore, this inhibition resulted in marked alteration in the mitochondrial phospho-proteome and suggests that TOR dependent phosphorylation of intramitochondrial proteins is part of the mechanism of TOR action.

Modulation of the mitochondrial permeability transition (PT) pore (also located at the junction of the mitochondrial inner and outer membranes) is regulated by the activity of GSK-3β, which is under convergent regulation by the protein kinase B/Akt and mTOR/p70s6k pathways [63]. This pathway has been described in cardiomyocytes and implicated in the cardioprotective pathway in response to hypoxic insult. In isolated mouse heart, inhibition of TOR signaling with rapamycin confers preconditioning-like protection against ischemia–reperfusion injury [110]. mTOR or its target(s) has been reported to play an important role in load-induced cardiac hypertrophy. Since systemic administration of rapamycin has been successfully used in the treatment of transplant rejection, it may be a useful therapeutic modality to suppress cardiac hypertrophy in human [111]. Also, inhibition of mTOR signaling with rapamycin regresses decompensated cardiac hypertrophy induced by pressure overload in mice, improving left ventricular end-systolic dimensions, fractional shortening, and ejection fraction [112].

Signaling at the Plasma Membrane

Sarcolemmal K_ATP Channel

ATP-sensitive potassium (K_{ATP}) channels link membrane excitability to metabolism [113]. They are regulated by intracellular nucleotides and by other factors including, membrane phospholipids, protein kinases, and phosphoprotein phosphatases. K_{ATP} channels comprise octamers of four Kir6 pore-forming subunits associated with four sulphonylurea receptor (SUR) subunits. K_{ATP} channels are targets for antidiabetic sulphonylurea blockers, and for channel opening drugs that are used as antianginals and antihypertensives. In vascular smooth muscle, K_{ATP} channels are regulated by diverse signaling pathways, and cause vasodilation contributing both to resting blood flow and vasodilator-induced increases in flow. In cardiac muscle, sarcolemmal K_{ATP} channels open to protect cells under stress conditions, such as ischemia and exercise, and appear central to the protection induced by ischemic preconditioning (IPC).

Signaling in the Mitochondria: Key Players

Nuclear Gene Activation

Nuclear transcriptional modulators that govern the expression of a wide array of mitochondrial proteins in response to diverse cellular stimuli and signals, have been identified. For instance, nuclear transcription factors such as NRF-1 and NRF-2 are implicated in activation of mitochondrial biogenesis [114–116]. These factors exert a direct effect on the synthesis of specific nuclear-encoded subunits of the mitochondrial respiratory enzymes as well as indirectly by up-regulating levels of mitochondrial transcription factor A (mtTFA), involved in both mitochondrial DNA replication and transcription (Fig. 7.6). In addition, a "master" transcription co-activator (PGC-1) activates expression of transcription factors NRF-1 and NRF-2 [117]. The nucleus also contains global regulatory transcription factors such as peroxisome proliferator-activated receptors and their transcriptional co-activators (i.e., PPARα, RXRα), which also play a pivotal regulatory role in the expression of mitochondrial FAO pathways, integral to bioenergetic metabolism [118, 119]. Transcriptional control by these activators is affected by hypoxia, ischemia, and HF [120, 121].

PGC-1 expression and mitochondrial biogenesis are modulated by the activation of a calcium/calmodulin-dependent protein kinase (CaMK), indicating that the calcium-regulated signaling pathway plays a significant role in transcriptional activation of genes governing mitochondrial biogenesis [122]. Moreover, these nuclear activators are modulated during cardiac development [123, 124]; activation of the NFAT gene has been shown to be crucial in early cardiac development and is required to maintain myocardial mitochondrial oxidative function. Targeted cardiac disruption of NFAT genes results in cardiomyocyte mitochondria ETC dysfunction, reduced ventricular size, and aberrant cardiomyocyte structure in mice embryo [124].

These nuclear transcriptional factors modulate the cardiac phenotype in transgenic animals bearing either mutations in specific transcriptional factors or over-expressed genes. Also, it has been found that specific nuclear transcription factors are essential for normal cardiac phenotype and mitochondrial function. For instance, cardiac-specific PGC-1 over-expression in transgenic mice results in uncontrolled mitochondrial proliferation and extensive loss of sarcomeric structure leading to DCM [117]. Myocardial over-expression of PPAR-α may lead to severe cardiomyopathy with both increased myocardial fatty acid uptake and mitochondrial FAO [125]. Similarly, mutations targeting mtTFA produce inactivation of myocardial mitochondrial gene expression and ETC dysfunction resulting in DCM and atrio-ventricular conduction defects [126].

Mitochondrial Receptors

Few, well-characterized heart mitochondrial receptors have been detected despite the large number of receptors that have been identified in other tissues/cell types. The thyroid hormone (TH) receptor Erb-Aα, which was identified as an "orphan" receptor [127, 128] interacting with mtDNA during targeted hormonal stimulation (Fig. 7.6), has not yet been documented in mitochondria from cardiac tissue, despite the known marked effect of TH in heart mitochondria. Moreover, a large number of nuclear transcription factors described and characterized in many other tissues/cell types as translocating to mitochondria, including P53, NF-κB, PPAR-α, RXR, and TR3, have also not yet been documented in heart mitochondria. No specific mitochondrial receptors have yet been found that bind TNF-α or various cytokines known to effect cardiac mitochondrial function, despite several recent studies demonstrating that TNF-α impacts cardiomyocyte mitochondria. Moreover, and in contrast to other tissues, there has been no characterization in heart mitochondria of anchoring proteins, which bind and concentrate protein kinases.

A common theme concerning signaling and activation includes the stimuli-generated translocation of specific cytosolic proteins into the mitochondria; the growing list of such translocated entities includes many of the pro-apoptotic proteins (e.g., BAX, BID) as well as protein kinases. Many of these appear to target specific proteins on the outer mitochondria membrane; others are imported as preproteins by recognizing a small set of specific receptors (translocases) on the mitochondrial outer membrane (TOM). The import of proteins into mitochondria is often mediated by heat shock proteins (e.g., HSP60, HSP70), which specifically interact with a complex mitochondrial protein import apparatus (including matrix proteases). Interestingly, a number of physiological stimuli and stresses, including temperature changes and hormone treatment (including TH), can result in regulation of the heart mitochondrial import apparatus [129].

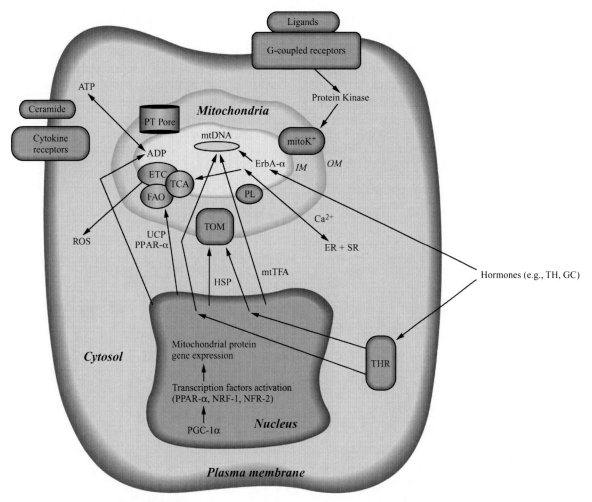

Fig. 7.6 Mitochondria receiving diverse signals from various cellular locations. A number of representative signaling pathways are shown that have impact on mitochondria including thyroid hormone (TH) and glucocorticoid hormone (GC) which targets both nuclear processes, influencing nuclear transcription of a large assortment of genes some of which will affect mitochondrial function, such as uncoupling proteins (UC) and mitochondrial transcription factor A (mtTFA), and more directly affecting mitochondria transcription of mtDNA via its orphan receptor (ErbA-α). Other signaling pathways shown include the nuclear transcription of PPAR-α which modulates mitochondrial fatty acid β oxidation (FAO), the ceramide pathway transducing cytokine signals impacting on complex III of electron transport chain (ETC), mitochondrial calcium import from ER and SR, and the outer membrane (OM) associated mitochondrial protein import apparatus via Translocator Outer Membrane (TOM) and heat shock proteins (HSPs). The cardioprotection pathway is also depicted involving the mitochondrial K_{ATP} channels in the inner membrane mediated by ROS, ligands binding to an assortment of membrane receptors (G-coupled), and the involvement of protein kinases

Reactive Oxidative Species

We have dealt with the generation of ROS and the effect of OS in HF in Chaps. 5 and 10 respectively. Here, we limit our discussion to some of the negative effects of ROS and signaling.

Negative Effects of ROS

Increased ROS generation resulting from myocardial ischemia/reperfusion (I/R), inflammation, impaired antioxidant defenses, and aging may cause profound effects on cells including elevated lipid peroxidation targeting membrane phospholipids and proteins. Protein modifications, such as carbonylation, nitration, and the formation of lipid peroxidation adducts e.g., 4-hydroxynonenal (HNE), are products of oxidative damage secondary to ROS [130]. ROS-mediated nitration, carbonylation, and HNE adduct formation reduces the enzymatic activity of myocardial respiratory complexes I to V as shown with in vitro studies [131]. Superoxide is also particularly damaging to the Fe–S centers of enzymes such as complex I, aconitase, and succinic dehydrogenase (SDH) causing inhibition of mitochondrial bioenergetic function. Moreover, the inactivation of mitochondrial aconitase by superoxide, which generates Fe (II) and H_2O_2, also increases hydroxyl radical formation through the Fenton reaction [132], thereby amplifying the deleterious effects of ROS production. Lipids and in particular the mitochondrial-specific phospholipid cardiolipin serve as a focal target for ROS damage. A large accumulation of superoxide radicals produced in vitro with submitochondrial particles from heart resulted in extensive cardiolipin peroxidation with a parallel loss of cytochrome c oxidase activity [133, 134]. Oxidative damage also targets nucleic acids, and in particular mtDNA by inducing single- and double-strand breaks base damage

and modification (including 8-oxoguanosine formation), resulting in the generation of point mutations and deletions in mtDNA. Inhibition of mitochondrial respiration by NO can result in further increases in mitochondrial ROS production; interaction with NO enhances the potency of superoxide (Fig. 7.7) as an inhibitor of respiration [135]. In addition, the highly reactive peroxynitrite irreversibly impairs mitochondrial respiration [136], since it inhibits complex I activity, largely by tyrosine nitration of several targeted subunits [137, 138], modifies cytochrome c structure and function [139], affects cytochrome c oxidase (COX) activity, inhibits

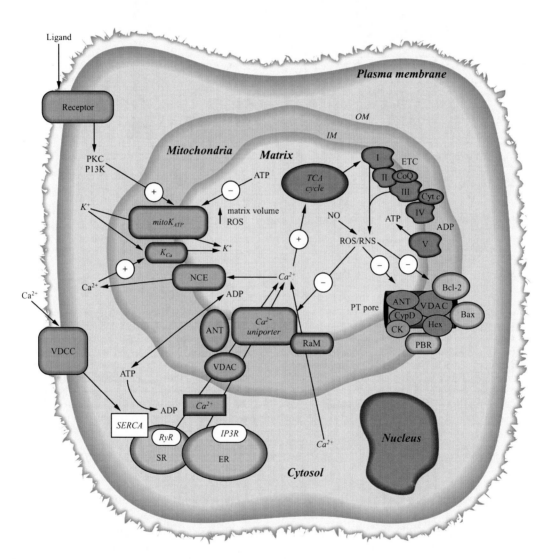

Fig. 7.7 Mitochondrial channels are pivotal signal transducers in myocardium. The cardioprotection pathway involving the mitochondrial K^+ channels (mitoK_{ATP}) is located in the inner membrane and is mediated by ROS, ligands binding to an assortment of G-coupled membrane receptors and protein kinases (PKC/PI3K). Calcium enters the mitochondria in response to a variety of stimuli via a complex of membrane proteins including, the outer-membrane (OM) voltage-dependent anion carrier (VDAC), the inner membrane (IM) proteins, RAM and the Ca^{2+} uniporter; high Ca^{2+} levels can be supplied from ryanodine release (RyR) and IP3 receptors (IP3R) located in the sarcoplasmic (SR) and endoplasmic (ER) reticuli respectively, and is coupled to the entry of calcium into the cardiomyocyte through the voltage-dependent Ca^{2+} channel (VDCC). Entry of high calcium levels into the mitochondria can increase activities of several enzymes of TCA cycle, electron transport chain (ETC) and complex V. Calcium also modulates the opening of the permeability transition (PT) pore shown with its accessory components including VDAC, adenine nucleotide translocator (ANT), hexokinase (HK), creatine kinase (CK), cyclophilin D (CpD) and cardiolipin (CL). Calcium efflux is primarily managed by the Na$^+$/Ca^{2+} exchanger

mitochondrial aconitase [140], and causes induction of the PT pore [141]. A number of peroxynitrite effects on its mitochondrial targets (e.g., the PT pore) are potentiated by increased calcium levels [142], and can be clearly distinguished from the effects of NO, which are often reversible [136].

Not surprisingly, mitochondria (a major site of intracellular ROS generation) are also a primary locus of its damaging effects. ROS-induced damage to mtDNA results in abnormalities of the mtDNA-encoded polypeptides of the respiratory complexes located in the inner membrane, with consequent decrease of electron transfer and further production of ROS, thus establishing a vicious cycle of OS, mitochondrial function, and bioenergetic decline.

It is worth noting that ROS produced by cellular sources, besides mitochondria, can have substantial effects on cardiovascular function. Superoxide radicals are generated from reactions of oxygen with microsomal cytochrome p450, which has an endogenous NAD(P)H oxidase activity, usually in the presence of metal ions. Phagocytic cells (present at sites of active inflammation), vascular endothelial cells, and SMCs have an NAD (P)H oxidase activity that can be induced by certain stimuli such as angiotensin II [143], TNF-α [144], and thrombin [145] to generate ROS. NAD(P)H oxidase also produces ROS in response to endothelin-1 in vascular SMCs and cardiac muscle cells. As a result, NAD(P)H oxidases may be a key source of ROS that participate in vascular oxidant-related signaling mechanisms under physiological and pathophysiological conditions. In addition, xanthine oxidase (XO), a primarily cytosolic enzyme involved in purine metabolism, is also a source of the superoxide radical. Notably, XO activity and its superoxide generation are markedly increased in the heart after I/R damage. Its location within the human myocardium is primarily in the endothelial cells of capillaries and smaller vessels [146]. Ischemia and hypoxia promote the accumulation of XO substrates, hypoxanthine, and xanthine. Numerous studies have shown that the XO inhibitor allopurinol can provide protection against the cardiac damage resulting from anoxia. A provocative link has been proposed between XO activity and abnormal cardiac energy metabolism in patients with idiopathic DCM, since inhibition of XO with allopurinol significantly improves myocardial function [147]. These toxic metabolic by-products, which are potent cell-damaging oxidants, are normally neutralized by antioxidant enzymes, some of which are mitochondrially located (e.g., Mn-SOD and glutathione peroxidase), while others are cytosolic (e.g., Cu-SOD and catalase).

Role of ROS in Cell Signaling

In addition to their cell-damaging effects, ROS generation and OS play a critical role in cell regulation and signaling. Oxidative species such as H_2O_2 and the superoxide anion can

be deployed as potent signals sent from mitochondria to other cellular sites rapidly and reversibly triggering an array of intracellular cascades leading to diverse physiological end-points for the cardiomyocyte, some negative (e.g., apoptosis and necrosis) and others positive (e.g., cardioprotection and cell proliferation). Mitochondrial-produced H_2O_2 exported to the cytosol (Fig. 7.8) is involved in several signal transduction pathways, including the activation of JNK1 and MAPK activities [148–150], and can impact the regulation of redox-sensitive K^+ channels affecting arteriole constriction [151]. The release of H_2O_2 from mitochondria and its subsequent cellular effects are increased in cardiomyocytes treated with antimycin and high Ca^{2+}, and further enhanced by treatment with CoQ. CoQ plays a dual role in the mitochondrial generation of intracellular redox signaling, by acting both as a prooxidant involved in ROS generation, and as an antioxidant [152]. Increased mitochondrial H_2O_2 generation and signaling also occur with NO modulation of the ETC [153], as well as with the induction of myocardial mitochondrial NO production, resulting from treatment with enalapril [154]. Furthermore, ROS plays a fundamental role in the cardioprotective signaling pathways of IPC, in oxygen sensing, and in the induction of stress responses that promote cell survival.

Mitochondrial K_{ATP} Channel

ATP-sensitive potassium channels of the inner mitochondrial membrane (mitoK$_{ATP}$) are blocked by ATP and have been implicated as potential mediators of cardioprotective mechanisms such as IPC [155]. This cardioprotective effect is partially mediated by attenuating Ca^{2+} overloading in the mitochondrial matrix, and by increased ROS generation during preconditioning, further leading to protein kinase activation and decreased ROS levels generated during reperfusion [156]. The mitoK$_{ATP}$ is also regulated by a variety of ligands (e.g., adenosine, opioids, bradykinin, acetylcholine), which bind sarcolemmal G-protein coupled receptors as shown in Fig. 7.6, with subsequent activation of calcium flux, tyrosine protein kinases, and the PI3K/Akt pathway [157, 158]. In addition, marked changes in mitochondrial matrix volume associated with mitoK$_{ATP}$ channel opening, may play a contributory role in the cytoprotection process [159], although this has been recently challenged [160]. Drugs such as diazoxide and nicorandil specifically activate the mitoK$_{ATP}$ opening, and can also inhibit H_2O_2-induced apoptotic progression in cardiomyocytes, suggesting that mitoK$_{ATP}$ channels may also play a significant role in mediating OS signals in the mitochondrial apoptotic pathway [161, 162]. Another ion channel (i.e., the calcium-activated K^+ channel) has recently been identified on the mitochondrial inner membrane, and has been shown

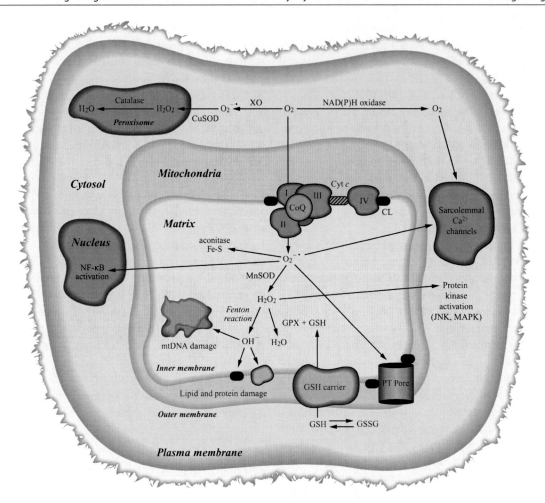

Fig. 7.8 ROS generation and signaling. Mitochondrial bioenergetic activity generates reactive oxygen species (ROS) including superoxide, hydroxyl radicals and hydrogen peroxide (H_2O_2). Sites of mitochondrial superoxide O_2^{-} radical (via respiratory complexes I, II, and III) and cytosolic O_2^{-} generation (by NAD(P)H oxidase or xanthine oxidase) are depicted. MnSOD (in mitochondria) and CuSOD (in cytosol) to form H_2O_2 are displayed. The H_2O_2 is then either further neutralized in the mitochondria by glutathione peroxidase (GPX) and glutathione, in the peroxisome by catalase, or in the presence of Fe^{2+} via the Fenton reaction, which forms the highly reactive OH$^{\cdot}$ radical, which can cause severe lipid peroxidation and extensive oxidative damage to proteins and mtDNA. Superoxide radicals produced in mitochondria can be delivered to the cytosol through anion channels (e.g., VDAC), and may impact sites far from its generation, including activation of transcription factor NF-κB

to have a cardioprotective function [163]. Nevertheless, the precise temporal order of events in the mitochondrial cardioprotection cascade, and the exact molecular nature of the mitoK$_{ATP}$ channel remain to be defined [164].

PT Pore

The opening of another mitochondrial membrane megachannel, the permeability transition (PT) pore, located at contact sites between the inner and outer membranes, has been suggested to cause a number of important changes in mitochondrial structure and metabolism, including increased mitochondrial matrix volume (leading to mitochondrial swelling), release of matrix Ca^{2+}, altered cristae, cessation of ATP production, primarily due to uncoupling of the ETC, and dissipation of the mitochondrial membrane potential. At the onset of reperfusion following an episode of myocardial ischemia, opening of this nonspecific pore is a critical determinant of myocyte death. Besides its role in the mitochondrial pathway of apoptosis, the opening of the PT pore, if unrestrained, leads to the loss of ionic homeostasis, and ultimately to necrotic cell death [165]. The PT pore appears to be composed of several mitochondrial membrane (see Figs. 5.2 and 5.4) proteins including the voltage-dependent anion channel (VDAC/porin), peripheral benzodiazepine receptor (PBR), the adenine nucleotide translocator (ANT), cytosolic proteins (e.g., hexokinase II, glycerol kinase), matrix proteins (e.g., cyclophilin D (CypD)), and from proteins of the intermembrane space such as creatine kinase. Fatty acids, high matrix Ca^{2+} levels, pro-oxidants, metabolic uncouplers, NO, and excessive mitochondrial ROS production (primarily from respiratory complex I and III) promote the opening of the PT pore. The PT pore may also be an important target of cardioprotection. New observations have showed that suppressing PT pore opening at the onset of reoxygenation can protect human myocardium against lethal hypoxia–reoxygenation injury [166]. The inhibition of PT pore opening can be mediated either directly by Cyclosporin A (CsA) and Sanglifehrin A (SfA), or indirectly by decreasing calcium loading and ROS levels.

Mitochondrial Kinases

Evidence has been gathered that mitochondria contain multiple protein substrates for protein kinases, and also that a number of protein kinases are translocated into heart mitochondria. This suggests that protein phosphorylation within the mitochondria is a critical component of the mitochondrial signaling pathways [167]. Protein kinases identified in heart mitochondria include pyruvate dehydrogenase kinase, PKA, PKC δ, and ε isoforms and JNK kinase (Table 7.2). Characterization of these proteins has provided new insights into the fundamental mechanisms regulating the mitochondrial response to diverse physiological stimuli and cardiovascular stresses.

In cardiomyocytes, isoforms of PKC (PKCs δ and ε) translocate from the cytoplasm to mitochondria for subsequent signal transduction [171]. PKC-ε, after translocation forms a "signaling module" by complexing with specific MAP kinases (e.g., ERK, p38 and JNK) resulting in phosphorylation of the

Table 7.2 Protein kinases identified in heart mitochondria

Protein kinase	References
PDH kinase	[168]
PKA	[169]
PKC δ	[170]
PKC ε	[171]
PKG	[172]
JNK	[173, 174]
p38 MAPK	[171]
Stress-activated protein kinase-3	[175]
ERK ½	[171]
MAP kinase kinase	[174]

PDH pyruvate dehydrogenase; *PKA* protein kinase A; *JNK* Jun N-terminal kinase; *MAPK* mitogen-activated protein kinase; *ERK* extracellular signal-regulated kinase

proapoptotic protein Bad. Also, PKC-ε forms physical interaction with components of the cardiac mitochondrial PT pore, in particular VDAC and ANT [176]. This interaction may inhibit pathological opening of the pore, including Ca^{2+}-induced opening, and subsequent mitochondrial swelling contributing to PKC-ε-induced cardioprotection. Activation of PKC in CP likely precedes mitoK$_{ATP}$ channel opening; nevertheless, a direct interaction of these kinases with the mitoK$_{ATP}$ channels has not yet been proved. Following diazoxide treatment, PKC-δ is translocated to cardiac mitochondria which triggers mitoK$_{ATP}$ channel opening leading to CP [170]. On the other hand, it has been shown that PKC-δ does not play a contributory role in the CP provided by IPC, although the role of PKC-ε translocation has been confirmed.

A mitochondrial cAMP-dependent protein kinase A (mtPKA), as well as its protein substrates have been localized to the matrix side of the inner mitochondrial membrane [169]. In cardiomyocytes, mtPKA phosphorylates the 18 kDa subunit of complex I (NDUFS4), and increased levels of cAMP promote NDUFS4 phosphorylation enhancing both complex I activity, and NAD-linked mitochondrial respiration/dephosphorylation mediated by a mitochondrial-localized phosphatase. In addition, PKA phosphorylation of several subunits of cytochrome *c* oxidase (COXI, III and Vb) at serine residues, modulates the activity of this important respiratory enzyme [177], and is considered to be a critical element of respiratory control. This cAMP-dependent phosphorylation occurs with high ATP/ADP ratios, resulting in the allosteric inhibition of COX activity. In the resting state, this regulatory control results in reduced membrane potential, and more efficient energy transduction. Conversely, increases in mitochondrial phosphatase (Ca^{2+}-induced) reverse the allosteric COX inhibition/respiratory control, resulting in increased membrane potential and ROS formation. Similarly, various stress stimuli leading to increased Ca^{2+} flux (activating the phosphatase) result in increased membrane potential and ROS formation.

New techniques of proteomic analysis have led to the identification of mitochondrial protein targets for these kinases. Interestingly, a group of proteins constituting a mitochondrial phosphoprotein proteome has been identified using a proteomic approach in bovine heart, and characterized as protein targets of kinase-mediated phosphorylation [178]. The majority of the identified phosphoproteins were involved in mitochondrial bioenergetic pathways, including the TCA cycle (e.g., aconitase, isocitrate and pyruvate dehydrogenases), and mitochondrial respiratory complexes, including NDUFA 10 (complex I), the flavoprotein subunit of SDH (Complex II), core I and III subunits (complex III), α and β subunits (complex V), while others are essential elements for the homeostasis of mitochondrial bioenergetics (e.g., creatine kinase and ANT).

Mitochondrial Translocation

An important subject concerning cell signaling and activation includes the stimuli-dependent translocation to, and incorporation of specific cytosolic proteins into the cardiomyocyte mitochondria. A growing list of such translocated molecules include several of the proapoptotic proteins (e.g., Bax, Bid), as well as some of the aforementioned protein kinases. Many of these proteins target or interact with specific proteins on the outer mitochondria membrane, and others are imported as preproteins by virtue of recognizing a small set of specific receptors (translocases) on the mitochondrial TOM (Fig. 7.6). Mitochondrial protein import is often mediated by heat shock proteins (e.g., HSP60, HSP70), which specifically interact with a complex mitochondrial protein import apparatus, including matrix proteases. As previously noted, physiological stimuli and stresses, including temperature changes and hormone treatment (e.g., thyroid hormone) impact the regulation of the heart mitochondrial import apparatus [179, 180].

Mitochondrial Retrograde Signaling

Mitochondrial retrograde signaling is a pathway of communication from mitochondria to the nucleus that influences many cellular activities under both normal and pathophysiological conditions. In both yeast and animal cells, retrograde signaling is linked to mTOR signaling, but the precise connections in cardiomyocytes have not yet been determined. In mammalian cells, mitochondrial dysfunction sets off signaling cascades through altered Ca^{2+} dynamics including calcineurin activation, which activates several protein kinase pathways (e.g., PKC and MAPK) and transcription factors such as NF-κB, calcineurin-dependent NFAT, CREB and ATF leading to stress protein expression (e.g., chaperone proteins) and activities [180]. These can result in alterations in both cell morphology and phenotype including proliferative growth, apoptotic signaling, and glucose metabolism.

Mitochondrial Calcium Signaling

Although calcium signaling will be further discussed in Chap. 9, at this time, it suffices to say that mitochondria also exert a significant regulatory role as a sensor of intracellular free Ca^{2+}. Several mechanisms of enhanced function of OXPHOS by Ca^{2+} have been reported, including stimulation of several dehydrogenases in the TCA cycle due to increases

in mitochondrial matrix Ca^{2+} [181, 182], and activation by Ca^{2+} of mitochondrial ATP synthase activity [183, 184]. Acute HF generated by manipulating calcium concentrations in perfused canine hearts was accompanied by a striking decrease in mitochondrial respiratory function [185].

The import of Ca^{2+} from cytosol into cardiac mitochondria is an important regulatory event in cell signaling. Mitochondrial calcium flux, particularly in cultured cardiomyocytes, has become detectable using advanced cell imaging techniques with fluorescent dyes, confocal microscopy, and recombinantly-derived Ca^{2+} sensitive photo-probes [186, 187]. Mitochondrial calcium influx is primarily provided by a Ca^{2+} pump uniporter located in the inner membrane, driven by the mitochondrial membrane potential, as well as by low matrix Ca^{2+} levels and can be blocked by ruthenium red [188]. Mitochondrial Ca^{2+} uptake is significantly and rapidly increased in cardiomyocytes during physiological Ca^{2+} signaling and is often accompanied by a highly localized transient mitochondrial depolarization [187]. Efflux of Ca^{2+} from cardiomyocyte mitochondria is mediated by a Na^+/Ca^{2+} exchanger linked to ETC proton pumping, although calcium efflux also occurs with PT pore opening. Activation of the PT pore and mitochondrial Ca^{2+} flux also occur in apoptosis and I/R and are involved in the generation of a calcium wave delivering system between adjacent mitochondria [189].

An important consequence of increased mitochondrial Ca^{2+} uptake is the up-regulation of energy metabolism and stimulation of mitochondrial oxidative phosphorylation. Elevated mitochondrial Ca^{2+} levels allosterically stimulate the activity of three TCA cycle enzymes including pyruvate, isocitrate and 2-oxoglutarate dehydrogenase [182, 190]. Activation of these enzymes by Ca^{2+} results in increased $NADH/NAD^+$ ratios, and ultimately leads to increased mitochondrial ATP synthesis. A thermokinetic model of cardiac bioenergetics described calcium-activation of the dehydrogenases as the rate-limiting determinant of respiratory flux regulating myocardial oxygen consumption, proton efflux, NADH and ATP synthesis [191]. In cardiomyocytes, mitochondrial ATP synthase activity can be directly modulated by increased mitochondrial Ca^{2+} levels [192, 193].

Intra-compartment Ca^{2+} signaling is recognized as a key mode of signal transduction and amplification in mitochondria [186, 187]. Using inositol phospholipids, such as IP3 as second messengers, a variety of cell-surface hormones and neurotransmitters signal the release of Ca^{2+} from ER and Golgi apparatus into the cytosol (Fig. 7.7).

The proximity of mitochondria to ER membranes appears to be a significant factor for ER Ca^{2+} release and mitochondrial Ca^{2+} uptake [184]. This dramatic increase in mitochondrial Ca^{2+} is rapidly mobilized from the ER-IP3 receptor channels, when in close contact to mitochondria, albeit the precise molecular mechanism of this transfer has not been fully established. Similarly, the sarcoplasmic reticulum ryanodine receptors are located near the cardiomyocytes mitochondria undergoing calcium release [194]. Proposed mechanisms for the rapid calcium mitochondrial import include, the involvement of diffusable cytosolic factors that stimulate the Ca^{2+} uniporter, activation of an entirely different channel in the heart mitochondrial membrane (RaM), and enhanced uptake by mitochondrial analogues of ryanodine receptors residing in the inner membrane [195–198]. Recently, VDAC has also been identified (see Fig. 7.7) as a component in Ca^{2+} transport from ER through the outer mitochondrial membrane [199].

Signals of Survival and Stress Impact Heart Mitochondria

The list of extracellular and intracellularly-generated signals which impact the mitochondrial organelle is increasing as reflected in Table 7.3. In addition to hormonal and cytokines stimuli (e.g., TH, TNF-α, interleukins), there are nutrient, serum, growth, and mitotic factors, as well as stress and metabolic stimuli. There are also pro/anti-apoptotic modulators that are discussed in detail in Chap. 5 (instrinsic pathway of apoptosis) and in Chap. 11 (extrinsic pathway of apoptosis).

Endoplasmic Reticulum

The endoplasmic reticulum (ER) is a multifunctional signaling organelle that contributes to the regulation of cellular processes such as the entry and release of Ca^{2+} (Fig. 7.7), sterol biosynthesis, apoptosis, and the release of arachidonic acid [209]. One of its primary functions is as a source of the Ca^{2+} signals that are released through either IP3 or ryanodine

receptors (RyRs) which are themselves Ca^{2+}-sensitive. The capability of ER in spreading signals throughout the cell mediated by a process of Ca^{2+}-induced Ca^{2+} release is particularly important in the control of cardiomyocyte function. The role of ER as an internal reservoir of Ca^{2+} is coordinated with its role in protein synthesis since a constant luminal level of Ca^{2+} is essential for protein folding. In order to achieve this regulation, the ER also contains several stress signaling pathways that can activate transcriptional cascades to regulate the luminal content of the Ca^{2+} dependent chaperones responsible for the folding and packaging of secretory proteins. Another significant function of the cardiomyocyte ER is to regulate apoptosis by operating in tandem with mitochondria. Antiapoptotic regulators of apoptosis such as Bcl-2 may act by reducing the ebb and flow of Ca^{2+} through ER/mitochondrial cross-talk.

P53 Pathways

The product of the p53 gene is a multifunctional protein that is involved in many cellular processes, the most important of which are cell cycle control and apoptosis in response to stress [210, 211]. p53 contains 393 amino acids and has functional domains such as transactivation and DNA binding domains, and several cellular protein binding sites such as MDM2 and viral protein binding sites [212]. Cellular levels of p53 are normally low in part due to its direct interaction with MDM2, a cellular proto-oncogene product that binds to p53 and inhibits its transactivating ability [213]. Increasing evidence showed that p53 is an important regulator of apoptotic cell death [214, 215], and specifically implicated p53 in cardiomyocyte apoptosis [216–218]. p53-mediated apoptotic cell death involves both its nuclear translocation and its

Table 7.3 Stimuli signaling heart mitochondria

Stimuli	Signaling pathway	Mitochondrial effect	References
IL-1	NO production	Decreased respiration	[180, 200]
TNF-α	Ceramide pathway	Decreased activities of PDH, complex I and II	[200]
Heat stress	Increased HSP 32,60,72 levels	Increased complex I–V activities	[201]
Low glucose	Myocardial apoptosis	Cytochrome c release	[202]
Low serum	Myocardial apoptosis	Cytochrome c release	[202]
Palmitate	Myocardial apoptosis ceramide increase	Decreased complex III and membrane potential, cytochrome c release, mitochondria swelling, UCP expression increased	[203]
Ceramide	Ceramide pathway	Complex III decrease	[204]
Electrical stimulation	Transcription factor activation (e.g., NRF-1)	Mitochondrial proliferation	[116]
Nitric oxide	peroxynitrite formation	Complex I and IV decrease, cytochrome c release	[205, 206]
Thyroid hormone	Receptor-mediated nuclear and mtDNA gene activation	Mitochondrial proliferation. Increased UCP and uncoupled OXPHOS	[207, 208]

well-characterized transcriptional activation of downstream pro-apoptotic proteins such as Bax, Noxa, and PUMA (p53 upregulated modulator of apoptosis) [219], as well as its capacity to directly activate Bax in permeabilizing mitochondria and triggering apoptosis in a transcription-independent manner [220]. Nonetheless, the sequence and mechanism of intracellular signaling events underlying the p53-activated cardiomyocyte apoptotic pathway in response to OS remain largely undefined.

Posttranscriptional modifications including phosphorylation are likely involved in activating p53 during cellular stress [221, 222]. In different cell types, p53 can be phosphorylated on multiple serine/threonine residues located at both the N- and the C-terminus by a variety of protein kinases in response to specific stressors. These include p38 MAP kinases [223], protein kinase C [224], casein kinase II [225], DNA-dependent protein kinase (DNA-PK) [226], Ataxia Telangiectasia mutated (ATM) kinase [227, 228], and the Ataxia Telangiectasia and rad-3-related (ATR) kinase [229]. Phosphorylation of serine-15 of the N-terminal region has been shown to enhance specific DNA binding and transcriptional activity of p53 through decreased binding of p53 to its negative regulator MDM2 [230], and increased binding to coactivator protein p300 [231]. Moreover, H_2O_2-mediated OS results in phosphorylation of serine-15, p53 activation and apoptosis in rat neural cells [232]. Gathered observations have shown that OS is a potent inducer of cardiomyocyte apoptosis and a mediator of HF [233, 234], and that multiple signaling pathways exist to regulate the OS-induced cardiomyocyte death. One of the signaling pathways may be controlled by p53, which plays a crucial role in cell cycle control and apoptosis [233]. Studies with isolated cardiomyocytes have shown that hypoxia or increased OS leads to an upregulation of p53 [233, 235], a finding that has been confirmed at both the transcript and protein level [234].

Activation of the protein p53 by site-specific phosphorylation at its serine residues in response to stress appears to be important for the regulation of p53 function [236, 237]; for example, phosphorylation of p53 at a functional site, serine-15, is critical for stabilization and functional activation of p53 during cellular stress [238]. Long et al. [234] have reported that H_2O_2-induced cardiomyocyte apoptosis is accompanied in cultured cardiomyocytes by enhanced phosphorylation of p53 at the serine-15; this represents a novel demonstration that OS enhances p53 phosphorylation at this functional site with evidence of its downstream activation of target genes. Using nonphospho-specific and phospho-specific p53 antibodies these investigators [234] have examined the levels of nonphospho-p53 and phospho-p53, respectively. H_2O_2 caused a rapid increase in the level of the phosphorylated p53 at the serine-15 in cardiomyocytes, but only a slight change in the level of nonphosphorylated p53 suggesting that the site-specific phosphorylation

of p53 is an important event in the process of cardiomyocyte apoptosis. Furthermore, phosphorylation of the serine-15 site results in activation of p53 function through decreased binding of p53 to its negative regulator MDM2 [230] and increased binding to the p300 coactivator protein [231]. Mutation at this site impairs the apoptotic activity of p53 [239]. These findings indicate that phosphorylation of the serine-15 is important for p53 activation and again in induction of apoptosis. In addition to H_2O_2, other DNA-damaging agents such as ultraviolet and ionizing radiation also increase phosphorylation of p53 at serine-15 [227, 228, 240]. Besides this critical phosphorylation site, it is important to note that other sites on p53 may be phosphorylated as well. However, observations in human umbilical vein endothelial cells have shown that H_2O_2 produces rapid phosphorylation of p53 specifically at serine-15, but not serine-9, 20, or 392 [241].

Protein phosphorylation is an important mechanism of signal transduction that plays a crucial role in many aspects of cellular function [242, 243]. In addition, the phosphorylation status of proteins is closely associated with activation of protein kinases, and the possible involvement of specific protein kinases in the phosphorylation of serine-15 on p53, using protein kinase inhibitors with different specificity has been studied [234]. The mitogen-activated protein kinase cascade (MAPK) is one of the major signaling pathways that are activated during OS [244], and in mammalian cells three distinct subgroups of MAPKs have been found: the extracellular-signal-regulated kinases (ERKs), the stress-activated c-Jun N-terminal kinase (JNK), and p38 kinase [245].

ERKs are primarily associated with cell growth and proliferation, while JNKs and p38 kinase mainly mediate cellular stress signals [246]. Serine-15 of p53 is phosphorylated in JB6 mouse epidermal cells in response to UV radiation [238], and ERKs and p38 kinase have been found to participate in the phosphorylation of this serine site [240]. In addition, p38 kinase can phosphorylate p53 at serine-33, serine-46, and serine-389 [223, 247]; however, it is not known whether MAPKs phosphorylate this serine-15 in cardiomyocytes in response to H_2O_2, leading to functional activation of p53. The effect of PD98059 (inhibitor of MEK), SB202190 (inhibitor of p38 kinase), and SP600125 (inhibitor of JNK) on phosphorylation of serine-15 has been assessed. H_2O_2-induced phosphorylation of p53 at serine-15 is unaffected by inhibition of the MAPK signaling pathway [234]. Although in some studies MAPKs was not found to be involved in the site-specific phosphorylation of p53, others observations have shown that this p53 serine residue can be a target for DNA-PK, ATM, and ATR [226–228], which are members of the phosphoinositide-3-kinase (PI3K)-related kinase superfamily. DNA-PK acts primarily during DNA repair [248], whereas ATM and ATR participate in the activation of cell cycle checkpoints induced by DNA damage [249].

In vitro studies have shown that DNA-PK directly phosphorylates p53 at serine-15 [239], and ATM and ATR have been reported to mediate phosphorylation of serine-15 in response to ionizing or UV radiation [228, 229]. Furthermore, defects in phosphorylation of serine-15 are observed in cells lacking DNA-PK or ATM after UV radiation [228, 229], and wortmannin or caffeine blocks the H_2O_2-induced phosphorylation of p53 at serine-15 in human umbilical vein endothelial cells [241]. No inhibition of H_2O_2-induced phosphorylation of serine-15 has been observed in cardiomyocytes treated with either wortmannin or caffeine suggesting that DNA-PK, ATM, and ATR may be less likely to mediate phosphorylation of p53 at serine-15 in cardiomyocytes during the H_2O_2 treatment [234]. Moreover, inhibition of protein kinase C by staurosporine or chelerythrine fails to attenuate the phosphorylation of this serine site of p53. Future studies should be aimed at examining the possible role of other kinase signaling pathways including the nonreceptor protein tyrosine kinases in the activation of p53 through site-specific phosphorylation in cardiomyocytes in response to H_2O_2. Furthermore, delineation of the specific intracellular sites at which serine-15 phosphorylated p53 is localized as well as which genes and/or proteins it may preferentially bind (using chromatin immunoprecipitation) should provide further information elucidating the role of p53 activation in the OS pathway.

Phosphorylation of serine-15 of p53 appears to be an important signaling event in H_2O_2-treated cardiomyocytes as reported in other cell-types [232]. Phosphorylation of serine-15 leads to stabilization of p53 by reducing its interaction with MDM2, a negative regulator of p53 function [213], and increases the ability of p53 to recruit the coactivator proteins CBP and p300 [231]. CBP/p300 acts as a coactivator of p53 through interaction with the N-terminus of p53 and increases the sequence-specific DNA binding of p53, thus providing a positive mechanism for increasing transcriptional activity of p53 [231]. Of interest, marked changes in the level of the upstream modifier MDM2 and p300 occur in cardiomyocytes exposed to H_2O_2 [234] with H_2O_2 up-regulating the expression of p300 but down-regulating the expression of MDM2 in cardiomyocytes, thus contributing to enhanced p53 function. In addition, gadd [250], one of the well-characterized downstream genes of p53 that are associated with cell growth arrest and induction of apoptosis in several cell types [239, 251], was markedly increased in cardiomyocytes during OS as was PUMA [234], a BH3-only member of the Bcl-2 protein family that have been identified as a player in myocardial cell death [252]. In addition, following cardiomyocytes H_2O_2 treatment, the level of p21, an inhibitor of cyclin-dependent kinases and downstream effector of p53, was increased [253].

Thus, both up-regulation and phosphorylation of p53 at serine-15 are important events in cardiomyocytes response

to OS. ROS, such as H_2O_2, cause oxidative damage to DNA, leading to activation of protein kinases. Phosphorylation of p53 at serine-15 by protein kinases enhances the sequence-specific DNA binding and transcriptional activity of p53 by increasing binding of the coactivator protein p300 and by reducing binding of MDM2. After being activated, the transcriptional factor p53 transactivates downstream effector genes, whose protein products may mediate cell growth arrest and apoptotic cell death, and may become an important contributor toward the development of HF. Therefore, targeting p53 could be a novel therapy option (Fig. 7.9). Besides its crucial role in cell cycle control and apoptosis, p53, through its negative effect on cardiac angiogenesis may also be a causative factor in the development of HF secondary to chronic pressure overload. Under sustained pressure overload, accumulation of p53 inhibits the activity of hypoxia inducible factor-1 (factor or family of factors), which affects genes that regulate important cellular processes such as cell metabolism, angiogenesis, and cell survival [254], and worsens cardiac angiogenesis and systolic function. In contrast, by increasing cardiac angiogenesis using angiogenic factors or through the inhibition of p53, hypertrophy secondary to chronic pressure overload develops further, but cardiac function is normalized [255]. Thus, the antiangiogenic property of p53 appears to play a significant role in the transition from cardiac hypertrophy to HF, and inhibition of p53 activity may be a new tool for the treatment of HF secondary to chronic pressure overload.

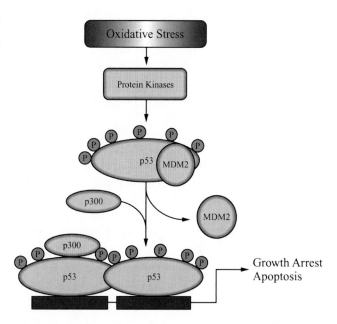

Fig. 7.9 p53 signaling pathway that mediates cell growth arrest and apoptosis. ROS cause oxidative damage to DNA, leading to activation of a variety of protein kinases that phosphorylate the p53 protein. Then, p53 transactivates several downstream effector genes whose protein products may result in cell growth arrest and apoptotic cell death

Conclusion

Post-genomic approaches currently available have implicated an increasing number of genes and their products as critical factors to cardiomyocyte signaling in both physiological and pathological conditions, including HF. While considerable progress has been made in the identification of the downstream targets of these genes and the pathways they constitute, the majority of targets and the complex interrelationships between the signaling pathways involved still remain largely undetermined. In particular, a large number of signaling interactions between cellular organelles remain to be identified.

Importantly, the cross-talk between mitochondria, plasma membrane receptors, exocytotic events, and excitable channels, with ER, Golgi bodies, peroxisomes, and with the nucleus in effecting nuclear import/export, regulatory gene expression, signaling cell cycle progression as well as the determination of cardiac-specific and developmentally-specific factors involved in myocardial signaling will require intensive research effort.

A driving force on the assessment of cardiovascular signaling is that it can enhance our understanding of the widening spectra of cardiac abnormalities, HF in particular, that may result from signaling dysfunction, as well as potentially contributing to the development of novel treatment modalities. The recognition that cytoprotective signaling plays an essential role in cardioprotection has generated great interest in the pharmacological manipulation of metabolism and signaling. However, several important caveats pertain to the application of targeting specific signaling molecules within the clinical setting. Many signaling molecules participate in multiple pathways. For instance, inhibiting ROS production might prove helpful in reducing the negative consequences of myocardial I/R, but could prove counterproductive in cardioprotection and in oxygen sensing. Secondly, the existence of redundant signaling pathways that trigger HF also poses challenges for therapeutic intervention.

Clearly, improved understanding of the precise order of intracellular events, their downstream consequences, the overall inter-relatedness, and regulation of these pathways will be critical to the discovery of new treatments for HF. Also, the development and characterization of reagents with high specificity to heart signaling pathways and technologies that may allow inhibition of stress signaling (e.g., specific kinase inhibitors) in cardiac and vascular cells may represent a breakthrough in the management of HF.

Summary

- Multiple signaling pathways regulate cardiomyocyte survival, growth, and proliferation. These are redundant mechanisms that typically involve serine/threonine kinases, which stimulate a series of sequential molecular and cellular events (cascades).
- The targeting and localization of signaling factors and enzymes to discrete subcellular compartments or substrates are important regulatory mechanisms that ensure specific signaling events in response to local stimuli.
- The molecular mechanisms underlying the proliferative growth of embryonic myocardium in vivo and adult cardiac myocyte hypertrophy in vivo remain largely undetermined, although considerable progress has been made using post-genomic analysis.
- In the regulation of cardiomyocyte growth and/or proliferation, there are several signals transduction acting as redundant mechanisms converging on one or several serine/threonine kinases. Several G-protein-coupled receptors (GPCRs) such as α-AR, β-AR, angiotensin II, and endothelin-1 are able to activate these signaling cascades, and induce changes in cell growth and proliferation.
- The PI3K/Akt pathway is a key regulator of four intersecting biological processes: cell growth and survival, cell cycle progression, and metabolism.
- Akt contributes to both pathological and physiological cardiac growth, myocyte survival, and contractile function.
- Akt expression confers protection from ischemia-induced cell death and cardiac dysfunction.
- Myocardial Akt levels have been found elevated in early heart failure (after 1–2 weeks of pacing) accompanied by increased levels of OS, TNF-α and free fatty acid accumulation, reduced activity levels of mitochondrial respiratory complex III and complex V, and apoptosis initiation.
- One potential downstream target of the Akt pathway is the shift in myocardial substrate utilization, including FAO.
- Akt activation can directly down-regulate the activity of cardiac AMPK, an energy sensor that acts to modulate glucose uptake and FAO.
- Akt acts as an antiapoptotic factor important in cardiomyocyte survival; one way it can modulate apoptotic progression is by phosphorylation of pro-apoptotic peptide factors (e.g., BAD).
- Several mechanisms and/or effectors by which the PI3K/Akt pathway stems apoptosis have been identified, and it appears likely that these effectors might be enhanced when applied in combination.
- The constitutive activation of PI3K led to an adaptive hypertrophy, and did not change into a maladaptive hypertrophy, consistent with a critical role for the PI3K/PDK-1/Akt pathway in regulating normal cardiac growth.
- Because its ability to improve flow-metabolism coupling, IGF-1 could indeed represent a new cardiovascular disease treatment option for many cardiac disorders such as ischemic heart disease and heart failure.

- Observations in animal models of myocardial ischemia–reperfusion revealed that the administration of IGF-1 can provide substantial cardioprotective effect.
- Cellular analyses revealed that IGF-1 inhibited characteristic cardiomyocyte elongation in dilated hearts and restored calcium dynamics comparable to that observed in normal cells.
- Overexpression of Sir2α protected cardiac myocytes from apoptosis in response to serum starvation and significantly increased the size of cardiac myocytes.
- Sir2α expression has been found increased in hearts from dogs with heart failure induced by rapid pacing superimposed on stable, severe hypertrophy.
- In HF, reduced Sir2α deacetylase activity and NAD$^+$ depletion mediate poly(ADP-ribose) polymerase-1 (PARP)-dependent cardiac myocyte cell death.
- A critical target of the SIR2 deacetylase activity is the FOXO forkhead transcription factors, shifting FOXO dependent responses away from cell death and toward cell survival contributing to enhanced longevity.
- Inhibition of mTOR signaling with rapamycin regresses decompensated cardiac hypertrophy induced by pressure overload in mice.
- In vascular smooth muscle, K_{ATP} channels are regulated by diverse signaling pathways, and cause vasodilation contributing both to resting blood flow and vasodilator-induced increases in flow.
- The nucleus contains global regulatory transcription factors such as peroxisome proliferator-activated receptors and their transcriptional co-activators (i.e., PPAR-α, RXR-α), which also play a pivotal regulatory role in the expression of mitochondrial FAO pathways, integral to bioenergetic metabolism.
- Lipids and in particular the mitochondrial-specific phospholipid cardiolipin serve as a focal target for ROS damage.
- It is worth noting that ROS produced from other cellular sources, besides mitochondria, can have substantial effects on cardiovascular function.
- A provocative link has been proposed between XO activity and abnormal cardiac energy metabolism in patients with idiopathic DCM, since inhibition of XO with allopurinol significantly improved myocardial function.
- Increased mitochondrial H_2O_2 generation and signaling occur with NO modulation of the ETC, as well as with the induction of myocardial mitochondrial NO production, resulting from treatment with enalapril.
- Mitochondrial retrograde signaling is a pathway of communication from mitochondria to the nucleus that influences many cellular activities under both normal and pathophysiological conditions.
- Acute HF generated by manipulating calcium concentrations in perfused canine hearts was accompanied by a striking decrease in mitochondrial respiratory function.
- Mitochondrial Ca^{2+} uptake is significantly and rapidly elevated in cardiomyocytes during physiological Ca^{2+} signaling and is often accompanied by a highly localized transient mitochondrial depolarization.
- Using inositol phospholipids, such as IP3 as second messengers, a variety of cell-surface hormones and neurotransmitters signal the release of Ca^{2+} from ER and Golgi apparatus into the cytosol.
- The capability of ER in spreading signals throughout the cell mediated by a process of Ca^{2+}-induced Ca^{2+} release is particularly important in the control of cardiomyocyte function.
- OS is a potent inducer of cardiomyocyte apoptosis and a mediator of HF. Multiple signaling pathways exist for regulating OS-induced cardiomyocyte death. One of the signaling pathways may be controlled by p53, which plays a crucial role in cell cycle control and apoptosis
- Activation of the protein p53 by site-specific phosphorylation at its serine residues in response to stress appears to be important for the regulation of p53 function.
- Transcriptional factor p53 transactivates downstream effector genes whose protein products may mediate cell growth arrest and apoptotic cell death, and may become an important contributor toward the development of HF.
- Antiangiogenic property of p53 appears to play a significant role in the transition from cardiac hypertrophy to HF, and inhibition of p53 activity may be a new tool for the treatment of HF secondary to chronic pressure overload.

References

1. Engel FB, Schebesta M, Duong MT, Lu G, Ren S, Madwed JB, Jiang H, Wang Y, Keating MT (2005) p38 MAP kinase inhibition enables proliferation of adult mammalian cardiomyocytes. Genes Dev 19:1175–1187
2. Tamamori-Adachi M, Ito H et al. (2003) Critical role of cyclin D1 nuclear import in cardiomyocyte proliferation. Circ Res 92: e12–e19
3. Pasumarthi KB, Kardami E, Cattini PA (1996) High and low molecular weight fibroblast growth factor-2 increase proliferation of neonatal rat cardiac myocytes but have differential effects on binucleation and nuclear morphology. Evidence for both paracrine and intracrine actions of fibroblast growth factor-2. Circ Res 78:126–136
4. Sheikh F, Jin Y, Pasumarthi KB, Kardami E, Cattini PA (1997) Expression of fibroblast growth factor receptor-1 in rat heart H9c2 myoblasts increases cell proliferation. Mol Cell Biochem 176:89–97
5. Sheng Z, Pennica D, Wood WI, Chien KR (1996) Cardiotrophin-1 displays early expression in the murine heart tube and promotes cardiac myocyte survival. Development 122:419–428
6. Kuwahara K, Saito Y, Kishimoto I et al (2000) Cardiotrophin-1 phosphorylates akt and BAD, and prolongs cell survival via a PI3K-dependent pathway in cardiac myocytes. J Mol Cell Cardiol 32:1385–1394
7. Huss JM, Kelly DP (2005) Mitochondrial energy metabolism in heart failure: a question of balance. J Clin Invest 115:547–555
8. Shiojima I, Walsh K (2006) Regulation of cardiac growth and coronary angiogenesis by the Akt/PKB signaling pathway. Genes Dev 20:3347–3365

9. Sugden PH (2003) Ras, Akt, and mechanotransduction in the cardiac myocyte. Circ Res 93:1179–1192

10. Chesley A, Lundberg MS, Asai T, Xiao RP, Ohtani S, Lakatta EG, Crow MT (2000) The beta(2)-adrenergic receptor delivers an anti-apoptotic signal to cardiac myocytes through G(i)-dependent coupling to phosphatidylinositol 3'-kinase. Circ Res 87:1172–1179

11. Ananthakrishnan R, Gordon WM, Goldenthal MJ, Marín-García J (2005) Akt signaling pathway in pacing-induced heart failure. Mol Cell Biochem 268:103–110

12. Pham FH, Sugden PH, Clerk A (2000) Regulation of protein kinase B and 4E-BP1 by oxidative stress in cardiac myocytes. Circ Res 86:1252–1258

13. Recchia FA, McConnell PI, Bernstein RD, Vogel TR, Xu X, Hintze TH (1998) Reduced nitric oxide production and altered myocardial metabolism during the decompensation of pacing-induced heart failure in the conscious dog. Circ Res 83:969–979

14. Osorio JC, Stanley WC, Linke A et al (2002) Impaired myocardial fatty oxidation and reduced protein expression of retinoid X receptor-alpha in pacing – induced heart failure. Circulation 106:606–612

15. Sack MN, Rader TA, Park S, Bastin J, McCune SA, Kelly DP (1996) Fatty acid oxidation enzyme gene expression is down regulated in the failing heart. Circulation 94:2837–2842

16. Cook SA, Matsui T, Li L, Rosenzweig A (2002) Transcriptional effects of chronic Akt activation in the heart. J Biol Chem 277: 22528–22533

17. Kovacic S, Soltys CL, Barr AJ, Shiojima I, Walsh K, Dyck JR (2003) Akt activity negatively regulates phosphorylation of AMP-activated protein kinase in the heart. J Biol Chem 278:39422–39427

18. Qin S, Chock PB (2003) Implication of phosphatidylinositol 3-kinase membrane recruitment in hydrogen peroxide-induced activation of PI3K and Akt. Biochemistry 42:2995–3003

19. Gudz T, Tserng K, Hoppel DL (1997) Direct inhibition of mitochondrial respiratory chain complex III by cell-permeable ceramide. J Biol Chem 272:24154–24158

20. Datta SR, Dudek H, Tao X, Masters S, Fu H, Gotoh Y, Greenberg ME (1997) Akt phosphorylation of BAD couples survival signals to the cell-intrinsic death machinery. Cell 91:231–241

21. Liu W, Akhand AA, Takeda K, Kawamoto Y, Itoigawa M, Kato M, Suzuki H, Ishikawa N, Nakashima I (2003) Protein phosphatase 2A-linked and -unlinked caspase-dependent pathways for down-regulation of Akt kinase triggered by 4-hydroxynonenal. Cell Death Differ 10:772–781

22. Kageyama K, Ihara Y, Goto S, Urata Y, Toda G, Yano K, Kondo T (2002) Overexpression of calreticulin modulates protein kinase B/Akt signaling to promote apoptosis during cardiac differentiation of cardiomyoblast H9c2 cells. J Biol Chem 277:19255–19264

23. Neumann J, Eschenhagen T, Jones LR, Linck B, Schmitz W, Scholz H, Zimmermann N (1997) Increased expression of cardiac phosphatases in patients with end-stage heart failure. J Mol Cell Cardiol 29:265–272

24. Nikolaidis LA, Sturzu A, Stolarski C, Elahi D, Shen YT, Shannon RP (2004) The development of myocardial insulin resistance in conscious dogs with advanced dilated cardiomyopathy. Cardiovasc Res 61:297–306

25. Matsui T, Li L, del Monte F, Fukui Y, Fukui Y, Franke TF, Hajjar RJ, Rosenzweig A (1999) adenoviral gene transfer of activated phospatidyl inositol 3- kinase and Akt inhibits apoptosis of hypoxic cardiomyocytes in vitro. Circulation 100:2373–2379

26. McMullen JR, Shioi T, Huang WY, Zhang L, Tarnavski O, Bisping E, Schinke M, Kong S, Sherwood MC, Brown J, Riggi L, Kang PM, Izumo S (2004) The insulin-like growth factor 1 receptor induces physiological heart growth via the phosphoinositide 3-kinase (p110alpha) pathway. J Biol Chem 279:4782–4793

27. Soltys CL, Buchholz L, Gandhi M, Clanachan AS, Walsh K, Dyck JR (2002) Phosphorylation of cardiac protein kinase B is regulated by palmitate. Am J Physiol Heart Circ Physiol 283:H1056–H1064

28. Leslie NR, Bennett D, Lindsay YE, Sterwart H, Gray A, Downes CP (2003) Redox regulation of PI 3-kinase signalling via inactivation of PTEN. EMBO J 22:5501–5510

29. Dorn GW 2nd, Force T (2005) Protein kinase cascades in the regulation of cardiac hypertrophy. J Clin Invest 115:527–537

30. Stokoe D, Stephens LR, Copeland T et al (1997) Dual role of phosphatidylinositol-3,4,5-trisphosphate in the activation of protein kinase B. Science 277:567–570

31. Sarbassov DD, Guertin DA, Ali SM, Sabatini DM (2005) Phosphorylation and regulation of Akt/PKB by the rictor-mTOR complex. Science 307:1098–1101

32. Wang L, Wang X, Proud CG (2000) Activation of mRNA translation in rat cardiac myocytes by insulin involves multiple rapamycin-sensitive steps. Am J Physiol Heart Circ Physiol 278:H1056–H1068

33. Gao X, Zhang Y, Arrazola P, Hino O, Kobayashi T, Yeung RS, Ru B, Pan D (2002) Tsc tumour suppressor proteins antagonize amino-acid-TOR signalling. Nat Cell Biol 4:699–704

34. Marygold SJ, Leevers SJ (2002) Growth signaling: TSC takes its place. Curr Biol 12:R785–R787

35. Zhang Y, Gao X, Saucedo LJ, Ru B, Edgar BA, Pan D (2003) Rheb is a direct target of the tuberous sclerosis tumour suppressor proteins. Nat Cell Biol 5:578–581

36. Tee AR, Manning BD, Roux PP, Cantley LC, Blenis J (2003) Tuberous sclerosis complex gene products, Tuberin and Hamartin, control mTOR signaling by acting as a GTPase-activating protein complex toward Rheb. Curr Biol 13:1259–1268

37. Badorff C, Ruetten H, Mueller S et al (2002) Fas receptor signaling inhibits glycogen synthase kinase 3 beta and induces cardiac hypertrophy following pressure overload. J Clin Invest 109:373–381

38. Haq S, Choukroun G, Kang ZB et al (2000) Glycogen synthase kinase-3beta is a negative regulator of cardiomyocyte hypertrophy. J Cell Biol 151:117–130

39. Morisco C, Zebrowski D, Condorelli G, Tsichlis P, Vatner SF, Sadoshima J (2000) The Akt-glycogen synthase kinase 3beta pathway regulates transcription of atrial natriuretic factor induced by beta-adrenergic receptor stimulation in cardiac myocytes. J Biol Chem 275:14466–14475

40. Proud CG (2004) Ras, PI3-kinase and mTOR signaling in cardiac hypertrophy. Cardiovasc Res 63:403–413

41. Haq S, Michael A, Andreucci M, Bhattacharya K, Dotto P, Walters B, Woodgett J, Kilter H, Force T (2003) Stabilization of beta-catenin by a Wnt-independent mechanism regulates cardiomyocyte growth. Proc Natl Acad Sci USA 100:4610–4615

42. Michael A, Haq S, Chen X, Hsich E, Cui L, Walters B, Shao Z, Bhattacharya K, Kilter H, Huggins G, Andreucci M, Periasamy M, Solomon RN, Liao R, Patten R, Molkentin JD, Force T (2004) Glycogen synthase kinase-3beta regulates growth, calcium homeostasis, and diastolic function in the heart. J Biol Chem 279:21383–21393

43. Liao W, Wang S, Han C, Zhang Y (2005) 14-3-3 proteins regulate glycogen synthase 3beta phosphorylation and inhibit cardiomyocyte hypertrophy. FEBS J 272:1845–1854

44. Chan AY, Soltys CL, Young ME, Proud CG, Dyck JR (2004) Activation of AMP-activated protein kinase inhibits protein synthesis associated with hypertrophy in the cardiac myocyte. J Biol Chem 279:32771–32779

45. Arsham AM, Howell JJ, Simon MC (2003) A novel hypoxia-inducible factor-independent hypoxic response regulating mammalian target of rapamycin and its targets. J Biol Chem 278:29655–29660

46. van Noort M, Meeldijk J, van der Zee R, Destree O, Clevers H (2002) Wnt signaling controls the phosphorylation status of beta-catenin. J Biol Chem 277:17901–17905

47. Aikawa R, Nawano M, Gu Y, Katagiri H, Asano T, Zhu W, Nagai R, Komuro I (2000) Insulin prevents cardiomyocytes from oxidative stress-induced apoptosis through activation of PI3 kinase/Akt. Circulation 102:2873–2879

48. Gao F, Gao E, Yue TL, Ohlstein EH, Lopez BL, Christopher TA, Ma XL (2002) Nitric oxide mediates the antiapoptotic effect of insulin in myocardial ischemia-reperfusion: the roles of PI3-kinase, Akt, and endothelial nitric oxide synthase phosphorylation. Circulation 105:1497–1502

49. Matsui T, Li L, del Monte F, Fukui Y, Franke TF, Hajjar RJ, Rosenzweig A (1999) Adenoviral gene transfer of activated phosphatidylinositol 3′-kinase and Akt inhibits apoptosis of hypoxic cardiomyocytes in vitro. Circulation 100:2373–2379

50. Yamashita K, Kajstura J, Discher DJ, Wasserlauf BJ, Bishopric NH, Anversa P, Webster KA (2001) Reperfusion-activated Akt kinase prevents apoptosis in transgenic mouse hearts overexpressing insulin-like growth factor-1. Circ Res 88:609–614

51. Craig R, Wagner M, McCardle T, Craig AG, Glembotski CC (2001) The cytoprotective effects of the glycoprotein 130 receptor-coupled cytokine, cardiotrophin-1, require activation of NF-kappa B. J Biol Chem 276:37621–37629

52. Negoro S, Oh H, Tone E, Kunisada K, Fujio Y, Walsh K, Kishimoto T, Yamauchi-Takihara K (2001) Glycoprotein 130 regulates cardiac myocyte survival in doxorubicin-induced apoptosis through phosphatidylinositol 3-kinase/Akt phosphorylation and Bcl-xL/caspase-3 interaction. Circulation 103:555–561

53. Tian B, Liu J, Bitterman P, Bache RJ (2003) Angiotensin II modulates nitric oxide-induced cardiac fibroblast apoptosis by activation of AKT/PKB. Am J Physiol Heart Circ Physiol 285:H1105–H1112

54. Clerk A, Sugden PH (1999) Activation of protein kinase cascades in the heart by hypertrophic G protein-coupled receptor agonists. Am J Cardiol 83:64H–69H

55. Krieg T, Landsberger M, Alexeyev MF, Felix SB, Cohen MV, Downey JM (2003) Activation of Akt is essential for acetylcholine to trigger generation of oxygen free radicals. Cardiovasc Res 58:196–202

56. Yin H, Chao L, Chao J (2004) Adrenomedullin protects against myocardial apoptosis after ischemia/reperfusion through activation of Akt-GSK signaling. Hypertension 43:109–116

57. Naga Prasad SV, Esposito G, Mao L, Koch WJ, Rockman HA (2000) Gbetagamma-dependent phosphoinositide 3-kinase activation in hearts with in vivo pressure overload hypertrophy. J Biol Chem 275:4693–4698

58. Mockridge JW, Marber MS, Heads RJ (2000) Activation of Akt during simulated ischemia/reperfusion in cardiac myocytes. Biochem Biophys Res Commun 270:947–952

59. Condorelli G, Drusco A, Stassi G et al (2002) Akt induces enhanced myocardial contractility and cell size in vivo in transgenic mice. Proc Natl Acad Sci USA 99:12333–12338

60. Liu Tj, Lai Hc, Wu W, Chinn S, Wang PH (2001) Developing a strategy to define the effects of insulin-like growth factor-1 on gene expression profile in cardiomyocytes. Circ Res 88:1231–1238

61. Bialik S, Cryns VL, Drincic A, Miyata S, Wollowick AL, Srinivasan A, Kitsis RN (1999) The mitochondrial apoptotic pathway is activated by serum and glucose deprivation in cardiac myocytes. Circ Res 85:403–414

62. Edinger AL, Thompson CB (2002) Akt maintains cell size and survival by increasing mTOR-dependent nutrient uptake. Mol Biol Cell 13:2276–2288

63. Juhaszova M, Zorov DB, Kim SH et al (2004) Glycogen synthase kinase-3beta mediates convergence of protection signaling to inhibit the mitochondrial permeability transition pore. J Clin Invest 113:1535–1549

64. Conti E, Musumeci MB, Assenza GE, Quarta G, Autore C, Volpe M (2008) Recombinant human insulin-like growth factor-1: a new cardiovascular disease treatment option? Cardiovasc Hematol Agents Med Chem 6:258–271

65. Noguchi S, Kashihara Y, Ikegami Y, Morimoto K, Miyamoto M, Nakao K (1993) Insulin-like growth factor-I ameliorates transient ischemia-induced acute renal failure in rats. J Pharmacol Exp Ther 267:919–926

66. Gluckman P, Klempt N, Guan J, Mallard C, Sirimanne E, Dragunow M, Klempt M, Singh K, Williams C, Nikolics K (1992) A role for IGF-1 in the rescue of CNS neurons following hypoxic-ischemic injury. Biochem Biophys Res Commun 182:593–599

67. Buerke M, Murohara T, Skurk C, Nuss C, Tomaselli K, Lefer AM (1995) Cardioprotective effect of insulin-like growth factor I in myocardial ischemia followed by reperfusion. Proc Natl Acad Sci USA 92:8031–8035

68. Davani EY, Brumme Z, Singhera GK, Cote HC, Harrigan PR, Dorscheid DR (2003) Insulin-like growth factor-1 protects ischemic murine myocardium from ischemia/reperfusion associated injury. Crit Care 7:R176–R183

69. Otani H, Yamamura T, Nakao Y, Hattori R, Kawaguchi H, Osako M, Imamura H (2000) Insulin-like growth factor-I improves recovery of cardiac performance during reperfusion in isolated rat heart by a wortmannin-sensitive mechanism. J Cardiovasc Pharmacol 35:275–281

70. Friehs I, Stamm C, Cao-Danh H, McGowan FX, del Nido PJ (2001) Insulin-like growth factor-1 improves postischemic recovery in hypertrophied hearts. Ann Thorac Surg 72:1650–1656

71. Yamamura T, Otani H, Nakao Y, Hattori R, Osako M, Imamura H (2001) IGF-I differentially regulates Bcl-xL and Bax and confers myocardial protection in the rat heart. Am J Physiol Heart Circ Physiol 280:H1191–H1200

72. Li Q, Li B, Wang X, Leri A, Jana KP, Liu Y et al (1997) Overexpression of insulin-like growth factor-1 in mice protects from myocyte death after infarction, attenuating ventricular dilation, wall stress, and cardiac hypertrophy. J Clin Invest 100:1991–1999

73. Fujio Y, Nguyen T, Wencker D, Kitsis RN, Walsh K (2000) Akt promotes survival of cardiomyocytes in vitro and protects against ischemia-reperfusion injury in mouse heart. Circulation 101:660–667

74. Ren J, Samson WK, Sowers JR (1999) Insulin-like growth factor I as a cardiac hormone: physiological and pathophysiological implications in heart disease. J Mol Cell Cardiol 31:2049–2061

75. Lai HC, Liu TJ, Ting CT, Sharma PM, Wang PH (2003) Insulin-like growth factor-1 prevents loss of electrochemical gradient in cardiac muscle mitochondria via activation of PI 3 kinase/Akt pathway. Mol Cell Endocrinol 205:99–106

76. Foncea R, Andersson M, Ketterman A, Blakesley V, Sapag-Hagar M, Sugden PH, LeRoith D, Lavandero S (1997) Insulin-like growth factor-I rapidly activates multiple signal transduction pathways in cultured rat cardiac myocytes. J Biol Chem 272:19115–19124

77. Vander Heiden MG, Chandel NS, Williamson EK, Schumacker PT, Thompson CB (1997) Bcl-xL regulates the membrane potential and volume homeostasis of mitochondria. Cell 91:627–637

78. Juhaszova M, Zorov DB, Kim SH, Pepe S, Fu Q, Fishbein KW, Ziman BD, Wang S, Ytrehus K, Antos CL, Olson EN, Sollott SJ (2004) Glycogen synthase kinase-3 beta mediates convergence of protection signaling to inhibit the mitochondrial permeability transition pore. J Clin Invest 113:1535–1549

79. Chao W, Matsui T, Novikov MS, Tao J, Li L, Liu H, Ahn Y, Rosenzweig A (2003) Strategic advantages of insulin-like growth factor-I expression for cardioprotection. J Gene Med 5:277–286

80. Pi Y, Goldenthal MJ, Marín-García J (2007) Mitochondrial involvement in IGF-1 induced protection of cardiomyocytes against hypoxia/reoxygenation injury. Mol Cell Biochem 301:181–189

81. Welch S, Plank D, Witt S et al (2002) Cardiac-specific IGF-1 expression attenuates dilated cardiomyopathy in tropomodulin-overexpressing transgenic mice. Circ Res 90:641–648

82. Kennedy BK, Austriaco NR Jr, Zhang J, Guarente L (1995) Mutation in the silencing gene SIR4 can delay aging in S. cerevisiae. Cell 80:485–496

83. Kaeberlein M, McVey M, Guarente L (1999) The SIR2/3/4 complex and SIR2 alone promote longevity in Saccharomyces cerevisiae by two different mechanisms. Genes Dev 13:2570–2580

84. Tissenbaum HA, Guarente L (2001) Increased dosage of a sir-2 gene extends lifespan in Caenorhabditis elegans. Nature 410:227–230

85. Rine J, Herskowitz I (1987) Four genes responsible for a position effect on expression from HML and HMR in Saccharomyces cerevisiae. Genetics 116:9–22

86. Sinclair DA, Guarente L (1997) Extrachromosomal rDNA circles – a cause of aging in yeast. Cell 91:1033–1042

87. Lin SJ, Ford E, Haigis M, Liszt G, Guarente L (2004) Calorie restriction extends yeast life span by lowering the level of NADH. Genes Dev 18:12–16

88. Alcendor RR, Kirshenbaum LA, Imai S, Vatner SF, Sadoshima J (2004) Silent information regulator 2alpha, a longevity factor and class III histone deacetylase, is an essential endogenous apoptosis inhibitor in cardiac myocytes. Circ Res 95:971–980

89. Pillai JB, Isbatan A, Imai S, Gupta MP (2005) Poly(ADP-ribose) polymerase-1-dependent cardiac myocyte cell death during heart failure is mediated by NAD+ depletion and reduced Sir2alpha deacetylase activity. J Biol Chem 280:43121–43130

90. Motta MC, Divecha N, Lemieux M et al (2004) Mammalian SIRT1 represses forkhead transcription factors. Cell 116:551–563

91. Brunet A, Sweeney LB, Sturgill JF et al (2004) Stress-dependent regulation of FOXO transcription factors by the SIRT1 deacetylase. Science 303:2011–2015

92. Daitoku H, Hatta M, Matsuzaki H, Aratani S, Ohshima T, Miyagishi M, Nakajima T, Fukamizu A (2004) Silent information regulator 2 potentiates Foxo1-mediated transcription through its deacetylase activity. Proc Natl Acad Sci USA 101:10042–10047

93. Wang C, Chen L, Hou X et al (2006) Interactions between E2F1 and SirT1 regulate apoptotic response to DNA damage. Nat Cell Biol 8:1025–1031

94. Nemoto S, Fergusson MM, Finkel T (2005) SIRT1 functionally interacts with the metabolic regulator and transcriptional coactivator PGC-1{alpha}. J Biol Chem 280:16456–16460

95. Bouras T, Fu M, Sauve AA, Wang F, Quong AA, Perkins ND, Hay RT, Gu W, Pestell RG (2005) SIRT1 deacetylation and repression of p300 involves lysine residues 1020/1024 within the cell cycle regulatory domain 1. J Biol Chem 280:10264–10276

96. Yang T, Fu M, Pestell R, Sauve AA (2006) SIRT1 and endocrine signaling. Trends Endocrinol Metab 17:186–191

97. Seymour EM, Parikh RV, Singer AA, Bolling SF (2006) Moderate calorie restriction improves cardiac remodeling and diastolic dysfunction in the Dahl-SS rat. J Mol Cell Cardiol 41:661–668

98. Rogina B, Helfand SL (2004) Sir2 mediates longevity in the fly through a pathway related to calorie restriction. Proc Natl Acad Sci USA 101:15998–16003

99. Chen D, Steele AD, Lindquist S, Guarente L (2005) Increase in activity during calorie restriction requires Sirt1. Science 310:1641

100. Picard F, Kurtev M, Chung N et al (2004) Sirt1 promotes fat mobilization in white adipocytes by repressing PPAR-gamma. Nature 429:771–776

101. Lee CK, Allison DB, Brand J, Weindruch R, Prolla TA (2002) Transcriptional profiles associated with aging and middle age-onset caloric restriction in mouse hearts. Proc Natl Acad Sci USA 99:14988–14993

102. Kaeberlein M, Powers RW 3rd, Steffen KK et al (2005) Regulation of yeast replicative life span by TOR and Sch9 in response to nutrients. Science 310:1193–1196

103. Kapahi P, Zid BM, Harper T, Koslover D, Sapin V, Benzer S (2004) Regulation of lifespan in Drosophila by modulation of genes in the TOR signaling pathway. Curr Biol 14:885–890

104. Powers RW 3rd, Kaeberlein M, Caldwell SD, Kennedy BK, Fields S (2006) Extension of chronological life span in yeast by decreased TOR pathway signaling. Genes Dev 20:174–184

105. Desai BN, Myers BR, Schreiber SL (2002) FKBP12-rapamycin-associated protein associates with mitochondria and senses osmotic stress via mitochondrial dysfunction. Proc Natl Acad Sci USA 99:4319–4324

106. Kim DH, Sarbassov DD, Ali SM, King JE, Latek RR, Erdjument-Bromage H, Tempst P, Sabatini DM (2002) mTOR interacts with raptor to form a nutrient-sensitive complex that signals to the cell growth machinery. Cell 110:163–175

107. Tokunaga C, Yoshino K, Yonezawa K (2004) mTOR integrates amino acid- and energy-sensing pathways. Biochem Biophys Res Commun 313:443–446

108. Nojima H, Tokunaga C, Eguchi S et al (2003) The mammalian target of rapamycin (mTOR) partner, raptor, binds the mTOR substrates p70 S6 kinase and 4E-BP1 through their TOR signaling (TOS) motif. J Biol Chem 278:15461–15464

109. Schieke SM, Phillips D, McCoy JP Jr, Aponte AM, Shen RF, Balaban RS, Finkel T (2006) The mammalian target of rapamycin (mTOR) pathway regulates mitochondrial oxygen consumption and oxidative capacity. J Biol Chem 281:27643–27652

110. Khan S, Salloum F, Das A, Xi L, Vetrovec GW, Kukreja RC (2006) Rapamycin confers preconditioning-like protection against ischemia-reperfusion injury in isolated mouse heart and cardiomyocytes. J Mol Cell Cardiol 41:256–264

111. Shioi T, McMullen JR, Tarnavski O, Converso K, Sherwood MC, Manning WJ, Izumo S (2003) Rapamycin attenuates load-induced cardiac hypertrophy in mice. Circulation 107:1664–1670

112. McMullen JR, Sherwood MC, Tarnavski O, Zhang L, Dorfman AL, Shioi T, Izumo S (2004) Inhibition of mTOR signaling with rapamycin regresses established cardiac hypertrophy induced by pressure overload. Circulation 109:3050–3055

113. Flagg TP, Nichols CG (2005) Sarcolemmal K(ATP) channels: what do we really know? J Mol Cell Cardiol 39:61–70

114. Scarpulla RC (2002) Nuclear activators and coactivators in mammalian mitochondrial biogenesis. Biochim Biophys Acta 1576:1–14

115. Goffart S, Wiesner RJ (2003) Regulation and co-ordination of nuclear gene expression during mitochondrial biogenesis. Exp Physiol 88:33–40

116. Xia Y, Buja LM, Scarpulla RC et al (1997) Electrical stimulation of neonatal cardio-myocytes results in sequential activation of nuclear genes governing mitochondrial proliferation and differentiation. Proc Natl Acad Sci USA 94:11399–11404

117. Lehman JJ, Barger PM, Kovacs A et al (2000) Peroxisome proliferator-activated receptor gamma coactivator-1 promotes cardiac mitochondrial biogenesis. J Clin Invest 106:847–856

118. Gilde AJ, van der Lee KA, Willemsen PH et al (2003) Peroxisome proliferator-activated receptor PPARalpha and PPARbeta/delta, but not PPARgamma, modulate the expression of genes involved in cardiac lipid metabolism. Circ Res 92:518–524

119. Barger PM, Kelly DP (2000) PPAR signaling in the control of cardiac energy metabolism. Trends Cardiovasc Med 10:238–245

120. Garnier A, Fortin D, Delomenie C et al (2003) Depressed mitochondrial transcription factors and oxidative capacity in rat failing cardiac and skeletal muscles. J Physiol 551:491–501

121. Huss JM, Levy FH, Kelly DP (2001) Hypoxia inhibits the peroxisome proliferator-activated receptor alpha/retinoid X receptor gene regulatory pathway in cardiac myocytes: a mechanism for O2-dependent modulation of mitochondrial fatty acid oxidation. J Biol Chem 276:27605–27612

122. Wu H, Kanatous SB, Thurmond FA et al (2002) Regulation of mitochondrial biogenesis in skeletal muscle by CaMK. Science 296:349–352

123. Sack MN, Harrington LS, Jonassen AK et al (2000) Coordinate regulation of metabolic enzyme encoding genes during cardiac development and following carvedilol therapy in spontaneously hypertensive rats. Cardiovasc Drugs Ther 14:31–39

124. Bushdid PB, Osinska H, Waclaw RR et al (2003) NFATc3 and NFATc4 are required for cardiac development and mitochondrial function. Circ Res 92:1305–1313

125. Finck BN, Lehman JJ, Leone TC et al (2002) The cardiac phenotype induced by PPARalpha overexpression mimics that caused by diabetes mellitus. J Clin Invest 109:121–130

126. Wang J, Wilhelmsson H, Graff C et al (1999) Dilated cardiomyopathy and atrioventricular conduction blocks induced by heart-specific inactivation of mtDNA gene expression. Nat Genet 21:133–137

127. Rapizzi E, Pinton P, Szabadkai G, Wieckowski MR, Vandecasteele G, Baird G et al (2002) Recombinant expression of the voltage dependent anion channel enhances the transfer of Ca2+ microdomains to mitochondria. J Cell Biol 159:613–624

128. Casas F, Rochard P, Rodier A, Cassar-Malek I, Marchal-Victorion S, Wiesner RJ et al (1999) A variant form of the nuclear triiodothyronine receptor c-ErbAalpha1 plays a direct role in regulation of mitochondrial RNA synthesis. Mol Cell Biol 19:7913–7924

129. Scheller K, Seibel P, Sekeris CE (2003) Glucocorticoid and thyroid hormone receptors in mitochondria of animal cells. Int Rev Cytol 222:1–61

130. Stadtman ER, Berlett BS (1998) Reactive oxygen-mediated protein oxidation in aging and disease. Drug Metab Rev 30:225–243

131. Choksi KB, Boylston WH, Rabek JP, Widger WR, Papaconstantinou J (2004) Oxidatively damaged proteins of heart mitochondrial electron transport complexes. Biochim Biophys Acta 1688:95–101

132. Vasquez-Vivar J, Kalyanaraman B, Kennedy MC (2000) Mitochondrial aconitase is a source of hydroxyl radical. An electron spin resonance investigation. J Biol Chem 275:14064–14069

133. Paradies G, Petrosillo G, Pistolese M, Ruggiero FM (2002) Reactive oxygen species affect mitochondrial electron transport complex I activity through oxidative cardiolipin damage. Gene 286:135–141

134. Petrosillo G, Ruggiero FM, Pistolese M, Paradies G (2001) Reactive oxygen species generated from the mitochondrial electron transport chain induce cytochrome c dissociation from beefheart submitochondrial particles via cardiolipin peroxidation: possible role in the apoptosis. FEBS Lett 509:435–438

135. Wolin MS, Ahmad M, Gupte SA (2005) Oxidant and redox signaling in vascular oxygen sensing mechanisms: basic concepts, current controversies, and potential importance of cytosolic NADPH. Am J Physiol Lung Cell Mol Physiol 289:L159–L173

136. Brown GC (1999) Nitric oxide and mitochondrial respiration. Biochim Biophys Acta 1411:351–369

137. Murray J, Taylor SW, Zhang B, Ghosh SS, Capaldi RA (2003) Oxidative damage to mitochondrial complex I due to peroxynitrite: identification of reactive tyrosines by mass spectrometry. J Biol Chem 278:37223–37230

138. Riobo NA, Clementi E, Melani M, Boveris A, Cadenas E, Moncada S, Poderoso JJ (2001) Nitric oxide inhibits mitochondrial NADH:ubiquinone reductase activity through peroxynitrite formation. Biochem J 359:139–145

139. Cassina AM, Hodara R, Souza JM, Thomson L, Castro L, Ischiropoulos H, Freeman BA, Radi R (2000) Cytochrome c nitration by peroxynitrite. J Biol Chem 275:21409–21415

140. Castro L, Rodriguez M, Radi R (1994) Aconitase is readily inactivated by peroxynitrite, but not by its precursor, nitric oxide. J Biol Chem 269:29409–29415

141. Packer MA, Scarlett JL, Martin SW, Murphy MP (1997) Induction of the mitochondrial permeability transition by peroxynitrite. Biochem Soc Trans 25:909–914

142. Brookes PS, Darley-Usmar VM (2004) Role of calcium and superoxide dismutase in sensitizing mitochondria to peroxynitrite-induced permeability transition. Am J Physiol Heart Circ Physiol 286:H39–H46

143. Griendling KK, Minieri CA, Ollerenshaw JD, Alexander RW (1994) Angiotensin stimulates NADH and NADPH oxidase activity in cultured vascular smooth muscle cells. Circ Res 74:1141–1148

144. De Keulenaer GW, Alexander RW, Ushio-Fukai M, Ishizaka N, Griendling KK (1998) Tumor necrosis factor activates a p22phox-based NADH oxidase in vascular smooth muscle. Biochem J 329:653–657

145. Patterson C, Ruef J, Madamanchi NR, Barry-Lane P, Hu Z, Horaist C, Ballinger CA, Brasier AR, Bode C, Runge MS (1999) Stimulation of a vascular smooth muscle cell NAD(P)H oxidase by thrombin: evidence that p47phox may participate in forming this oxidase in vitro and in vivo. J Biol Chem 274:19814–19822

146. Hellsten-Westing Y (1993) Immunohistochemical localization of xanthine oxidase in human cardiac and skeletal muscle. Histochemistry 100:215–222

147. Cappola TP, Kass DA, Nelson GS, Berger RD, Rosas GO, Kobeissi ZA, Marban E, Hare JM (2001) Allopurinol improves myocardial efficiency in patients with idiopathic dilated cardiomyopathy. Circulation 104:2407–2411

148. Nemoto S, Takeda K, Yu ZX, Ferrans VJ, Finkel T (2000) Role for mitochondrial oxidants as regulators of cellular metabolism. Mol Cell Biol 20:7311–7318

149. Cadenas E (2004) Mitochondrial free radical production and cell signaling. Mol Aspects Med 25:17–26

150. Bogoyevitch MA, Ng DC, Court NW, Draper KA, Dhillon A (2000) Abas L Intact mitochondrial electron transport function is essential for signalling by hydrogen peroxide in cardiac myocytes. J Mol Cell Cardiol 32:1469–1480

151. Archer SL, Wu XC, Thebaud B, Moudgil R, Hashimoto K, Michelakis ED (2004) O2 sensing in the human ductus arteriosus: redox-sensitive K+ channels are regulated by mitochondria-derived hydrogen peroxide. Biol Chem 385:205–216

152. Yamamura T, Otani H, Nakao Y, Hattori R, Osako M, Imamura H, Das DK (2001) Dual involvement of coenzyme Q10 in redox signaling and inhibition of death signaling in the rat heart mitochondria. Antioxid Redox Signal 3:103–112

153. Brookes PS, Levonen AL, Shiva S, Sarti P, Darley-Usmar VM (2002) Mitochondria: regulators of signal transduction by reactive oxygen and nitrogen species. Free Radic Biol Med 33:755–764

154. Boveris A, D'Amico G, Lores-Arnaiz S, Costa LE (2003) Enalapril increases mitochondrial nitric oxide synthase activity in heart and liver. Antioxid Redox Signal 5:691–697

155. O'Rourke B (2000) Myocardial KATP channels in preconditioning. Circ Res 87:845–855

156. Lebuffe G, Schumacker PT, Shao ZH, Anderson T, Iwase H, Vanden Hoek TL (2003) ROS and NO trigger early preconditioning: relationship to mitochondrial KATP channel. Am J Physiol Heart Circ Physiol 284:H299–H308

157. Oldenburg O, Cohen MV, Yellon DM, Downey JM (2002) Mitochondrial K(ATP) channels: role in cardioprotection. Cardiovasc Res 55:429–437

158. Ardehali H, O'Rourke B (2005) Mitochondrial K(ATP) channels in cell survival and death. J Mol Cell Cardiol 39:7–16

159. Garlid KD, Dos Santos P, Xie ZJ, Costa AD, Paucek P (2003) Mitochondrial potassium transport: the role of the mitochondrial ATP-sensitive K(+) channel in cardiac function and cardioprotection. Biochim Biophys Acta 1606:1–21

160. Das M, Parker JE, Halestrap AP (2003) Matrix volume measurements challenge the existence of diazoxide/glibencamide-sensitive KATP channels in rat mitochondria. J Physiol 547:893–902

161. Akao M, Teshima Y, Marban E (2002) Antiapoptotic effect of nicorandil mediated by mitochondrial atp-sensitive potassium channels in cultured cardiac myocytes. J Am Coll Cardiol 40:803–810

162. Nagata K, Obata K, Odashima M, Yamada A, Somura F, Nishizawa T, Ichihara S, Izawa H, Iwase M, Hayakawa A, Murohara T, Yokota M (2003) Nicorandil inhibits oxidative stress-induced apoptosis in cardiac myocytes through activation of mitochondrial ATP-sensitive potassium channels and a nitrate-like effect. J Mol Cell Cardiol 35:1505–1512

163. Xu W, Liu Y, Wang S, McDonald T, Van Eyk JE, Sidor A, O'Rourke B (2002) Cytoprotective role of Ca2+- activated K+ channels in the cardiac inner mitochondrial membrane. Science 298:1029–1033

164. Hanley PJ, Daut J (2005) K(ATP) channels and preconditioning: a re-examination of the role of mitochondrial K(ATP) channels and an overview of alternative mechanisms. J Mol Cell Cardiol 39:17–50

165. Halestrap AP, Clarke SJ, Javadov SA (2004) Mitochondrial permeability transition pore opening during myocardial reperfusion – a target for cardioprotection. Cardiovasc Res 61:372–385

166. Shanmuganathan S, Hausenloy DJ, Duchen MR, Yellon DM (2005) Mitochondrial permeability transition pore as a target for cardioprotection in the human heart. Am J Physiol Heart Circ Physiol 289:H237–H242

167. Thomson M (2002) Evidence of undiscovered cell regulatory mechanisms: phospho-proteins and protein kinases in mitochondria. Cell Mol Life Sci 59:213–219

168. Sugden MC, Orfali KA, Fryer LG, Holness MJ, Priestman DA (1997) Molecular mechanisms underlying the long-term impact of dietary fat to increase cardiac pyruvate dehydrogenase kinase: regulation by insulin, cyclic AMP and pyruvate. J Mol Cell Cardiol 29:1867–1875

169. Technikova-Dobrova Z, Sardanelli AM, Stanca MR, Papa S (1994) cAMP-dependent protein phosphorylation in mitochondria of bovine heart. FEBS Lett 350:187–191

170. Wang Y, Hirai K, Ashraf M (1999) Activation of mitochondrial ATP-sensitive K(+) channel for cardiac protection against ischemic injury is dependent on protein kinase C activity. Circ Res 85:731–741

171. Baines CP, Zhang J, Wang GW, Zheng YT, Xiu JX, Cardwell EM, Bolli R, Ping P (2002) Mitochondrial PKCepsilon and MAPK form signaling modules in the murine heart: enhanced mitochondrial PKCepsilon-MAPK interactions and differential MAPK activation in PKCepsilon-induced cardioprotection. Circ Res 90:390–397

172. Garlid KD, Costa AD, Cohen MV, Downey JM, Critz SD (2004) Cyclic GMP and PKG activate mito K(ATP) channels in isolated mitochondria. Cardiovasc J S Afr 15:S5

173. He H, Li HL, Lin A, Gottlieb RA (1999) Activation of the JNK pathway is important for cardiomyocyte death in response to simulated ischemia. Cell Death Differ 6:987–991

174. Aoki H, Kang PM, Hampe J, Yoshimura K, Noma T, Matsuzaki M, Izumo S (2002) Direct activation of mitochondrial apoptosis machinery by c-Jun N-terminal kinase in adult cardiac myocytes. J Biol Chem 277:10244–10250

175. Court NW, Kuo I, Quicley O, Bogoyevitch MA (2004) Phosphorylation of the mitochondrial protein Sab by stress-activated protein kinase 3. Biochem Biophys Res Commun 319:130–137

176. Baines CP, Song CX, Zheng YT, Wang GW, Zhang J, Wang OL, Guo Y, Bolli R, Cardwell EM, Ping P (2003) Protein kinase Cepsilon interacts with and inhibits the permeability transition pore in cardiac mitochondria. Circ Res 92:873–880

177. Lee I, Bender E, Kadenbach B (2002) Control of mitochondrial membrane potential and ROS formation by reversible phosphorylation of cytochrome c oxidase. Mol Cell Biochem 234–235:63–70

178. Schulenberg B, Aggeler R, Beechem JM, Capaldi RA, Patton WF (2003) Analysis of steady-state protein phosphorylation in mitochondria using a novel fluorescent phosphosensor dye. J Biol Chem 278:27251–27255

179. Hood DA, Joseph AM (2004) Mitochondrial assembly: protein import. Proc Nutr Soc 63:293–300

180. Colavecchia M, Christie LN, Kanwar YS, Hood DA (2003) Functional consequences of thyroid hormone-induced changes in the mitochondrial protein import pathway. Am J Physiol Endocrinol Metab 284:E29–E35

181. Gibbs C (1999) Respiratory control in normal and hypertrophic hearts. Cardiovasc Res 42:567–570

182. McCormack JG, Halestrap AP, Denton RM (1990) Role of calcium ions in regulation of mammalian intramitochondrial metabolism. Physiol Rev 70:391–425

183. Harris DA, Das AM (1991) Control of mitochondrial ATP synthesis in heart. Biochem J 280:561–573

184. Territo PR, Mootha VK, French SA, Balaban RS (2000) Ca2+ activation of heart mitochondrial phosphorylation: role of the F_0/F_1-ATPase. Am J Physiol Cell Physiol 278:C423–C435

185. Takaki M, Zhao DD, Zhao LY, Araki J, Mori M, Suga H (1995) Suppression of myocardial mitochondrial respiratory function in acute failing hearts made by a short term Ca2+ free, high Ca2+ coronary perfusion. J Mol Cell Cardiol 27:2009–2013

186. He H, Chen M, Scheffler NK et al (2001) Phosphorylation of mitochondrial elongation factor Tu in ischemic myocardium: basis for chloramphenicol-mediated cardioprotection. Circ Res 89:461–467

187. Rutter GA, Rizzuto R (2000) Regulation of mitochondrial metabolism by ER Ca+ release:an intimate connection. Trends Biochem Sci 25:215–222

188. Duchen M (1999) Contributions of mitochondria to animal physiology: from homeostatic sensor to calcium signalling and cell death. J Physiol 516:1–17

189. Griffiths EJ (2000) Use of ruthenium red as an inhibitor of mitochondrial Ca(2+) uptake in single rat cardiomyocytes. FEBS Lett 486:257–260

190. Pacher P (2001) Hajnoczky G Propagation of the apoptotic signal by mitochondrial waves. EMBO J 20:4107–4121

191. Robb-Gaspers LD, Burnett P, Rutter GA et al (1998) Integrating cytosolic calcium signals into mitochondrial metabolic responses. EMBO J 17:4987–5000

192. Cortassa S, Aon MA, Marban E et al (2003) An integrated model of cardiac mitochondrial energy metabolism and calcium dynamics. Biophys J 84:2734–2755

193. Das AM, Harris DA (1991) Control of mitochondrial ATP synthase in rat cardiomyocytes: effects of thyroid hormone. Biochim Biophys Acta 1096:284–290

194. Rizzuto R (1998) Close contacts with the endoplasmic reticulum as determinants of mitochondrial Ca+ responses. Science 280:1763–1766

195. Csordas G, Thomas AP, Hajnoczky G (2001) Calcium signal transmission between ryanodine receptors and mitochondria in cardiac muscle. Trends Cardiovasc Med 11:269–275

196. Gunter TE, Gunter KK (2001) Uptake of calcium by mitochondria: transport and possible function. IUBMB Life 52:197–204

197. Buntinas L, Gunter KK, Sparagna GC et al (2001) The rapid mode of calcium uptake into heart mitochondria (RaM): comparison to RaM in liver mitochondria. Biochim Biophys Acta 1504:248–261

198. Crompton M, Costi A, Hayat L (1987) Evidence for the presence of a reversible Ca2+-dependent pore activated by oxidative stress in heart mitochondria. Biochem J 245:915–918

199. Hajnoczky G, Csordas G, Yi M (2002) Old players in a new role: mitochondria-associated membranes, VDAC, and ryanodine receptors as contributors to calcium signal propagation from endoplasmic reticulum to the mitochondria. Cell Calcium 32:363–377

200. Oddis CV, Finkel MS (1995) Cytokine-stimulated nitric oxide production inhibits mitochondrial activity in cardiac myocytes. Biochem Biophys Res Commun 213:1002–1009

201. Zell R, Geck P, Werdan K et al (1997) TNF-alpha and IL-1 alpha inhibit both pyruvate dehydrogenase activity and mitochondrial function in cardiomyocytes: evidence for primary impairment of mitochondrial function. Mol Cell Biochem 177:61–67

202. Sammut IA, Harrison JC (2003) Cardiac mitochondrial complex activity is enhanced by heat shock proteins. Clin Exp Pharmacol Physiol 30:110–115

203. Bialik S, Cryns VL, Drincic A et al (1999) The mitochondrial apoptotic pathway is activated by serum and glucose deprivation in cardiac myocytes. Circ Res 85:403–414

204. Sparagna GC, Hickson-Bick DL, Buja LM et al (2001) Fatty acid-induced apoptosis in neonatal cardiomyocytes: redox signaling. Antioxid Redox Signal 3:71–79

205. Xia Y, Buja LM, Scarpulla RC, McMillin JB (1997). Electrical stimulation of neonatal cardio-myocytes results in sequential activation of nuclear genes governing mitochondrial proliferation and differentiation. Proc Natl Acad Sci USA 94:11399–11404

206. Riobo NA, Clementi E, Melani M et al (2001) Nitric oxide inhibits mitochondrial NADH:ubiquinone reductase activity through peroxynitrite formation. Biochem J 359:139–145

207. Poderoso JJ, Peralta JG, Lisdero CL et al (1998) Nitric oxide regulates oxygen uptake and hydrogen peroxide release by the isolated beating rat heart. Am J Physiol 274:C112–C119

208. Wiesner RJ, Hornung TV, Garman JD et al (1999) Stimulation of mitochondrial gene expression and proliferation of mitochondria following impairment of cellular energy transfer by inhibition of phosphocreatine circuit in rat hearts. J Bioenerg Biomembr 31:559–567

209. Berridge MJ (2002) The endoplasmic reticulum: a multifunctional signaling organelle. Cell Calcium 32:235–249

210. Kastan MB, Canman CE, Leonard CJ (1995) p53, cell cycle control and apoptosis: implications for cancer. Cancer Metastasis Rev 14:3–15

211. Agarwal ML, Taylor WR, Chernov MV, Chernova OB, Stark GR (1998) The p53 network. J Biol Chem 273:1–4

212. Kussie PH, Gorina S, Marechal V, Elenbaas B, Moreau J, Levine AJ, Pavletich NP (1996) Structure of the MDM2 oncoprotein bound to the p53 tumor suppressor transactivation domain. Science 274:948–953

213. Thut CJ, Goodrich JA, Tjian R (1997) Repression of p53-mediated transcription by MDM2: a dual mechanism. Genes Dev 11:1974–1986

214. Moll UM, Zaika A (2001) Nuclear and mitochondrial apoptosis pathways of p53. FEBS Lett 493:65–69

215. Moll UM, Marchenko N, Zhang XK (2006) p53 and Nur77/TR3 – transcription factors that directly target mitochondria for cell death induction. Oncogene 25:4725–4743

216. Pierzchalski P, Reiss K, Cheng W, Cirielli C, Kajstura J, Nitahara JA, Rizk M, Capogrossi MC, Anversa P (1997) p53 Induces myocyte apoptosis via the activation of the renin-angiotensin system. Exp Cell Res 234:57–65

217. Long X, Crow MT, Sollott SJ, O'Neil L, Menees DS, Hipolito ML, Boluyt MO, Asai T, Lakatta EG (1998) Enhanced expression of p53 and apoptosis induced by blockade of the vacuolar proton ATPase in cardiomyotes. J Clin Invest 101:1453–1461

218. Leri A, Claudio PP, Li Q, Wang X, Reiss K, Wang S, Malhotra A, Kajstura J, Anversa P (1998) Stretch-mediated release of angiotensin II induces myocyte apoptosis by activating p53 that enhances the local renin-angiotensin system and decreases the Bcl-2-to-Bax protein ratio in the cell. J Clin Invest 101:1326–1342

219. Liu G, Chen X (2006) Regulation of the p53 transcriptional activity. J Cell Biochem 97:448–458

220. Chipuk JE, Kuwana T, Bouchier-Hayes L, Droin NM, Newmeyer DD, Schuler M, Green DR (2004) Direct activation of Bax by p53 mediates mitochondrial membrane permeabilization and apoptosis. Science 303:1010–1014

221. Steegenga WT, van der Eb AJ, Jochemsen AG (1996) How phosphorylation regulates the activity of p53. J Mol Biol 263:103–113

222. Giaccia AJ, Kastan MB (1998) The complexity of p53 modulation: emerging patterns from divergent signals. Genes Dev 12:2973–2983

223. Huang C, Ma WY, Maxiner A, Sun Y, Dong Z (1999) p38 kinase mediates UV-induced phosphorylation of p53 protein at serine 389. J Biol Chem 274:12229–12235

224. Takenaka I, Morin F, Seizinger BR, Kley N (1995) Regulation of the sequence-specific DNA binding function of p53 by protein kinase C and protein phosphatases. J Biol Chem 270:5405–5411

225. Meek DW, Simon S, Kikkawa U, Eckhart W (1990) The p53 tumor suppressor protein is phosphorylated at serine 389 by casein kinase II. EMBO J 9:3253–3260

226. Lees-Miller SP, Sakaguchi K, Ullrich SJ, Appella E, Anderson CW (1992) Human DNA-activated protein kinase phosphorylates serine 15 and 37 in the amino-terminal transactivation domain of human p53. Mol Cell Biol 12:5041–5049

227. Banin S, Moyal L, Shieh S-Y, Taya Y, Anderson CW, Chessa L, Smorodinsky NI, Prives C, Reiss Y, Shiloh Y, Ziv Y (1998) Enhanced phosphorylation of p53 by ATM in response to DNA damage. Science 281:1674–1677

228. Canman CE, Lim D-S, Cimprich KA, Taya Y, Tamai K, Sakaguchi K, Appella E, Kastan MB, Siliciano JD (1998) Activation of the ATM kinase by ionizing radiation and phosphorylation of p53. Science 281:1677–1679

229. Tibbetts RS, Brumbaugh KM, Williams JM, Sarkaria JN, Cliby WA, Shieh S-Y, Taya Y, Prives C, Abraham RT (1999) A role for ATR in the DNA damage-induced phosphorylation of p53. Genes Dev 13:152–157

230. Shieh S-Y, Ikeda M, Taya Y, Prives C (1997) DNA damage-induced phosphorylation of p53 alleviates inhibition by MDM2. Cell 91:325–334

231. Lambert PF, Kashanchi F, Radonovich MF, Shiekhattar R, Brady JN (1998) Phosphorylation of p53 serine 15 increases interaction with CBP. J Biol Chem 273:33048–33053

232. McNeill-Blue C, Wetmore BA, Sanchez JF, Freed WJ, Alex Merrick B (2006) Apoptosis mediated by p53 in rat neural AF5 cells following treatment with hydrogen peroxide and staurosporine. Brain Res 1112:1–15

233. von Harsdorf R, Li PF, Dietz R (1999) Signaling pathways in reactive oxygen species-induced cardiomyocyte apoptosis. Circulation 99:2934–2941

234. Long X, Goldenthal MJ, Wu GM, Marin-Garcia J (2004) Mitochondrial Ca2+ flux and respiratory enzyme activity decline are early events in cardiomyocyte response to H2O2. J Mol Cell Cardiol 37:63–70

235. Chandel NS, Vander Heiden MG, Thompson CB, Schumacker P (2000) Redox regulation of p53 during hypoxia. Oncogene 19:3840–3848

236. Ashcroft M, Kubbutat MH, Vousden KH (1999) Regulation of p53 function and stability by phosphorylation. Mol Cell Biol 19:1751–1758

237. Unger T, Sionov RV, Moallem E, Yee CL, Howley PM, Oren M, Haupt Y (1999) Mutations in serines 15 and 20 of human p53 impair its apoptotic activity. Oncogene 18:3205–3212

238. Siliciano JD, Canman CE, Taya Y, Sakaguchi K, Appella E, Kastan MB (1997) DNA damage induces phosphorylation of the amino terminus of p53. Genes Dev 11:3471–3481

239. Sheikh MS, Hollander MC, Fornance AJ (2000) Role of Gadd45 in apoptosis. Biochem Pharmacol 59:43–45

240. She QB, Chen N, Dong Z (2000) ERKs and p38 kinase phosphorylate p53 protein at serine 15 in response to UV radiation. J Biol Chem 275:20444–20449

241. Chen K, Albano A, Ho A, Keaney JF (2003) Activation of p53 by oxidative stress involves platelet-derived growth factor-beta receptor-mediated ataxia telangiectasia mutated (ATM) kinase activation. J Biol Chem 278:39527–39533

242. Karin M, Hunter T (1995) Transcriptional control by protein phosphorylation: signal transmission from the cell surface to the nucleus. Curr Biol 5:747–757

243. Hunter T (1995) Protein kinases and phosphatases: the yin and yang of protein phosphorylation and signaling. Cell 80:225–236

244. Guyton KZ, Liu Y, Gorospe M, Xu Q, Holbrook NJ (1996) Activation of mitogen-activated protein kinase by H2O2. Role in cell survival following oxidant injury. J Biol Chem 271:4138–4142

245. Treisman R (1996) Regulation of transcription by MAP kinase cascades. Curr Opin Cell Biol 8:205–215

246. Cobb MH, Goldsmith EJ (1995) How MAP kinases are regulated. J Biol Chem 270:14843–14846

247. Bulavin DV, Saito S, Hollander MC, Sakaguchi K, Anderson CW, Appella E, Fornace AJ (1999) Phosphorylation of human p53 by

p38 kinase coordinates N-terminal phosphorylation and apoptosis in response to UV radiation. EMBO J 18:6845–6854

248. Jackson SP (1997) DNA-dependent protein kinase. Int J Biochem Cell Biol 29:935–938

249. Keith CT, Schreiber SL (1995) PIK-related kinases: DNA repair, recombination, and cell cycle checkpoints. Science 270:50–51

250. Jimenez GS, Bryntesson F, Torres-Arzayus MI et al (1999) DNA-dependent protein kinase is not required for the p53-dependent response to DNA damage. Nature 400:81–83

251. Zhan Q, Carrier F, Fornace AJ (1993) Induction of cellular p53 activity by DNA-damaging agents and growth arrest. Mol Cell Biol 13:4242–4250

252. Toth A, Jeffers JR, Nickson P, Min JY, Morgan JP, Zambetti GP, Erhardt P (2006) Targeted deletion of Puma attenuates cardiomyocyte death and improves cardiac function during ischemia-reperfusion. Am J Physiol Heart Circ Physiol 291:H52–H60

253. Kemp TJ, Causton HC, Clerk A (2003) Changes in gene expression induced by H_2O_2 in cardiac myocytes. Biochem Biophys Res Commun 307:416–421

254. Shohet RV, Garcia JA (2007) Keeping the engine primed: HIF factors as key regulators of cardiac metabolism and angiogenesis during ischemia. J Mol Med 85:1309–1315

255. Sano M, Komuro I (2008) P53 and its role in the development of heart failure. Nippon Rinsho 66:1013–1021

Chapter 8
Cyclic Nucleotides Signaling (Second Messengers) and Control of Myocardial Function: Effects of Heart Failure

Overview

Nerves (sympathetic and parasympathetic) and neurohumoral agents can provide beat-to-beat control of myocardial function. They operate through the generation of second messengers in cardiac myocytes. Nitric oxide and natriuretic peptides increase production of the second messenger cyclic GMP through activation of guanylyl cyclases. Cyclic GMP reduces myocardial contractility and these effects are mediated through changes in protein phosphorylation; cyclic GMP affects cyclic AMP phosphodiesterases, ion channels, and cytosolic calcium levels. Moreover, cyclic GMP is degraded by phosphodiesterases. As the heart begins to fail, cyclic GMP levels increase partly in response to increased sympathetic activity. However, downstream signaling from this signal transduction system is reduced.

Sympathetic activation stimulates both myocardial α adrenergic and β adrenergic receptors although β adrenergic receptors are more important in cardiac myocytes. Activation of β adrenergic receptors leads to the stimulation of adenylyl cyclase (AC) through a G-protein to produce the second messenger cyclic AMP. Cyclic AMP is degraded by several phosphodiesterases. This second messenger produces positive inotropic effects in the heart primarily through activation of a cyclic AMP-dependent protein kinase. In heart failure (HF), there are changes in receptor subtypes, coupling, and downstream signaling.

In this chapter, we will discuss second messenger systems that increase and decrease myocyte contractility, their cellular mechanisms of action, and how these signal transduction systems are altered as the heart begins to fail. In addition, suggestions are made as to the ways in which these second messengers systems may be improved to increase their effectiveness in HF.

Introduction

The main function of the heart is to pump blood, and this ability is controlled by both internal and external forces. Internally, cardiac function is controlled by the contractile machinery and excitation–contractile coupling. External signals from nerves, etc. also affect myocardial function (rate and contractility), with these external signals acting through second messenger systems in cardiac myocytes to control function. Changes in the level of these second messengers can rapidly increase or decrease myocardial function. During the progression of the heart into failure, both internal and external control systems become less effective in the regulation of myocardial function. In this chapter, we will examine the effects of second messengers on the control of cardiac function and how these control systems change, in terms of activity and function, during the progression toward HF.

Second Messengers and Contractile Function

Second messengers have both positive and negative effects on contractile function. Parasympathetic activity, nitric oxide (NO), natriuretic peptides, and the second messenger cyclic GMP reduce contractile force, heart rate, and myocardial oxygen consumption. Sympathetic activity and the second messenger cyclic AMP increase these factors. In addition, there are minor effects of the protein kinase C-inositol 1,4,5-trisphosphate second messenger system. Significant interactions exist between these second messenger systems in normal hearts, and both positive and negative effects of these messengers are reduced in HF. Since positive factors, such as cyclic AMP signaling have been extensively reviewed previously [1–3] we will focus in this chapter on the negative factors. Later, how these second messenger systems are affected by HF, the occurrence of changes in their levels, and how they loose their ability to affect cardiac function as the heart fails will be discussed.

Cyclic GMP

NO, natriuretic peptides and parasympathetic activity reduce cardiac function in the normal heart [4, 5]. This effect is mainly related to the production of the second messenger cyclic GMP. The actions of cyclic GMP are mediated through changes in protein phosphorylation, cyclic GMP affected cyclic AMP phosphodiesterases, ion channels, and cytosolic calcium levels [5–9]. Furthermore, cyclic GMP can reduce the rise of intracellular calcium in cardiac myocytes [10] and can also reduce myocardial contractility and metabolism [5, 11].

There is direct evidence that increases in cyclic GMP reduce the responses of myofilaments to calcium in intact cardiac myocytes [7]. Some of these effects may be by direct or indirect inhibition of L-type calcium channels through the action of the cyclic GMP protein kinase [12, 13]. The interaction between nitric oxide, natriuretic peptides, and the actions of cyclic GMP is shown in Fig. 8.1. Cyclic GMP also antagonizes the positive inotropic effects of catecholamines in the heart [13, 14]. This may be related to its effects on the cyclic GMP-dependent cyclic AMP phosphodiesterases [2, 8]. Moreover, some of the effects of cyclic GMP are related to its influence on cyclic AMP [2, 15, 16].

Cyclic GMP Production: Activation of Guanylyl Cyclase

Cyclic GMP is produced by activation of a particulate or soluble guanylyl cyclase. There are three important members of the natriuretic peptide family in the heart: atrial natriuretic peptide (ANP), brain natriuretic peptide (BNP), and C-type natriuretic peptide (CNP). The particulate forms of guanylyl cyclases are also part of the receptors for these natriuretic peptides. ANP and BNP are produced mainly in the atrium and ventricle and are ligands for natriuretic peptide receptor A (NPR1). CNP is predominantly located in the central nervous system, anterior pituitary, kidney, and vascular endothelial cells and binds the type B receptor (NPR2). Binding of these natriuretic peptides to their receptors activates particulate guanylyl cyclase, leading to an elevation in intracellular cyclic GMP [17, 18]. These increases in cyclic GMP lead to decreases in myocardial function.

NO is produced by three isoforms of nitric oxide synthase: neuronal nitric oxide synthase (NOS1, nNOS), inducible

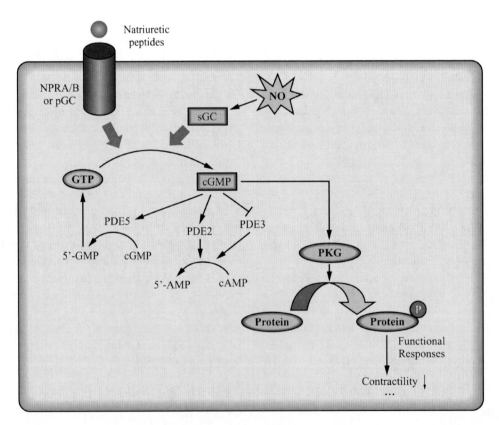

Fig. 8.1 Effects of nitric oxide (NO) and natriuretic peptides on the heart. Natriuretic peptides activate receptors (NPRA and NPRB), which contain a particulate guanylyl cyclase (pGC). Nitric oxide activates a soluble guanylyl cyclase (sGC). Guanylyl cyclase converts GTP to cyclic GMP, which is broken down by a phosphodiesterase (PDE5). Cyclic GMP acts on cyclic GMP affected cyclic AMP phosphodiesterases to control the level of cyclic AMP. The major effect of cyclic GMP in reducing cardiac myocyte function is through a cyclic GMP protein kinase (PKG). This kinase phosphorylates several proteins that help reduce cardiac function

nitric oxide synthase (NOS2, iNOS), and endothelial nitric oxide synthase (NOS3, eNOS) and activates the soluble form of guanylyl cyclase. In the normal heart, NOS3 plays a more important role than NOS1, and differential effects of activation of NOS1 and NOS3 on cardiac myocyte function may be present [19, 20]. This may be related to their distinct subcellular localization [21].

Cyclic GMP Degradation

Cyclic GMP is degraded by Cyclic GMP-phosphodiesterases. In the heart, this is primarily by PDE5 although there is some controversy on this subject [22]. Importantly, the balance between the activity of guanylyl cyclases and cyclic GMP-phosphodiesterases controls the level of cyclic GMP in the heart.

Cyclic GMP Effectors: Cyclic GMP Protein Kinase and Cyclic GMP Affected Cyclic AMP Phosphodiesterases

The cyclic GMP-dependent protein kinase has major effects on the heart [8, 12]. This kinase phosphorylates a variety of distinct myocardial proteins and controls the regulation of L-type calcium channels and calcium sensitivity [6, 9, 12, 13]. This protein kinase may also affect gap junctions, calcium release channels, Ca^{2+}-ATPase, and potassium channels [8, 23]. Both the β-adrenergic and nitric oxide–natriuretic peptide system phosphorylate phospholamban to activate the sarcoplasmic reticulum Ca^{2+}-ATPase [23, 24]. This speeds the reuptake of calcium into the sarcoplasmic reticulum.

There are also interactions between cyclic GMP- and cyclic AMP-dependent protein kinases [13]. Protein phosphorylation caused by the cyclic GMP-dependent protein kinase may be the major mechanism through which the second messenger cyclic GMP causes its negative functional effects on the heart. Probably, changes in the degree and specificity of protein phosphorylation caused by the cyclic GMP-dependent protein kinase will prove to be an important mechanism for the loss of the functional effects of NO and natriuretic peptides in cardiac hypertrophy and failure.

Cyclic GMP Also Affects the Levels of Cyclic AMP

When β-adrenoceptors are stimulated, a series of post receptor events occur which lead to the increased production of cyclic AMP [25]. Once the signal from these surface receptors is transduced into the cell, conformational changes in membrane bound GTP-binding proteins (major effects through Gs and Gi) occur [26]. These G proteins affect AC activity [27].

The level of cyclic AMP is also controlled by cyclic AMP phosphodiesterase that catalyzes its degradation; agents that alter phosphodiesterase activity greatly affect myocardial function [28, 29]. Some of cyclic AMP phosphodiesterases are significantly affected by the level of cyclic GMP [2, 30]. The activity of two forms of these cyclic AMP phosphodiesterases, cyclic GMP-stimulated cyclic AMP phosphodiesterase (PDE2), and cyclic GMP-inhibited cyclic AMP phosphodiesterase (PDE3) are regulated by the intracellular level of cyclic GMP and are important in the control of cardiac function [16, 31, 32]. In the myocardium, a small increase in cyclic GMP levels predominantly inhibits PDE3 [4], and this could lead to increases in cyclic AMP and may limit the negative functional effects of cyclic GMP. Moreover, interaction between these two second messenger systems can increase or decrease the functional effects of cyclic GMP.

Myocardial Hypertrophy and Failure

Cardiac hypertrophy develops as a basic response of the heart to chronic increases in cardiac work and elevated oxygen consumption. If this increased workload continues, the heart hypertrophies and when the work load is reduced, the hypertrophy regresses [33, 34]. As long as the degree of hypertrophy does not exceed a certain critical size, this represents a useful adaptive mechanism. In cardiac hypertrophy, myocardial O_2 balance is essentially normal [35]. However, during increased work, this balance can be more adversely affected than in normal hearts [36]. One of the key responses to increased cardiac needs is an enhanced sympathetic activity and increases in myocardial cyclic AMP. However, with most forms of pressure-overload cardiac hypertrophy, there is usually a loss of β-adrenoceptors and a reduction in muscarinic receptor levels [37, 38]. There are also increases in cyclic GMP [39, 40]. These increases in cyclic GMP may be a protective response to increases in cyclic AMP. The interaction between cyclic AMP and cyclic GMP appear to be altered in pressure-overload hypertrophy [41]. The ability of the heart to respond to stress is reduced under these circumstances.

Alterations in Cyclic GMP and Natriuretic Peptide Levels

The importance and actions of natriuretic peptides and cyclic GMP in cardiac hypertrophy and failure have been of much recent interest. It is known that circulating levels of cyclic GMP and natriuretic peptide can be used as an index of the degree of HF in man [39, 40, 42]. Elevated levels of cyclic GMP have also been reported in experimental models of HF and hypertrophy [43–45]. These changes may be a protective response to the increased levels of cyclic AMP and sympathetic activity observed in HF. In addition, there are changes in the ability of cyclic GMP to affect myocardial function after cardiac hypertrophy [46].

Cyclic GMP Has Been Implicated in Both the Process of Hypertrophy and HF

Understanding the effect of cyclic GMP will be important in the treatment of HF [47–50]. In some experimental models of cardiac hypertrophy, increases in the level of NO or natriuretic peptides may prove to be beneficial [48, 51–53]. While blockade of cyclic GMP production can cause cardiac hypertrophy [54], increasing the level of ANP or cyclic GMP has been reported to lead to regression of pressure overload cardiac hypertrophy in mice [55, 56]. There appears to be significant changes in the ability of NO and natriuretic peptides to affect function in the failing cardiac myocytes; it is possible that manipulation of the NO–natriuretic peptide-cyclic GMP signal transduction system may prove to be of significant therapeutic benefit in HF.

Effects of Nitric Oxide

Changes in NO and its myocardial effects are linked to HF [57, 58], in which significant endothelial dysfunction and reduced nitric oxide levels may be present [59]. Both NO and natriuretic peptides (NPs) increase myocardial cyclic GMP levels.

A recombinant form of human BNP has been approved for the treatment of HF in the United States [57, 60]; however, BNP may worsen renal function in patients with HF [61]. Nonetheless, it has been suggested that direct cardiac administration may be of significant benefit [62]. NPs are released from the failing heart and their level correlates with its severity [40, 42, 63, 64]. They are also released during ischemia and reperfusion, and exogenous peptide may prove beneficial in protecting the ischemic myocardium [17, 65, 66]. These NPs act almost exclusively through the generation of cyclic GMP. Interestingly, NPs and NO may exert some of their beneficial effects by counteracting the enhanced sympathetic activity occurring during HF [14], with increases in NO, NPs, and the second messenger cyclic GMP likely happening in response to the loss of downstream signaling effects of this system in the failing heart.

Changes in Downstream Cyclic GMP Signaling

During cardiac hypertrophy and failure, there is a loss of ability of the cyclic GMP-dependent protein kinase to affect myocardial function and phosphorylate proteins in the heart [8, 67]. Thus, despite high levels of NPs and cyclic GMP, this signal transduction system's effects are significantly depressed in hypertrophy and HF [67, 68]. This would affect the system's ability to increase phosphorylation of L-type calcium channels, ryanodine receptors, and phospholamban, and may cause significant loss of the downstream signaling and function of the system. Furthermore, the actions of the cyclic GMP-dependent cyclic AMP phosphodiesterases are of reduced significance in myocardial hypertrophy and failure [69]. This would restrict the role of cyclic GMP in the control of the level of cyclic AMP. These losses of downstream effects of this signal transduction system may partly explain the higher levels of this second messenger in HF. Understanding the role that cyclic GMP signal transduction system plays in the development of HF will be of great significance to develop new therapies. Potential therapeutic approaches to improve cardiac myocyte function in the failing heart may include changes in the guanylyl cyclase, cyclic GMP-dependent protein kinase, or the cyclic GMP-dependent cyclic AMP phosphodiesterases.

Cyclic AMP and β-Adrenergic Receptors

The normal human heart expresses both β1- and β2-adrenergic receptors and both subtypes increase heart rate and contractility, although there are more β1-receptors in the healthy heart [37, 70]. A diagram depicting the mechanism of action of β-adrenergic signaling through cyclic AMP in cardiac myocytes is shown in Fig. 8.2. Interestingly, myocardial β3-receptors have also been described, but their role remains uncertain. All three subtypes are found in cardiac myocytes, but they seem to possess distinct intracellular signaling and functional properties [71, 72]; and this may be related to distinct receptor and downstream signaling domains [73]. Activity of these receptors is partially controlled by phosphorylation through specific receptor kinases [74].

β1-adrenergic receptors are coupled to the G-protein Gs to activate AC, which leads to the production of the second messenger cyclic AMP. β2-adrenergic receptors are coupled to Gs as well as to the inhibitory Gi [75]; and they also increase cyclic AMP levels. On the other hand, parasympathetic activity and muscarinic receptor activation coupled to Gi inhibits AC, leading to a lower cyclic AMP level. Cyclic AMP production by AC leads to increased cardiac function.

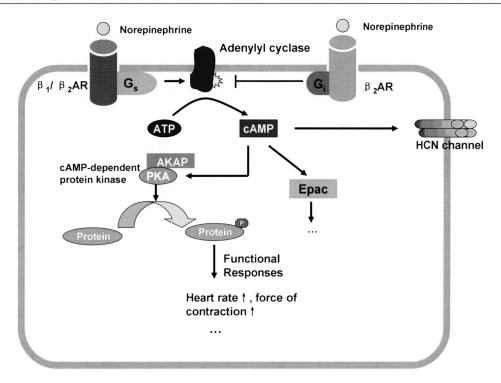

Fig. 8.2 Effects of norepinephrine on the heart. The main effect of norepinephrine is to activate β adrenergic receptors (AR) in the heart. The receptors act to produce cyclic AMP from ATP. Cyclic AMP activates hyperpolarization-activated cyclic G protein to primarily activate (Gs) or secondarily inhibit (Gi) adenylyl cyclase to nucleotide gated channels (HCN), and exchange proteins directly activated by cyclic AMP (epac). However, the primary mechanism is that cyclic AMP activates a cyclic AMP protein kinase (PKA). This protein kinase phosphorylates several proteins that lead to an increase in cardiac function. The intracellular location of PKA is controlled by cyclic AMP protein kinase anchoring proteins (AKAP)

Cyclic AMP Effectors

Cyclic AMP activates three effectors in cardiac cells: cyclic AMP-dependent protein kinase (PKA), HCN channels (hyperpolarization-activated cyclic nucleotide-gated channels), and Epac (exchange protein directly activated by cyclic AMP). The cyclic AMP-dependent protein kinase phosphorylates a myriad of proteins including ones that increase cardiac myocyte function [76]. This protein kinase is the major mechanism of cyclic AMP's functional effects on myocytes and leads to significant increases in cardiac function. Cyclic AMP-dependent protein kinase anchoring proteins (AKAPs) contribute to the specificity of cyclic AMP signaling by limiting the distribution of cyclic AMP effects within the cardiac cell [77]. In addition, β-adrenergic receptor distribution may be limited by their presence in cell membrane invaginations called caveolae [3]. These various scaffolding and signaling pathways lend complexity to the effects of cyclic AMP. In addition, the cyclic AMP signaling system may also affect the role of the cyclic GMP signaling system. However, this cyclic AMP signaling pathway is the major external drive to increase heart rate and myocardial contractility.

Changes in Cyclic AMP Signaling in Myocardial Hypertrophy and Failure

The β-adrenergic receptor system plays a major role in HF. This signaling system is activated by many stresses, such as pressure load, that eventually lead to HF. Activation of this signaling system can lead to cardiac hypertrophy, as can genetic alterations in the receptors [78, 79]. This signaling system is usually activated in patients with HF [80]. In addition, while cardiac β1-adrenergic receptors are downregulated in human HF [37, 70], cardiac β2-adrenergic receptors are upregulated. It is noteworthy that some polymorphic forms of these receptors are more likely to lead to HF [78], and shifts in the subcellular distribution of these receptors may occur within the failing heart [3]. Many of these changes may also be related to abnormalities in the activity of the β-adrenergic receptor kinases [74].

A large number of the remaining β-adrenergic receptors are uncoupled from Gs, presumably via increased activity of receptor kinases [81]. Furthermore, an increase in Gi in the failing heart can antagonize the degree of β-adrenergic signaling [82].

The use of β-adrenergic receptor antagonists in HF is now part of the standard treatment [70, 83]. This helps to reduce excess myocardial adrenergic activity and the work load of the failing heart. Moreover, alterations in β-adrenergic signaling during the progression toward HF may provide several targets for gene therapy [84].

α-Adrenergic Receptor Signaling

Cardiac myocytes express α_1-adrenergic receptors, but not α_2-adrenergic receptors. Although α_1-adrenergic receptors are not generally considered major regulators of cardiac function under physiological conditions, they have been thought to exert more influence under some pathological circumstances [85]. Activation of these receptors generally lead to increased myocardial contractile responses [86]. The heart of most species studied express both α_{1A}- and α_{1B}-adrenergic receptors at the protein level [75]. The α_{1B}-adrenergic receptor subtype predominates in rodents, whereas the α_{1A}-adrenergic receptor is the major subtype in the human heart [85, 87]. Both of these subtypes couple via the heterotrimeric G-protein G_q to the phospholipase C β isoform and should cause activation of protein kinase C. This would significantly affect Ca^{2+} signaling via generation of both diacylglycerol and inositol 1,4,5-trisphosphate (IP$_3$) [86]. Major differences in downstream signaling have not been reported between these subtypes, and α_{1A}- and α_{1B}-adrenergic receptors would be expected to induce similar functional effects in the myocardium. However, major functional differences have been observed when the two receptor subtypes were overexpressed in different transgenic mouse models [88]. Hearts overexpressing α_{1B} demonstrated a depressed contractile function compared to wild type mice [89]. In marked contrast, hearts overexpressing α_{1A}-adrenergic receptors have substantially heightened contractile responses [85, 90]. The signaling pathways responsible for these differences in functional effects of these two receptor subtypes remain to be determined. Some of these effects may be related to specific AKAPs or their distribution [91]. Similar to chronic β-adrenergic stimulation, chronic activation of α-adrenergic receptors also leads to cardiac hypertrophy [92].

Changes in α-Adrenergic Receptor Signaling in Myocardial Hypertrophy and Failure

There have been several attempts to treat the failing heart with α-adrenergic blocking agents [86, 93]. This could reduce the work load in the failing human heart. However, little benefit has been found for these agents in several clinical

trials. In fact, some negative effects have been observed [93]. The combination of α and β adrenergic blockade has proven to be more useful.

It has been reported that α-adrenergic receptors are little changed in HF [37, 94]. On the other hand, it has been suggested that the function of specific α-adrenergic receptor subtypes may be markedly altered in the failing heart [88]. Although this signaling system appears to be of minor importance in the normal human heart, there may be changes in the transition to failure. Clearly, further work is necessary to understand the importance of the α-adrenergic signaling system in HF.

Conclusions

In this chapter, we have discussed the signaling systems that affect cardiac myocyte function. For example, the NO–natriuretic peptide-cyclic GMP signaling system normally acts as a brake on cardiac function; on the other hand, the β-adrenergic-cyclic AMP and the α-adrenergic-IP$_3$ signaling systems generally increase cardiac function. These pathways interact in the normal heart, in a not completely understood manner, and clearly further research will be necessary to fully understand their interaction.

As the heart undergoes the transition from hypertrophy to failure, these signaling systems change dramatically. In general, their ability to affect function (either up or down) decreases. There is evidence for a decreased ability of the cyclic GMP-dependent protein kinase and cyclic GMP-regulated cyclic AMP phosphodiesterases to act on cellular contractility. Cyclic GMP and natriuretic peptide levels increase in HF; perhaps as a partial compensatory mechanism. In addition, the β-adrenergic system loses its ability to increase function, and there are changes in receptor subtype, receptor kinases, and G proteins. To help these systems operate better in the failing heart, generalized drugs have been used. Hopefully, as our understanding of the true defects in these systems increase, it is possible that newer, more specific treatments can be devised. Furthermore, by understanding these systems better, it is possible that specific gene therapies can be devised. This would help to restore control of myocardial function to the failing heart.

Summary

- There are both negative (nitric oxide, natriuretic peptides, and parasympathetic nerves) and positive (sympathetic nerves) external signals that affect cardiac myocyte function. The effectiveness of these signaling systems is reduced in heart failure. They operate through the generation of several second messengers.

- Cyclic GMP, produced by particulate and soluble guanylyl cyclase, leads to negative functional and metabolic effects on myocytes. This reduces heart work and metabolic costs.
- Cyclic GMP is degraded by cyclic GMP phosphodiesterases.
- Cyclic GMP-dependent protein kinase is the major effector for the second messenger cyclic GMP. It phosphorylates several proteins involved in the control of cytoplasmic calcium levels. This leads to a reduction in cytoplasmic calcium.
- Cyclic GMP also interacts with cyclic GMP-dependent cyclic AMP phosphodiesterases to change the level of cyclic AMP in cardiac myocytes. This could increase or decrease metabolic and functional effects depending on whether they lead to increases or decreases in cyclic AMP level.
- During the transition to heart failure, the levels of cyclic GMP and natriuretic peptides increase dramatically. However, the effects of nitric oxide and natriuretic peptides are reduced.
- Downstream signaling of the cyclic GMP system is significantly reduced in failure. The effects and protein levels of the cyclic GMP-dependent protein kinase are reduced. There is also a shift in the actions of the cyclic GMP-regulated cyclic AMP phosphodiesterases. These changes lead to a reduced negative metabolic and functional effect of this signaling system in heart failure.
- Activation of the sympathetic nervous system and the increased production of norepinephrine lead to activation of both α and β adrenergic receptors in cardiac myocytes.
- Activation of β adrenergic receptors leads to increased production of cyclic AMP. This increase in cyclic AMP occurs by activation of adenylyl cyclase through the actions of a G protein.
- Cyclic AMP is degraded by several cyclic AMP phosphodiesterases.
- Cyclic AMP-dependent protein kinase is the major effector for the second messenger cyclic AMP. This protein kinase phosphorylates several proteins involved in the control of cytoplasmic calcium levels.
- Cyclic AMP also affects HCN channels (hyperpolarization-activated cyclic nucleotide-gated channels), and Epac (exchange protein directly activated by cyclic AMP). These effects may be compartmentalized within the cell. All of these actions of the second messenger cyclic AMP lead to increases in cardiac function and metabolic costs.
- During the transition to heart failure, the level of sympathetic activity increases as do the levels of circulating catecholamines.
- There are shifts in the distribution of β adrenergic receptor subtypes in failure. These receptors may also become uncoupled from their G proteins. The subcellular distribution of these receptors may also change. These changes ultimately reduce the degree of positive functional and metabolic effects caused by these receptors.
- Activation of α adrenergic receptors leads to increases in myocyte function via generation of both diacylglycerol and inositol 1,4,5-trisphosphate (IP_3). This system plays a minor role in the normal heart.
- Agents that affect α adrenergic signaling system have not proven effective in the treatment of heart failure. There may be some shifts in receptor function and signaling, but further work is necessary to determine whether the importance of α adrenergic receptors increases in heart failure.
- The changes in signaling for both the cyclic AMP and cyclic GMP signaling systems in heart failure may provide important new targets for potential treatments. For the cyclic GMP system, the losses of downstream signaling provide new targets. For the cyclic AMP system, there are shifts in receptor subtypes, connections, and distribution. These may also provide new targets. Replacement of missing or damaged elements of these signaling systems may help the damaged heart.

References

1. Sucharov CC (2007) Beta-adrenergic pathways in human heart failure. Expert Rev Cardiovasc Ther 5:119–124
2. Zaccolo M, Movsesian MA (2007) cAMP and cGMP signaling cross-talk: role of phosphodiesterases and implications for cardiac pathophysiology. Circ Res 100:1569–1578
3. Saucerman JJ, McCulloch AD (2006) Cardiac beta-adrenergic signaling: from subcellular microdomains to heart failure. Ann N Y Acad Sci 1080:348–361
4. Kojda G, Kottenberg K (1999) Regulation of basal myocardial function by NO. Cardiovasc Res 41:514–523
5. Casadei B, Sears CE (2003) Nitric-oxide-mediated regulation of cardiac contractility and stretch responses. Prog Biophys Mol Biol 82:67–80
6. Francis SH, Blount MA, Zoraghi R, Corbin JD (2005) Molecular properties of mammalian proteins that interact with cGMP: protein kinases, cation channels, phosphodiesterases, and multi-drug anion transporters. Front Biosci 10:2097–2117
7. Shah AM, MacCarthy PA (2000) Paracrine and autocrine effects of nitric oxide on myocardial function. Pharmacol Ther 86:49–86
8. Yan L, Zhang Q, Scholz PM, Weiss HR (2003) Cyclic GMP protein kinase activity is reduced in thyroxine-induced hypertrophic cardiac myocytes. Clin Exp Pharmacol Physiol 30:943–950
9. Fischmeister R, Castro L, Abi-Gerges A, Rochais F, Vandecasteele G (2005) Species- and tissue-dependent effects of NO and cyclic GMP on cardiac ion channels. Comp Biochem Physiol 142:136–143
10. Gallo MP, Malan D, Bedendi I, Biasin C, Alloatti G, Levi RC (2001) Regulation of cardiac calcium current by NO and cGMP-modulating agents. Pflugers Arch 441:621–628
11. Bergemann C, Loken C, Becker C, Graf B, Hamidizadeh M, Fischer Y (2001) Inhibition of glucose transport by cyclic GMP in cardiomyocytes. Life Sci 69:1391–1406

12. Jiang LH, Gawler DJ, Hodson N et al (2000) Regulation of cloned cardiac L-type calcium channels by cGMP-dependent protein kinase. J Biol Chem 275:6135–6143

13. Klein G, Drexler H, Schroder F (2000) Protein kinase G reverses all isoproterenol induced changes of cardiac single L-type calcium channel gating. Cardiovasc Res 48:367–374

14. Luchner A, Schunkert H (2004) Interactions between the sympathetic nervous system and the cardiac natriuretic peptide system. Cardiovasc Res 63:443–449

15. Senzaki H, Smith CJ, Juang GJ et al (2001) Cardiac phosphodiesterase 5 (cGMP-specific) modulates beta-adrenergic signaling in vivo and is down-regulated in heart failure. FASEB J 15:1718–1726

16. Weiss HR, Lazar MJ, Punjabi K, Tse J, Scholz PM (2003) Negative functional effects of cyclic GMP are altered by cyclic AMP phosphodiesterases in rabbit cardiac myocytes. Eur J Pharmacol 481:25–31

17. Baxter GF (2004) Natriuretic peptides and myocardial ischaemia. Bas Res Cardiol 99:90–93

18. Kuhn M (2005) Cardiac and intestinal natriuretic peptides: insights from genetically modified mice. Peptides 26:1078–1085

19. Martin SR, Emanuel K, Sears CE, Zhang YH, Casadei B (2006) Are myocardial eNOS and nNOS involved in the beta-adrenergic and muscarinic regulation of inotropy? A systematic investigation. Cardiovasc Res 70:97–106

20. Khan SA, Skaf MW, Harrison RW et al (2003) Nitric oxide regulation of myocardial contractility and calcium cycling: independent impact of neuronal and endothelial nitric oxide synthases. Circ Res 92:1322–1329

21. Seddon M, Shah AM, Casadei B (2007) Cardiomyocytes as effectors of nitric oxide signalling. Cardiovasc Res 75:315–326

22. Stehlik J, Movsesian MA (2006) Inhibitors of cyclic nucleotide phosphodiesterase 3 and 5 as therapeutic agents in heart failure. Expert Opin Investig Drugs 15:733–742

23. Zhang Q, Yan L, Weiss HR, Scholz PM (2002) Cyclic GMP-induced reduction in cardiac myocyte function is partially mediated by activation of the sarcoplasmic reticulum Ca(2+)-ATPase. Pharmacology 64:106–112

24. Brittsan AG, Ginsburg KS, Chu G et al (2003) Chronic SR Ca2+-ATPase inhibition causes adaptive changes in cellular Ca2+ transport. Circ Res 92:769–776

25. Breitwieser GE (1991) G protein-mediated ion channel activation. Hypertension 17:684–692

26. Gilman AG (1987) G proteins: transducers of receptor-generated signals. Annu Rev Biochem 56:615–649

27. Fleming JW, Watanabe AM (1988) Muscarinic cholinergic-receptor stimulation of specific GTP hydrolysis related to adenylate cyclase activity in canine cardiac sarcolemma. Circ Res 63:340–350

28. Sharma RK (1995) Signal transduction: regulation of cAMP concentration in cardiac muscle by calmodulin-dependent cyclic nucleotide phosphodiesterase. Mol Cell Biochem 149–150:241–247

29. Tse J, Cimini C, Kedem J, Rodriquez E, Gonzalez M, Weiss HR (1993) Role of ischemia-reperfusion on myocardial cyclic AMP and cyclic AMP phosphodiesterase: effects of amrinone on regional myocardial force and shortening. J Cardiothorac Vasc Anesth 7:566–572

30. Hove-Madsen L, Mery PF, Jurevicius J, Skeberdis AV, Fischmeister R (1996) Regulation of myocardial calcium channels by cyclic AMP metabolism. Basic Res Cardiol 91:1–8

31. Leone RJ Jr, Straznicka M, Scholz PM, Weiss HR (2000) Cyclic GMP attenuates cyclic AMP-stimulated inotropy and oxygen consumption in control and hypertrophic hearts. Basic Res Cardiol 95:28–38

32. Gustafsson AB, Brunton LL (2002) Attenuation of cAMP accumulation in adult rat cardiac fibroblasts by IL-1beta and NO: role of cGMP-stimulated PDE2. Am J Physiol 283:C463–C471

33. Francis GS (2001) Pathophysiology of chronic heart failure. Am J Med 110 Suppl 7A:37S–46S

34. Russell B, Motlagh D, Ashley WW (2000) Form follows function: how muscle shape is regulated by work. J Appl Physiol 88:1127–1132

35. Cimini CM, Upsher ME, Weiss HR (1989) Myocardial O2 supply and consumption in early cardiac hypertrophy of renal hypertensive rabbits. Basic Res Cardiol 84:13–21

36. Cimini CM, Weiss HR (1990) Isoproterenol and myocardial O2 supply/consumption in hypertension-induced myocardial hypertrophy. Am J Physiol 259:H346–H351

37. Brodde OE, Leineweber K (2004) Autonomic receptor systems in the failing and aging human heart: similarities and differences. Eur J Pharmacol 500:167–176

38. Scholz PM, Grover GJ, Mackenzie JW, Weiss HR (1990) Regional oxygen supply and consumption balance in experimental left ventricular hypertrophy. Basic Res Cardiol 85:575–584

39. Jakob G, Mair J, Pichler M, Puschendorf B (1995) Ergometric exercise testing and sensitivity of cyclic guanosine 3′, 5′-monophosphate (cGMP) in diagnosing asymptomatic left ventricular dysfunction. Br Heart J 73:145–150

40. Lubien E, DeMaria A, Krishnaswamy P et al (2002) Utility of B-natriuretic peptide in detecting diastolic dysfunction: comparison with Doppler velocity recordings. Circulation 105:595–601

41. Kotchi Kotchi E, Weisselberg T, Rohnert P et al (1998) Nitric oxide inhibits isoprenaline-induced positive inotropic effects in normal, but not in hypertrophied rat heart. Naunyn-Schmiedebergs Arch Pharmacol 357:579–583

42. Morrison LK, Harrison A, Krishnaswamy P, Kazanegra R, Clopton P, Maisel A (2002) Utility of a rapid B-natriuretic peptide assay in differentiating congestive heart failure from lung disease in patients presenting with dyspnea. J Am Coll Cardiol 39:202–209

43. Guo X, Kedem J, Weiss HR, Tse J, Roitstein A, Scholz PM (1996) Effect of cyclic GMP reduction on regional myocardial mechanics and metabolism in experimental left ventricular hypertrophy. J Cardiovasc Pharmacol 27:392–400

44. Roitstein A, Kedem J, Cheinberg B, Weiss HR, Tse J, Scholz PM (1994) The effect of intracoronary nitroprusside on cyclic GMP and regional mechanics is altered in a canine model of left ventricular hypertrophy. J Surg Res 57:584–590

45. Seymour AA, Burkett DE, Asaad MM, Lanoce VM, Clemons AF, Rogers WL (1994) Hemodynamic, renal, and hormonal effects of rapid ventricular pacing in conscious dogs. Lab Anim Sci 44:443–452

46. Tajima M, Bartunek J, Weinberg EO, Ito N, Lorell BH (1998) Atrial natriuretic peptide has different effects on contractility and intracellular pH in normal and hypertrophied myocytes from pressure-overloaded hearts. Circulation 98:2760–2764

47. Paulus WJ, Frantz S, Kelly RA (2001) Nitric oxide and cardiac contractility in human heart failure: time for reappraisal. Circulation 104:2260–2262

48. Rosenkranz AC, Hood SG, Woods RL, Dusting GJ, Ritchie RH (2003) B-type natriuretic peptide prevents acute hypertrophic responses in the diabetic rat heart: importance of cyclic GMP. Diabetes 52:2389–2395

49. Silberbach M, Roberts CT Jr (2001) Natriuretic peptide signaling: molecular and cellular pathways to growth regulation. Cell Signal 13:221–231

50. Simko F, Simko J (2000) The potential role of nitric oxide in the hypertrophic growth of the left ventricle. Physiol Res 49:37–46

51. Fagan JM, Rex SE, Hayes-Licitra SA, Waxman L (1999) L-arginine reduces right heart hypertrophy in hypoxia-induced pulmonary hypertension. Biochem Biophys Res Commun 254:100–103

52. Padilla F, Garcia-Dorado D, Agullo L et al (2001) Intravenous administration of the natriuretic peptide urodilatin at low doses

during coronary reperfusion limits infarct size in anesthetized pigs. Cardiovasc Res 51:592–600

53. Wollert KC, Drexler H (2002) Regulation of cardiac remodeling by nitric oxide: focus on cardiac myocyte hypertrophy and apoptosis. Heart Fail Rev 7:317–325

54. Devlin AM, Brosnan MJ, Graham D et al (1998) Vascular smooth muscle cell polyploidy and cardiomyocyte hypertrophy due to chronic NOS inhibition in vivo. Am J Physiol 274:H52–H59

55. Bubikat A, De Windt LJ, Zetsche B et al (2005) Local atrial natriuretic peptide signaling prevents hypertensive cardiac hypertrophy in endothelial nitric-oxide synthase-deficient mice. J Biol Chem 280:21594–21599

56. Takimoto E, Champion HC, Belardi D et al (2005) cGMP catabolism by phosphodiesterase 5A regulates cardiac adrenergic stimulation by NOS3-dependent mechanism. Circ Res 96:100–109

57. Burger AJ, Horton DP, LeJemtel T et al (2002) Effect of nesiritide (B-type natriuretic peptide) and dobutamine on ventricular arrhythmias in the treatment of patients with acutely decompensated congestive heart failure: the PRECEDENT study. Am Heart J 144:1102–1108

58. Winter WE, Elin RJ (2004) The role and assessment of ventricular peptides in heart failure. Clin Lab Med 24:235–274

59. Parodi O, De Maria R, Roubina E (2007) Redox state, oxidative stress, and endothelial dysfunction in heart failure: the puzzle of nitrate-thiol interaction. J Cardiovasc Med (Hagerstown, MD) 8:765–774

60. Silver MA, Horton DP, Ghali JK, Elkayam U (2002) Effect of nesiritide versus dobutamine on short-term outcomes in the treatment of patients with acutely decompensated heart failure. J Am Coll Cardiol 39:798–803

61. Sackner-Bernstein JD, Skopicki HA, Aaronson KD (2005) Risk of worsening renal function with nesiritide in patients with acutely decompensated heart failure. Circulation 111:1487–1491

62. Nishikimi T, Maeda N, Matsuoka H (2006) The role of natriuretic peptides in cardioprotection. Cardiovasc Res 69:318–328

63. Richards AM (2004) The natriuretic peptides in heart failure. Basic Res Cardiol 99:94–100

64. Wu AH, Smith A (2004) Biological variation of the natriuretic peptides and their role in monitoring patients with heart failure. Eur J Heart Fail 6:355–358

65. Asada J, Tsuji H, Iwasaka T, Thomas JD, Lauer MS (2004) Usefulness of plasma brain natriuretic peptide levels in predicting dobutamine-induced myocardial ischemia. Am J Cardiol 93:702–704

66. D'Souza SP, Davis M, Baxter GF (2004) Autocrine and paracrine actions of natriuretic peptides in the heart. Pharmacol Ther 101:113–129

67. Su J, Zhang Q, Moalem J, Tse J, Scholz PM, Weiss HR (2005) Functional effects of C-type natriuretic peptide and nitric oxide are attenuated in hypertrophic myocytes from pressure-overloaded mouse hearts. Am J Physiol Heart Circ Physiol 288:H1367–H1373

68. Katz E, Zhang Q, Weiss HR, Scholz PM (2006) T4-induced cardiac hypertrophy disrupts cyclic GMP mediated responses to brain natriuretic peptide in rabbit myocardium. Peptides 27:2276–2283

69. Zhang Q, Lazar M, Molino B et al (2005) Reduction in interaction between cGMP and cAMP in dog ventricular myocytes with hypertrophic failure. Am J Physiol Heart Circ Physiol 289:H1251–H1257

70. Lohse MJ, Engelhardt S, Eschenhagen T (2003) What is the role of beta-adrenergic signaling in heart failure? Circ Res 93:896–906

71. Nikolaev VO, Bunemann M, Schmitteckert E, Lohse MJ, Engelhardt S (2006) Cyclic AMP imaging in adult cardiac myocytes reveals far-reaching beta1-adrenergic but locally confined beta2-adrenergic receptor-mediated signaling. Circ Res 99:1084–1091

72. Steinberg SF (1999) The molecular basis for distinct beta-adrenergic receptor subtype actions in cardiomyocytes. Circ Res 85:1101–1111

73. Steinberg SF, Brunton LL (2001) Compartmentation of G protein-coupled signaling pathways in cardiac myocytes. Annu Rev Pharmacol Toxicol 41:751–773

74. Penela P, Murga C, Ribas C, Tutor AS, Peregrin S, Mayor F Jr (2006) Mechanisms of regulation of G protein-coupled receptor kinases (GRKs) and cardiovascular disease. Cardiovasc Res 69:46–56

75. Xiang Y, Kobilka BK (2003) Myocyte adrenoceptor signaling pathways. Science 300:1530–1532

76. Vandecasteele G, Rochais F, Abi-Gerges A, Fischmeister R (2006) Functional localization of cAMP signalling in cardiac myocytes. Biochem Soc Trans 34:484–488

77. McConnachie G, Langeberg LK, Scott JD (2006) AKAP signaling complexes: getting to the heart of the matter. Trends Mol Med 12:317–323

78. Brodde OE (2008) Beta1- and beta2-adrenoceptor polymorphisms and cardiovascular diseases. Fundam Clin Pharmacol 22:107–125

79. Metrich M, Lucas A, Gastineau M et al (2008) Epac mediates beta-adrenergic receptor-induced cardiomyocyte hypertrophy. Circ Res 102:959–965

80. Lymperopoulos A, Rengo G, Koch WJ (2007) Adrenal adrenoceptors in heart failure: fine-tuning cardiac stimulation. Trends Mol Med 13:503–511

81. Ping P, Anzai T, Gao M, Hammond HK (1997) Adenylyl cyclase and G protein receptor kinase expression during development of heart failure. Am J Physiol 273:H707–H717

82. Bohm M, Gierschik P, Jakobs KH et al (1990) Increase of Gi alpha in human hearts with dilated but not ischemic cardiomyopathy. Circulation 82:1249–1265

83. Bristow MR (2000) beta-adrenergic receptor blockade in chronic heart failure. Circulation 101:558–569

84. Vinge LE, Raake PW, Koch WJ (2008) Gene therapy in heart failure. Circ Res 102:1458–1470

85. Woodcock EA (2007) Roles of alpha1A- and alpha1B-adrenoceptors in heart: insights from studies of genetically modified mice. Clin Exp Pharmacol Physiol 34:884–888

86. Lamba S, Abraham WT (2000) Alterations in adrenergic receptor signaling in heart failure. Heart Fail Rev 5:7–16

87. Hawrylyshyn KA, Michelotti GA, Coge F, Guenin SP, Schwinn DA (2004) Update on human alpha1-adrenoceptor subtype signaling and genomic organization. Trends Pharmacol Sci 25:449–455

88. Du XJ (2008) Distinct role of adrenoceptor subtypes in cardiac adaptation to chronic pressure overload. Clin Exp Pharmacol Physiol 35:355–360

89. Zuscik MJ, Chalothorn D, Hellard D et al (2001) Hypotension, autonomic failure, and cardiac hypertrophy in transgenic mice over-expressing the alpha 1B-adrenergic receptor. J Biol Chem 276:13738–13743

90. Lin F, Owens WA, Chen S et al (2001) Targeted alpha(1A)-adrenergic receptor overexpression induces enhanced cardiac contractility but not hypertrophy. Circ Res 89:343–350

91. Appert-Collin A, Cotecchia S, Nenniger-Tosato M, Pedrazzini T, Diviani D (2007) The A-kinase anchoring protein (AKAP)-Lbc-signaling complex mediates alpha1 adrenergic receptor-induced cardiomyocyte hypertrophy. Proc Natl Acad Sci U S A 104:10140–10145

92. O'Connell TD, Ishizaka S, Nakamura A et al (2003) The alpha(1A/C)- and alpha(1B)-adrenergic receptors are required for physiological cardiac hypertrophy in the double-knockout mouse. J Clin Invest 111:1783–1791

93. Shannon R, Chaudhry M (2006) Effect of alpha1-adrenergic receptors in cardiac pathophysiology. Am Heart J 152:842–850

94. Woodcock EA, Du XJ, Reichelt ME, Graham RM (2008) Cardiac alpha 1-adrenergic drive in pathological remodelling. Cardiovasc Res 77:452–462

Chapter 9
Calcium Signaling: Receptors, Effectors, and Other Signaling Pathways

Overview

HF could be described, among many definitions, as a disorder of cell signaling, with determination of the way in which signals are coupled to their effectors/receptors – at the center of the most innovative work on HF pathophysiology and pathogenesis.

Previously in Chap. 8, the role of cyclic nucleotides, second messengers signaling in the control of myocardial function and their effects on HF has been discussed. In this chapter, we continue the discussion on other second messengers such as calcium-mediated signaling, followed by an appraisal of some receptor/effector factors and other relevant signaling cascades as they relate to the pathogenesis and pathophysiology of HF.

Introduction

The heart is a dynamic transmitter and receiver of a variety of intracellular and extracellular stimuli, and an integrator of numerous interacting transducers. Protein modifiers that lead to downstream activation or deactivation of specific transcription factors, modulate specific gene expression affecting a broad spectrum of cellular events. The modulation of gene expression can be fostered as well by effectors that modulate chromatin structure, and histone proteins (e.g., acetylases and deacetylases). These effectors can also directly target proteins involved in metabolic pathways, ion transport, Ca^{2+} regulation and handling, which affect contractility and excitability, as well as cardiomyocyte apoptosis and cell survival.

Protein kinases and effectors, the G-proteins, and small G-protein activators are critically influenced by their position within the cell. Several G-protein-coupled receptors (GPCRs), including the α- and β-adrenergic receptors (previously discussed in Chap. 8), angiotensin II, and endothelin-1 are able to activate a series of sequential molecular and cellular events (cascades). Other receptors, pivotal in cardiac and cardiovascular signaling include protease-activated, toll-like receptors, receptor tyrosine kinases (RTK). Regulatory control of the receptors is exerted by phosphorylation (by either protein kinase A (PKA) or other kinases), which can lead to receptor internalization and desensitization to the agonist.

In this chapter, a group of specific cell signaling cascades of great significance in HF including, calcium, effector/receptors, stress, metabolic, and extracellular/matrix signals are discussed.

Ca²⁺-Mediated Signaling

Since Ca^{2+} functions as a second messenger activating multiple signaling cascades, it has been suggested that in addition to the effects of altered Ca^{2+} handling on cardiac contractile parameters, Ca^{2+} may directly affect gene expression in the heart [1]. Key components of the cardiomyocyte calcium-handling pathway show characteristic changes in HF. Changes in Ca^{2+} transport and metabolism are known to occur in HF. At the molecular level, marked reductions in the levels of phospholamban mRNA and both sarcoplasmic reticulum Ca^{2+}-ATPase (SERCA) mRNA and enzyme activity (see Chap. 5), as well as increased levels of sarcolemmal Na^+–Ca^{2+} exchanger have been reported [2–5]. In the myocardium, the principal SERCA protein is the SERCA2a isoform the activity of which is regulated by a closely associated protein, phospholamban (PLB) (Fig. 9.1), in a manner that is dependent on its phosphorylation status [6, 7]. When phosphorylated, PLB enhances Ca^{2+} uptake into the sarcoplasmic reticulum, generally leading to increased Ca^{2+} release and contractile force. In the dephosphorylated state, PLB exerts an inhibitory action on SERCA2a, slowing its enzymatic rate. When PLB is phosphorylated, this inhibitory action is lost, and SERCA activity increases. This occurs in the context of adrenergic activation with a resultant hastening of relaxation due to heightened SERCA activity. Also, at the physiological level, there is prolonged action potential and Ca^{2+} transient, decreased Ca^{2+} uptake and reduced Ca^{2+}

J. Marín-García, *Heart Failure*, Contemporary Cardiology,
DOI 10.1007/978-1-60761-147-9_9, © Springer Science+Business Media, LLC 2010

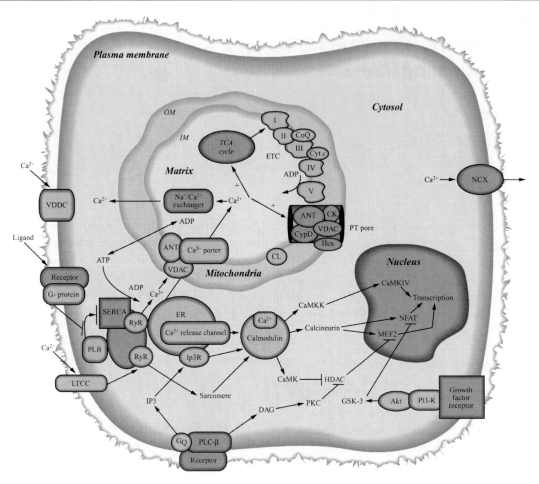

Fig. 9.1 Ca^{2+}-mediated kinase signaling. Depiction of the major cardiac Ca^{2+}/CaM dependent enzymes includes Ca^{2+}/CaM dependent protein kinase (CaMK), myosin light chain kinase (MLCK), and the phosphatase calcineurin. These signaling pathways, including Ca^{2+}/CaM regulated kinase, phosphatase pathways, and PKC isozymes are directly activated by Ca^{2+} and they are sufficient to promote the development of cardiac hypertrophy. SERCA, in particular SERCA2a isoform, activity is regulated by a closely associated protein, phospholamban (PLB)

release by the sarcoplasmic reticulum, and increased diastolic Ca^{2+} concentration [5]. Notwithstanding, it is not clear whether these are primary or secondary changes to other events happening in HF.

Ca²⁺/Sarcolemmal/Stress-Dependent Signaling Pathways

Ca^{2+} is a major intracellular messenger involved in the activation of Ca^{2+}-dependent signaling pathways where it regulates cardiac growth and function by activation of kinases and phosphatases as well as playing a pivotal role in excitation–contraction coupling (ECC) discussed in Chap. 2. The Ca^{2+} signal inducing contraction in cardiac muscle originates from two sources. In response to depolarization of the sarcolemma, Ca^{2+} enters the cell through voltage dependent L-type Ca^{2+} channels (VDCC). This Ca^{2+} binds to and activates Ca^{2+} release

channels (ryanodine receptors) of the sarcoplasmic reticulum (SR) through a Ca^{2+} induced Ca^{2+} release (CICR) process increasing intracellular Ca^{2+} concentration by more than tenfold to induce contraction. Entry of Ca^{2+} with each contraction requires an equal amount of Ca^{2+} extrusion within a single heartbeat to maintain Ca^{2+} homeostasis and to ensure relaxation. Removal of Ca^{2+} from the cytosol is mainly affected by the sarcolemmal Na^+/Ca^{2+} exchanger and by the SR ATP dependent Ca^{2+} pump (Ca^{2+} ATPase) or SERCA. These transport systems are important determinants of the intracellular Ca^{2+} level and cardiac contractility. Altered intracellular Ca^{2+} handling is one factor contributing to impaired contractility in HF.

In response to disease-causing stimuli (many of them remain to be identified), neuroendocrine secreted growth factors and/or cytokines induce ventricular remodeling, hypertrophic enlargement of cardiomyocytes, and alterations in the viability of cardiomyocytes. Many of these neuroendocrine factors (e.g., angiotensin II and endothelin-1) signal cardiomyocytes through G-protein-coupled receptors (GPCRs) to induce phospholipase C (PLC) activation, which in turn generates inositol 1,4,5-trisphosphate (InsP3) and diacylglycerol (DAG). InsP3 generation in turn leads to the release of Ca²⁺ from the endoplasmic and sarcoplasmic reticulum through the InsP3R channels and ryanodine receptor (RyR)/intracellular Ca²⁺ release channels.

Neuroendocrine factors and cytokines have been implicated in the development of hypertrophy and HF, in part by promoting the activation of a number of intracellular signaling pathways in cardiac myocytes, including MAPK, protein kinase C (PKC), the Ca²⁺ regulated phosphatase calcineurin, calcium/calmodulin-dependent protein kinase (CaMK), and IGF-1 pathway constituents. Interestingly, three of these signaling factors, calcineurin, CaMK, and PKC, require increases in Ca²⁺ to become activated, and both calcineurin and CaMK are potent inducers of the myocardial hypertrophic response. Chronic hyperactivity of the β-adrenergic signaling pathway results in PKA-hyperphosphorylation of the cardiac (RyR)/intracellular Ca²⁺ release channels.

There is a growing interest in the intersection of these two aspects of Ca²⁺: increase in Ca²⁺ that drives the larger contractions may be responsible for switching on a second process of signalosome remodeling to down-regulate the Ca²⁺ signaling pathway, and Ca²⁺ transient transmits information responsible for remodeling of the cardiac gene transcription program that leads first to hypertrophy and then to HF [8].

Ca²⁺ associated stress response pathways also control cardiac gene expression by modulating the activities of chromatin-remodeling enzymes, which have been shown to act as global regulators of the cardiac genome during pathological remodeling of the heart. Deacetylation of nucleosomal histones in chromatin by histone deacetylases (HDACs) results in transcriptional repression due to chromatin condensation. Several lines of evidence from transgenic mice have strongly implicated class II HDACs in preventing myocyte hypertrophy in response to diverse agonists. Moreover, in stressed animals, class II HDACs are shuttled out of the nucleus, dependent on phosphorylation by GPCR-activated kinases, including CaMK and the kinase PKD. In addition to kinase regulation of cardiac gene expression controlling hypertrophy through negative effects on HDACs, phosphoprotein phosphatases also play an equally important role in the regulation of chromatin structure and gene expression during cardiac remodeling. For example, the calcium and calmodulin-dependent phosphoprotein phosphatase calcineurin is activated in response to cardiac stress signaling, and its activation has been shown to be sufficient for pathological cardiac hypertrophy. Calcineurin dephosphorylates members of the NFAT family of transcription factors, which enable them to translocate into the nucleus, where they activate transcription in cooperation with other transcription factors, including MEF2 and GATA4. NFAT factors activate myocardial gene expression, in part, by recruiting histone acetyltransferases (HATs) to gene regulatory elements containing NFAT and MEF2 binding sites.

Calcineurin/Calmodulin

Many of the actions of Ca²⁺ are mediated via its interaction with calmodulin (CaM), which is an intracellular Ca²⁺ sensor and selectively activates downstream signaling pathways in response to local changes in Ca²⁺ (see Fig. 9.1) [9].

Major signaling pathways that are both, directly activated by Ca²⁺ and are sufficient to contribute to the development of cardiac hypertrophy, include Ca²⁺/CaM regulated kinase and phosphatase pathways, and PKC isozymes [10]. Major cardiac Ca²⁺/CaM dependent enzymes include Ca²⁺/CaM dependent protein kinase (CaMK), myosin light chain kinase (MLCK), and the phosphoprotein phosphatase calcineurin [10]. In the heart, the main CaMKII isoform is CaMKIIδ localized in the nucleus, whereas other isoforms are localized in the SR [11]. Increased intracellular [Ca²⁺] results in autophosphorylation of CaMKII, which switches it to a Ca²⁺-independent state and prolongs its activation. CaMKI, which is ubiquitously expressed, and CaMKIV, mainly expressed in testis and brain, are activated by upstream Ca²⁺/CaM dependent protein kinases [10]. CaMKII isoforms associated with SR are capable of phosphorylating Ca²⁺-cycling proteins, and hence altering Ca²⁺ re-uptake and release. In cultured cardiac myocytes, pharmacological inhibitors of CaMKII have been found to attenuate both, ET-1 induced hypertrophy [12] and mechanically stretch activated BNP gene transcription [13]. Moreover, overexpression of CaMKIIδ in the heart of transgenic mice is sufficient to promote hypertrophic growth [14], as well as cardiac-specific overexpression of either CaMKI or CaMKIV [15]. Furthermore, MLCK is activated by Ca²⁺/CaM leading to subsequent phosphorylation of its single main substrate, ventricular specific isoform of myosin light chain-2 (MLC-2).

Besides cardiac kinases, Ca²⁺/CaM activates phosphoprotein phosphatases, including calcineurin [16]. Activated calcineurin dephosphorylates NFAT3 transcription factors, inducing their nuclear translocation and interaction with the cardiac-restricted transcription factor GATA4, resulting in the synergistic activation of embryonic cardiac genes and a hypertrophic response. Transgenic mice expressing constitutively activated calcineurin develop LVH that can be prevented by administration of the calcineurin inhibitors cyclosporin and FK506. These findings promoted interest in the role of elevated Ca²⁺ and the calcineurin-signaling pathway in the pathogenesis of LVH.

Activation of calcineurin by the Ca²⁺/CaM complex results in dephosphorylation of its substrates, including nuclear factor of activated T-cells (NFAT) or Ets-like gene-1

(Elk-1). Importantly, in the failing human heart there is interaction of Ca^{2+}/CaM and calcineurin, and in experimental animal models of cardiac hypertrophy increased levels of cardiac calcineurin activity have been reported [17]. Furthermore, calcineurin is sufficient to produce cardiac hypertrophy when overexpressed in the heart of transgenic mice [16]. The human hypertrophied heart in comparison to normal controls, exhibits higher calcineurin activity [18], and patients maintained with partially inhibited calcineurin activity still can develop cardiac hypertrophy. This is probably related to the presence of additional pathways making calcineurin signaling not indispensable for hypertrophy [19, 20].

Other Kinases and Phosphatases

Protein Kinase A

PKA, also known as cAMP-dependent protein kinase, is a regulatory holoenzyme the activity of which in cardiomyocytes rises sharply in response to exercise and various stresses. PKA is structurally organized as a heterotetramer composed of 2 regulatory (R) subunits that upon binding the 2 catalytic (C) subunits maintain the overall complex in a dormant state. The binding of two cyclic AMP molecules to tandem sites on each R subunit results in the release of the C subunits and the activation of their enzymatic activity. The dissociated C subunits phosphorylate serine or threonine residues on target proteins in the nucleus and cytoplasm leading to changes in cardiomyocyte metabolism, ion channel function, growth and gene expression. The catalytic subunits are encoded by three different genes ($C\alpha$, $C\beta$, and $C\gamma$), while the regulatory subunits are encoded by four genes ($RI\alpha$, $RI\beta$, $RII\alpha$, and $RII\beta$). The regulatory subunit contains an N-terminal dimerization domain, an autophosphorylation site that also comprises the primary site for catalytic subunit binding, and two tandem cAMP binding sites.

Compartmentalization of these enzymes can be achieved through association with anchoring or adaptor proteins that target them to subcellular organelles or tether them directly to target substrates via protein–protein interactions. Specific PKA anchoring proteins (AKAPs) serve as important regulators of PKA function and signaling by directing the subcellular localization of PKA, by binding to its regulatory (R) subunits, in effect concentrating PKA at specific intracellular locations. Using a variety of experimental approaches, including yeast two hybrid screening, proteomic analysis and interaction cloning, two major anchoring proteins for PKA, MAP2, and AKAP75, and over 13 different AKAPs

have been found in the heart [21]. Targeting of AKAPs to specific sites within the cell is governed by sequences in the AKAP. Interestingly, despite their diverse structure, the AKAPs all contain an amphipathic helical region of 14–18 amino acids that binds to the N-terminus of the RII subunit, underlying their interaction with PKA. Besides PKA, AKAPs also interact with other signaling components, including phosphodiesterase inhibitors, phosphatases, and PKA substrates [22]. Myocyte AKAPs have been identified in association with specific plasma membrane ion channels (e.g., delayed rectifier K^+ channel (KCNQ1), dihydropyridine receptor (L-type Ca^{2+} channel)), the β-AR complex, and the sodium–calcium exchanger (NCX1), in association with ryanodine-sensitive Ca^{2+} release channel (RyR) at both the sarcoplasmic reticulum (SR) and T-tubule junction. In addition, AKAPs have been found on the nuclear membrane, and in association with the mitochondrial outer membrane. The precise functional role of a number of the identified AKAPs in the cardiac myocyte has not yet been established.

Also a novel role for leucine zipper motifs in targeting kinases and phosphatases via anchoring proteins has been identified. Several cardiac ion channels contain a domain to anchor phosphoprotein phosphorylation modulatory proteins to the channel, essentially allowing the formation of a scaffolding structure for regulatory proteins. Ion channels such as the RyR, L-type Ca^{2+} channel, KCNQ1, all contain a modified leucine zipper termed a LIZ (leucine/isoleucine zipper), which promotes protein–protein interaction, and protein oligomerization [23].

Protein Kinase C

The serine/threonine protein kinase C (PKC) has been implicated as the intracellular mediator of a variety of factors acting through multiple signal transduction pathways. The PKC family of isozymes is increasingly recognized as playing a pivotal role in the cardiac phenotype expressed during postnatal growth and development and in response to pathologic stimuli and in the development of cardiac hypertrophy and HF. The expression of multiple PKC isoforms contributes to both a broad spectrum of adaptive and maladaptive cardiac responses with significantly different responses provided by each isoform [24]. While over 12 isoforms of PKC have been reported, in the heart the four most functionally significant members of the PKC family are PKC α and β (both calcium- and DAG-activated), and PKC δ and ε (DAG-activated with no requirement for calcium). These PKC isoforms are activated by membrane receptors coupled to PLC via G_q/G_{11} heterotrimeric G-proteins. Activation of PKC-dependent phosphorylation is conditioned upon translocation from the cytosol to the site of action (e.g., to the plasma membrane and to the mitochondria). PKC has an N-terminal regulatory region and a C-terminal catalytic region; protein–lipid interactions are implicated in PKC targeting with the N-terminus, which is required for PKC interaction with the second messenger DAG and Ca^{2+}.

Anchoring proteins recruit PKC to specific sites, and receptors for activated C-kinase (RACKs) have been found to be operative in the translocation of PKCε in cardiomyocyte growth signaling [25].

Protein Kinase G

cGMP-dependent protein kinase (PKG) modulates several targets involved in muscular contraction. In contrast to the multisubunit nature of other protein kinases, PKG is composed of a single polypeptide sequence containing both regulatory and catalytic domains. In comparison to protein kinases A, B, and C, the role of cGMP/PKG-mediated signaling in cardiac tissue has been less documented.

Natriuretic peptide binding to type I receptors (NPRA and NPRB) on target cells activates their intrinsic guanylyl cyclase (GC) activity, resulting in a rapid increase in cGMP. Diffusible cGMP acts as a second messenger primarily by stimulating PKG, the primary mediator of cGMP-induced smooth muscle relaxation [26]. Downstream effects that have been directly linked to activated PKG include modulation of the L-type calcium channel, and cross-talk with heterologous receptors, such as GPCRs. PKG substrates are membrane-bound, cytosolic, and intranuclear. Evidence indicates that the membrane-bound GC, but not the soluble guanylyl cyclases that are activated by NO, has potent effects on plasma membrane control of the calcium ATPase pump, suggesting that NO- and natriuretic peptide-mediated effects are compartmentalized in cells. Moreover, using a cytosolic yeast two-hybrid system employing PKG as bait, PKG was found to directly interact with NPRA [27].

NO donors increase heart rate through a GC-dependent stimulation of the pacemaker current I_f, without affecting basal I_{Ca-L}. NO signaling via cGMP and cGMP-dependent protein kinase type I (PKG I), has been recognized as a negative regulator of cardiac myocyte hypertrophy. Calcineurin, promotes hypertrophy partly by activating NFAT transcription factors that promote the expression of hypertrophic genes, including BNP. Activation of PKG I by NO/cGMP suppressed NFAT transcriptional activity, BNP induction, and cell enlargement. PKG I inhibits cardiomyocyte hypertrophy by targeting the calcineurin-NFAT signaling pathway, and provides a framework for understanding how NO inhibits cardiomyocyte hypertrophy [28]. The NO/PKG I signal transduction pathway also plays an important role in vascular biology, regulating smooth muscle tone by decreasing

Ca^{2+} release from intracellular stores, and by reducing calcium sensitivity of the contractile apparatus together with SMC proliferation and differentiation. PKG I also regulates endothelial cell permeability, motility, and platelet aggregation. Also, insulin-induced relaxation of vascular SMCs is mediated via NO/cGMP/PKG inhibition of RhoA [29]. PKG regulates gene expression both at the transcriptional and post-transcriptional level, increasing the expression of several genes, including c-fos, heme oxygenase, and MAP kinase phosphatase 1, and decreasing the expression of others, such as thrombospondin, gonadotropin-releasing hormone, and soluble GC [30–33].

NO can directly influence cardiac contractile function. In the absence of stimulation by extrinsic agonists, both endothelium-derived NO and exogenous NO donors accelerate myocardial relaxation, and/or reduce diastolic pressure. NO can also modulate the myocardial inotropic state; however, whether it is positively or negatively modulated may depend on several factors, including the concentration of NO, the rate of NO release, and/or the presence of β-adrenergic stimulation.

Elevation of intracellular cGMP in cardiac myocytes can potentially influence several different pathways, including PKG activation, and inhibition or stimulation of cAMP phosphodiesterase activity and consequent changes in cAMP levels. It is also feasible that high levels of cGMP could induce changes in contractility via cross-activation of PKA. Rat ventricular myocytes are known to express low levels of PKG (approximately tenfold lower than in smooth muscle) [34]. In spite of these low levels, evidence suggests that myocardial PKG mediates the cGMP-induced reduction in the L-type Ca^{2+} current following cAMP stimulation.

The intracellular signaling mechanisms responsible for the contractile effects of NO in cardiac myocytes are not known. It is possible that phosphorylation of troponin I by PKG may have comparable effects to PKA-induced phosphorylation. Furthermore, PKG can phosphorylate troponin I in vitro, and the contractile effects of NO may be related to troponin I phosphorylation [35]. Earlier, in vitro observations suggested that PKG phosphorylates cardiac troponin I at the same sites (Ser23/24) as those phosphorylated by PKA. Moreover, reduction in myofilament Ca^{2+} responsiveness produced by NO is also mediated by PKG-dependent phosphorylation of troponin I at the same site(s) as those phosphorylated by PKA.

Whereas the signal transduction pathways promoting cardiomyocyte hypertrophy have been increasingly well characterized, information concerning signaling pathways that oppose cardiomyocyte hypertrophy is more limited. NO, through activation of soluble GC and cGMP formation, attenuates the hypertrophic response to growth factor stimulation in cardiomyocytes. In addition to its antihypertrophic effect, NO promotes apoptosis in cardiomyocytes in a dose-dependent manner. On the other hand, the role of cGMP in the proapoptotic effects of NO is rather controversial since cGMP analogs may or may not induce cardiomyocyte apoptosis.

In general, cGMP effectors include cGMP-regulated phosphodiesterases, cGMP-regulated ion channels, and PKGs [36]. Two PKG genes have been identified in mammalian cells, encoding PKG type I (including α- and β-splice variants), and PKG type II. In cardiomyocytes, PKG I has been suggested to mediate negative inotropic effects of NO/cGMP, possibly through regulation of the L-type Ca^{2+} channel and troponin I, thereby reducing Ca^{2+} influx and myofilament Ca^{2+} sensitivity. However, a role for PKG I in controlling cardiomyocyte hypertrophy and/or apoptosis has not been reported.

Potential targets for PKG I in cardiomyocytes include Ca^{2+} dependent signaling pathways, RhoA, and VASP [37, 38]. Localization of VASP at intercalated disks in cardiomyocytes suggests that VASP may be involved in PKG I regulation of electrical coupling.

Ca^{2+} dependent signaling pathways, such as calcineurin and Ca^{2+}/calmodulin-dependent kinases, are crucial regulators of the hypertrophic response in cardiomyocytes. PKG I regulates intracellular Ca^{2+} at multiple levels, including the L-type Ca^{2+} channel and the InsP3 receptor. PKG I-dependent inhibition of the L-type Ca^{2+} current may mediate negative inotropic effects of NO/cGMP in cardiomyocytes. Importantly, Ca^{2+} influx through the L-type Ca^{2+} channel has also been implicated in the regulation of cardiomyocyte hypertrophy. Therefore, antihypertrophic effects of PKG I may be mediated in part through inhibition of Ca^{2+} dependent signaling pathways in cardiomyocytes. The low-molecular-weight GTPase RhoA, which is required for α1-AR signaling in cardiomyocytes, may represent an additional PKG I target. PKG I has recently been shown to phosphorylate RhoA, and inhibits its biological activity in vascular SMCs, suggesting that inhibition of RhoA may also contribute to the antihypertrophic effects of PKG I. Notwithstanding the above observations, further research is needed to identify which of its many molecular targets PKG I uses to inhibit cardiomyocyte hypertrophy.

G-Protein Regulated Kinases

The regulation of myocardial adrenergic receptors, like that of most GPCRs, involves a desensitization mechanism characterized by a rapid loss of receptor responsiveness despite the continued presence of agonist. The desensitization process has been particularly well characterized using the β2-AR system promoted by a phosphorylation event targeting only the agonist-occupied receptors by a serine/threonine kinase known as β-ARK. β-ARK1 and a highly homologous isozyme β-ARK2 are two of the most studied members of the G-protein regulated kinase (GRK) family, which currently consists of six members. Desensitization of GPCRs requires not only GRK-mediated phosphorylation, but also the binding of a second class of inhibitory proteins, the β-arrestins (β-arrestin-1 and β-arrestin-2), which bind to phosphorylated receptors and sterically restrict the further activation of G-proteins, in part by their displacement from the receptors resulting in receptor-G-protein uncoupling [39]. The GRKs shown to be expressed in the heart are β-ARK1 (the most abundant), β-ARK2, GRK5, and GRK6. Since β1-AR is the most critical receptor mediating acute changes in myocardial rate and contractility, it is important to realize that three of these GRKs (β-ARK1, β-ARK2, and GRK5) have been shown to phosphorylate and desensitize β1-ARs in vitro [40].

Like most GRKs, β-ARK1 is a cytosolic enzyme that has to be translocated to the plasma membrane in order to phosphorylate the activated receptor substrate. The mechanism for translocation of β-ARK1 and β-ARK2 involve the physical interaction between the kinase and the membrane-bound β subunits of G-proteins (G_β). G_β, anchored to the membrane through a lipid modification on the C-terminus of the subunit (termed prenylation), is available to interact with β-ARK after G-protein activation and dissociation. The region of β-ARK responsible for binding G_β has been mapped to a 125-amino acid domain located within the C-terminus of the enzyme. Recently, peptides derived from the G_β-binding domain of β-ARK have been shown to act as in vitro β-ARK inhibitors by competing for G_β and preventing β-ARK translocation [41].

A pathophysiological role for GRKs can be inferred from recent studies on HF as well as from the observation that chronic treatment with various agonists or antagonists for G-protein-coupled receptors results in alterations of GRK expression [42, 43]. Furthermore, β-adrenergic receptor desensitization and uncoupling are further induced by HF-induced increases in the level of GRKs [44]. Increased myocardial levels of the most abundant GRK, β-ARK-1 precede HF development in several animal models and are present in HF patients and may be a key factor in the transition from compensatory cardiac hypertrophy to overt HF [45].

MAP Kinases

The MAPK cascade consists of a series of successively acting protein kinases that include three well-characterized branches, the extracellular signal-regulated kinases (ERKs), the c-Jun N-terminal kinases (JNKs), and the p38 MAPKs. Signaling through each of these MAPK branches is initiated by diverse stress and mitogenic stimuli localized to the cell membrane or within the cytoplasm. Activation of ERKs, JNKs, and p38 MAPKs facilitates the phosphorylation of multiple transcriptional regulators such as myocyte enhancer factor-2 (MEF2), activating transcription factor-2 (ATF-2), p53, NFAT, c-Jun, and c-Myc. MAPK-mediated phosphorylation of these and other transcriptional regulators profoundly influences adaptive and inducible gene expression in many cell types. Members of the MAPK signaling cascade are also important regulators of cardiomyocyte hypertrophy, although the downstream transcriptional mechanisms that alter cardiac gene expression have not been characterized.

Signaling the Receptors

Adrenergic Receptors

ARs, members of the G-protein-coupled receptor superfamily, interface between the sympathetic nervous system and the cardiovascular system, and have integral roles in the rapid regulation of myocardial function. In HF, chronic catecholamine stimulation of adrenoceptors has been linked to pathological cardiac remodeling, including cardiomyocyte apoptosis and hypertrophy; PKC activation of ERK has been implicated in the α1-adrenoceptor stimulation of cardiomyocyte hypertrophy, and the human myocardium contains a relatively small number of α1-ARs with a β/α-AR ratio of 10:1. In the failing heart, with diminished β-AR levels, there is an increase in the α1-AR-to β-AR ratio, suggesting that α1-AR may assume a greater functional role by providing a secondary inotropic system in the failing heart.

It has been demonstrated that α2-adrenoceptors (α2-ARs) are receptors for endogenous catecholamine agonists (e.g., norepinephrine and epinephrine), which mediate a number of physiological and pharmacological responses including changes in blood pressure and heart rate. Three distinct subtypes of α2-ARs, denoted α2A-, α2B-, and α2C-AR, have been characterized and cloned [46], and screening of human populations from various ethnic backgrounds has shown that α2-AR genes are polymorphic. Functional changes in G-protein coupling, in agonist-promoted receptor phosphorylation and desensitization, have been found in heterologous systems such as CHO and COS-7 cells, which express these genetic polymorphisms in comparison to wild-type receptors [47].

Muscarinic Receptors

Muscarinic acetylcholine receptors (mAChR) mediate a variety of cellular responses, including inhibition of adenylyl cyclase (AC), modulation of K+ channels, and increased phosphoinositide breakdown [48]. These diverse effects of mAChR activation elicit both negative and positive inotropic and chronotropic effects in the heart. In human ventricular myocardium, however, the negative inotropic effect can be only achieved when basal force of contraction has been prestimulated by cyclic AMP-elevating agents such as β-adrenoceptor agonists, forskolin or phosphodiesterase inhibitors (indirect effect); this has been shown in various in vitro and in vivo studies. Accumulative evidence has shown that vagal activity in chronic HF is decreased. On the other hand, cardiac muscarinic M2 receptor density and functional responsiveness (inhibition of AC activity and negative inotropic effects) in the failing heart are not significantly changed when compared with nonfailing hearts, but cardiac Gi-activity is increased [49]. Positive inotropic effects of cholinergic agonists are present only at high agonist concentration (>10 μmol/L), and tend to be pertussis toxin (PTX)-insensitive in contrast to the negative inotropic effects observed at lower agonist concentrations, which are sensitive to inactivation by PTX. These dual effects of mAChR activation in heart may be a result of the presence of multiple subtypes of mAChRs [50]. Thus far, five mAChR subtypes (M1–M5) have been identified, and each subtype is encoded by a different gene. The mAChR proteins contain seven transmembrane spanning domains, and are coupled to G-proteins of the G_i and G_q families to inhibit AC and activate PLC respectively. While M2 receptors have been considered to be the only functional mAChRs in the myocardium, several observations revealed that M3 receptors are also present in the hearts of various species [51].

Stimulation of muscarinic acetylcholine receptors results in the activation of an inward rectifier K+ current termed I_{KACh} in cardiac myocytes, primarily mediated by the M2 subtype of mAChR. However, a novel delayed rectifier-like K+ current designated I_{KM3}, which is distinct from I_{KACh} and other known K+ currents, and which is mediated by the activation of the cardiac M3 receptors, has been identified [52]. While I_{KACh} is known to be a G_i-protein-gated K+ channel, I_{KM3} represents the first G_q-protein-coupled K+ channel described in cardiomyocytes. Interestingly, the regulation of these channels is fundamentally different during atrial fibrillation; the atrial levels of I_{KM3} are increased in both animal models and human hearts, whereas the atrial M2 receptor density decreased, indicating down-regulation [53].

Neurohumoral Signaling

A cascade of intracellular events have been identified in cardiomyocytes, which appear to be important in mediating the progression of HF. Hormones such as angiotensin II, endothelin 1, and norepinephrine, which bind and activate cardiomyocyte membrane receptors, coupled to the G_q-proteins have been implicated in the development of cardiac hypertrophy and ultimate decompensation [54].

Endothelin

Endothelin-1 is known to be an agonist involved in the stimulation of phosphoinositide-generated second messengers and protein kinases in cardiac signal transduction leading to myocyte remodeling and hypertrophy [55, 56]. Effects on kinase-phosphorylation, which could activate or deactivate specific enzyme subunits/active sites or specific allosteric regulators, may be involved. Such regulatory modifications could be rapidly generated in response to a variety of stimuli, and direct reversible modifications in the enzymes responsible for generating the bulk of mitochondrial ATP. Questions have been posited regarding if endothelin directly interacts with mitochondria, either the mitochondrial inner or the outer membrane. To the best of our knowledge there is no definitive evidence for a direct interaction of endothelin or endothelin receptors with the mitochondrial organelle. Three endothelin (ET) signaling peptides, ET-1, ET-2, and ET-3 with well-established effects on the cardiomyocyte, including modulation of contractile function and growth stimulation, have been identified [57]. ET-1, a vasoconstrictor peptide produced by vascular endothelial cells, binds to the ET(A) receptor on the cell surface, coupled to the G_q class of GTP binding proteins, and stimulates hydrolysis of phosphatidylinositol 4′, 5′-bisphosphate to DAG and InsP3. DAG remains in the plane of the membrane causing translocation and activation of PKC δ- and ε-isoforms. This is followed by activation of the small G-protein Ras and by an ERK cascade. Over a longer time course, two protein kinase cascades related to the ERK1/2 cascade, the JNK and p38 MAP kinase cascades also become activated. Downstream activation of nuclear transcription factors (e.g., GATA-4, c-Jun), protein kinases (e.g., 90-kDa ribosomal protein S6 kinase, MAPK-activated protein kinase 2), and ion exchangers/channels (e.g., the Na^+/H^+ exchanger 1) follows. These changes are responsible for the overall biological effects of ET isopeptides on the cardiomyocyte [58].

Drimal et al. [59] have questioned whether ET-1 is primarily responsible for increased myocardial ET-1 expression and release with resultant inotropic effects, or for the induction of myocardial hypertrophy and HF. To find the answer to these questions these investigators evaluated in the isolate rat heart, the subtype-selective mechanisms underlying the inotropic response to ET-1 and to its ET(B) receptor-selective fragment (8-21)ET-1. They found that both peptides, ET-1 and its (8-21)ET-1 fragment, significantly reduced coronary blood flow in nmolar and higher concentrations. The concomitant negative inotropic and chronotropic effects were significant after ET-1, while the infusion of the (8-21)ET-1 fragment produced a slight but significant positive inotropic effect. Among the four endothelin antagonists tested in continuous infusion only the nonselective PD145065 and ET(B1/B2) selective BQ788 (in nmolar concentrations) slightly reduced the early contractile dysfunction of the heart induced

by ischemia, whereas ET(A)-selective antagonist PD155080 partially protected the rat heart on reperfusion.

Besides myocardial cells, ET-1 can be produced by vascular and endocardial endothelium. Activation of endothelin receptors modulates a wide variety of biological processes, including vascular tone, growth, and myocardial contractile function. Since increased levels of cardiac and circulating ET-1 have been linked to the development of cardiac dysfunction and severity of HF, renew interest has sprung toward the development of endothelin antagonists (ET receptor and converting enzyme inhibitors) because of the potential benefits that might derive from their use in clinical cardiology [60].

The role of the norepinephrine pathway has a well-characterized association with increased myocyte apoptosis [61, 62]; the extensive left ventricular remodeling, and resulting deterioration of cardiac function that accompanies apoptosis can be stemmed in response to treatment with the ET(A) receptor blockade using LU 135252 inhibitor [63]. When compared to paced untreated animals, treatment with LU 135252 resulted in significantly lowered levels of plasma norepinephrine [64]. Furthermore, endothelin activation may be involved in the myocardial dysfunction and specific mitochondrial enzyme deficiencies found in pacing-induced HF. Thus, elucidating the precise role of endothelin in myocardial dysfunction will be critical in the development of ET(A) antagonists as novel therapeutic agents to stop the progression of HF [65].

Angiotensin

Angiotensin converting enzyme (ACE), a central element of the renin–angiotensin system, converts the decapeptide angiotensin I to the potent pressor octapeptide angiotensin II (Ang II), mediating peripheral vascular tone, as well as glomerular filtration in the kidney. In addition to its direct effect on blood flow, Ang II directly causes changes in cell phenotype, cell growth, and apoptosis, and regulates gene expression of a broad range of bioactive molecules (e.g., vasoactive hormones, growth factors, extracellular matrix components, and cytokines). In addition, Ang II activates multiple intracellular signaling cascades, involving numerous transduction components such as MAP kinases, tyrosine kinases and various transcription factors in cardiomyocytes, fibroblasts, vascular endothelial, smooth muscle cells (SMCs), and renal cells [66]. Ang II also promotes cardiomyocyte enlargement and protein synthesis, as well as hypertrophy-associated alterations in the cardiac gene expression program through specific cellular receptor subtypes AT1 and AT2. AT1 is more abundant in the adult heart, and has been linked to both hypertrophy and apoptosis control in the cardiomyocyte.

In a model of renal dysfunction-associated HF, Li et al. [67] have recently studied in AT1 knockout (AT1KO) and wild-type mice (WT) the mechanism underlying the beneficial effects of AT1 blockade on cardiac function. Twelve weeks after nephrectomy, WT showed significant LV dilatation and dysfunction accompanied by cardiomyocyte hypertrophy, fibrosis, and reduced capillary density. These changes were less significant in AT1KO. Nephrectomy led to upregulation of myocardial expression of AT1, transforming growth factor-β1 (TGF-β1), matrix metalloproteinase (MMP)-2, MMP-9, tissue inhibitor of metalloproteinase-1 (TIMP-1), and phosphorylated Akt (p-Akt), and also led to increased oxidative damage in cardiomyocytes. In AT1KO, TGF-β1, TIMP-1, oxidative damage levels were lower, whereas MMPs and p-Akt levels were higher. Furthermore, nephrectomized WT mice treated with valsartan (an AT1 blocker), but not hydralazine, AT1 expression was down-regulated with improved cardiac function and altered molecular signaling in a manner similar to that seen in AT1KO mice.

Through the G$_q$ proteins, the AT1 receptor is coupled to a variety of intracellular signals, including the generation of oxygen free radicals, the activation of Ras, and the ERK/MAPK protein kinase family [68]. Ang II activates NF-κB-dependent transcription in other cell types, likely through its effects on the cellular redox state [69]. These actions contribute to the pathophysiology of cardiac hypertrophy and remodeling, HF, vascular thickening, and atherosclerosis [70]. Furthermore, regarding their role on the modulation of diastolic function, neurohumoral mediators like angiotensin-II and endothelin-1 have been found to have only severe side effects (e.g., cardiac hypertrophy and fibrosis). In contrast, newly published data suggest that several peptides may have a novel role on the acute modulation of cardiac diastolic function because in the acute setting, these mediators potentially induce an adaptive cardiac response [71].

Several studies have demonstrated that the AT2 receptor acts in opposition to AT1, although the myocardial AT2 receptor is less well understood. Using gain-of-function gene transfer, Nakajima et al. [72] found that the angiotensin II type 2 (AT2) receptor antagonizes the growth effects of the AT1 receptor. In rats the AT2 receptor can modulate the growth of vascular smooth muscle cells by transfecting an AT2 receptor expression vector into the balloon-injured carotid artery, and overexpression of the AT2 receptor attenuated neointimal formation. In cultured smooth muscle cells, AT2 receptor transfection reduced proliferation and inhibited mitogen-activated protein kinase activity. Furthermore, the AT2 receptor mediated the developmentally regulated decrease in aortic DNA synthesis at the latter stages of gestation. Taken together, these findings suggest that the AT2 receptor exerts an antiproliferative effect, counteracting the growth action of AT1 receptor.

To ameliorate cardiac function in myocardial infarct (MI)-induced Wistar rats, direct AT2 receptor stimulation has been tried using a novel nonpeptide AT2 receptor agonist compound 21 (C21). C21 significantly improved systolic and diastolic ventricular function and decreased scar size in the C21-treated rats. At the molecular level, C21 reduced MI-induced Fas-ligand and caspase-3 expression in the peri-infarct zone, indicating an antiapoptotic effect. Phosphorylation of the ERKs and p38 MAPK, both involved in the regulation of cell survival, was strongly reduced after MI but nearly rescued by C21 treatment. Furthermore, C21 decreased inflammation as suggested by decreased MI-induced serum monocyte chemoattractant protein-1 and myeloperoxidase as well as cardiac interleukin-6, interleukin-1β, and interleukin-2 expression [73]. Also, overexpression of AT2 receptors along with inhibition of ERKs have been associated with the cardioprotective effects of rosiglitazone (i.e., an agonist of PPARs, primarily γ receptors), in the cell nucleus, that besides its effect on insulin resistance, it appears to have an anti-inflammatory effect (NFκB levels decrease and inhibitor (IκB) levels increase) against myocardial ischemia–reperfusion injury [74–76].

Growth Transcription Factors

Coordinated regulation of progrowth and antigrowth mechanisms is required for cardiomyocyte hypertrophy. The extracellular signal-regulated kinases 1/2 (ERK1/2) are activated in cardiomyocytes by G$_q$-protein-coupled receptors, and are associated with the induction of hypertrophy. Recently, the requirement of ERK1/2 signaling in mediating the cardiac hypertrophic growth response in Erk1(−/−) and Erk2(+/−) mice, as well as in transgenic mice with inducible expression of an ERK1/2-inactivating dual-specificity phosphatase 6 in the heart, have been studied by Purcell et al. [77]. Although inducible expression of dual-specificity phosphatase 6 in the heart eliminated ERK1/2 phosphorylation at baseline, and after stimulation, without affecting any other MAPK, it did not diminish the hypertrophic response to pressure overload stimulation, neuroendocrine agonist infusion, or exercise. Similarly, Erk1(−/−) and Erk2(+/−) mice showed no reduction in pathologic or physiologic stimulus-induced cardiac growth in vivo. However, blockade or deletion of cardiac ERK1/2 did predispose to HF after long-term pressure overload in conjunction with an increase in myocyte TUNEL. Taken together, ERK1/2 signaling is not required for mediating physiologic or pathologic cardiac hypertrophy in vivo, although it does play a protective role in response to pathologic stimuli. On the other hand, in primary cardiomyocyte cultures, platelet-derived growth factor (PDGF), epidermal growth factor (EGF), and fibroblast growth factor (FGF) promoted receptor-coupled Erk1 activation and significantly increased cardiomyocyte size. This contrasts to insulin, IGF-1 and nerve growth factor (NGF), which had little effect.

Peptide growth factors activate phospholipase Cγ1 (PLCγ1), and PKC. In cardiomyocytes, only PDGF stimulated tyrosine phosphorylation of PLCγ1 and PKC. Furthermore, activation of ERK1/2 by PDGF, but not EGF, required PKC activity. In contrast, EGF substantially increased Ras-GTP with rapid activation of c-Raf, whereas stimulation of Ras-GTP loading by PDGF was minimal, and activation of c-Raf was delayed suggesting differential coupling of PDGF and EGF receptors to the ERK1/2 cascade [78].

FOXO (Forkhead O) transcription factors Foxo1 (also known as FKHR), Foxo3a (also known as FKHRL1), and Foxo4 (also known as AFX) play key roles in transmitting insulin signaling downstream of Akt [79], which contribute to cardiomyocyte remodeling and through inhibition of calcineurin signaling these factors blunt cardiac hypertrophy. Ni et al. [80] have shown that expression of either Foxo1 or Foxo3 in cardiomyocytes attenuates calcineurin phosphatase activity and inhibits agonist-induced hypertrophic growth. FOXO proteins decrease calcineurin phosphatase activity and repress both basal and hypertrophic agonist-induced expression of MCIP1.4, a direct downstream target of the calcineurin/NFAT pathway, and hearts from Foxo3-null mice exhibit increased MCIP1.4 abundance and a hypertrophic phenotype with normal systolic function at baseline. These findings suggest that FOXO proteins repress cardiac growth at least in part through inhibition of the calcineurin/NFAT pathway. Furthermore, multiple hypertrophic agonists triggered inactivation of FOXO proteins in cardiomyocytes through a mechanism requiring the PI3K/Akt pathway (see Fig. 7.1), and both Foxo1 and Foxo3 are phosphorylated and consequently inactivated in hearts undergoing hypertrophic growth induced by hemodynamic stress. This study suggests that inhibition of the calcineurin/NFAT signaling cascade by FOXO and the release of this repressive action by the PI3K/Akt pathway are important mechanisms for FOXO factors to regulate cardiomyocyte growth. Furthermore, besides playing a significant role in the cell survival pathway (see Chap. 7) FOXO proteins, in particular Foxo1 and Foxo3, have been found in the developing myocardium from embryonic to neonatal stages together with increased cyclin kinase inhibitor expression. Embryonic cardiomyocytes were found to be responsive to IGF-1 stimulation, which results in the induction of the PI3K/AKT pathway, cytoplasmic localization of FOXO proteins, and increased myocyte proliferation [81].

Toll-Like Receptors

There is evidence that Toll-like receptors (TLR) activation contributes to the development and progression of athero-sclerosis, cardiac dysfunction in sepsis, and congestive HF [82]. However, the role that individual members of the TLR family play in the pathophysiology of cardiovascular diseases remains unknown.

Increased expression of innate immune response proteins, including IL-1β, TNF-α, and the cytokine-inducible isoform of nitric oxide synthase (iNOS) has been detected in the failing heart of human and experimental animals, regardless of etiology (see Chap. 12). Transmembrane signaling proteins of the TLR constitute key signaling elements in both macrophages and in atherosclerotic lesions. The Toll-like receptor 4 (TLR4) is highly expressed in the heart, and this expression is strongly up-regulated in mice with cardiac ischemia (relative to controls), in patients with DCM and in the myocardium of patients with advanced HF [83, 84], and is consistent with the activation of signaling pathways leading to the expression of proinflammatory cytokines, which have been implicated in the etiology of DCM. Furthermore, myocardial TLR4 levels were positively correlated with the levels of enteroviral replication in DCM [85]. In normal murine and human myocardium, TLR4 expression is diffused but predominantly confined to cardiac myocytes; in myocardium from patients with advanced HF, however, there are focal areas of intense TLR4 staining. Notwithstanding, the cause and mechanism of this change in TLR4 expression in the failing myocardium remain unknown; interestingly, IRAK1 as well as NFκB (key components of TLR signaling) are activated by cardiac ischemia, as seen in experimental models and in human HF secondary to myocardial infarction [86, 87].

That TLR4 serves a proinflammatory role in ischemia-reperfusion (I/R) injury, has been provided by observations that TLR4-deficient mice sustain smaller infarctions, and exhibit less inflammation after myocardial I/R injury [88]. Systemic administration of lipopolysaccharide (LPS), a TLR4 agonist, confers a cardioprotective effect against ischemic injury and myocardial infarction (MI) [89]. On the other hand, data from chimeric mice have implicated TLR4 effect on leukocytes (not on cardiac myocytes), as an important factor for cardiac myocyte impairment during endotoxemia [90]. Furthermore, the Toll-like receptor 2 (TLR2) is directly involved in mediating the response of cardiomyocytes to OS (e.g., H_2O_2) [91], and OS-induced cytotoxicity and apoptosis are enhanced by blocking TLR2.

In addition, the TLR signaling cascade appears to play an important role in hypertrophy as suggested by the Tlr4 knockout mice, which compared to wild type, present less severe cardiac hypertrophy after pressure overload secondary to aortic banding [92]; also critical in the hypertrophic growth are the phosphoinositide 3-kinase (PI3K), protein kinase B (Akt), and mammalian target of rapamycin (mTOR) since inhibition of mTOR results in further decrease in the degree of cardiac hypertrophy in Tlr4 knockout mice. This indicates that TLR-mediated and mTOR-mediated hypertrophy follow separate pathways [93]. Also, mice with cardio-myocyte-restricted expression of a NFκB superrepressor had impaired angiotensin-II-induced cardiac hypertrophy and isoproterenol-induced hypertrophy without increasing the susceptibility to apoptosis [94] confirming that the TLR pathway has an important role in hypertrophic growth in addition to mTOR signaling.

Protease Activated Receptors

A number of signaling events are critical factors in the cardiac remodeling process with the development of hypertrophy first and HF later. A novel class of protease-activated receptors (PAR-1, PAR-2, PAR-3, and PAR-4), containing seven transmembrane G-protein-coupled domains, has been identified as an important participant in distinct cardiac signaling pathways. These receptors are activated by cleavage with serine proteases such as thrombin and trypsin [95]. Extracellular proteolytic activation of protease activated receptors results in: (1) cleavage of specific sites in the extracellular domain; (2) formation of a new N-terminus (often containing the sequence SFLLRN), which functions as a tethered ligand, and binds to an exposed site in the second transmembrane loop triggering G-protein binding; (3) intracellular signaling.

PAR-1, a high-affinity receptor for thrombin, is expressed by a variety of cell types in the heart, including cardiomyocytes and cardiac fibroblasts. Chronic/persistent PAR-1 activation leads to cardiomyocyte hypertrophy and cardiac fibroblast proliferation [96], with PAR-1-dependent growth responses in these two types of cells happening through distinct signaling mechanisms. In cardiomyocytes expressing PAR-1, agonist binding and activation of PAR leads to InsP3 accumulation, stimulation of extracellular signal-regulated (ERK) protein kinase, and modulated contractile function. Coexpression in cardiomyocytes of PAR-2, activated by trypsin/tryptase but not thrombin, with PAR-1 leads to a more extensive signaling response including InsP3 accumulation, stimulation of MAP kinases (both ERK and p38 MAP kinase), elevated Ca^{2+} levels and contractile function as well as the activation of JNK and Akt, associated with growth and/or survival pathways and induction of both cardiomyocyte hypertrophy and elongation [97]. While PAR-1 evokes a significant increase in ERK, p38 MAPK, and Akt, and increases DNA synthesis through an epidermal growth factor receptor (EGFR) transactivation pathway in cardiac fibroblasts, PAR-1 in cardiomyocytes activates ERK (and induces only a minor increase in Akt) by a mechanism that does not require EGFR kinase activity [98].

Interestingly, PAR-1, PAR-2, and PAR-4 have been implicated in vascular development, as well as in a variety of other biological processes, including apoptosis and remodeling [97]. In mice with chronic HF the expression of PAR-1 can be normalized following the administration of cardiospecific tissue inhibitor of metalloproteinase-4 (TIMP-4/CIMP); also, amelioration was noted in oxidative-proteolytic stress and endothelial-myocyte uncoupling [99]. Furthermore, in PAR-1$^{+/-}$ mice bred to generate PAR-1$^{+/+}$ and PAR-1$^{-/-}$ littermate mice [100] deficiency of PAR-1 decreased dilatation of the left ventricle and ameliorated left ventricular (LV) function after I/R injury. Activation of ERK1/2 was also increased in injured PAR-1$^{-/-}$ mice compared with wild-type mice; however, PAR-1 deficiency did not affect infarct size. While cardiomyocyte-specific overexpression of PAR-1 in mice induced eccentric hypertrophy and DCM, deletion of the tissue factor gene reduced the eccentric hypertrophy [101]. On the other hand, it has been shown that a competitive inhibitor of PAR-1 (SCH 79797) protects the rat's heart against acute I/R injury [102], and the possibility that another PAR, such as PAR-4 is compensating for the PAR-1 deficiency has been suggested [103].

Receptor Tyrosine Kinases

Over 20 Receptor tyrosine kinase (RTK) classes have been identified in this large family of receptors, all of which share a similar structure that includes a ligand binding extracellular domain, a single transmembrane domain, and an intracellular tyrosine kinase domain. This large protein family includes the receptors for many growth factors and for insulin. Most of the RTK subfamilies are defined by the extracellular region containing the ligand binding domains, which exhibit variable length and subdomain composition with highly conserved structural motifs, including domains that are immunoglobulin-binding, cysteine-rich, ephrin-binding, and fibronectin repeats [104].

Except in the case of the insulin receptor, which exists as a dimer in the absence of ligand, ligand binding to the extracellular portion of these receptors results in receptor dimerization, which facilitates the trans-autophosphorylation of specific tyrosine residues in the highly conserved cytoplasmic portion (Fig. 9.2). The phosphotyrosine residues enhance the receptor catalytic activity, and can provide docking sites for downstream signaling proteins. The creation of docking sites allows the recruitment to the receptor kinase complex of a variety of proteins containing specific binding domains, such as Src homology 2 and 3 or phosphotyrosine binding domains, which can broaden the signaling capacity of the RTKs. For instance, GPCRs which lack an intrinsic kinase activity possessed by RTKs, such as PDGFR or EGFR have been shown to activate RTKs in response to stimulation by cytokines, cell adhesion, and stress stimuli. In this way,

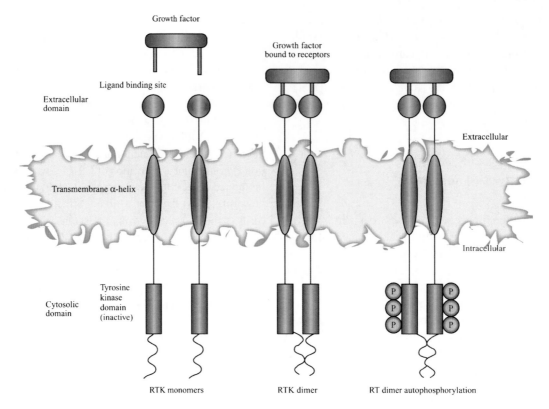

Fig. 9.2 Receptor tyrosine kinases. Ligand binding to the extracellular portion of these receptors results in receptor dimerization, which facilitates the trans-autophosphorylation of specific tyrosine residues in the highly conserved cytoplasmic portion. RTKs are phosphorylated in response to stimulation by cytokines, cell adhesion and stress stimuli

RTKs can function in integrating a large array of stimuli from diverse environmental and intracellular inputs.

Phosphorylation, although necessary, may not be sufficient to fully activate many RTKs. Oligomerization-induced conformational changes may be necessary to modulate the kinetic properties of RTKs, and render them fully functional. Because of the critical roles played by RTKs in cellular signaling processes, their catalytic activity is normally under tight control by a variety of intrinsic regulatory mechanisms as well as by protein phosphotyrosine phosphatases (PTPs).

Although cardiomyocyte signaling pathways may activate tyrosine kinases, the role of specific PTPs in these pathways is unknown. Recently, Kontaridis et al. [105] reported that deletion of Ptpn11 (Shp2) in cardiomyocyte causes DCM via effects on the extracellular signal-regulated kinase/mitogen-activated protein kinase and RhoA signaling pathways. Interestingly, mice with muscle-specific deletion of Ptpn11, rapidly develop a phenotype of compensated DCM without an intervening hypertrophic phase, with cardiac dysfunction appearing by the second postnatal month. Shp2-deficient primary cardiomyocytes are defective in extracellular signal-regulated kinase/mitogen-activated protein kinase (Erk/MAPK) activation in response to a variety of soluble agonists and

pressure overload, but show hyperactivation of the RhoA signaling pathway. The response to treatment of primary cardiomyocytes with ERK1/2- and RhoA pathway-specific inhibitors suggested that both abnormal Erk/MAPK and RhoA activities contribute to the dilated cardiomyopathy phenotype of Shp2-deficient hearts.

A number of RTKs have been shown to play essential roles in early cardiac development as well as in the growth, repair, and survival of adult cardiomyocytes as part of a signaling network. For example, the erbB2 RTK is known to have a critical role in cardiac development. In addition, erbB2 participates in an important pathway that involves neuregulins, cell–cell signaling proteins that are ligands for RTKs of the ErbB family, and the neuregulin receptor erbB4. Two of the neuregulins (NRG-1 and NRG-2) and their receptors (erbB2 and erbB4) are essential for normal cardiac development, and can mediate hypertrophic growth and enhance the survival of embryonic, postnatal, and adult ventricular cardiomyocytes. Targeting the neuregulin receptors to caveolae microdomains, within cardiac myocytes, has been shown to be a viable approach to regulate neuregulin signaling in the heart [106, 107]. New evidence for the involvement of neuregulin-1/ErbB signals in HF is emerging. Recently, changes in NRG-1 expression, ErbB receptor phosphorylation and downstream activation of intracellular ErbB targets during rapid pacing and progressive ventricular dysfunction in the dog have been reported by Doggen et al. [108]. mRNA expression was measured in ventricular biopsies using quantitative PCR, and activation of NRG-1/ErbB signaling and of downstream targets were investigated using immunoprecipitation and/or Western blotting. Over the course of 7 weeks of pacing, ventricular levels of NRG-1, but not of other ErbB4 ligands, and of ADAM19, a protease promoting NRG-1 release, progressively increased. Also, levels of activated ErbB2 and ErbB4, phosphorylated at tyrosine residues 877/1248 and 1284, respectively, became progressively higher, and levels of total and phosphorylated PI3 kinase increased. In contrast with activation of downstream targets of ErbB receptors in normal hearts, Akt and ERK1/2, remained inactivated. Taken together these findings suggest that ventricular ErbB2 and ErbB4 receptors become activated during the development of pacing-induced HF, but that the downstream signaling is, at least partly, abrogated; nonetheless, the underlying mechanisms for these findings remain to be established. Interestingly, new data from animal studies as well as preliminary data from human seem to reinforce the concept that NRG-1 has a remarkable effect on the recovery of the pumping function of the failing heart, and has prompted the investigation on the possible use of NRG-1 as a novel treatment of HF. So far, the available animal data and preliminary human findings seem to hold the promise that human recombinant NRG may have a positive effect in the management of HF [109].

RTKs also play a pivotal role in the growth responses of vascular cells. RTKs include the VEGF receptors, Eph receptors, Tie1, and Tie2, all of which are expressed on vascular endothelial cells, as well as the PDGF receptors, which are expressed on vascular SMCs [110, 111]. While all of these RTKs activate many similar effector molecules, some of the signals initiated appear to be distinct. This could explain, at least in part, how different RTKs expressed in the developing vasculature can direct unique biological functions.

Using PTP inhibitors, improvement of peripheral endothelial dysfunction in HF has been reported by Vercauteren et al. [112]. In mice with chronic HF, the PTP1B inhibitors AS279, AS098, and AS713 restored blood flow to levels similar to those of control normal mice. This flow restoration was reduced by inhibitors of eNOS and PI3K. Polymerase chain reaction and Western blotting showed that arteries express PTP1B, and this expression was not affected by HF. Immunolocalization revealed the presence of PTP1B in the endothelium and the adventitia. PTP1B inhibition stimulated early eNOS phosphorylation and increased phosphorylation of Akt. Taken together these findings demonstrated that PTP1B inhibitors may be a potent treatment to restore endothelial function in HF.

G-Proteins

Chapter 8 dealt with G-protein coupled receptors in the context that β1-adrenergic receptors are coupled to the G-protein G_s to activate AC, and produce second messenger, cyclic AMP. Also, β2-adrenergic receptors are coupled to G_s as well as the inhibitory G_i, and they also increase cyclic AMP levels. Furthermore, parasympathetic activity and muscarinic receptor activation of coupled to G_i inhibits AC, leading to a lower cyclic AMP level. Cyclic AMP production by adenylyl cyclase leads to increased cardiac function.

A number of hormones and neurotransmitters exert their physiological effects through activation of G-protein-coupled receptors (GPCRs). Approximately, 1,000 GPCR genes are present in the human genome and these represent a primary target for drug development. Because GPCRs play a central role in cardiac regulation, the identification of new G-proteins with physiologic and pathophysiologic significance is a work in progress, mainly on the potential discovery of drugs that can act upon these GPCRs. Our overall hypothesis is that there are novel GPCRs that can be targeted in HF, representing new directions in both translational research and experimental therapeutics. Several laboratories are investing significant resources in developing new animal models and in vitro systems where novel GPCR, targeted to HF can be found. Alternatively, these novel GPCRs could be used as biomarkers in the diagnosis and prognostication of human HF. Furthermore, to accelerate the discovery of drugs targeting GPCRs across diverse therapeutic areas, including HF, broad-based technological platform are currently being employed.

Interestingly, upon activation with the appropriate ligands, GPCRs, also known as seven transmembrane domain receptors, are converted into the active conformation, and are able to complex with and activate heterotrimeric G-proteins [113]. The heterotrimeric G-proteins are composed of three subunits: the α subunit, which carries the guanine–nucleotide binding site, and the β and γ subunits, which form a tightly bound dimer. Inactive G-proteins are heterotrimers composed of a GDP-bound α subunit associated with the $G_{\beta\gamma}$ dimer, which serves to anchor the heterotrimeric G-protein to the membrane. The activated GPCRs function as GDP/GTP exchange factors, and promote the release of GDP and the binding of GTP to the α subunits leading to dissociation of the α subunit and the $G_{\beta\gamma}$ dimer. As noted previously, GTP-G_α and $G_{\beta\gamma}$ can interact with a variety of effectors, such as AC and PLC, in order to modulate cellular signaling pathways. The deactivation of GPCR signaling occurs at several levels. Importantly, the G_α subunit has an innate GTPase activity, which hydrolyses GTP to GDP, and promotes reassociation with $G_{\beta\gamma}$ to form the inactive heterotrimer. In addition, ligand dissociation from the GPCRs converts the receptors back to their inactive state.

Heterotrimeric G-proteins are classified into subclasses according to the α subunit, with each subfamily designated by its corresponding downstream signaling effect. The $G_{\alpha s}$ or more simply G_S-proteins are stimulatory regulators of AC, linking receptor stimulation (e.g., β-AR) to the accumulation of the second messenger, cyclic AMP (cAMP). The G_S subunit is a target of covalent modification by cholera toxin (CTX), which slows GTP hydrolysis, locking G_S in an active GTP-bound form that constitutively stimulates AC. In contrast, the $G_{\alpha i/o}$ or $G_{i/o}$ proteins inhibit AC activity. These proteins are targets for ADP-ribosylation by the pertussis toxin (PTX), which prevents their interaction with receptors, and inhibits their downstream signaling. The other two subfamilies, G_q and $G_{12/13}$ proteins are insensitive to PTX and CTX. The GTP-bound $G_{\alpha q}$-protein activates phosphoinositide phospholipase C-β (PLC-β), leading to generation of InsP3 and DAG, accompanied by the mobilization of calcium and the activation of PKC, respectively. Dissociated $G_{\beta\gamma}$ can activate small GTP binding protein Ras and initiate a tyrosine kinase cascade leading to the activation of MAPK. Furthermore, G_q may activate MAPK independently of $G_{\beta\gamma}$ via a mechanism that is PKC dependent [62].

Hormones such as angiotensin II, endothelin 1, and norepinephrine, which bind and activate cardiomyocyte membrane receptors coupled to the G_q-proteins, have been implicated in the development and ultimate decompensation of cardiac hypertrophy [54].

Regulators of G-protein signaling (RGS) proteins are a family of proteins that accelerate intrinsic GTP hydrolysis on α subunits of heterotrimeric G-proteins [114]. They play crucial roles in the physiological regulation of G-protein-mediated cell signaling. In addition, the small G-proteins are a superfamily of guanine nucleotide-binding proteins with a size ranging from 20 to 25 kDa, including several subfamilies such as Ras, Rho, Rab, Ran, and ADP ribosylation factor(s). These small G-proteins act as molecular switches to regulate numerous cellular responses, including cardiac myocyte hypertrophy and cell survival associated with cell growth and division, multiple changes in the cytoskeleton, vesicular transport, and myofibrillar apparatus. They share some features with the heterotrimeric G-proteins, including activation by the exchange of GDP to GTP, and inactivation by their return to a GDP-bound state, which is enhanced by GTPase activating proteins. Not surprisingly, there are regions of homology shared between these proteins and the G_α subunit. Modification of these proteins by isoprenylation promotes their attachment to the membrane. However, the activation of the small G-proteins differs from that of the heterotrimeric G-proteins in one critical respect. With the heterotrimeric G-proteins, ligand binding to a GPCR is the primary stimulus that promotes GDP release from GDP binding to the α subunit, whereas an association with ago-nist-occupied receptors is not found with small G-proteins (e.g., Ras and Rho). Instead, activation by the release of GDP from the small G-proteins is primarily mediated by the activation of guanine nucleotide exchange factors (GEFs). Hearts from transgenic mice expressing activated Ras develop features consistent with myocardial hypertrophy, whereas mice overexpressing RhoA develop lethal HF. In isolated neonatal rat cardiac myocytes, transfection or infection with activated Ras, RhoA, or Rac1 induces features of hypertrophy. Interestingly, overexpression of the G-protein $G_{\alpha q}$ or constitutively active components of its signaling pathway have been shown in transgenic studies to lead to increased cardiac mass, cardiomyocyte hypertrophy, contractile dysfunction and ventricular remodeling (a list of several identified gene mutations in cardiac signaling proteins is shown in Chap. 7).

G-proteins and second messenger pathways function differently in cardiac fibroblasts from those in cardiac myocytes. Cardiac fibroblasts are important cellular components of the myocardial responses to injury, and to hypertrophic stimuli. In cardiac fibroblasts, agonists such as bradykinin stimulate inositol phosphate production, and increased intracellular Ca^{2+} levels, while endothelin-1 and norepinephrine do not, in contrast to their action in cardiac myocytes. Cardiac fibroblasts express functional G-protein-linked receptors that couple to G_q and G_s, with little or no coupling to G_i. The expression of receptors and their coupling to G_q but not to G_i-linked responses distinguishes the signaling in cardiac fibroblasts from that in myocytes. Furthermore, agonists that activate G_q in fibroblasts also potentiate the stimulation of G_s, an example of signaling cross talk not previously observed in adult cardiomyocytes [115]. Representing new directions in both translational research and experimental therapeutics, it is plausible that the discovery of novel GPCRs can be targeted in HF.

Nuclear Receptor Transcription Factors

Nuclear receptor transcription factors are important regulatory players governing the cardiac metabolic gene program [116]. This superfamily of receptors has been previously described as ligand-dependent transcription factors, which is in fact the case for nearly 50% of those characterized [117]. Such ligand-activated receptors include the classical endocrine receptors that respond to steroid or thyroid hormones. Interestingly, a number of receptors have been identified (without prior insight to their ligands), that respond to dietary-derived lipid intermediates, including long-chain fatty acids (LCFAs) and bile acids. These receptors generally participate in the regulation of pathways involved in the metabolism of the activating ligands. On the other hand, a group of "orphan" nuclear receptors have no identifiable ligands (although modulating ligands may be soon identified for some of these receptors).

Of particular interest are the peroxisome proliferator-activated receptors (PPARs), fatty acid-activated nuclear receptors, increasingly recognized as key regulators of cardiac fatty acid metabolism. The PPAR-α isoform has been characterized as the central regulator of mitochondrial fatty acid catabolism, including fatty acid oxidation (FAO), whereas PPAR-γ primarily regulates lipid storage [116]. Moreover, orphan nuclear receptors that serve new roles in the regulation of cardiac energy metabolism have been identified.

The nuclear receptors bind to regulatory DNA elements in target genes as homodimers, heterodimers, or in some cases as monomers. Unlike the classic steroid receptors that function as homodimers, a number of the nuclear receptors involved in nutrient sensing and metabolic regulation (e.g., PPARs, TR, RAR) heterodimerize with the retinoid X receptor (RXR). The interaction of these receptors with regulatory DNA elements is within the 5' regulatory region of their target genes that are composed of variably spaced hexameric half-sites (AGGTCA) arranged as direct, indirect, or everted repeats. Once bound to their specific response element, the receptors recruit coactivator proteins often in concert with the displacement of corepressor proteins. One such adaptor/coactivator, the PPAR gamma coactivator-1 (PGC-1), serves as a key link between physiological cues and metabolic regulation in heart.

Effectors Signaling

Adenylyl Cyclase

Since the role that adenylyl cyclase (AC) plays on cardiac β-adrenergic signaling had been addressed in Chap. 8; here, it is suffice to say that increased AC, independent of β-AR number and G-protein content, provides a means to regulate cardiac responsiveness to β-AR stimulation [118]. Overexpressing an effector such as AC does not alter transmembrane signaling except when receptors are activated, in contrast to receptor/G-protein overexpression, which promotes continuous activation with detrimental consequences [119, 120]. This suggests that AC overexpression may be a novel target for safely increasing cardiac responsiveness to β-AR stimulation [118].

Expression of type V AC isoform is restricted to the heart and brain, and generates the major AC isoform found in the adult heart. Type V AC is potently activated through PKC-mediated phosphorylation, and the degree of this activation is greater than that achieved by forskolin, the most potent AC agonist. Furthermore, the two PKC isoenzymes are additive

in their capacity to activate AC. In contrast, PKA-mediated phosphorylation inhibits type V AC. Thus, type V AC is subject to dual regulation by phosphorylation: activation by PKC and inhibition by PKA, mediated via phosphorylation at unique residues within the type V molecule [121].

PKA-mediated inactivation of AC creates a feedback system within the cAMP-signaling pathway, analogous to PKC-mediated inhibition of the phospholipase C pathway. Catecholamine stimulation in the heart activates both the phospholipase C/PKC pathway via α-adrenoreceptors, and the AC/PKA pathway via β-adrenergic receptors. Regulation of AC by PKC and PKA may play a key role in the integration of these two principal signal transduction pathways, modulating neuronal and hormonal input to the heart.

Phospholipase C

Diverse and distinct hormonal stimuli engage specific surface receptors of the cardiomyocyte to initiate the hydrolysis of inositol phospholipids, mediated by the effector phospholipase C (PLC), while changes in intracellular levels of InsP3 and inositol 1,3,4,5-tetrakisphosphate, DAG and Ca^{2+} result in the specific phosphorylation of cellular proteins by various protein kinases such as the PKC family, Ca^{2+}-calmodulin-dependent kinase, and MAPK. Four classes of PLC isozymes are considered to underlie these signaling responses [122].

A myriad of seven transmembrane-spanning receptors activate isozymes of the PLC-β class through the release of α-subunits of the G_q family of heterotrimeric G-proteins. A subset of PLC-β isozymes can also be activated by $G_{\beta\gamma}$. PLC-γ isozymes are activated by protein phosphorylation following the activation of RTKs. Another class of PLC isozymes (PLC-ϵ) has been found to be involved in signaling [123], and exhibits a novel pattern of regulation mediated by the Ras oncoprotein and $G_{\alpha12}$-subunits of heterotrimeric G-proteins.

Phospholipase D2 (PLD2) is the major PLD isozyme associated with the cardiac sarcolemmal (SL) membrane. It hydrolyses phosphatidylcholine to produce phosphatidic acid, an important phospholipid signaling molecule known to influence cardiac function [124].

Expression of PLD isozyme mRNA, protein contents and activities have been measured in rat congestive HF secondary to myocardial infarction. In the failing heart SL PLD1 and PLD2 protein contents, were elevated in the viable LV tissue, but SL PLD1 activity was significantly decreased and SL PLD2 activity was significantly increased. In the scar tissue PLD2 protein and activity were detected, but not PLD1 protein. Thus, differential changes in PLD isozymes may contribute to the pathophysiology of CHF and may be involved in the processes of scar remodeling [125].

Caveolae/Caveolins

It has been established that mechanical unloading ameliorates cardiac adrenergic responsiveness and lipid metabolism, and these processes seem to be regulated by caveolar function. Uray et al. [126] have tested the hypothesis that mechanical unloading in patients receiving left ventricle assisting devices (LVADs), as a bridge to cardiac transplantation, alters the expression of caveolins and these changes are linked to altered the expression of markers of reverse remodeling. Paired myocardial samples were obtained and transcript levels were measured using real-time Q-RT-PCR in prepared RNA. Caveolin-1 and -3 protein levels were determined by Western blots and caveolin-3 localization was determined by immunohistochemistry. Caveolin-1 protein levels were upregulated in all LVAD-patients after mechanical unloading, and caveolin-1 mRNA was increased in 76% of the patients. Interestingly, the higher induction of caveolin-1 was associated with greater suppression of ANF. Caveolin-3 transcript levels increased in 82% of the cohort, along with a 2.5-fold induction of caveolin-2. Sarcolemmal caveolin-3 staining was increased after LVAD-support, although no change in total caveolin-3 protein was detected. The mRNA levels of the caveolin-associated CD36 (thrombospondin receptor) also increased with unloading. Patients with ischemic cardiomyopathy showed greater induction of CD36 than nonischemic cases, as well as highly correlated changes in the expression of caveolin isoforms. Thus, mechanical unloading in HF patients induces the expression of caveolins and CD36; the enhanced caveolin expression may be related to reverse remodeling of lipid metabolism, NO production and adrenergic signaling.

Caveolae are small organelles (50–100 nm), invagination-like plasma membranes, present in many cell types, and particularly abundant in cells of the cardiovascular system, including endothelial cells, SMCs, macrophages, cardiac myocytes, and fibroblasts. In these cell types, caveolae function both in protein trafficking and signal transduction. In vertebrates, the caveolin family of proteins is integrated by three members of similar structure: caveolin-1, caveolin-2, and caveolin-3. These proteins (primarily caveolin-2, and caveolin-3 in cardiomyocytes) are both necessary, and sufficient for the formation of caveolae membrane domains. Caveolin forms oligomers and associates with cholesterol and sphingolipids in certain areas of the cell membrane, leading to the formation of caveolae. In a number of ways, caveolins serve both to compartmentalize and to concentrate key signaling proteins, thereby regulating cardiomyocyte signaling. Furthermore, caveolin-1 has also been shown to play a role in the integrins (i.e., cell surface receptors that interact with the extracellular matrix and mediate various intracellular signals from it) signaling. Multiple components of signaling cascades including β-ARs, G-proteins, AC, the Rho family of small GTPases, PKCα, PKCε, and ERK have been localized to caveolae [127, 128]. Colocalization of G-protein pathway signaling molecules may be a contributory factor in both the spatial and temporal regulation of cardiomyocyte signal transduction.

Studies on caveolin-deficient mouse models demonstrated that caveolae and caveolins can promote a number of pathological phenotypes, including atherosclerosis, cardiac hypertrophy and cardiomyopathy, pulmonary hypertension, and neointimal hyperplasia (smooth muscle cell proliferation) [129].

Regulatory Players: Transcription Factors

NF-κB

NF-κB is a pleiotropic family of transcription factor implicated in the regulation of diverse biological phenomena, including apoptosis, cell survival, growth, division and differentiation, innate immunity, and the responses to stress, hypoxia, stretch and ischemia. In the heart, NF-κB is activated in atherosclerosis, myocarditis, during transplant rejection, after myocardial I/R, in congestive HF, DCM, after ischemic and pharmacological preconditioning, heat shock, and in hypertrophy of isolated cardiomyocytes. In addition to being activated by cytokine-mediated pathways, NF-κB is modulated by many of the signal transduction cascades associated with the development of cardiac hypertrophy, and response to oxidative stress. Many of these signaling cascades activate NF-κB by activating the IκB kinase (IKK) complex. These signaling interactions primarily involve the MAP kinase/ERK kinases (MEKKs) that are components of MAPK signaling pathways. In addition, other signaling factors directly activate NF-κB via IκB or via direct phosphorylation of NF-κB subunits. Combinatorial interactions have been reported at the level of the promoter between NF-κB, its coactivators, and other transcription factors, several of which are activated by MAPK and cytokine signaling pathways. In addition to being a major mediator of cytokine effects in the heart, NF-κB represents a signaling integrator, functioning as a key regulator of cardiac gene expression programs, downstream of multiple signal transduction cascades in a variety of physiological, and pathophysiological states. Genetic blockade of NF-κB can reduce the size of infarcts resulting from I/R in the murine heart, consistent with its role as a major determinant of cell death after I/R, and suggests that NF-κB may constitute an important therapeutic target in specific cardiovascular diseases [130].

PPAR-α and Cofactors (RXR and PGC)

For further discussion on these nuclear transcription factors, critical regulatory players controlling the heart metabolic gene program, the reader is addressed to the above section "Nuclear Receptor Transcription Factors" and Chap. 5.

Stress and Metabolic Signaling

The list of extracellular influences and intracellular-generated signals, which impact the cardiomyocyte, continues to grow. In addition to hormonal and cytokines stimuli, such as TH, TNF-α and interleukins, there are also pro/antiapoptotic modulators, nutrient, serum, growth, and mitotic factors, as well as stress and metabolic stimuli which we will describe in more detail in this section.

Stress Signals

Stresses in cardiac hypertrophy (e.g., mechanical) and ischemia/hypoxia (e.g., oxidative) elicit a variety of adaptive responses at the tissue, cellular, and molecular levels. A current model displaying the cardiac physiological response to hypoxia suggests the existence of a mitochondrial O_2 sensor coupled to a signal transduction system, which in turn activates a functional response [131]. As pointed out in Chap. 5, myocardial mitochondria may function as O_2 sensors by increasing their generation of ROS during hypoxia and with their abundant heme proteins (e.g., cytochrome c oxidase), which reversibly bind oxygen. Similarly, mitochondria in cultured cells from pulmonary artery function as O_2 sensors which underlie hypoxic pulmonary vasoconstriction [132]. Respiratory inhibitors such as rotenone abolish the hypoxic vasoconstriction; ROS plays a significant role in the mitochondrial signaling in the hypoxic response. Oxidant signals such as ROS act as second messengers initiating signaling cascades and are prominent features in both adaptive responses to hypoxia and mechanically-stressed heart. Down-regulation of cytochrome c oxidase (COX) activity contributes to the increased ROS generation and signaling observed in cardiomyocytes during hypoxia [133]. Also, hypoxia stimulates NO synthesis in cardiomyocytes [134], and NO down-regulates COX activity with subsequent mitochondrial H_2O_2 production. This event has been proposed to provide a mitochondrial-generated signal for further regulating redox-sensitive signaling pathways, including apoptosis and can proceed even in the absence of marked changes in ATP levels [134]. Interestingly, although NOS has been iden-

tified in heart mitochondria its role in regulating OXPHOS is not clear [135]; also mitochondrial ROS has been shown to activate p38 MAPK in hypoxic cardiomyocytes [136]. Longer term responses to hypoxia have been shown to include increased gene expression of hypoxia-induced factors (HIF) and the activation of transcription factors such as NF-κB which have also been implicated in the complex regulation of cardiac hypertrophy and inflammatory cytokines (e.g., TNF-α, IL-1) (see Chap. 13). Although increased ROS has been shown to be an important element in NF-κB gene activation, there is evidence that cardiomyocyte HIF gene activation can also occur in the absence of ROS [137].

It is worth noting, that human HF may be associated with alterations in multiple components of the IL-6-glycoprotein (gp) 130 receptor system, which suggests that they play an important role in cardiac pathophysiology. Experimental studies have shown that the common receptor subunit of IL-6 cytokines is phosphorylated in response to pressure overload and myocardial infarction and activates at least three different downstream signaling pathways: The signal transducers and activators of transcription 1 and 3 (STAT1/3), the Src-homology tyrosine phosphatase 2 (SHP2)-Ras-ERK, and the PI3K-Akt system [138]. Gp130 receptor-mediated signaling promotes cardiomyocyte survival, induces hypertrophy, and modulates cardiac extracellular matrix and cardiac function. Thus, the gp130 receptor system and its main downstream mediator STAT3 play a key role in survival and cardioprotection.

Metabolic Signals

The cardiomyocyte responds to changes in cellular levels of key metabolites such as adenosine, ATP, ADP, oxygen, NADH, as well as numerous substrates and coenzymes. After birth, cardiac FAO becomes critical as a bioenergetic substrate and source of electrons/NADH for the TCA cycle and respiratory chain function [139]. Fatty acids also physically interact with mitochondrial membranes affecting membrane structure and function, such as transport and excitability. Increased accumulation of intermediary metabolites of fatty acids, which occur with defective mitochondrial FAO and transport, is considered responsible for cardiac dysrhythmias and also contribute to HF and sudden death [140]. Long-chain fatty acids (LCFAs), for example palmitate, can modulate the proton conductance of the inner mitochondrial membrane (increased uncoupling) and affect the opening of the PT pore, determining the release of apoptogenic proteins into the cytosol [141]. Major myocardial targets of hormone signaling (thyroid hormone) as well as of LCFAs such as palmitate include the uncoupling proteins (UCP1–UCP5), carrier proteins located within the inner mitochondrial membrane, which functions to dissipate the proton gradient across the membrane. These proteins are upregulated transcriptionally in the presence of palmitate and T3 [142, 143]. Interestingly, cardiac expression of one of the uncoupling protein genes (UCP3) has been reported to be PPAR-α-dependent [144]. In addition, increased expression of uncoupling proteins in cardiac muscle results in increased uncoupling of OXPHOS from respiration, decreased myocardial efficiency and mitochondrial membrane potential [143]. Recently, Murray et al. [145] have studied whether increased mitochondrial UCP levels contribute to decreased energetics in HF, by measuring UCPs and respiration in mitochondria isolated from the viable myocardium of chronically infarcted rat hearts, and also by measuring efficiency (hydraulic work/O_2 consumption) in the isolated, working rat's heart. After 10 weeks postinfarction, UCP3 levels were increased by 53% in the infarcted, failing hearts (ejection fractions below 45%), and cardiac UCP3 levels correlated positively with nonfasting plasma FFAs. Mitochondria coupling (measuring ADP/O ratio) in HF animals was below that in control hearts. Furthermore, the decreased ADP/O ratio was reflected in lower efficiency in the failing hearts when perfused with 1 mM palmitate, compared to controls. Taken together these findings showed that the failing heart has increased UCP3 levels associated with high circulating FFA concentrations, mitochondrial uncoupling, and decreased cardiac efficiency, suggesting that respiratory uncoupling may underlie the abnormal energetics and decreased efficiency found in the failing heart; although, whether these alterations are maladaptive or adaptive could not be determined. A discussion on role of UCPs in cardiac remodeling is presented in Chap. 11.

Extracellular Signals and Matrix

Besides providing structural and mechanical support, the heart extracellular matrix (ECM) plays a critical role in cellular signaling [146]. This signaling becomes most apparent during myocardial remodeling, which may develop as either a physiological or pathological response as it occurs in cardiac hypertrophy and in the progression to HF.

An important link exists between the ECM and the cardiomyocyte cytoskeleton, since during the progression to HF, changes in ECM and cardiomyocytes will lead to a change in the interaction between these two; this interaction is essential for mechanotransduction. One class of cell-surface receptor molecules that constitute part of that link are the transmembrane integrins, which act as signaling molecules and transducers of mechanical force [147]. Interestingly, integrins are expressed in all cellular components of the cardiovascular system, including the vasculature, blood, cardiac myocytes and nonmuscle cardiac cells. In response to specific changes in their micro-environment, these receptors become activated and form focal adhesions, areas of attachment of the cells to ECM proteins involving the colocalization of cytoskeletal proteins, intracellular signaling molecules, and growth factor receptors. Growth factor-mediated integrin activation can stimulate cell growth, gene expression and adhesion in cardiac fibroblasts [148]. In addition, a large number of bioactive signaling molecules and growth factors, proteases, and structural proteins have been identified that influence cell–matrix interactions. ECM proteins can be degraded by matrix metalloproteinases (MMPs), the activation of which is associated with ventricular remodeling. The dynamic balance of degradative enzymes, the MMPs, their regulation by multifunctional endogenous inhibitors, the TIMPs, and their highly regulated synthesis largely determines ECM remodeling.

In response to biochemical and physical stimuli, myocardial fibroblasts, the most abundant cell type in the heart and a critical component in the structure of myocardial ECM, can rapidly proliferate and their gene expression program significantly contributes to the remodeling process occurring with cardiac pathologies such as MI. For instance, myocardial ECM collagen is markedly increased with pressure overload hypertrophy due to a combination of increased synthesis and deposition by fibroblasts, and decreased collagen degradation. Fibrosis is stimulated by pro-fibrotic factors such as norepinephrine, angiotensin II, and endothelin-1 by modulating collagen synthesis and MMP/TIMP activity. In contrast, other bioactive molecules including natriuretic peptides (e.g., BNP) and NO, show anti-fibrotic action by inhibiting collagen synthesis and by stimulating MMP activity. These molecules signal primarily via the second messenger cGMP/PKG pathway. The resultant formation and activation of specific MMPs targeted to the cell membrane as well as released into the local interstitial space, has an amplification effect on MMP activity; the targeting of MMPs to the membrane can stimulate the release of extracellular signaling molecules such as TNF-α. A variety of signaling systems can be integrated to effect ECM turnover and ventricular remodeling. These findings support the use of pharmacological intervention to adjust the level of bioactive molecules as a therapeutic strategy to attenuate the adverse ventricular remodeling associated with HF (for further discussion on remodeling see Chap. 11).

Conclusion

There is increasing awareness that critical information about the nature of the signaling processes can be ascertained from the study of the multi-protein complexes involved in signaling. Postgenomic analysis has increasingly focused on these macromolecular aggregates and the delineation of protein–protein interactions, and subproteomic analysis has resulted in identification of the protein components within tyrosine kinase modules, G-protein complexes, ion, and PT pore channels. Identification of kinases, ligands, and second messengers, and the panoply of docking proteins, scaffolding proteins that organize the aggregate structure, and the numerous modulators, which affect the signaling processes will eventually allow a three-dimensional architecture of cardiomyocyte signaling. Manipulation of these components within the hearts of transgenic animals, and in cardiomyocytes grown in vitro is already possible using advanced techniques of gene transfer and RNAi to target specific gene expression. Nonetheless, the development of techniques to reconstitute functional complexes within artificial membranes has shown less success in signaling studies, underlining the view that the context of molecular interactions that constitute the cardiomyocyte signaling environment can be lost in such reductionist schemes.

Clearly, a better understanding of the precise order of the intracellular events, downstream consequences, and overall inter-relatedness and regulation of these pathways will be necessary to advance the development and characterization of reagents with high specificity to heart signaling pathways, and new technologies that could allow specific inhibition of stress signaling (e.g., specific kinase inhibitors) in cardiac and vascular cells.

Summary

- The heart is a dynamic transmitter and receiver of many intracellular and extracellular stimuli, and an integrator of numerous interacting transducers.
- Ca^{2+} is a major intracellular messenger involved in the activation of Ca^{2+}-dependent signaling pathways where it regulates cardiac growth and function by activation of kinases and phosphatases as well as playing a pivotal role in excitation–contraction coupling.
- Removal of Ca^{2+} from the cytosol is mainly affected by the sarcolemmal Na^+-Ca^{2+} exchanger and by the SR ATP dependent Ca^{2+} pump (Ca^{2+} ATPase or SERCA).
- In the heart, the principal SERCA protein is the SERCA2a isoform the activity of which is regulated by a closely associated protein, phospholamban (PLB), in a manner that is dependent on its phosphorylation status.
- Increase in Ca^{2+} that drives the larger contractions may be responsible for switching on a second process of signalosome remodeling to down-regulate the Ca^{2+} signaling pathway.
- Ca^{2+} associated stress response pathways also control cardiac gene expression by modulating the activities of chromatin-remodeling enzymes, which have been shown to act as global regulators of the cardiac genome during pathological remodeling of the heart.
- Major signaling pathways that are both, directly activated by Ca^{2+} and sufficient to promote the development of cardiac hypertrophy, include Ca^{2+}/CaM regulated kinase and phosphatase pathways, and PKC isozymes.
- Interaction of Ca^{2+}/CaM and calcineurin has been found to increase in the failing human heart, and increased levels of cardiac calcineurin activity have been reported in experimental animal models of cardiac hypertrophy.
- Multiple signaling pathways regulate cardiomyocyte growth and proliferation. These redundant mechanisms typically involve serine/threonine kinases, which stimulate a series of sequential molecular and cellular events (cascades).
- These cascades usually are initiated by signals received at the plasma membrane receptors and transmit via coupled G-proteins and bound second messengers to a wide-spectrum of protein kinases and phosphatases. These include protein kinase A, B, C, and G, the latter which operates in conjunction with cyclic GMP.
- Several G-protein-coupled receptors (GPCRs), including the α- and β-adrenergic receptors, angiotensin II, and endothelin-1 are able to activate these signaling cascades. Other receptors pivotal in cardiac and cardiovascular signaling include protease-activated, Toll-like receptors, and receptor tyrosine kinases (RTKs).
- These activated protein modifiers can lead to downstream activation or deactivation of specific transcription factors (e.g., NF-κB), which modulate specific gene expression affecting a broad spectrum of cellular events.
- The modulation of gene expression can be fostered as well by effectors that modulate chromatin structure and histone proteins (e.g., acetylases and deacetylases).
- Effectors also can target directly proteins involved in metabolic pathways, ion transport, Ca^{2+} regulation and handling, which affect contractility and excitability, as well as cardiomyocyte apoptosis and cell survival.
- Adrenoceptors (ARs) are members of the GPCR superfamily, interfacing between the sympathetic nervous system and the cardiovascular system, with integral roles in the rapid regulation of myocardial function.
- Stimulation of β1-adrenergic receptors (the predominant subtype found in both neonatal and adult ventricular myocytes) results in the activation of stimulatory G-protein and adenylyl cyclase (AC) with increased intracellular cAMP, and induction of protein kinase A (PKA). This leads to the downstream phosphorylation of key target proteins, including L-type calcium channels, phospholamban, troponin I, and ryanodine receptors resulting in the modulation of cardiac contractility in both neonatal and adult ventricular myocytes.

- Regulatory control of receptors is exerted by phosphorylation (by either PKA or other kinases), which can lead to receptor internalization and desensitization to the agonist. Chronic β-AR stimulation causes down-regulation of the receptors.
- Upon stimulation with agonists such as noradrenaline and adrenaline, α1-ARs activate G_q-proteins and subsequently activate phospholipase Cβ resulting in increased levels of second messengers InsP3 and DAG which promote an increase in intracellular Ca^{2+} levels, and protein PKC activation. They are involved in both modulating cardiac contractility and cardiomyocyte hypertrophy.
- A variety of G-proteins plays an essential role in mediating signal transduction from receptor to effector, and can either be stimulatory or inhibitory.
- Small GTP binding proteins as well as effectors of GTP hydrolysis can modulate the activity of heterotrimeric G-proteins.
- Specific proteins can organize the signaling complexes within microdomains at the plasma membrane, caveolae. Other proteins serve to enhance and orchestrate the signaling complexes, including anchoring adaptor and scaffolding proteins interacting with diverse stimuli.
- Stress, metabolic, and mitotic stimuli can act through signaling pathways and share a variety of signaling components. Survival pathways involving Akt and PI3K, PKA, and PKC can be utilized by these different stimuli.
- Stresses in cardiac hypertrophy (e.g., mechanical) and ischemia/hypoxia (e.g., oxidative) elicit a variety of adaptive responses at the tissue, cellular, and molecular levels.
- Long term responses to hypoxia have been shown to include increased gene expression of hypoxia-induced factors (HIF) and the activation of transcription factors, such as NF-κB, which have also been implicated in the complex regulation of cardiac hypertrophy and inflammatory cytokines.
- The failing heart has increased UCP3 levels associated with high levels of circulating FFA, mitochondrial uncoupling, and decreased cardiac efficiency, suggesting that respiratory uncoupling may underlie the abnormal energetics and decreased efficiency found in the failing heart.
- Besides providing structural and mechanical support, the heart extracellular matrix (ECM) plays a critical role in cellular signaling.
- An important link exists between the ECM and the cardiomyocyte cytoskeleton, since during the progression of HF, changes in ECM and cardiomyocytes will lead to a change in interaction between these two. This interaction is essential for mechanotransduction. Parts of the link are the transmembrane integrins, which act as signaling molecules and transducers of mechanical force.

References

1. Nicol RL, Frey N, Olson EN (2000) From the sarcomere to the nucleus: role of genetics and signaling in structural heart disease. Annu Rev Genomics Hum Genet 1:179–223
2. Studer R, Reinecke H, Bilger J (1994) Gene expression of the cardiac Na+-Ca++ exchanger in end stage human heart failure. Circ Res 75:443–453
3. Takahashi T, Allen PD, Lacro RV, Marks AR, Dennis AR, Schoen FJ, Grossman W, Marsh JD, Izumo S (1992) Expression of dihydropyridine receptor (Ca2+ channel) and calsequestrin genes in the myocardium of patients with end-stage heart failure. J Clin Invest 90:927–935
4. Takahashi T, Allen P, Izumo S (1992) Expression of A-, B-, and C-type natriuretic peptide genes in failing and developing human ventricles. Correlation with expression of the Ca2+-ATPase gene. Circ Res 71:9–17
5. Linck B, Boknik P, Eschenhagen T, Muller FU, Neumann J, Nose M, Jones LR, Schmitz W, Scholz H (1996) Messenger RNA expression and immunological quantification of phospholamban and SR-Ca ATPase in failing and nonfailing human heart. Cardiovasc Res 31:625–632
6. MacLennan DH, Kranias EG (2003) Phospholamban: a crucial regulator of cardiac contractility. Nat Rev Mol Cell Biol 4: 566–577
7. Tada M, Toyofuku T (1998) Molecular regulation of phospholamban function and expression. Trends Cardiovasc Med 8:330–340
8. Berridge MJ (2006) Remodelling Ca^{2+} signalling systems and cardiac hypertrophy. Biochem Soc Trans 34:228–231
9. Chin D, Means AR (2000) Calmodulin: a prototypical calcium sensor. Trends Cell Biol 10:322–328
10. Frey N, McKinsey TA, Olson EN (2000) Decoding calcium signals involved in cardiac growth and function. Nat Med 6:1221–1227
11. Zhang T, Johnson EN, Gu Y, Morissette MR, Sah VP, Gigena MS, Belke DD, Dillmann WH, Rogers TB, Schulman H, Ross J Jr, Brown JH (2002) The cardiac-specific nuclear delta(B) isoform of Ca2+/calmodulin-dependent protein kinase II induces hypertrophy and dilated cardiomyopathy associated with increased protein phosphatase 2A activity. J Biol Chem 277:1261–1267
12. Zhu W, Zou Y, Shiojima I, Kudoh S, Aikawa R, Hayashi D, Mizukami M, Toko H, Shibasaki F, Yazaki Y, Nagai R, Komuro I (2000) Ca2+/calmodulin-dependent kinase II and calcineurin play critical roles in endothelin-1-induced cardiomyocyte hypertrophy. J Biol Chem 275:15239–15245
13. Liang F, Wu J, Garami M, Gardner DG (1997) Mechanical strain increases expression of brain natriuretic peptide gene in rat cardiac myocytes. J Biol Chem 272:28050–28056
14. Zhang T, Maier LS, Dalton ND, Miyamoto S, Ross J Jr, Bers DM, Brown JH (2003) The deltaC isoform of CaMKII is activated in cardiac hypertrophy and induces dilated cardiomyopathy and heart failure. Circ Res 92:912–919
15. Passier R, Zeng H, Frey N, Naya FJ, Nicol RL, McKinsey TA, Overbeek P, Richardson JA, Grant SR, Olson EN (2000) CaM kinase signaling induces cardiac hypertrophy and activates the MEF2 transcription factor in vivo. J Clin Invest 105:1395–1406
16. Molkentin JD (2004) Calcineurin-NFAT signaling regulates the cardiac hypertrophic response in coordination with the MAPKs. Cardiovasc Res 63:467–475
17. Olson EN, Molkentin JD (1999) Prevention of cardiac hypertrophy by calcineurin inhibition: hope or hype? Circ Res 84:623–632
18. Haq S, Choukroun G, Lim H, Tymitz KM, del Monte F, Gwathmey J, Grazette L, Michael A, Hajjar R, Force T, Molkentin JD (2001) Differential activation of signal transduction pathways in human hearts with hypertrophy versus advanced heart failure. Circulation 103:670–677

19. McKinsey TA, Olson EN (2005) Toward transcriptional therapies for the failing heart: chemical screens to modulate genes. J Clin Invest 115:538–546

20. Chen M, Li X, Dong Q, Li Y, Liang W (2005) Neuropeptide Y induces cardiomyocyte hypertrophy via calcineurin signaling in rats. Regul Pept 125:9–15

21. Ruehr ML, Russell MA, Bond M (2004) A-kinase anchoring protein targeting of protein kinase A in the heart. J Mol Cell Cardiol 37:653–656

22. Dodge KL, Khouangsathiene S, Kapiloff MS, Mouton R, Hill EV, Houslay MD, Langeberg LK, Scott JD (2001) mAKAP assembles a protein kinase A/PDE4 phosphodiesterase cAMP signaling module. EMBO J 20:1921–1930

23. Hulme JT, Scheuer T, Catterall WA (2004) Regulation of cardiac ion channels by signaling complexes: role of modified leucine zipper motifs. J Mol Cell Cardiol 37:625–631

24. Sabri A, Steinberg SF (2003) Protein kinase C isoform-selective signals that lead to cardiac hypertrophy and the progression of heart failure. Mol Cell Biochem 251:97–101

25. Mochly-Rosen D, Wu G, Hahn H, Osinska H, Liron T, Lorenz JN, Yatani A, Robbins J, Dorn GW 2nd (2000) Cardiotrophic effects of protein kinase C epsilon: analysis by in vivo modulation of PKCepsilon translocation. Circ Res 86:1173–1179

26. Zhuang D, Ceacareanu AC, Ceacareanu B, Hassid A (2005) Essential role of protein kinase G and decreased cytoplasmic Ca2+ levels in NO-induced inhibition of rat aortic smooth muscle cell motility. Am J Physiol Heart Circ Physiol 288:H1859–H1866

27. Airhart N, Yang YF, Roberts CT Jr, Silberbach M (2003) Atrial natriuretic peptide induces natriuretic peptide receptor-cGMP-dependent protein kinase interaction. J Biol Chem 278:38693–38698

28. Fiedler B, Lohmann SM, Smolenski A, Linnemuller S, Pieske B, Schroder F, Molkentin JD, Drexler H, Wollert KC (2002) Inhibition of calcineurin-NFAT hypertrophy signaling by cGMP-dependent protein kinase type I in cardiac myocytes. Proc Natl Acad Sci USA 99:11363–11368

29. Begum N, Sandu OA, Duddy N (2002) Negative regulation of rho signaling by insulin and its impact on actin cytoskeleton organization in vascular smooth muscle cells: role of nitric oxide and cyclic guanosine monophosphate signaling pathways. Diabetes 51:2256–2263

30. Suzuki YJ, Nagase H, Day RM, Das DK (2004) GATA-4 regulation of myocardial survival in the preconditioned heart. J Mol Cell Cardiol 37:1195–1203

31. Gudi T, Chen JC, Casteel DE, Seasholtz TM, Boss GR, Pilz RB (2002) cGMP-dependent protein kinase inhibits serum-response element-dependent transcription by inhibiting rho activation and functions. J Biol Chem 277:37382–37393

32. Gudi T, Huvar I, Meinecke M, Lohmann SM, Boss GR, Pilz RB (1996) Regulation of gene expression by cGMP-dependent protein kinase. Transactivation of the c-fos promoter. J Biol Chem 271:4597–4600

33. Immenschuh S, Hinke V, Ohlmann A, Gifhorn-Katz S, Katz N, Jungermann K, Kietzmann T (1998) Transcriptional activation of the haem oxygenase-1 gene by cGMP via a cAMP response element/activator protein-1 element in primary cultures of rat hepatocytes. Biochem J 334:141–146

34. Mery PF, Lohmann SM, Walter U, Fischmeister R (1991) Ca2+ current is regulated by cyclic GMP-dependent protein kinase in mammalian cardiac myocytes. Proc Natl Acad Sci USA 88:1197–1201

35. Kaye DM, Wiviott SD, Kelly RA (1999) Activation of nitric oxide synthase (NOS3) by mechanical activity alters contractile activity in a Ca2+-independent manner in cardiac myocytes: role of troponin I phosphorylation. Biochem Biophys Res Commun 256:398–403

36. Layland J, Li JM, Shah AM (2002) Role of cyclic GMP-dependent protein kinase in the contractile response to exogenous nitric oxide in rat cardiac myocytes. J Physiol 540:457–467

37. Becker EM, Schmidt P, Schramm M, Schroder H, Walter U, Hoenicka M, Gerzer R, Stasch JP (2000) The vasodilator-stimulated phosphoprotein (VASP): target of YC-1 and nitric oxide effects in human and rat platelets. J Cardiovasc Pharmacol 35:390–397

38. Sporbert A, Mertsch K, Smolenski A, Haseloff RF, Schonfelder G, Paul M, Ruth P, Walter U, Blasig IE (1999) Phosphorylation of vasodilator-stimulated phosphoprotein: a consequence of nitric oxide- and cGMP-mediated signal transduction in brain capillary endothelial cells and astrocytes. Brain Res Mol Brain Res 67:258–266

39. Pi M, Oakley RH, Gesty-Palmer D, Cruickshank RD, Spurney RF, Luttrell LM, Quarles LD (2005) Beta-arrestin- and G protein receptor kinase-mediated calcium-sensing receptor desensitization. Mol Endocrinol 19:1078–1087

40. Hata JA, Williams ML, Koch WJ (2004) Genetic manipulation of myocardial beta-adrenergic receptor activation and desensitization. J Mol Cell Cardiol 37:11–21

41. Koch WJ, Rockman HA, Samama P, Hamilton RA, Bond RA, Milano CA, Lefkowitz RJ (1995) Cardiac function in mice overexpressing the beta-adrenergic receptor kinase or a beta ARK inhibitor. Science 268:1350–1353

42. Metaye T, Gibelin H, Perdrisot R, Kraimps JL (2005) Pathophysiological roles of G-protein-coupled receptor kinases. Cell Signal 17:917–928

43. Vinge LE, Oie E, Andersson Y, Grogaard HK, Andersen G, Attramadal H (2001) Myocardial distribution and regulation of GRK and beta-arrestin isoforms in congestive heart failure in rats. Am J Physiol Heart Circ Physiol 281:H2490–H2499

44. Penela P, Murga C, Ribas C, Tutor AS, Peregrín S, Mayor F Jr (2006) Mechanisms of regulation of G protein-coupled receptor kinases (GRKs) and cardiovascular disease. Cardiovasc Res 69:46–56

45. Hata JA, Koch WJ (2003) Phosphorylation of G protein-coupled receptors: GPCR kinases in heart disease.Mol Interv 3:264–272; Molkentin JD (2006) Dichotomy of Ca^{2+} in the heart: contraction versus intracellular signaling. J Clin Invest 116:623–626

46. O'Rourke MF, Iversen LJ, Lomasney JW, Bylund DB (1994) Species orthologs of the alpha-2A adrenergic receptor: the pharmacological properties of the bovine and rat receptors differ from the human and porcine receptors. J Pharmacol Exp Ther 27:735–740

47. Flordellis C, Manolis A, Scheinin M, Paris H (2004) Clinical and pharmacological significance of alpha2-adrenoceptor polymorphisms in cardiovascular diseases. Int J Cardiol 97:367–372

48. Brodde OE, Michel MC (1999) Adrenergic and muscarinic receptors in the human heart. Pharmacol Rev 51:651–690

49. Giessler C, Dhein S, Pönicke K, Brodde OE (1999) Muscarinic receptors in the failing human heart. Eur J Pharmacol 375:197–202

50. Ness J (1996) Molecular biology of muscarinic acetylcholine receptors. Crit Rev Neurobiol 10:69–99

51. Wang Z, Shi H, Wang H (2004) Functional M3 muscarinic acetylcholine receptors in mammalian hearts. Br J Pharmacol 142:395–408

52. Shi H, Wang H, Yang B, Xu D, Wang Z (2004) The M3 receptor-mediated K(+) current (IKM3), a G(q) protein-coupled K(+) channel. J Biol Chem 279:21774–21778

53. Shi H, Wang H, Li D, Nattel S, Wang Z (2004) Differential alterations of receptor densities of three muscarinic acetylcholine receptor subtypes and current densities of the corresponding K+ channels in canine atria with atrial fibrillation induced by experimental congestive heart failure. Cell Physiol Biochem 14:31–40

54. Dorn GW 2nd, Brown JH (1999) Gq signaling in cardiac adaptation and maladaptation. Trends Cardiovasc Med 9:26–34

55. van Heugten HA, Eskildsen-Helmond YE, de Jonge HW, Bezstarosti K, Lamers JM (1996) Phosphoinositide-generated messengers in cardiac signal transduction. Mol Cell Biochem 157:5–14

56. Bogoyevitch MA, Glennon PE, Andersson M, Clerk A, Lazou A, Marshall CJ, Parker PJ, Sugden PH (1994) Endothelin-1 and fibroblast growth factors stimulate the mitogen-activated protein kinase signaling cascade in cardiac myocytes. The potential role of the cascade in the integration of two signaling pathways leading to myocyte hypertrophy. J Biol Chem 269:1110–1119

57. Giannessi D, Del Ry S, Vitale RL (2001) The role of endothelins and their receptors in heart failure. Pharmacol Res 43:111–126

58. Sugden PH (2003) An overview of endothelin signaling in the cardiac myocyte. J Mol Cell Cardiol 35:871–886

59. Drímal J, Knezl V, Drímal J Jr, Drímal D, Bauerová K, Kettmann V, Doherty AM, Stefek M (2003) Cardiac effects of endothelin-1 (ET-1) and related C terminal peptide fragment: increased inotropy or contribution to heart failure? Physiol Res 52:701–708

60. Leite-Moreira AF (2008) Myocardial effects of endothelin-1. Rev Port Cardiol 27:925–951

61. Communal C, Singh K, Pimentel DR, Colucci WS (1998) Norepinephrine stimulates apoptosis in adult rat ventricular myocytes by activation of the beta-adrenergic pathway. Circulation 98:1329–1334

62. Adams JW, Brown JH (2001) G-proteins in growth and apoptosis: lessons from the heart. Oncogene 20:1626–1634

63. Mulder P, Richard V, Bouchart F, Derumeaux G, Munter K, Thuillez C (1998) Selective ETA receptor blockade prevents left ventricular remodeling and deterioration of cardiac function in experimental heart failure. Cardiovasc Res 39:600–608

64. Moe GW, Albernaz A, Naik GO, Kirchengast M, Stewart DJ (1998) Beneficial effects of long-term selective endothelin type A receptor blockade in canine experimental heart failure. Cardiovasc Res 39:571–579

65. Marín-García J, Goldenthal MJ, Moe GW (2002) Selective endothelin receptor blockade reverses mitochondrial dysfunction in canine heart failure. J Card Fail 8:326–332

66. Dinh DT, Frauman AG, Johnston CI, Fabiani ME (2001) Angiotensin receptors: distribution, signalling and function. Clin Sci (Lond) 100:481–492

67. Li Y, Takemura G, Okada H, Miyata S, Maruyama R, Esaki M, Kanamori H, Li L, Ogino A, Ohno T (2007) Molecular signaling mediated by angiotensin II type 1A receptor blockade leading to attenuation of renal dysfunction-associated heart failure. J Card Fail 13:155–162

68. Saito Y, Berk BC (2002) Angiotensin II-mediated signal transduction pathways. Curr Hypertens Rep 4:167–171

69. Brasier AR, Jamaluddin M, Han Y, Patterson C, Runge MS (2000) Angiotensin II induces gene transcription through cell-type-dependent effects on the nuclear factor-kappaB (NF-kappaB) transcription factor. Mol Cell Biochem 212:155–169

70. Chen Y, Arrigo AP, Currie RW (2004) Heat shock treatment suppresses angiotensin II-induced activation of NF-kappaB pathway and heart inflammation: a role for IKK depletion by heat shock? Am J Physiol Heart Circ Physiol 287:H1104–H1114

71. Ladeiras-Lopes R, Ferreira-Martins J, Leite-Moreira AF (2009) Acute neurohumoral modulation of diastolic function. Peptides 30: 419–425

72. Nakajima M, Hutchinson HG, Fujinaga M, Hayashida W, Morishita R, Zhang L, Horiuchi M, Pratt RE, Dzau VJ (1995) The angiotensin II type 2 (AT2) receptor antagonizes the growth effects of the AT1 receptor: gain-of-function study using gene transfer. Proc Natl Acad Sci USA 92:10663–10667

73. Kaschina E, Grzesiak A, Li J, Foryst-Ludwig A, Timm M et al (2008) Angiotensin II type 2 receptor stimulation: a novel option of therapeutic interference with the renin-angiotensin system in myocardial infarction? Circulation 118:2523–2532

74. Yki-Järvinen H (2004) Thiazolidinediones. N Engl J Med 351:1106–1118

75. Mohanty P, Aljada A, Ghanim H, Hofmeyer D, Tripathy D, Syed T, Al-Haddad W, Dhindsa S, Dandona P (2004) Evidence for a potent antiinflammatory effect of rosiglitazone. J Clin Endocrinol Metab 89:2728–2735

76. Molavi B, Chen J, Mehta JL (2006) Cardioprotective effects of rosiglitazone are associated with selective overexpression of type 2 angiotensin receptors and inhibition of p42/44 MAPK. Am J Physiol Heart Circ Physiol 291:H687–H693

77. Purcell NH, Wilkins BJ, York A, Saba-El-Leil MK, Meloche S, Robbins J, Molkentin JD (2007) Genetic inhibition of cardiac ERK1/2 promotes stress-induced apoptosis and heart failure but has no effect on hypertrophy in vivo. Proc Natl Acad Sci USA 104: 14074–14079

78. Clerk A, Aggeli IK, Stathopoulou K, Sugden PH (2006) Peptide growth factors signal differentially through protein kinase C to extracellular signal-regulated kinases in neonatal cardiomyocytes. Cell Signal 18:225–235

79. Daitoku H, Hatta M, Matsuzaki H, Aratani S, Ohshima T, Miyagishi M, Nakajima T, Fukamizu A (2004) Silent information regulator 2 potentiates Foxo1-mediated transcription through its deacetylase activity. Proc Natl Acad Sci USA 101:10042–10047

80. Ni YG, Berenji K, Wang N, Oh M, Sachan N, Dey A, Cheng J, Lu G, Morris DJ, Castrillon DH, Gerard RD, Rothermel BA, Hill JA (2006) Foxo transcription factors blunt cardiac hypertrophy by inhibiting calcineurin signaling. Circulation 114:1159–1168

81. Evans-Anderson HJ, Alfieri CM, Yutzey KE (2008) Regulation of cardiomyocyte proliferation and myocardial growth during development by FOXO transcription factors. Circ Res 102:686–694

82. Frantz S, Ertl G, Bauersachs J (2007) Mechanisms of disease: toll-like receptors in cardiovascular disease. Nat Clin Pract Cardiovasc Med 4:444–454

83. Frantz S, Kobzik L, Kim YD, Fukazawa R, Medzhitov R, Lee RT, Kelly RA (1999) Toll4 (TLR4) expression in cardiac myocytes in normal and failing myocardium. J Clin Invest 104:271–280

84. Birks EJ, Felkin LE, Banner NR, Khaghani A, Barton PJ, Yacoub MH (2004) Increased toll-like receptor 4 in the myocardium of patients requiring left ventricular assist devices. J Heart Lung Transplant 23:228–235

85. Satoh M, Nakamura M, Akatsu T, Shimoda Y, Segawa I, Hiramori K (2004) Toll-like receptor 4 is expressed with enteroviral replication in myocardium from patients with dilated cardiomyopathy. Lab Invest 84:173–181

86. Frantz S, Hu K, Bayer B, Gerondakis S, Strotmann J, Adamek A, Ertl G, Bauersachs J (2006) Absence of NF-kappaB subunit p50 improves heart failure after myocardial infarction. FASEB J 20:1918–1920

87. Tillmanns J, Carlsen H, Blomhoff R, Valen G, Calvillo L, Ertl G, Bauersachs J, Frantz S (2006) Caught in the act: in vivo molecular imaging of the transcription factor NF-kappaB after myocardial infarction. Biochem Biophys Res Commun 342:773–774

88. Oyama J, Blais C Jr, Liu X, Pu M, Kobzik L, Kelly RA, Bourcier T (2004) Reduced myocardial ischemia-reperfusion injury in toll-like receptor 4-deficient mice. Circulation 109:784–789

89. Wang YP, Sato C, Mizoguchi K, Yamashita Y, Oe M, Maeta H (2002) Lipopoly-saccharide triggers late preconditioning against myocardial infarction via inducible nitric oxide synthase. Cardiovasc Res 56:33–42

90. Tavener SA, Long EM, Robbins SM, McRae KM, Van Remmen H, Kubes P (2004) Immune cell Toll-like receptor 4 is required for cardiac myocyte impairment during endotoxemia. Circ Res 95:700–707

91. Frantz S, Kelly RA, Bourcier T (2001) Role of TLR-2 in the activation of nuclear factor kappaB by oxidative stress in cardiac myocytes. J Biol Chem 276:5197–5203

92. Ha T, Li Y, Gao X, McMullen JR, Shioi T, Izumo S, Kelley JL, Zhao A, Haddad GE, Williams DL, Browder IW, Kao RL, Li C (2005) Attenuation of cardiac hypertrophy by inhibiting both mTOR and NFkappaB activation in vivo. Free Radic Biol Med 39:1570–1580

93. Ha T, Li Y, Hua F, Ma J, Gao X, Kelley J, Zhao A, Haddad GE, Williams DL, William Browder I, Kao RL, Li C (2005) Reduced cardiac hypertrophy in toll-like receptor 4-deficient mice following pressure overload. Cardiovasc Res 68:224–234

94. Freund C, Schmidt-Ullrich R, Baurand A, Dunger S, Schneider W, Loser P, El-Jamali A, Dietz R, Scheidereit C, Bergmann MW (2005) Requirement of nuclear factor-kappaB in angiotensin II- and isoproterenol-induced cardiac hypertrophy in vivo. Circulation 111:2319–2325

95. Coughlin SR, Camerer E (2003) PARticipation in inflammation. J Clin Invest 111:25–27

96. Sabri A, Short J, Guo J, Steinberg SF (2002) Protease-activated receptor-1-mediated DNA synthesis in cardiac fibroblast is via epidermal growth factor receptor transactivation: distinct PAR-1 signaling pathways in cardiac fibroblasts and cardiomyocytes. Circ Res 91:532–539

97. Sabri A, Muske G, Zhang H, Pak E, Darrow A, Andrade-Gordon P, Steinberg SF (2000) Signaling properties and functions of two distinct cardiomyocyte protease-activated receptors. Circ Res 86:1054–1061

98. Obreztchikova M, Elouardighi H, Ho M, Wilson BA, Gertsberg Z, Steinberg SF (2006) Distinct signaling functions for Shc isoforms in the heart. J Biol Chem 281:20197–20204

99. Moshal KS, Tyagi N, Henderson B, Ovechkin AV, Tyagi SC (2005) Protease-activated receptor and endothelial-myocyte uncoupling in chronic heart failure. Am J Physiol Heart Circ Physiol 288:H2770–H2777

100. Darrow AL, Fung-Leung W-P, Ye RD, Santulli RJ, Cheung W-M, Derian CK, Burns CL, Damiano BP, Zhou L, Keenan CM, Peterson PA, Andrade-Gordon P (1996) Biological consequences of thrombin receptor deficiency in mice. Thromb Haemost 76:860–866

101. Pawlinski R, Tencati M, Hampton CR, Shishido T, Bullard TA, Casey LM, Andrade-Gordon P, Kotzsch M, Spring D, Luther T, Abe J, Pohlman TH, Verrier ED, Blaxall BC, Mackman N (2007) Protease-activated receptor-1 contributes to cardiac remodeling and hypertrophy. Circulation 116:2298–2306

102. Strande JL, Hsu A, Su J, Fu X, Gross GJ, Baker JE (2007) SCH 79797, a selective PAR1 antagonist, limits myocardial ischemia/reperfusion injury in rat hearts. Basic Res Cardiol 102:350–358

103. Strande JL (2008) Letter regarding article "Protease-activated receptor-1 contributes to cardiac remodeling and hypertrophy". Circulation 117:e495, author reply e496

104. Grassot J, Mouchiroud G, Perriere G (2003) RTKdb: database of receptor tyrosine kinase. Nucleic Acids Res 31:353–358

105. Kontaridis MI, Yang W, Bence KK, Cullen D et al (2008) Deletion of Ptpn11 (Shp2) in cardiomyocytes causes dilated cardiomyopathy via effects on the extracellular signal-regulated kinase/mitogen-activated protein kinase and RhoA signaling pathways. Circulation 117:1423–1435

106. Zhao YY, Feron O, Dessy C, Han X, Marchionni MA, Kelly RA (1999) Neuregulin signaling in the heart. Dynamic targeting of erbB4 to caveolar microdomains in cardiac myocytes. Circ Res 84:1380–1387

107. Zhao YY, Sawyer DR, Baliga RR, Opel DJ, Han X, Marchionni MA, Kelly RA (1998) Neuregulins promote survival and growth of cardiac myocytes. Persistence of ErbB2 and ErbB4 expression in neonatal and adult ventricular myocytes. J Biol Chem 273:10261–10269

108. Doggen K, Ray L, Mathieu M, McEntee K, Lemmens K, De Keulenaer GW (2008) Direct evidence for activation of the neuregulin-1/ErbB system inmyocardium of dogs with pacing-induced heart failure. Eur J Heart Fail Suppl 7:1

109. Xu Y, Li X, Zhou M (2009) Neuregulin-1/ErbB signaling: a druggable target for treating heart failure. Curr Opin Pharmacol 9:214–219

110. Lee HJ, Koh GY (2003) Shear stress activates Tie2 receptor tyrosine kinase in human endothelial cells. Biochem Biophys Res Commun 304:399–404

111. Becker E, Huynh-Do U, Holland S, Pawson T, Daniel TO, Skolnik EY (2000) Nck-interacting Ste20 kinase couples Eph receptors to c-Jun N-terminal kinase and integrin activation. Mol Cell Biol 20:1537–1545

112. Vercauteren M, Remy E, Devaux C, Dautreaux B et al (2007) Improvement of peripheral endothelial dysfunction by protein tyrosine phosphatase inhibitors in heart failure. Circulation 115:e648

113. Hamm HE (1998) The many faces of G protein signaling. J Biol Chem 273:669–672

114. Clerk A, Sugden PH (2000) Small guanine nucleotide-binding proteins and myocardial hypertrophy. Circ Res 86:1019–1023

115. Meszaros JG, Gonzalez AM, Endo-Mochizuki Y, Villegas S, Villarreal F, Brunton LL (2000) Identification of G protein-coupled signaling pathways in cardiac fibroblasts: cross talk between G(q) and G(s). Am J Physiol Cell Physiol 278:C154–C162

116. Huss JM, Kelly DP (2004) Nuclear receptor signaling and cardiac energetics. Circ Res 95:568–578

117. Chawla A, Repa JJ, Evans RM, Mangelsdorf DJ (2001) Nuclear receptors and lipid physiology: opening the X-files. Science 294:1866–1870

118. Gao MH, Lai NC, Roth DM, Zhou J, Zhu J, Anzai T, Dalton N, Hammond HK (1999) Adenylyl cyclase increases responsiveness to catecholamine stimulation in transgenic mice. Circulation 99:1618–1622

119. Lai NC, Roth DM, Gao MH, Tang T, Dalton N, Lai YY, Spellman M, Clopton P, Hammond HK (2004) Intracoronary adenovirus encoding adenylyl cyclase VI increases left ventricular function in heart failure. Circulation 110:330–336

120. Roth DM, Gao MH, Lai NC, Drumm J, Dalton N, Zhou JY, Zhu J, Entrikin D, Hammond HK (1999) Cardiac-directed adenylyl cyclase expression improves heart function in murine cardiomyopathy. Circulation 99:3099–3102

121. Iwami G, Kawabe J, Ebina T, Cannon PJ, Homcy CJ, Ishikawa Y (1995) Regulation of adenylyl cyclase by protein kinase A. J Biol Chem 270:12481–12484

122. Rhee SG (2001) Regulation of phosphoinositide-specific phospholipase C. Annu Rev Biochem 70:281–312

123. Wing MR, Bourdon DM, Harden TK (2003) PLC-epsilon: a shared effector protein in Ras-, Rho-, and G alpha beta gamma-mediated signaling. Mol Interv 3:273–280

124. Yu CH, Panagia V, Tappia PS, Liu SY, Takeda N, Dhalla NS (2002) Alterations of sarcolemmal phospholipase D and phosphatidate phosphohydrolase in congestive heart failure. Biochim Biophys Acta 1584:65–72

125. Dent MR, Singal T, Dhalla NS, Tappia PS (2004) Expression of phospholipase D isozymes in scar and viable tissue in congestive heart failure due to myocardial infarction. J Cell Mol Med 8:526–536

126. Uray IP, Connelly JH, Frazier OH, Taegtmeyer H, Davies PJ (2003) Mechanical unloading increases caveolin expression in the failing human heart. Cardiovasc Res 59:57–66

127. Rybin VO, Xu X, Steinberg SF (1999) Activated protein kinase C isoforms target to cardiomyocyte caveolae: stimulation of local protein phosphorylation. Circ Res 84:980–988

128. Head BP, Patel HH, Roth DM, Lai NC, Niesman IR, Farquhar MG, Insel PA (2005) G-protein coupled receptor signaling components localize in both sarcolemmal and intracellular caveolin-3-associated microdomains in adult cardiac myocytes. J Biol Chem 280:31036–31044

129. Williams TM, Lisanti MP (2004) The Caveolin genes: from cell biology to medicine. Ann Med 36:584–595

130. Jones WK, Brown M, Ren X, He S, McGuinness M (2003) NF-kappaB as an integrator of diverse signaling pathways: the heart of myocardial signaling? Cardiovasc Toxicol 3:229–254

131. Chandel NS, Schumacker PT (2000) Cellular oxygen sensing by mitochondria: old questions, new insight. J Appl Physiol 88:1880–1889

132. Waypa GB, Marks JD, Mack MM, Boriboun C, Mungai PT, Schumacker PT (2002) Mitochondrial reactive oxygen species trigger calcium increases during hypoxia in pulmonary arterial myocytes. Circ Res 91:719–726

133. Duranteau J, Chandel NS, Kulisz A, Shao Z, Schumacker PT (1998) Intracellular signaling by reactive oxygen species during hypoxia in cardiomyocytes. J Biol Chem 273:11619–11624

134. Kacimi R, Long CS, Karliner JS (1997) Chronic hypoxia modulates the interleukin-1β stimulated inducible nitric oxide synthase pathway in cardiac myocytes. Circulation 96:1937–1943

135. French S, Giulivi C, Balaban RS (2001) Nitric oxide synthase in porcine heart mitochondria: evidence for low physiological activity. Am J Physiol Heart Circ Physiol 280:H2863–H2867

136. Kulisz A, Chen N, Chandel NS, Shao Z, Schumacker PT (2002) Mitochondrial ROS initiate phosphorylation of p38 MAP kinase during hypoxia in cardiomyocytes. Am J Physiol Lung Cell Mol Physiol 282:L1324–L1329

137. Enomoto N, Koshikawa N, Gassmann M, Hayashi J, Takenaga K (2002) Hypoxic induction of hypoxia-inducible factor-1alpha and oxygen-regulated gene expression in mitochondrial DNA-depleted HeLa cells. Biochem Biophys Res Commun 297:346–352

138. Fischer P, Hilfiker-Kleiner D (2007) Survival pathways in hypertrophy and heart failure: the gp130-STAT3 axis. Basic Res Cardiol 102:393–411

139. Lopaschuk GD, Collins-Nakai RL, Itoi T (1992) Developmental changes in energy substrate use by the heart. Cardiovasc Res 26:1172–1180

140. Bonnet D, Martin D, De Lonlay P et al (1999) Arrhythmias and conduction defects as presenting symptoms of fatty acid oxidation disorders in children. Circulation 100:2248–2253

141. Sparagna GC, Hickson-Bick DL, Buja LM, McMillin JB (2001) Fatty acid-induced apoptosis in neonatal cardiomyocytes: redox signaling. Antioxid Redox Signal 3:71–79

142. Lanni A, De Felice M, Lombardi A, Moreno M, Fleury C, Ricquier D, Goglia F (1997) Induction of UCP2 mRNA by thyroid hormones in rat heart. FEBS Lett 418:171–174

143. Boehm EA, Jones BE, Radda GK, Veech RL, Clarke K (2001) Increased uncoupling proteins and decreased efficiency in palmitate-perfused hyperthyroid rat heart. Am J Physiol Heart Circ Physiol 280:H977–H983

144. Young ME, Patil S, Ying J, Depre C, Ahuja HS, Shipley GL, Stepkowski SM, Davies PJ, Taegtmeyer H (2001) Uncoupling protein 3 transcription is regulated by peroxisome proliferator-activated receptor (alpha) in the adult rodent heart. FASEB J 15:833–845

145. Murray AJ, Cole MA, Lygate CA, Carr CA, Stuckey DJ, Little SE, Neubauer S, Clarke K (2008) Increased mitochondrial uncoupling proteins, respiratory uncoupling and decreased efficiency in the chronically infarcted rat heart. J Mol Cell Cardiol 44:694–700

146. Spinale FG (2002) Bioactive peptide signaling within the myocardial interstitium and the matrix metalloproteinases. Circ Res 91:1082–1084

147. Ross RS, Borg TK (2001) Integrins and the myocardium. Circ Res 88:1112–1119

148. Iwami K, Ashizawa N, Do YS, Graf K, Hsueh WA (1996) Comparison of ANG II with other growth factors on Egr-1 and matrix gene expression in cardiac fibroblasts. Am J Physiol 270:H2100–H2107

Chapter 10
Oxidative Stress and Heart Failure

Overview

Heart failure (HF) is a complex clinical syndrome whose pathogenesis includes an interplay of neurohormonal and inflammatory processes at the cellular and molecular levels. Oxidative stress (OS) may represent the common pathway for cell death/apoptosis, cardiac remodeling, and dysfunction. There is increasing evidence to indicate that reactive oxygen species (ROS) play an important role in the development and progression of HF. However, while levels of ROS are elevated in HF, the relative contribution of the different intracellular sources of ROS and the precise mechanisms of this increase remains unclear. Further delineation of the downstream signaling pathways involved in ROS accumulation is important, in order to improve our understanding of these processes and also for the development of new therapies. Indeed, despite previously disappointing results from using antioxidants in human studies, it is likely that modulation of endogenous antioxidants in human HF will continue to have the potential for both, treatment and prevention. In this chapter, we will look at how changes in the cellular redox state of cardiovascular tissue affect the development and progression of HF. In addition, the potential sources of ROS involved in the HF syndrome will be discussed.

Introduction

Independent of its etiology, ROS play an important role in the development and progression of HF. Oxygen is the critical terminal electron acceptor in the mitochondrial electron transport chain (ETC); in its absence, the ETC shuts down and the cardiac demands for ATP are not met. Molecular oxygen is also central in both the formation of nitric oxide (NO), a primary determinant of both vascular tone and cardiac contractility, and in the generation of ROS and subsequent induction of OS as a significant by-product of energy metabolism during its sequential acceptance of electrons in the mitochondrial ETC. These short-lived intermediates can act either as important signaling molecules or induce irreversible oxidative damage to proteins, lipids and nucleic acids, thus, ROS and oxygen exert both beneficial and deleterious effects. ROS have been implicated in the development of agonist-induced cardiac hypertrophy, cardiomyocyte apoptosis, and in the remodeling processes of the failing heart. Changes in HF phenotype are driven by redox sensitive gene expression, and in this way ROS may act as potent intracellular second messengers. It is important to remember that ROS can be generated in the heart and endothelial tissues by non-mitochondrial reactions as well, including the involvement of xanthine oxidase (XO), NAD(P)H oxidases, and cytochrome P450 [1]. Furthermore, after myocardial infarction (MI), ROS-induced mitochondrial DNA (mtDNA) damage may result in mitochondrial dysfunction, which will contribute to progressive left ventricular (LV) remodeling and HF.

ROS Production

The major ROS are the superoxide radical $O_2^{\cdot-}$, hydrogen peroxide (H_2O_2), and the hydroxyl radical $OH^\cdot$. The superoxide anion ($O_2^{\cdot-}$) is formed when oxygen accepts an electron. Superoxide is in equilibrium with its more reactive protonated form, $^\cdot HO_2$, which is favored in acidosis (such as occurs with ischemia). The rates of mitochondrial $O_2^{\cdot-}$ generation are known to be inversely correlated with the maximum lifespan potential of different mammalian species [2]. The production of the $OH^\cdot$ (which is the most reactive form of ROS) is primarily responsible for the damage to cellular macromolecules such as proteins, DNA, and lipids. Formation of the highly reactive $OH^\cdot$ comes from reactions involving the other ROS species (e.g., the Fenton reaction) in which ubiquitous metal ions, such as Fe (II) or Cu (I), react with H_2O_2. The high reactivity of the hydroxyl radical and its extremely short physiological half-life of 10^{-9} s restrict its damage to a small radius from where it is generated, since it is too short-lived to diffuse far from its origin [3]. The location of free metal ions can determine the initiation of free radical damage. In contrast, the less reactive superoxide radicals produced in mitochondria can be delivered to the cytosol through anion channels (e.g., VDAC) and thereby may impact sites far from their generation,

J. Marín-García, *Heart Failure*, Contemporary Cardiology,
DOI 10.1007/978-1-60761-147-9_10, © Springer Science+Business Media, LLC 2010

including activation of transcription factors such as NF-κB among other effects [4]. Similarly, the freely diffusible H_2O_2 generated in mitochondria can be delivered to the cytosol, where it contributes to increased levels of cellular ROS. An accurate quantification of mitochondrial ROS flux inside living cells is very difficult since the turnover of several ROS species (particularly the OH· radical) is extremely rapid. Indirect strategies, including the use of gene knockout and overexpression studies [5], have been used to demonstrate the presence and involvement of mitochondrial ROS.

Under normal physiological conditions, the primary source of ROS is the mitochondrial ETC, where oxygen can be activated to superoxide radical by a nonenzymatic process. This production of ROS is a by-product of normal metabolism and occurs from electrons produced (or leaked) from the ETC at complexes I, II, and III. There is evidence that semiquinones generated within complexes I and III are the most likely donors of electrons to molecular oxygen, providing a constant source of superoxide [6, 7]; also, a supportive role for complex II in ROS production has been suggested [8]. Mitochondrial ROS generation can be amplified in cells with abnormal respiratory chain function as well as, under physiological and pathological conditions such as HF, where oxygen consumption is increased.

Besides mitochondria, other cellular sources for generating superoxide radicals include the reactions of oxygen with microsomal cytochrome p450 and with reduced flavins (e.g., NAD(P)H), usually in the presence of metal ions. In addition, xanthine oxidase (XO), a primarily cytosolic enzyme involved in purine metabolism, is also a source of the superoxide radical. Notably, XO activity and its superoxide generation are markedly increased in the heart post-ischemia/reperfusion damage. Its location within the human myocardium is primarily in the endothelial cells of capillaries and smaller vessels [9, 10]. A number of studies have shown that the XO inhibitor allopurinol protects against the cardiac damage resulting from anoxia. Recently, Cappola et al. demonstrated a provocative link between XO activity and abnormal cardiac energy metabolism in patients with idiopathic DCM, since inhibition of XO with allopurinol significantly improved myocardial function [11].

In the presence of the enzyme superoxide dismutase (SOD), superoxide radicals can be converted to H_2O_2 that can further react via the Fenton reaction to form the hydroxyl radical. Superoxide can also react with NO to form peroxynitrite, which is also a highly reactive and deleterious free radical species (Fig. 10.1).

Abnormal ROS Effects

ROS cause deleterious effects on cells including extensive peroxidative damage to membrane phospholipids and proteins. Protein modifications, such as carbonylation, nitration,

and the formation of lipid peroxidation adducts (e.g., 4-hydroxynonenal (HNE)), which are products of oxidative damage secondary to ROS [12]. Significantly, changes in the myocardial respiratory complexes I to V by ROS-mediated nitration, carbonylation, and HNE adduct, with associated decline in their enzymatic activity, have been reported in both in vitro and in vivo studies [13]. Superoxide is also especially damaging to the Fe–S centers of enzymes (e.g., complex I, aconitase, and succinate dehydrogenase). Moreover, the inactivation of mitochondrial aconitase by superoxide, which generates Fe (II) and H_2O_2, also increases hydroxyl radical formation through the Fenton reaction [14].

Lipids and in particular the mitochondrial-specific cardiolipin serve as a focal target for free radical damage. A large accumulation of superoxide radicals produced in vitro, with sub-mitochondrial particles from heart results in extensive cardiolipin peroxidation, with a parallel loss of cytochrome c oxidase activity [15, 16]. Oxidative damage also affects nucleic acids and in particular mtDNA by the induction of single- and double-strand breaks, base damage, and modification (including 8-oxoguanosine formation), resulting in the generation of point mutations and deletions [17–19].

In addition, the highly reactive peroxynitrite irreversibly impairs mitochondrial respiration [20] since it inhibits complex I activity, largely by tyrosine nitration of several targeted subunits [21–23], modifies cytochrome c structure and function [22], affects cytochrome c oxidase activity, inhibits mitochondrial aconitase [24], and causes induction of the PT pore [25]. Some of the effects of peroxynitrite on mitochondrial targets (e.g., the PT pore) are potentiated by increased calcium levels [26]. Notably, the effects of peroxynitrite on mitochondria can be clearly distinguished from the effects of NO, which often are reversible [20]. Taken together, mitochondria, the primary site of intracellular ROS generation, are also a primary locus of its damaging effects. Specifically, damage to mtDNA induces abnormalities in the mtDNA-encoded polypeptides of the respiratory complexes located in the inner membrane, with consequent decrease of electron transfer and further production of ROS, thus establishing a vicious cycle of OS, mitochondrial dysfunction, and bioenergetic decline.

ROS and Cell Signaling

In addition to the cell-damaging effects of ROS, mitochondrial ROS generation and the OS they engender play a major role in cell regulation and signaling. Oxidative species such as H_2O_2 and the superoxide anion can be used as potent signals sent from mitochondria to other cellular sites rapidly and reversibly, triggering an array of intracellular cascades leading to diverse physiological end-points for the cardiomyo-

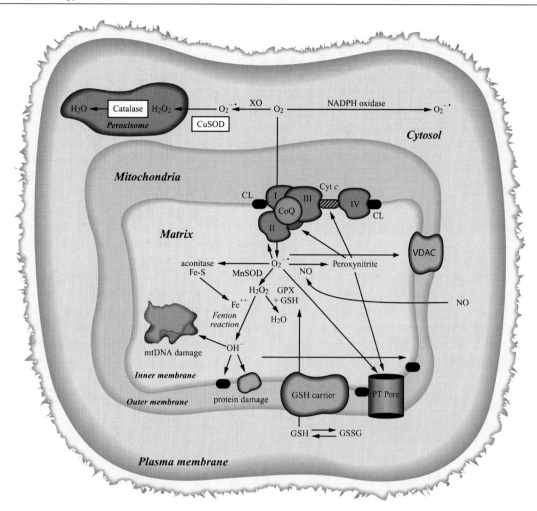

Fig. 10.1 Cellular ROS generation and metabolism. Sites of mitochondrial superoxide $O_2^{\cdot-}$ radical (via respiratory complexes I, II, and III) and cytosolic $O_2^{\cdot-}$ generation (by NAD(P)H oxidase or xanthine oxidase) are depicted. Also shown are reactions of the $O_2^{\cdot-}$ radical with NO to form the highly reactive peroxynitrite, which can target PT pore opening and the inactivation of mitochondrial aconitase by $O_2^{\cdot-}$. MnSOD (in mitochondria) and CuSOD (in cytosol) to form H_2O_2 are also displayed. The H_2O_2 is then either further neutralized in the mitochondria by glutathione peroxidase (GPx) and glutathione, in the peroxisome by catalase, or in the presence of Fe^{2+} via the Fenton reaction, which forms the highly reactive OH˙ radical that can cause severe lipid peroxidation and extensive oxidative damage to proteins and mtDNA

cyte, some negative (e.g., apoptosis and necrosis) and others positive (e.g., cardioprotection and cell proliferation). H_2O_2 produced by mitochondria and sent to the cytosol is involved in several signal transduction pathways, including the activation of c-Jun N-terminal kinase (JNK1) and mitogen-activated protein kinases (MAPK) [27–29], and can impact the regulation of redox-sensitive K^+ channels affecting arteriole constriction [30]. The release of H_2O_2 from mitochondria and its subsequent cellular effects are increased in cardiomyocytes treated with antimycin and high Ca^{2+} and further enhanced by treatment with CoQ. CoQ plays a dual role in the mitochondrial generation of intracellular redox signaling, by acting both as a prooxidant involved in ROS generation and as an antioxidant by inhibiting the PT pore, cytochrome c release, and also by increasing ATP synthesis [31]. Increased mitochondrial H_2O_2 generation and signaling occur with NO modulation of the respiratory chain [28, 32],

as well as with the induction of myocardial mitochondrial NO production, resulting from treatment with enalapril [33]. ROS play a fundamental role in the cardioprotective signaling pathways of ischemic preconditioning, in critical oxygen sensing, and in the induction of stress responses that promote cell survival. These phenomena are further examined in Chaps. 5 and 11.

ROS and Cardiac Pathology

Generation of ROS together with impaired antioxidant defenses is observed in the failing heart as well as in myocardial ischemia and reperfusion (I/R). During the first moments of reperfusion and myocardial injury, a burst of ROS occurs that is associated with changes in mitochondria (e.g., PT pore opening) [34]. The source of ROS generation during early reperfusion has not been clearly determined; it may be of either mitochondrial or cytoplasmic origin. On the other hand, during ischemia (and likely in the early/acute pathway of ischemic preconditioning) the source of ROS generated clearly involves the mitochondrial ETC, and this may be different from the source of ROS generated in early reperfusion [35, 36]. As it turns out, mitochondria are central in the myocardial failing process since ROS generation by mitochondria impacts the expression of genes encoding key elements of the apoptotic pathway (Fig. 10.2), including mitochondrial PT pore components (i.e., ANT and porin) and the associated mitochondrial creatine kinase in response to HF (J. Marín-García unpublished data).

A number of studies have shown that in the failing heart, cardioprotective interventions may prevent or slowdown ROS production via antioxidants like MnSOD and target apoptosis. Furthermore, when exposed to an insult, cardiomyocytes are able to mount a cardioprotective response. Also chemical, metabolic, and even physical stressors have been shown to generate cardioprotective responses that share

elements of the ischemic preconditioning (IPC) model and in these responses mitochondria are the key factors. Besides regulating the cellular bioenergetic supply in the form of adenosine triphosphate (ATP), the organelle has many roles (see Chap. 5). A participant in the trigger and mediation of cardioprotective responses, mitochondria house and regulate pivotal early events in the apoptotic pathway. This plasticity enables the organelle to function both as a target and as a player in myocardial signal transduction events and in the generation of ROS in response to a variety of cellular insults providing an appropriate antioxidant response (Table 10.1).

The time course of MnSOD induction, a mitochondrial-specific protective response to ROS-mediated damage, correlates well with the appearance of ischemic tolerance. However, the activities of other cellular anti-oxidants, i.e., catalase and CuSOD are not similarly affected.

In the canine model of pacing-induced HF, there is a marked increase of aldehyde in left ventricle tissue that suggests elevated free radical-induced damage [37, 38]. The increased levels of OS correlated with the onset of reduced cardiac complex III and V activities. This has been

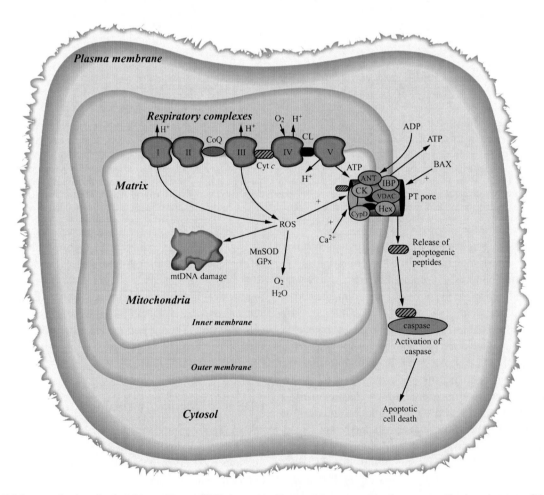

Fig. 10.2 ROS generation by mitochondria produces mtDNA damage and impacts the expression of genes encoding key elements of the apoptotic pathway

Table 10.1 Mitochondrial functional plasticity allows modulation of:

Cell respiration

Ion (K^+, Ca^{2+}) transport

ATP production

Cytochrome c release

Redox state

ROS generation

Antioxidant response (e.g., MnSOD)

Cardiac protection with K_{ATP} channel openers (e.g., diazoxide and nicorandil)

corroborated by measurements of ROS levels compared in paced and unpaced dogs, revealing that both $O_2^{\cdot-}$ and OH$^\cdot$ radicals generated from mitochondrial-produced H_2O_2 are increased in the failing heart and correlated with the severity of left ventricular dysfunction [39, 40]. OS also appears to be involved in the generation of large-scale myocardial mtDNA deletions that have been shown in pacing-induced HF [37], as well as in studies of ameroid constriction-mediated myocardial ischemia in the dog [41]. Furthermore, neonatal cardiac myocytes treated with TNF-α displayed a significant increase in ROS levels, accompanied by an overall decline in mtDNA copy number and decreased complex III activity [42]. The TNF-α mediated decline in mtDNA copy number might result from an increase in mtDNA deletions. ROS-induced mtDNA damage, resulting in respiratory complex enzyme dysfunction, contributes to the progression of left ventricular (LV) remodeling and failure after myocardial infarction (MI). In a murine model of MI and remodeling created by ligation of the left anterior descending coronary artery, increased ROS production (e.g., OH$^\cdot$ level) was found in association with decreased levels of mtDNA and ETC activities, suggesting impairment of mitochondrial function [43]. In addition, chronic release of ROS has been linked to the development of left ventricular hypertrophy, ECM remodeling, and HF. Thus, blocking/reducing ROS production may be an important target in the treatment of HF. Indeed, recent observations have suggested that overexpression of the genes for peroxiredoxin-3 (Prx-3), a mitochondrial antioxidant, or mitochondrial transcription factor A (TFAM), might prevent the decline in mtDNA copy number (likely secondary to mtDNA damage (i.e., increased deletions)) and also the mitochondrial dysfunction observed in HF [44]. Thus, preventing OS and mtDNA damage may be a significant approach in HF treatment.

Besides chronic ROS generation from the mitochondrial organelle, ROS can also derive from nonmitochondrial NAD(P)H oxidase, which in endothelial cells is activated by cytokines, neurohormones, and growth factors (e.g., angiotensin II, norepinephrine, and TNF-α) [45, 46]. Furthermore, long-term alterations in cardiac phenotype can be driven by redox-sensitive gene expression, and

in this way, ROS may act as potent intracellular second messengers. In cardiac myocytes, NAD(P)H oxidase plays a prominent role in the hypertrophic pathway [47–49]. In addition, NAD(P)H oxidase activity is significantly increased in the failing versus nonfailing myocardium [50]. It has been reported that statins (i.e., 3-hydroxyl-3-methylglutaryl coenzyme A (HMG-CoA) reductase inhibitors), by modulating the ROS-generating activity of NAD(P)H oxidase, can inhibit cardiac hypertrophy by cholesterol-independent mechanisms [51, 52]. Statins block the isoprenylation and activation of members of the Rho guanosine triphosphatase (GTPase) family such as Rac1, an essential component of NAD(P)H oxidase. Taken together, it appears that blocking ROS production with statins may be beneficial to patients with myocardial hypertrophy and chronic HF.

Oxidative Stress, Myocardial Ischemia, and HF

Myocardial ischemia, an important cause of HF in human can produce changes in the endogenous defense mechanisms against oxygen free radicals, mainly through a reduction in the activity of mitochondrial superoxide dismutase (SOD) and a decline in tissue content of reduced glutathione [53]. Increased ROS production in both mitochondria and white blood cells (WBC) and toxic oxygen metabolite production are exacerbated by re-admission of oxygen during post-ischemic reperfusion. Furthermore, OS resulting from both increased ROS generation and diminished antioxidant reserve promotes the oxidation of thiol groups in proteins and lipid peroxidation leading first to reversible damage, and eventually to necrosis.

Mitochondria of circulating WBC and platelets sense OS during capillary passage and react by producing ROS. While a number of observations have shown that severe HF is associated with OS, the mediator role of WBC and platelets OS in HF has only been recently investigated. Ijsselmuiden et al. have studied a group of HF patients and healthy volunteers (control group) [54]. WBCs and platelets of both arterial and venous blood samples were quantitatively analyzed with respect to the development of cytoplasmic and mitochondrial OS using fluorescent dyes. The increased number and percentage of cells with both cytosolic and mitochondrial fluorescence indicated the extensive presence of OS and was significantly greater than that found in control samples. Moreover, myocardial OS production (gauged by coronary sinus sampling) exceeded systemic production (gauged by peripheral venous sampling). Furthermore, partial pulmonary clearance of OS containing cells was identified in controls by the reduction in arterial compared to venous samples;

in contrast, no significant difference (between arterial and venous samples) was found in OS-containing cells in severe HF patients suggesting defective pulmonary clearance in these cases. Thus, in severe HF, the proportion of WBC and platelets that are ROS-positive is raised, possibly because cytosolic ROS-positive WBC and platelets are normally cleared in the lungs and this function appears to be deficient in severe HF while mitochondrial ROS production is increased. The raised numbers of circulating ROS-positive WBC and platelets amplify OS in HF. Ideally, a more rigorous approach could have been employed by first carry out the study in an animal model that might eliminate the concerns raised by the numerous drug treatments, and the potential heterogeneity of HF etiology, which may impact on these findings.

Since coronary artery disease (CAD), with consequent myocardial ischemia and necrosis, is a well-recognized leading cause of HF worldwide, it is relevant to note here that ROS play an integral role in the genesis and progression of CAD and HF. In the vessel wall ROS contribute to the formation of oxidized LDL, a major player in the pathogenesis of atherosclerosis and ROS-mediated activation of matrix metalloproteinases (MMPs) may play a contributory role in vessel plaque rupture, initiating coronary thrombosis, and occlusion [55–57].

Observations in vitro and animal studies have shown that in the failing heart, ROS influence several components of the cardiac phenotype and its remodeling, including contractile function, interstitial fibrosis, endothelial dysfunction, and myocyte hypertrophy. ROS contribute to the remodeling processes in a number of ways, including activating MMPs that participate in the reconfiguration of the extracellular matrix (ECM); acting as signaling molecules in the development of compensatory hypertrophy; and contributing to myocyte loss via apoptosis signaling.

Excessive production of NO has also been implicated in the pathogenesis of chronic HF [58, 59]. Uncoupling of constitutive nitric oxide synthase (NOS) leads to the overproduction of superoxide ($O_2^{.-}$) and peroxynitrite ($ONOO^-$), two extremely potent oxidants. Peroxynitrite produced from the reaction of highly reactive NO with the superoxide anion impairs cardiovascular function through multiple mechanisms, including activation of MMPs and nuclear enzyme poly (ADP-ribose) polymerase (PARP). Increased OS resulting from the overproduction of superoxide also mediates the dysregulation of S-nitrosylation of proteins at specific cysteine residues by reactive nitrogen species (RNS), a more selective modification of proteins than found with protein oxidation. This redox mechanism has been demonstrated to lead to altered myocardial excitation–contractility and vascular reactivity [60, 61].

ROS in the Aging Failing Heart

In the failing aging heart, increased OS is mainly related to augmentation of electron leak thru impaired complex I, II, and III (Fig. 10.3), although both normal aging human and animal hearts have increased levels of ROS and nitrogen species (RNS). The balance between ROS/RNS generating enzymes and scavenger enzyme systems can be disrupted in a number of pathologic conditions, including degenerative diseases [62], diabetes mellitus [63], endothelial dysfunction, atherosclerosis, and hypertension [64].

While antioxidant mechanisms may be enhanced in the myocardium with aging, these compensatory mechanisms appears not to be completely effective in stemming ROS accumulation. Protein oxidation, lipid oxidation, and mitochondrial DNA damage increase with aging whereas chronic ROS stress acts as a trigger of matrix fibrosis. With aging and in the failing heart the increased oxidative damage of proteins by ROS or RNS is characterized by protein carboxylation and nitration.

Mitochondria are not only considered as the major source of ROS but they are also the targets of ROS during the aging process, and increased mitochondrial ROS formation would be expected to cause mitochondrial protein oxidative damage in the senescent animals [65–67].

ANT has been found to be one of the mitochondrial proteins most susceptible to ROS during aging [68], and this ANT oxidative damage is mostly displayed as carbonylation. Increased ANT carbonyl modification has also been found in aged houseflies [68] as well as in aging mammalian animals [69–71]. ANT contains three redox-sensitive cysteine residues on loops projecting into the matrix compartment. These residues are particularly susceptible to oxidation by sulfenic acid moieties and mixed disulfides if the normally high intramitochondrial glutathione (GSH)/glutathione disulfide (GSSG) ratio is not maintained during periods of OS [72]. Indeed, GSH/GSSG ratio is significantly reduced during aging [73–77].

ANT carbonyl modification is associated with a reduced capability to exchange ADP/ATP across the inner membrane, which may cause the inhibition or uncoupling of OXPHOS and the collapse of $\Delta\Psi m$, turning mitochondrial ATP synthesis into hydrolysis (see Fig. 10.3). ANT oxidation may also shift from its native state as a gated pore (mediating ADP/ATP exchange) into a non-selective pore, allowing free permeation of small ions and metabolites across the mitochondria inner membrane. Furthermore, ANT conformation conversion is affected by cyclophilin-D (CyP-D) in the mitochondrial matrix. CyP-D contains a relatively high proportion of polyunsaturated fatty acids that could be oxidized by ROS to generate highly reactive lipid fragments

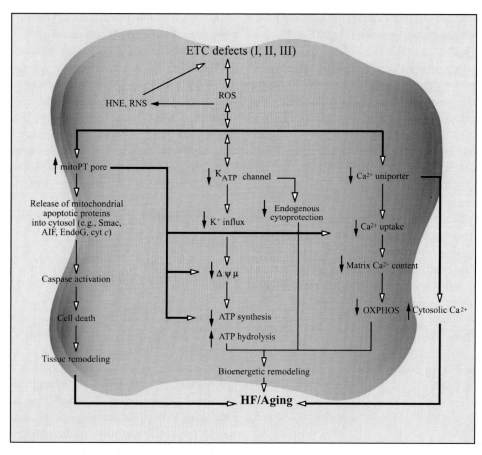

Fig. 10.3 Flow-chart of remodeling resulting from aging/HF-modulation of mitochondrial ion function. Mitochondrial ETC defects result in electron leak, ROS overproduction followed by formation of reactive nitrogen species (RNS), and lipid peroxidation (e.g., HNE). Increased oxidative stress, in turn, damages mitochondrial ion channel function. Sensitized mitoPTP causes loss of mitochondrial Ca^{2+}, decreased Ca^{2+} uptake, and reduced $\Delta\Psi m$, which in turn reduces OXPHOS and ATP synthesis. Increased mitoPTP also promotes increased mitochondrial vulnerability to Ca^{2+} loading and release of apoptogenic factors (e.g., AIF, cyt c) from mitochondria which sets into motion the apoptotic pathway including caspase activation, leading to cell death. Mitochondrial K_{ATP} is also targeted in aging and HF, resulting in reduced cardiac tolerance to stress and loss of preconditioning cytoprotection; moreover, decreased K^+ influx and electrochemical gradient results in diminished OXPHOS. Reduced Ca^{2+} uniporter activity not only decreases mitochondrial Ca^{2+} uptake, dampening Ca^{2+} stimulatory effects on bioenergetic metabolism, but also exaggerates intracellular Ca^{2+} disturbance, leading to elevated cytosolic Ca^{2+} levels. MitoK$_{ATP}$ and mitoPTP channel modulation can trigger ROS production, which can further target ETC activities, as does increased HNE (indicated by *double-headed arrows*). ETC Electron transport chain, HNE 4-hydroxyl-2-nonal, mitoPTP mitochondrial permeability transition pore, cyt c cytochrome c, AIF apoptosis-inducing factor, $\Delta\Psi m$ mitochondrial membrane potential. *Solid vertical arrows* indicate reduced or increased levels, whereas *unfilled arrows* denote relationship within a pathway

such as 4-hydroxy-2-nonenal (HNE) and 4-hydroxyhexenal (HHE). These lipid peroxidation byproducts may interact with or modify specific thiol groups on ANT leading to adduct formation, thereby inhibiting ANT activity [78], and also increasing CyP-D binding to ANT [79, 80], thereby destabilizing ANT and sensitizing mitoPTP to calcium [81].

With aging, VDAC is also particularly vulnerable to oxidative damage because the tyrosine residue of VDAC is subject to conversion into 3-nitrotyrosine (3-NT) by reactive nitrogen species (RNS) including NO and peroxynitrite (ONOO⁻), which are normally produced under physiologic conditions and increased with aging. This nitration of tyrosine can compromise the functional and/or structural integrity of the target protein [82]. Interestingly, proteomic analysis using 2-D gel electrophoresis combined with nano-electrospray ionization-tandem mass spectrometry (NSI-MS/ MS) technique showed that there is an age-dependent nitration of VDAC in mitochondria [83]. Increased VDAC nitration is very likely related to excessive OS in mitochondria since similar changes have been found in diabetic hearts which exhibit increased OS [84]. Although it has not yet been established whether oxidative modification of tyrosine residues directly alters the property of VDAC or sensitize VDAC to its regulators, it has been found that superoxide anion ($O_2^{\cdot-}$) could induce VDAC-dependent rapid and massive cytochrome c release and enhance mitoPTP to Ca^{2+} in permeabilized HepG2 cells [85].

Ca^{2+} is the key trigger for PT pore formation, possibly by binding to the negatively charged cardiolipin head groups on the inner face of the inner membrane, thereby disrupting the stabilizing interactions between cardiolipin and ANT [86]. Since mitochondrial Ca^{2+} content tends to decrease with aging, the impaired mitochondrial Ca^{2+} handling and reduced threshold of mitoPTP to Ca^{2+} may be more critical than Ca^{2+} itself in mediating mitoPTP in the aging failing heart. For instance, in response to stress such as ischemia/reperfusion, heart mitochondrial Ca^{2+} significantly increased (about two-fold greater with senescence). Taking these findings together with the evidence of increased lipid peroxidation (HNE formation) in senescent hearts on reperfusion, it seems that the aging hearts are increasingly vulnerable to reperfusion damage brought about by increased mitochondrial Ca^{2+} [87], increased creatine kinase nitration [88, 89], age-dependent decreased hexokinase [87], and decreased nucleotide pool [69], which may also facilitate the formation of ANT-VDAC complex, sensitize PTP, or cause the permeability transition in the aging failing heart.

Oxidative Stress and Apoptosis

Both the generation of ROS and the onset of apoptotic cell death are important and often related events in cell homeostasis. Increased OS and ROS accumulation can lead to myocyte hypertrophy, interstitial fibrosis (through matrix metalloproteinases activation), and apoptosis. Apoptosis can be blocked or delayed by treatment with antioxidants and thiol reductants [90]. Moreover, overexpression of antioxidant proteins (e.g., MnSOD, glutathione peroxidase, and metallothionein) can block apoptotic progression [91–93]. Attenuation of apoptosis by overexpression of the antiapoptotic protein Bcl-2 was associated with protection against ROS and OS [94]. Cells from transgenic mice containing ablated genes encoding antioxidant proteins (e.g., glutathione peroxidase) have both increased OS levels and increased apoptosis [95, 96].

Agents that induce apoptosis (e.g., TNF-α) also promote high levels of mitochondrial-generated ROS [97]. In addition, ROS production can target an array of signal transducers (e.g., JNK, TNF-α and MAPK), which interface with the apoptotic machinery. This includes both activation of the proapoptotic Bcl-2 family and mediators (e.g., TNF-α), as well as the modulation of their gene expression by activation of specific transcription factors (e.g., NF-κB).

It is worth noting that an important model system has emerged to study the induction of OS and apoptosis using H_2O_2 treated cultured cardiomyocytes [98]. This approach allowed molecular and biochemical appraisal of cellular and mitochondrial events presaging, accompanying and following the induction of cardiomyocyte apoptosis. In addition, it allowed the study of short-lived signaling intermediates, as well as the use of various treatments (e.g., antioxidants) to stem the development of cardiomyocyte OS and apoptotic progression [99, 100]. Not all cardiomyocyte apoptosis is triggered by OS and ROS generation. Gathered observations have shown no evidence of ROS (or NO) involvement in the palmitate-mediated induction of apoptosis in neonatal rat cardiomyocytes [101], illustrating the complex, multiforked, and parallel nature of signals in the apoptotic pathway.

Nitric Oxide and HF

Oxygen serves as the critical terminal electron acceptor in the ETC; in its absence the ETC shuts down and cardiac demands for ATP are not met. Molecular oxygen is also central in both the formation of nitric oxide (NO), a primary determinant of both vascular tone and cardiac contractility and in the generation of ROS (and subsequent OS) as a significant by-product of energy metabolism during its sequential acceptance of electrons in the mitochondrial ETC. The end results of NO/redox disequilibrium have implications for cardiac and vascular homeostasis and may result in the development of atherosclerosis, myocardial tissue remodeling, and hypertrophy. ROS/RNS generation is also attributed to the transit from hypertrophic to apoptotic phenotypes, a possible mechanism of myocardial failure [102].

Endothelial dysfunction in advanced HF patients (see Chap. 12) is a critical component in the systemic vasoconstriction and reduced peripheral perfusion that characterizes these patients [103]. Endothelial regulation of vascular tone is mediated mainly by NO. Increased OS in patients with HF may be related to decreased bioavailability of NO secondary to reduced expression of endothelial NOs and increased generation of ROS. These react with NO in the setting of decreased antioxidant defenses that would normally clear these radicals, culminating in attenuated endothelium-dependent vasodilation in patients with advanced HF. Moreover, abnormal production and/or distribution of ROS and reactive nitrosative species in blood creates oxidative and/or nitrosative stresses in the failing myocardium and endothelium. As previously noted, the uncoupling of constitutive NOS leads to increased generation of superoxide ($O_2^{\cdot-}$) and peroxynitrite ($ONOO^-$). Peroxynitrite affects cardiovascular function and contributes to the pathogenesis of cardiac and endothelial dysfunction associated with myocardial infarction, chronic HF, diabetes, atherosclerosis, hypertension, aging, and various forms of shock. Moreover, pharmacological inhibition of xanthine oxidase-derived superoxide formation, as well as neutralization of peroxynitrite, or inhibition of PARP, provide significant benefit in various forms of cardiovascular injury [104]. Increased OS resulting from the overproduction of superoxide mediates the dysregulation of S-nitrosylation of proteins at specific cysteine residues by RNS, a more selective modification of proteins than found with protein oxidation. This redox mechanism has been found to lead to altered myocardial excitation–contractility and vascular reactivity [60, 61].

Antioxidant Defense

It is important to notice that ROS and cellular redox states regulate an extensive number of vital pathways in the myocardium, including energy metabolism, survival and stress responses, apoptosis, inflammatory response, and oxygen sensing. Gathered observations have shown that ROS role in ischemia and reperfusion injury, as well as the role that antioxidants therapy may play, varies significantly whether one use whole organ and animal models or isolated cell models; findings are often contradictory in providing insights into why clinical trials of antioxidants frequently have shown mixed results.

The powerful cell-damaging ROS oxidants can be neutralized by an array of protective antioxidant scavenger enzymes, as well as by various lipid and water-soluble compounds including ascorbic acid, glutathione, thioredoxin, and α-tocopherol. The antioxidant enzymes are located in a variety of cellular compartments including the mitochondria (e.g., MnSOD, glutathione peroxidase, thioredoxin reductase), peroxisomes (e.g., catalase), microsomes (e.g., cytochrome P450), and in the cytosol (e.g., CuSOD and cytosolic thioredoxin reductase). In general, there are significantly lower levels of antioxidants in myocardial mitochondria than in liver mitochondria, but the consensus opinion is that the antioxidant capacity of the heart is generally sufficient to handle the normal levels of ROS production, although insufficient to meet the greater ROS accumulation that occurs in myocardial ischemia [105].

A mitochondrial isoform of catalase with low specific activity has been found in rats [106, 107]. This mitochondrial catalase activity was detected in the heart but not in liver or skeletal muscle and it appears to increase during caloric-restricted (CR) diets and in the diabetic heart [108–110]. The role that this enzyme plays has not been fully determined although there is evidence of its participation in the prevention of excess lipid peroxidation in myocardial ischemia [111]. On the other hand, a mitochondria-specific catalase has not been found in the heart of transgenic mice even after overexpression of the catalase gene [112].

While superoxide dismutases catalyze the removal of superoxide radicals by the formation of H_2O_2, glutathione peroxidase (GPx) catalyzes the breakdown of H_2O_2 to water and oxidized glutathione (GSSG) by using reduced glutathione (GSH) as depicted in Fig. 10.1. Since GPx is located in both the mitochondria and cytosol, H_2O_2 can be removed from either compartment depending on the availability of glutathione. A small fraction of the total cellular pool of GSH is sequestered in mitochondria by the action of a carrier that transports GSH from cytosol to the mitochondrial matrix [113]. Upon exposure to increased exogenous ROS, isolated, perfused rat hearts are rapidly depleted of their antioxidant reserves, including those of SOD and GSH, rendering them more vulnerable to the action of oxidative injury [114].

Another important mechanism in the antioxidant reactions is the sequestering of iron and copper ions to keep them from reacting with superoxide or H_2O_2. The antioxidant dexrazoxane prevents site-specific iron-based oxygen radical damage by chelating free and loosely bound iron. In addition, it has been used as a cardioprotective drug against doxorubicin-induced oxidative damage to myocardial mitochondria in both humans and animals [115, 116]. The antioxidant metal-binding protein metallothionein (MT) also provides cardioprotection by directly reacting with ROS produced by ischemia/reperfusion and doxorubicin treatment, as found in studies with a cardiac-specific MT-overexpressing transgenic mouse model [117]. MT expression is also inducible within the heart (and other tissues) by TNF-α, IL-6, doxorubicin, and metals such as cadmium and Zn [117–119], although its cardioprotective role has not been determined.

The uncoupling of mitochondrial respiration from OXPHOS ATP production, by either artificial uncouplers such as 2,4-dinitrophenol (e.g., DNP) or natural uncouplers (e.g., laurate), fatty acids, and mitochondrial uncoupling (UCP) proteins – strongly inhibits $O_2^{\cdot-}$ and H_2O_2 formation in mitochondria [120–122]. ROS production is favored when the mitochondrial membrane potential is above a specific threshold. Under conditions where the mitochondrial membrane potential is at its peak (e.g., state 4 respiration), ROS production is increased. It is noteworthy that increased mitochondrial membrane potential slows electron transport through the respiratory chain, resulting in increased half-life of the ubiquinone free radical and the likelihood that electrons will interact with oxygen to form ROS [123]. Uncouplers prevent the transmembrane electrochemical H^+ potential difference (Δm_H) from being above a threshold critical for ROS formation by respiratory complexes I and III. This has been corroborated in transgenic mice in which UCP3 protein is lacking, resulting in enhanced ROS production and increased OS in heart and skeletal muscle [124], in transgenic mice with UCP1 overexpression [125], and in cardiomyocytes with UCP2 overexpression, in which ROS is markedly attenuated [126].

Pharmacological inhibition of xanthine oxidase-derived superoxide formation and neutralization of peroxynitrite or inhibition of poly(ADP-ribose) polymerase (PARP) have been reported to provide significant benefit in various forms of cardiovascular injury [104]. Using rat and mouse models of HF, the beneficial effects of a novel ultrapotent PARP inhibitor was studied by Pacher et al. [127]. The effect of INO-1001 on the development of HF induced by permanent ligation of the left anterior descending coronary artery was assessed, as well as in HF induced by doxorubicin, and acute myocardial dysfunction induced by bacterial endotoxin. In the coronary ligation model, significantly depressed left ventricular performance and impaired vascular relaxation of aortic rings were found; PARP inhibition significantly improved both cardiac function and vascular relaxation. In the doxorubicin model, a single injection of doxorubicin induced high mortality and a significant decrease in left ventricular systolic pressure, $+dP/dt$, $-dP/dt$, stroke volume, stroke work, ejection fraction, and cardiac output. Treatment with the PARP inhibitor reduced doxorubicin-induced mortality and markedly improved cardiac function; on the other hand, PARP inhibition did not interfere with doxorubicin's antitumor effect. In the endotoxin model of cardiac dysfunction, PARP inhibition attenuated the reduction in myocardial contractility elicited by endotoxin. Taken together, these data support the view that PARP inhibition may be an effective approach in the experimental treatment of various forms of acute and chronic HF.

Antioxidants Therapy

Mitochondrial ROS and OS are implicated in the pathogenesis of the cardiac damage elicited by ischemia/reperfusion and the cardiomyopathies associated with FRDA and doxorubicin-induction [128, 129]. Several oxygen radical scavengers, including CoQ_{10}, vitamin E, dexrazoxane, and idebenone, have been used in their treatment [130–132]. In doxorubicin-induced cardiomyopathy, the free-radical scavenger dexrazoxane has been shown to protect the heart from doxorubicin-associated oxidative damage, and has been recommended for clinical use to attenuate the myocardial damage that may occur in children with acute lymphoblastic leukemia treated with doxorubicin chemotherapy [116]. Both CoQ_{10} and idebenone have been found to markedly improve cardiac function and reduce cardiac hypertrophy in patients with FRDA [133–135]. Interestingly, ataxia and other CNS symptoms occurring in FRDA are less affected by the administration of these antioxidants than is the cardiac phenotype. In addition, Idebenone seems to improve the cardiac dysfunction observed in mitochondrial cardiomyopathy [136]. CoQ_{10}, besides its role as an antioxidant, also serves multiple cellular functions, including participation as an electron carrier in the respiratory chain and as an activating cofactor for mitochondrial uncoupling proteins. In addition, CoQ_{10} appears to have a beneficial effect in several neurological disorders with cardiac involvement, including MELAS and KSS syndromes [137]. Moreover, a significant reduction in the incidence of cardiac conduction abnormalities seen in patients with KSS or CPEO syndromes has been reported using CoQ_{10} at relatively high doses ranging (60–150 mg/day) [138]. Also, clinical improvement was observed in patients with advanced HF after CoQ_{10} supplementation to standard therapy [139]. Nonetheless, because the sample size and the design used in these studies raised concerns as to the validity of systematic clinical use of CoQ_{10} in treating HF, presently a large double-blind multisite clinical trial is underway to test its efficacy [140, 141].

Since increased plasma catecholamines and sympathetic stimulation may lead in HF patients to increased production of ROS, and possibly to endothelial damage/dysfunction and atheroma formation, treatment with β-blockers and ACE inhibitors have been recommended. The beneficial anti-oxidative effects of carvedilol, a vasodilating β-blocker with antioxidant activity, in HF remains controversial. Whereas some groups found a reduction of OS in HF patients treated with carvedilol [142] others did not [143]. Using immunohistochemistry, Nakamura et al. [144] evaluated the expression of 4-hydroxy-2-nonenal (HNE)-modified protein (a major lipid peroxidation product) in endomyocardial biopsy tissues from 23 patients with DCM and 13 control subjects with normal cardiac function; whether levels of lipid peroxides were elevated in the myocardium of patients with DCM, and whether carvedilol reduces lipid peroxidation level. Expression of HNE-modified protein was found in all myocardial tissue samples from patients with DCM. Expression was distinctive in cardiomyocytes cytosol. Myocardial HNE-modified protein levels in patients with DCM were significantly increased compared with the levels in control subjects. In addition, biopsy samples from 11 patients with DCM were examined before and after treatment with carvedilol (5–30 mg/day; mean dosage, 22 ± 8 mg/day). Following treatment, myocardial HNE-modified protein levels decreased by 40% with improvement in HF. Taken together, this study confirmed that OS is elevated in HF and the administration of carvedilol resulted in reduction of OS and improvement in cardiac function. These investigators have also studied whether levels of 8-hydroxy-2-deoxyguanosine (8-OHdG), a marker of oxidative DNA damage, were elevated in the serum and myocardium of patients with DCM, and whether carvedilol could decrease 8-OHdG [145]. Serum 8-OHdG was measured by enzyme immunoassay in 56 patients with DCM and in 20 control subjects. DCM patients had significantly increased levels of 8-OHdG compared to control subjects. Interestingly, immunohistochemically positive 8-OHdG staining was detected in the nuclei of cardiomyocytes from DCM endomyocardial tissue patients, but not in controls. After treatment with carvedilol, the serum levels of 8-OHdG in DCM patients decreased by 19%, together with improvement in HF. Thus, levels of 8-OHdG are elevated in serum and myocardium of HF patients and carvedilol seems to be an effective way to reduce oxidative DNA damage.

The anti-oxidative properties of carvedilol and ACE inhibitors in severe HF have been studied by Chin et al. [146]. From a group of 66 outpatients with HF, 46 patients that were on an established treatment with ACE inhibitor were started on β-blocker, and 20 patients not previously on ACE-inhibitors were treated with lisinopril. Baseline parameters were compared to 22 healthy control subjects. Serum lipid hydroperoxides (LHP) and total antioxidant capacity (TAC) were determined as indices of oxidative damage and antioxidant defense, and plasma von Willebrand factor (vWf) as an index of endothelial damage/dysfunction. The baseline indices for the measures of oxidative damage and endothelial function in the 66 CHF patients were significantly higher than healthy control subjects. After 3 months of maintenance therapy with β-blockers, a significant reduction in LHP levels occurred, but not TAC or vWf. ACE inhibitor therapy also significantly reduced vWf levels, but failed to have any statistically significant effects on LHP or TAC. This pilot study suggests that OS in advanced, severe HF may be due to increased free radical production or inefficient free radical clearance by scavengers and that β-blockers, but not ACE inhibitors, reduced lipid peroxidation (although no relation was found between a reduction in oxidative damage and endothelial damage/dysfunction).

Treatment with ACE inhibitors, angiotensin, aldosterone, and endothelin–antagonists has been shown to beneficially modulate endothelial dysfunction in severe HF. As pointed out by Bauersachs and Widder [147], these therapies increase NO bioactivity by either modulation of ROS generation, thereby preventing the interaction of superoxide anions with NO, and/or increasing endothelial NO synthase (eNOS) expression/activity. Experiments in rats after large myocardial infarction treatment with AVE9488, a novel eNOS transcription enhancer, attenuates cardiac remodeling and endothelial dysfunction. Furthermore, antioxidants, L-arginine, cofactors of endothelial NO-synthase, and exercise training positively modulate endothelial function [148].

Conclusion

Molecular oxygen is central in both the formation of nitric oxide (NO), a primary determinant of both vascular tone and cardiac contractility, and in the generation of ROS (and subsequent OS), as a significant by-product of energy metabolism during its sequential acceptance of electrons in the mitochondrial ETC. Since these short-lived intermediates can act either as an important signaling molecule or induce irreversible oxidative damage to proteins, lipids and nucleic acids, both ROS and oxygen exert both beneficial and deleterious effects.

ROS play an integral role not only in the genesis of CAD but also in its progression. Several in vitro and animal studies have demonstrated that in the failing heart, ROS influence several components of the cardiac phenotype and cardiac remodeling, including contractile function, interstitial fibrosis, endothelial dysfunction, and myocyte hypertrophy. Furthermore, ROS contribute to the remodeling processes in a number of ways including activation of MMPs that participate in reconfiguration of the ECM, acting as signaling molecules in the development of compensatory hypertrophy and contributing to myocyte loss via apoptosis signaling.

It is important to keep in mind that ROS can be generated in the heart and endothelial tissues by non-mitochondrial reactions, including the involvement of xanthine oxidase (XO), NAD(P)H oxidases, and cytochrome P450. Furthermore, increased ROS and toxic oxygen metabolite production in both the myocardial mitochondrial organelle and leukocytes are exacerbated by re-admission of oxygen during post-ischemic reperfusion. OS, resulting from both increased ROS generation and diminished antioxidant protection promotes the oxidation of thiol groups in proteins and lipid peroxidation leading initially to reversible damage, and finally to necrosis.

Significantly, reduced bioavailability of NO and increased generation of ROS within the vascular wall are key determinants in endothelial dysfunction, and this imbalance between NO and ROS mainly results from neurohumoral activation associated with HF. Furthermore, the excessive activation of the renin–angiotensin aldosterone and endothelin systems plays a central role. While the use of scavengers to treat OS has been considered for quite sometime, the success of this approach has been questionable to the least. Nonetheless, there is increasing evidence that HF-related generation of ROS/RNS may be ameliorated by targeting ROS/RNS-generating enzymes and upstream mediators. β-blockers, but not ACE inhibitors, appears to reduce lipid peroxidation although so far no relation has been demonstrated between a reduction in oxidative damage and endothelial damage/dysfunction. Nevertheless, therapies that ameliorate endothelial function in HF patients have been shown to improve exercise tolerance and outcomes making endothelial dysfunction an important target to develop novel therapies (Table 10.2).

Table 10.2 Metabolic and antioxidant treatments for mitochondrial-based cardiac disorders

Treatment	Primary mechanism	Disorder
Coenzyme Q	Antioxidant/ETC carrier	HF, FRDA, MELAS, KSS
Dichloroacetate	Increased PDH activity; decreased FAO	KSS, MELAS, lactic acidosis, diabetic cardiomyopathy
Idebenone	Antioxidant	FRDA, mitochondrial cardiomyopathy
Carnitine	Increased fatty acid transport	Cardiomyopathy and HF
Etomoxir	FAO inhibitor	FAO disorders
Trimetazidine	FAO inhibitor; increased phospholipid turnover	FAO disorders, myocardial ischemia/angina, diabetic cardiomyopathy
Ranolazine	Partial FAO inhibitor	FAO disorders, myocardial ischemia/angina
Perhexilene	FAO inhibitor	Dysrhythmia
N-3 PUFA	Reduced FAO	Dysrhythmia
Copper supplement	Assist in COX subunit assembly	HCM due to SCO_2 mutation
Dexrazoxane	Antioxidant	Doxorubicin-induced cardiomyopathy
Carvedilol	β-adrenergic blocker; FAO shift to glucose	CHF
Diltiazem	Inhibits release of mitochondrial Ca^{2+}	Dysrhythmia
		Myocardial ischemia

FRDA Friedreich ataxia; *HF* heart failure; *CHF* congestive HF; *HCM* hypertrophic cardiomyopathy; *KSS* Kearns–Sayre syndrome; *MELAS* mitochondrial encephalomyopathy, lactic acidosis and stroke-like episodes

Summary

- ROS play an important role in the development and progression of HF, namely by direct damage and as intracellular second messengers.
- The major ROS are the superoxide radical $O_2^{\cdot-}$, hydrogen peroxide (H_2O_2), and the hydroxyl radical $OH^{\cdot}$.
- The production of the hydroxyl radical (which is the most reactive form of ROS) is primarily responsible for the damage to cellular macromolecules such as proteins, DNA, and lipids.
- Under normal conditions, the primary source of ROS is the mitochondrial ETC, where oxygen can be activated to superoxide radical by a nonenzymatic process. This production of ROS is a by-product of normal metabolism and occurs from electrons leaked from the ETC, at complexes I, II, and III.
- Lipids and in particular the mitochondrial-specific cardiolipin serve as a focal target for free radical damage.
- Highly reactive peroxynitrite irreversibly impairs mitochondrial respiration since it inhibits complex I activity and mitochondrial aconitase, and causes induction of the PT pore.
- Mitochondrial ROS generation can be amplified in cells with abnormal respiratory chain function as well as, under physiological and pathological conditions such as HF, where oxygen consumption is increased.
- Besides mitochondria, other cellular sources for generating superoxide radicals include the reactions of oxygen with microsomal cytochrome p450 and with reduced flavins (e.g., NAD(P)H), usually in the presence of metal ions. In addition, xanthine oxidase (XO), a primarily cytosolic enzyme involved in purine metabolism, is also a source of the superoxide radical.
- In addition to the cell-damaging effects of ROS, mitochondrial ROS generation and the OS they engender play a major role in cell regulation and signaling.
- Increased mitochondrial H_2O_2 generation and signaling occur with NO modulation of the respiratory chain as well as with the induction of myocardial mitochondrial NO production, resulting from treatment with enalapril.
- ROS play a fundamental role in the cardioprotective signaling pathways of ischemic preconditioning, in critical oxygen sensing, and in the induction of stress responses that promote cell survival.
- Generation of ROS together with impaired antioxidant defenses increase in the failing heart as well as in myocardial ischemia and reperfusion.
- In the failing heart, cardioprotective interventions may prevent or slowdown ROS production via antioxidants like MnSOD and target apoptosis.
- The time course of MnSOD induction, a mitochondrial-specific protective response to ROS mediated damage, correlates well with the appearance of ischemic tolerance. However, the activities of other cellular anti-oxidants i.e., catalase and CuSOD are not similarly affected.
- Mitochondria of circulating WBC and platelets sense OS during capillary passage and react by producing ROS. The raised numbers of circulating ROS-positive WBC and platelets amplify OS in HF.
- Uncoupling of constitutive nitric oxide synthase (NOS) leads to overproduction of superoxide (O_2^-) and peroxynitrite ($ONOO^-$), two extremely potent oxidants.
- Peroxynitrite produced from the reaction of highly reactive NO with the superoxide anion impairs cardiovascular function through multiple mechanisms, including activation of MMPs and nuclear enzyme poly (ADP-ribose) polymerase (PARP).

- Both the generation of ROS and the onset of apoptotic cell death are important and often related events in cell homeostasis. Increased OS and ROS accumulation can lead to myocyte hypertrophy, interstitial fibrosis (through matrix metalloproteinases activation), and apoptosis.

- Increased OS in patients with HF may be related to decreased bioavailability of NO secondary to reduced expression of endothelial NOS and increased generation of ROS.

- The powerful cell-damaging ROS oxidants can be neutralized by an array of protective antioxidant scavenger enzymes, as well as by various lipid and water-soluble compounds including ascorbic acid, glutathione, thioredoxin, and α-tocopherol.

- Pharmacological inhibition of xanthine oxidase derived superoxide formation, neutralization of peroxynitrite, or inhibition of poly(ADP-ribose) polymerase (PARP) have been reported to provide significant benefit in various forms of cardiovascular injury.

- In doxorubicin-induced cardiomyopathy, the free-radical scavenger dexrazoxane has been shown to protect the heart from doxorubicin-associated oxidative damage and has been recommended for clinical use.

- Since in HF patients increased plasma catecholamines and sympathetic stimulation may lead to increased production of ROS, and possibly to endothelial damage/dysfunction and atheroma formation, treatment with β-blockers and ACE inhibitors have been recommended.

- The beneficial anti-oxidative effects of carvedilol, a vasodilating β-blocker with antioxidant activity in HF remains controversial.

- There is increasing evidence that HF-related generation of ROS/RNS may be ameliorated by targeting ROS/RNS-generating enzymes and upstream mediators.

- β-blockers, but not ACE inhibitors, appear to reduce lipid peroxidation although no relation has been found between reduction in oxidative damage and endothelial damage/dysfunction.

- Therapies that ameliorate endothelial function in HF patients have been shown to improve exercise tolerance and outcomes making endothelial dysfunction an important target to develop novel therapies.

References

1. Giordano FJ (2005) Oxygen, oxidative stress, hypoxia, and heart failure. J Clin Invest 115:500–508
2. Sohal RS, Svensson I, Sohal BH, Brunk UT (1989) Superoxide anion radical production in different animal species. Mech Ageing Dev 49:129–135
3. Pryor WA (1986) Oxy-radicals and related species: their formation, lifetimes, and reactions. Annu Rev Physiol 48:657–667
4. Han D, Antunes F, Canali R, Rettori D, Cadenas E (2003) Voltage-dependent anion channels control the release of the superoxide anion from mitochondria to cytosol. J Biol Chem 278:5557–5563
5. Wallace DC (2002) Animal models for mitochondrial disease. Methods Mol Biol 197:3–54
6. Chen Q, Vazquez EJ, Moghaddas S, Hoppel CL, Lesnefsky EJ (2003) Production of reactive oxygen species by mitochondria: central role of complex III. J Biol Chem 278:36027–36031
7. Herrero A, Barja G (2000) Localization of the site of oxygen radical generation inside the complex I of heart and nonsynaptic brain mammalian mitochondria. J Bioenerg Biomembr 32:609–615
8. McLennan HR, Degli Esposti M (2000) The contribution of mitochondrial respiratory complexes to the production of reactive oxygen species. J Bioenerg Biomembr 32:153–162
9. Hellsten-Westing Y (1993) Immunohistochemical localization of xanthine oxidase in human cardiac and skeletal muscle. Histochemistry 100:215–222
10. Moriwaki Y, Yamamoto T, Suda M, Nasako Y, Takahashi S, Agbedana OE, Hada T, Higashino K (1993) Purification and immunohistochemical tissue localization of human xanthine oxidase. Biochim Biophys Acta 1164:327–330
11. Cappola TP, Kass DA, Nelson GS, Berger RD, Rosas GO, Kobeissi ZA, Marban E, Hare JM (2001) Allopurinol improves myocardial efficiency in patients with idiopathic dilated cardiomyopathy. Circulation 104:2407–2411
12. Stadtman ER, Berlett BS (1998) Reactive oxygen-mediated protein oxidation in aging and disease. Drug Metab Rev 30:225–243
13. Choksi KB, Boylston WH, Rabek JP, Widger WR, Papaconstantinou J (2004) Oxidatively damaged proteins of heart mitochondrial electron transport complexes. Biochim Biophys Acta 1688:95–101
14. Vasquez-Vivar J, Kalyanaraman B, Kennedy MC (2000) Mitochondrial aconitase is a source of hydroxyl radical. An electron spin resonance investigation. J Biol Chem 275:14064–14069
15. Petrosillo G, Ruggiero FM, Pistolese M, Paradies G (2001) Reactive oxygen species generated from the mitochondrial electron transport chain induce cytochrome c dissociation from beef-heart submitochondrial particles via cardiolipin peroxidation: possible role in the apoptosis. FEBS Lett 509:435–438
16. Paradies G, Petrosillo G, Pistolese M, Ruggiero FM (2002) Reactive oxygen species affect mitochondrial electron transport complex I activity through oxidative cardiolipin damage. Gene 286:135–141
17. Shen Z, Wu W, Hazen SL (2000) Activated leukocytes oxidatively damage DNA, RNA, and the nucleotide pool through halide-dependent formation of hydroxyl radical. Biochemistry 39:5474–5482
18. LeDoux SP, Wilson GL (2001) Base excision repair of mitochondrial DNA damage in mammalian cells. Prog Nucleic Acid Res Mol Biol 68:273–284
19. Yakes FM, Van Houten B (1997) Mitochondrial DNA damage is more extensive and persists longer than nuclear DNA damage in human cells following oxidative stress. Proc Natl Acad Sci USA 94:514–519
20. Brown GC (1999) Nitric oxide and mitochondrial respiration. Biochim Biophys Acta 1411:351–369
21. Riobo NA, Clementi E, Melani M, Boveris A, Cadenas E, Moncada S, Poderoso JJ (2001) Nitric oxide inhibits mitochondrial NADH:ubiquinone reductase activity through peroxynitrite formation. Biochem J 359:139–145
22. Murray J, Taylor SW, Zhang B, Ghosh SS, Capaldi RA (2003) Oxidative damage to mitochondrial complex I due to peroxynitrite: identification of reactive tyrosines by mass spectrometry. J Biol Chem 278:37223–37230
23. Cassina AM, Hodara R, Souza JM, Thomson L, Castro L, Ischiropoulos H, Freeman BA, Radi R (2000) Cytochrome c nitration by peroxynitrite. J Biol Chem 275:21409–21415

24. Castro L, Rodriguez M, Radi R (1994) Aconitase is readily inactivated by peroxynitrite, but not by its precursor, nitric oxide. J Biol Chem 269:29409–29415

25. Packer MA, Scarlett JL, Martin SW, Murphy MP (1997) Induction of the mitochondrial permeability transition by peroxy-nitrite. Biochem Soc Trans 25:909–914

26. Brookes PS, Darley-Usmar VM (2004) Role of calcium and superoxide dismutase in sensitizing mitochondria to peroxynitrite-induced permeability transition. Am J Physiol Heart Circ Physiol 286:H39–H46

27. Nemoto S, Takeda K, Yu ZX, Ferrans VJ, Finkel T (2000) Role for mitochondrial oxidants as regulators of cellular metabolism. Mol Cell Biol 20:7311–7318

28. Cadenas E (2004) Mitochondrial free radical production and cell signaling. Mol Aspects Med 25:17–26

29. Bogoyevitch MA, Ng DC, Court NW, Draper KA, Dhillon A, Abas L (2000) Intact mitochondrial electron transport function is essential for signalling by hydrogen peroxide in cardiac myocytes. J Mol Cell Cardiol 32:1469–1480

30. Archer SL, Wu XC, Thebaud B, Moudgil R, Hashimoto K, Michelakis ED (2004) O2 sensing in the human ductus arteriosus: redox-sensitive K+ channels are regulated by mitochondria-derived hydrogen peroxide. Biol Chem 385:205–216

31. Yamamura T, Otani H, Nakao Y, Hattori R, Osako M, Imamura H, Das DK (2001) Dual involvement of coenzyme Q10 in redox signaling and inhibition of death signaling in the rat heart mitochondria. Antioxid Redox Signal 3:103–112

32. Brookes PS, Levonen AL, Shiva S, Sarti P, Darley-Usmar VM (2002) Mitochondria: regulators of signal transduction by reactive oxygen and nitrogen species. Free Radic Biol Med 33:755–764

33. Boveris A, D'Amico G, Lores-Arnaiz S, Costa LE (2003) Enalapril increases mitochondrial nitric oxide synthase activity in heart and liver. Antioxid Redox Signal 5:691–697

34. Hess ML, Manson NH (1984) Molecular oxygen: friend and foe. The role of the oxygen free radical system in the calcium paradox, the oxygen paradox and ischemia/reperfusion injury. J Mol Cell Cardiol 16:969–985

35. Becker LB (2004) New concepts in reactive oxygen species and cardiovascular reperfusion physiology. Cardiovasc Res 61:461–470

36. Becker LB, vanden Hoek TL, Shao ZH, Li CQ, Schumacker PT (1999) Generation of superoxide in cardiomyocytes during ischemia before reperfusion. Am J Physiol 277:H2240–H2246

37. Marin-Garcia J, Goldenthal MJ, Moe GW (2001) Abnormal cardiac and skeletal muscle mitochondrial function in pacing-induced cardiac failure. Cardiovasc Res 52:103–110

38. Moe GW, Marin-Garcia J, Konig A, Goldenthal M, Lu X, Feng Q (2004) In vivo tumor necrosis factor alpha inhibition ameliorates cardiac mitochondrial dysfunction, oxidative stress and apoptosis in experimental heart failure. Am J Physiol Heart Circ Physiol 287:H1813–H1820

39. Ide T, Tsutsui H, Kinugawa S et al (2000) Direct evidence for increased hydroxyl radicals originating from superoxide in the failing myocardium. Circ Res 6:152–157

40. Ide T, Tsutsui H, Kinugawa S, Utsumi H et al (1999) Mitochondrial electron transport complex I is a potential source of oxygen free radicals in the failing myocardium. Circ Res 85:357–363

41. Marin-Garcia J, Goldenthal MJ, Ananthakrishnan R, Mirvis D (1996) Specific mitochondrial DNA deletions in canine myocardial ischemia. Biochem Mol Biol Int 40:1057–1065

42. Suematsu N, Tsutsui H, Wen J et al (2003) Oxidative stress mediates tumor necrosis factor-alpha-induced mitochondrial DNA damage and dysfunction in cardiac myocytes. Circulation 107:1418–1423

43. Ide T, Tsutsui H, Hayashidani S et al (2001) Mitochondrial DNA damage and dysfunction associated with oxidative stress in failing hearts after myocardial infarction. Circ Res 88:529–535

44. Tsutsui H, Kinugawa S, Matsushima S (2009) Mitochondrial oxidative stress and dysfunction in myocardial remodeling. Cardiovasc Res 81:449–456

45. Sorescu D, Griendling K (2002) Reactive oxygen species, mitochondria, and NAD(P)H oxidases in the development and progression of heart failure. Congest Heart Fail 8:132–140

46. Griendling KK, Sorescu D, Ushio-Fukai M (2000) NAD(P)H oxidase: role in cardiovascular biology and disease. Circ Res 86:494–501

47. Sabri A, Hughie HH, Lucchesi PA (2003) Regulation of hypertrophic and apoptotic signaling pathways by reactive oxygen species in cardiac myocytes. Antioxid Redox Signal 5:731–740

48. Li JM, Gall NP, Grieve DJ, Chen M, Shah AM (2002) Activation of NADPH oxidase during progression of cardiac hypertrophy to failure. Hypertension 40:477–484

49. Xiao L, Pimentel DR, Wang J, Singh K, Colucci WS, Sawyer DB (2002) Role of reactive oxygen species and NAD(P)H oxidase in alpha(1)-adrenoceptor signaling in adult rat cardiac myocytes. Am J Physiol Cell Physiol 282:C926–C934

50. Heymes C, Bendall JK, Ratajczak P, Cave AC, Samuel JL, Hasenfuss G, Shah AM (2003) Increased myocardial NADPH oxidase activity in human heart failure. J Am Coll Cardiol 41:2164–2171

51. Nakagami H, Liao JK (2004) Statins and myocardial hypertrophy. Coron Artery Dis 15:247–250

52. Maack C, Kartes T, Kilter H, Schafers HJ, Nickenig G, Bohm M, Laufs U (2003) Oxygen free radical release in human failing myocardium is associated with increased activity of rac1-GTPase and represents a target for statin treatment. Circulation 108:1567–1574

53. Ferrari R, Guardigli G, Mele D, Percoco GF, Ceconi C, Curello S (2004) Oxidative stress during myocardial ischaemia and heart failure. Curr Pharm Des 10:1699–1711

54. Ijsselmuiden AJ, Musters RJ, de Ruiter G et al (2008) Circulating white blood cells and platelets amplify oxidative stress in heart failure. Nat Clin Pract Cardiovasc Med 5:811–820

55. Witztum JL, Steinberg D (1991) Role of oxidized low density lipoprotein in atherogenesis. J Clin Invest 88:1785–1792

56. Rajagopalan S, Meng XP, Ramasamy S, Harrison DG, Galis ZS (1996) Reactive oxygen species produced by macrophage-derived foam cells regulate the activity of vascular matrix metalloproteinases in vitro. Implications for atherosclerotic plaque stability. J Clin Invest 98:2572–2579

57. Khatri JJ, Johnson C, Magid R et al (2004) Vascular oxidant stress enhances progression and angiogenesis of experimental atheroma. Circulation 109:520–525

58. Malinski T (2005) Understanding nitric oxide physiology in the heart: a nanomedical approach. Am J Cardiol 96:13i–24i

59. Ungvari Z, Gupte SA, Recchia FA, Batkai S, Pacher P (2005) Role of oxidative-nitrosative stress and downstream pathways in various forms of cardiomyopathy and heart failure. Curr Vasc Pharmacol 3:221–229

60. Hare JM, Stamler JS (2005) NO/redox disequilibrium in the failing heart and cardiovascular system. J Clin Invest 115:509–517

61. Martinez-Ruiz A, Lamas S (2004) S-nitrosylation: a potential new paradigm in signal transduction. Cardiovasc Res 62:43–52

62. Lodi R, Tonon C, Calabrese V, Schapira AH (2006) Friedreich's ataxia: from disease mechanisms to therapeutic interventions. Antioxid Redox Signal 8:438–443

63. Kaneto H, Katakami N, Kawamori D et al (2007) Involvement of oxidative stress in the pathogenesis of diabetes. Antioxid Redox Signal 9:355–366

64. Cave AC, Brewer AC, Narayanapanicker A, Ray R, Grieve DJ, Walker S, Shah AM (2006) NADPH oxidases in cardiovascular health and disease. Antioxid Redox Signal 8:691–728

65. Lucas DT, Szweda LI (1998) Cardiac reperfusion injury: aging, lipid peroxidation, and mitochondrial dysfunction. Proc Natl Acad Sci USA 95:510–514

66. Nohl H, Hegner D (1978) Do mitochondria produce oxygen radicals in vivo? Eur J Biochem 82:563–567

67. Sohal RS, Arnold LA, Sohal BH (1990) Age-related changes in antioxidant enzymes and prooxidant generation in tissues of the rat with special reference to parameters in two insect species. Free Radic Biol Med 9:495–500

68. Yan LJ, Sohal RS (1998) Mitochondrial adenine nucleotide translocase is modified oxidatively during aging. Proc Natl Acad Sci USA 95:12896–12901

69. Nohl H, Kramer R (1980) Molecular basis of age-dependent changes in the activity of adenine nucleotide translocase. Mech Aging Dev 14:137–144

70. Kim JH, Shrago E, Elson CE (1988) Age-related changes in respiration coupled to phosphorylation. II. Cardiac mitochondria. Mech Aging Dev 46:279–290

71. Kim JH, Woldgiorgis G, Elson CE, Shrago E (1988) Age-related changes in respiration coupled to phosphorylation. I. Hepatic mitochondria. Mech Aging Dev 46:263–277

72. Hashimoto M, Majima E, Goto S, Shinohara Y, Terada H (1999) Fluctuation of the first loop facing the matrix of the mitochondrial ADP/ATP carrier deuced from intermolecular cross linking of Cys56 residues by bifunctional dimaleimides. Biochemistry 38:1050–1056

73. Yokozawa T, Satoh A, Cho EJ (2004) Ginsenoside-Rd attenuates oxidative damage related to aging in senescence-accelerated mice. J Pharm Pharmacol 56:107–113

74. Zhu Y, Carvey PM, Ling Z (2006) Age-related changes in glutathione and glutathione-related enzymes in rat brain. Brain Res 1090:35–44

75. Judge S, Jang YM, Smith A, Hagen T, Leeuwenburgh C (2005) Age-associated increases in oxidative stress and antioxidant enzyme activities in cardiac interfibrillar mitochondria: implications for the mitochondrial theory of aging. FASEB J 19:419–421

76. Suh JH, Heath SH, Hagen TM (2003) Two subpopulations of mitochondria in the aging rat heart display heterogenous levels of oxidative stress. Free Radic Biol Med 5:1064–1072

77. Mo JQ, Hom DG, Andersen JK (1995) Decreases in protective enzymes correlates with increased oxidative damage in the aging mouse brain. Mech Aging Dev 81:73–78

78. Chen JJ, Bertrand H, Yu BP (1995) Inhibition of adenine nucleotide translocator by lipid peroxidation products. Free Radic Biol Med 19:583–590

79. Pepe S (2005) Effect of dietary polyunsaturated fatty acids on age-related changes in cardiac mitochondrial membranes. Exp Gerontol 40:751–758

80. Kristal BS, Park BK, Yu BP (1996) 4-Hydroxyhexenal is a potent inducer of the mitochondrial permeability transition. J Biol Chem 271:6033–6038

81. Hansford RG, Castro F (1982) Effect of senescence on Ca-ion transport by heart mitochondria. Mech Aging Dev 19:5–13

82. Beckman JS, Koppenol WH (1996) Oxidative damage and tyrosine nitration from peroxynitrite. Chem Res Toxicol 9:836–844

83. Kanski J, Behring A, Pelling J, Schoneich C (2005) Proteomic identification of 3- nitrotyrosine-containing rat cardiac proteins: effects of biological aging. Am J Physiol 288:H371–H381

84. Turko IV, Li L, Aulak KS, Stuehr DJ, Chang JY, Murad F (2003) Protein tyrosine nitration in the mitochondria from diabetic mouse heart. Implications to dysfunctional mitochondria in diabetes. J Biol Chem 278:33972–33977

85. Madesh M, Hajnoczky G (2001) VDAC-dependent permeabilization of the outer mitochondrial membrane by superoxide induces rapid and massive cytochrome c release. J Cell Biol 155:1003–1015

86. Hoffman B, Stockl A, Schame M, Beyer K, Klingenberg M (1994) Reconstituted ADP/ATP carrier has an absolute requirement for cardiolipin as shown in cysteine mutants. J Biol Chem 269:1940–1949

87. Nehal M, Azam M, Baquer NZ (1990) Changes in the levels of catecholamines, hexokinase and glucose 6-phosphate dehydrogenase in red cell aging. Biochem Int 22:517–522

88. Kanski J, Schoneich C (2005) Protein nitration in biological aging: proteomic and tandem mass spectrometric characterization of nitrated sites. Methods Enzymol 396:160–171

89. Pastoris O, Boschi F, Verri M, Baiardi P, Felzani G, Vecchiet J, Dossena M, Catapano M (2000) The effects of aging on enzyme activities and metabolite concentrations in skeletal muscle from sedentary male and female subjects. Exp Gerontol 35:95–104

90. Kannan K, Jain SK (2000) Oxidative stress and apoptosis. Pathophysiology 7:153–163

91. Keller JN, Kindy MS, Holtsberg FW et al (1998) Mitochondrial manganese superoxide dismutase prevents neural apoptosis and reduces ischemic brain injury: suppression of peroxynitrite production, lipid peroxidation, and mitochondrial dysfunction. J Neurosci 18:687–697

92. Shiomi T, Tsutsui H, Matsusaka H et al (2004) Overexpression of glutathione peroxidase prevents left ventricular remodeling and failure after myocardial infarction in mice. Circulation 109:544–549

93. Kang YJ, Zhou ZX, Wu H, Wang GW, Saari JT, Klein JB (2000) Metallothionein inhibits myocardial apoptosis in copper-deficient mice: role of atrial natriuretic peptide. Lab Invest 80:745–757

94. Lud Cadet J, Harrington B, Ordonez S (2000) Bcl-2 overexpression attenuates dopamine-induced apoptosis in an immortalized neural cell line by suppressing the production of reactive oxygen species. Synapse 35:228–233

95. Kokoszka JE, Coskun P, Esposito LA, Wallace DC (2001) Increased mitochondrial oxidative stress in the Sod2 (+/-) mouse results in the age-related decline of mitochondrial function culminating in increased apoptosis. Proc Natl Acad Sci USA 98:2278–2283

96. Fu Y, Porres JM, Lei XG (2001) Comparative impacts of glutathione peroxidase-1 gene knockout on oxidative stress induced by reactive oxygen and nitrogen species in mouse hepatocytes. Biochem J 359:687–695

97. Goossens V, Stange G, Moens K, Pipeleers D, Grooten J (1999) Regulation of tumor necrosis factor-induced, mitochondria- and reactive oxygen species-dependent cell death by electron flux through electron transport chain complex I. Antioxid Redox Signal 1:285–295

98. von Harsdorf R, Li PF, Dietz R (1999) Signaling pathways in reactive oxygen species-induced cardiomyocyte apoptosis. Circulation 99:2934–2941

99. Akao M, O'Rourke B, Teshima Y, Seharaseyon J, Marban E (2003) Mechanistically distinct steps in the mitochondrial death pathway triggered by oxidative stress in cardiac myocytes. Circ Res 92:186–194

100. Long X, Goldenthal MJ, Wu GM, Marin-Garcia J (2004) Mitochondrial Ca2+ flux and respiratory enzyme activity decline are early events in cardiomyocyte response to H(2)O(2). J Mol Cell Cardiol 37:63–70

101. Hickson-Bick DL, Sparagna GC, Buja LM, McMillin JB (2002) Palmitate-induced apoptosis in neonatal cardiomyocytes is not dependent on the generation of ROS. Am J Physiol Heart Circ Physiol 282:H656–H664

102. Elahi MM, Naseem KM, Matata BM (2007) Nitric oxide in blood. The nitrosative-oxidative disequilibrium hypothesis on the pathogenesis of cardiovascular disease. FEBS J 274:906–923

103. Sharma R, Davidoff MN (2002) Oxidative stress and endothelial dysfunction in heart failure. Congest Heart Fail 8:165–172

104. Ungvári Z, Gupte SA, Recchia FA, Bátkai S, Pacher P (2005) Role of oxidative-nitrosative stress and downstream pathways in various forms of cardiomyopathy and heart failure. Curr Vasc Pharmacol 3:221–229

105. Chen Y, Saari JT, Kang YJ (1994) Weak antioxidant defenses make the heart a target for damage in copper-deficient rats. Free Radic Biol Med 17:529–536

106. Radi R, Turrens JF, Chang LY, Bush KM, Crapo JD, Freeman BA (1991) Detection of catalase in rat heart mitochondria. J Biol Chem 266:22028–22034

107. Antunes F, Han D, Cadenas E (2002) Relative contributions of heart mitochondria glutathione peroxidase and catalase to H2O2 detoxification in vivo conditions. Free Radic Biol Med 33: 1260–1267

108. Phung CD, Ezieme JA, Turrens JF (1994) Hydrogen peroxide metabolism in skeletal muscle mitochondria. Arch Biochem Biophys 315:479–482

109. Judge S, Judge A, Grune T, Leeuwenburgh C (2004) Short-term CR decreases cardiac mitochondrial oxidant production but increases carbonyl content. Am J Physiol Regul Integr Comp Physiol 286:R254–R259

110. Turko IV, Murad F (2003) Quantitative protein profiling in heart mitochondria from diabetic rats. J Biol Chem 278:35844–35849

111. Radi R, Bush KM, Freeman BA (1993) The role of cytochrome c and mitochondrial catalase in hydroperoxide-induced heart mitochondrial lipid peroxidation. Arch Biochem Biophys 300: 409–415

112. Zhou Z, Kang YJ (2000) Cellular and subcellular localization of catalase in the heart of transgenic mice. J Histochem Cytochem 48:585–594

113. Fernandez-Checa JC, Garcia-Ruiz C, Colell A, Morales A, Mari M, Miranda M, Ardite E (1998) Oxidative stress: role of mitochondria and protection by glutathione. Biofactors 8:7–11

114. Vaage J, Antonelli M, Bufi M et al (1997) Exogenous reactive oxygen species deplete the isolated rat heart of antioxidants. Free Radic Biol Med 22:85–92

115. Hasinoff BB, Schnabl KL, Marusak RA, Patel D, Huebner E (2003) Dexrazoxane protects cardiac myocytes against doxorubicin by preventing damage to mitochondria. Cardiovasc Toxicol 3:89–99

116. Lipshultz SE, Rifai N, Dalton VM, Levy DE et al (2004) The effect of dexrazoxane on myocardial injury in doxorubicin-treated children with acute lymphoblastic leukemia. N Engl J Med 351:145–153

117. Kang YJ (1999) The antioxidant function of metallothionein in the heart. Proc Soc Exp Biol Med 222:263–273

118. Nath R, Kumar D, Li T, Singal PK (2000) Metallothioneins, oxidative stress and the cardiovascular system. Toxicology 155:17–26

119. Ali MM, Frei E, Straub J, Breuer A, Wiessler M (2002) Induction of metallothionein by zinc protects from daunorubicin toxicity in rats. Toxicology 179:85–93

120. Okuda M, Lee HC, Kumar C, Chance B (1992) Comparison of the effect of a mitochondrial uncoupler, 2, 4-dinitrophenol and adrenaline on oxygen radical production in the isolated perfused rat liver. Acta Physiol Scand 145:159–168

121. Korshunov SS, Korkina OV, Ruuge EK, Skulachev VP, Starkov AA (1998) Fatty acids as natural uncouplers preventing generation of O2- and H2O2 by mitochondria in the resting state. FEBS Lett 435:215–218

122. Casteilla L, Rigoulet M, Penicaud L (2001) Mitochondrial ROS metabolism: modulation by uncoupling proteins. IUBMB Life 52:181–188

123. Papa S, Skulachev VP (1997) Reactive oxygen species, mitochondria, apoptosis and aging. Mol Cell Biochem 174:305–319

124. Vidal-Puig AJ, Grujic D, Zhang CY et al (2000) Energy metabolism in uncoupling protein 3 gene knockout mice. J Biol Chem 275:16258–16266

125. Hoerter J, Gonzalez-Barroso MD, Couplan E et al (2004) Mitochondrial uncoupling protein 1 expressed in the heart of transgenic mice protects against ischemic-reperfusion damage. Circulation 110:528–533

126. Teshima Y, Akao M, Jones SP, Marban E (2003) Uncoupling protein-2 overexpression inhibits mitochondrial death pathway in cardiomyocytes. Circ Res 93:192–200

127. Pacher P, Liaudet L, Mabley JG, Cziráki A, Haskó G, Szabó C (2006) Beneficial effects of a novel ultrapotent poly(ADP-ribose) polymerase inhibitor in murine models of heart failure. Int J Mol Med 17:369–375

128. Cooper JM, Schapira AH (2003) Friedreich's ataxia: disease mechanisms, antioxidant and Coenzyme Q10 therapy. Biofactors 18:163–171

129. Santos DL, Moreno AJ, Leino RL, Froberg MK, Wallace KB (2002) Carvedilol protects against doxorubicin-induced mitochondrial cardiomyopathy. Toxicol Appl Pharmacol 185:218–227

130. Lerman-Sagie T, Rustin P, Lev D et al (2001) Dramatic improvement in mitochondrial cardiomyopathy following treatment with idebenone. J Inherit Metab Dis 24:28–34

131. Sayed-Ahmed M, Salman T, Gaballah H, Abou El-Naga SA, Nicolai R, Calvani M (2001) Propionyl-L-carnitine as protector against adriamycin-induced cardiomyopathy. Pharmacol Res 43:513–520

132. Shite J, Qin F, Mao W, Kawai H, Stevens SY, Liang C (2001) Antioxidant vitamins attenuate oxidative stress and cardiac dysfunction in tachycardia-induced cardiomyopathy. J Am Coll Cardiol 38:1734–1740

133. Geromel V, Darin N, Chretien D, Benit P, DeLonlay P, Rotig A, Munnich A, Rustin P (2002) Coenzyme Q(10) and idebenone in the therapy of respiratory chain diseases: rationale and comparative benefits. Mol Genet Metab 77:21–30

134. Hausse AO, Aggoun Y, Bonnet D, Sidi D, Munnich A, Rotig A, Rustin P (2002) Idebenone and reduced cardiac hypertrophy in Friedreich's ataxia. Heart 87:346–349

135. Rustin P, Munnich A, Rotig A (1999) Quinone analogs prevent enzymes targeted in Friedreich ataxia from iron-induced injury in vitro. Biofactors 9:247–251

136. Lerman-Sagie T, Rustin P, Lev D, Yanoov M, Leshinsky-Silver E, Sagie A, Ben-Gal T, Munnich A (2001) Dramatic improvement in mitochondrial cardiomyopathy following treatment with idebenone. J Inherit Metab Dis 24:28–34

137. Shoffner JM, Wallace DC (1994) Oxidative phosphorylation diseases and mitochondrial DNA mutations: diagnosis and treatment. Annu Rev Nutr 14:535–568

138. Ogasahara S, Yorifuji S, Nishikawa Y et al (1985) Improvement of abnormal pyruvate metabolism and cardiac conduction defect with coenzyme Q10 in Kearns-Sayre syndrome. Neurology 35: 372–377

139. Mortensen SA, Vadhanavikit S, Baandrup U, Folkers K (1985) Long-term coenzyme Q10 therapy: a major advance in the management of resistant myocardial failure. Drugs Exp Clin Res 11:581–593

140. Hargreaves IP (2003) Ubiquinone: cholesterol's reclusive cousin. Ann Clin Biochem 40:207–218

141. Mortensen SA (2003) Overview on coenzyme Q10 as adjunctive therapy in chronic heart failure: rationale, design and end-points of "Q-symbio" a multinational trial. Biofactors 18:79–89

142. Castro P, Vukasovic JL, Chiong M et al (2005) Effects of carvedilol on oxidative stress and chronotropic response to exercise in patients with chronic heart failure. Eur J Heart Fail 7: 1033–1039

143. Chin BS, Gibbs CR, Blann AD, Lip GY (2003) Neither carvedilol nor bisoprolol in maximally tolerated doses has any specific

advantage in lowering chronic heart failure oxidant stress: implications for beta-blocker selection. Clin Sci (Lond) 105: 507–512

144. Nakamura K, Kusano K, Nakamura Y et al (2002) Carvedilol decreases elevated oxidative stress in human failing myocardium. Circulation 105:2867–2871

145. Kono Y, Nakamura K, Kimura H et al (2006) Elevated levels of oxidative DNA damage in serum and myocardium of patients with heart failure. Circ J 70:1001–1005

146. Chin BS, Langford NJ, Nuttall SL, Gibbs CR, Blann AD, Lip GY (2003) Anti-oxidative properties of beta-blockers and angiotensin-converting enzyme inhibitors in congestive heart failure. Eur J Heart Fail 5:171

147. Bauersachs J, Widder JD (2008) Endothelial dysfunction in heart failure. Pharmacol Rep 60:119–126

148. Bauersachs J, Schäfer A (2004) Endothelial dysfunction in heart failure: mechanisms and therapeutic approaches. Curr Vasc Pharmacol 2:115–124

Chapter 11
Cardiac Remodeling and Cell Death in Heart Failure

Overview

Remodeling may be defined as changes in the morphology, structure, and function of the heart related to alterations in loading conditions and/or cardiac injury. This process is critical to the progression of HF, and understanding its mechanism may allow us to better understand the pathophysiology of HF. In this chapter, we will discuss the potential mechanisms conducive to remodeling in the failing heart, available animal models, therapies currently used, and emerging therapies to stop and/or reverse the remodeling process.

Introduction

A crucial step in the progression of left ventricular (LV) dysfunction and HF is cardiac remodeling [1, 2]. Remodeling involves alterations in both the myocytes and the cardiac extracellular matrix (ECM), the latter includes the activation of proteolytic enzymes leading to the degradation and reorganization of collagens [3–6]. The morphological patterns that often accompany cardiac remodeling include hypertrophy and subsequent chamber dilatation with associated progressive impairment in function [2]. On the other hand, the heart might respond to environmental stimuli not only by growth with increasing myocardial mass, but also by shrinkage (atrophy) with a dynamic range that has been estimated to be of at least 100% [7]. Indeed, progressive cardiac remodeling results in the onset of LV dilatation with relatively proportional increases in LV mass, a process sometimes named eccentric hypertrophy [8]. These events are more characteristic in patients with initially compensated LV dysfunction but later with development of clinically overt HF mainly triggered by the marked ventricular dilatation that occurs once the resources from the myocardial hypertrophic response are exhausted [9]. With end-stage disease and clinically overt HF, profound LV dilatation occurs without comparable levels of hypertrophy, resulting in relative wall thinning from the disproportional increases in LV chamber size. In addition, excessive LV dilatation alters the overall shape of the LV from a normal ellipsoid configuration to a more spherical shape.

While hypertrophy is considered by some investigators as an adaptive response to increased workload and is accompanied by alterations in metabolism [10], for others, whether left-ventricular hypertrophy is adaptive or maladaptive is rather a controversial concept, as suggested by the patterns of signaling pathways, transgenic models, and clinical findings in aortic stenosis [11].

At least some of the cytoplasmic signaling pathways thought to be responsible for pathological hypertrophy are mediated through increased levels of growth factors signaling through G-protein coupled cell-surface receptors (GPCR) [12]. In addition, atrial natriuretic peptide (ANP), through its guanylyl cyclase-A (GC-A) receptor, locally moderates cardiomyocyte growth. To characterize the anti-hypertrophic effects of ANP, the possible contribution of Na^+/H^+ exchanger (NHE-1) to cardiac remodeling was recently examined in a model of GC-A-deficient (GC-A$^{-/-}$) mice [13]. Fluorometric measurements in the cardiomyocytes demonstrated that cardiac hypertrophy in GC-A$^{-/-}$ mice was associated with enhanced NHE-1 activity, alkalinization of intracellular pH, and increased Ca^{2+} levels. Chronic treatment of GC-A$^{-/-}$ mice with the NHE-1 inhibitor cariporide, normalized cardiomyocyte pH and Ca^{2+} levels and regressed cardiac hypertrophy and fibrosis. Activity of four prohypertrophic signaling pathways – the mitogen-activated protein kinases (MAPK), the serine–threonine kinase Akt, calcineurin/NFAT, and Ca^{2+}/calmodulin-dependent kinase II (CaMKII), were activated in GC-A$^{-/-}$ mice, but only CaMKII and Akt activity regressed upon reversal of the hypertrophic phenotype following cariporide. By contrast, the MAPK and calcineurin/NFAT signaling pathways remained activated during regression of hypertrophy. These observations suggest that the ANP/GC-A system modulates the cardiac growth response to pressure overload during remodeling by preventing excessive activation of NHE-1 and subsequent increases in cardiomyocyte intracellular pH, Ca^{2+} and CaMKII as well as Akt activity.

J. Marín-García, *Heart Failure*, Contemporary Cardiology,
DOI 10.1007/978-1-60761-147-9_11, © Springer Science+Business Media, LLC 2010

Progression of Cardiac Remodeling and Transition to Overt HF

The mechanisms of cardiac remodeling, particularly those underlying the transition from stable hypertrophy to cardiac dilatation and ultimately to overt HF remain unclear. Many factors including neurohormonal and cytokine activation and impaired Ca^{2+} handling are thought to play a contributory role, particularly following MI (Fig. 11.1) [14, 15]. In addition, with increased work load the adult heart develops pathological growth and activation of the fetal program of gene expression followed by LV dilatation, thinning of the wall, and pump failure. In a transgenic mouse model, it has been demonstrated that activation of the fetal gene program and pathological remodeling of the heart can be achieved with overexpression of myocyte enhancer factor-2 (MEF2D), a transcription factor that serve as targets of the signaling pathway that drive pathological remodeling [16]. Also, it has been demonstrated that class II histone deacetylases (HDACs) suppress stress-dependent remodeling of the heart through their association with MEF2 transcription factor, and that protein kinase D (PKD), a stress-responsive kinase that phosphorylates class II HDACs, dissociate MEF2 resulting in activation of MEF2

target genes. A mouse model with a conditional PKD1-null allele has been recently developed by Fielitz et al. [17]. Mice with cardiac specific deletion of PKD1 exhibited improved cardiac function and diminished hypertrophy in response to pressure overload and angiotensin II signaling, confirming that PKAD1 is a key transducer of stress stimuli involved in the abnormal remodeling of the heart. Previously, Harrison et al. [18] have observed that activation of PKD1 in cardiomyocytes occurs through PKC-dependent and -independent mechanisms, and in vivo cardiac PKD1 is activated in rodent models of pathological cardiac remodeling. Moreover, PKD1 activation correlates with phosphorylation-dependent nuclear export of HDAC5, and reduction of endogenous PKD1 expression with siRNA suppresses HDAC5 shuttling and associated cardiomyocyte growth. In contrast, ectopic overexpression of constitutively active PKD1 in mouse heart leads to DCM. Thus, PKD1 has a significant role in the control of pathological remodeling of the heart by its ability to phosphorylate and neutralize HDAC5.

Diacylglycerol, a lipid second messenger accumulates in cardiomyocytes when stimulated by $Gq\alpha$, protein-coupled receptor (GPCR) agonists such as angiotensin II and phenylephrine. GPCR signaling pathway, which includes dia-

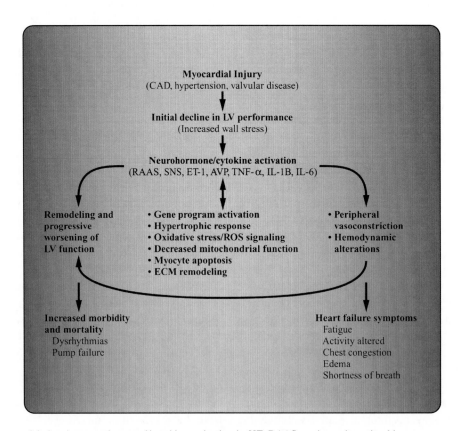

Fig. 11.1 Flow-chart model showing neurohormonal/cytokine activation in HF. RAAS, renin-angiotensin-aldosterone system; SNS, sympathetic nervous system; ET-1, endothelin-1; AVP, arginine vasopressin; TNF-α, tumor necrosis factor-alpha; IL-1B, interleukin-1β; IL-6, interleukin-6.

cylglycerol (DAG) and protein kinase C (PKC), plays a critical role in the development of cardiac hypertrophy and HF. DAG kinase (DGK) phosphorylates DAG and controls cellular DAG levels, thus acting as a regulator of GPCR signaling. Furthermore, DGK inhibits GPCR agonist-induced activation of the DAG-PKC signaling and subsequent cardiomyocyte hypertrophy. To determine whether DGK modifies the development of cardiac hypertrophy induced by pressure overload, Harada et al. [19] assessed the effect of thoracic aortic stenosis on the heart of transgenic mice with cardiac-specific overexpression of DGKzeta (DGKzeta-TG) and in wild-type (WT) mice. While the WT mice showed increases in interventricular septal thickness, LV dilatation, decreases in LV systolic function, cardiac fibrosis and up-regulation of profibrotic genes, such as transforming growth factor-β1, collagen type I, and collagen type III at 4 weeks post-surgery, the DGKzeta-TG mice heart weight appeared to decrease. Furthermore, cardiac fibrosis and gene induction of type I and type III collagens, but not transforming growth factor-β1, were blocked in the DGKzeta-TG mice. Taken together, these data confirm that DGKzeta suppresses cardiac hypertrophy and fibrosis and prevents LV systolic dysfunction caused by pressure overload. Interestingly, in neonatal rat, cardiomyocytes DGKzeta inhibits PKC activation and subsequent hypertrophic programs in response to endothelin-1 (ET-1). DGKzeta blocks cardiac hypertrophy induced by G protein-coupled receptor agonists and pressure overload in vivo. Moreover, DGKzeta attenuates ventricular remodeling and improves survival after myocardial infarction [20].

Pressure and volume overload have been known to be accompanied by increased glucose uptake and glycolysis and decreased FAO [21]. Alterations in energy status and metabolism have been proposed to play a role in the transition from stable cardiac hypertrophy to overt HF, at least based on observations from animal studies [10, 22, 23].

Based on a number of observations, the general concept that emerged is that myocardial substrate selection is relatively normal during the early stages of HF but later on there is a downregulation in FAO, increased glycolysis and glucose oxidation, reduced respiratory chain activity, and impaired reserve for mitochondrial oxidative flux. In a recent review article on metabolic remodeling of the failing heart, van Bilsen et al. [24] wondered if metabolic remodeling is beneficial or detrimental to the heart. From a therapeutic point of view, for the failing heart, it is considered preferable to further stimulate glucose oxidation rather than to normalize substrate metabolism by stimulating FA utilization; however, if this also applies to the earlier stages of HF is not known. The therapeutic potential of acute and long-term manipulation of cardiac substrate metabolism in HF remains to be determined.

In HF, changes in myocardial energy metabolism correlates inversely with plasma free-fatty-acid concentrations, and mitochondrial uncoupling proteins (UCPs) may play a significant role in its regulation. Murray et al. [25] investigated the link between energetic and metabolic abnormalities in 39 patients undergoing coronary artery bypass graft surgery. When plasma free-fatty-acid concentrations were raised, cardiac mitochondrial UCPs increased (isoforms UCP2 and UCP3) and those of glucose transporter (GLUT4) protein decreased (in cardiac and skeletal muscle). These findings suggest that energy deficiency in HF might result from increased mitochondrial UCPs (i.e., less efficient ATP synthesis) and depleted GLUT4 (i.e., reduced glucose uptake). Therefore, simultaneous lowering of plasma free fatty acids and finding an alternative energy source may be warranted.

Mitochondrial UCP-2 gene expression has been correlated with changes in cardiac performance and ATP biosynthesis in a rat model of aortic valve regurgitation (AR) progressing to HF. Noma et al. [26] have reported that while in the early stages of HF development following AR, LV ANP mRNA expression was increased in proportion to chamber enlargement, UCP-2 mRNA expression was suppressed (no difference in comparison to sham rats), and TNF-α mRNA expression showed no changes during the early post-operative stage. However, at 30–100 days post-AR surgery while the LV ANP mRNA displayed further increases, also the levels of UCP-2 mRNA and TNF-α progressively increased. On the other hand, no differences were observed between AR and sham rats for UCP-2 mRNA in skeletal muscle, nor in cardiac ATP levels; however, cardiac CRP was significantly reduced in the very late stages (at 100 days) after AR operation. Taken together, these findings suggest that mitochondrial UCP-2 gene expression experienced serial changes in rats volume overload HF, and suppression of its expression may be reflected by the cellular energy state. Furthermore, a decrease in UCP-2 may lead to suppression or reduction of mitochondrial proton leakage, and cardiac oxygen utilization may shift from heat production to ATP biosynthesis. Interestingly, in the late stage of AR, there was a significant increase in TNF-α expression not observed in the early stage, suggesting that up-regulation of TNF-α may be a potential explanation for the induction of UCP-2 in the advanced stage of AR. Based upon the aforementioned data, cardiac UCP expression in chronic HF provides a likely explanation for the reversible LV dysfunction/remodeling observed in patients with AR. Also, the in vivo role of UCP2 in the heart has been studied in the Dahl salt-sensitive rat HF model. UCP2 mRNA level was significantly upregulated together with proapoptotic protein Bcl-2 and 19-kDa interacting protein 3 (BNIP3). It appeared that UCP2 increases sensitivity of adult rat cardiac myocytes to hypoxia–reoxygenation by way of ATP depletion and acidosis, which in turn causes accumulation of prodeath protein BNIP3 [27].

Myocardial Metabolism and Neurohormonal Signaling in Cardiac Remodeling

Insights from Transgenic Models

Some of the recent research conducted on the relationship between myocardial metabolism and cardiac remodeling using transgenic models have been discussed elsewhere in this volume (see Chaps. 4 and 6). In this section, it suffices to mention that the creation of transgenic mice with altered expression of genes involved in carbohydrate and lipid metabolism has provided unique insights into the fine balance within the heart, to maintain energy status and function, as well as to evaluate the cause–effect relationships between mitochondrial function and myocardial disease [28]. A list of transgenic models of metabolic modification in the heart that associated with cardiac dysfunction and/or HF phenotype is shown in Table 11.1.

Loss-of-function model systems, which disrupt mitochondrial metabolism, exhibit different cardiac phenotypes. One genetically engineered mouse model having a causal relationship between a mitochondrial energetic defect and cardiomyopathy is the Ant1 null mouse. The adenine nucleotide translocators (ANT) are a family of proteins that exchange mitochondrial ATP for cytosolic ADP, providing new ADP substrate to the mitochondria while delivering ATP to the cytoplasm for cellular work. Mice express two isoforms of this enzyme; with tissue-specific expression patterns [29]. Ant1 is expressed in skeletal muscle, heart, and the brain, while Ant2 is expressed in all tissues except skeletal muscle. The Ant1 gene deficient mice exhibit mitochondrial abnormalities including a partial deficit in ADP-stimulated respiration, consistent with impairment in the translocation of ADP into mitochondria in both skeletal muscle and heart. The skeletal muscle respiratory defect was profound, presumably because Ant2 can partially compensate for the loss of Ant1 in heart, but not in skeletal muscle. Ant1$^{-/-}$ mice exhibit a progressive cardiac hypertrophic phenotype coincident with the proliferation of mitochondria [30]. The mitochondrial biogenic response has therefore been hypothesized to be a compensatory mechanism to correct the energy deficit, but could also contribute to cardiac remodeling. Transgenic models of specific defects in the mitochondrial FAO pathways have also been developed (Table 11.2). Two distinct mouse models with genetic deletion of the second step in the mitochondrial FAO pathway, a fatty acid chain-length-specific dehydrogenase enzyme (VLCAD and LCAD), display a cardiomyopathic phenotype [31, 32]. Furthermore, mice null for the PPAR-α gene also exhibit diminished

Table 11.1 Transgenic models of metabolopathies associated with cardiac remodeling and HF

Gene	Manipulation	Cardiac phenotype
GLUT4	Global KO	Hypertrophy, ↑ expression of MCAD and LCAD, ↑ glycogen synthesis, interstitial fibrosis
	Heterozygous KO	Diabetic cardiomyopathy
	Cardiac specific KO	Hypertrophy, ↑ BNP, glucose uptake
IR	Cardiac specific KO	↓ myocyte size, ↓ basal glucose uptake, impaired cardiac function
IGF-R	Cardiac overexpression	Cardiac hypertrophy
IGF-1	Overexpression	Cardiac hypertrophy, attenuation of cardiac dysfunction following myocardial infarct
PI3Kα	Constitutively active	Cardiac hypertrophy with no alterations in cardiac function or fibrosis
	Dominant negative	Smaller hearts with normal cardiac function
PTEN	Cardiac specific KO	Cardiac hypertrophy and impaired contractility
PTEN	Constitutively active	Cardiac hypertrophy, concentric LV hypertrophy, ↓ infarct size following I/R, altered contractility
PDK1	Cre/LoxP KO	Sudden death due to HF
AMPKα2	Inactive kinase	↓ heart weight and in vivo LV dP/dt, impaired glucose uptake, glycolysis and FAO, ↑ apoptosis and impaired LV recovery in response to ischemia
MEF2	Overexpression	Pathological cardiac remodeling
PFK2	Cardiac specific kinase deficient	Multiple cardiac pathologies, fibrosis, ↓ contractility, impaired glycolysis
G6PDH	Global KO	Myocardial dysfunction

KO knock-out; *IR* insulin receptor; *IGF* insulin like growth factor; *MCAD* medium chain acyl-CoA dehydrogenase; *PDK* pyruvate dehydrogenase kinase; *I/R* ischemia/reperfusion; *LCAD* long chain acyl-CoA dehydrogenase; *MEF2* myocyte enhancer factor-2; *PFK2* phosphofructokinase 2; *G6PDH* glucose 6 phosphate dehydrogenase; *AMPK* adenosine monophosphate kinase; *PTEN* phosphatase and tensin homologue deleted on chromosome 10; *GLUT* glucose transporter; *BNP* B-type or brain natriuretic peptide; *PI3K* phosphatidylinositol-3-kinase; *FAO* fatty acid oxidation

Table 11.2 Transgenic models of fatty acid defects and HF

PPAR-α	Global KO	↑ myocardial fibrosis; ↓ LV fractional shortening;↓ cardiac contractile performance under basal and under stimulation of β1 adrenergic receptors; ↓ cardioprotection to I/R
	Cardiac specific overexpression	Diabetic cardiomyopathy; ↑ FAO, ↓ glucose uptake and oxidation
FAT/CD36	Global KO	DCM; ↓ cardiac fatty acid uptake and triglyceride
FAT/CD36	Overexpression	↑ FAO; ↓ plasma triglyceride + fatty acid; no cardiac pathology; ↑ glucose
H-FABP	Global KO	Hypertrophy, ↑ANF expression, ↓ LCFA utilization
FATP-1	Cardiac-specific overexpression	Lipotoxic CM
ACS1	Cardiac-specific overexpression	Cardiomyopathy, hypertrophy, LV dysfunction, HF, intramyocellular triglyceride accumulation
LpL	Cardiac-specific KO	DCM; ↑ triglyceride; ↓ FAO; ↑ Glut expression and glucose uptake
LCAD	Global ablation	Cardiomyopathy, lipid accumulation, myocardial fibrosis
Leptin (ob)	Null	↑ FAO , fatty acid uptake, triglyceride + lipid accumulation; ↑ diastolic dysfunction
DGK zeta-TG	Overexpression	↓ Hypertrophy and fibrosis; blocks cardiac dysfunction and gene induction of type I and type III collagens, but not transforming growth factor-β1

FATP fatty acid transport protein; *ACS* long-chain acyl-CoA synthetase; *Lp* lipoprotein lipase; *LCAD* long-chain acyl-coenzyme A dehydrogenase; *FAT/CD36* fatty acid translocase; *H-FABP* heart-type fatty acid binding protein; *LCFA* long chain fatty acids; *FAO* fatty acid oxidation; Glut glucose transporter; *I/R* ischemia/reperfusion; *ANF* atrial natriuretic factor; *PPAR* peroxisome proliferator-activated receptor; *DGK* zeta-TG diacylglycerol kinase transgenic

myocardial fat catabolic capacity and mild cardiomyopathic phenotype that accompanies aging [33].

Besides "loss of function" models, "gain of function" overexpression strategies have also shed light on the relation between mitochondrial dysfunction and cardiac dysfunction, particularly in a poorly characterized entity of cardiomyopathy associated with diabetes. The healthy heart generates ATP using both carbohydrate utilization and mitochondrial FAO pathways as shown in transgenic mice (see Table 11.2), the diabetic heart derives a preponderance of ATP from FAO [34].

The cardiac PPAR-α/PGC-1α system is activated in diabetes mellitus [35]. This metabolic shift associated with high level of fatty acid import and oxidation may eventually lead to pathological mitochondrial and cardiac remodeling. Transgenic mice with cardiac restricted overexpression of PPAR-α (the MHC-PPAR-α mice) exhibit increased expression of genes encoding enzymes involved in multiple steps of mitochondrial FAO with strong reciprocal down-regulation of glucose transporter (GLUT4) and glycolytic enzyme gene expression. Myocardial fatty acid uptake and mitochondrial fatty acid β-oxidation are markedly increased in MHC-PPAR-α hearts, whereas glucose uptake and oxidation are profoundly diminished in MHC-PPAR-α mice [36]. Echocardiographic assessment identified LV hypertrophy and dysfunction in the MHC-PPAR-α mice in a transgene expression-dependent manner, and sequential studies showed that both high fat diet and insulinopenia induced further remodeling accompanied by signs of HF. The HF phenotype caused by the HF chow was completely reversed by resumption of standard chow.

To test the hypothesis that mismatch between myocardial fatty acid uptake and utilization leads to the accumulation of cardiotoxic lipid species, transgenic mouse lines that overexpress long-chain acyl-CoA synthetase in the heart (MHC-ACS) have been developed by Chiu et al. [37]. The MHC-ACS plays an important role in vectorial fatty acid transport across the plasma membrane, and this model displays cardiac-restricted expression of the transgene and marked cardiac myocyte triglyceride and phospholipids accumulation. These increases were observed in the presence of normal serum glucose and lipid levels and in the absence of underlying defects in myocardial fatty acid β-oxidation. Lipid accumulation was associated with cardiac hypertrophy initially followed by LV dysfunction and premature death. This novel mouse model may provide significant information on the role that alterations in myocardial lipid metabolism play in the pathogenesis of inherited and acquired HF.

Neurohormonal Changes and Cytokines

Besides abnormal lipid metabolism, diverse neurohormonal signals acting through interwoven signal transduction pathways can lead to pathological cardiac hypertrophy and HF (see Fig. 11.1). Many such agonists act through cell surface receptors coupled with G-proteins to mobilize intracellular calcium, with consequent activation of downstream kinases and the calcium-and calmodulin-dependent phosphatase calcineurin. MAPK signaling pathways are also interconnected at multiple levels with calcium-dependent kinases and calcineurin [38]. β-adrenergic agonists influence cardiac growth and function through the generation of cAMP, which activates protein kinase A (PKA) and other downstream effectors [39]. These signaling pathways target a variety of substrates in the cardiomyocyte, including components of the contractile apparatus, calcium channels, and their regulatory proteins.

Contractile Elements

Although HF that is secondary to altered loading conditions may not be associated with reduced intrinsic contractile function until the late stages, in general an important hallmark of HF is reduced myocardial contractility, with defective intracellular Ca^{2+} handling playing a crucial role in the pathogenesis of these contractile abnormalities. Individual cardiomyocytes intrinsic contractile ability is impaired during the evolving HF process and reflects important cellular changes that include altered expression of membrane and contractile proteins, altered energy metabolism, and impaired excitation–contraction coupling [40]. Cell isolation and function studies have demonstrated that the reduction in contractile performance in these failing cells is not simply a consequence of associated wall stresses, ischemia, or myocardial perfusion defects [41, 42]. However, there is no direct evidence to support that depressed contractility has a causative role in the initiation and progression of human HF, nor that remodeling in HF may occur in the absence of depressed myocyte contractility [41, 43]. Although alterations in cardiomyocyte contractility contribute to cardiac dysfunction, it cannot adequately account for the profound structural changes occurring in both, the cells and the surrounding ECM that characterize cardiac remodeling. The progressive cytoskeletal stiffness, the contractile dysfunction, and fibrosis typical of the failing heart may be partly explained by the up-regulation of many genes encoding cytoskeletal proteins, sarcomeric, and ECM proteins. In their review on the role that the cytoskeleton plays in HF, Hein et al. [44] found that in chronic HF secondary to DCM there is a morphological basis of reduced contractile function: the cytoskeletal and membrane-associated proteins are disorganized and increased in amount confirming experimental reports. On the other hand, the contractile myofilaments and the proteins of the sarcomeric skeleton including titin, alpha-actinin, and myomesin are significantly decreased. The investigators presented a hypothesis assuming that changes occurred in stages: (1) The early and reversible stage characterized by accumulation of cytoskeletal proteins to counteract an increased strain without loss of contractile material, and (2) increased accumulation of microtubules and desmin to compensate for the increasing loss of myofilaments and titin. This last stage represents the late clinical and irreversible state. Based on structural basis for HF, they suggest an integrative view which closes the gap between changes within cardiac myocytes and the involvement of the extracellular matrix (ECM), including the development of fibrosis. Further discussion on the interaction between the cystoskeleton and ECM are presented in a later section.

Cellular Hypertrophy

The hypertrophy of cardiomyocytes is a well-recognized remodeling response to increased hemodynamic load [45]. Myocyte hypertrophy is likely an adaptive mechanism designed to improve pump function by expanding the number of contractile units while simultaneously reducing wall stress by increasing wall thickness. When excessive or prolonged, myocyte hypertrophy is maladaptive. Hypertrophy can directly result in HF, as evidenced by patients with HCM [46]. In the failing heart, excessive LV hypertrophy is associated with reduced chamber compliance, myocardial fibrosis, and lethal dysrhythmias [47, 48]. However, the time frame of transition from adaptive to maladaptive hypertrophy is not known. Experimental evidence indicates that targeted increases in wall thickness in the absence of concomitant increases in LV volume can have beneficial effects on cardiac performance and the progression of HF [49].

The first stimulus to induce myocyte hypertrophy is usually mechanical, such as hemodynamic overload, although neurohormones and cytokines also play an important role in its maintenance [50, 51]. Transduction of mechanical stress and other environmental signals is believed to occur through integrin proteins, transmembrane receptors that couple extracellular matrix components directly to the intracellular cytoskeleton and nucleus [52, 53]. In general, the signal for hypertrophy is mediated by a complex cascade of signaling systems within the cardiomyocyte, resulting in gene reprogramming [54]. These signaling mechanisms have been discussed in other chapters; in brief, diverse neurohumoral signals acting through many interrelated signal transduction pathways lead to pathological cardiac hypertrophy and HF [54]. Moreover, activated hypertrophy-related genes induce the synthesis of new contractile proteins that are organized into new sarcomeres. Thus, extensive remodeling of the complete intracellular contractile apparatus is characteristic of the failing heart.

Recent experimental observations have shown that the introduction of functional miRNA (e.g., miRNA-21 or miRNA-18b) into cardiomyocytes (see Chap. 3) represses myocyte hypertrophy. The role miRNAs play in cardiac remodeling and HF, has been recently reviewed by Divakaran and Mann [55]. Alterations in the expression or activity, or both, of myofilament regulatory proteins are potential mechanisms for the decrease in cardiac contractile function in HF, including changes in myosin light chains and the troponin–tropomyosin complex. While some studies have implicated a role for miRNA-21 in the regulation of cardiomyocytes hypertrophic growth, others did not. This discrepancy between studies could be explained on findings that the modulation of hypertrophic growth by miRNA-21 in myocytes is achieved through an indirect mechanism, rather than a direct targeting effect of miR-21 on hypertrophy-related genes. So far, miRNA-21 has no confirmed gene targets that are related to cardiomyocyte hypertrophy. Therefore, its role in cardiomyocyte hypertrophy remains unknown, since exogenously administered premiRNA-21 (i.e., primary transcripts to short stem-loop structures that become a messenger RNA after processing) fails to be processed in myocytes, resulting in a lack of capacity to overexpress mature miRNA-21 in these cells. Finally, based on current knowledge, we agree that the role that miRNAs play in HF is rather limited, and is based largely on studies that have examined the miRNA expression profiles on explanted hearts from HF patients or from studies that have examined miRNA microarrays in experimental animal models that develop remodeling or from stimulated cardiomyocytes cell culture.

Cell Death and Renewal

Environmental stress and injury produce cell death by apoptosis, necrosis, and perhaps autophagy. Little is known about the role of necrosis and autophagy in HF (see Chap. 5). On the other hand, a conceptual framework has been developed for apoptosis, a highly regulated cell suicide process that is hard-wired into all metazoan cells. Chronic cardiac remodeling response and transition to overt HF have been associated with modestly increased apoptosis [56–58], although the actual burden of chronic cell loss attributable to apoptosis is not clear. Measures of actual rates are highly variable and depend on the species, type of injury, timing, location, and method of assessment. When viewed in absolute terms, the rate of apoptosis is quite low [59], however, when the relatively low rates are viewed in the context of months or years, it is entirely plausible that the apoptotic burden could be substantial. Unfortunately, the timing of the apoptotic process is not well defined and the assessment of the true rates and their consequences is still quite limited.

Apoptosis is a complex process and its regulation is not completely defined. An important signaling pathway for myocardial apoptosis during the transition to HF is mediated by the balance of the proapoptotic protein Bax relative to the antiapoptotic protein Bcl-2 [60]. These proteins can stimulate or suppress the action of the caspases, which carry out the characteristic biochemical and morphological changes of apoptosis. Other key pathways include the expression of the death receptor Fas, which is up-regulated in failing cardiomyocytes and activates downstream caspases, resulting in apoptosis [61, 62]. In short, apoptosis is mediated by two evolutionarily conserved central death pathways: the extrinsic pathway, which utilizes cell surface death receptors; and the intrinsic pathway (see Chap. 5), involving mitochondria and the ER (Fig. 11.2) [63]. In the extrinsic pathway, death ligands (e.g., FasL) initiate apoptosis by binding their cognate receptors [64]. This stimulates the recruitment of the adaptor protein Fas-associated via death domain (FADD), which then recruits procaspase-8 into the death-inducing signaling complex (DISC) [65]. Procaspase-8 is activated by dimerization within this complex and subsequently cleaves and activates procaspase-3 and other downstream procaspases [66].

As discussed in Chap. 5, the intrinsic pathway transduces a wide variety of extracellular and intracellular signaling stimuli including loss of survival/trophic factors, toxins, radiation, hypoxia, OS, myocardial ischemia/reperfusion (I/R) injury, and DNA damage. Although a number of peripheral pathways connect these signals with the central death machinery, each ultimately feeds into a variety of proapoptotic Bcl-2 related proteins that possess only Bcl-2 homology domain 3 (BH3-only proteins, including Bid, Bad, Noxa, Puma, Bim and Bmf, all have only the short BH3 motif) and the proapoptotic multidomain Bcl-2 proteins Bax and Bak [67]. These proteins undergo activation through diverse mechanisms to trigger the release of mitochondrial apoptogens, such as cytochrome c, Smac, EndoG, and AIF into the cytoplasm [68–71]. Once in the cytoplasm, cytochrome c binds Apaf-1 along with dATP. This stimulates Apaf-1 to homo-oligomerize and recruits procaspase-9 into the multiprotein complex called the apoptosome [72–75]. Within the apoptosome, procaspase-9 is activated by dimerization, after which it cleaves and activates downstream procaspases. Bid unites the extrinsic and intrinsic pathways; following cleavage by caspase-8, Bid's C-terminal portion translocates to the mitochondria and triggers further apoptogen release [76, 77].

The extrinsic and intrinsic pathways are regulated by a variety of endogenous inhibitors of apoptosis (see Fig. 11.2). FLICE-like (Fas-associated death domain protein-like-interleukin-1-converting enzyme-like) inhibitory protein (FLIP), whose expression is highly enriched in striated muscle, binds to and inhibits procaspase-8 in the DISC [78]. Antiapoptotic Bcl-2 proteins, such as Bcl-2 and Bcl-xL, inhibit mitochondrial apoptogen release through biochemical mechanisms that are still incompletely understood. Ku-70 and humanin bind Bax and block its conformational activation

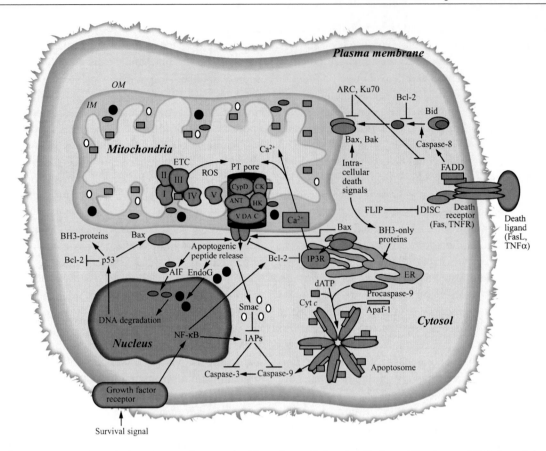

Fig. 11.2 The extrinsic and survival pathways of apoptosis. The extrinsic pathway is initiated by ligand binding to death receptors leading to recruitment of FADD and DISC which stimulates the activation of caspase 8 resulting in caspase 3 activation and Bid cleavage (a C-terminal fragment of Bid targets mitochondria). FLIP, ARC, and Ku70 can stem this pathway's progression at specific points. Intracellular stimuli trigger ER release of Ca^{2+} through both Bax and BH3-protein interactions. Also depicted is the survival pathway triggered by survival stimuli, mediated by growth factor receptors, transcription factor activation (e.g., NF-κB), and enhanced expression of IAPs and Bcl-2. Also shown is the intrinsic pathway (previously discussed in Chap. 5)

and translocation to the mitochondria [79]. X-linked inhibitor of apoptosis (XIAP) and related proteins, which contain baculovirus inhibitor of apoptosis repeats, bind to and inhibit already activated caspases-9, -3, and -7, as well as interfering with procaspase-9 dimerization and activation [80, 81]. Each of these inhibitors acts on circumscribed portions of either the extrinsic or intrinsic pathway. By contrast, the apoptosis repressor with caspase recruitment domain (ARC), which is expressed preferentially in striated muscle and some neurons, antagonizes both the intrinsic and extrinsic apoptosis pathways [82]. The extrinsic pathway is inhibited by ARC's direct interactions with Fas, FADD, and procaspase-8, which prevent DISC assembly, while the intrinsic pathway is inhibited by ARC's direct binding and inhibition of Bax's interaction with the mitochondrial membrane [83, 84].

In the failing human heart, the expression of protooncogenes that regulate programmed cell death is increased and is associated with increased cardiomyocyte apoptosis [85].

To assess the role of apoptosis in human HF, patients with acute myocardial infarction (MI) were assessed for the rate of cardiomyocyte apoptosis relative to indices of structural LV remodeling. Within the infarct area and in areas remote from the site of injury, the rate of myocardial apoptosis was increased and was strongly associated with maladaptive LV remodeling in addition to adverse clinical outcomes [86]. The most common form of HF that has been associated with significant levels of apoptosis is associated with DCM [87]. Apoptosis is also correlated with the clinical severity of DCM and the subsequent need for cardiac transplantation [88]. Despite the demonstration that apoptosis occurs in cardiac remodeling and HF, it is not clear whether apoptosis is a cause or consequence of transition to HF. Experimental models of progressive LV dysfunction and HF provide an opportunity to regulate apoptosis and examine the resultant influence on LV structure and function. In rabbits with coronary artery ligation, the administration of a viral antiapoptotic Bcl-2 gene to the heart limited apoptosis and simultaneously attenuated LV dilatation and dysfunction [89]. In addition, bioactive peptides such as insulin-like growth factor-1 (IGF-1) can protect cardiomyocytes from apoptosis [90]. The overexpression of IGF-1 in a mouse coronary artery ligation model limited cell death and correspondingly attenuated maladaptive remodeling and the transition to HF [91]. In a canine model of HF, exogenously administered IGF-1 attenuated wall thinning and improved function in association with reduced apoptosis [92]. These observations in animal models lend support to the concept that apoptosis may play a contributory role in cardiac remodeling and the transition to HF.

A new concept of cardiomyocyte regeneration has been proposed. This concept is based on the premise that myocyte death and regeneration are homeostatic mechanisms intrinsic to both the normal and diseased heart [93, 94]. Estimates of the rates of cell death would suggest that an innate system of cardiomyocyte replacement might be present to account for the maintenance of cardiac muscle mass over a lifetime [95]. Although some investigators believe that significant regeneration are not observed in conditions where myocytes are extensively lost, myocardial tumors are rare, and the current evidence supporting cell renewal in the heart is preliminary and controversial [96]. Findings of cyclin and cyclin-dependent kinase up-regulation in both normal and pathological myocardium, as well as increased telomerase activity in cardiomyocytes, have been proposed to be evidence of myocyte renewal. Opposing viewpoints dismiss these observations as nonspecific biochemical events of hypertrophy and not as evidence of cardiomyocyte hyperplasia [96]. Direct evidence for the concept of myocyte regeneration was obtained by Anversa et al. examining normal and post-MI left ventricular myocardium for the presence of cytological and biochemical markers of cell replication in cardiomyocytes. Measurements of Ki67 and the mitotic index indicated that cardiomyocyte replication occurred in normal myocardium and was increased in diseased myocardium, particularly in the border zone between infarcted and viable myocardium [92, 97, 98]. These investigators hypothesize that the majority of adult cardiomyocytes are indeed terminally differentiated and only a small proportion of cardiomyocytes retains the ability to reenter the cell cycle, becoming particularly prolific when the myocardium is injured and cell losses were incurred. Based on the magnitude and rate at which these events are hypothesized to occur, the proponents of the cell renewal theory estimate that the entire LV could be regenerated in a period of 6 months, and as such, the generation of new myocytes likely contributes to remodeling the failing heart [99]. Unfortunately, these mechanisms of cell renewal do not appear capable of regenerating the burden of cells lost within an area of infarction and are limited to the restoration of cells lost in the remaining viable myocardium.

While evidence does exist in support of a limited population of cardiomyocyte stem cells in the myocardium, the possibility exists that a population of extracardiac stem cells, perhaps from the bone marrow, is capable of regenerating cardiomyocytes lost to injury [100–103]. In transplanted human hearts, chimerism has been observed, supporting the possibility that extracardiac progenitor cells exist and serve to regenerate cardiomyocytes in the heart [104, 105]. Moreover, chimerism has also been demonstrated in the heart after bone-marrow transplantation [106].

The Extracellular Matrix

A fundamental process in cardiac remodeling is the myocardial extracellular matrix (ECM) dynamic interaction with the various cellular and acellular components of the heart, including cardiomyocytes, collagen, soluble factors, and mechanical cues that provide both positive and negative signals generated by various physiologic conditions.

Also, critical to this cardiac remodeling dynamic process are several classes of transmembrane receptors that provide both inside-out and outside-in signaling [107]. ECM translates the force generated by individual myocytes into organized ventricular contraction and prevents myocyte slippage. ECM surrounds and interconnects cardiac myocytes, myofibrils, muscle fibers, and the coronary circulation [52, 108], and because of the high tensile strength of fibrillar collagen and its close association with the functioning components of the myocardium, alterations in the ECM can significantly influence the size, shape, and function of the cardiac chamber.

As previously noted, there is an important link between the ECM and the cardiomyocyte cytoskeleton; one class of cell-surface receptor molecules that constitute part of that link are the transmembrane integrins which act as signaling molecules and transducers of mechanical force [109]. Interestingly, integrins are expressed in all cellular components of the cardiovascular system, including the vasculature, blood, cardiac myocytes, and nonmuscle cardiac cells. In response to specific changes in their micro-environment, these receptors become activated and form focal adhesions, areas of attachment of the cells to ECM proteins involving the colocalization of cytoskeletal proteins, intracellular signaling molecules, and growth factor receptors. Growth factor-mediated integrin activation can stimulate cell growth, gene expression, and adhesion in cardiac fibroblasts [110]. In addition, a large number of bioactive signaling molecules and growth factors, proteases, and structural proteins have been identified that influence cell–matrix interactions. For example, small G proteins act as molecular switches to regulate numerous cellular responses including cardiac myocyte hypertrophy and cell survival associated with cell growth and division, multiple changes in the cytoskeleton, vesicular transport, and myofibrillar apparatus. Extensive cardiac remodeling may occur prior to the development of symptomatic HF. For example, pressure overloading during the compensated phase leads to concentric hypertrophy that is characterized by an increase in myocyte cross-sectional area (CSA). On the other hand, volume overloading during the compensated phase of HF leads to an increase in chamber diameter/wall thickness, which is characterized by increased myocyte length and CSA. Excessive myocyte lengthening without changes in CSA appears to be the primary cellular alteration leading to chamber dilatation in the progression to HF [106].

The classical perspective that the ECM is an inert biomaterial and passive structural support mechanism has been replaced by the new concept that the ECM is a dynamic entity that is in equilibrium with the cellular components of the heart, and that it alters its composition and organization in response to environmental cues and tissue injury [111]. Furthermore, myocardial ECM has considerable plasticity such that the components of the ECM are actively degraded and replaced [108, 112, 113].

Metalloproteinases

Physiologic degradation of matrix elements is primarily the result of the coordinated activity of the proteolytic enzymes. A family of zinc-dependent enzymes capable of degrading the ECM of biological tissues, which play a fundamental role in ECM remodeling in normal and disease states, are the matrix metalloproteinases (MMPs) [114, 115]. Among the 20 species reported, MMPs can be divided into two principal types: those that are secreted into the extracellular space and those that are membrane bound. The secreted MMPs comprise the majority of known MMP species and are released into the extracellular space in a latent or proenzyme state (proMMP). Activation of these latent MMPs is required for proteolytic activity, achieved through enzymatic cleavage of the propeptide domain. Serine proteases such as plasmin as well as other MMP species can convert proMMPs to active enzyme. Rapid amplification of MMP activity therefore occurs after an initial enzymatic step. The secreted MMPs bind to specific ECM proteins based on the sequence of the C-terminus of the enzyme and therefore they are in very close juxtaposition to the future proteolytic substrate, providing a means for rapid induction of proteolytic activity. The activated MMPs subsequently undergo autocatalysis, resulting in lower molecular weight forms and ultimately inactive protein fragments. The classification of MMPs was originally determined by substrate specificity, but as the

characterization of this enzyme system proceeded, a great deal of substrate crossover between MMP classes and species has been identified. Nevertheless, a general classification has been developed for the MMPs and discussed in several reviews [116, 117]. In brief, the interstitial collagenases such as MMP-1, MMP-13, the stromelysins, MMP-3, and the gelatinases, MMP-2 and MMP-9 have been observed within the myocardium [3, 118, 119]. A second and novel class of MMPs is the membrane-type MMPs (MT-MMPs), which are membrane bound and therefore provide a focal substrate for ECM proteolytic degradation [120]. During trafficking to cell membrane, MT-MMPs undergo intracellular activation through a proprotein convertase pathway. Thus, unlike other classes of MMPs, MT-MMPs are proteolytically active once inserted into the cell membrane. Finally, MT-MMPs contain substrate recognition site for other MMP species and therefore constitute an important pathway for activation of other MMPs [117, 121]. Type 1 MT-MMP (MT1-MMP) proteolytically processes the proforms of the gelatinase MMP-2 and the interstitial collagenase MMP-13. MT-MMPs do not appear to be under the influence of local inhibitory control because the tissue inhibitors of the MMPs (TIMPs), including TIMP-1, fail to effectively bind to MT-MMPs [121, 122]. Six different MT-MMPs have been cloned and appear to be expressed in both normal and diseased heart. A number of cell types within the myocardium express MT-MMPs, including fibroblasts, vascular smooth muscle, and cardiac myocytes. The best characterized MT-MMP is MT1-MMP and it has been the focus of several studies [120]. It has been shown that MT1-MMP degrades fibrillar collagens and a wide range of ECM glycoproteins and proteoglycans. MT-MMPs therefore likely play a key role in ECM degradation localized to basement membrane and cell–cell contact points.

An important control point of MMP activity is through the presence of an endogenous class of low molecular weight TIMPs [122]. To date, four different TIMP species have been identified and are known to bind to activated MMPs in a 1:1 stoichiometric ratio. The four TIMP species all bind and inactivate the various MMPs, including MMP-2 and MMP-9, but with different affinities. TIMP-3 is a more potent inhibitor of MMP-9 than the other TIMPs [123]. Certain MMPs bind to proMMPs and thereby form MMP–TIMP complexes. The functional significance of these proMMP–TIMP complexes is not completely understood but may actually facilitate MMP activation. One of the better-characterized TIMPs is TIMP-1, which binds with great affinity to activated MMPs, and as discussed earlier does not effectively bind and inhibit MT-MMPs. TIMP-4 appears to have a predominant distribution within the myocardium [124]. However, the significance of the myocardial expression of TIMP-4 remains to be determined. Besides to binding to MMPs, TIMPs appear also to influence cell growth and metabolism in vitro [122]. Thus, TIMPs may have multiple biological effects with respect to MMP activity within the myocardium that would be relevant to the cardiac remodeling process. An important emerging concept in the biology of MMPs is that MMP can alter the bioactive properties and signaling capacity of the ECM through the activation and release of growth factors, and other biologically active matrix elements including the collagen degradation products [116].

The ADAMs (a disintegrin and metalloproteinase) are a unique and novel class of enzymes from the metalloproteinase family that degrade ECM components and simultaneously activate key biopeptides in the interstitial microenvironment [125]. ADAMs are believed to be able to modify cell–cell and cell–matrix interactions via integrin receptors and may therefore influence issue architecture and remodeling by reorganizing cells within their matrix. ADAMs may also activate biologically active peptides, cytokines, and growth factor resulting in biological effects [125]. Although ADAMs have been implicated in cardiac disease and remodeling [50, 126–128], their specific profile and their role in HF remain to be evaluated.

There is ample evidence to incriminate a pathophysiologic role for MMPs in LV remodeling and HF; and the topic has been the subject of several recent reviews [129, 130]. In brief, increased MMP expression has been found in patients with end-stage HF and in animal models of HF due to LV dysfunction [118, 124, 131–134], and a cause and effect relationship between MMPs and LV remodeling have been established through the use of transgenic models and the use of pharmacologic MMP inhibitors [5, 133, 135–138]. For example, a loss of MMP inhibitory control through TIMP-1 gene deletion has been shown to produce LV chamber dilation in mice [138]. Cardiac restricted overexpression of the MMP-1 (interstitial collagenase) resulted in a loss of collagen abundance with transition to LV dysfunction [136]. Moreover, deletion of the MMP-9 gene in mice reduces the rate of cardiac rupture and alters the course of LV remodeling following MI [133].

Changes in collagen phenotypes, MMPs, TIMPs, lysyl oxidase (LOX), and the role of TGF-β in the induction of type III collagen in cardiac fibroblast have been recently the subject of appraisal by Sivakumar et al. [139], both in DCM and in non-failing human heart. In DCM, the heart collagen concentration was markedly elevated compared to that of the non-failing hearts associated with an increase in Type I (18%) and Type III (33%) collagen. In comparison with non-failing hearts the content of MMP-2 and MMP-9 was significantly increased in DCM. Transcriptional level of LOX, TIMP 1, and 2 were markedly upregulated in DCM. Furthermore, a significant increase in the transcript levels of cytokines, notably IFN, IL-6, TNF-α, and TGF-β superfamily was observed in all DCM hearts. The addition of TGF-β

to cardiac fibroblasts caused a dose dependent increase in type III collagen. Taken together, these data support the concept that defects in collagen, MMPs, various cytokines, and LOX are contributory to the cardiac remodeling process leading to HF.

Electrical Remodeling Secondary to Ventricular Dysrhythmias

Although a detailed analysis on the incidence and types of dysrhythmias occurring as a consequence of or concomitant with HF is addressed in Chap. 13, in this section, we will briefly comment only on LV remodeling associated with ventricular dysrhythmias.

Defective electrical activation of the heart secondary to pacing or HF may induce marked ventricular electrical remodeling. According to Marrus and Nerbonne, cardiac myocytes, in response to these electrical or mechanical perturbations, exhibit remarkable changes in the expression and/or the function of sarcolemmal ion channels, a process that is broadly described as electrical remodeling [140]. This remodeling has beneficial, as well as adverse, effects on myocardial function, including increased risk of fatal dysrhythmias. One specific example of cardiac electrical remodeling is cardiac memory, a phenomenon induced in the heart after abnormal myocardial activation patterns produced by artificial pacemakers. Based on recent observations, Jeyaraj et al. [141] have presented the intriguing similarities between cardiac memory and HF. In both situations, abnormal mechanical stretch of the myocardium results in direct alterations in ion channel properties, as well as in the activation of angiotensin-dependent signaling cascades. With time, altered gene transcription and protein synthesis lead to persistent changes in ion channel levels and activities, changes that can significantly impact normal cardiac function and increase dysrhythmias susceptibility.

Defective electrical activation of the heart secondary to pacing or HF may induce marked ventricular electrical remodeling, which may be manifested electrocardiographically as T-wave memory, and ultimately as deleterious mechanical remodeling from heterogeneous strain [141]. Although T-wave memory is associated with altered expression of sarcolemmal ion channels, the biophysical mechanisms responsible for triggering remodeling of cardiac ion channels have not been established.

The study by St. John Sutton et al. [142] has addressed the relationship of ventricular dysrhythmias (premature ventricular contractions > 10/h) and ventricular tachycardia (VT) to measures of LV remodeling, following acute myocardial infarction (AMI). They found that both premature ventricular contractions (PVCs) and ventricular tachycardia

(VT) are related to LV mass area at the mid papillary muscle level (LVMA) and cavity area change (LVΔ) at baseline, 1, and 2 years. A change in LV size and function from baseline to 2 years was predictive of both PVCs and VT. In addition, there was an increased likelihood of PVCs and VT with each quintile of LV size and function at baseline, at 1 and 2 years. Thus, adverse LV remodeling, defined as higher LVMA and greater LV volume, and decreased systolic function, is associated with higher grade of ventricular dysrhythmias including VT. The likely mechanism is that LV remodeling is associated with greater areas of myocardial fibrosis that results in the substrate for ventricular dysrhythmias; however, this study has significant limitations since it did not provide conclusive information regarding the potential success of treatment, and also it was limited to ventricular dysrhythmias.

Reversing Cardiac Remodeling

Insights from Patients with Left Ventricular Assist Device

In the last few years, new knowledge has emerged on the basic mechanisms of ventricular remodeling from studies of HF patients supported by mechanical left-ventricular assist devices (LVADs). LVADs, used as a "bridge to transplant" for some HF patients, can induce profound cardiac unloading and have been shown to be associated with reverse cardiac remodeling on a structural and functional level [143]. These devices offer a unique setting to study the molecular mechanisms underlying cardiac remodeling. To analyze this reverse remodeling at a transcriptional level, a series of studies have been performed using cardiac tissue from patients before and after placement of an LVAD [144, 145]. One study analyzed six HF patients with different etiologies using oligonucleotide microarrays [141]. Paired test analysis revealed numerous genes that were regulated, including a down-regulation of several previously studied genes. Further analysis revealed that the overall gene expression profiles could significantly distinguish pre- and post-LVAD status. Importantly, the data also identified two distinct groups among the pre-LVAD failing hearts, in which there was blind segregation of patients based on HF etiology. In addition to the substantial divergence in genomic profiles for these two HF groups, there were significant differences in their corresponding LVAD-mediated regulation of gene expression, with an association between the process of reverse remodeling and changes in cellular metabolic pathways [144]. Another study analyzed seven patients with DCM. On average, 1,374 (±155) genes were reported as "increased" and 1,629 (±45)

as "decreased" after LVAD support. Up-regulated genes included a large proportion of transcription factors, genes related to cell growth/apoptosis/DNA repair, cell structural proteins, metabolism, and cell signaling/communication. LVAD support resulted in down-regulation of genes for a group of cytokines [146]. In another study, analysis of a gene expression library of 19 paired human failing heart samples from different etiologies harvested at the time of LVAD implant, and again at explant revealed a high percentage of genes involved in the regulation of vascular networks including neuropilin-1 (a VEGF receptor), FGF9, Sprouty1, stromal-derived factor 1, and Endomucin, suggesting that mechanical unloading alters the regulation of vascular organization and migration in the heart. In addition to vascular signaling networks, GATA4 binding protein, a critical mediator of myocyte hypertrophy, was significantly down-regulated following mechanical unloading. In summary, these findings may have important implications for defining the role of mechanical stretch and load on autocrine/paracrine signals directing vascular organization in the failing human heart and the role of GATA4 in orchestrating reverse myocardial remodeling [145].

The impact of LVADs support on reversing the remodeling process has been recently reviewed by Klotz et al. [147]. It appears that the clinical outcome following the use of LVADs have not always been favorable, since some patients treated with LVADs often progressed rapidly back to HF. Nonetheless, important information have emerged from studies of LVAD implantation (with the intention of a "bridge to transplant" for some HF patients) that provides insights into the basic mechanisms of ventricular remodeling, and also in establishing the possible limits of ventricular recovery. These studies generated the concept of reverse remodeling, now recognized as an important goal of many HF treatment modalities. As pointed out by these investigators, there are important structural and functional elements that do not necessarily regress toward normal during treatment with LVADs, including abnormal extracellular matrix metabolism, increased tissue angiotensin levels, myocardial stiffening, and partial recovery of gene expression involved with metabolism. Notwithstanding these findings, LVADs studies have led to understand that an unprecedented degree of myocardial recovery is possible, when given sufficient mechanical unloading and restoration of more normal neurohormonal milieu. Also, Sopa et al. have reviewed LVADs- induced molecular changes in the failing myocardium [148]. In both patients and experimental models, improved myocardial function was associated with alterations in several key pathways including cell survival, cytokine signaling, calcium handling, adrenergic receptor signaling, cytoskeletal and contractile proteins, energy metabolism, extracellular matrix, and endothelial and microvascular functions. The unique research opportunities offered by LVADs analysis are beginning to distinguish changes associated with recovery from those of mechanical unloading alone, allowing the establishment of potential predictors and novel therapeutic targets capable of improving myocardial repair.

Remodeling and CRT

Although more detailed information about the use of cardiac resynchronization therapy (CRT) in HF patients is presented in Chap. 20, here it will suffice to comment only on the positive and negative side of using this methodology in relation to New York Heart Association NYHA functional class, and its effect in remodeling. Acquired information from extensive databases and hand searches directed to evaluate the efficacy, effectiveness, and safety of CRT in patients with LV systolic dysfunction showed that CRT reduces morbidity and mortality in patients with LV systolic dysfunction, prolonged QRS duration, and NYHA class 3 or 4 symptoms, when combined with optimal pharmacotherapy. However, the incremental benefits of combined CRT plus implantable cardioverter-defibrillator devices vs. CRT-alone devices in patients with LV systolic dysfunction remain uncertain [149]. On the other hand, based on the concept that CRT improves LV structure and function and clinical outcomes in NYHA functional class III and IV HF with prolonged QRS, the European REVERSE study group have carried out a randomized trial of cardiac resynchronization in mildly symptomatic HF, and in asymptomatic patients with LV dysfunction and previous HF symptoms [150]. This study consisted of a cohort of 610 patients with NYHA functional class I or II HF with a QRS ≥ 120 ms and a LV ejection fraction ≤40% that received a CRT device (±defibrillator), and were randomly assigned to active CRT (CRT-ON; n = 419) or control (CRT-OFF; n = 191) for 12 months. The HF clinical composite response end point showed that 16% worsened in CRT-ON compared with 21% in CRT-OFF. CRT-ON patients experienced a greater improvement in LV end-systolic volume index and other measures of LV remodeling. Time-to-first HF hospitalization was significantly delayed in CRT-ON. Taken together, the REVERSE trial demonstrates that CRT, in combination with optimal medical therapy (±defibrillator), reduces the risk for hospitalization in HF patients and improves ventricular remodeling in NYHA functional class II as well as in NYHA functional class I patients with previous HF symptoms. What makes this study particularly interesting is that the REVERSE is the first randomized study designed to evaluate the results of using CRT in patients with NYHA class I–II HF symptoms and abnormal LV function. Notwithstanding, the benefits of CRT in patients with mild HF may require a longer period of time to become apparent. Furthermore, caution is needed before definitive conclusions can be reached concerning the use of CRT in mild HF, keeping in mind not only the cost of CRT devices but also their potential side effects (e.g., ventricular dysrhythmias) and other complications.

Other Approaches to Remodeling Therapy

Critical to the current treatment of HF is the ability to favorably reverse the chronic processes by which the failing heart remodels. Reverse remodeling can be induced by pharmacological and non-pharmacological therapy. The CARMEN (Carvedilol ACE Inhibitor Remodeling Mild CHF) study have explored the need for combined treatment for remodeling and order of introduction by comparing angiotensin-converting enzyme (ACE) against carvedilol, a β-adrenergic antagonist with vasodilatory properties (α1-antagonism), and their combination. These studies demonstrated that carvedilol could be safely administered before starting ACE inhibitor treatment, but that patients presenting with mild HF should receive a combination of carvedilol and an ACE inhibitor at the initiation of therapy to help slow disease progression [151]. More recently, it has been argued that carvedilol alone not only attenuate LV remodeling and improve clinical outcomes in patients with LV dysfunction and/or HF following acute myocardial infarction, but that in comparative studies with metoprolol, carvedilol may be associated with greater survival benefit in HF patients [152].

In 1999 the RESOLVD pilot study [153], a prospective, multinational study of 768 randomized patients with New York Heart Association class II to IV heart failure (ischemic heart disease was present in 71% of them), distributed these patients to receive an angiotensin II receptor antagonist (candesartan), ACE inhibitor (enalapril), or candesartan plus enalapril for 43 weeks. It was found that ACE inhibitors can substantially reduce morbidity and mortality in HF patients, that angiotensin II (AII) levels raised despite treatment, and also that the event rates remained high. Furthermore, the study also demonstrated that combining an ACE inhibitor with an AII-receptor blocker may be more effective in reducing LV remodeling than either agent alone. However, while end-diastolic and end-systolic volumes showed lesser increases with combination therapy than with candesartan or enalapril alone, the higher mortality rate associated with the combination therapy finally forced cancellation of the study, 6 weeks prior to completion. More recently, a follow up study in RESOLVD [154] has addressed the applicability of temporal changes in neurohormones as markers of ventricular remodeling and also its use for prognostication in patients with LV systolic dysfunction and HF, who were treated with either candesartan, enalapril, or both. Temporal changes in plasma renin, angiotensin-II, aldosterone, epinephrine, norepinephrine, B-type natriuretic peptide (BNP), and N-terminal atrial natriuretic peptide (NT-ANP) were measured at baseline and at 17 and 43 weeks after randomization. These measurements were examined regarding their relations with concurrent changes in LV ejection fraction (LVEF), cardiac volumes, and risk for subsequent adverse clinical outcomes. Increasing BNP and NT-ANP over time were associated with concurrent decreasing in LVEF, increasing end-diastolic volume (EDV), and increasing end-systolic volume. In multivariable analysis, changes in BNP and NT-ANP were independent predictors of the changes in ESV and EDV, whereas the change in BNP also predicted the change in EF. Patients who died or experienced HF hospitalization had higher increases in NT-ANP and lesser decreases in norepinephrine. Increasing NT-ANP and norepinephrine over time independently predicted increased risk for subsequent death or HF hospitalization. Taken together, this study showed that in treated patients with HF, increasing NT-ANP and BNP over time predict a decreasing EF and LV dilatation, while increasing NT-ANP and norepinephrine independently predict greater mortality and morbidity. Thus, serial measurements of these neurohormones may serve as useful substitute markers of ventricular remodeling and prognosticators for clinical risk stratification.

Besides pharmacotherapy, LVADs, containment devices and new methods to restore synchronous contraction have been added to the treatment of chronic HF, and in some cases significant improvement in both symptoms and mortality have been achieved. LVADs in advanced HF cases might allow significant unloading to the failing ventricle; but when weaning from LVADs should be carried out, if persistent functional improvement continues in HF patients, is questionable. Nonetheless, as previously mentioned, besides its role as a therapeutic modality, LVADs have provided remarkable insights into the molecular and cellular basis of cardiac remodeling (since the procedure allows access to collection of heart tissue). In the future, genetic and cellular approaches, as well as new small molecule targets, may provide alternative avenues to reverse the remodeling process, improving symptoms and disease outcome [155].

Conclusions and Future Directions

LV remodeling is a critical process in the progression of HF, and understanding its mechanism(s) may allow understanding of the pathophysiology of HF. Recently, the assessment of this process have significantly evolved to include not only changes in heart size and shape, but also intriguing new information on cellular and molecular remodeling, mainly as

the heart undergoes evolutionary changes toward failure. There is an ongoing debate whether reverse remodeling in HF can be used as a surrogate endpoint; however, the information available in this regard and at this point is rather conflictive.

While LV dilatation and dysfunction are major negative prognostic markers in patients with HF, changes in LV dimensions rather than in ejection fraction are considered the major markers to monitor remodeling. LVEF can be influenced by transient loading conditions and by agents that stimulate contractility at the expense of increased oxygen demand, whereas dimensional changes bring about specific structural modifications in the myocardium [156]. Of importance, neurohormonal antagonists that reduce mortality and morbidity in HF, are also able to inhibit or reverse remodeling; reversing remodeling, β-blockers appear to be superior to the other classes of drugs, exhibiting a stronger correlation between dose and effect. Nonetheless, β-blockers have been used mainly in addition to background therapy, including ACE inhibitors. As mentioned earlier, nonpharmacological methodologies such as LVEDs and CRT are also capable to achieve functional improvement and reverse remodeling in mildly symptomatic HF patients, asymptomatic patients with LV dysfunction and previous HF symptoms, as well as in patients with advanced HF.

In HF subcellular remodeling or remodeling of cellular organelles that include the ECM, sarcoplasmic reticulum, myofibrils, mitochondria, and nucleus undergo varying degrees of changes in their biochemical composition and molecular structure, which might induce cardiac dysfunction [157]. We have addressed most of these changes in earlier chapters, and in general we concur with the concept that subcellular remodeling may be related to alterations in cardiac gene expression as well as to activation of different proteases and phospholipases in the failing heart. Opie et al. have addressed some of the controversies on remodeling [11]. They pointed out that the transition from apparently compensated hypertrophy to HF suggests a changing balance between metalloproteinases and their inhibitors, effects of ROS, and death-promoting and profibrotic neurohumoral responses. Although these alterations are rather evasive therapeutic targets, a number of potential novel therapies for these disorders are being developed, including sildenafil, an unexpected option for anti-transition therapy; surgery for increased sphericity caused by chronic volume overload of mitral regurgitation; an antifibrotic peptide to inhibit the fibrogenic effects of transforming growth factor β, mechanical intervention in advanced HF cases, and gene and stem-cell therapy. These approaches together with novel small molecule targets are some of the methodologies that may become available to reverse the remodeling process, improving symptoms and disease outcome.

Summary

- A crucial change in the progression of LV dysfunction and HF is cardiac remodeling.
- Remodeling involves alterations in both the myocytes and the cardiac extracellular matrix (ECM), the latter includes the activation of proteolytic enzymes leading to the degradation and re-organization of collagens.
- The development of overt HF is mainly triggered by the marked ventricular dilatation that occurs once the resources from myocardial hypertrophic response are exhausted.
- Many factors including neurohormonal and cytokine activation and impaired Ca^{2+} handling are thought to play a contributory role in remodeling.
- With increased work load the adult heart develops pathological growth and activation of the fetal program of gene expression followed by LV dilatation, thinning of the wall, and pump failure.
- Mice with cardiac specific deletion of PKD1 exhibited improve cardiac function and diminish hypertrophy in response to pressure overload and angiotensing II signaling, confirming that PKAD1 is a key transducer of stress stimuli involved in the abnormal remodeling of the heart.
- Alterations in energy status and metabolism are proposed to play a role in the transition from stable cardiac hypertrophy to overt HF.
- In HF changes in myocardial energy metabolism correlates inversely with plasma free-fatty-acid concentrations, and mitochondrial uncoupling proteins (UCPs) may play a significant role in its regulation.
- The creation of transgenic mice with altered expression of genes involved in carbohydrate and lipid metabolism has provided unique insights into the fine balance within the heart to maintain energy status and function, as well as to evaluate the cause–effect relationships between mitochondrial function and myocardial disease.
- Besides abnormal lipid metabolism, diverse neurohormonal signals acting through interwoven signal transduction pathways can lead to pathological cardiac hypertrophy and HF.
- An important hallmark of HF is reduced myocardial contractility, with defective intracellular Ca^{2+} handling playing a crucial role in the pathogenesis of these contractile abnormalities.
- The progressive cytoskeletal stiffness, the contractile dysfunction, and fibrosis typical of the failing heart may be partly explained by the up-regulation of many genes encoding cytoskeletal proteins, sarcomeric proteins, and extracellular matrix (ECM) proteins.
- Myocyte hypertrophy is likely an adaptive mechanism designed to improve pump function by expanding the number of contractile units while simultaneously reducing wall stress by increasing wall thickness.
- In the failing heart, excessive LV hypertrophy is associated with reduced myocardial compliance, myocardial fibrosis, and lethal dysrhythmias. However, the time frame of transition from adaptive to maladaptive hypertrophy is not known.
- Recent experimental observations have shown that the introduction of functional miRNA (e.g., miRNA-21 or miRNA-18b) into cardiomyocytes represses myocyte hypertrophy.
- Chronic cardiac remodeling response and transition to overt HF have been associated with modestly increased apoptosis, although the actual burden of chronic cell loss attributable to apoptosis is not clear.
- It is not clear whether apoptosis is a cause or consequence of transition to HF.
- A fundamental process in cardiac remodeling is the myocardial ECM dynamic interaction with the various cellular and acellular components of the heart, including cardiomiocytes, collagen, soluble factors, and mechanical cues that provide both positive and negative signals generated by various physiologic conditions.
- The classical perspective that the ECM is an inert biomaterial and passive structural support mechanism has been replaced by the new concept that the ECM is a dynamic entity that is in equilibrium with the cellular components of the heart, and that it alters its composition and organization in response to environmental cues and tissue injury.
- A family of zinc-dependent enzymes capable of degrading the ECM of biological tissues and that play a fundamental role in ECM remodeling in normal and disease states are the matrix metalloproteinases (MMPs).
- A cause and effect relationship between MMPs and LV remodeling appear to have been established through the use of transgenic models and through the use of pharmacologic MMP inhibitors.
- Defective electrical activation of the heart secondary to pacing or HF may induce marked ventricular electrical remodeling.
- Left-ventricular assist devices, used as a "bridge to transplant" for some HF patients, can induce profound cardiac unloading and have been shown to be associated with reverse cardiac remodeling on a structural and functional level.
- CRT reduces morbidity and mortality in patients with LV systolic dysfunction, prolonged QRS duration, and NYHA class 3 or 4 symptoms, when combined with optimal pharmacotherapy.
- Caution is needed before definitive conclusions can be reached concerning the use of CRT in mild HF, keeping in mind not only the cost of CRT devices but also their

potential side effects (e.g., ventricular dysrhythmias) and complications.

- Besides pharmacotherapy, LVADs, containment devices, and new methods to restore synchronous contraction have been added to the chronic HF treatment, and in some cases, significant improvement in both symptoms and mortality have occurred.
- Potential novel therapies to slow or reverse the process of LV remodeling are in the developmental stage, including: surgery for increased sphericity caused by chronic volume overload of mitral regurgitation, an antifibrotic peptide to inhibit the fibrogenic effects of transforming growth factor β, mechanical intervention in advanced HF cases, and gene and stem-cell therapy.

References

1. Cohn JN (2004) New therapeutic strategies for heart failure: left ventricular remodeling as a target. J Card Fail 10:S200–S201
2. Cohn JN, Ferrari R, Sharpe N (2000) Cardiac remodeling – concepts and clinical implications: a consensus paper from an international forum on cardiac remodeling. Behalf of an International Forum on Cardiac Remodeling. J Am Coll Cardiol 35:569–582
3. Gunja-Smith Z, Morales AR, Romanelli R, Woessner JF Jr (1996) Remodeling of human myocardial collagen in idiopathic dilated cardiomyopathy. Role of metalloproteinases and pyridinoline cross-links. Am J Pathol 148:1639–1648
4. Spinale FG, Tomita M, Zellner JL, Cook JC, Crawford FA, Zile MR (1991) Collagen remodeling and changes in LV function during development and recovery from supraventricular tachycardia. Am J Physiol 261:H308–H318
5. Spinale FG, Coker ML, Thomas CV, Walker JD, Mukherjee R, Hebbar L (1998) Time-dependent changes in matrix metalloproteinase activity and expression during the progression of congestive heart failure: relation to ventricular and myocyte function. Circ Res 82:482–495
6. Weber KT, Pick R, Janicki JS, Gadodia G, Lakier JB (1988) Inadequate collagen tethers in dilated cardiopathy. Am Heart J 116:1641–1646
7. Hill JA, Olson EN (2008) Cardiac plasticity. N Engl J Med 358:1370–1380
8. Carabello BA (2002) Concentric versus eccentric remodeling. J Card Fail 8:S258–S263
9. Brower GL, Janicki JS (2001) Contribution of ventricular remodeling to pathogenesis of heart failure in rats. Am J Physiol Heart Circ Physiol 280:H674–H683
10. Sambandam N, Lopaschuk GD, Brownsey RW, Allard MF (2002) Energy metabolism in the hypertrophied heart. Heart Fail Rev 7:161–173
11. Opie LH, Commerford PJ, Gersh BJ, Pfeffer MA (2006) Controversies in ventricular remodelling. Lancet 367:356–367
12. Molkentin JD, Dorn GW II (2001) Cytoplasmic signaling pathways that regulate cardiac hypertrophy. Annu Rev Physiol 63:391–426
13. Kilic A, Velic A, De Windt LJ, Fabritz L, Voss M, Mitko D, Zwiener M, Baba HA (2005) van EM, Schlatter E, Kuhn M. Enhanced activity of the myocardial Na+/H+ exchanger NHE-1 contributes to cardiac remodeling in atrial natriuretic peptide receptor-deficient mice. Circulation 112:2307–2317
14. del Monte F, Hajjar RJ (2003) Targeting calcium cycling proteins in heart failure through gene transfer. J Physiol 546:49–61
15. Fedak PW, Verma S, Weisel RD, Li RK (2005) Cardiac remodeling and failure. From molecules to man (Part II). Cardiovasc Pathol 14:49–60
16. Kim Y, Phan D, van Rooij E et al (2008) The MEF2D transcription factor mediates stress-dependent cardiac remodeling in mice. J Clin Invest 118:124–132
17. Fielitz J, Kim MS, Shelton JM, Qi X, Hill JA, Richardson JA, Bassel-Duby R, Olson EN (2008) Requirement of protein kinase D1 for pathological cardiac remodeling. Proc Natl Acad Sci USA 105:3059–3063
18. Harrison BC, Kim MS, van Rooij E et al (2006) Regulation of cardiac stress signaling by protein kinase d1. Mol Cell Biol 26:3875–3888
19. Harada M, Takeishi Y, Arimoto T, Niizeki T, Kitahara T, Goto K, Walsh RA, Kubota I (2007) Diacylglycerol kinase zeta attenuates pressure overload-induced cardiac hypertrophy. Circ J 71:276–282
20. Takeishi Y, Goto K, Kubota I (2007) Role of diacylglycerol kinase in cellular regulatory processes: a new regulator for cardiomyocyte hypertrophy. Pharmacol Ther 115:352–359
21. Leong HS, Brownsey RW, Kulpa JE, Allard MF (2003) Glycolysis and pyruvate oxidation in cardiac hypertrophy – why so unbalanced? Comp Biochem Physiol A Mol Integr Physiol 135:499–513
22. Garnier A, Fortin D, Delomenie C, Momken I, Veksler V, Ventura-Clapier R (2003) Depressed mitochondrial transcription factors and oxidative capacity in rat failing cardiac and skeletal muscles. J Physiol 551:491–501
23. Ananthakrishnan R, Moe GW, Goldenthal MJ, Marin-Garcia J (2005) Akt signaling pathway in pacing-induced heart failure. Mol Cell Biochem 268:103–110
24. van Bilsen M, van Nieuwenhoven FA, van der Vusse GJ (2009) Metabolic remodelling of the failing heart: beneficial or detrimental? Cardiovasc Res 81:420–428
25. Murray AJ, Anderson RE, Watson GC, Radda GK, Clarke K (2004) Uncoupling proteins in human heart. Lancet 364:1786–1788
26. Noma T, Nishiyama A, Mizushige K et al (2001) Possible role of uncoupling protein in regulation of myocardial energy metabolism in aortic regurgitation model rats. FASEB J 15:1206–1208
27. Bodyak N, Rigor DL, Chen YS, Han Y, Bisping E, Pu WT, Kang PM (2007) Uncoupling protein 2 modulates cell viability in adult rat cardiomyocytes. Am J Physiol Heart Circ Physiol 293:H829–H835
28. Hartil K, Charron MJ (2005) Genetic modification of the heart: transgenic modification of cardiac lipid and carbohydrate utilization. J Mol Cell Cardiol 39:581–593
29. Stepien G, Torroni A, Chung AB, Hodge JA, Wallace DC (1992) Differential expression of adenine nucleotide translocator isoforms in mammalian tissues and during muscle cell differentiation. J Biol Chem 267:14592–14597
30. Graham BH, Waymire KG, Cottrell B, Trounce IA, MacGregor GR, Wallace DC (1997) A mouse model for mitochondrial myopathy and cardiomyopathy resulting from a deficiency in the heart/muscle isoform of the adenine nucleotide translocator. Nat Genet 16:226–234
31. Exil VJ, Roberts RL, Sims H, McLaughlin JE, Malkin RA, Gardner CD, Ni G, Rottman JN, Strauss AW (2003) Very-long-chain acyl-coenzyme a dehydrogenase deficiency in mice. Circ Res 93:448–455
32. Kurtz DM, Rinaldo P, Rhead WJ et al (1998) Targeted disruption of mouse long-chain acyl-CoA dehydrogenase gene reveals crucial roles for fatty acid oxidation. Proc Natl Acad Sci USA 95:15592–15597
33. Watanabe K, Fujii H, Takahashi T et al (2000) Constitutive regulation of cardiac fatty acid metabolism through peroxisome proliferator-activated receptor alpha associated with age-dependent cardiac toxicity. J Biol Chem 275:22293–22299

34. Lopaschuk GD (2002) Metabolic abnormalities in the diabetic heart. Heart Fail Rev 7:149–159

35. Finck BN, Lehman JJ, Leone TC et al (2002) The cardiac phenotype induced by PPARalpha overexpression mimics that caused by diabetes mellitus. J Clin Invest 109:121–130

36. Finck BN, Han X, Courtois M, Aimond F, Nerbonne JM, Kovacs A, Gross RW, Kelly DP (2003) A critical role for PPARalpha-mediated lipotoxicity in the pathogenesis of diabetic cardiomyopathy: modulation by dietary fat content. Proc Natl Acad Sci USA 100: 1226–1231

37. Chiu HC, Kovacs A, Ford DA, Hsu FF, Garcia R, Herrero P, Saffitz JE, Schaffer JE (2001) A novel mouse model of lipotoxic cardiomyopathy. J Clin Invest 107:813–822

38. Sugden PH, Clerk A (1998) "Stress-responsive" mitogen-activated protein kinases (c-Jun N-terminal kinases and p38 mitogen-activated protein kinases) in the myocardium. Circ Res 83:345–352

39. Rockman HA, Koch WJ, Lefkowitz RJ (2002) Seven-transmembrane-spanning receptors and heart function. Nature 415:206–212

40. Houser SR, Margulies KB (2003) Is depressed myocyte contractility centrally involved in heart failure? Circ Res 92:350–358

41. Davies CH, Davia K, Bennett JG, Pepper JR, Poole-Wilson PA, Harding SE (1995) Reduced contraction and altered frequency response of isolated ventricular myocytes from patients with heart failure. Circulation 92:2540–2549

42. Harding SE, MacLeod KT, Davies CH, Wynne DG, Poole-Wilson PA (1995) Abnormalities of the myocytes in ischaemic cardiomyopathy. Eur Heart J 16:74–81

43. Anand IS, Liu D, Chugh SS, Prahash AJ, Gupta S, John R, Popescu F, Chandrashekhar Y (1997) Isolated myocyte contractile function is normal in postinfarct remodeled rat heart with systolic dysfunction. Circulation 96:3974–3984

44. Hein S, Kostin S, Heling A, Maeno Y, Schaper J (2000) The role of the cytoskeleton in heart failure. Cardiovasc Res 45:273–278

45. Sugden PH (1999) Signaling in myocardial hypertrophy: life after calcineurin? Circ Res 84:633–646

46. Maron BJ (2002) Hypertrophic cardiomyopathy: a systematic review. JAMA 287:1308–1320

47. Swynghedauw B (1999) Molecular mechanisms of myocardial remodeling. Physiol Rev 79:215–262

48. Weber KT, Jalil JE, Janicki JS, Pick R (1989) Myocardial collagen remodeling in pressure overload hypertrophy. A case for interstitial heart disease. Am J Hypertens 2:931–940

49. Litwin SE, Raya TE, Anderson PG, Litwin CM, Bressler R, Goldman S (1991) Induction of myocardial hypertrophy after coronary ligation in rats decreases ventricular dilatation and improves systolic function. Circulation 84:1819–1827

50. Asakura M, Kitakaze M, Takashima S et al (2002) Cardiac hypertrophy is inhibited by antagonism of ADAM12 processing of HB-EGF: metalloproteinase inhibitors as a new therapy. Nat Med 8:35–40

51. Liao JK (2002) Shedding growth factors in cardiac hypertrophy. Nat Med 8:20–21

52. Ross RS, Borg TK (2001) Integrins and the myocardium. Circ Res 88:1112–1119

53. Terracio L, Rubin K, Gullberg D, Balog E, Carver W, Jyring R, Borg TK (1991) Expression of collagen binding integrins during cardiac development and hypertrophy. Circ Res 68:734–744

54. Frey N, Olson EN (2003) Cardiac hypertrophy: the good, the bad, and the ugly. Annu Rev Physiol 65:45–79

55. Divakaran V, Mann DL (2008) The emerging role of microRNAs in cardiac remodeling and heart failure. Circ Res 103:1072–1083

56. Li Z, Bing OH, Long X, Robinson KG, Lakatta EG (1997) Increased cardiomyocyte apoptosis during the transition to heart failure in the spontaneously hypertensive rat. Am J Physiol 272:H2313–H2319

57. Mani K, Kitsis RN (2003) Myocyte apoptosis: programming ventricular remodeling. J Am Coll Cardiol 41:761–764

58. Moe GW, Naik G, Konig A, Lu X, Feng Q (2002) Early and persistent activation of myocardial apoptosis, bax and caspases: insights into mechanisms of progression of heart failure. Pathophysiology 8:183–192

59. Kang PM, Izumo S (2000) Apoptosis and heart failure: a critical review of the literature. Circ Res 86:1107–1113

60. Condorelli G, Morisco C, Stassi G et al (1999) Increased cardiomyocyte apoptosis and changes in proapoptotic and antiapoptotic genes bax and bcl-2 during left ventricular adaptations to chronic pressure overload in the rat. Circulation 99:3071–3078

61. Schulze-Osthoff K, Ferrari D, Los M, Wesselborg S, Peter ME (1998) Apoptosis signaling by death receptors. Eur J Biochem 254:439–459

62. Yue TL, Ma XL, Wang X et al (1998) Possible involvement of stress-activated protein kinase signaling pathway and Fas receptor expression in prevention of ischemia/reperfusion-induced cardiomyocyte apoptosis by carvedilol. Circ Res 82:166–174

63. Danial NN, Korsmeyer SJ (2004) Cell death: critical control points. Cell 116:205–219

64. Ashkenazi A, Dixit VM (1998) Death receptors: signaling and modulation. Science 281:1305–1308

65. Muzio M, Chinnaiyan AM, Kischkel FC et al (1996) FLICE, a novel FADD-homologous ICE/CED-3-like protease, is recruited to the CD95 (Fas/APO-1) death – inducing signaling complex. Cell 85:817–827

66. Boatright KM, Renatus M, Scott FL et al (2003) A unified model for apical caspase activation. Mol Cell 11:529–541

67. Crow MT, Mani K, Nam YJ, Kitsis RN (2004) The mitochondrial death pathway and cardiac myocyte apoptosis. Circ Res 95:957–970

68. Du C, Fang M, Li Y, Li L, Wang X (2000) Smac, a mitochondrial protein that promotes cytochrome c-dependent caspase activation by eliminating IAP inhibition. Cell 102:33–42

69. Li LY, Luo X, Wang X (2001) Endonuclease G is an apoptotic DNase when released from mitochondria. Nature 412:95–99

70. Liu X, Kim CN, Yang J, Jemmerson R, Wang X (1996) Induction of apoptotic program in cell-free extracts: requirement for dATP and cytochrome c. Cell 86:147–157

71. Susin SA, Lorenzo HK, Zamzami N et al (1999) Molecular characterization of mitochondrial apoptosis-inducing factor. Nature 397:441–446

72. Acehan D, Jiang X, Morgan DG, Heuser JE, Wang X, Akey CW (2002) Three-dimensional structure of the apoptosome: implications for assembly, procaspase-9 binding, and activation. Mol Cell 9:423–432

73. Hu Y, Ding L, Spencer DM, Nunez G (1998) WD-40 repeat region regulates Apaf-1 self-association and procaspase-9 activation. J Biol Chem 273:33489–33494

74. Qin H, Srinivasula SM, Wu G, Fernandes-Alnemri T, Alnemri ES, Shi Y (1999) Structural basis of procaspase-9 recruitment by the apoptotic protease-activating factor 1. Nature 399:549–557

75. Zou H, Henzel WJ, Liu X, Lutschg A, Wang X (1997) Apaf-1, a human protein homologous to C. elegans CED-4, participates in cytochrome c-dependent activation of caspase-3. Cell 90:405–413

76. Gross A, Yin XM, Wang K et al (1999) Caspase cleaved BID targets mitochondria and is required for cytochrome c release, while BCL-XL prevents this release but not tumor necrosis factor-R1/Fas death. J Biol Chem 274:1156–1163

77. Luo X, Budihardjo I, Zou H, Slaughter C, Wang X (1998) Bid, a Bcl2 interacting protein, mediates cytochrome c release from mitochondria in response to activation of cell surface death receptors. Cell 94:481–490

78. Peter ME (2004) The flip side of FLIP. Biochem J 382:e1–e3

79. Guo B, Zhai D, Cabezas E, Welsh K, Nouraini S, Satterthwait AC, Reed JC (2003) Humanin peptide suppresses apoptosis by interfering with Bax activation. Nature 423:456–461

80. Shiozaki EN, Chai J, Rigotti DJ et al (2003) Mechanism of XIAP-mediated inhibition of caspase-9. Mol Cell 11:519–527

81. Sun C, Cai M, Meadows RP, Xu N, Gunasekera AH, Herrmann J, Wu JC, Fesik SW (2000) NMR structure and mutagenesis of the third Bir domain of the inhibitor of apoptosis protein XIAP. J Biol Chem 275:33777–33781

82. Nam YJ, Mani K, Ashton AW et al (2004) Inhibition of both the extrinsic and intrinsic death pathways through nonhomotypic death-fold interactions. Mol Cell 15:901–912

83. Gustafsson AB, Tsai JG, Logue SE, Crow MT, Gottlieb RA (2004) Apoptosis repressor with caspase recruitment domain protects against cell death by interfering with Bax activation. J Biol Chem 279:21233–21238

84. Olivetti G, Abbi R, Quaini F et al (1997) Apoptosis in the failing human heart. N Engl J Med 336:1131–1141

85. Abbate A, Biondi-Zoccai GG, Bussani R et al (2003) Increased myocardial apoptosis in patients with unfavorable left ventricular remodeling and early symptomatic post-infarction heart failure. J Am Coll Cardiol 41:753–760

86. Schaper J, Lorenz-Meyer S, Suzuki K (1999) The role of apoptosis in dilated cardiomyopathy. Herz 24:219–224

87. Saraste A, Pulkki K, Kallajoki M et al (1999) Cardiomyocyte apoptosis and progression of heart failure to transplantation. Eur J Clin Invest 29:380–386

88. Chatterjee S, Stewart AS, Bish LT et al (2002) Viral gene transfer of the antiapoptotic factor Bcl-2 protects against chronic postischemic heart failure. Circulation 106:I212–I217

89. Ren J, Samson WK, Sowers JR (1999) Insulin-like growth factor I as a cardiac hormone: physiological and pathophysiological implications in heart disease. J Mol Cell Cardiol 31:2049–2061

90. Li Q, Li B, Wang X, Leri A, Jana KP, Liu Y, Kajstura J, Baserga R, Anversa P (1997) Overexpression of insulin-like growth factor-1 in mice protects from myocyte death after infarction, attenuating ventricular dilation, wall stress, and cardiac hypertrophy. J Clin Invest 100:1991–1999

91. Lee WL, Chen JW, Ting CT, Ishiwata T, Lin SJ, Korc M, Wang PH (1999) Insulin-like growth factor I improves cardiovascular function and suppresses apoptosis of cardiomyocytes in dilated cardiomyopathy. Endocrinology 140:4831–4840

92. Nadal-Ginard B, Kajstura J, Leri A, Anversa P (2003) Myocyte death, growth, and regeneration in cardiac hypertrophy and failure. Circ Res 92:139–150

93. Nadal-Ginard B, Kajstura J, Anversa P, Leri A (2003) A matter of life and death: cardiac myocyte apoptosis and regeneration. J Clin Invest 111:1457–1459

94. Anversa P, Nadal-Ginard B (2002) Myocyte renewal and ventricular remodelling. Nature 415:240–243

95. Soonpaa MH, Field LJ (1998) Survey of studies examining mammalian cardiomyocyte DNA synthesis. Circ Res 83:15–26

96. Anversa P, Kajstura J (1998) Ventricular myocytes are not terminally differentiated in the adult mammalian heart. Circ Res 83:1–14

97. Beltrami AP, Urbanek K, Kajstura J et al (2001) Evidence that human cardiac myocytes divide after myocardial infarction. N Engl J Med 344:1750–1757

98. Kajstura J, Leri A, Finato N, Di LC, Beltrami CA, Anversa P (1998) Myocyte proliferation in end-stage cardiac failure in humans. Proc Natl Acad Sci USA 95:8801–8805

99. Orlic D, Kajstura J, Chimenti S et al (2001) Bone marrow cells regenerate infarcted myocardium. Nature 410:701–705

100. Orlic D, Kajstura J, Chimenti S et al (2001) Mobilized bone marrow cells repair the infarcted heart, improving function and survival. Proc Natl Acad Sci USA 98:10344–10349

101. Orlic D, Kajstura J, Chimenti S, Bodine DM, Leri A, Anversa P (2001) Transplanted adult bone marrow cells repair myocardial infarcts in mice. Ann N Y Acad Sci 938:221–229

102. Orlic D, Hill JM, Arai AE (2002) Stem cells for myocardial regeneration. Circ Res 91:1092–1102

103. Laflamme MA, Myerson D, Saffitz JE, Murry CE (2002) Evidence for cardiomyocyte repopulation by extracardiac progenitors in transplanted human hearts. Circ Res 90:634–640

104. Quaini F, Urbanek K, Beltrami AP et al (2002) Chimerism of the transplanted heart. N Engl J Med 346:5–15

105. Deb A, Wang S, Skelding KA, Miller D, Simper D, Caplice NM (2003) Bone marrow-derived cardiomyocytes are present in adult human heart: a study of gender-mismatched bone marrow transplantation patients. Circulation 107:1247–1249

106. Goldsmith EC, Borg TK (2002) The dynamic interaction of the extracellular matrix in cardiac remodeling. J Card Fail 8:S314–S318

107. Janicki JS, Brower GL (2002) The role of myocardial fibrillar collagen in ventricular remodeling and function. J Card Fail 8:S319–S325

108. Weber KT, Anversa P, Armstrong PW et al (1992) Remodeling and reparation of the cardiovascular system. J Am Coll Cardiol 20:3–16

109. Iwami K, Ashizawa N, Do YS, Graf K, Hsueh WA (1996) Comparison of ANG II with other growth factors on Egr-1 and matrix gene expression in cardiac fibroblasts. Am J Physiol 270:H2100–H2107

110. Gerdes AM (2002) Cardiac myocyte remodeling in hypertrophy and progression to failure. J Card Fail 8:S264–S268

111. Libby P, Lee RT (2000) Matrix matters. Circulation 102: 1874–1876

112. Bonnin CM, Sparrow MP, Taylor RR (1981) Collagen synthesis and content in right ventricular hypertrophy in the dog. Am J Physiol 241:H708–H713

113. Weber KT (1989) Cardiac interstitium in health and disease: the fibrillar collagen network. J Am Coll Cardiol 13:1637–1652

114. Benjamin IJ (2001) Matrix metalloproteinases: from biology to therapeutic strategies in cardiovascular disease. J Investig Med 49:381–397

115. Vu TH, Werb Z (2000) Matrix metalloproteinases: effectors of development and normal physiology. Genes Dev 14:2123–2133

116. Nagase H (1997) Activation mechanisms of matrix metalloproteinases. Biol Chem 378:151–160

117. Nelson AR, Fingleton B, Rothenberg ML, Matrisian LM (2000) Matrix metalloproteinases: biologic activity and clinical implications. J Clin Oncol 18:1135–1149

118. Spinale FG, Coker ML, Heung LJ et al (2000) A matrix metalloproteinase induction/activation system exists in the human left ventricular myocardium and is upregulated in heart failure. Circulation 102:1944–1949

119. Thomas CV, Coker ML, Zellner JL, Handy JR, Crumbley AJ III, Spinale FG (1998) Increased matrix metalloproteinase activity and selective upregulation in LV myocardium from patients with end-stage dilated cardiomyopathy. Circulation 97:1708–1715

120. Knauper V, Murphy G (1998) Membrane-type matrix metalloproteinases and cell surface-associated activation cascades for matrix metalloproteinases. In: Parks WC, Mecham RP (eds) Matrix metalloproteinases. Academic, San Diego, pp 199–218

121. Woessner JF, Nagase H (2003) Activation of the zymogen forms of MMPs. In: Woessner JF, Nagase H (eds) Matrix metalloproteinases and TIMPs. Oxford University Press, Oxford, pp 72–86

122. Woessner JF, Nagase H (2000) Function of the TIMPs. Matrix metalloproteinases and TIMPs. Oxford University Press, Oxford, pp 130–135

123. Sternlicht MD, Werb Z (2001) How matrix metalloproteinases regulate cell behavior. Annu Rev Cell Dev Biol 17:463–516

124. Li YY, Feldman AM, Sun Y, McTiernan CF (1998) Differential expression of tissue inhibitors of metalloproteinases in the failing human heart. Circulation 98:1728–1734

125. Schlondorff J, Blobel CP (1999) Metalloprotease-disintegrins: modular proteins capable of promoting cell-cell interactions and triggering signals by protein-ectodomain shedding. J Cell Sci 112:3603–3617

126. Amour A, Slocombe PM, Webster A et al (1998) TNF-alpha converting enzyme (TACE) is inhibited by TIMP-3. FEBS Lett 435:39–44

127. Leco KJ, Khokha R, Pavloff N, Hawkes SP, Edwards DR (1994) Tissue inhibitor of metalloproteinases-3 (TIMP-3) is an extracellular matrix-associated protein with a distinctive pattern of expression in mouse cells and tissues. J Biol Chem 269:9352–9360

128. Woessner JF Jr (2001) That impish TIMP: the tissue inhibitor of metalloproteinases-3. J Clin Invest 108:799–800

129. Shastry S, Hayden MR, Lucchesi PA, Tyagi SC (2003) Matrix metalloproteinase in left ventricular remodeling and heart failure. Curr Cardiol Rep 5:200–204

130. Sierevogel MJ, Pasterkamp G, De Kleijn DP, Strauss BH (2003) Matrix metalloproteinases: a therapeutic target in cardiovascular disease. Curr Pharm Des 9:1033–1040

131. Bradham WS, Moe G, Wendt KA et al (2002) TNF-alpha and myocardial matrix metalloproteinases in heart failure: relationship to LV remodeling. Am J Physiol Heart Circ Physiol 282:H1288–H1295

132. Coker ML, Thomas CV, Clair MJ, Hendrick JW, Krombach RS, Galis ZS, Spinale FG (1998) Myocardial matrix metalloproteinase activity and abundance with congestive heart failure. Am J Physiol 274:H1516–H1523

133. Rohde LE, Ducharme A, Arroyo LH et al (1999) Matrix metalloproteinase inhibition attenuates early left ventricular enlargement after experimental myocardial infarction in mice. Circulation 99:3063–3070

134. Spinale FG, Coker ML, Krombach SR et al (1999) Matrix metalloproteinase inhibition during the development of congestive heart failure: effects on left ventricular dimensions and function. Circ Res 85:364–376

135. Bauvois B (2001) Transmembrane proteases in focus: diversity and redundancy? J Leukoc Biol 70:11–17

136. Kim HE, Dalal SS, Young E, Legato MJ, Weisfeldt ML, D'Armiento J (2000) Disruption of the myocardial extracellular matrix leads to cardiac dysfunction. J Clin Invest 106:857–866

137. Peterson JT, Hallak H, Johnson L et al (2001) Matrix metalloproteinase inhibition attenuates left ventricular remodeling and dysfunction in a rat model of progressive heart failure. Circulation 103:2303–2309

138. Roten L, Nemoto S, Simsic J et al (2000) Effects of gene deletion of the tissue inhibitor of the matrix metalloproteinase-type 1 (TIMP-1) on left ventricular geometry and function in mice. J Mol Cell Cardiol 32:109–120

139. Sivakumar P, Gupta S, Sarkar S, Sen S (2008) Upregulation of lysyl oxidase and MMPs during cardiac remodeling in human dilated cardiomyopathy. Mol Cell Biochem 307:159–167

140. Marrus SB, Nerbonne JM (2008) Mechanisms linking short- and long-term electrical remodeling in the heart...is it a stretch? Channels 2:125–129

141. Jeyaraj D, Wilson LD, Zhong J, Flask C, Saffitz JE, Deschênes I, Yu X, Rosenbaum DS (2007) Mechanoelectrical feedback as novel mechanism of cardiac electrical remodeling. Circulation 115:3145–3155

142. St John Sutton M, Lee D, Rouleau JL, Goldman S, Plappert T, Braunwald E, Pfeffer MA (2003) Left ventricular remodeling and ventricular arrhythmias after myocardial infarction. Circulation 107:2577–2582

143. Margulies KB (2002) Reversal mechanisms of left ventricular remodeling: lessons from left ventricular assist device experiments. J Card Fail 8:S500–S505

144. Blaxall BC, Tschannen-Moran BM, Milano CA, Koch WJ (2003) Differential gene expression and genomic patient stratification following left ventricular assist device support. J Am Coll Cardiol 41:1096–1106

145. Hall JL, Grindle S, Han X et al (2004) Genomic profiling of the human heart before and after mechanical support with a ventricular assist device reveals alterations in vascular signaling networks. Physiol Genomics 17:283–291

146. Chen Y, Park S, Li Y et al (2003) Alterations of gene expression in failing myocardium following left ventricular assist device support. Physiol Genomics 14:251–260

147. Klotz S, Jan Danser AH, Burkhoff D (2008) Impact of left ventricular assist device (LVAD) support on the cardiac reverse remodeling process. Prog Biophys Mol Biol 97:479–496

148. Soppa GK, Barton PJ, Terracciano CM, Yacoub MH (2008) Left ventricular assist device-induced molecular changes in the failing myocardium. Curr Opin Cardiol 23:206–218

149. McAlister FA, Ezekowitz J, Hooton N et al (2007) Cardiac resynchronization therapy for patients with left ventricular systolic dysfunction: a systematic review. JAMA 297:2502–2514

150. Linde C, Abraham WT, Gold MR, St John Sutton M, Ghio S, Daubert C; REVERSE (REsynchronization reVErses Remodeling in Systolic left vEntricular dysfunction) Study Group (2008) Randomized trial of cardiac resynchronization in mildly symptomatic heart failure patients and in asymptomatic patients with left ventricular dysfunction and previous heart failure symptoms. J Am Coll Cardiol 52:1834–1843

151. Remme WJ, Riegger G, Hildebrandt P et al (2004) The benefits of early combination treatment of carvedilol and an ACE-inhibitor in mild heart failure and left ventricular systolic dysfunction. The carvedilol and ACE-inhibitor remodelling mild heart failure evaluation trial (CARMEN). Cardiovasc Drugs Ther 18:57–66

152. Doughty RN, White HD (2007) Carvedilol: use in chronic heart failure. Expert Rev Cardiovasc Ther 5:21–31

153. McKelvie RS, et al. The RESOLVD Pilot Study Investigators (1999) Comparison of candesartan, enalapril, and their combination in congestive heart failure: Randomized Evaluation of Strategies for Left Ventricular Dysfunction (RESOLVD) pilot study. Circulation 100:1056–1064

154. Yan RT, White M, Yan AT et al Randomized Evaluation of Strategies for Left Ventricular Dysfunction (RESOLVD) Investigators (2005) Usefulness of temporal changes in neurohormones as markers of ventricular remodeling and prognosis in patients with left ventricular systolic dysfunction and heart failure receiving either candesartan or enalapril or both. Am J Cardiol 96:698–704

155. Mudd JO, Kass DA (2007) Reversing chronic remodeling in heart failure. Expert Rev Cardiovasc Ther 5:585–598

156. Frigerio M, Roubina E (2005) Drugs for left ventricular remodeling in heart failure. Am J Cardiol 96:10L–18L

157. Dhalla NS, Saini-Chohan HK, Rodriguez-Leyva D, Elimban V, Dent MR, Tappia PS (2009) Subcellular remodelling may induce cardiac dysfunction in congestive heart failure. Cardiovasc Res 81:429–438

Section VI
Peripheral Changes and Co-morbid Conditions in Heart Failure

Chapter 12
Heart Failure and Changes at the Periphery: Vascular, Inflammation, Neurohormonal, and Renal Systems

Overview

The clinical syndrome of chronic heart failure (HF) has traditionally been linked to malfunction of the heart as a pump, usually caused by insults to the myocardium. In recent years, there is mounting evidence to support the concept that the complex pathophysiology of heart failure begins with an abnormality of the heart, but then involves dysfunction of most body organs, including the cardiac, peripheral vascular, renal, neurohormonal, immune, as well as the inflammatory systems [1, 2]. The magnitude of these abnormalities has been related to disease progression and subsequent mortality. Less clear, however, is the origin of these derangements and the sequence of triggering mechanisms in the course of the natural history of HF [3]. One of the known abnormalities associated with the complex clinical syndrome of HF is the profound disturbance in the regulation of the autonomic nervous system [4]. The link between peripheral systems activated in HF and the central nervous system as a source of neurohumoral drive has therefore received increasing attention. The key abnormality in HF is the kidneys' perception of an inadequate circulating volume by various sensors located on critical sites within the circulation. As a result, the normal relationship between intravascular volume and holding capacity, as perceived by these sensing mechanisms, is perturbed. This leads to the activation of various effector mechanisms whose aim is to increase intravascular volume and maintain blood pressure. The kidney is therefore the central site of action for these effectors that increase intravascular volume, and therefore plays a major pathogenetic role in the sodium and water retention in HF. Renal insufficiency is common in patients with HF and is an adverse prognostic factor [5, 6].

Over the last several decades, substantial evidence has been accumulated to support the concept that peripheral afferent systems innervating the heart and vascular tree are altered in HF. Furthermore, recently, a vascular component has been recognized to contribute to HF. Increased peripheral vasoconstriction in response to exercise and impaired vasodilatation after stimulation with agonists are the hallmarks of endothelial dysfunction in the setting of HF. Among the most studied vascular mechanisms that might contribute to the development of HF has been the reduced production of nitric oxide (NO) or the reduced bioactivity of NO associated with both basic models of HF and disease in patients [7]. According to Linke et al. [8] the evolving concept that HF is a cytokine-activated state has focused attention on the possibility that cytokine driven isoform of NO synthase (NOS), iNOS, may produce enough amount of NO to suppress cardiac myocyte function, thus contributing to the reduced inotropic state in the failing heart.

Introduction

Despite recent therapeutic advances, the prognosis for patients with HF remains poor. The importance of neurohormonal activation in the causation and progression of HF is now recognized. Unopposed neurohormonal excitation is believed to be a critical element in the progressive clinical deterioration associated with the HF syndrome[9], and its peripheral manifestations have become the principal targets for intervention. Maladaptive changes in the periphery largely account for the symptomatology of patients with HF. A decline in the systolic function of the left ventricle precipitates activation of neural and humoral systems to provide circulatory support. These include sympathetic release of norepinephrine, increases in angiotensin II, elevated levels of circulating arginine vasopressin, and impairment of the counterregulatory function of the natriuretic peptides. The resultant circulatory changes are ultimately responsible for the declining function of the peripheral vasculature and skeletal muscles of patients with HF. In the peripheral vasculature, impaired vasodilatory capacity results from excess vessel wall stiffness, endothelial dysfunction, and structural abnormalities. The skeletal muscles develop poor aerobic capacity as a result of a change in predominant fiber type and excess reliance on metabolic pathways. Physical deconditioning induced by symptoms tends to further promote these peripheral changes. Therapeutic interventions with symptomatic and prognostic benefits have

J. Marín-García, *Heart Failure*, Contemporary Cardiology,
DOI 10.1007/978-1-60761-147-9_12, © Springer Science+Business Media, LLC 2010

still been targeted mostly at the periphery. Angiotensin converting enzyme inhibitors may act by normalizing electrolyte and water balance, improving vascular endothelial function, and reversing structural changes in peripheral vessels. Exercise training appears to exert its benefit at the level of the vascular endothelium. Recent advances in the therapy of HF have therefore depended in part on the understanding of changes at the periphery, which are the topics of discussion in this chapter.

Central and Autonomic Nervous System Perturbations

One of the known abnormalities associated with the complex clinical syndrome of HF is the profound disturbance in the regulation of the autonomic nervous system [4]. Over the last several decades, substantial evidence has been accumulated to support the concept that peripheral afferent systems innervating the heart and vascular tree are altered in HF. Dysfunction has been described in all components of the reflexes mediated by these cardiovascular afferent systems – the afferent fibers themselves, the central processing of the afferent signals, the efferent innervation of the end organs, and the end organs themselves. In general, the influence of low- and high-pressure baroreceptors [10] that normally restrain sympathetic drive and vasopressin release is diminished, whereas the excitatory influences of arterial chemoreceptors [11] and cardiac sympathetic afferent fibers [12] are enhanced.

Autonomic imbalance, favoring increased sympathetic tone, which is accompanied by depleted vagal drive, occurs at an early stage in the natural history of HF, and precedes other key derangements, including immune and hormonal pathologies. In the experimental canine model of tachycardia-induced HF, parasympathetic tone, expressed as high-frequency component of spectral analysis of heart rate variability, decreased on the third day after induction of cardiac dysfunction [13], and preceded sympathetic activation [14]. In patients with asymptomatic left ventricular dysfunction, neurohormonal activation, as evidenced by increased levels of norepinephrine, precedes the development of symptoms and is related to poor survival [15, 16]. On the other hand, increased sympathetic tone and depleted parasympathetic drive are present at the early stage of symptomatic HF, when left ventricular function is only mildly impaired [17]. Changes in autonomic balance are seen irrespectively of HF etiology [18, 19]. Moreover, in healthy subjects, the heart rate profile during exercise and recovery, reflecting depleted parasympathetic tone (i.e., an increased resting heart rate, an insufficient heart rate response to exercise, an insufficient reduction of heart rate

after cessation of exercise), is strongly related to increased mortality due to sudden death, which itself is frequently the first manifestation. The clinical and prognostic significance of the overactivation of the sympathetic nervous system has been clearly established [20]. β-adrenergic blockade is now a standard therapy in patients with HF and systolic dysfunction [21]. In contrast, the reduction in parasympathetic tone in HF, although demonstrated over three decades ago [22], has received less attention. Reduced parasympathetic tone, i.e., blunted baroreflex gain, impaired indices of heart rate variability, predict poor outcome in patients with HF and in subjects after myocardial infarction [23]. In a canine experimental model, pharmacological blockade of the vagal reflexes with atropine, results in a worsening of existing ventricular dysrhythmias leading to sudden cardiac death [24], whereas vagal activation due to direct electrical stimulation of efferent vagal fibers prevents ventricular fibrillation and sudden cardiac death during induction of acute myocardial ischemia [25].

Humoral Heart–Brain Signaling

Central nervous system (CNS) neurons affecting cardiovascular regulation respond to humoral as well neural signals. It is now recognized that blood–borne neuroactive peptides, too large to readily cross the blood–brain barrier, may influence the brain by activating sensory neurons at specific sites in hindbrain and forebrain that lack a blood–brain barrier [26] or by inducing the release of mediators that do penetrate the barrier [27]. Importantly, the cardiovascular regions of forebrain that sense and respond to circulating peptides [28] also process the signals originating in cardiovascular afferent nerves [29] and are capable of modulating cardiovascular reflexes [30].

The constellation of centrally driven autonomic abnormalities in HF, augmented sympathetic drive in the face of vasoconstriction, salt, and water retention in the presence of volume overload, suggests dysfunction of the forebrain neurons that regulate these systems. In a pioneering study, Patel et al. demonstrated that metabolic activity was increased in the parvicellular and magnocellular regions of the paraventricular nucleus PVN in rats with HF induced by coronary artery ligation [31]. More recently, Vahid-Ansari and Leenen demonstrated that Fra-like immunoreactivity, an indicator of long-term neuronal activation, was increased in these same regions in rats with large myocardial infarctions [32]. Other investigators also demonstrated that manipulations within the forebrain region affect the regulation of sympathetic drive in the rat coronary artery ligation model [33, 34]. Particularly pertinent to the HF syndrome are those neurons of the PVN of the hypothalamus that produce and release arginine vasopression and corticotrophin-releasing factor [35], and those that project to the principal centers of sympathetic drive, the rostral ventrolateral medulla (RVLM) and the intermediolateral cell column (IML) of the spinal cord [36]. PVN neurons receive and integrate signals from the hindbrain regions related to pressure and volume within the cardiovascular system [29] and signals from forebrain regions including the circumventricular organs of the lamina terminalis, which lack a blood–brain barrier and thus sense the presence of blood–borne neuroactive peptides [37]. In normal rats, the PVN and related forebrain nuclei play a prominent role in thirst, sodium appetite, and humoral release. The role of the PVN in driving the sympathetic nervous system is less clear. In the anesthetized rat, for example, electrical stimulation of the PVN elicits only a small pressor response [38]. Similarly, the cardiovascular response of normal rats to activation of the forebrain region with angiotensin II is small [39] and is restrained by the baroreceptor input. Under normal conditions, the PVN is under the potent inhibitory influence of GABA and NO, as demonstrated by the increase in sympathetic drive that can be elicited by local injection of bicuculline or inhibitors of

nitric oxide synthase (NOS) [40]. In certain disease conditions, including HF, heightened sympathetic drive emanating from the PVN may become an important pathophysiological determinant.

In rats with HF induced by coronary artery ligation monitored continuously by telemetry over 6-week period, heart rates were higher and blood pressures lower than sham-operated controls. Sympathetic nerve activity in conscious HF rats is increased, with a characteristic pattern of unsuppressed yet still pulse-related bursting, suggesting some degree of continued baroreceptor modulation. As shown in Fig. 12.1, the pulse-triggered average of sympathetic discharge is higher in the HF rats. Baroreflex regulation of renal sympathetic nerve activity (RSNA) is blunted [41].

To evaluate the importance of the forebrain as an active participant in the pathophysiology of HF, as opposed to a passive sensor of adverse peripheral events, MI was induced in rats 6 weeks after they have fully recovered from a lesion in the anteroventral third ventricle (AV3V) region, which included the organum vasculosum as well as the pathways connecting the circumventricular organs of the lamina terminalis to PVN [42]. There were several important findings. First, the characteristic features of HF that were present in

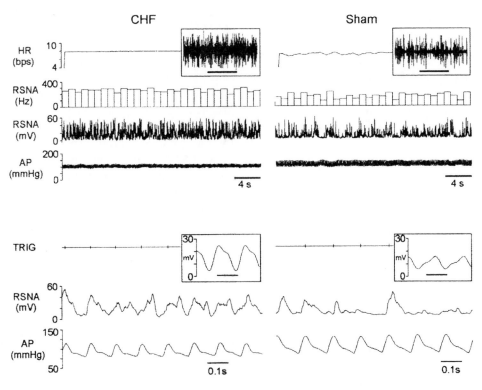

Fig. 12.1 RSNA is increased in congestive heart failure (CHF) induced by coronary artery ligation. Tracings of integrated RSNA (mV) and AP (mmHg) taken from conscious rats 6 weeks after coronary ligation or sham operation. *Top insets* show raw tracings of RSNA. TRIG, trigger generated by the peak of the AP tracing, used to obtain a triggered average of the integrated RSNA voltage over a 2-min interval. Bottom insets show the triggered average of RSNA voltage for these two rats. The pulse-locked quality of the integrated RSNA signal in both conditions, indicating that some degree of baroreceptor modulation persists in heart failure but the loss of a more general modulatory influence that may be respiratory related (respiration was not monitored in these experiments). Triggered average shows that RSNA is increased in the CHF rat on a beat-by-beat basis, unrelated to differences in HR (Reprinted from Francis et al. [41]. With permission from the American Physiological Society)

MI rats with sham AV3V lesion, increased sodium appetite, the decreased sodium and water excretion, and augmented sympathetic drive with blunted baroreflex, were dramatically attenuated in animals with an AV3V lesion. Second, the expected increase in plasma renin activity (PRA) did not occur in the AV3V-lesioned MI rats. These findings suggest that the forebrain may be an active participant in the progression of HF and further suggest that the renin response to renal underperfusion after MI may be largely dependent on sympathetic efferent regulation emanating from the forebrain. There appears to be some precedent for that suggestion in the previous work demonstrating that electrical stimulation of PVN can increase renin release from the kidney [43] and facilitate the renin response to other usual stimuli [44]. The most important was a third finding, the survival of the AV3V-lesioned MI rats was compromised to the extent that most had died 3 weeks after MI, in contrast to MI rats with sham-AV3V lesion and AV3V-lesioned rats with sham MI (Fig. 12.2). Thus, the AV3V lesion identified the forebrain as important not only to the centrally mediated (e.g., thirst and sodium appetite) mechanisms in HF but also to remote peripheral manifestations (e.g., renal sodium and water handling and renin release). Furthermore, forebrain mechanisms appear to confer a survival benefit in HF that cannot be ascribed simply to the ability to mount a stress response.

Does enhanced activity of the renin–angiotensin–aldosterone system (RAAS) drive forebrain mechanisms in HF? Angiotensin II (ANG II) and aldosterone, active products of the RAAS, can both act on receptors in the forebrain to induce changes in volume regulation [45] and sympathetic drive [46]. Both peptides can also be produced within the

blood–brain barrier [47, 48]. Furthermore, aldosterone increases the binding of ANG II to AT_1 receptors in the subfornical organ and the PVN [49] and also increases mRNA for vasopressin in PVN and vasopressin release. Aldosterone has been shown to promote the activity of angiotensin converting enzyme (ACE) [50]. ACE is present in the forebrain and is particularly abundant in the circumventricular organs of the forebrain [51]. Thus, it is conceivable that aldosterone may amplify the influences of circulating as well as intrinsically produced ANG II. Whereas most of these potential interactions have yet to be tested in the brain in HF, there is evidence for increased AT_1 receptors in the forebrain of rats with high-output HF [52]. The influences of the RAAS on forebrain neurons in rats with chronic HF have also been studied [53]. Single-unit recordings were made from PVN neurons in anesthetized rats 4–6 weeks after MI. HF was documented by echocardiography. Drugs were administered by the intracarotid route, directed centrally, an approach that has been shown to preferentially influence the ipsilateral forebrain while sparing the hindbrain [54]. The activity of PVN neurons was on average increased in rats with HF, although the discharge rate of some neurons remained within the range of normal. Neurons with high discharge frequencies were tested for the effects of selectively blocking several components of the RAAS. The effects of the AT_1 receptor blocker losartan, the ACE inhibitor captopril, and the mineralocorticoid (MC) receptor blocker spironolactone were tested. Both losartan and captopril transiently reduced the discharge rate of PVN neurons and arterial pressure. Spironolactone also reduced the discharge rate of PVN neurons but with a longer latency and without affecting arterial pressure. Thus, despite a chronic high discharge rate in HF, PVN neurons remain responsive to acute manipulations of the RAAS. This latter point may have important implications for the clinical management of HF – acute interventions can have substantial impact on central neural mechanisms in the presence of chronic HF.

Mineralcorticoid receptors have well-known effects in the brain to increase sodium appetite [55], ANG II binding in subfornical organ and PVN [49], AVP production and its release into the circulation [56], and sympathetic drive [57]. The effect of chronic central administration of spironolactone on volume regulation and sympathetic drive was tested in rats with HF induced by coronary artery ligation [58]. Central MC receptor blockade produced the behavioral effect of reduced salt intake in the HF rats. Within the first week of treatment, urinary sodium and water excretion had normalized in the MI rats treated with intracerebroventricular spironolactone, whereas these variables remained abnormally low in the MI rats treated with intraperitoneal spironolactone. However, 2 weeks into the protocol, rats receiving intraperitoneal spironolactone also experienced normalization of sodium appetite and renal handling of sodium and water.

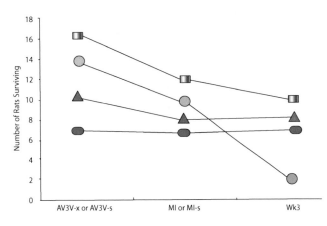

Fig. 12.2 Survival after myocardial infarction is compromised in rats with a forebrain lesion. Data indicate numbers of rats surviving a lesion of the anteroventral 3rd ventricle (AV3V-x) or sham lesion (AV3V-s), a MI induced by coronary ligation or a sham MI (MI-s) performed 6 weeks later, and the subsequent 3 weeks (Wk3) of the study protocol. Rats with AV3V lesion had a decidedly poorer survival after MI, compared with all other groups, ▢ AV3V-s/MI; ⬤ AV3V-x/MI; ▲ AV3V-x/MI-s; ⬤ AV3V-s/MI-s. (Adapted with permission from Francis et al. [42])

After 4 weeks of treatment by either route, the spironolactone-treated MI rats had a reduction in sympathetic discharge and some, although not complete, improvement in baroreflex function. These results indicate that spironolactone acts centrally on MC receptors to reduce sympathetic drive in HF. This mechanism may account at least in part for the beneficial effect of spironolactone observed in the clinical setting.

The Cytokine-CNS Connection

Increased level of proinflammatory cytokines in the circulation has numerous potential deleterious peripheral effects [59], including depression of myocardial function [60], activation of ROS [61], and stimulation of the renin–angiotensin system by impairing feedback regulation by circulating ANG II [62]. With relevance to the current discussion, the cytokines also act on the CNS [27, 63]. Although the cytokines may be too large to readily cross the blood–brain barrier, they nevertheless activate the hypothalamic–pituitary–adrenal (HPA) axis [27] to augment sympathetic drive [64] and increase the release of vasopressin and ACTH [63, 65], all components of a feedback inhibitory mechanism that restrains the peripheral inflammatory response. In a series of functional anatomical studies, Ericsson et al. [66, 67] provided evidence that interleukin 1β (IL-1β) elicits these responses indirectly by activating its receptors on endothelial cells in cerebral circulation that in turn release PGE2. PGE2 diffuses across the blood–brain barrier and appears to preferentially activate receptors on neurons in the ventrolateral medulla [66]. These investigators further demonstrated that an ascending pathway from the ventrolateral medulla is a critical element of the PVN response to systemically administered IL-1β [66] and that stimulation of C1 catecholaminergic neurons in RVLM with PGE2 provides excitatory input to PVN, simulating the response to intravenous cytokine administration [67].

This model of immune activation of the forebrain is interesting when considered in the context of HF. In HF, cytokine production persists [68] despite this combined HPA and sympathetic feedback pathway, and the pro-inflammatory cytokines act on the same general classes of neurons, CRF, AVP, and presympathetic, that mediate the central effects of the RAAS. Moreover, PGE2 production is increased generally in HF, in which its vasodilator properties counterbalance the vasoconstrictor effects of such peptides as ANG II, vasopressin, and endothelin. Such convergence of immune system mediators and RAAS mediators, seemingly affecting the same general populations of neurons in the forebrain, led to further studies of several elements of the proposed mechanism of cytokine-induced HPA axis activation, but in the

context of cardiovascular regulation [69]. Ipsilateral carotid artery (ICA) TNF-α increases RSNA, mean arterial pressure (MAP), heart rate, and the discharge rate of anesthetized RVLM neurons in the PVN rats. The cardiovascular and sympathetic responses to TNF-α were not different in rats that had undergone bilateral cervical vagotomy 1 h before testing, confirming that the acute cardiovascular responses to blood–borne TNF-α are not dependent upon vagal afferent activation. The effects of intravenous TNF-α on RSNA, MAP, and heart rate in intact rats and rats that had undergone a mid-collicular decerebration 1 h before study were compared. The decerebrate rats had no response to TNF-α, suggesting an involvement of higher centers; however, a significant increase in the baseline values also rendered these data inconclusive at the time [69].

The effects of the putative diffusible cytokine mediator PGE2 on sympathetic nerve discharge, arterial pressure, and HR, and simultaneously recorded PVN or RVLM neuronal activity have been assessed. PGE2 administered intracerebroventricularly increased the activity of PVN neurons as well as all three measures of sympathetic drive; PGE2 microinjected into PVN increased the activity of RVLM neurons and the indexes of sympathetic drive [69]. These results suggest that if PGE2 is produced in the forebrain region during cytokine stimulation, it may directly activate the sympathoexcitatory PVN neurons. Finally, the cyclooxygenase inhibitor ketorolac, administered intracerebroventricularly, blocked the increases in PVN neuronal discharge and RSNA and the pressor response to ICA TNF-α. These results strongly support the general hypothesis that PGE2 is a critical mediator of the central influences of TNF-α on sympathetic drive, but also suggest that the cardiovascular and autonomic responses to TNF-α may ultimately be dependent on prostaglandin production by cyclooxygenase within the CNS rather than in perivascular cells of the bloodbrain barrier [27, 67]. A similar mechanism has also been proposed for activation of splenic nerve activity by peripheral endotoxin [70], a stimulus to cytokine production. Extrapolating these concepts and findings to the HF setting, one might speculate that cytokine signaling of the HPA, which under normal circumstances serves to regulate the immune system, targets a population of PVN neurons that are already strongly driven in HF by excessive activity of the RAAS.

Renal Adaptation and Alterations

From the standpoint of extracellular (ECF) volume homeostasis, the key abnormality in HF is the kidneys' perception of an inadequate circulating volume by various sensors located on critical sites within the circulation. As a result, the normal relationship between intravascular volume and holding capacity as perceived by these sensing mechanisms is perturbed. This leads to the activation of various effector mechanisms whose aim is to increase intravascular volume and maintain blood pressure. The kidney is therefore the central site of action for these effectors that increase intravascular volume, and therefore plays a major pathogenetic role in the sodium and water retention in HF.

Abnormalities in Sensing Mechanisms

Alterations in the signals emanating from sensing mechanisms involved in the afferent limb for volume homeostasis represent the primary disturbance in ECF volume homeostasis in HF consequent to the perturbed relationship between intravascular volume and holding capacity of the circulation. Considerable evidence has accrued in human and animal studies that the renal responses to both high output and low-output cardiac failure are quite similar. Therefore, the disturbances in the afferent signaling must be necessary and sufficient to initiate a state of sodium retention in both hemodynamic situations.

Indeed, a common denominator for all forms of HF with renal sodium retention is a diminution in blood flow at several critical sites of the arterial circuit with pressure- and flow-sensing capabilities. This occurs as a result of either an absolute decrease in cardiac output (low-output HF) or diversion of blood flow through anatomic or physiologic arteriovenous shunts (high-output HF). The presence of afferent signals for sodium retention emanating from these sites has been demonstrated in several experimental HF models. Priebe et al. studied the relationship of diminished cardiac output to the development of sodium retention induced by thoracic vena cava obstruction [71]. In this study, the positive sodium balance was mitigated when cardiac output was restored to normal by means of autologous blood transfusion, in spite of the fact that systemic venous pressure was still elevated. Based on these observations, it was concluded that reduction of cardiac output, rather than venous congestion, was the principal hemodynamic disturbance leading to salt retention. Similarly, Witte et al. have studied the impact of venous congestion on sodium retention in patients with HF [72]. In these patients, the cervical thoracic ducts were cannulated. Upon venting of the lymph, clinical signs of right-sided HF abated, but urinary sodium excretion did not increase. Therefore, the authors concluded that cardiac output was a more important determinant of urinary sodium excretion than the systemic venous pressure. Epstein et al., in a classical study [73], demonstrated that diversion of blood flow from the arterial to the venous circuit resulted in decreased urinary sodium excretion. Based on these

observations, it appears that diminished blood flow in the arterial circuit can induce sufficient perturbations in the afferent limb of volume homeostasis to initiate renal sodium retention in HF. The volume sensors in the arterial circuit serve the function of avoiding under filling of the circulation. On the other hand, a second set of volume sensors in the venous circuit serve the function of detecting overfilling of the circulation. Indeed, in addition to absolute or relative diminution in cardiac output, systemic or pulmonary venous congestion represents the other major disturbance in circulatory function in HF. Under normal circumstances, overfilling of the venous circuit initiates afferent signals emanating from various venous volume-sensing sites (e.g., the cardiac atria, the hepatic sinusoids), aiming ultimately to induce natriuresis and thereby relieve circulatory congestion. Therefore, the blunted natriuresis associated with HF in the face of venous congestion and elevated cardiac filling pressures reflects a disturbance in afferent signaling mechanisms emanating from these venous volume-sensing sites. Evidence from several experimental and clinical studies of HF has suggested that a disturbance in the normal relationship between volume and holding capacity at these sites in HF results in a perturbation in the afferent signaling mechanisms. In dogs with a surgically created shunt between the left atrium and the left subclavian artery, systemic venous pressure remained normal despite elevated left ventricular end-diastolic pressure [74]. As long as systemic venous pressure remained normal, sodium retention did not occur even after saline challenge. These results were interpreted as reflecting a causal relationship between increased systemic venous pressure and sodium retention in HF. A similar conclusion was reached in a study of patients with severe valvular heart disease [75]. In this study, it was found that patients with edema had an impaired ability to excrete a sodium load when compared with that of patients without edema. Furthermore, when several hemodynamic variables were compared, the only parameter that clearly distinguished the two groups was right ventricular end-diastolic pressure, which was significantly higher in patients with edema.

The mechanisms by which altered pressure–volume relationships in the cardiac atria and intrathoracic vessels contribute to the pathogenesis of sodium retention in HF have been evaluated. Greenberg et al. [76] studied the firing of atrial stretch receptors in dogs with chronic HF induced by pulmonic valve stenosis and tricuspid regurgitation. When compared with this mechanism in normal dogs, the tiring of atrial receptors in response to saline infusion was markedly attenuated in dogs with chronic HF. In an aortocaval fistula canine model of HF, Zucker et al. [77] demonstrated reduced firing of type B left atrial receptors in response to dextran volume expansion in dogs with HF when compared with that in the control dogs. In addition, sonomicrometry of the left

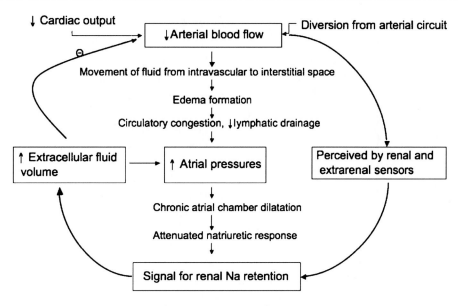

Fig. 12.3 Sensing mechanisms that initiate and maintain sodium retention in heart failure

atrial appendage demonstrated reduced atrial compliance, and microscopy indicated loss of end arborization. These data suggest that reduced atrial compliance and structural alterations of the atria in chronic HF may account for the decreased sensitivity. The disturbances in the sensing mechanisms that initiate and maintain renal sodium retention in HF are summarized in Fig. 12.3.

A decrease in cardiac output or a diversion of systemic blood flow (anatomic or physiologic) diminishes the blood flow to the critical sites of the arterial circuit with pressure- and flow-sensing capabilities. The perception of diminished blood flow culminates in renal sodium retention, mediated by effector mechanisms, to be described. An increase in systemic venous pressure promotes the transudation of fluid from the intravascular to the interstitial compartments by increasing the peripheral transcapillary hydraulic pressure gradient. The transudation is further enhanced by the transmission of elevated venous pressures to the thoracic duct ostium, resulting in reduced lymphatic drainage [78]. Furthermore, increments in systemic venous pressure are associated with a resetting of precapillary and postcapillary resistance, eventuating in an overall decrement in peripheral resistance [79]. These processes augment the perceived loss of volume and flow in the arterial circuit. In addition, distortion of the pressure volume relationships due to chronic dilatation in the cardiac atria attenuates the normal natriuretic response to central venous congestion. This attenuation is predominantly manifested as diminished neural response to atrial stretch, with a possible altered plasma natriuretic peptide-atrial stretch relationship.

Abnormalities in Effector Mechanisms

Abnormalities in effector mechanisms of volume homeostasis acting to promote sodium retention at the level of the kidney are themselves a consequence of the primary disturbance in afferent-sensing mechanisms, outlined in the previous section. For the most part, these effector mechanisms for salt and water retention are not distinguishable from those that govern renal function in states of true sodium depletion. These include adjustments in glomerular hemodynamics and tubule transport, which in turn are brought about by alterations in neural and humoral effector input.

Glomerular Hemodynamics

The global renal hemodynamic changes consistently observed in HF include a decrease in renal plasma flow (RPF) and a proportionately smaller decrease in glomerular filtration rate (GFR). These changes result in an increase in the filtration fraction [80, 81]. These changes were also observed at the single nephron level in the rat model of HF induced by coronary artery ligation [82]. When compared with normal rats, in rats with HF, single nephron filtration rate (SNGFR) was lower, but single nephron plasma flow was disproportionately reduced such that single nephron filtration fraction was markedly elevated. In the HF rats, both afferent and efferent arteriolar resistances were elevated, thus accounting for the diminished single nephron glomerular

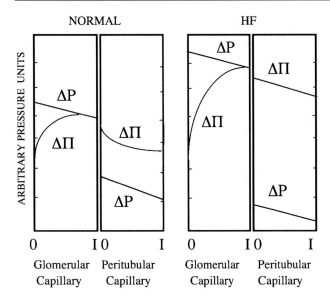

Fig. 12.4 The glomerular and peritubular microcirculations in heart failure

plasma flow, and the ultrafiltration coefficient was diminished. However, the disproportionate increase in efferent arteriolar resistance accounted for the rise in single nephron filtration fraction. In Fig. 12.4, a comparison of the glomerular capillary hemodynamic profile in the normal (left panel) versus HF state (right panel) is illustrated on the left graph of each panel. First, the transmural hydraulic pressure gradient (ΔP) declines along the distance of the glomerular capillary in both the normal and the HF states, but when compared with the normal state, ΔP in the HF state is much higher as a result of the increased efferent arteriolar resistance. Second, the transmural plasma colloid oncotic pressure gradient ($\Delta \Pi$) increases over the length of the glomerular capillary in both states, as fluid is filtered in Bowman's space, but increases to a greater extent in HF because of the increased filtration fraction. It is therefore evident that a major component of the glomerular hemodynamic alterations in HF originates from the disproportionate increase in efferent as compared with afferent arteriolar resistance. This alteration is mediated principally by the action of angiotensin II (Ang II).

The aim of the adjustment in glomerular hemodynamics is to preserve normalcy of GFR in the face of reduced RPF. A study by Cody et al. [83] emphasized the importance of this mechanism in the regulation of glomerular filtration in patients with chronic HF. In these patients, the failure to maintain GFR was correlated with a diminished RPF as well as an impaired ability to maintain an adequately high filtration fraction in the face of diminished RPF. Thus, individuals with the greatest impairment of GFR had the greatest increase in overall renal vascular resistance and the lowest filtration fraction.

Physical Factors

A direct consequence of the glomerular hemodynamic alterations previously outlined is an increase in the fractional reabsorption of filtered sodium at the level of the proximal tubule. In Fig. 12.4, a comparison of the peritubular capillary hemodynamic profile between the normal state (left panel) and the HF state (right panel) is shown on the right graph of each panel. When compared with the normal state, the average value of $\Delta \Pi$ along the peritubular capillary is increased in HF, whereas that of ΔP is decreased. This favors fluid movement into the capillary and may also reduce backleak of fluid into the tubule via paracellular pathways, promoting overall net reabsorption. The contribution of enhanced fractional proximal sodium reabsorption in HF and its dependence on abnormal glomerular hemodynamics has been demonstrated in a number of experimental and clinical studies. Using clearance techniques, it was shown that the infusion of mannitol led to a greater increase in free water excretion in patients with HF than in normal subjects [84]. Since the site of action of mannitol is largely proximal to the diluting segment of the nephron, it was inferred that proximal tubule sodium reabsorption is raised above normal levels in patients with HF and that distal delivery is restored after the administration of mannitol. Bennett et al. [85] showed that proximal fractional sodium reabsorption (as measured during pharmacologic blockade of distal nephron sodium transport) was increased in patients with HF, when compared with that in normal subjects at any given level of extracellular fluid volume. Johnston et al. [86] administered desoxycorticosterone acetate to normal dogs and dogs with arteriovenous fistulas. The sodium and potassium balance in the dogs with fistulas did not escape from the sodium-retaining effects of the mineralocorticoid hormone, and the animals did not become hypokalemic; when compared with proximal tubule sodium reabsorption and a consequent decrease in delivery of sodium to more distal sodium/potassium, exchange sites accounted for the lack of increased urinary potassium excretion in the experimental group. The most direct evidence for the dependence of enhanced proximal fractional sodium reabsorption on altered glomerular hemodynamics in HF was obtained by Ichikawa et al. [82] in the coronary ligation model of myocardial infarction in rats. When the increased single nephron filtration fraction was restored toward normal with the use of an ACE inhibitor, there was a pari passu normalization of proximal peritubular capillary Starling forces and sodium reabsorption.

Distal nephron sites also participate in the enhanced tubule sodium reabsorption in experimental models of HF. Micropuncture studies performed in dogs with arteriovenous fistulas [87], pericardial constriction [88], or chronic partial thoracic vena caval obstructions [89] have documented an enhanced distal nephron sodium reabsorption. Levy has shown that the inability of dogs with chronic vena caval obstruction to excrete a sodium load is a consequence of enhanced reabsorption of sodium at the loop of Henle [90]. Furthermore, the mechanism leading to the augmented reabsorption of sodium by the loop of Henle in dogs with constriction of the vena cava seems to involve physical factors determined by renal hemodynamics, much as in the case of the proximal tubule [91]. Specifically, the combined effects of renal vasodilatation and elevation of renal perfusion pressure in dogs with caval constriction served to prevent the enhanced reabsorption of filtrate by the loop of Henle, thereby permitting a normal natriuretic response to saline loading. One other consistent observation in clinical and experimental HF is an attenuated natriuretic response to atrial natriuretic peptide (ANP). Since the natriuretic action of ANP is not entirely dependent on its actions on glomerular function [92], it is therefore possible that resistance to the actions of ANP at the level of the collecting tubule can contribute to sodium retention in HF.

Another perspective of the altered distal nephron function in HF has been reported in dogs with thoracic caval constriction [93]. In this model, it was shown that activation of tubuloglomerular feedback by intrarenal infusion of hypertonic saline was significantly blunted when compared with the response seen in normal dogs. The extent of reduction in tubuloglomerular feedback paralleled the degree of impairment of baseline renal function. In this respect, the caval-constricted dogs behaved in a manner analogous to that observed in the states of volume depletion. Indeed, all the abnormalities in distal nephron function described in HF appear to be similar to those reported in states of severe volume depletion. The precise relative contribution of proximal versus distal nephron sites to avid sodium reabsorption in HF probably depends on the magnitude of the perceived decline in arterial blood flow and the extent of impairment in renal hemodynamics. This applies in states of both true volume depletion as well as "perceived" volume depletion in the case of HF.

Humoral Mechanisms

Despite a marked impairment of renal blood flow, GFR is usually preserved in patients with HF until the terminal stage. The preservation of filtering function of the kidney is mediated in part by the release of vasoactive hormones within the kidney, namely Ang II, prostaglandins, and natriuretic peptides, in response to decreased renal perfusion, and/or increased renal sympathetic nerve activity, or both [94]. The vasoactive and vasodilator hormonal systems have opposite intrarenal hemodynamic effects: the appropriate balance of their effects serves to maintain GFR. The natriuretic peptides, particularly ANP also plays a counterregulatory role to Ang II and other vasoconstrictors in maintaining intrarenal hemodynamic homeostasis [95].

Sympathetic Nervous System

The observation that cardiac catecholamine stores are markedly reduced in HF [96] has long suggested that the sympathetic nervous system is involved in HF. Indeed, increased plasma norepinephrine levels are frequently observed and have been thought to be a prognostic marker in patients with HF [4]. Direct intraneural recordings in patients with HF have also documented increased neural traffic that correlated with the increased plasma norepinephrine level [96]. The kidney is richly innervated by postganglionic neurons of the sympathetic nervous system [97]. Indeed, catecholamines produce changes in glomerular hemodynamics quite similar to those observed in HF and with the administration of AII [98]. Studies on isolated perfused proximal tubules and cortical collecting ducts have demonstrated that catecholamines can increase sodium reabsorption that may be blocked by propranolol [99]. Besides their renal hemodynamic and tubule effects, the catecholamines also stimulate the secretion of renin and may antagonize the counterregulatory actions of the vasodilator neurohormone: both may contribute to unopposed influence of Ang II and increased fluid retention [100]. In dogs with low cardiac output induced by caval constriction, administration of a ganglionic blocker resulted in a marked increase in sodium excretion [101]. In rats with HF induced by coronary artery ligation, renal denervation resulted in an increase in RPF and SNGFR, and a decrease in afferent and efferent arteriolar resistance [102]. Similar changes were observed in water-deprived rats but not euvolemic rats. In patients with HF, switching from the low- to the high-sodium diet resulted in a suppression of the elevated catecholamine level [103]. These experimental and clinical data therefore indicate that the sympathetic nervous system plays an important role in the regulation of glomerular hemodynamics in situations, in which there is volume depletion or reduced cardiac output.

Renin–Angiotensin–Aldosterone System

The renin–angiotensin–aldosterone system (RAAS) may not play a major part in volume homeostasis when renal perfusion is normal. However, in sodium-depleted states, intrarenal angiotensin is activated and exerts a renal vasoconstrictor effect predominantly on the efferent arteriole [98, 104], such that glomerular capillary hydraulic pressure and filtration fraction are increased [98]. The resulting changes in peritubular hydraulic and oncotic pressure gradients lead to enhanced tubule sodium and fluid reabsorption [105]. The glomerular microcirculatory changes act to preserve GFR in the presence of reduced renal perfusion pressure. Accordingly, renal function may deteriorate in sodium-depleted states if the actions of Ang II are abolished either experimentally [90] or clinically [106]. The observation that the microcirculatory changes described in HF are almost identical to those seen in sodium-depleted states and during infusions of Ang II, suggests that Ang II plays a crucial role in mediating the alterations in renal function in HF. This is supported by evidence derived from a study using the rat coronary artery ligation model [82]. In this study, the abnormalities in single nephron glomerular hemodynamics and corresponding adjustments in proximal tubule function could be entirely abrogated by the administration of teprotide, an angiotensin-converting enzyme (ACE) inhibitor.

Whereas several studies have related renal sodium retention in HF to elevated levels of renin, Ang II, or aldosterone [107, 108], in other studies, no consistent relationship could be established [109]. In this regard, data from several experimental and clinical studies that explored the relationship between the renin–angiotensin–aldosterone axis and sodium balance at different stages of HF are worthy of discussion. In dogs with pulmonary artery or thoracic inferior vena cava constriction, the RAAS was activated to a striking degree during the early phase of constriction and was necessary for the support of systemic blood pressure; administration of the converting enzyme inhibitor captopril resulted in systemic hypotension. Over subsequent days, sodium retention and ECF volume expansion were pronounced, and inhibition of ACE was no longer accompanied by significant hypotension. However, animals with severe impairment in cardiac output remained sensitive to the hypotensive effects of ACE inhibition. Similarly, among patients with HF, plasma renin activity and levels of vasoconstrictor hormones were most elevated in those with acute, severe, and poorly compensated HF [110]. However, levels of these hormones were not elevated in patients with chronic stable HF. Furthermore, the levels declined when the patients with acute, decompensated HF became stable in the chronic stage. In a recent study with careful measurement of sodium balance, Cody et al. [103] examined the relationship of the RAAS to shifts in salt intake in patients with chronic HF. Sodium intake was 10–100 mmol/day. The maneuver was accompanied by weight gain and increased sodium excretion but not by an increase in blood volume. Plasma renin activity was greater with the 10 mmol/day diet and was suppressed with the 100 mmol/day diet. During both diets, plasma renin activity (PRA) was correlated with urinary sodium excretion. Of interest, systemic vascular

resistance remained elevated on the 100 mmol/day diet and could not be lowered by captopril. However, systemic vascular resistance could be lowered by captopril while the patient was receiving the 10 mmol/day diet. There was heterogeneity among the patients in their ability to achieve salt balance. One group was capable of achieving neutral salt balance while receiving the 100 mmol/day diet, whereas the second group displayed continued avid sodium retention. The avid sodium retention in the latter group could not be attributed to measurable differences in blood volume or other hemodynamic parameters. However, there was greater activation of the RAAS in the avid sodium retainers. Therefore, the foregoing experimental and clinical data indicate that the importance of the RAAS in maintaining circulatory homeostasis depends on the stage of HF and status of the ECF volume. Its influence is most pronounced in acute and decompensated HF and least in chronic stable HF and during states of sodium excess. Overall, the net effect of Ang II receptor blockade or converting enzyme inhibition on renal function in HF depends on a multiplicity of interacting factors. On the one hand, renal blood flow may improve as a result of lower efferent arteriolar resistance. Systemic vasodilatation may be associated with a rise in cardiac output. Under such circumstances, reversal of hemodynamically mediated effects of Ang II on sodium reabsorption would promote natriuresis. On the other hand, the aim of AII-induced elevation of single nephron filtration fraction is to preserve GFR in the face of diminished RPF. In those patients with precarious renal hemodynamics, a fall in systemic arterial pressure below the autoregulatory range combined with removal of the Ang II effect on glomerular hemodynamics may cause severe deterioration in renal function. The net result depends on the integrated sum of these physiologic effects, which in turn is dependent on the severity and stage of the heart disease. In addition to its hemodynamically mediated effects on renal sodium handling, there are other effects of Ang II that may be operative in promoting sodium retention in HF. Angiotensin II has a dose-dependent direct epithelial effect on the proximal tubule that favors active sodium reabsorption [111]. The predominant effect of the RAAS on distal nephron function is mediated by the action of aldosterone on cortical and medullary portions of the collecting duct to enhance sodium reabsorption. Here, aldosterone increases net sodium reabsorption and diminishes sodium back leak. The effect of a given circulating level of aldosterone on overall sodium excretion also depends on the volume of filtrate reaching the collecting duct and the composition of luminal and intracellular fluids. This delivery of filtrate is influenced by other effector mechanisms (i.e., Ang II, sympathetic nerve activity, and peritubular physical forces) acting at more proximal nephron sites. Numerous studies have reported elevated plasma aldosterone concentration or urinary aldosterone secretion or the effects of pharmacologic aldosterone antagonists in animal models and human subjects with HF [107, 108].

Variability in the relative importance of mineralocorticoid action in the sodium retention of HF that emerged from these reports should be interpreted in light of the very same considerations regarding stage and severity of disease that were noted with respect to the hemodynamic actions of angiotensin II.

Prostaglandins

When renal blood flow is impaired, hypoperfusion of the kidney, the activation of the RAAS, or both, stimulate the release of prostaglandins (PG) [112, 113]. Under these circumstances, prostaglandins exert a vasodilator effect that counteracts renal vasoconstriction locally. This vasodilatory effect may occur predominantly at the level of the afferent arteriole [114, 115]. The effects of the efferent arteriole are complex and are confounded by concomitant prostaglandin-mediated renin release and consequent Ang II production. As a result, the net effect is to counteract the decrease in RPF, with variable effects on filtration. Besides the hemodynamic effects, prostaglandins may also produce sodium and water retention through other mechanisms; they can directly inhibit sodium transport in the collecting tubule [116]; they may antagonize the dipsogenic action of Ang II [117]; they may oppose the effects of AVP on the collecting tubule [116]; and they may inhibit active sodium transport by the medullary thick ascending limb of Henle [116, 118]. Gathered observations in both experimental and human HF [119, 120] have demonstrated a direct linear relationship between the plasma renin activity and Ang II concentrations and levels of circulating and urinary prostaglandin E, and I, metabolites. This correlation probably reflects both a stimulation of prostaglandins synthesis by Ang II and an increased release of renin induced by prostaglandins. A similar counterregulatory role of prostaglandins with respect to the other major vasoconstrictors (catecholamines, AVP) may also be inferred. An inverse correlation between serum sodium concentrations and plasma levels of PGE, metabolites has been demonstrated [120]. In two experimental models of HF, inhibition of prostaglandin synthesis has been associated with adverse renal hemodynamic consequence [82, 119]. In one of these studies using a rat myocardial infarction model, administration of indomethacin to rats with HF was associated with a further rise in the already elevated efferent arteriolar resistance and a fall in glomerular plasma flow and SNGFR. Based on these observations, it is not surprising to find that patients with hyponatremia accompanied by the most striking activation of the sympathetic and the renin–angiotensin systems were most susceptible to adverse glomerular hemodynamic consequences following the administration of indomethacin [120].

Natriuretic Peptides

The natriuretic peptides such as ANP oppose the systemic vasoconstricting effect of Ang II [121], inhibits Ang II-stimulated proximal tubule sodium reabsorption, and opposes the dipsogenic of Ang II as well as the ability of the latter to stimulate thirst and secretion of aldosteronone [121]. Based on these observations, one may conceive that the high plasma level of ANP in HF should result in natriuresis. However, studies administering synthetic ANP to experimental models [122, 123] and patients with HF [103, 124] have consistently demonstrated attenuated renal response when compared with that in normal control subjects. The mechanisms for the attenuated renal effects of ANP in HF are unclear, although several possibilities are worthy of consideration [125]. First, the ability of ANP to antagonize the renal effects of Ang II may be limited in the presence of markedly impaired renal blood flow [126]. Second, it is possible that the activation of the sympathetic nervous system, Ang II and AVP in HF may have antagonized the renal effects of ANP [100]. Third, enhanced activity of neutral endopeptidase (NEP) in HF may reduce the availability of natriuretic peptides in the kidney [125].

In summary, the perturbations in the efferent limb of volume homeostasis in HF are a result of a complex interplay of the sympathetic nervous system and several other neurohormonal mechanisms on the glomeruli and the renal tubules. These interactions are summarized in Fig. 12.5.

Renal insufficiency is common in patients with HF and is an adverse prognostic factor [5, 6]. Mechanisms that mediate increased risk when HF and renal disease coexist include a higher burden of comorbidities, increased toxicities from diagnostic procedures or therapies, accelerated atherosclerosis, or less use of proven efficacious therapies in patients with both conditions [127]. Renal insufficiency as a comorbid condition in HF is discussed in Chap. 13. A large number of patients admitted to hospital have various degrees of heart and kidney dysfunction. Primary disorders of one of these two organs often result in secondary dysfunction or injury to the other [128]. Such interactions represent the pathophysiological basis for a clinical entity called cardiorenal syndrome [129].

Cardiorenal Syndrome

The term cardiorenal syndrome (CRS) has been increasingly utilized in clinical practice but often without a consistent or well-accepted definition [130]. Ronco et al. recently presented a classification of the cardiorenal syndrome of five subtypes that reflect the pathophysiology, the time-frame,

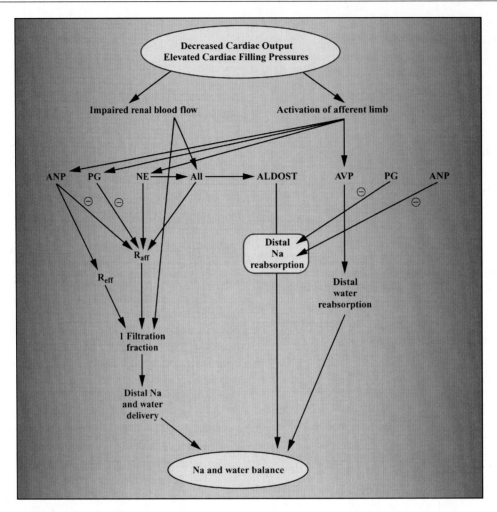

Fig. 12.5 Efferent limb of volume homeostasis in heart failure. Effector mechanisms that initiate and maintain renal sodium retention. *ANP* atrial natriuretic peptide; *PG* prostaglandins; *NE* norepinephrine; *AII* angiotensin II; *ALDOST* aldosterone; *AVP* arginine vasopressin; *Raff* afferent arteriolar resistance; *Reff* efferent arteriolar resistance; *minus sign* inhibitory effects

and the nature of concomitant cardiac and renal dysfunction [129]. CRS is defined as a pathophysiologic disorder of the heart and kidneys whereby acute or chronic dysfunction of one organ induces acute or chronic dysfunction of the other. Type 1 CRS reflects an abrupt worsening of cardiac function (e.g., acute cardiogenic shock or decompensated HF) leading to acute kidney injury. Type 2 CRS comprises chronic abnormalities in cardiac function leading to progressive chronic kidney disease. Type 3 CRS consists of an abrupt worsening of renal function (e.g., acute kidney ischemia or glomerulonephritis) causing acute cardiac dysfunction (e.g., dysrhythmia, ischemia). Type 4 CRS describes a state of chronic kidney disease (e.g., chronic glomerular disease) contributing to decreased cardiac function, cardiac hypertrophy, and/or increased risk of adverse cardiovascular events. Type 5 CRS reflects a systemic condition (e.g., sepsis) causing both cardiac and renal dysfunction. As the mechanisms mediating the subtypes of CRS may be different, the management strategies may not be the same either. For example, type 1 CRS is characterized by a rapid worsening of cardiac function, leading to acute kidney injury (AKI) (Fig. 12.6).

As more than 1 million patients in the United States are admitted to a hospital every year with either de novo acute HF or acutely decompensated chronic HF [130], type 1 CRS must be very common. Among these patients, premorbid chronic renal dysfunction is a common occurrence and predisposes them to acute kidney injury. In acute HF, kidney injury is more severe in patients with impaired LV systolic function compared with those with preserved LV function [131]. Furthermore, impaired renal function is consistently found as an independent risk factor for 1-year mortality in acute HF, including patients with ST-segment elevation myocardial infarction [132]. A plausible reason for this independent effect might be that an acute decline in renal function does not simply act as a marker of illness severity but also carries an associated acceleration in cardiovascular pathophysiology through activation of inflammatory pathways discussed elsewhere in this chapter [133].

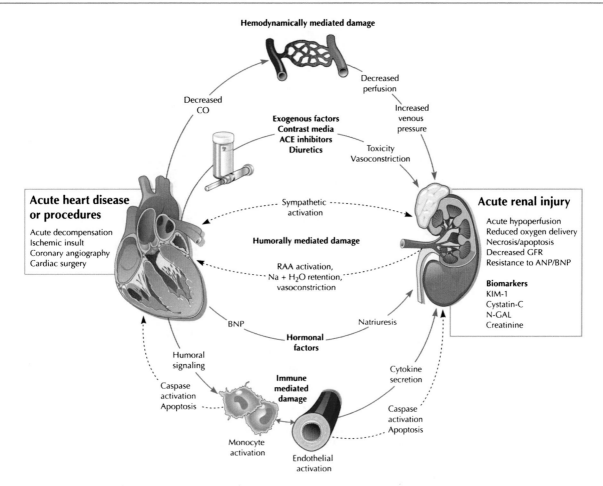

Fig. 12.6 Pathophysiological interactions between heart and kidney in type 1 cardiorenal syndrome. *ACE* angiotensin-converting enzyme; *ANP* atrial natriuretic peptide; *BNP* B-type natriuretic peptide; *CO* cardiac output; *GFR* glomerular filtration rate; *KIM* kidney injury molecule; *N-GAL* neutrophil gelatinase-associated lipocalin; *RAA* renin–angiotensin–aldosterone (Reproduced from Ronco et al. [129], with permission from Elsevier)

On the other hand, type 3 CRS is characterized by an abrupt and primary worsening of kidney function (e.g., acute kidney injury and ischemia, or glomerulonephritis), leading to acute cardiac dysfunction (e.g., HF, dysrhythmia and ischemia). Type 3 CRS may be less common than type 1 CRS, but this may only be due to the fact that, unlike type 1 CRS, it has not been studied as well. Acute kidney injury is a common disorder in hospital and ICU patients. When the RIFLE (risk, injury, and failure; loss; and end-stage kidney disease) consensus definition is used, acute kidney injury has been identified in close to 9% of hospital patients [134]. Acute kidney injury can affect the heart through several pathways (Fig. 12.7), whose hierarchy is not yet established. Fluid overload can contribute to the development of pulmonary edema. Hyperkalemia can contribute to dysrhythmias and may cause cardiac arrest. Untreated uremia affects cardiac contractility through the accumulation of myocardial depressant factors and pericarditis [135]. Acidemia produces pulmonary vasoconstriction, which can significantly contribute to right-sided HF. Acidemia appears to have a negative inotro-

pic effect and might, together with electrolyte imbalances, contribute to an increased risk of dysrhythmias [136].

Endothelial Dysfunction

Increased peripheral vasoconstriction in response to exercise and impaired vasodilatation after stimulation with agonists are the hallmarks of endothelial dysfunction in the setting of HF. The disruption of endothelial cell function has been attributed to the activation of the sympathetic nervous system, the renin–angiotensin system, as well as the vasopressin system [7]. Experimental and some clinical studies indicate that impaired endothelium-dependent relaxation is related, at least to a great extent, to impaired availability of NO [137].

Recent data demonstrated that expression of endothelial NO synthase (eNOS) is reduced in an experimental model of HF. On the other hand, a 10-day training program resulted in an increase in the expression of eNOS [138]. The expression

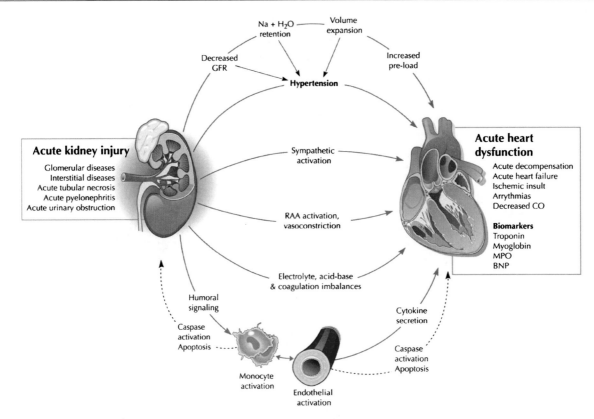

Fig. 12.7 Pathophysiologic interactions between heart and kidney in type 3 CRS or abrupt worsening of renal function. *MPO* myeloperoxidase; other abbreviations as in Fig. 12.6 (Reprinted from Ronco et al. [129]. With kind permission from Elsevier Limited)

of eNOs is increased by shear stress in isolated endothelial cells [139]. Therefore, impaired endothelium-dependent relaxation in HF may be related in part to reduced peripheral blood flow, which in turn may be restored by repetitive increases in blood flow by physical training, resulting in intermittent enhanced shear stress and, consequently, increased expression and activity of eNOS. In this regard, it has been shown that a training protocol confined to one extremity in patients with HF results in enhanced flow-dependent, endothelium-mediated dilation, whereas endothelial function of the untrained extremity remains unchanged [140]. These observations suggest that local mechanical forces play an important role in the beneficial effect of training. In addition to the regulation of eNOS, other shear-dependent mechanisms may be involved as well; i.e., shear stress upregulated the expression of Cu/Zn superoxide dismutase, a radical scavenging enzyme [141], but suppressed the expression of ACE [142]. There is evidence that HF is associated with increased oxidative stress [143]. Thus, increased expression and activity of endothelial superoxide dismutase may be protective via the scavenging of radicals, thereby reducing the inactivation of NO. The local activity of radical scavenging enzymes and radical-producing enzymes

in the periphery has not been assessed in patients with HF. There is evidence that endothelial dysfunction in patients with HF can be improved and normalized by the antioxidant vitamin C, which supports the notion that chronic HF is associated with increased radical formation that in turn affects endothelium-mediated vasomotor tone [144]. Shear-stress-mediated suppression of ACE may have an impact on endothelium-dependent relaxation by affecting local concentrations of bradykinin, because ACE is identical to kininase II, which degrades bradykinin into inactive products. Bradykinin is a strong stimulus for the release of NO from the endothelium. Experimental and clinical data suggest that bradykinin or the B2 receptor is involved in flow-dependent, endothelium-mediated dilation [145]. Moreover, ACE inhibition improves endothelium-dependent relaxation by bradykinin/bradykinin B_2 receptor-mediated mechanisms [138]. Taken together, impaired endothelium-dependent relaxation in HF may be a secondary event in response to alterations in peripheral hemodynamics. Alterations in shear stress related to impaired blood flow may play an important role in the development of endothelial dysfunction in this setting, although other factors such as increased levels of cytokines likely play a contributory role as well.

Immune and Cytokine Activation

A feature of HF is immune activation [146], with proinflammatory cytokines (e.g., TNF-α, IL-1, IL-6) overexpressed both in the systemic circulation [147] as well as locally in the failing myocardium [148]. Sustained overexpression of inflammatory mediators contributes to the development of central and peripheral manifestations of the syndrome of HF [146, 147, 149]. The cytokine hypothesis of HF [150] proposes that HF progresses because the cytokine cascade activated after myocardial injury exerts deleterious effects on the heart and circulation. This hypothesis implies that the overexpression of cytokines contributes to the progression of HF once LV dysfunction is present, but it does not mean that cytokines per se initiate heart HF. After an initial myocardial injury by myocardial infarction, hemodynamic overload, or inflammation, various secondary mediators such as cytokines and neurohormones act on the myocardium and stimulate myocardial remodeling through myocyte hypertrophy, apoptosis, and altered gene expression in cardiac myocytes.

There have been several hypotheses that address the source of proinflammatory cytokines in HF. One hypothesis is that activation of the immune system is responsible for cytokine elaboration, which happens in response to some forms of tissue injury (as described above) or possibly some unknown stimulus to the immune system. A second hypothesis is that the failing heart itself may be the source of TNF-α production in HF and that elevated levels of TNF-α represent spillover of cytokines that were produced locally within the myocardium, leading to secondary activation of the immune system [151]. This then is capable of amplifying the cytokine signal in the periphery. The third hypothesis is that decreased cardiac output in HF leads to the elaboration of TNF-α by underperfusion of systemic tissues. An extension of this hypothesis is that gut wall edema allows translocation of endotoxin, which activates cytokine production [152].

The effect of cytokines on the heart is initiated by specific receptors on the myocyte. In the case of TNF-α, ligand-receptor signaling is initiated by binding of TNF-α to a lower-affinity, 55-kD receptor (TNFR1) or a higher affinity, 75-kD receptor (TNFR2). TNF receptors in HF are capable of receptor shedding; that is, they are cleaved from the cell membrane and subsequently exist in the circulation as circulating soluble receptors, referred to as sTNFR1 and sTNFR2. In cell cultures, these soluble receptors have been shown to retain their ability to bind to TNF-α and inhibit its cytotoxic activity. It is believed that the role of circulating soluble binding proteins (such as TNF-binding proteins) in vivo is to serve as biologic buffers capable of neutralizing the highly cytotoxic activities of cytokines [151].

Several aspects of HF have been linked to the biological effects of cytokines. Some of the proposed mechanisms by which cytokines damage the heart are based on the hypothesis that TNF-α is a mediator of sepsis-induced alterations in the diastolic mechanical properties of the myocardium. Administration of TNF-α suppresses myocyte contractility, increases apoptosis, and decreases interstitial matrix [153]. This promotes LV dysfunction [154], pulmonary edema, and cardiomyopathy in humans and LV remodeling in dogs [153]. Although the most consistently increased cytokines in HF have been IL-6 and TNF-α, other cytokines, such as IL-1β and IL-2, have also been associated with the pathogenesis of HF [155].

High blood levels of TNF-α have been found to correspond to the severity of HF symptoms. Investigators for the Studies of Left Ventricular Dysfunction (SOLVD) in patients with HF reported a trend toward increasing mortality with increasing levels of TNF-α [156]. In vitro studies have shown that TNF-α produces negative inotropic effects in isolated contracting cardiac myocytes by altering calcium homeostasis. Soluble TNF receptors (sTNFR1 and sTNFR2) that bind to TNF-α can both prevent and reverse the negative inotropic effects of TNF-α in isolated contracting cardiac myocytes. However, elevated levels of sTNFR2 have also been shown to correlate with adverse short-term clinical outcomes in hospitalized HF patients [157]. The significance of this finding is unclear because soluble TNF receptors may also be considered protective of the heart because they bind to TNF-α and inactivate it. In a study on the prognostic importance of proinflammatory cytokines, investigators found that increased levels of TNF-α, sTNFR1, sTNFR2, and IL-6 predicted 24-month mortality in 152 patients with HF. sTNFR1 was found to be the strongest and most accurate prognosticator, independent of established markers of HF severity [158]. The Vesnarinone Multicenter Trial (VEST), which involved 1,200 patients, revealed that cytokines (TNF and IL-6) and their cognate soluble receptors (sTNFR1 and sTNFR2) were independent predictors of increased mortality in patients with advanced HF and that levels of cytokines were modified by age, sex, and cause of HF. The investigators also reported that cytokines were consistently higher in patients with ischemic cardiomyopathy than in patients with dilated cardiomyopathy [68].

Because it has been shown that cytokine production and activity can be antagonized e.g., high amounts of soluble TNF receptors function as specific inhibitors of TNF activity, one natural question that arises is whether cytokine bioactivity can be modulated as a treatment modality in patients with HF. Treatment with two TNF blockers, etanercept (soluble TNF-α) and infliximab (chimeric antibody), has been shown to have strikingly beneficial effects in patients with rheumatoid arthritis [159, 160]. In an experimental study, investigators found that a soluble p75 TNF receptor fusion protein (etanercept) that binds to TNF and functionally inactivates TNF can reverse some of the cardiotoxic effects of TNF in vitro and in vivo [60]. In a canine model of pacing-induced

HF, concomitant with etanercept reduced LV end-diastolic volume and LV tissue metalloproteinase (MMP) [161]. These finding were implemented in a phase I, double-blind clinical trial of patients with NYHA class III HF, and it was shown that TNF-α bioactivity was significantly decreased 2 weeks after treatment with a single intravenous infusion of etanercept (Enbrel). Improvements were particularly seen in increased ejection fraction, physical function as measured by a 6-min walk test, and an overall improvement in quality-of-life scores. Etanercept was found to be safe and well tolerated in this small group of HF patients [162]. However, the two subsequent large multicenter phase II and III clinical trials, RENAISSANCE (Randomized Etanercept North American Strategy to Study Antagonism of Cytokines) in the United States and RECOVER (Research into Enbrel: Cytokine Antagonism in Ventricular Dysfunction) in Europe, were stopped because of a lack of evidence of clinical benefit from etanercept [163]. Furthermore, in the anti-TNF Therapy Against Congestive Heart Failure (ATTACH) trial short-term TNF-α antagonism with a chimeric monoclonal antibody infliximab did not improve, and at high doses, adversely affected the clinical condition of patients with moderate-to-severe chronic HF [164].

Conclusions

The clinical syndrome of chronic HF has evolved from traditionally being primarily a malfunction of the heart as a pump to that of the periphery including peripheral vascular, renal, neurohormonal, as well as the inflammatory system. However, the mechanisms underlying the myriad of changes in the periphery in chronic HF, such as those discussed in this chapter, are complex and remain inadequately addressed by existing therapies. Particularly unclear is the origin of these derangements and the sequence of triggering mechanisms in the course of the natural history of HF. Still, recent advances in the therapy of HF have depended to a large extent on the understanding of changes at the periphery.

Summary

- The link between peripheral systems activated in HF and the central nervous system as a source of neurohumoral drive has therefore received increasing attention.
- The forebrain and particularly the paraventricular nucleus of the hypothalamus have emerged as sites that sense humoral signals generated peripherally in response to the stresses of HF and contribute to the altered volume regulation and augmented sympathetic drive that characterize the HF syndrome.
- Recent experimental studies have confirmed a critical role for the forebrain in the pathogenesis of HF. Peripheral systems adapting to myocardial injury and reduced cardiac output release humoral factors that enlist the forebrain to help restore volume and pressure within the cardiovascular system.
- Unrestrained by the usual negative feedback mechanisms, peripheral and central compensatory systems persist in a futile effort to restore homeostasis.
- The clinical approach to the HF syndrome is complicated by the fact that these compensatory mechanisms are initially supportive but are ultimately detrimental.
- The challenge is to develop therapeutic strategies that recognize the wisdom of adaptive mechanisms but prevent the excesses that promote clinical deterioration.
- A rational approach will modulate but will not eliminate these mechanisms. The forebrain may be a prime target for such interventions.
- From the standpoint of extracellular fluid volume homeostasis, the key abnormality in HF is the perception of an inadequate circulating volume by various sensors located on critical sites within the circulation. As a result, the normal relationship between intravascular volume and holding capacity as perceived by these sensing mechanisms is perturbed. This leads to the activation of various effector mechanisms, whose aim is to increase intravascular volume and maintain blood pressure.
- Abnormalities in effector mechanisms of volume homeostasis acting to promote sodium retention at the level of the kidney are themselves a consequence of the primary disturbance in afferent-sensing mechanisms.
- The perturbations in the efferent limb of volume homeostasis in HF are a result of a complex interplay of the sympathetic nervous system and several other neurohormonal mechanisms on the glomeruli and the renal tubules.
- Renal insufficiency is common in patients with HF and is a poor prognostic factor. Mechanisms that mediate increased risk when HF and renal disease coexist include a higher burden of comorbidities, increased toxicities from diagnostic procedures or therapies, and accelerated atherosclerosis.
- A large number of patients admitted to hospital have various degrees of heart and kidney dysfunction. Primary disorders of one of the two organs often result in secondary dysfunction or injury to the other. Such interactions represent the pathophysiological basis for a clinical entity called cardiorenal syndrome.
- A vascular component has been recognized to contribute to HF.
- The most studied vascular mechanisms that might contribute to the development of HF is the reduced produc-

tion of nitric oxide (NO) or the reduced bioactivity of NO seen in basic models of HF and disease in patients.

• The concept that HF is a cytokine activated state has, in addition, focused attention on the possibility that the cytokine driven isoform of NO synthase (NOS), iNOS, may produce sufficient quantities of NO to suppress cardiac myocyte function contributing to the reduced inotropic state in the already failing heart.

• The view of the role of NO in the development of HF has evolved from simply a reduction in production of NO in blood vessels, to altered substrate availability (i.e. L-arginine), to increased scavenging of NO by superoxide anion, to increased production of NO from iNOS. As these concepts develop, the approach to the therapeutics of HF has also progressed with the recognition of the need to develop treatments directed towards addressing one or more of these etiologies.

• Proinflammatory cytokines (interleukin-1, interleukin-2, interleukin-6, interleukin-10, and tumor necrosis factor) are involved in cardiac depression and in the complex syndrome of HF.

• Proinflammatory cytokines exert deleterious effects on the heart. Overproduction of cytokines contributes to the progression of HF, and it may be a marker of more severe or more active disease. However, the use of monoclonal antibodies directed against specific cytokines has not been found to be useful to reverse the downhill progression of HF.

References

1. Braunwald E, Bristow MR (2000) Congestive heart failure: fifty years of progress. Circulation 102:IV14–IV23
2. Mann DL (1999) Mechanisms and models in heart failure: a combinatorial approach. Circulation 100:999–1008
3. Jankowska EA, Ponikowski P, Piepoli MF, Banasiak W, Anker SD, Poole-Wilson PA (2006) Autonomic imbalance and immune activation in chronic heart failure – pathophysiological links. Cardiovasc Res 70:434–445
4. Francis GS, Cohn JN (1986) The autonomic nervous system in congestive heart failure. Annu Rev Med 37:235–247
5. Al-Ahmad A, Rand WM, Manjunath G, Konstam MA, Salem DN, Levey AS, Sarnak MJ (2001) Reduced kidney function and anemia as risk factors for mortality in patients with left ventricular dysfunction. J Am Coll Cardiol 38:955–962
6. McAlister FA, Ezekowitz J, Tonelli M, Armstrong PW (2004) Renal insufficiency and heart failure: prognostic and therapeutic implications from a prospective cohort study. Circulation 109: 1004–1009
7. Drexler H (1998) Endothelium as a therapeutic target in heart failure. Circulation 98:2652–2655
8. Linke A, Recchia F, Zhang X, Hintze TH (2003) Acute and chronic endothelial dysfunction: implications for the development of heart failure. Heart Fail Rev 8:87–97
9. Packer M (1993) How should physicians view heart failure? The philosophical and physiological evolution of three conceptual models of the disease. Am J Cardiol 71:3C–11C

10. DiBona GF, Sawin LL (1994) Reflex regulation of renal nerve activity in cardiac failure. Am J Physiol 266:R27–R39
11. Sun SY, Wang W, Zucker IH, Schultz HD (1999) Enhanced activity of carotid body chemoreceptors in rabbits with heart failure: role of nitric oxide. J Appl Physiol 86:1273–1282
12. Ma R, Zucker IH, Wang W (1997) Central gain of the cardiac sympathetic afferent reflex in dogs with heart failure. Am J Physiol 273:H2664–H2671
13. Ishise H, Asanoi H, Ishizaka S, Joho S, Kameyama T, Umeno K, Inoue H (1998) Time course of sympathovagal imbalance and left ventricular dysfunction in conscious dogs with heart failure. J Appl Physiol 84:1234–1241
14. Motte S, Mathieu M, Brimioulle S, Pensis A, Ray L, Ketelslegers JM, Montano N, Naeije R, van de BP, Entee KM (2005) Respiratory-related heart rate variability in progressive experimental heart failure. Am J Physiol Heart Circ Physiol 289:H1729–H1735
15. Francis GS, Benedict C, Johnstone DE, Kirlin PC, Nicklas J, Liang CS, Kubo SH, Rudin-Toretsky E, Yusuf S (1990) Comparison of neuroendocrine activation in patients with left ventricular dysfunction with and without congestive heart failure. A substudy of the Studies of Left Ventricular Dysfunction (SOLVD). Circulation 82:1724–1729
16. Benedict CR, Shelton B, Johnstone DE, Francis G, Greenberg B, Konstam M, Probstfield JL, Yusuf S (1996) Prognostic significance of plasma norepinephrine in patients with asymptomatic left ventricular dysfunction. SOLVD Investigators. Circulation 94: 690–697
17. Grassi G, Seravalle G, Bertinieri G, Turri C, Stella ML, Scopelliti F, Mancia G (2001) Sympathetic and reflex abnormalities in heart failure secondary to ischaemic or idiopathic dilated cardiomyopathy. Clin Sci (Lond) 101:141–146
18. Binkley PF, Nunziata E, Haas GJ, Nelson SD, Cody RJ (1991) Parasympathetic withdrawal is an integral component of autonomic imbalance in congestive heart failure: demonstration in human subjects and verification in a paced canine model of ventricular failure. J Am Coll Cardiol 18:464–472
19. Jouven X, Empana JP, Schwartz PJ, Desnos M, Courbon D, Ducimetiere P (2005) Heart-rate profile during exercise as a predictor of sudden death. N Engl J Med 352:1951–1958
20. Floras JS (2003) Sympathetic activation in human heart failure: diverse mechanisms, therapeutic opportunities. Acta Physiol Scand 177:391–398
21. Arnold JM, Liu P, Demers C, Dorian P, Giannetti N, Haddad H, Heckman GA, Howlett JG, Ignaszewski A, Johnstone DE, Jong P, McKelvie RS, Moe GW, Parker JD, Rao V, Ross HJ, Sequeira EJ, Svendsen AM, Teo K, Tsuyuki RT, White M (2006) Canadian Cardiovascular Society consensus conference recommendations on heart failure 2006: diagnosis and management. Can J Cardiol 22:23–45
22. Eckberg DL, Drabinsky M, Braunwald E (1971) Defective cardiac parasympathetic control in patients with heart disease. N Engl J Med 285:877–883
23. Ponikowski P, Anker SD, Chua TP, Szelemej R, Piepoli M, Adamopoulos S, Webb-Peploe K, Harrington D, Banasiak W, Wrabec K, Coats AJ (1997) Depressed heart rate variability as an independent predictor of death in chronic congestive heart failure secondary to ischemic or idiopathic dilated cardiomyopathy. Am J Cardiol 79:1645–1650
24. De Ferrari GM, Vanoli E, Stramba-Badiale M, Hull SS Jr, Foreman RD, Schwartz PJ (1991) Vagal reflexes and survival during acute myocardial ischemia in conscious dogs with healed myocardial infarction. Am J Physiol 261:H63–H69
25. Vanoli E, De Ferrari GM, Stramba-Badiale M, Hull SS Jr, Foreman RD, Schwartz PJ (1991) Vagal stimulation and prevention of sudden death in conscious dogs with a healed myocardial infarction. Circ Res 68:1471–1481

26. Brody MJ (1988) Central nervous system and mechanisms of hypertension. Clin Physiol Biochem 6:230–239

27. Rivest S (2001) How circulating cytokines trigger the neural circuits that control the hypothalamic-pituitary-adrenal axis. Psychoneuroendocrinology 26:761–788

28. McKinley MJ, McAllen RM, Pennington GL, Smardencas A, Weisinger RS, Oldfield BJ (1996) Physiological actions of angiotensin II mediated by AT1 and AT2 receptors in the brain. Clin Exp Pharmacol Physiol Suppl 3:S99–S104

29. McKellar S, Loewy AD (1981) Organization of some brain stem afferents to the paraventricular nucleus of the hypothalamus in the rat. Brain Res 217:351–357

30. Bealer SL (1995) Preoptic recess ablation selectively increases baroreflex sensitivity to angiotensin II in conscious rats. Peptides 16:1197–1201

31. Patel KP, Zhang PL, Krukoff TL (1993) Alterations in brain hexokinase activity associated with heart failure in rats. Am J Physiol 265:R923–R928

32. Vahid-Ansari F, Leenen FH (1998) Pattern of neuronal activation in rats with CHF after myocardial infarction. Am J Physiol 275: H2140–H2146

33. Sato T, Yoshimura R, Kawada T, Shishido T, Miyano H, Sugimachi M, Sunagawa K (1998) The brain is a possible target for an angiotensin-converting enzyme inhibitor in the treatment of chronic heart failure. J Card Fail 4:139–144

34. Zhang K, Li YF, Patel KP (2002) Reduced endogenous GABA-mediated inhibition in the PVN on renal nerve discharge in rats with heart failure. Am J Physiol Regul Integr Comp Physiol 282: R1006–R1015

35. Sawchenko PE (1987) Evidence for differential regulation of corticotropin-releasing factor and vasopressin immunoreactivities in parvocellular neurosecretory and autonomic-related projections of the paraventricular nucleus. Brain Res 437:253–263

36. Sawchenko PE, Swanson LW (1982) Immunohistochemical identification of neurons in the paraventricular nucleus of the hypothalamus that project to the medulla or to the spinal cord in the rat. J Comp Neurol 205:260–272

37. McKinley MJ, Allen AM, Burns P, Colvill LM, Oldfield BJ (1998) Interaction of circulating hormones with the brain: the roles of the subfornical organ and the organum vasculosum of the lamina terminalis. Clin Exp Pharmacol Physiol Suppl 25:S61–S67

38. Porter JP, Brody MJ (1986) A comparison of the hemodynamic effects produced by electrical stimulation of subnuclei of the paraventricular nucleus. Brain Res 375:20–29

39. Wei SG, Felder RB (2002) Forebrain renin-angiotensin system has a tonic excitatory influence on renal sympathetic nerve activity. Am J Physiol Heart Circ Physiol 282:H890–H895

40. Zhang K, Mayhan WG, Patel KP (1997) Nitric oxide within the paraventricular nucleus mediates changes in renal sympathetic nerve activity. Am J Physiol 273:R864–R872

41. Francis J, Weiss RM, Wei SG, Johnson AK, Felder RB (2001) Progression of heart failure after myocardial infarction in the rat. Am J Physiol Regul Integr Comp Physiol 281:R1734–R1745

42. Francis J, Wei SG, Weiss RM, Beltz T, Johnson AK, Felder RB (2002) Forebrain-mediated adaptations to myocardial infarction in the rat. Am J Physiol Heart Circ Physiol 282:H1898–H1906

43. Porter JP (1988) Electrical stimulation of paraventricular nucleus increases plasma renin activity. Am J Physiol 254:R325–R330

44. Porter JP (1988) The renin response to aortic occlusion is enhanced by stimulation of the hypothalamus. Hypertension 12:52–58

45. Johnson AK, Thunhorst RL (1997) The neuroendocrinology of thirst and salt appetite: visceral sensory signals and mechanisms of central integration. Front Neuroendocrinol 18:292–353

46. Lappe RW, Brody MJ (1984) Mechanisms of the central pressor action of angiotensin II in conscious rats. Am J Physiol 246:R56–R62

47. Bunnemann B, Fuxe K, Ganten D (1992) The brain renin-angiotensin system: localization and general significance. J Cardiovasc Pharmacol 19 Suppl 6:S51–S62

48. Moe GW (2006) B-type natriuretic peptide in heart failure. Curr Opin Cardiol 21:208–214

49. De Nicola AF, Seltzer A, Tsutsumi K, Saavedra JM (1993) Effects of deoxycorticosterone acetate (DOCA) and aldosterone on Sar1-angiotensin II binding and angiotensin-converting enzyme binding sites in brain. Cell Mol Neurobiol 13:529–539

50. Harada E, Yoshimura M, Yasue H, Nakagawa O, Nakagawa M, Harada M, Mizuno Y, Nakayama M, Shimasaki Y, Ito T, Nakamura S, Kuwahara K, Saito Y, Nakao K, Ogawa H (2001) Aldosterone induces angiotensin-converting-enzyme gene expression in cultured neonatal rat cardiocytes. Circulation 104:137–139

51. Sakaguchi K, Chai SY, Jackson B, Johnston CI, Mendelsohn FA (1988) Inhibition of tissue angiotensin converting enzyme. Quantitation by autoradiography. Hypertension 11:230–238

52. Yoshimura R, Sato T, Kawada T, Shishido T, Inagaki M, Miyano H, Nakahara T, Miyashita H, Takaki H, Tatewaki T, Yanagiya Y, Sugimachi M, Sunagawa K (2000) Increased brain angiotensin receptor in rats with chronic high-output heart failure. J Card Fail 6:66–72

53. Zhang ZH, Francis J, Weiss RM, Felder RB (2002) The renin-angiotensin-aldosterone system excites hypothalamic paraventricular nucleus neurons in heart failure. Am J Physiol Heart Circ Physiol 283:H423–H433

54. Haywood JR, Fink GD, Buggy J, Phillips MI, Brody MJ (1980) The area postrema plays no role in the pressor action of angiotensin in the rat. Am J Physiol 239:H108–H113

55. De Nicola AF, Grillo C, Gonzalez S (1992) Physiological, biochemical and molecular mechanisms of salt appetite control by mineralocorticoid action in brain. Braz J Med Biol Res 25:1153–1162

56. Saravia FE, Grillo CA, Ferrini M, Roig P, Lima AE, de Kloet ER, De Nicola AF (1999) Changes of hypothalamic and plasma vasopressin in rats with deoxycorticosterone-acetate induced salt appetite. J Steroid Biochem Mol Biol 70:47–57

57. Gomez AM, Valdivia HH, Cheng H, Lederer MR, Santana LF, Cannell MB, McCune SA, Altschuld RA, Lederer WJ (1997) Defective excitation-contraction coupling in experimental cardiac hypertrophy and heart failure. Science 276:800–806

58. Francis J, Weiss RM, Wei SG, Johnson AK, Beltz TG, Zimmerman K, Felder RB (2001) Central mineralocorticoid receptor blockade improves volume regulation and reduces sympathetic drive in heart failure. Am J Physiol Heart Circ Physiol 281:H2241–H2251

59. Meldrum DR (1998) Tumor necrosis factor in the heart. Am J Physiol 274:R577–R595

60. Bozkurt B, Kribbs SB, Clubb FJ Jr, Michael LH, Didenko VV, Hornsby PJ, Seta Y, Oral H, Spinale FG, Mann DL (1998) Pathophysiologically relevant concentrations of tumor necrosis factor-alpha promote progressive left ventricular dysfunction and remodeling in rats. Circulation 97:1382–1391

61. Das UN (2000) Free radicals, cytokines and nitric oxide in cardiac failure and myocardial infarction. Mol Cell Biochem 215:145–152

62. Antonipillai I, Wang Y, Horton R (1990) Tumor necrosis factor and interleukin-1 may regulate renin secretion. Endocrinology 126: 273–278

63. Turnbull AV, Lee S, Rivier C (1998) Mechanisms of hypothalamic-pituitary-adrenal axis stimulation by immune signals in the adult rat. Ann N Y Acad Sci 840:434–443

64. Saindon CS, Blecha F, Musch TI, Morgan DA, Fels RJ, Kenney MJ (2001) Effect of cervical vagotomy on sympathetic nerve responses to peripheral interleukin-1beta. Auton Neurosci 87:243–248

65. Dunn AJ (2000) Cytokine activation of the HPA axis. Ann N Y Acad Sci 917:608–617

66. Ericsson A, Kovacs KJ, Sawchenko PE (1994) A functional anatomical analysis of central pathways subserving the effects of interleukin-1 on stress-related neuroendocrine neurons. J Neurosci 14:897–913

67. Ericsson A, Arias C, Sawchenko PE (1997) Evidence for an intramedullary prostaglandin-dependent mechanism in the activation of stress-related neuroendocrine circuitry by intravenous interleukin-11. J Neurosci 17:7166–7179

68. Deswal A, Petersen NJ, Feldman AM, Young JB, White BG, Mann DL (2001) Cytokines and cytokine receptors in advanced heart failure: an analysis of the cytokine database from the Vesnarinone trial (VEST). Circulation 103:2055–2059

69. Felder RB, Francis J, Zhang ZH, Wei SG, Weiss RM, Johnson AK (2003) Heart failure and the brain: new perspectives. Am J Physiol Regul Integr Comp Physiol 284:R259–R276

70. MacNeil BJ, Jansen AH, Janz LJ, Greenberg AH, Nance DM (1997) Peripheral endotoxin increases splenic sympathetic nerve activity via central prostaglandin synthesis. Am J Physiol 273: R609–R614

71. Priebe HJ, Heimann JC, Hedley-Whyte J (1980) Effects of renal and hepatic venous congestion on renal function in the presence of low and normal cardiac output in dogs. Circ Res 47:883–890

72. Witte MH, Dumont AE, Clauss RH, Rader B, Levine N, Breed ES (1969) Lymph circulation in congestive heart failure: effect of external thoracic duct drainage. Circulation 39:723–733

73. Epstein FH, Post RS, McDowell M (1953) The effects of an arteriovenous fistula on renal hemodynamics and electrolyte excretion. J Clin Invest 32:233–241

74. Friedberg CK, Lasser RP, Allen DF, Furst SE, Gabor GE (1964) Production of chronic elevation of left ventricular end diastolic pressure in dogs: hemodynamic and renal studies. Circ Res 15:1–10

75. Hollander W, Judson WE (1956) The relationship of cardiovascular and renal hemodynamic function to sodium excretion in patients with severe heart disease but without edema. J Clin Invest 35: 970–979

76. Greenberg TT, Richmond WH, Stocking RA, Gupta PD, Meehan JP, Henry JP (1973) Impaired atrial receptor responses in dogs with heart failure due to tricuspid insufficiency and pulmonary artery stenosis. Circ Res 32:424–433

77. Zucker IH, Earle AM, Gilmore JP (1977) The mechanism of adaptation of left atrial stretch receptors in dogs with chronic congestive heart failure. J Clin Invest 60:323–331

78. Wegria R, Entrup RW, Jue J, Hughes M (1967) A new factor in pathogenesis of edema of cardiac origin 465. Am J Physiol 213:94–101

79. Mellander S, Oberg B (1967) Transcapillary fluid absorption and other vascular reactions in the human forearm during reduction of the circulating blood volume. Acta Physiol Scand 71:37–46

80. Merrill AJ (1949) Mechanisms of salt and water retention in heart failure. Am J Med 6:357–367

81. Vander AJ, Wilde WS, Malvin RL, Sullivan LP (1958) Re-examination of salt and water retention in congestive heart failure: significance of renal filtration fraction. Am J Med 25:497–502

82. Ichikawa I, Pfeffer JM, Pfeffer MA, Hostetter TH, Brenner BM (1984) Role of angiotensin II in the altered renal function of congestive heart failure. Circ Res 55:669–675

83. Cody RJ, Ljungman S, Covit AB, Kubo SH, Sealey JE, Pondolfino K, Clark M, James G, Laragh JH (1988) Regulation of glomerular filtration rate in chronic congestive heart failure patients. Kidney Int 34:361–367

84. Bell NH, Schedl HP, Bartter FC (1964) An explanation for abnormal water retention and hypoosmolality in congestive heart failure. Am J Med 36:351–360

85. Bennett WM, Bagby GC Jr, Antonovic JN, Porter GA (1973) Influence of volume expansion on proximal tubular sodium reabsorption in congestive heart failure. Am Heart J 85:55–64

86. Johnston CI, Davis JO, Robb CA, Mackenzie JW (1968) Plasma renin in chronic experimental heart failure and during renal sodium "escape" from mineralocorticoids. Circ Res 22:113–125

87. Kirchheim HR, Finke R, Hackenthal E, Lowe W, Persson P (1985) Baroreflex sympathetic activation increases threshold pressure for the pressure-dependent renin release in conscious dogs. Pflugers Arch 405:127–135

88. Mandin H, Davidman M (1978) Renal function in dogs with acute cardiac tamponade. Am J Physiol 234:F117–F122

89. Auld RB, Alexander EA, Levinsky NG (1971) Proximal tubular function in dogs with thoracic caval constriction. J Clin Invest 50:2150–2158

90. Levy M (1972) Effects of acute volume expansion and altered hemodynamics on renal tubular function in chronic caval dogs. J Clin Invest 51:922–938

91. Friedler RM, Belleau LJ, Martino JA, Earley LE (1967) Hemodynamically induced natriuresis in the presence of sodium retention resulting from constriction of the thoracic inferior vena cava. J Lab Clin Med 69:565–583

92. Zeidel ML, Brenner BM (1987) Actions of atrial natriuretic peptides on the kidney. Semin Nephrol 7:91–97

93. Johnson MD, Malvin RL (1977) Stimulation of renal sodium reabsorption by angiotensin II. Am J Physiol 232:F298–F306

94. Schrier RW, Abraham WT (1999) Hormones and hemodynamics in heart failure. N Engl J Med 341:577–585

95. Chidsey CA, Braunwald E, Morrow AG (1965) Catecholamine excretion and cardiac stores of norepinephrine in congestive heart failure. Am J Med 39:442–451

96. Leimbach WN Jr, Wallin BG, Victor RG, Aylward PE, Sundlof G, Mark AL (1986) Direct evidence from intraneural recordings for increased central sympathetic outflow in patients with heart failure. Circulation 73:913–919

97. Barajas L, Powers K, Wang P (1984) Innervation of the renal cortical tubules: a quantitative study. Am J Physiol 247:F50–F60

98. Myers BD, Deen WM, Brenner BM (1975) Effects of norepinephrine and angiotensin II on the determinants of glomerular ultrafiltration and proximal tubule fluid reabsorption in the rat. Circ Res 37:101–110

99. Bello-Reuss E (1980) Effect of catecholamines on fluid reabsorption by the isolated proximal convoluted tubule. Am J Physiol 238:F347–F352

100. Packer M (1988) Neurohormonal interactions and adaptations in congestive heart failure. Circulation 77:721–730

101. Gill JR Jr, Carr AA, Fleischmann LE, Casper AG, Bartter FC (1967) Effects of pentolinium on sodium excretion in dogs with constriction of the vena cava. Am J Physiol 212:191–196

102. Kon V, Yared A, Ichikawa I (1985) Role of renal sympathetic nerves in mediating hypoperfusion of renal cortical microcirculation in experimental congestive heart failure and acute extracellular fluid volume depletion. J Clin Invest 76:1913–1920

103. Cody RJ, Atlas SA, Laragh JH, Kubo SH, Covit AB, Ryman KS, Shaknovich A, Pondolfino K, Clark M, Camargo MJ (1986) Atrial natriuretic factor in normal subjects and heart failure patients. Plasma levels and renal, hormonal, and hemodynamic responses to peptide infusion. J Clin Invest 78:1362–1374

104. Edwards RM (1983) Segmental effects of norepinephrine and angiotensin II on isolated renal microvessels. Am J Physiol 244: F526–F534

105. Brenner BM, Troy JL, Daugharty TM, MacInnes RM (1973) Quantitative importance of changes in postglomerular colloid osmotic pressure in mediating glomerulotubular balance in the rat. J Clin Invest 52:190–197

106. Murphy BF, Whitworth JA, Kincaid-Smith P (1984) Renal insufficiency with combinations of angiotensin converting enzyme inhibitors and diuretics. Br Med J (Clin Res Ed) 288:844–845

107. Brown JJ, Davies DL, Johnson VW, Lever AF, Robertson JI (1970) Renin relationships in congestive cardiac failure, treated and untreated. Am Heart J 80:329–342

108. Genest J, Granger P, De CJ, Boucher R (1968) Endocrine factors in congestive heart failure. Am J Cardiol 22:35–42

109. Chonko AM, Bay WH, Stein JH, Ferris TF (1977) The role of renin and aldosterone in the salt retention of edema. Am J Med 63:881–889

110. Dzau VJ, Colucci WS, Hollenberg NK, Williams GH (1981) Relation of the renin-angiotensin-aldosterone system to clinical state in congestive heart failure. Circulation 63:645–651

111. Harris PJ, Young JA (1977) Dose-dependent stimulation and inhibition of proximal tubular sodium reabsorption by angiotensin II in the rat kidney. Pflugers Arch 367:295–297

112. Jackson EK, Gerkens JF, Brash AR, Branch RA (1982) Acute renal artery constriction increases renal prostaglandin I2 biosynthesis and renin release in the conscious dog. J Pharmacol Exp Ther 222:410–413

113. Schor N, Ichikawa I, Brenner BM (1981) Mechanisms of action of various hormones and vasoactive substances on glomerular ultrafiltration in the rat. Kidney Int 20:442–451

114. De Forrest JM, Davis JO, Freeman RH, Seymour AA, Rowe BP, Williams GM, Davis TP (1980) Effects of indomethacin and meclofenamate on renin release and renal hemodynamic function during chronic sodium depletion in conscious dogs. Circ Res 47:99–107

115. Edwards RM (1985) Effects of prostaglandins on vasoconstrictor action in isolated renal arterioles. Am J Physiol 248:F779–F784

116. Stokes JB, Kokko JP (1977) Inhibition of sodium transport by prostaglandin E2 across the isolated, perfused rabbit collecting tubule. J Clin Invest 59:1099–1104

117. Perez Guaita MF, Chiaraviglio E (1980) Effect of prostaglandin E1 and its biosynthesis inhibitor indomethacin on drinking in the rat. Pharmacol Biochem Behav 13:787–792

118. Iino Y, Imai M (1978) Effects of prostaglandins on Na transport in isolated collecting tubules. Pflugers Arch 373:125–132

119. Oliver JA, Sciacca RR, Pinto J, Cannon PJ (1981) Participation of the prostaglandins in the control of renal blood flow during acute reduction of cardiac output in the dog. J Clin Invest 67:229–237

120. Dzau VJ, Packer M, Lilly LS, Swartz SL, Hollenberg NK, Williams GH (1984) Prostaglandins in severe congestive heart failure. Relation to activation of the renin–angiotensin system and hyponatremia. N Engl J Med 310:347–352

121. Laragh JH (1985) Atrial natriuretic hormone, the renin-aldosterone axis, and blood pressure-electrolyte homeostasis. N Engl J Med 313:1330–1340

122. Kohzuki M, Hodsman GP, Johnston CI (1989) Attenuated response to atrial natriuretic peptide in rats with myocardial infarction. Am J Physiol 256:H533–H538

123. Scriven TA, Burnett JC Jr (1985) Effects of synthetic atrial natriuretic peptide on renal function and renin release in acute experimental heart failure. Circulation 72:892–897

124. Moe GW, Canepa-Anson R, Armstrong PW (1992) Atrial natriuretic factor: pharmacokinetics and cyclic GMP response in relation to biologic effects in severe heart failure. J Cardiovasc Pharmacol 19:691–700

125. Charloux A, Piquard F, Doutreleau S, Brandenberger G, Geny B (2003) Mechanisms of renal hyporesponsiveness to ANP in heart failure. Eur J Clin Invest 33:769–778

126. Sosa RE, Volpe M, Marion DN, Atlas SA, Laragh JH, Vaughan ED Jr, Maack T (1986) Relationship between renal hemodynamic and natriuretic effects of atrial natriuretic factor. Am J Physiol 250:F520–F524

127. McCullough PA (2002) Cardiorenal risk: an important clinical intersection. Rev Cardiovasc Med 3:71–76

128. Schrier RW (2007) Cardiorenal versus renocardiac syndrome: is there a difference? Nat Clin Pract Nephrol 3:637

129. Ronco C, House AA, Haapio M (2008) Cardiorenal syndrome: refining the definition of a complex symbiosis gone wrong. Intensive Care Med 34:957–962

130. Haldeman GA, Croft JB, Giles WH, Rashidee A (1999) Hospitalization of patients with heart failure: National Hospital Discharge Survey, 1985 to 1995. Am Heart J 137:352–360

131. Jose P, Skali H, Anavekar N, Tomson C, Krumholz HM, Rouleau JL, Moye L, Pfeffer MA, Solomon SD (2006) Increase in creatinine and cardiovascular risk in patients with systolic dysfunction after myocardial infarction. J Am Soc Nephrol 17:2886–2891

132. Goldberg A, Hammerman H, Petcherski S, Zdorovyak A, Yalonetsky S, Kapeliovich M, Agmon Y, Markiewicz W, Aronson D (2005) Inhospital and 1-year mortality of patients who develop worsening renal function following acute ST-elevation myocardial infarction. Am Heart J 150:330–337

133. Berl T, Henrich W (2006) Kidney-heart interactions: epidemiology, pathogenesis, and treatment. Clin J Am Soc Nephrol 1:8–18

134. Uchino S, Bellomo R, Goldsmith D, Bates S, Ronco C (2006) An assessment of the RIFLE criteria for acute renal failure in hospitalized patients1. Crit Care Med 34:1913–1917

135. Meyer TW, Hostetter TH (2007) Uremia. N Engl J Med 357:1316–1325

136. McCullough PA, Sandberg KR (2004) Chronic kidney disease and sudden death: strategies for prevention. Blood Purif 22:136–142

137. Drexler H (1997) Endothelial dysfunction: clinical implications. Prog Cardiovasc Dis 39:287–324

138. Sessa WC, Pritchard K, Seyedi N, Wang J, Hintze TH (1994) Chronic exercise in dogs increases coronary vascular nitric oxide production and endothelial cell nitric oxide synthase gene expression. Circ Res 74:349–353

139. Nishida K, Harrison DG, Navas JP, Fisher AA, Dockery SP, Uematsu M, Nerem RM, Alexander RW, Murphy TJ (1992) Molecular cloning and characterization of the constitutive bovine aortic endothelial cell nitric oxide synthase. J Clin Invest 90:2092–2096

140. Hornig B, Maier V, Drexler H (1996) Physical training improves endothelial function in patients with chronic heart failure. Circulation 93:210–214

141. Inoue N, Ramasamy S, Fukai T, Nerem RM, Harrison DG (1996) Shear stress modulates expression of Cu/Zn superoxide dismutase in human aortic endothelial cells. Circ Res 79:32–37

142. Rieder MJ, Carmona R, Krieger JE, Pritchard KA Jr, Greene AS (1997) Suppression of angiotensin-converting enzyme expression and activity by shear stress. Circ Res 80:312–319

143. Belch JJ, Bridges AB, Scott N, Chopra M (1991) Oxygen free radicals and congestive heart failure. Br Heart J 65:245–248

144. Hornig B, Arakawa N, Kohler C, Drexler H (1998) Vitamin C improves endothelial function of conduit arteries in patients with chronic heart failure. Circulation 97:363–368

145. Groves P, Kurz S, Just H, Drexler H (1995) Role of endogenous bradykinin in human coronary vasomotor control. Circulation 92:3424–3430

146. Mann DL (2002) Inflammatory mediators and the failing heart: past, present, and the foreseeable future. Circ Res 91:988–998

147. Levine B, Kalman J, Mayer L, Fillit HM, Packer M (1990) Elevated circulating levels of tumor necrosis factor in severe chronic heart failure. N Engl J Med 323:236–241

148. Torre-Amione G, Kapadia S, Lee J, Durand JB, Bies RD, Young JB, Mann DL (1996) Tumor necrosis factor-alpha and tumor necrosis factor receptors in the failing human heart. Circulation 93:704–711

149. Aukrust P, Gullestad L, Ueland T, Damas JK, Yndestad A (2005) Inflammatory and anti-inflammatory cytokines in chronic heart failure: potential therapeutic implications1. Ann Med 37:74–85

150. Seta Y, Shan K, Bozkurt B, Oral H, Mann DL (1996) Basic mechanisms in heart failure: the cytokine hypothesis. J Card Fail 2:243–249

151. Kapadia S, Dibbs Z, Kurrelmeyer K, Kalra D, Seta Y, Wang F, Bozkurt B, Oral H, Sivasubramanian N, Mann DL (1998) The role of cytokines in the failing human heart. Cardiol Clin 16:645–656, viii

152. Rauchhaus M, Coats AJ, Anker SD (2000) The endotoxin-lipoprotein hypothesis. Lancet 356:930–933

153. Pagani FD, Baker LS, Hsi C, Knox M, Fink MP, Visner MS (1992) Left ventricular systolic and diastolic dysfunction after infusion of tumor necrosis factor-alpha in conscious dogs. J Clin Invest 90:389–398

154. Finkel MS, Oddis CV, Jacob TD, Watkins SC, Hattler BG, Simmons RL (1992) Negative inotropic effects of cytokines on the heart mediated by nitric oxide. Science 257:387–389

155. Blum A, Miller H (2001) Pathophysiological role of cytokines in congestive heart failure. Annu Rev Med 52:15–27

156. Torre-Amione G, Kapadia S, Benedict C, Oral H, Young JB, Mann DL (1996) Proinflammatory cytokine levels in patients with depressed left ventricular ejection fraction: a report from the Studies of Left Ventricular Dysfunction (SOLVD). J Am Coll Cardiol 27:1201–1206

157. Ferrari R, Bachetti T, Confortini R, Opasich C, Febo O, Corti A, Cassani G, Visioli O (1995) Tumor necrosis factor soluble receptors in patients with various degrees of congestive heart failure. Circulation 92:1479–1486

158. Rauchhaus M, Doehner W, Francis DP, Davos C, Kemp M, Liebenthal C, Niebauer J, Hooper J, Volk HD, Coats AJ, Anker SD (2000) Plasma cytokine parameters and mortality in patients with chronic heart failure. Circulation 102:3060–3067

159. Maini R, St Clair EW, Breedveld F, Furst D, Kalden J, Weisman M, Smolen J, Emery P, Harriman G, Feldmann M, Lipsky P (1999) Infliximab (chimeric anti-tumour necrosis factor alpha monoclonal antibody) versus placebo in rheumatoid arthritis patients receiving concomitant methotrexate: a randomised phase III trial. ATTRACT Study Group. Lancet 354:1932–1939

160. Weinblatt ME, Kremer JM, Bankhurst AD, Bulpitt KJ, Fleischmann RM, Fox RI, Jackson CG, Lange M, Burge DJ (1999) A trial of etanercept, a recombinant tumor necrosis factor receptor: Fc fusion protein, in patients with rheumatoid arthritis receiving methotrexate. N Engl J Med 340:253–259

161. Bradham WS, Moe G, Wendt KA, Scott AA, Konig A, Romanova M, Naik G, Spinale FG (2002) TNF-alpha and myocardial matrix metalloproteinases in heart failure: relationship to LV remodeling. Am J Physiol Heart Circ Physiol 282:H1288–H1295

162. Deswal A, Bozkurt B, Seta Y, Parilti-Eiswirth S, Hayes FA, Blosch C, Mann DL (1999) Safety and efficacy of a soluble P75 tumor necrosis factor receptor (Enbrel, etanercept) in patients with advanced heart failure. Circulation 99:3224–3226

163. Mann DL, McMurray JJ, Packer M, Swedberg K, Borer JS, Colucci WS, Djian J, Drexler H, Feldman A, Kober L, Krum H, Liu P, Nieminen M, Tavazzi L, van Veldhuisen DJ, Waldenstrom A, Warren M, Westheim A, Zannad F, Fleming T (2004) Targeted anticytokine therapy in patients with chronic heart failure: results of the Randomized Etanercept Worldwide Evaluation (RENEWAL). Circulation 109:1594–1602

164. Chung ES, Packer M, Lo KH, Fasanmade AA, Willerson JT (2003) Randomized, double-blind, placebo-controlled, pilot trial of infliximab, a chimeric monoclonal antibody to tumor necrosis factor-alpha, in patients with moderate-to-severe heart failure: results of the anti-TNF Therapy Against Congestive Heart Failure (ATTACH) trial. Circulation 107:3133–3140

Chapter 13
Comorbidities in Heart Failure

Overview

Comorbidity complicates the care of patients with heart failure (HF) and is prevalent in one form or another for the majority of elderly patients with HF. A wide range of comorbidities, which includes respiratory comorbidities, diabetes, obesity, renal dysfunction, anemia, arthritis, cognitive dysfunction, and depression, contributes to the progression of the disease and may alter the response to treatment. Polypharmacy is inevitable in these patients. In addition, dysrhythmias, particularly atrial fibrillation (AF) is particularly common in patients with HF. The aim of this chapter is to discuss the recognition and management of several comorbid conditions that are commonly encountered in patients with chronic HF.

Introduction

Comorbidity is frequently defined as a chronic condition that coexists in an individual with another condition that is being described. HF is an increasingly common condition in North America, with a lifetime risk of approximately 20% for those 40 years of age and older [1]. Because HF incidence and prevalence increase with advancing age, HF is also more likely to occur in the setting of other illnesses. Indeed, the average patient with HF suffers from five or six concomitant medical conditions [2]. Physicians and other healthcare workers caring for patients with chronic HF need to be vigilant to comorbid conditions that may complicate the care of these patients. However, patients with increased comorbid disease burden, especially in the elderly and those hospitalized, are less likely to be enrolled in randomized clinical trials, and as such, have not been specifically addressed in published HF practice guidelines. As the global population ages, there is an accompanying increase in the prevalence of both atrial fibrillation (AF) and HF alone, as well as combined. The development of AF in patients with existing HF, and vice versa, is associated with clinical deterioration and worsening prognosis. Although one condition usually predates the other, one in five participants in the Framingham Heart Study who developed both HF and AF were diagnosed with both conditions on the same day. There are multiple pathophysiological mechanisms to explain how either condition contributes to the de novo development of the other. A better understanding of these links results in targeted treatments aimed at interrupting the development and progression of AF in HF and vice versa.

Prevalence of Comorbidities in Heart Failure

Data on the presence and effect of comorbidities on HF were derived from clinical trials and geographically limited studies of relatively small numbers of patients such as the Framingham cohort [3]. However, data from these trials may not always be reflective of the real-world experience as they are largely derived from younger patients with few or no comorbidities. More recently, studies have utilized databases to examine the impact of comorbidity in larger groups of elderly patients with chronic HF.

In the United States (US), National Heart Failure project from the Centers for Medicare and Medicaid Services found that comorbidity was common among 34,587 Medicare elderly patients aged >65 years, hospitalized with a principal diagnosis of HF [4]. About a third had chronic obstructive pulmonary disease (COPD), 18% had a history of stroke and 9.2% had dementia. More recently, Braunstein et al. reported the findings of a cross sectional analysis of 122,630 individuals aged >65 years with HF identified through a 5% random sample of all US Medicare beneficiaries [5]. Nearly 40% of patients with HF had >5 noncardiac comorbidities and this group accounted for 81% of the total inpatient hospital days experienced by patients with HF. The top ten most common non-cardiac conditions were COPD/bronchiectasis (26%), osteoarthritis (16%), chronic respiratory failure, or other lower respiratory disease excluding COPD/bronchiectasis (14%), thyroid disease (14%), Alzheimer's disease/dementia

J. Marín-García, *Heart Failure*, Contemporary Cardiology,
DOI 10.1007/978-1-60761-147-9_13, © Springer Science+Business Media, LLC 2010

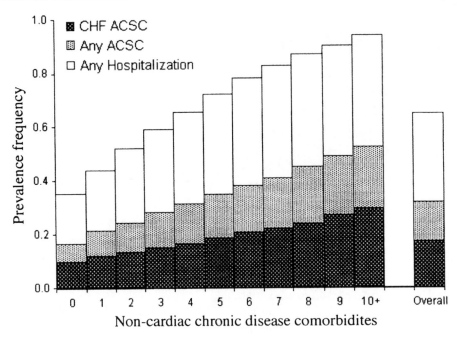

Fig. 13.1 Impact of non-cardiac comorbidity burden on the annual probability of a Medicare beneficiary with chronic heart failure (CHF) experiencing a hospitalization due to any cause. *P*<0.001 for linear trend for all outcomes. *ACSC* ambulatory care sensitive conditions (Reprinted from Braunstein et al. [5], copyright 2003. With permission from The American College of Cardiology Foundation)

(9%), depression (8%), chronic renal failure (7%), asthma (5%), osteoporosis (5%) and anxiety (3%). The risk of hospitalization and potentially preventable hospitalizations strongly increased with the number of chronic conditions (Fig. 13.1).

After controlling for demographic factors and other diagnoses, comorbidities that were associated consistently with higher risks for HF hospitalizations and mortality included COPD/bronchiectasis, renal failure, diabetes, depression, and lower respiratory diseases. Several factors may explain why older patients with HF with greater comorbidity may experience more adverse events that lead to preventable hospitalizations. These include underutilization of effective HF treatments in the presence of other conditions because of safety concerns e.g., use of β-blockers in asthma or ACE inhibitors in renal insufficiency, patient non-adherence to or inability to recall complex medication regimens, inadequate postdischarge care, failed social support and failure to promptly seek medical attention during symptom recurrence. Psychological stress from chronically poor health may also predispose to bad outcomes. Finally, elderly patients with multiple comorbidities and polypharmacy are also susceptible to poor coordination of care and are also at an increased risk for experiencing adverse drug reactions from drug–drug interactions. The association between comorbidity and healthcare costs has also been examined in a Medicare healthcare expenditure study. Patients with HF having expensive comorbidities included those with chronic pulmonary disease (33% of patients, mean total annual expenditure $23,104 per patient), renal disease (8% of patients, mean total annual expenditure $33,014 per patient), rheumatological disease (5% of patients, mean total annual expenditure, $20,527 per patient), and dementia (15% of patients, mean total annual expenditure, $26,263 per patient). Using data from 27,477 Scottish morbidity records listing HF, Brown et al. [6] reported that 12% of HF admissions were associated with chronic airways obstruction, 8% with chronic or acute renal failure, and 5% with cerebrovascular accident.

Diabetes Mellitus

Diabetes mellitus is a well-established risk factor for coronary artery disease. Diabetes prevalence is increasing world wide with prevalence of diabetes among patients with HF increasing at an even faster pace [7, 8]. Diabetes is present in more than 40% of patients with HF [9]. Despite advances in therapy for HF, mortality remains 40–80% higher for diabetics with HF than non-diabetics [7,10]. Diabetes has a particularly pernicious impact among women for the development of HF [11]. While multiple mechanisms are likely to be responsible for development of HF in diabetics, ischemic heart disease and comorbidities such as obesity and hypertension likely play a major role as well [7].

It is now recognized that diabetes mellitus may also produce HF independent of coronary artery disease by causing a diabetic cardiomyopathy [12,13]. At the molecular level, hyperglycemia-induced activation of protein kinase C has been implicated in some of the maladaptive changes seen at the cellular level in diabetes mellitus. Protein kinase C activation leads to changes in contractile protein function, stimulation of angiotensin converting enzymes (ACE) genes, and inducible nitric oxide synthase activity. Increased ACE activity in diabetes leads to many of the maladaptive changes seen in the diabetic patients with heart and vascular complications. These include apoptosis and necrosis of cardiomyocytes and endothelial cells and increased interstitial fibrosis. Animal and human studies show that chronic hyperglycemia leading to glycation of collagen and raised serum levels of advanced glycation end products result in increased myocardial stiffness. Further, at the cellular level, impairment of calcium homoeostasis is frequently seen in diabetic cardiomyocytes. These changes have been extensively studied in animal models. Derangements in calcium homoeostasis lead to decreased rates of release and reuptake of calcium into the sarcoplasmic reticulum. Changes at the receptor level are seen as decreased expression of sarcolemmal sodium–calcium exchanger. Preferential use of free fatty acids by the diabetic heart over time may lead to lipid accumulation in the myocardium, resulting in cell damage and destruction. There is evidence for the development of a distinct cardiomyopathy in diabetes independent of coexisting conditions such as coronary disease and hypertension and explains why diabetic subjects develop HF even in the absence of epicardial coronary artery disease [14].

Data from the National Health Examination Survey I [15] as well as the Framingham study [16] have shown the incidence of HF in patients with diabetes mellitus to be two- and fourfold higher, respectively, than in patients without diabetes. While an increase in glycosylated hemoglobin (HbA1C) among patients with diabetes is a recognized risk factor for the development of HF [17–20], no study to date has demonstrated that improved glycemic control significantly reduces the incidence of HF [21]. In this regard, the Canadian Diabetes Association 2003 Clinical Practice Guidelines for the Prevention and Management of Diabetes in Canada [22] does recommend that most patients with type 1 or type 2 diabetes be targeted to achieve an HbA1C level of 7.0% or lower.

Management of Patients with Heart Failure and Diabetes

Although prospective studies specifically dealing with heart HF in diabetes may be lacking, extrapolation of data from recent large trials has shed light on the management of HF in diabetes [7]. The Canadian Cardiovascular Society Consensus Conference Recommendations on Heart Failure Update 2007 [23] recommends that elevated blood glucose in patients with HF should be treated according to current Canadian Diabetes Association guideline recommendations – aim for a target HbA1C level of 7.0% or fasting/preprandial blood glucose of 4.4–7.0 mmol/L (class I, level A).

Treatment choices in patients with HF and diabetes involve dietary therapy, metformin, thiazoladinediones, biguanides, sulphonylureas, and insulin, all of which have their advantages and disadvantages. Metformin is an effective oral antidiabetic agent. Due to the presumed effects on pyruvate metabolism, metformin is approved for use under the "black box" warning in the setting of "hypoxic" conditions, such as renal insufficiency, HF, liver disease, and COPD. This warning is based on isolated case reports and a biochemical rationale that these conditions predispose patients to lactic acidosis (a condition associated with decreased serum bicarbonate levels), anion gap acidosis and systemic lactate level >5 mmol/L, with a mortality of 40–60%. In addition, two large meta-analyses and a smaller case series have evaluated the outcomes and occurrence of lactic acidosis associated with use of metformin compared with placebo (nonrandomized) or other antidiabetic agents, such as sulphonylureas and insulin [24–26]. The combined number of patients in these analyses was in excess of 40,000 and included those with HF, COPD, and renal disease. There was no increase in the occurrence of lactic acidosis and in addition cardiovascular outcomes of patients with HF taking metformin were better than those taking other antidiabetic therapies. While a precise renal function cut-off point for use of metformin was not apparent from these data, in general, only those with a serum creatinine level up to 150 μmol/L were included in the meta-analyses and those with serum creatinine levels up to 200 μmol/L were included in a smaller, single-centre study. Current evidence suggests that patients with HF and/or mild to moderate renal dysfunction (estimated glomerular filtration rate (eGFR) > 30 mL/min which correlates reasonably with a serum creatinine greater than 150 μmol/L in women and greater than 180 μmol/L in men unless at extremes of age or body weight) fare at least as well, if not better, with metformin than with other antidiabetic agents and metformin should still be considered as first-line therapy in HF patients with mild to moderate renal dysfunction [24–26]. Thiazolidinediones have been known to cause fluid retention, although this is generally mild. Recent studies suggest this is not a direct toxic effect on the myocardium. The recently reported Prospective Pioglitazone Clinical Trial in Macrovascular Events (PROACTIVE) study [27], in which pioglitazone was administered to diabetic patients at risk for cardiac ischemic events, showed that thizoladinedione was associated with fewer cardiac ischemic events, but with an increase in HF hospitalizations (2% absolute excess over 2.8 years, or less than 1% per year). The recently completed Diabetes Reduction Assessment with Ramipril and Rosiglitazone Medication (DREAM) study (2×2 factorial design) tested whether development of diabetes could be prevented by rosiglitazone and/or ramipril. In more than 5,000 patients, a significant reduction of new glucose intolerance and CV events (absolute 0.8% reduction) was seen with rosiglitazone, but a small excess of new-onset HF was also observed (absolute 0.4%) [28], which was similar to the PROACTIVE study. A recently completed randomized trial that compared the efficacy of rosiglitazone, metformin, or glyburide monotherapy in type 2 diabetics reported a significantly greater failure rate of monotherapy with glyburide or metformin than with rosiglitazone, but showed an increase in reported HF with rosiglitazone. When only adjudicated events were considered, there was no significant difference in cardiovascular or HF-related mortality in any arm [29]. Recent reports suggest that the fluid retention with this drug class may be safely managed with careful observation, taking care not to increase diuretic therapy in the absence of either symptoms or signs of central volume overload (rather than just peripheral edema) [25,26]. As such, this medication remains a viable choice for glycemic control in stable HF patients without fluid retention, but such patients should be followed more closely for signs of fluid retention and pulmonary congestion.

Pulmonary Disorders

The interaction between HF and concomitant pulmonary disease is common and important. Indeed, patients with HF are often misdiagnosed as having air flow obstruction on the basis of overlapping symptoms (and vice versa). In patients with established chronic obstructive airway disease, HF has been recognized in up to 30% of these patients [30]. In patients presenting to the emergency department with dyspnea, both B-type natriuretic peptide (BNP) and N-terminal prohormone BNP (NT-proBNP) have been shown to be useful in improving the diagnostic accuracy of HF [31]. Recently, in a controlled study of the use of both BNP and NT-proBNP in 306 patients with suspected HF referred to rapid access HF clinics [32], both tests proved useful, in particular when the results were normal. When both HF and respiratory disorders coexist, it may be important to quantify the relative contribution of cardiac and pulmonary components to the

disability. Exercise testing with simultaneous gas exchange or blood gas measurements may be helpful in this regard. Optimum assessment and management of these patients therefore necessitate careful consideration of the possibility that cardiac and respiratory disease may coexist in the individual patient.

Obstructive Airway Disease

Chronic obstructive airway disease (COPD) is a frequent concomitant disease in patients with HF and it is an independent short-term prognostic indicator of mortality and cardiovascular comorbidity in patients who have been admitted to hospital for HF [33]. In a recently published observational study based on longitudinal information from administrative registers, 1,020 patients who were chronically treated for and hospitalized with HF were identified and followed-up for major events up to 1 year. Half of the patients were female and 241 patients (23.6%) had concomitant COPD. There were no differences in the prevalence of cardiovascular and non-cardiovascular comorbidities between HF patients with or without COPD. However, COPD patients were more often male (60.6% vs. 46.3%), more frequently treated with diuretics (95.9% vs. 91.5%) but less often exposed to β-blockers (16.2% vs. 22.0%). Significantly higher adjusted in-hospital (hazard ratio 1.50 (95% confidence interval 1.00–2.26)) and out-of-hospital (1.42 (1.09–1.86)) mortality rates were found in HF patients with concomitant COPD. A higher occurrence of non-fatal myocardial infarction/stroke/rehospitalization for HF (1.26 (1.01–1.58)) as well as hospitalization for HF (1.35 (1.00–1.82)) was associated with COPD.

Diagnosing COPD in the presence of HF may be challenging. Some of the abnormalities observed on spirometry, such as reduced pulmonary diffusing capacity for carbon monoxide (DLCO), may be common to both COPD and HF [34]. To assess whether DLCO and its subdivisions, alveolar–capillary membrane conductance (DM) and pulmonary capillary blood volume (Vc) were sensitive to changes in intravascular volume, the effects of volume loading on airflow rates were examined [35]. In patients with left ventricular dysfunction (LVD), infusion of 10 mL/kg body weight of 0.9% saline acutely reduced DM (12.0±3.3 vs. 10.4±3.5 mmol/min/kPa, $P<0.005$), FEV1 (2.3±0.4 vs. 2.1±0.4 L, $P<0.0005$), and PEFR (446±55 vs. 414±56 L/min, $P<0.005$). All pulmonary function tests returned to baseline values 24 h later. In normal subjects, saline infusion had no measurable effect on lung function. Acute intravascular volume expansion therefore impairs alveolar–capillary membrane function and increases airflow obstruction in patients with LVD but not in normal subjects. Thus, the abnormalities of pulmonary diffusion in HF, which were believed to be fixed previously, may also have a variable component that could be amenable to therapeutic intervention.

β-blockers are deemed to be contraindicated in patients with HF and air flow obstruction; in practice, because of the overwhelming benefits of these agents in HF due to systolic dysfunction, many patients with fixed or limited airways reversibility are given them, and they tolerate them surprisingly well. Whether β-1 selective agents offer advantages over non-selective agents such as carvedilol remains unclear [36, 37]. In a direct comparison of carvedilol and bisoprolol on lung function on 57 patients with HF [38], FEV1 and FVC were similar; after salbutamol FEV1 was higher with bisoprolol ($P = 0.04$). Absolute values for DLCO, DLCO subcomponents, and alveolar volume are shown in Fig. 13.2.

The higher DLCO value with bisoprolol was due to an improvement in DM. Twenty-two subjects had a DLCO value, 80% of which are predicted with either carvedilol (20 cases) or bisoprolol (17 cases). In these subjects, DLCO was 15.9 ± 3.4 mL/min/mmHg ($63 \pm 14\%$) and 17.7 ± 3.1 ($72 \pm 12\%$) ($P = 0.02$ for both absolute values and %) with carvedilol and bisoprolol, respectively. Thus, in terms of DLCO only, response to salbutamol challenge and exercise capacity, this study shows a superior effect of bisoprolol over carvedilol in HF patients. Over all, cardioselective β-blockers given in mild to moderate reversible airway disease do not produce adverse respiratory effects in the short term and the effects of β-2 agonists do not appear to be attenuated by selective β-1 blockade. Given their demonstrated benefit in HF, β-blockers should not be withheld from such patients, but long-term safety (especially, their impact during an acute exacerbation) still needs to be established.

Heart Failure and Renal Dysfunction

The close relationship between cardiovascular and renal function in normal physiology is also apparent in the diseases involved in these organs. The mechanism for renal dysfunction in the context of HF was discussed in Chap. 12. The importance of renal dysfunction in the setting of HF is increasingly being recognized [39]. Several studies have shown renal function to be one of the strongest predictors of adverse outcomes in HF patients [40]. A recent study from Canada has shown that renal dysfunction is particularly highly prevalent in patients with HF than previously reported and is an independent prognostic factor in diastolic and systolic dysfunction (see Fig. 13.2) [41]. Indeed, given the relationship between renal function and cardiac output, renal dysfunction is an adverse prognostic marker, and also a strong predictor of poor outcome in HF than functional class [42]. In general, adverse vascular events increase once GFR falls below 60 mL/min. [39] As a consequence of accelerated atherosclerotic coronary artery disease, concomitant hypertension and fluid retention, patients with primary renal disease are at high risk of HF. Conversely, many patients with HF have evidence of renal dysfunction in the absence of intrinsic renal disease. About 40% of patients with HF have chronic kidney disease, defined as a serum creatinine level of >133 mmol/L or a creatinine clearance rate of <60 mL/min. [42] The observed low glomerular filtration rate in HF is a consequence of diminished cardiac output, with decreased renal perfusion and intrarenal vasoconstriction accompanied by sodium and water retention, medications (NSAIDs and others) as well as diabetes and intrinsic renal disorders. Multiple theories have been offered to explain the excess

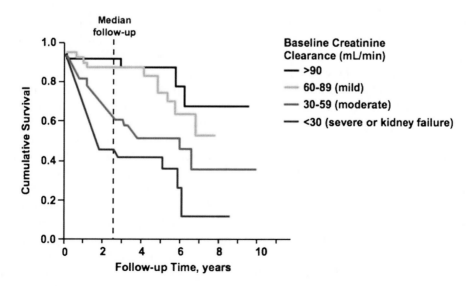

Fig. 13.2 Baseline creatinine clearance and survival in acute heart failure (Adapted from McAlister et al. [41]. With permission from Wolters Kluwer)

risks in patients with HF with renal dysfunction including more advanced coronary atherosclerosis. However, recent data from 6,427 patients with HF with documented coronary angiography showed that the adverse prognostic influence of renal dysfunction was independent of atherosclerotic burden and left ventricular systolic function [42].

Management of Patients with Heart Failure and Renal Dysfunction

The effects of HF drugs on patients with HF with concomitant renal dysfunction have not been well studied. Patients with renal hypoperfusion or intrinsic renal disease show an impaired response to diuretics and ACE inhibitors [43] and are at an increased risk of adverse effects during treatment with digitalis. Most HF trials have studied patients with normal renal function with only a few reporting subgroup analyses of patients with renal dysfunction. In a post hoc analysis of the Cardiac Insufficiency Bisoprolol Study, those with moderate to severe renal failure showed a similar benefit on mortality and hospitalization from bisoprolol treatment to those with normal renal function [44]. The most impressive effect of a β-blocker in HF and end-stage renal failure was recently reported by Cice et al. [45]. A total of 114 dialysis patients with dilated cardiomyopathy were randomized to receive either carvedilol or a placebo in addition to standard therapy. At 2 years, the carvedilol group had smaller cavity diameters in both systole and diastole and had higher ejection fractions. By 2 years, 51.7% of the patients in the carvedilol group had died, whereas 73.2% in the placebo group had died. There were significantly fewer cardiovascular deaths and fewer hospital admissions among the patients receiving carvedilol. All these data strongly support the use of such drugs in patients with HF with chronic kidney disease. In view of the extremely high cardiovascular morbidity and mortality in chronic kidney disease and end-stage renal disease, there is a need for routine use of such cardioprotective agents in these patients. Unfortunately, in the "real world" population, prescription rates for such HF drugs are inversely related to renal function [42]. Recent guidelines recommended that HF patients with stable renal function (serum creatinine levels <200 μmol/L) should receive standard therapy with an ACE inhibitor, angiotensin receptor blocker, or spironolactone, but monitoring of serum potassium and creatinine levels should be more frequent, especially if combination therapy is used or in the case of an acute concomitant illness that causes dehydration (class I, level B) [23].

As the renal vasoconstriction that develops in the setting of reduced cardiac output depends on angiotensin II, treatment with an ACE inhibitor or angiotensin-receptor blocker

may lead to an (generally, clinically unimportant) increase in the serum creatinine concentration. Generally, these slight rises in serum creatinine levels are reversible and are only infrequently the cause of drug discontinuation. Most patients with HF tolerate mild to moderate degrees of functional renal impairment without difficulty. However, if the serum creatinine increases >220 mmol/L, the presence of renal dysfunction can severely limit the efficacy and enhance the toxicity of established treatments. An arbitrary creatinine cut-off value to define renal insufficiency (serum creatinine >220 mmol/L) for spironolactone has been suggested in published guidelines [46]. However, this may not be appropriate in the elderly because of the competing age-related decline in creatinine as a result of decline in muscle mass and rise in creatinine as a result of decline in glomerular filtration rate. Indeed, in a prescription linked study, Juurlink et al. [47] found that immediately after the publication of the Randomized Aldactone Evaluation Study, the prescription rate in Canada rose sharply and that this was associated with an increase in the rate of admission for hyperkalemia, from 2.4 per 1,000 patients in 1994 to 11 per 1,000 patients in 2001 ($P=0.001$), and the associated mortality rose from 0.3 per 1,000 to 2 per 1,000 patients ($P=0.001$). However, it should be noted that there were several differences in this real-patient population study from the cohort in the Randomized Aldactone Evaluation Study (RALES) trial. These older patients received a higher dose of spironolactone without close attention to serum creatinine and follow-up. In the study of Medicare beneficiaries aged >65 years discharged after hospitalization for HF, spironolactone was prescribed to 22.8% of patients with serum potassium >5 mmol/L, to 14.1% with a serum creatinine value >220 mmol/L and to 17.3% with severe renal dysfunction (glomerular filtration rate <30 mL/min/1.73 m^2) [48]. In multivariate analysis, factors associated with such prescribing patterns included advanced age and non-cardiovascular morbidities. There is a need for greater vigilance and care to be given to frequent monitoring of electrolytes and renal parameters in patients with HF with renal dysfunction.

It is important to recognize worsening renal function early because there is a critical time period during which correction of reversible causes may re-establish stability. Several reversible factors have been known to frequently contribute to worsening renal function. The most important are systemic hypotension and volume depletion. In addition, concomitant drugs may contribute if they have a risk for adverse renal effects such as renin–angiotensin–aldosterone system inhibitors, ARBs and spironolactone, hypotensive agents (especially vasodilators), NSAIDs, and cyclooxygenase 2 inhibitors [49]. Systemic factors such as sepsis and urinary obstruction are also important. Mild fluctuations in renal function are common in HF patients, but these usually do not exceed 30% of the baseline creatinine level and should simply be observed. However, oliguria or larger increases in serum creatinine levels should prompt action and increased surveillance. In a subset of patients with increased creatinine levels and severe volume overload, diuresis may actually result in improved renal function, presumably due to a left shift from the extreme right of the Starling curve, which allows stroke volume to increase.

Anemia and Heart Failure

Anemia is common in patients with HF with a prevalence ranging from 4 to 55% [26]. Reasons for this wide variation include differences in the population with HF studied, in study methods, and in the definition of anemia used. Although the most commonly accepted definition of anemia is that of the World Health Organization (hemoglobin <13 g/dL in men and <12 g/dL in women), studies have varied considerably in the criteria used to classify patients as anemic. In general, the prevalence of anemia is greater in less selected populations (such as insurance claims data) and lower in highly selected populations such as patients enrolled in clinical trials. Anemia appears to be more common in patients with more severe disease, with a reported prevalence in patients with New York Heart Association (NYHA) functional class IV populations as high as 79%. Multiple potential mechanisms of interaction exist between anemia and the clinical syndrome of HF. HF is a disease of the elderly, a population where the prevalence of anemia is high irrespective of cardiac status. Multiple comorbid conditions are common in patients with HF, in particular, renal insufficiency, which is closely associated with the development of anemia. Other potential contributing factors include hemodilution, proinflammatory cytokines, malnutrition due to right-sided HF, and decreased perfusion to the bone marrow. With respect to hemodilution, expansion of plasma volume is a characteristic of the HF syndrome, and, therefore, some anemia may be dilutional rather than due to a true decrease in red blood cell mass. In a study of thirty seven patients with HF, it has been shown that true anemia i.e., a decrease in red blood cell mass was present in 54%, and hemodilution was present in 46%. Notably, in this study, both hemodilution and true anemia were associated with adverse survival, with the worst survival seen in patients with hemodilution [50]. Another study on 100 consecutive patients with chronic HF also explored the determinants of anemia (iron parameters, erythropoietin, hepcidin and kidney function) including red cell volume (RCV) as well as related markers and plasma volume [51]. Plasma volumes were significantly higher in anemic HF patients and was the best predictor of hemoglobin concentrations in the regression model. In practice, it is likely that several of these mechanisms are active

simultaneously, and that anemia in HF is the result of a complex interaction between cardiac performance, neurohormonal and inflammatory activation, renal function and bone marrow responsiveness. A prospective ongoing study including both specialty and community sites, the Study of Anemia in a Heart Failure Population registry, is evaluating the prevalence, etiologies and mechanisms of anemia in a broad population of patients with HF. While the optimal hemoglobin level is not known, increased adverse events are seen when the plasma hemoglobin level is lower than 110 g/L or hematocrit lower than 35%. The increased event rate seems to be inversely related to hemoglobin below these levels [52, 53].

The association of anemia with adverse clinical outcomes in HF has led to substantial interest in anemia as a potential therapeutic target. Preliminary data involving small groups of patients with HF suggest that attempts to correct of anemia may result in a significant symptomatic improvement in HF [50, 54]. A previous study evaluated the effect of 3 months of erythropoietin treatment on exercise capacity in single-blind placebo controlled study of twenty six patients with anemia and NYHA functional class III–IV HF [54]. This study demonstrated significant improvements in mean±SD peak oxygen consumption with erythropoietin treatment (from 11 ± 0.8 to 12.7 ± 2.8 in the recombinant human erythropoietin (rHuEPO)-treated patients ($P > 0.05$) vs. no significant change in the control patients). A significant correlation was observed between increases in hemoglobin with rHuEPO treatment and increased peak oxygen consumption. Notably, the improvement in exercise performance with rHuEPO treatment was observed whether the anemia was found to be from decreased red blood cell mass or from hemodilution. These studies used rHuEPO in a regimen similar to the one used in patients with end-stage renal disease. Newer erythropoietin analogs have been developed (such as darbepoetin) that have a longer half-life and require less frequent administration, potentially making them more attractive for HF treatment. It should also be noted that aggressive treatment of anemia may also be associated with an increased risk of hypertension or thrombosis. Multiple ongoing studies will provide definitive data on the balance of risks and benefits of anemia treatment in chronic HF. Results from the recently published Study of Anemia in Heart Failure-Heart Failure Trial (STAMINA-HeFT) [55] suggest an improvement in symptoms and treadmill exercise time, but an uncertain effect on death and hospitalization. Similar strategies for patients with chronic kidney disease but without HF have also not shown benefit [56]. It has been suggested that increasing hemoglobin aggressively may be associated with thrombotic events. The ongoing, multicentre, randomized study, Reduction of Events with Darbepoetin α in Heart Failure (RED-HF), will address these issues and is powered for morbidity and mortality.

Cognitive Dysfunction and Heart Failure in the Elderly

An abnormal prevalence of cognitive dysfunction ranging from 35 to 50% has been reported in patients with HF [57]. Reduced cardiac output as a result of HF may further compromise cerebral blood flow in a patient with borderline perfusion of the brain. Furthermore, HF is largely driven by vascular disease and cerebrovascular disease is an important contributor to multi-infarct dementia. Among elderly patients with HF, cognitive dysfunction has been associated with a fivefold increase in the risk of mortality and a sixfold increase in the probability of dependence for the activities of daily living [58].

Reducing the burden of cognitive dysfunction potentially allows for substantial gains in terms of survival rates, quality of life, and resource consumption. However, no interventions are yet known to improve cognitive performance largely because of the incomplete knowledge about the pathophysiology of cognitive dysfunction in these patients. It should be noted that measures of cognitive function have rarely been used in HF trials, unlike hypertension trials such as Systolic Hypertension in Europe and Study on Cognition and Prognosis in the Elderly. Given the consistent reporting of impaired cognitive function in cross sectional studies of patients with HF, this parameter should be considered as an endpoint for future trials of HF pharmacotherapy.

Depression is a common and often overlooked comorbidity in patients with chronic HF. Depending on the methodology used to diagnose depression, between 17 and 37% of patients with HF have been found to be clinically significantly depressed [59]. Depression increases in prevalence with HF severity, as assessed by New York Heart Functional class and other measures [60]. The comorbid presence of depression portends an even poorer prognosis than the already high mortality associated with chronic HF per se [61]. A recent meta-analysis suggested a risk ratio of 2.1 for death and secondary events in comparison with HF alone [60]. This was associated with an increased burden on the healthcare system because of high rates of hospitalization and emergency department visits. The presence of concomitant depression may also influence the course of HF disease progression. Mechanistic studies have demonstrated increases in proinflammatory cytokine activity as well as evidence of alteration in platelet function, hypothalamic–pituitary–adrenal axis activation, and autonomic stimulation in depressed patients [62]. All these pathophysiologic changes may contribute adversely to the ventricular remodeling process that accompanies HF. In this setting, the influence of drug therapy for treatment of both HF and depression on pathophysiologic mechanisms and clinical outcomes is important. What is remarkable, however, is how little research has been done in this area. For example, it is not known whether treating the

HF and improving a patient's functional status has a major impact on concomitant depression. Furthermore, little is known when the question is asked the other way around, that is, will treating depression favorably affect the course of a patient's HF?

The Canadian Cardiovascular Society heart failure guidelines recommend that elderly or frail HF patients who present with acute illness should be assessed for evidence of delirium and, before discharge, cognitive impairment (class IIa, level C) [23]. A relatively simple score can be used to characterize frail elderly patients who are clinically stable (Fig. 13.3) [63]. It may be useful to identify high risk patients who require more careful and detailed development of a multidisciplinary care plan. When frail elderly patients present with either an exacerbation of HF itself or another medical condition, they often appear confused. This may be due to acute delirium, chronic dementia, or a combination of both. The relative contributions of each may be difficult to determine during acute illness, and may become apparent only when the aggravating illness is controlled. Delirium should be suspected in the setting of an acute illness accompanied by an altered and fluctuating level of consciousness and/or cognition, and can be screened for using available tools [64, 65]. In many cases, discussion and development of complex treatment plans are delayed or made increasingly difficult when evidence of patient

---

The CSHA Frailty Scale

1 *Very fit*— robust, active, energetic, well motivated and fit; these people commonly exercise regularly and are in the most fit group for their age

2 *Well*— without active disease, but less fit than people in category 1

3 *Well, with treated comorbid disease*— disease symptoms are well controlled compared with those in category 4

4 *Apparently vulnerable*— although not frankly dependent, these people commonly complain of being "slowed up" or have disease symptoms

5 *Mildly frail*— with limited dependence on others for instrumental activities of daily living

6 *Moderately frail*— help is needed with both instrumental and non-instrumental activities of daily living

7 *Severely frail*— completely dependent on others for the activities of daily living, or terminally ill

Note: CSHA = Canadian Study of Health and Aging.

Fig. 13.3 A simple score that can be used to characterize clinically stable frail elderly patients (Reprinted from Rockwood et al. [63]. With permission from the Canadian Medical Association)

cognitive impairment becomes apparent. In addition, cognitive impairment may persist well beyond the resolution of the acute precipitating illness.

To screen for persistent cognitive impairment in clinically stable patients, several instruments have been developed that require varying degrees of time, effort, and expertise to administer. The Mini Mental Status Examination requires approximately 20 min for administration. It has been validated and is moderately sensitive and specific, although some aspects of executive function are not well identified [66]. The Montreal Cognitive Assessment test [67] has been developed to specifically identify mild cognitive impairment, especially if related to vascular disease, and is endorsed by the Canadian Stroke Network. It requires little training to administer and the short form may be performed in about 5 min. This short form includes the Montreal Cognitive Assessment subtests (five word memory task tests – registration, recall, recognition – six item orientation tests and one letter phonemic fluency test) and can be downloaded free for noncommercial purposes [67]. Because these instruments have been validated in medically stable patients, they may be best used once the HF patient is stabilized to choose appropriate care plans and discharge planning. Other instruments, according to the clinical need (i.e., screening, documentation of mental status, complete neuropsychiatric evaluation), may be found in the National Institute of Neurological Disorders publication [66].

Dysrhythmias in Heart Failure

Patients with HF are at increased risk for the development of both atrial and ventricular tachydysrhythmias. Ventricular tachydysrhythmias predispose to sudden cardiac death and are associated with the extent and severity of myocardial dysfunction [68]. As such, ventricular arrhythmias should be regarded more as a complication of HF rather than a comorbid condition and the topic will therefore be discussed in other chapters. On the other hand, atrial tachyarrhythmias, particularly atrial fibrillation and HF are two disease processes that propagate the development and the progression of the other. Atrial fibrillation is therefore considered in detail in this chapter.

Atrial Fibrillation in Heart Failure

Atrial fibrillation (AF) is the most frequent sustained dysrhythmia encountered in clinical practice [69, 70]. The presence of AF increases the morbidity and mortality in the general population even after adjusting for preexisting con-

ditions [71]. AF is particularly prevalent in patients with HF [72, 73]. Indeed, AF and HF are two global epidemics of cardiovascular disease that often interact, resulting in significant morbidity and mortality and with a reciprocal causal relationship existing between them [74]. Chronic HF affects more than 50% of patients with AF [75]. The prevalence of AF increases in proportion to the severity of chronic HF [76]. Recent data have shown that the total proportion of HF with AF develop HF at any time was 41% while 42% with AF at some point during their lifetime [3]. These conditions also affect the elderly disproportionately with the incidence of each conditions doubling for every successive decade of age [77].

Animal studies have demonstrated that atrial dilation through various mechanisms results in a shortened atrial refractory period and a prolonged atrial conduction time [78–81]. Programmed electrical stimulation subsequently resulted in an increased vulnerability to atrial tachydysrhythmias when compared to control groups. This inducibility of AF with premature stimuli is directly related to atrial pressure. Thus atrial stretch has been shown to change atrial electrical properties in these animal models, resulting in increased frequency of atrial adysrhythmias. Indeed, a substantial number of antecedent risk factors including hypertension, diabetes, coronary heart disease, and valvular disease are common for both AF and HF. Each condition is associated with neurohormonal activation, myocardial cellular and extracellular alterations and electrophysiologic alterations that form the substrate that predisposes a person to the development and maintenance of both AF and HF (Table 13.1) [73].

The development of AF is in turn associated with increased mortality in patients with HF including those with impaired or preserved systolic function [3, 82, 83]. Data from the Studies of Left Ventricular Dysfunction (SOLVD) database has shown that the presence of AF in patients with asymptomatic and symptomatic left ventricular systolic dysfunction is associated with an increased risk for all-cause mortality, largely explained by an increased risk for pump-failure death. This analysis suggests that AF is associated with progression of left ventricular systolic dysfunction. An increase in sudden cardiac death was not observed [83]. In an analysis of the Framingham Heart Study data, the subsequent development of HF in patients with AF was found to be associated with a hazard ratio for mortality of 2.7 in men and 3.1 in women. The development of subsequent AF in patients with HF was associated with a hazard ratio for mortality of 1.6 in men and 2.7 in women. The authors conclude that the development of the second condition has a deleterious impact on survival [3]. In a recent post hoc analysis of the Candesartan in Heart failure-Assessment of Reduction in Mortality and morbidity (CHARM) study [82], a total of 670 (17%) patients in the low ejection fraction group and 478 (19%) in the preserved ejection fraction group had AF at baseline. Atrial

Table 13.1 Common risk factors for atrial fibrillation and heart failure

Risk factors	Atrial fibrillation	Heart failure
Hypertension	Irregular ventricular rhythm	Atrial stretch
Diabetes mellitus	Absence of atrial transport	Atrial fibrosis
Coronary heart disease	Diminished cardiac output	Altered atrial refractory periods and conduction velocities
Valvular heart disease	Structural changes of cardiac myocytes, leading to tachycardia-induced cardiomyopathy	Neurohormonal activation

Table 13.2 Risk of baseline atrial fibrillation (AF) for cardiovascular (CV) events based on ejection fraction (EF) in patients with congestive heart failure (CHF) in the CHARM study [82]

	AF	No AF
CV-death or hospitalization due to CHF		
Preserved EF	161/478 (34%)	538/2,545 (21%)
Low EF	299/670 (45%)	1,462/3,906 (37%)
CV-death		
Preserved EF	83/478 (17%)	257/2,545 (10%)
Low EF	204/670 (30%)	916/3,906 (23%)
Hospitalization due to CHF		
Preserved EF	115/478 (24%)	402/2,545 (16%)
Low EF	199/670 (30%)	959/3,906 (25%)
All-cause mortality		
Preserved EF	117/478 (24%)	364/2,545 (14%)
Low EF	248/670 (37%)	1,102/3,906 (28%)
Fatal or non-fatal stroke		
Preserved EF	25/478 (5%)	96/2,545 (4%)
Low EF	39/670 (6%)	127/3,906 (3%)
CV-death or hospitalization due to CHF or non-fatal stroke		
Preserved EF	169/478 (35%)	589/2,545 (23%)
Low EF	313/670 (47%)	1,504/3,906 (39%)

fibrillation predicted a high risk of cardiovascular morbidity and mortality regardless of baseline ejection fraction. Patients with AF and low ejection fraction had the highest absolute risk for adverse cardiovascular outcomes. However, AF was associated with greater relative increased risk of the major outcomes in patients with preserved ejection fraction than in patients with low ejection fraction. The same held true for the risk of all-cause mortality (Table 13.2).

The loss of atrial transport and an irregular ventricular rhythm may both make important contributions to the worsening of cardiac output and other hemodynamic parameters. The subsequent hemodynamic changes may then explain the clinical alterations that are observed in this population. Such observations argue for the maintenance of sinus rhythm in patients with HF. The clinical and hemodynamic consequences of developing AF was investigated in HF patients in sinus rhythm undergoing evaluation for cardiac transplantation [84]. Subjects underwent right heart catheterization, cardiopulmonary exercise testing, and two-dimensional echocardiography. There was no difference in any clinical or hemodynamic variables between patients who developed AF and those who remained in sinus rhythm.

In clinical practice, rate control versus rhythm control for AF in HF represents a dynamic interplay between the neutral results of population trials on clinical outcomes and the symptomatic deterioration sometimes attributed to recurrent AF in selected individuals. Data from the earlier Atrial Fibrillation Follow-up Investigation of Rhythm Management (AFFIRM) investigators suggests that a rate-control strategy should be considered a superior approach to patients with AF when compared with rhythm-control [85]. However, only about 26% of all patients in this study had an ejection fraction of less than 50%, and only 23% had a history of HF. The AFFIRM study was therefore not adequately designed to examine treatment approaches in the subset of patients with HF.

The recently-published Atrial Fibrillation in Congestive Heart Failure (AF-CHF) study is a prospective randomized controlled trial designed to determine whether restoring and maintaining sinus rhythm reduces cardiovascular mortality compared with a rate control strategy in patients with AF and HF [86]. 1367 patients were randomized from 130 centers in Canada, United States, South America, Europe, and Israel. Patients had NYHA class II to IV symptoms and left ventricular ejection fraction <35% (NYHA class I patients with prior hospitalization for HF or ejection fraction <25% are also eligible) and a documented clinically significant episode of AF within the past 6 months to one of two treatment strategies:

1. Rhythm control with the use of electrical cardioversion combined with antidysrhythmic drugs (amiodarone or other class III agents), and additional nonpharmacological therapy in resistant patients.
2. Rate control with the use of β-blockers, digoxin or pacemaker, and AV node ablation if necessary.

The primary endpoint was cardiovascular mortality. At the end, 682 patients were randomized to rhythm control and 694 to rate control. At baseline, 31% of patients had NYHA class III or IV symptoms. Mean ejection fraction was 27%. Atrial fibrillation was paroxysmal in 31% of patients and persistent in 69%. By trial design, rhythm control was predominantly achieved with amiodarone (82%) with less use of sotalol (1.8%) and dofetilide (0.4%) in the rhythm control cohort. In the rate control group, β-blockers were used in 88% of patients and digoxin in 75%. Crossover from rhythm to rate control occurred in 21% of the rhythm group and from rate to rhythm control in 10% of the rate group. There was no difference in the primary endpoint of between the groups (26.7% of the rhythm control group vs. 25.2% of the rate control group, hazard ratio (HR) 1.06, 95% CI 0.86–1.30, $P=0.59$). There was also no difference in total mortality (31.8% vs. 32.9%, $P=0.73$), stroke (2.6% vs. 3.6%, $P=0.32$), worsening HF (27.6% vs. 30.8%, $P=0.17$) or the composite of CV death, stroke, or worsening HF (42.7% vs. 45.8%, $P=0.20$) for rhythm control vs. rate control, respectively. In the rhythm control group, 39% had cardioversion compared with 8% of the rate control group ($P=0.0001$). Bradydysrhythmias were more common in the rhythm control group (8.5% vs. 4.9%, $P=0.007$). Among patients with HF and AF, the use of rhythm control was not associated with differences in cardiovascular mortality compared with rate control through a mean follow-up of 3 years. The results of this landmark trigger the following new recommendation in the 2009 Canadian Cardiovascular Society Consensus Conference guidelines in HF [87]:

- In patients with stable HF and asymptomatic AF, rate control is an acceptable management strategy and routine rhythm control is not required (class I, level II).

Data from large clinical trials to date therefore suggest that routine rhythm control does not confer a benefit in clinical outcomes in patients with AF and HF. However, in patients whom the physicians are reasonably certain the patients are symptomatic from AF, attempt for rhythm control should still be pursued.

Conclusions

Non-cardiac comorbidity frequently complicates the care of patients with HF especially in the elderly patients. These comorbid conditions include diabetes chronic lung disease, renal dysfunction, anemia, and dysrythmias including AF. The presence of these comorbid conditions also increases the mortality of these patients. They are also the same patients that are most likely encountered in real world clinical practice. Exclusion of patients with comorbidities in large HF clinical trials makes generalization of trial findings to these patients somewhat difficult. Clinical research must therefore adapt to ensure its relevance, and trials need to include not just young patients with systolic dysfunction and little comorbidity. Ongoing studies enrolling the often ignored group of elderly patients and those with preserved systolic function are an encouraging trend but only represent the beginning of a necessary trend. Future trials must also focus on optimal strategies for the comprehensive management of the patient with HF with multiple comorbidities rather than the isolated effects of single drugs in younger patients with few or no comorbidities.

Summary

- Over 40% of patients with HF also have diabetes. While the prevalence of diabetes is increasing world wide, the prevalence of diabetes among patients with HF is increasing at a faster pace.
- It is now recognized that diabetes mellitus may also produce HF independent of coronary artery disease by causing a diabetic cardiomyopathy.
- The Canadian Cardiovascular Society Consensus Conference Recommendations on Heart Failure Update 2007 [23] recommends that elevated blood glucose in patients with HF should be treated according to current Canadian Diabetes Association guideline recommendations – aim for a target HbA1C level of 7.0% or fasting/preprandial blood glucose of 4.4–7.0 mmol/L (class I, level A).
- Treatment choices in patients with HF and diabetes involve dietary therapy, metformin, thiazoladinediones, biguanides, sulphonylureas, and insulin, all of which have their advantages and disadvantages.
- Chronic obstructive airway disease (COPD) is a frequent concomitant disease in patients with HF and it is an independent short-term prognostic indicator of mortality and cardiovascular comorbidity in patients who have been admitted to hospital for HF.
- When both HF and respiratory disorders coexist, it may be important to quantify the relative contribution of cardiac and pulmonary components to the disability.
- Exercise testing with simultaneous gas exchange or blood gas measurements may be helpful in this regard.
- B-type natriuretic peptide (BNP) and N-terminal prohormone BNP (NT-proBNP) have been shown to be useful in improving the diagnostic accuracy of HF.
- Optimum assessment and management of these patients therefore necessitate careful consideration of the possibility that cardiac and respiratory disease may coexist in the individual patient.
- Given their demonstrated benefit in HF, β-blockers should not be withheld from patients with HF and COPD, but long-term safety (especially, their impact during an acute exacerbation) still needs to be established.
- The importance of renal dysfunction in the setting of HF is increasingly being recognized and many studies have shown renal function to be one of the strongest predictors of adverse outcomes in HF failure patients.
- Renal dysfunction is typically multifactorial, and is frequently related to poor renal perfusion, vascular disease and effects of chronic hypertension and medications e.g., NSAIDs as well as diabetes and intrinsic renal disorders.
- It is important to recognize worsening renal function early because there is a critical time period during which correction of reversible causes may re-establish stability.

- Several reversible factors frequently contribute to worsening renal function. The most important ones are systemic hypotension and volume depletion. In addition, concomitant drugs may contribute if they have a risk for adverse renal effects. In general, slight rises in serum creatinine levels are reversible and are only infrequently the cause of drug discontinuation.
- Most patients with HF tolerate mild to moderate degrees of functional renal impairment without difficulty. However, if the serum creatinine increases >220 mmol/L, the presence of renal insufficiency can severely limit the efficacy and enhance the toxicity of established treatments.
- Anemia is frequently observed in patients with chronic HF. Prevalence of anemia depends both on the severity of HF and diagnostic criteria used to define it, but may be as high as 50% in selected patient cohorts.
- Anemia is not only prevalent in the HF population, but several studies in different patient populations found an association with anemia, impaired cardiac function, healthcare utilization, and morbidity. In addition, numerous studies have assessed associations between anemia and mortality in HF.
- Early clinical trials have been performed with bone marrow-stimulating agents, such as erythropoietin and darbepoetin, in patients with HF. To date, studies suggest an improvement in symptoms and treadmill exercise time, but an uncertain effect on death and hospitalization. Similar strategies for patients with chronic kidney disease but without heart failure have also not shown benefit.
- It has been suggested that increasing hemoglobin aggressively may be associated with thrombotic events. The ongoing, multicentre, randomized study, Reduction of Events with Darbepoetin alfa in Heart Failure (RED-HF), will address these issues and is powered for morbidity and mortality.
- A relatively high prevalence of cognitive dysfunction ranging from 35 to 50% has been reported in patients with HF. Among elderly patients with HF, cognitive dysfunction has been associated with a fivefold increase in the risk of mortality.
- Reducing the burden of cognitive dysfunction potentially allows for substantial gains in terms of survival rates, quality of life, and resource consumption. However, no interventions are yet known to improve cognitive performance largely because of the incomplete knowledge about the pathophysiology of cognitive dysfunction in these patients.
- Given the consistent reporting of impaired cognitive function in cross sectional studies of patients with HF, this parameter should be considered as an endpoint for future trials of HF pharmacotherapy.
- Atrial fibrillation (AF) and HF are two disease processes that propagate the development and the progression of the

other. For this reason, they often coexist in the same patient. Indeed, chronic HF affects more than 50% of patients with atrial fibrillation.
- The presence of AF worsens the prognosis of patients with heart failure. The emergence of agents such as dofetilide and amiodarone has led to the suggestion that a rhythm-control strategy may be reasonably safe and effective in this subset of patients.
- The optimal management of these patients remains controversial although the results of a recent landmark trial have not suggested that a strategy of rhythm-control does not seem to offer benefit in clinical outcome over a rate-control strategy.

References

1. Lloyd-Jones DM, Larson MG, Leip EP et al (2002) Lifetime risk for developing congestive heart failure: the Framingham Heart Study. Circulation 106:3068–3072
2. Howlett JG, Johnstone DE, Sketris I, O'Reilly M, Horne GS, Cox JL (2003) Identifying opportunities to address the congestive heart failure burden: the Improving Cardiovascular Outcomes in Nova Scotia (ICONS) study. Can J Cardiol 19:439–444
3. Wang TJ, Larson MG, Levy D et al (2003) Temporal relations of atrial fibrillation and congestive heart failure and their joint influence on mortality: the Framingham Heart Study. Circulation 107:2920–2925
4. Havranek EP, Masoudi FA, Westfall KA, Wolfe P, Ordin DL, Krumholz HM (2002) Spectrum of heart failure in older patients: results from the National Heart Failure project. Am Heart J 143:412–417
5. Braunstein JB, Anderson GF, Gerstenblith G, Weller W, Niefeld M, Herbert R, Wu AW (2003) Noncardiac comorbidity increases preventable hospitalizations and mortality among Medicare beneficiaries with chronic heart failure. J Am Coll Cardiol 42:1226–1233
6. Brown AM, Cleland JG (1998) Influence of concomitant disease on patterns of hospitalization in patients with heart failure discharged from Scottish hospitals in 1995. Eur Heart J 19:1063–1069
7. Kamalesh M (2007) Heart failure in diabetes and related conditions. J Card Fail 13:861–873
8. Kamalesh M (2009) Diabetes and prognosis: are systolic and diastolic heart failure different? Heart 95:178–179
9. Adams KF Jr, Fonarow GC, Emerman CL et al (2005) Characteristics and outcomes of patients hospitalized for heart failure in the United States: rationale, design, and preliminary observations from the first 100,000 cases in the Acute Decompensated Heart Failure National Registry (ADHERE). Am Heart J 149:209–216
10. Kamalesh M, Subramanian U, Sawada S, Eckert G, Temkit M, Tierney W (2006) Decreased survival in diabetic patients with heart failure due to systolic dysfunction. Eur J Heart Fail 8:404–408
11. Mosterd A, Hoes AW (2007) Clinical epidemiology of heart failure. Heart 93:1137–1146
12. Bell DS (2003) Heart failure: the frequent, forgotten, and often fatal complication of diabetes. Diabetes Care 26:2433–2441
13. Spector KS (1998) Diabetic cardiomyopathy. Clin Cardiol 21:885–887
14. Fang ZY, Prins JB, Marwick TH (2004) Diabetic cardiomyopathy: evidence, mechanisms, and therapeutic implications. Endocr Rev 25:543–567

15. He J, Ogden LG, Bazzano LA, Vupputuri S, Loria C, Whelton PK (2001) Risk factors for congestive heart failure in US men and women: NHANES I epidemiologic follow-up study. Arch Intern Med 161:996–1002

16. Kannel WB, Hjortland M, Castelli WP (1974) Role of diabetes in congestive heart failure: the Framingham study. Am J Cardiol 34: 29–34

17. Johansson S, Wallander MA, Ruigomez A, Garcia Rodriguez LA (2001) Incidence of newly diagnosed heart failure in UK general practice. Eur J Heart Fail 3:225–231

18. Nichols GA, Gullion CM, Koro CE, Ephross SA, Brown JB (2004) The incidence of congestive heart failure in type 2 diabetes: an update. Diabetes Care 27:1879–1884

19. Vaur L, Gueret P, Lievre M, Chabaud S, Passa P (2003) Development of congestive heart failure in type 2 diabetic patients with microalbuminuria or proteinuria: observations from the DIABHYCAR (type 2 DIABetes, Hypertension, CArdiovascular Events and Ramipril) study. Diabetes Care 26:855–860

20. Iribarren C, Karter AJ, Go AS, Ferrara A, Liu JY, Sidney S, Selby JV (2001) Glycemic control and heart failure among adult patients with diabetes. Circulation 103:2668–2673

21. Intensive blood-glucose control with sulphonylureas or insulin compared with conventional treatment and risk of complications in patients with type 2 diabetes (UKPDS 33). UK Prospective Diabetes Study (UKPDS) Group. Lancet 1998; 352:837–853

22. Canadian Diabetes Association (2003) Canadian Diabetes Association 2003 clinical practice guidelines for the prevention and management of diabetes in Canada. Can J Diabetes 27: S21–S23

23. Arnold JM, Howlett JG, Dorian P et al (2007) Canadian Cardiovascular Society Consensus Conference recommendations on heart failure update 2007: prevention, management during intercurrent illness or acute decompensation, and use of biomarkers. Can J Cardiol 23:21–45

24. Eurich DT, Majumdar SR, McAlister FA, Tsuyuki RT, Johnson JA (2005) Improved clinical outcomes associated with metformin in patients with diabetes and heart failure. Diabetes Care 28:2345–2351

25. Masoudi FA, Wang Y, Inzucchi SE, Setaro JF, Havranek EP, Foody JM, Krumholz HM (2003) Metformin and thiazolidinedione use in Medicare patients with heart failure. JAMA 290:81–85

26. Masoudi FA, Inzucchi SE, Wang Y, Havranek EP, Foody JM, Krumholz HM (2005) Thiazolidinediones, metformin, and outcomes in older patients with diabetes and heart failure: an observational study. Circulation 111:583–590

27. Dormandy JA, Charbonnel B, Eckland DJ et al (2005) Secondary prevention of macrovascular events in patients with type 2 diabetes in the PROactive Study (PROspective pioglitAzone Clinical Trial In macroVascular Events): a randomised controlled trial. Lancet 366: 1279–1289

28. Bosch J, Yusuf S, Gerstein HC et al (2006) Effect of ramipril on the incidence of diabetes. N Engl J Med 355:1551–1562

29. Kahn SE, Haffner SM, Heise MA et al (2006) Glycemic durability of rosiglitazone, metformin, or glyburide monotherapy. N Engl J Med 355:2427–2443

30. Rutten FH, Moons KG, Cramer MJ, Grobbee DE, Zuithoff NP, Lammers JW, Hoes AW (2005) Recognising heart failure in elderly patients with stable chronic obstructive pulmonary disease in primary care: cross sectional diagnostic study. BMJ 331:1379

31. Mueller T, Gegenhuber A, Poelz W, Haltmayer M (2005) Diagnostic accuracy of B type natriuretic peptide and amino terminal proBNP in the emergency diagnosis of heart failure. Heart 91:606–612

32. Zaphiriou A, Robb S, Murray-Thomas T, Mendez G, Fox K, McDonagh T, Hardman SM, Dargie HJ, Cowie MR (2005) The diagnostic accuracy of plasma BNP and NTproBNP in patients referred from primary care with suspected heart failure: results of the UK natriuretic peptide study. Eur J Heart Fail 7:537–541

33. Macchia A, Monte S, Romero M, D'Ettorre A, Tognoni G (2007) The prognostic influence of chronic obstructive pulmonary disease in patients hospitalised for chronic heart failure. Eur J Heart Fail 9:942–948

34. Johnson M, Rennard S (2001) Alternative mechanisms for long-acting beta(2)-adrenergic agonists in COPD. Chest 120:258–270

35. Puri S, Dutka DP, Baker BL, Hughes JM, Cleland JG (1999) Acute saline infusion reduces alveolar-capillary membrane conductance and increases airflow obstruction in patients with left ventricular dysfunction. Circulation 99:1190–1196

36. Kotlyar E, Keogh AM, Macdonald PS, Arnold RH, McCaffrey DJ, Glanville AR (2002) Tolerability of carvedilol in patients with heart failure and concomitant chronic obstructive pulmonary disease or asthma. J Heart Lung Transplant 21:1290–1295

37. Salpeter SR, Ormiston TM, Salpeter EE (2002) Cardioselective beta-blockers in patients with reactive airway disease: a meta-analysis. Ann Intern Med 137:715–725

38. Agostoni P, Contini M, Cattadori G, Apostolo A, Sciomer S, Bussotti M, Palermo P, Fiorentini C (2007) Lung function with carvedilol and bisoprolol in chronic heart failure: is beta selectivity relevant? Eur J Heart Fail 9:827–833

39. McCullough PA (2002) Cardiorenal risk: an important clinical intersection. Rev Cardiovasc Med 3:71–76

40. Bongartz LG, Cramer MJ, Doevendans PA, Joles JA, Braam B (2005) The severe cardiorenal syndrome: 'Guyton revisited'. Eur Heart J 26:11–17

41. McAlister FA, Ezekowitz J, Tonelli M, Armstrong PW (2004) Renal insufficiency and heart failure: prognostic and therapeutic implications from a prospective cohort study. Circulation 109:1004–1009

42. Ezekowitz J, McAlister FA, Humphries KH, Norris CM, Tonelli M, Ghali WA, Knudtson ML (2004) The association among renal insufficiency, pharmacotherapy, and outcomes in 6, 427 patients with heart failure and coronary artery disease. J Am Coll Cardiol 44:1587–1592

43. Philbin EF, Santella RN, Rocco TA Jr (1999) Angiotensin-converting enzyme inhibitor use in older patients with heart failure and renal dysfunction. J Am Geriatr Soc 47:302–308

44. Erdmann E, Lechat P, Verkenne P, Wiemann H (2001) Results from post-hoc analyses of the CIBIS II trial: effect of bisoprolol in high-risk patient groups with chronic heart failure. Eur J Heart Fail 3:469–479

45. Cice G, Ferrara L, D'Andrea A, D'Isa S, Di BA, Cittadini A, Russo PE, Golino P, Calabro R (2003) Carvedilol increases two-year survival in dialysis patients with dilated cardiomyopathy: a prospective, placebo-controlled trial. J Am Coll Cardiol 41:1438–1444

46. Hunt SA, Abraham WT, Chin MH et al (2005) ACC/AHA 2005 Guideline Update for the Diagnosis and Management of Chronic Heart Failure in the Adult – Summary Article: a Report of the American College of Cardiology/American Heart Association Task Force on Practice Guidelines (Writing Committee to Update the 2001 Guidelines for the Evaluation and Management of Heart Failure): developed in collaboration with the American College of Chest Physicians and the International Society for Heart and Lung Transplantation: endorsed by the Heart Rhythm Society. Circulation 112:1825–1852

47. Juurlink DN, Mamdani MM, Lee DS, Kopp A, Austin PC, Laupacis A, Redelmeier DA (2004) Rates of hyperkalemia after publication of the Randomized Aldactone Evaluation Study. N Engl J Med 351:543–551

48. Masoudi FA, Gross CP, Wang Y, Rathore SS, Havranek EP, Foody JM, Krumholz HM (2005) Adoption of spironolactone therapy for older patients with heart failure and left ventricular systolic dysfunction in the United States, 1998–2001. Circulation 112:39–47

49. Merlo J, Broms K, Lindblad U et al (2001) Association of outpatient utilisation of non-steroidal anti-inflammatory drugs and hospitalised heart failure in the entire Swedish population. Eur J Clin Pharmacol 57:71–75

50. Androne AS, Katz SD, Lund L, LaManca J, Hudaihed A, Hryniewicz K, Mancini DM (2003) Hemodilution is common in patients with advanced heart failure. Circulation 107:226–229

51. Adlbrecht C, Kommata S, Hulsmann M et al (2008) Chronic heart failure leads to an expanded plasma volume and pseudoanaemia, but does not lead to a reduction in the body's red cell volume. Eur Heart J 29:2343–2350

52. Silverberg DS, Wexler D, Sheps D et al (2001) The effect of correction of mild anemia in severe, resistant congestive heart failure using subcutaneous erythropoietin and intravenous iron: a randomized controlled study. J Am Coll Cardiol 37:1775–1780

53. Silverberg DS, Wexler D, Blum M, et al (2002) The correction of anemia in severe resistant heart failure with erythropoietin and intravenous iron prevents the progression of both the heart and the renal failure and markedly reduces hospitalization. Clin Nephrol 58 Suppl 1:S37–S45

54. Mancini DM, Katz SD, Lang CC, LaManca J, Hudaihed A, Androne AS (2003) Effect of erythropoietin on exercise capacity in patients with moderate to severe chronic heart failure. Circulation 107:294–299

55. Ghali JK, Anand IS, Abraham WT et al (2008) Randomized double-blind trial of darbepoetin alfa in patients with symptomatic heart failure and anemia. Circulation 117:526–535

56. Singh AK, Szczech L, Tang KL, Barnhart H, Sapp S, Wolfson M, Reddan D (2006) Correction of anemia with epoetin alfa in chronic kidney disease. N Engl J Med 355:2085–2098

57. Almeida OP, Flicker L (2001) The mind of a failing heart: a systematic review of the association between congestive heart failure and cognitive functioning. Intern Med J 31:290–295

58. Zuccala G, Pedone C, Cesari M et al (2003) The effects of cognitive impairment on mortality among hospitalized patients with heart failure. Am J Med 115:97–103

59. Freedland KE, Rich MW, Skala JA, Carney RM, vila-Roman VG, Jaffe AS (2003) Prevalence of depression in hospitalized patients with congestive heart failure. Psychosom Med 65:119–128

60. Jiang W, Kuchibhatla M, Clary GL et al (2007) Relationship between depressive symptoms and long-term mortality in patients with heart failure. Am Heart J 154:102–108

61. Rutledge T, Reis VA, Linke SE, Greenberg BH, Mills PJ (2006) Depression in heart failure a meta-analytic review of prevalence, intervention effects, and associations with clinical outcomes. J Am Coll Cardiol 48:1527–1537

62. Joynt KE, Whellan DJ, O'Connor CM (2004) Why is depression bad for the failing heart? A review of the mechanistic relationship between depression and heart failure. J Card Fail 10:258–271

63. Rockwood K, Song X, MacKnight C, Bergman H, Hogan DB, McDowell I, Mitnitski A (2005) A global clinical measure of fitness and frailty in elderly people. CMAJ 173:489–495

64. Inouye SK, van Dyck CH, Alessi CA, Balkin S, Siegal AP, Horwitz RI (1990) Clarifying confusion: the confusion assessment method. A new method for detection of delirium. Ann Intern Med 113:941–948

65. McCusker J, Cole M, Bellavance F, Primeau F (1998) Reliability and validity of a new measure of severity of delirium. Int Psychogeriatr 10:421–433

66. Hachinski V, Iadecola C, Petersen RC et al (2006) National Institute of Neurological Disorders and Stroke-Canadian Stroke Network vascular cognitive impairment harmonization standards. Stroke 37:2220–2241

67. Nasreddine ZS, Phillips NA, Bedirian V et al (2005) The Montreal Cognitive Assessment, MoCA: a brief screening tool for mild cognitive impairment. J Am Geriatr Soc 53:695–699

68. Kjekshus J (1990) Arrhythmias and mortality in congestive heart failure. Am J Cardiol 65:42I–48I

69. Allessie MA, Boyden PA, Camm AJ et al (2001) Pathophysiology and prevention of atrial fibrillation. Circulation 103:769–777

70. Krahn AD, Manfreda J, Tate RB, Mathewson FA, Cuddy TE (1995) The natural history of atrial fibrillation: incidence, risk factors, and prognosis in the Manitoba Follow-Up Study. Am J Med 98:476–484

71. Benjamin EJ, Wolf PA, D'Agostino RB, Silbershatz H, Kannel WB, Levy D (1998) Impact of atrial fibrillation on the risk of death: the Framingham Heart Study. Circulation 98:946–952

72. Knight BP (2003) Atrial fibrillation in patients with congestive heart failure. Pacing Clin Electrophysiol 26:1620–1623

73. Maisel WH, Stevenson LW (2003) Atrial fibrillation in heart failure: epidemiology, pathophysiology, and rationale for therapy. Am J Cardiol 91:2D–8D

74. Efremidis M, Pappas L, Sideris A, Filippatos G (2008) Management of atrial fibrillation in patients with heart failure. J Card Fail 14:232–237

75. Feinberg WM, Blackshear JL, Laupacis A, Kronmal R, Hart RG (1995) Prevalence, age distribution, and gender of patients with atrial fibrillation. Analysis and implications. Arch Intern Med 155:469–473

76. Packer M, Bristow MR, Cohn JN, Colucci WS, Fowler MB, Gilbert EM, Shusterman NH (1996) The effect of carvedilol on morbidity and mortality in patients with chronic heart failure. U.S. Carvedilol Heart Failure Study Group. N Engl J Med 334:1349–1355

77. Kannel WB, Wolf PA, Benjamin EJ, Levy D (1998) Prevalence, incidence, prognosis, and predisposing conditions for atrial fibrillation: population-based estimates. Am J Cardiol 82:2N–9N

78. Ravelli F, Allessie M (1997) Effects of atrial dilatation on refractory period and vulnerability to atrial fibrillation in the isolated Langendorff-perfused rabbit heart. Circulation 96:1686–1695

79. Laurent G, Moe GW, Hu X et al (2008) Simultaneous right atrio-ventricular pacing: a novel model to study atrial remodeling and fibrillation in the setting of heart failure. J Card Fail 14:254–262

80. Laurent G, Moe G, Hu X et al (2008) Experimental studies of atrial fibrillation: a comparison of two pacing models. Am J Physiol Heart Circ Physiol 294:H1206–H1215

81. Moe GW, Laurent G, Doumanovskaia L, Konig A, Hu X, Dorian P (2008) Matrix metalloproteinase inhibition attenuates atrial remodeling and vulnerability to atrial fibrillation in a canine model of heart failure. J Card Fail 14:768–776

82. Olsson LG, Swedberg K, Ducharme A et al (2006) Atrial fibrillation and risk of clinical events in chronic heart failure with and without left ventricular systolic dysfunction: results from the Candesartan in Heart failure-Assessment of Reduction in Mortality and morbidity (CHARM) program. J Am Coll Cardiol 47:1997–2004

83. Dries DL, Exner DV, Gersh BJ, Domanski MJ, Waclawiw MA, Stevenson LW (1998) Atrial fibrillation is associated with an increased risk for mortality and heart failure progression in patients with asymptomatic and symptomatic left ventricular systolic dysfunction: a retrospective analysis of the SOLVD trials. Studies of Left Ventricular Dysfunction. J Am Coll Cardiol 32:695–703

84. Pozzoli M, Cioffi G, Traversi E, Pinna GD, Cobelli F, Tavazzi L (1998) Predictors of primary atrial fibrillation and concomitant clinical and hemodynamic changes in patients with chronic heart failure: a prospective study in 344 patients with baseline sinus rhythm. J Am Coll Cardiol 32:197–204

85. Wyse DG, Waldo AL, DiMarco JP et al (2002) A comparison of rate control and rhythm control in patients with atrial fibrillation. N Engl J Med 347:1825–1833

86. Roy D, Talajic M, Nattel S et al (2008) Rhythm control versus rate control for atrial fibrillation and heart failure. N Engl J Med 358:2667–2677

87. Howlett JG, McKelvie RS, Arnold JM et al (2009) Canadian Cardiovascular Society Consensus Conference guidelines on heart failure, update 2009: diagnosis and management of right-sided heart failure, myocarditis, device therapy and recent important clinical trials. Can J Cardiol 25:85–105

Chapter 14
Mechanisms and Clinical Recognition and Management of Heart Failure in Infants and Children

Overview

Compared to heart failure (HF) in the adult, a paucity of both basic science and clinical research exists for pediatric-related HF. The etiology of HF in this population differs, and presentation and management are affected by developmental changes in physiology and biochemistry. This chapter on Heart Failure in Children will provide focus on specific areas of interest in the field, which differ from HF in adults. Issues in development mechanisms are highlighted, as well as different treatment modalities.

Introduction

Since the 1960s rheumatic heart disease has declined in the United States and developed countries. Rheumatic valve disease has almost disappeared as a cause of HF in these populations, although it maintains high prevalence in certain developing countries. Although they occur in children, ischemic and primary cardiomyopathies are also relatively rare causes of congestive HF. Instead, congenital heart defects (CHD) cause the majority of HF cases in the pediatric age group. The mechanisms of HF then differ substantially from the adult population. Ventricular volume and pressure overload are major contributors and alter responses to stress and to medications in children. In 2002, the U.S. Congress passed the Best Pharmaceuticals for Children Act. Although, the intent of this legislation was to spur a significant increase in the number of pediatric studies of pharmaceuticals, the majority of cardiovascular drugs are used off-label in children, and research lags behind pharmaceuticals for adults. Nevertheless, important progress has been made, particularly in the areas of mechanical circulatory support and cardiac transplant.

Etiology of Heart Failure in Children

There are numerous and diverse etiologies for congestive heart failure in children, which differ substantially from the primary causes in adults. CHD is the principal cause in the pediatric population. CHD represents a fairly heterogeneous group of defects with variable presentations. Large left to right shunts caused by ventricular septal defects (VSD), either isolated or in combination with other heart anomalies, predominate. Isolated VSDs are surgically correctable and HF is often reversible after intervention. Left- or right-sided obstructive lesions can also cause HF in this age group. Subsets of these lesions are not totally correctable, and may be treated with palliative staged surgeries. Chronic HF can ensue, sometimes years after surgical correction. Primary cardiomyopathies are the etiology for HF in a relatively small subset of children. This is a heterogeneous group and will be reviewed later. Collagen vascular disease, drug-induced cardiomyopathy (anthracycline), and infection-induced (HIV) syndrome all occur in children. These will not be discussed in this chapter except when they relate to specific management issues in children. HF from ischemic cardiomyopathy occurs only rarely in children, and results mainly from Kawasaki disease, an inflammatory coronary vasculitis, or rarely from anomalous origin of the left coronary artery.

The principles of treatment for congestive HF (CHF) in infants, children, and even adolescents differ substantially from those operative in adults. These differences relate to altered mechanisms of HF and extend to the goals of therapy. Treatment in adults is directed toward reducing the risk of mortality and improving the quality of life. However, childhood is a period of growth and development, and therapy is also directed at maintaining these at normal rates. Quality of life is an issue, but in some cases it is poorly defined. Clinical HF scoring schemes have limited utility in children. Neither the New York Heart Association classification nor The American Heart Association and the American College of Cardiology Classification of Heart Failure are generally applicable to infants and children. Furthermore, quality of life is often judged from the parent's perspective as opposed to the patient's.

Validation of quality-of-life measures need to be age-specific and developmentally specific. The heterogeneity of the population and the etiology of HF in children make validation difficult. Most children with HF also undergo surgery

J. Marín-García, *Heart Failure*, Contemporary Cardiology,
DOI 10.1007/978-1-60761-147-9_14, © Springer Science+Business Media, LLC 2010

for CHD. Therefore, it is difficult to separate out surgical factors causing CHF. Classification in pediatric patients is also difficult to establish because the range of age encompasses different developmental ages with widely diverse exercise capabilities and cardiovascular physiology. In 1992, Ross and associates suggested a scoring system for infants incorporating feeding patterns and physical examination findings [1]. The Ross classification (Tables 14.1–14.3) evolved into a more sophisticated classification, which paralleled the New York Heart Association classification scheme. This classification corresponds to incremental increases in plasma norepinephrine level, which decreased on resolution by surgical or medical therapy. Reithman et al. developed another HF score for a wider range of age groups, which included clinical values and showed significantly decreased post-receptor adenylate cyclase activity in children with scores greater than 6 [2]. The Reithman and Ross methods have been merged and used in clinical research investigations, though not in any clinical trials. Attempts have been made to correlate levels of N-terminal pro-brain peptide with these scores [3]. Recent data show that changes in these scores do correlate with serial changes in echocardiographic indices and brain natriuretic peptide (BNP), although the absolute numbers show great variability [4, 5].

Table 14.1 Ross scoring system of heart failure in infants

	0 points	1 point	2 points
Volume per feed (oz)	>3.5	2.5–3.5	<2.5
Time per feed (min)	<40 min	>40 min	
Respiratory rate	<50/min	50–60/min	>60/min
Respiratory pattern	Normal	Abnormal	
Peripheral perfusion	Normal	Decreased	
S_3 or diastolic rumble	Absent	Present	
Liver edge form costal margin	<2 cm	2–3 cm	>3 cm
Totals			
No CHF	0–2 points		
Mild CHF	3–6 points		
Moderate CHF	7–9 points		
Severe CHF	10–12 points		

CHF congestive heart failure

Table 14.2 Ross classification of heart failure in infants

Class I	No limitations or symptoms
Class II	Mild tachypnea or diaphoresis with feeding in infants Dyspnea on exertion in older children
Class III	No growth failure Marked tachypnea or diaphoresis with feeds or exertion Prolonged feeding times Growth failure from CHF
Class IV	Symptoms at rest with tachypnea, retractions, grunting, or diaphoresis

CHF congestive heart failure

Table 14.3 Pediatric clinical heart failure score

	Score (points)		
	0	1	2
History			
Diaphoresis	Head only	Head and body during exercise	Head and body at rest
Tachypnea	Rare	Several times	Frequent
Physical examination			
Breathing	Normal	Retractions	Dyspnea
Respiratory rate/min			
0–1 year	<50	50–60	>60
1–6 years	<35	35–45	>45
7–10 years	<25	25–35	>35
11–14 years	<18	18–28	>28
Heart			
0–1 year	<160	160–170	>170
1–6 years	<105	105–115	>115
7–10 years	<90	90–100	>100
11–14 years	<80	80–90	>90
Liver edge from costal margin	<2 cm	2–3 cm	>3 cm

Growth and Nutrition

In contrast to clinical grading systems, growth is an objective benchmark of HF in childhood. Growth retardation in infancy has been defined as underweight <10 percentile for age. In some cases, a dramatic drop off in the weight for age curve indicates growth retardation. Treatment of CHF, particularly in infancy and childhood is directed at maintaining somatic growth and development at normal or near normal rates. The prevalence of malnutrition and growth retardation in infants and children with heart disease is fairly high. In infancy growth failure occurs commonly with large left to right shunts. Growth retardation has been studied in specific subgroups of children and infants with CHD and CHF [6]. Relatively little study has occurred in children with cardiomyopathy. The etiology of growth failure, even in nonsyndromic children with CHF, is multifactorial. Poor calorie intake may be responsible [7]. However, total daily energy expenditure is increased in infants with CHF between 2 and 8 months of age [8]. Furthermore, these infants lose a substantial calorie content through vomiting, approximately 12% of calories measured in one study. The increase in children with CHD and CHF in total daily energy expenditure can vary and may depend on superimposing factors such as hypoxia and anemia, which reduce oxygen-carrying capacity. For instance, Leitch et al. found mean total daily energy expenditure to be increased by 29%.

Multiple mechanisms are responsible for this increase in total daily energy expenditure in infants and children with CHF, although some require further clarification. Infants with

CHF exhibit higher fat-free mass, which has greater energy expenditure per gram than fat mass. However, this disproportionate mass can be explained somewhat by higher total body water in infants with CHF. Alternatively, disturbances in metabolism may contribute to growth retardation. Lundell et al. found increased insulin secretion in combination with low plasma insulin after glucose loading in infants with VSD [9]. Those results imply that enhanced insulin extraction or peripheral binding occur in these patients [9]. Children with CHF, which was caused by a VSD, showed disturbances in fatty acid metabolism or clearance after intravenous lipid loading. In particular, linoleic acid remained fairly high after loading, illustrating a defect in fatty acid transport into tissue [10]. However, the cellular and endocrine mechanisms contributing to growth failure in children with CHF caused by congenital heart defects still require elucidation.

Growth retardation plays a major role in determining management strategy for patients with CHD with CHF. Early surgical correction is indicated for some defects. The elevations in total daily energy expenditure and growth retardation can be reversed by successful surgical repair [6]. However, for those who are not early surgical repair candidates, increased energy intake above that for normal children is required to accommodate for elevated energy expenditure and calorie loss through vomiting. For many infants and children these requirements cannot be met orally and nasogastric feeding is required.

As noted, cardiomyopathy is relatively rare in children. Epidemiological data collection is ongoing by the Pediatric Cardiomyopathy Registry (PCMR) funded by the National Institutes of Health [11]. Currently, data from more than 3,000 children with cardiomyopathy have been entered in the PCMR database with annual follow-up continuing until death, heart transplant, or loss-to-follow up. Using PCMR data, the incidence of cardiomyopathy in two large regions of the United States was estimated to be 1.13 cases per 100,000 children at the last published report [11]. Only 1/3 of children had a known etiology at the time of cardiomyopathy diagnosis. The published reports do not define the clinical status of the patients. However, freedom from death and mortality for dilated cardiomyopathy (DCM) is shown in Figs. 14.1–14.3.

Five-year freedom from death and transplant was lowest for patients from the idiopathic subgroup. Children aged 6 years or older were more likely to die or receive heart transplant compared with younger children ($p < 0.001$). Using multivariate Cox regression modeling, after exclusion of patients with neuromuscular disease and inborn metabolic errors, DCM patients with an idiopathic diagnosis (compared to known diagnosis), the presence of CHF at diagnosis, and decreased left ventricular shortening fraction z-score were significant predictors of the composite endpoint of death or receive heart transplantation.

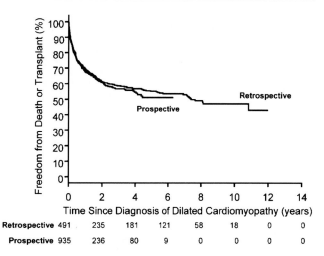

| Retrospective | 491 | 235 | 181 | 121 | 58 | 18 | 0 | 0 |
| Prospective | 935 | 236 | 80 | 9 | 0 | 0 | 0 | 0 |

Fig. 14.1 Estimated freedom from death or transplant for patients with pure dilated cardiomyopathy. ($p = 0.710$) by cohort (retrospective: diagnosed 1990 to 1995, 491 patients; prospective: diagnosed 1996 to 2002, 935 patients) (From Wilkinson et al. [11]. Reprinted with kind permission from Elsevier)

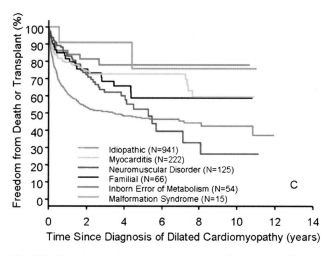

Fig. 14.2 Freedom from death or transplantation for patients with pure dilated cardiomyopathy by diagnosis (From Wilkinson et al. [11]. Reprinted with kind permission from Elsevier)

The investigators concluded that outcomes for children with DCM depend on cause, age at diagnosis, and HF at presentation. Unfortunately most children do not have a defined cause for DCM, which limits the application of disease-specific therapy.

Clinical outcomes (death or heart transplantation) were reported based on an analysis of 849 patients with hypertrophic cardiomyopathy (HCM). The causal subgroups were idiopathic (75%), malformation syndromes (9%), inborn errors of metabolism (9%), and neuromuscular disorders (8%). For HCM, survival was significantly lower for patients less than 1 year of age at diagnosis in the inborn errors of metabolism and idiopathic groups (Fig. 14.3) compared with

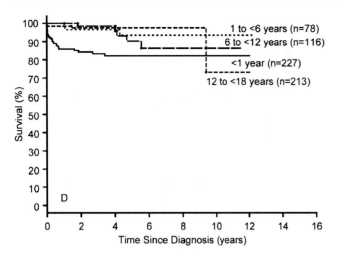

Fig. 14.3 Survival rates by age at diagnosis from the diagnosis of idiopathic hypertrophic cardiomyopathy (From Wilkinson et al. [11]. Reprinted with kind permission from Elsevier)

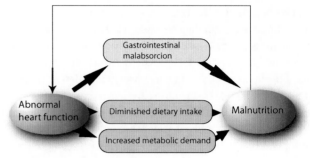

Fig. 14.4 The vicious cycle (Reprinted from Miller et al. [12]. With kind permission from Elsevier)

those aged 1 year or older. For the total cohort of HCM cases, there was a large peak in mortality between 0 and 2 years of age with a smaller peak for patients aged 12–16 years. In conclusion, children diagnosed at less than 1 year of age have the poorest outcomes and the widest spectrum of etiologies. For children who survive beyond 1 year of age, the annual mortality rate (1%) is lower than has been previously reported in children and is similar to results from adult studies.

Although the etiology of growth failure in CHD has been examined, a paucity of work exists for pediatric cardiomyopathy. This relates to issues noted above concerning disease specific research. Nevertheless, growth failure is recognized as a significant clinical problem for children with cardiomyopathy. Miller et al. stated that one-third of children with this disorder manifest some degree of growth failure during the course of their illness [12]. In a recent international study, Azevedo determined that progressive weight z-score was positively and independently correlated with survival in a chart review of 165 children with DCM between 1979 and 2003. Other than that study little information regarding nutritional state and clinical outcome exists for cardiomyopathy.

In adults chronic HF is associated with marked insulin resistance, characterized by both fasting and stimulated hyperinsulinemia. Insulin resistance increases in advanced HF, but this is not directly mediated through ventricular dysfunction or increased catecholamine levels. A decrease in skeletal muscle glucose-transporter-4 may be partially responsible for this HF-induced peripheral insulin resistance, noted in nondiabetic patients.

The underlying cause of growth failure is usually due to persistent CHF as a result of an overall poor response to medical treatment. Significant cardiac dysfunction in these children can result in increased metabolic demands, decreased

food intake, and malabsorption of important nutrients. Growth failure or malnutrition in children can lead to problems in virtually every organ system, with many of the effects only partially reversible [12]. Thus cardiomyopathy may lead to growth problems, but growth problems can lead to further complications that may directly or indirectly impact on heart function, leading to a vicious downward cycle (Fig. 14.4).

These clinical manifestations indicate that growth patterns may be an important predictor of the outcomes among cardiomyopathy patients or an important indicator of the severity of their cardiomyopathy. If this is so, then it becomes apparent that clinicians should be vigilant regarding treatment issues surrounding growth. The relationship between growth patterns and echocardiographic findings is unknown.

Clinical Signs and Symptoms

The clinical signs and symptoms of HF vary according to age. These signs become similar to those apparent in the adult as adolescence approaches, and these are discussed in other chapters. Here, we focus on the particular specific clinical presentation of CHF in the younger age groups. The age of HF presentation varies according to the specific etiology. Volume overload from extracardiac and intracardiac left to right lesions or pressure overload from obstructive lesions predominates as the cause for CHF in the first year of life. However, other primary etiologies include intrinsic cardiac muscle abnormalities, rhythm disturbances such as supraventricular tachycardia or atrioventricular conduction block. Systemic abnormalities which cause abnormalities in metabolic demand such as anemia, hypoxia, or sepsis can also cause HF in children.

Fetal Heart Failure

Decreased fetal movement can be noted when the fetus is in HF, and represents one of the few apparent clinical signs, which can be detected by the mother. Hydrops fetalis, excess fetal water associated with pleural and pericardial effusions with or without ascites, and identified by ultrasound indicates end-stage HF. However, clinical recognition of HF in the fetus depends primarily on accurate assessment by Doppler and echocardiography. The primary etiologies for CHF in the fetus are noted in Table 14.4 [13].

Table 14.4 Etiology of fetal heart failure

	Proportion of all cases (%)
Cause of hydrops unclear	26.3
Isoimmunization	4.5
Rh isoimmunization	4.2
Other	
Nonimmune	69.2
Congenital heart disease	13.7
Cardiomyopathy	3.8
Ebstein anomaly	2.3
Complex congenital heart disease (specific abnormality not reported)	1.3
Coarctation of aorta	1.2
Hypoplastic left heart	0.8
Hypoplastic right heart	0.8
Other heart defects	
Dysrhythmias	10.4
Supraventricular tachycardia	7.2
Fetal dysrhythmias	1.3
Wolff–Parkinson–White syndrome	1
Other heart rate anomalies	
Twin-to-twin transfusion	9
Congenital anomalies	8.7
Syndrome not defined	3.5
Cystic hygroma	1.7
Other anomalies	
Chromosomal abnormality	7.5
Trisomy 21g	5
Other chromosomal anomalies	
Anemia	5
Unknown cause for anemia (nonimmune)	3
Fetal-maternal transfusion	1.2
Thalassemia	0.8
Congenital chylothorax	3.2
Other	5
Fetal demise of twin or triplet	0.8
Inborn error of metabolism	0.8
Other	
Viral	6.7
Viral infection reported but organism not reported	2.8
Parvovirus	1.5
Cytomegalovirus	1.3
Other viral	1.4

Congenital cardiomegaly, $n=4$; aortic valve stenosis, $n=3$; atrioventricular canal, $n=3$; pulmonary valve atresia, $n=2$; pulmonary valve stenosis, $n=2$; truncus arteriosus, $n=2$; double-outlet right ventricle, $n=1$; right ventricular hypertrophy, $n=1$; single ventricle, $n=1$; total anomalous pulmonary venous return, $n=1$

Fetal circulation differs from postnatal as the ventricles pump in parallel with the left ventricle supplying the aorta and upper body and the right ventricle pumping to the ductus arteriosus and the lower body and placenta (Fig. 14.5).

The pulmonary vascular bed has high resistance in utero and the placenta supplies oxygenated blood through the ductus venous. Distribution of combined cardiac ventricular output in utero is noted in Fig. 14.6.

The parallel vascular circuits intersect at the aortic isthmus. In the case of obstruction from either side, the other side usually accommodates by increasing work. In the past except in rare cases, such as severe regurgitation associated with Ebstein's anomaly of the tricuspid valve, hearts with congenital malformations were thought to accommodate in utero. However, in recent years, ultrasound studies of human fetuses and experimental studies of fetal lambs with simulated lesions have demonstrated that congenital cardiac anomalies may drastically affect the fetal circulation and fetal development and even survival [14]. In some cases, fetal intervention has been attempted such as atrial septectomy for severely restrictive atrial septum in hypoplastic left heart syndrome [15].

Studies in animal models indicate that the fetal heart reacts differently in response to preload and afterload changes. The fetal myocardium exhibits reduced compliance and operates

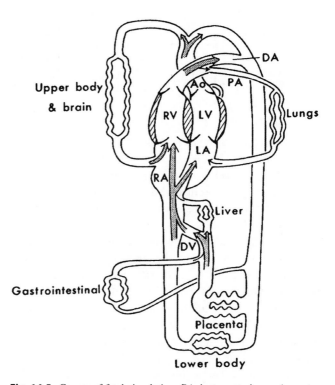

Fig. 14.5 Course of fetal circulation. *DA* ductus arteriosus; *Ao* aorta; *PA* pulmonary artery; *RV* right ventricle; *LA* left atrium; *RA* right atrium; *DV* ductus venosus (Reprinted from Rudolph AM (1977) Pediatrics. Appleton Century-Crofts, New York, p 1351. With kind permission of McGraw-Hill)

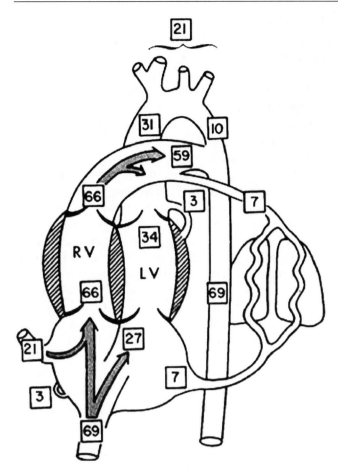

Fig. 14.6 Percentage of combined ventricular output ejected by the left ventricle (LV) and right ventricle (RV) and passing through major vascular channels are shown (numbers in *squares*) (Modified from Rudolph AM (1977) Pediatrics. Appleton Century-Crofts, New York, p 1351. With kind permission of McGraw-Hill)

near the peak of the Frank–Starling curve [16]. The fetal heart is also extremely sensitive to changes in afterload. The right ventricular afterload is determined mainly by the vascular bed of the placenta. Animal studies also show that the fetal myocardium develops less active tension than adult at similar fiber lengths. This reduction in fetal animals is attributed to structural differences such as fewer t-tubules and less organized myofibrils, as well as alterations in calcium handling. In human fetus, shifts in myosin heavy chain (MHC) profile from adult may explain some of these differences in contractility and active tension. The fetal heart shows predominance of MHC-β, which also achieves more prominence in the failing adult heart [17]. Accordingly, the fetal heart demonstrates reduced ability to increase ventricular stroke volume in response to stress. This leaves heart rate variation as the major mechanism for adjusting cardiac output. The fetal heart rate ranges between 50 and 200 beats/min.

As the right ventricle contributes the major work output in the fetus, the earliest signs of altered function relate to right heart hemodynamics. The right ventricle shows varying responses to heart rate change, which depend on mode of stimulation. While pacing the right or left atrium actually decreases end-diastolic and stroke volume, spontaneous elevations in heart rate increase both these parameters, thereby increasing cardiac output [18]. The fetal heart does demonstrate adrenoreceptor responsiveness although autonomic innervation develops throughout gestation. Thus the physiological response to stress may differ according to gestational age.

The factors noted above affect the development and presentation of fetal heart failure. Reduced contractility, compliance, adrenergic responsiveness, and greater dependence on heart rate to increase cardiac output all contribute to enhanced susceptibility of the fetus for development of HF. As noted, fetal hydrops is the major sign for end-staged HF in the fetus. However, data show that 13.7% of hydrops is caused by CHD or cardiomyopathy with another 10.4% caused by a rhythm disorder (see Table 14.4).

Several features contribute to fluid accumulation in fetal tissue and lead to elevation in ventricular end-diastolic pressure, atrial pressure, and central venous pressure. Umbilical venous pressure elevation correlates with cardiothoracic ratio. Therefore, any modest increase in this pressure moderates cardiac function. As the foramen ovale provides a large communication between the left atrium and systemic veins, the volume loading causes systemic venous hypertension regardless of whether there is insufficiency of a mitral, a tricuspid, or a common atrioventricular valve [19]. The systemic venous pressure hypertension coupled with low colloid osmotic pressure promotes edema and hydrops in the fetus. The physiologic low fetal serum albumin level may be further lowered by decreased hepatic albumin formation in the presence of retrograde inferior vena caval flow and loss of albumin into the extravascular space. The finding of umbilical venous pulsations by echocardiography is the most useful predictor of impending perinatal death in fetal hydrops.

While assessing the fetus, it is usually not adequate to evaluate for the signs and severity of HF, even though the final common pathway leading to fetal demise may be cardiac dysfunction. Hofstaetter et al. have recommended combining the cardiovascular profile score (CVPS) [20] with selected parameters of the biophysical profile [21, 22]. The CVPS is composed of 2 points in each of five categories used in serial studies to provide a method of uniform physiological assessment. A score of ten indicates no abnormality, and points are deducted to a maximum of two for each of five categories. Abnormalities in the cardiovascular profile may occur before hydrops fetalis is recognized. The five categories are: (1) hydrops, (2) umbilical venous Doppler, (3) heart size, (4) abnormal myocardial function, (5) arterial Doppler.

Hydrops

Hydrops may manifest with ascites, pleural effusion, pericardial effusion, or a combination of these. Advanced hydrops is accompanied by skin edema seen over the scalp and abdominal wall.

Umbilical Venous Doppler

Alterations in central venous flow blood velocity patterns reflect abnormalities in cardiac hemodynamics. Increased velocity of blood flow reversal away from the heart during atrial contraction occurs in the fetus with CHF and may indicate increased ventricular end-diastolic pressure. Pulsed Doppler sampling should be obtained in inferior vena cava (IVC), ductus venosus, the umbilical vein in the abdomen and the umbilical cord vein. The CVPS allows deductions for abnormal venous Doppler flow with 1 point deducted for ductus venosus atrial reversal and 2 points for umbilical venous pulsations.

Heart Size

Cardiomegaly occurs in the fetus as a consistent sign of CHF, although the mechanism for cardiac enlargement is not totally understood. The right atrium is the common chamber noted to dilate as the final pathway for blood flow returning to the heart, and can be enlarged in several clinical scenarios including foramen obstruction, volume overload, and tricuspid regurgitation. Right atrial dilation may occur secondary to increased right ventricular end-diastolic pressure. Small heart size can occur with external compression and is also a poor prognostic sign. Cardiomegaly by two-dimensional echocardiography is heart chest area ratio greater than 0.35 at any time in gestation (−1 point), and severe cardiomegaly defined as >0.5 (−2 points).

The CVPS incorporates a scoring component for myocardial function, although this assessment remains somewhat qualitative (a fetal CPVS profile is presented in Figure 14.7). Huhta et al. [22] have suggested subtraction based on points relating to valvular regurgitation and shortening fraction of both right and left ventricles. Nevertheless, shortening fraction depends on ventricular geometry, which does not fit adult configuration in utero. Myocardial performance index (MPI), known as the Tei index, provides assessment of right or left ventricular performance. This Doppler derived index encompasses both systolic and diastolic performance, is not subject to changes in ventricular dimension, and is afterload independent. The Tei index is the isovolemic time divided by the ejection time. The isovolemic time is determined by subtracting the ejection time of either the left or right ventricle (aortic or pulmonary outflow) by atrioventricular valve inflow time (time of AV valve closure to opening). The MPI has been validated for both systemic and pulmonary vascular circuits, and can be used for assessment of fetal right heart function. Less quantitative analyses include Doppler indication of tricuspid regurgitation. Trivial regurgitation in utero shows no prognostic significance, while holosystolic regurgitation implies severe but potentially reversible CHF in some clinical scenarios such as anemia or supraventricular tachycardia. Holosystolic mitral regurgitation implies severe left ventricular dysfunction in utero, and can be noted with cardiomyopathy or rhythm disturbance. Importantly, color Doppler indication of valve dysfunction requires substantiation by careful pulse Doppler interrogation. Right or left ventricular

Category	Score 2	Score 1	Score 0
Hydrops	None	Ascites, pleural or pericardial effusion	Skin edema
Cardiomegaly (cardiac/thoracic area)	> 0.20 and < 0.35	0.35-0.50	> 0.5 or < 0.20
Cardiac function	Normal TV and MV biphasic diastolic filling	Holosystolic TR	Holosystolic MR, monophasic diastolic filling
Arterial Umbilical Doppler	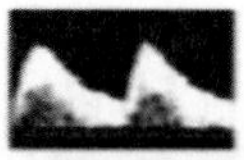	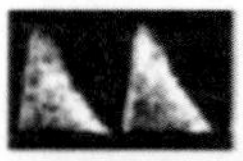	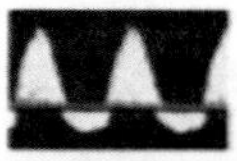
Venous Doppler UV and DV	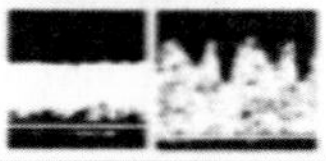	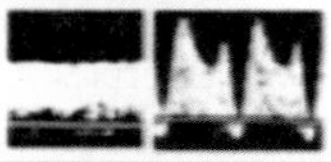	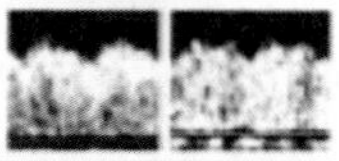

TV: Tricuspid Valve; MV: Mitral valve; TR: Tricuspid regurgitation; UV: Umbilical vein
DV: Ductus venosus

Fig. 14.7 Fetal Cardiovascular profile adapted from Hofstaetter et al [20]

diastolic function similar to postnatal heart can be assessed by comparing the A and E filling patterns. The A Doppler wave is normally higher than the E wave, and reversal implies abnormality in diastolic filling with a monophasic filling wave indicating severe diastolic dysfunction, these components are all considered in the CVPS under the cardiac function component, but still remain subjective and require considerable validation.

Arterial Doppler remains the final component for the CVPS. Elevations in umbilical arterial resistance will reduce diastolic inflow. Substantial increases in this resistance with brain sparing defined by absent diastolic flow with elevated diastolic velocity in the middle cerebral artery are signs of impending HF and together score −1 point on the CVPS. Reversed end-diastolic flow in the umbilical artery scores −2 points.

Treatment of Fetal Heart Failure

Medical management of fetal HF obviously depends on the etiology. Systemic etiologies of HF include anemia secondary to isoimmunization or twin to twin transfusion. In the latter the twin receiving transfusion also displays a high output state leading to failure due to increased blood volume, polycythemia, and elevated umbilical arterial impedance. Fetal interventional procedures such as laser treatment are currently being performed, as is umbilical venous transfusion for the anemic twin. Medical management does include maternal treatment with digoxin with variable response in high output HF states including fetal to fetal transfusion and arteriovenous fistula. Huhta et al. [22] recommends 0.2 mg orally two to four times a day based on maternal drug levels and suggest a trough level 1–2 ng/dl. These recommendations are based on anecdotal experience rather than evidence through clinical trials. Some benefits may exist for failure with ventricular volume overloading generated by severe semilunar or atrioventricular valve regurgitation.

As noted previously, catheter induced interventions have been used with variable success in the fetus for some CHD. Technical problems have not been totally solved and indications are yet unclear and need to be more fully developed.

Neonatal Heart Failure

Multiple physiological and bioenergetic mechanisms operate together in determining timing and impact of increased stress on the newborn and infant heart. Timing of HF in infants, particularly for CHD, depends substantially on decline in pulmonary vascular resistance (PVR) and other postnatal physiological changes. The first postnatal breath reduces pulmonary compliance and initiates the normal drop in pulmonary vascular resistance which decreases 50% by day 1 with progressive decline to adult levels at 2–6 weeks. Though drop in PVR is initiated mechanically by filling lungs with the first breath, which reduces compression of the pulmonary vasculature, it is also modulated by changing concentrations of vasoactive substances such as bradykinin, endothelin, prostaglandins and nitric oxide, as well as increased concentration of oxygen in blood. The alterations in circulation led to an increase in pulmonary venous return and left atrial pressure. Systemic vascular resistance concomitantly increases as the ductus arteriosus closes generally within the first 12–18 h after birth. Some of these circulatory changes are delayed in CHD associated with high pressure transmission to the pulmonary bed, most notably large VSD. Delay in the postnatal drop in PVR also occurs with cyanotic lesions due to decreased oxygen concentration. Thus, transposition of the great arteries or tricuspid atresia with large VSD or truncus arteriosus all show marked persistence of high pulmonary vascular resistance.

The eventual drop in PVR increases flow to the pulmonary bed and left atrium. These changes elevate alveolar capillary bed hydrostatic pressure and promote fluid movement across the interstitium and into the alveolar space. Additionally, engorged pulmonary arterial vessels can compress small airways in infants leading to actelectasis. These changes result in tachypnea and systemic desaturation, which are the hallmark symptoms of CHF in the neonate.

Echocardiography is the principal mode of diagnosis, and identifies structural and functional abnormalities in the neonate and older children. It should be noted that echocardiographic measures of systolic and diastolic function change with age and body surface area. The period of most rapid change occurs during the first 4 years of life. In normal healthy children, age and heart rate have been shown to account for variations in the mitral E/A velocity ratio, peak A velocity, and atrial filling contribution. These developmental changes should be considered in any evaluation for HF in infants or children and standardization data for age and body surface area are available in the literature [23–25].

A number of changes occur in myocardial structure and function during fetal and neonatal life, which modify the ability of the heart to deal with stress including volume and pressure overload. However, data documenting these changes are somewhat inconsistent, due to variability in species and experimental conditions. Data in lambs show that the ability of the heart to increase output in response to volume loading increases with age. This implies reduced ventricular compliance in the newborn lamb [26] and a reduced capability to compensate to volume or pressure stress. The neonatal heart also shortens more slowly against the same afterload as the adult. This may be due to differences within single fibers, as sarcomere shortening velocities are greater in the adult myocyte than in the neonatal [27].

Ventricular interdependence differs markedly in the newborn considering the dominance and size of the right ventricle. Ventricular interdependence relates to the change in performance of one ventricle caused by changes in the other ventricle via displacement of the septum. Developmental changes in ventricular interdependence are particularly important during pressure or volume loading caused by CHD. There are several operative mechanisms for ventricular interdependence. The heart is enclosed in the minimally compliant pericardial sac with little free space to accommodate ventricular dilation. As a result dilation of either ventricle limits filling of the other to the point that diastolic indices are modified. In a rabbit model under anesthesia and open pericardial exposure elevation in right ventricular (RV) diastolic volume decreased left ventricular (LV) diastolic volume secondary to decreased diastolic compliance, but with no change in systolic performance [28]. These relationships have been worked out in patients with right ventricular volume overloading, though no specific study in left ventricular volume loading associated with left to right shunts has been published to date. Diastolic filling abnormalities occur with right ventricular volume overloading occurring through atrial septal defects. The relaxation constant tau for the left ventricle is prolonged in patients with large shunts providing chronic right ventricular volume overload [29]. However, Walker et al. evaluated the acute alterations in interdependence caused by transcatheter closure of atrial septal defects [30]. This model provided was ideal for studying acute reductions in RV volume overload without the confounding factors of surgery including anesthesia and with intact pericardium. LV systolic function also improves acutely after removing the RV volume load. The study indicated that the mechanisms for decreased LV performance associated with RV volume overload include the mechanical disadvantage of a noncircular short-axis configuration and changes in chamber and myocardial preload. Septal occlusion increased LV end-diastolic volume and circumference, the latter a surrogate of myocardial preload. Septal occlusion eliminated inefficiency in energy expenditure caused by geometric reconfiguration during systole. Thus, the developing heart with limited systolic and diastolic functional reserve is also stressed by geometric changes induced by abnormal ventricular interdependence.

Developmental Changes in Cardiac Energy Metabolism

Reduced efficiency in energy utilization caused by relatively poor ventricular compliance and geometric changes associated with ventricular interdependence in the newborn are further complicated by changes in cardiac energy metabolism, which occur during transition after birth. These transitions in regulation of myocardial ATP production and substrate utilization can modify the ability of the newborn heart to adapt to stress.

The lamb heart has been the primary model for studying myocardial energy metabolism in vivo during development. Myocardial oxidative phosphorylation and mitochondrial membrane transport systems efficiently supply ATP for use by energy-consuming processes in the cardiomyocyte. ATP production rate generally matches the overall rate of ATP hydrolysis in the mature heart in vivo if carbon substrate and oxygen supplies are ample [31, 32]. At near maximal workloads in the mature heart, the phosphorylation potential [ATP/(ADP + Pi)] diminishes, indicating that a transition in respiratory control occurs [31, 32]. The reduction in phosphorylation potential presumably represents a shift to ADP dependent respiratory regulation through the adenine nucleotide translocator (ANT), the site of ATP/ADP exchange[33], and is not caused by limited oxygen supply [34–36]. The standard free energy of ATP hydrolysis ($\Delta G0'$) is directly related to phosphorylation potential by:

$$\Delta G0' = -2.303\ RT \operatorname{Log} [\text{ATP}] / ([\text{ADP}]\,[\text{Pi}])$$

Therefore, at near maximal work state in the mature heart, a somewhat lower amount of free energy is made available during the release of a phosphate from ATP at various ATPase sites within the myocyte: $\text{ATP} \rightarrow \text{ADP} + \text{Pi}$. [ADP] increases and phosphorylation potential declines with only moderate myocardial oxygen consumption (MVO_2) elevation in the developing heart [33] and the relationship between MVO_2 and ADP emulates a respiratory control pattern consistent with first order Michaelis–Menton kinetics. Transition to the mature and less ADP-dependent type respiratory control occurs in the first month of development and parallels accumulation of ANT in the mitochondrial membrane, suggesting that alterations in ADP/ATP exchange kinetics are responsible for this pattern in newborns.

The phosphorylation potential and $\Delta G0'$ therefore depend in part on ANT function. The ADP/ATP exchange rate must increase in concert with an increase in ATP hydrolysis at ATPase sites. Any diminution in ANT capacity would result in elevated cytosolic ADP concentration with phosphorylation potential and $\Delta G0'$ reduction. Qualitative or quantitative deficiencies in ANT and shifts to ADP-dependent respiration occur not only in the developing heart, but also during CHF in a porcine model in vivo [33]. The ATP hydrolysis efficiency is markedly diminished at very high work states in the mature heart and at more moderate work states in the developing heart due to the logarithmic nature of the relationship between $\Delta G0'$ and phosphorylation potential. The decrease in efficiency may not be problematic under conditions where the heart can maintain high levels of ATP synthesis. However, under stress or conditions that reduce efficiency of energy utilization, such as volume or pressure overload, the decreased efficiency of

ATP hydrolysis can limit energy supply to cellular processes including the contractile apparatus.

Even a transient decrease in oxygen supply to the developing heart substantially reduces phosphorylation potential, efficiency of mitochondrial ATP synthesis, and efficiency of oxidative phosphorylation–mechanical function coupling in vivo [37]. In sheep studies, graded hypoxia stimulated a stress response including a catecholamine surge and stimulation of contractile function. Though cardiac power and work were maintained through hypoxia, phosphocreatine rapidly declined, ATP dropped, ADP increased, and overall phosphorylation potential dropped once hemoglobin saturation dipped below a threshold value. Reoxygenation reestablished PCr levels at a rate much slower than predicted implying a reduction in efficiency of ATP synthesis (ADP phosphorylated per oxygen molecule) and/or ATP hydrolysis. In the recovery period, despite maintenance of PCr and ATP levels, efficiency of coupling between cardiac oxygen consumption and mechanical work was markedly reduced. Thus, even a transient limitation in oxygen supply initiating a stress response contributes to mitochondrial dysfunction in a model in vivo. Interestingly, although metabolically mature sheep maintain significantly higher myocardial ATP utilization rates during hypoxic stress than exhibited by immature lambs, the degree of mitochondrial dysfunction during reoxygenation was similar between the two groups. Accordingly, one can surmise that immature sheep, and possibly human infants, are more sensitive to energy stresses than their mature counterpart. These issues are compounded by exposure to hypoxia, such as occurs with cyanotic heart diseases.

The lamb heart in vivo exhibits a marked decrease in carbohydrate oxidation within 3 days after birth in conjunction with a substantial increase in oxidation of free fatty acids [38–40]. The increase in fatty acid oxidation (FAO) relates partially from changes in circulating levels of fatty acids after birth, as even the fetal heart can increase FAO in response to fat loading. Nevertheless, the lamb heart increases the ability to oxidize fatty acids within a week regardless of substrate supply [38–40]. Ketone bodies provide approximately 7% of acetyl-CoA in newborn lambs, although this proportion is highly dependent on supply, which increases during periods of stress. In the aerobic isovolemic perfused rabbit heart, glycolysis is the primary substrate source immediately after birth with a rapid shift occuring toward lactate and fatty acid utilization by 7 days of age. Isovolemic isolated newborn pig hearts show similar patterns of transition in substrate use [38–41]. Carnitine palmitoyl transferase I (CPTI) is considered a key regulator of fatty acid oxidation. However, stimulation of this neonatal metabolic transition appears to involve a decrease in malonyl-CoA production by acetyl-CoA carboxylase (ACC) rather than decreased sensitivity of carnitine palmitoyl transferase I to malonyl-CoA inhibition. The inhibition of ACC occurs in association with increased adenomonophosphate activated protein kinase

(AMPK) shortly after birth. This response has been linked to a nadir in insulin after birth, which should increase AMPK activity and initiate a cascade decreasing ACC activation, thereby diminishing malonyl-CoA and disinhibiting CPTI. There does appear to be some species variability in function of this cascade or perhaps differences relate to isovolemic heart versus physiology in situ. For instance, Bartelds et al. detected in sheep postnatal increases in CPTI activity, which were much lower than the increase in the rate of long chain fatty acid (LCFA) oxidation in vivo in the same animals. Furthermore, they found relatively high rates of CPTI activity in fetal lambs [40]. Therefore, alterations in CPTI activity do not totally explain the large postnatal increases in FAO in all species or in vivo. Modulation in activity for malonyl-CoA decarboxylase, responsible for regulating malonyl-CoA levels, might explain this discrepancy [42, 43]. Although capacity for FAO increases during the neonatal transition period, some data exist suggesting that carbohydrate oxidative capacity does not similarly expand [44]. Glucose oxidation produces more ATP molecules per carbon and is considered more energy efficient than fat. Many models of compensated cardiac hypertrophy show increased relative carbohydrate to FAO. In a neonatal pig model with persistent patent ductus arteriosus [45], volume overload hypertrophy delayed the maturational increase in acetyl-CoA carboxylase activity, which generally prompts the increase in FAO [45]. The concomitant inability to increase glucose oxidation in response to stress, may in fact further contribute to cardiac energy failure and CHF in the newborn (Fig. 14.8).

Right Ventricular Dysfunction in Congenital Heart Disease

Etiologies of right ventricular failure (RVF) differ substantially in children from those noted in adults. RVF in children occurs from various types of CHD, and through different pressure or volume loading stresses. RVF in the clinical scenarios of elevated pulmonary vascular resistance, acute respiratory distress syndrome, and sepsis will not be discussed in this chapter.

Though the left ventricle has a well defined shape, right ventricular geometry is more difficult to characterize through geometric models. The right ventricle has in the past been considered a passive conduit for systemic venous return based on preliminary studies showing that abolition of contractile function of the RV free wall did not seem to influence cardiac output. However, newer data dispute this theory. Afterload has a major influence on short and long term right ventricular function. In the short term, the right ventricle responds to acute changes in afterload, such as an increase in pulmonary artery pressure, generated by constriction or

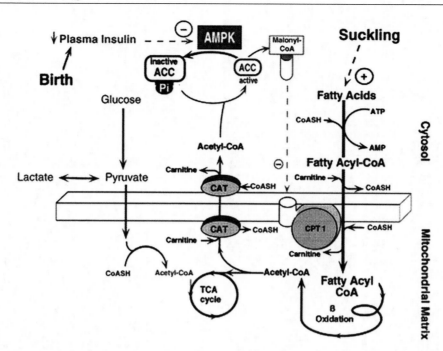

Fig. 14.8 Changes in energy balance and fatty acid oxidation in the newborn heart. Dominant pathways are indicated by *darker typeface*, and *bold arrows*; those indicated in *gray* are diminished. The inner mitochondrial membrane has been omitted for clarity. *ACC* acetyl CoA carboxylase; *AMP* adenosine monophosphate; *AMPK* 5'-AMP-activated protein kinase; *ATP* adenosine triphosphate; *CAT* carnitine acyl transferase; *CoA* coenzyme A; *CoASH* uncombined CoA; *CPT 1* carnitine palmitoyl transferase-1; *Pi* inorganic phosphate; *TCA* tricarboxylic acid. After birth, a fall in plasma insulin (which is an inhibitor of AMPK expression) levels, together with a decrease in available glucose and lactate substrate lead to a rise in AMPK activity. 5'-Adenosine mono- phosphate-activated protein kinase phosphorylates and inactivates ACC, resulting in a decrease in malonyl CoA production. Malonyl CoA in turn has a key role in inhibiting the activity of CPT 1, the rate limiting translocating protein which allows acylated long chain fatty acids to enter the mitochondrion. Thus the heart is prepared to utilize fatty acids in the postnatal period, as the level of malonyl CoA, the inhibitor effect of CPT 1, is greatly reduced. With the onset of suckling, a pronounced rise in plasma fatty acid levels, together with these low levels of malonyl CoA, facilitate the influx of fatty acyl-CoA into the mitochondrion, and an increase in β-oxidation occurs (Reprinted from Kantor et al. [45]. With kind permission from Elsevier)

embolism, with a decrease in stroke volume and cardiac output [46], creating a setting for acute RVF.

The right ventricle is normally highly compliant, but morphology changes rapidly according to chronic loading and interaction with the left ventricle (discussed in other sections). The normally thin-walled right ventricle poorly compensates for increased pulmonary artery pressure and undergoes progressive dilation. Chronic increases in preload also lead to dilation. The right ventricle preload is highly dependent on respiratory variation. Inspiration decreases intrathoracic pressure leading to increased venous return and preload, which in turn provides an elevation in stroke volume with a prolonged ejection time. Respiratory variation is more pronounced in diseased states. This includes patients with Fontan operation who have passive systemic venous return to the pulmonary artery circuit. Exaggerated respiratory variation can also be seen in patients with restrictive physiology, where diastolic function is impaired, such as some postoperative Tetralogy of Fallot patients [47].

In children with CHD, it is often difficult to separate volume overload lesions from pressure overload and restrictive lesions. The classic abnormality is repaired Tetralogy of Fallot with pulmonary regurgitation, which exhibits all those components. These patients often have no effective pulmonary valve. The degree of right ventricular dilation and failure exhibited by these patients appears to be highly variable and difficult to predict. However, Kilner et al. have recently shown that elevated pulmonary artery compliance noted with expansive pulmonary arteries promotes an increase in regurgitant fraction [48]. This is illustrated by a magnetic resonance imaging and function example in two patients with no functional pulmonary valve (Fig. 14.9) but very different pulmonary regurgitant volume and pulmonary artery capacity.

These same patients may also have residual obstruction or pulmonary artery narrowing, which can contribute to pressure overload. Children now rarely if ever undergo the atrial switch operation for transposition of the great arteries. Therefore, problems with chronic pressure loading of the right ventricle often seen with the Senning or Mustard operation, no longer occur in the pediatric population. However, patients with congenitally corrected transposition of the great arteries (atrioventricular and ventriculoarterial discordance) do show issues with prolonged afterload and eventual right

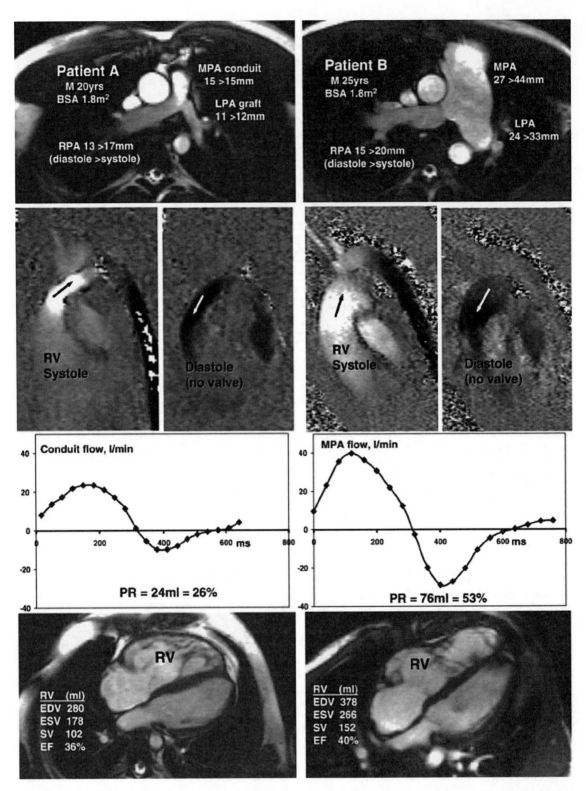

Fig. 14.9 Cardiovascular magnetic resonance studies in two patients, neither with an effective pulmonary valve, but with different amounts of pulmonary regurgitation. Patient A (*left panels*) born with tetralogy of Fallot, palliated with a right Blalock–Taussig shunt and subsequently repaired at 8 years with a homograft right ventricle to pulmonary artery conduit and graft augmentation of the proximal left pulmonary artery. Patient B (*right panels*) born with pulmonary and sub-pulmonary stenosis and a ventricular septal defect, who had patch reconstruction of the right ventricular outflow tract aged 2 years. Cine imaging (*upper row*) showed marked differences of size and expansion of the proximal pulmonary arteries, replaced by a conduit and graft in patient A, but dilated and expansile in patient B, as indicated by the end diastolic > peak systolic diameter measurements shown. In-plane, vertically encoded velocity maps aligned with the right ventricular outflow tract (second row) show no effective valve action in diastole. Flow curves (third row) were plotted from retrospectively gated acquisitions of velocities through planes transecting the proximal MPA or conduit, giving the regurgitant volumes and fractions shown. The peak systolic velocity was 3 m/s in the conduit of patient A and 1 m/s in the MPA of patient B. Patient A had a higher heart rate and a less dilated right ventricle as shown by the four-chamber cines and right ventricular volume measurements (*bottom row*). *M* male; *BSA* body surface area; *MPA* main pulmonary artery; *RPA* right pulmonary artery; *LPA* left pulmonary artery; *RV* right ventricle; *PR* pulmonary regurgitation; *EDV* end diastolic volume, *ESV* end systolic volume; *SV* stroke volume, *EF* ejection fraction (Reprinted from Kilner et al. [48]. With kind permission from Elsevier)

ventricular dysfunction. Right ventricular end systolic volume and diastolic volume slowly increase with chronic volume overload, such as occurs with atrial septal defect, pulmonary regurgitation, and tricuspid regurgitation. These changes preserve cardiac output and cardiac function [49]. The right ventricle also responds to chronic increases in afterload with preservation of function. However, over time the right ventricle undergoes dilation and hypertrophy, which can lead to myocardial fibrosis and failure. The time of progression or transition to failure is often unpredictable and represents a particular management problem for pediatric cardiologists. Recent data show that regional abnormalities in the right ventricular outflow tract in postoperative Tetralogy of Fallot patients contribute substantially to global dysfunction and may have important implications for patient management, including right ventricular outflow tract reconstruction [50].

Medical management for RVF associated with congenital heart lesions is limited. Some inotropic agents show improvement in right ventricular contractility in animal models [46]. Volume expansion may increase preload and maximize stretch and contractile function, but these measures are not supported by evidence-based studies. Surgical or catheter based management of these abnormalities is the hallmark of treatment. Percutaneous placement of pulmonary valves is currently under study and offers substantial promise for patients with pulmonary regurgitation or obstruction.

Single Ventricle and Heart Failure

Assessment and management of heart failure in children with single ventricle (SV) physiology represents a tremendous challenge. These patients represent a heterogenous group anatomically and functionally, and most are subjected to palliative surgery or transplant. The nature of the SV involves volume overloading, though pressure overloading is also not uncommon. Initial surgical intervention depends on the type of SV and associated abnormalities. For specifics regarding early surgical intervention the reader is referred to the major texts in Pediatric Cardiovascular Surgery. The Fontan type reconstruction or bidirectional cavopulmonary anastomosis was originally described by Fontan and Baudet [51] as a novel surgical repair for tricuspid atresia. The procedure has undergone a substantial number of modifications over the years and is now generally performed as a two stage-operation. The first stage is the bidirectional cavopulmonary anastomosis. This is a superior vena cava to pulmonary anastomosis with exclusion of blood flow to the atrium. The ventricle does not have access to the pulmonary artery and is partially volume unloaded. Patients remain cyanotic as only part of the systemic venous return enters the lungs. This intermediate procedure was proposed as hemodynamic deterioration occurred postoperatively when some studies showed that increased stress to the

ventricular wall occurs if the Fontan procedure was performed without this step [52]. Diastolic ventricular compliance issues were thought to play an important role. The ventricular thickness to chamber dimension ratio also acutely increased when the Fontan was performed without the intermediate step.

Before performance of the Fontan procedure, chronic ventricular loading is a major factor. The SV, especially the morphological right ventricle does not appear to tolerate the volume overload over the long term. Additional stressors include systemic arterial desaturation, ventricular hypertrophy, and altered afterload. Hypertrophy occurs to compensate in part for increased wall stretch due to volume overload, which can be exacerbated by atrioventricular or semilunar valve dysfunction and regurgitation. Neurohumoral abnormalities occur due to the excess volume loading. Patients before bidirectional cavopulmonary anastomosis demonstrate higher brain and atrial natriuretic peptide levels than occur in controls or patients after bidirectional cavopulmonary anastomosis. The noncompensated hypertrophy and possible irreversible effects of chronic volume overloading were instrumental in surgical decisions to complete Fontan procedures by 2 years of age. Kirklin et al. noted ventricular hypertrophy to be a significant risk factor for death after Fontan [53]. However, atrial dysrhythmias secondary to extensive atrial surgery also adversely affected outcome with Fontan modification. Accordingly, there is a recent impetus to exclude atrial tissue from Fontan completion. This latest modification is known as the extracardiac conduit type, which includes interposition of a polytetrafluoroethylene graft conduit between the inferior vena cava and the underside of the pulmonary artery (Fig. 14.9).

As noted, prior to staging with the bidirectional cavopulmonary anastomosis the acute change in volume unloading associated with the Fontan was thought to adversely influence outcome. Although, the bidirectional cavopulmonary anastomosis seems to improve clinical outcome, it did not change the mass/volume postoperatively. An echocardiographic study showed an increase up to 111% in wall thickness to ventricular volume after bidirectional cavopulmonary anastomosis [54]. However, this phenomenon is not permanent as an MRI study showed no difference in mass/volume between patients before and 6–9 months after bidirectional cavopulmonary anastomosis [52].

The Fontan reconstruction elicits major changes on hemodynamics and placing the circulations in series rather than in parallel. Firstly, systemic saturation is improved, ventricular volume loading is reduced, and peripheral perfusion presumably improved by eliminating shunting to the low resistance pulmonary vascular bed. However, central venous pressure is uniformly elevated in Fontan patients, and this may promote symptoms of venous congestion in part by increasing capillary hydrostatic pressure [55]. Additionally, systemic vascular resistance is elevated relative to the previous stage by placing the circulation in series. Accordingly, patients with SV after Fontan have low cardiac output and

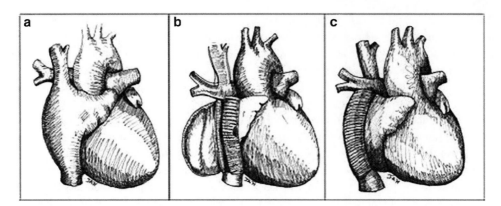

Fig. 14.10 Artist's rendering of the various modifications of the Fontan operation. (**a**) Initial total cavopulmonary connection performed by Fontan and Baudet in 1971. Valved homograft to proximal right pulmonary artery. Valve at inferior vena cava to right atrial (RA) junction. Unidirectional Glenn. (**b**) Lateral tunnel Fontan as described by De Leval et al. (**c**) Extracardiac Fontan (Courtesy of JA AboulHosn MD, Ahmanson-UCLA Adult Congenital Heart Disease Center, Los Angeles, CA)

reduced exercise capacity [52, 56]. Senzaki et al. evaluated ventricular–vascular coupling in SV and Fontan patients and SV after systemic to pulmonary artery shunt [57]. The Fontan patients were found at rest and with dobutamine stress to have elevation in the pulsatile component of ventricular afterload and in vascular resistance. These elevations in load were closely associated with decreased cardiac index. Szabo and Bahrle have also described that small but complex changes in of preload, afterload, and myocardial contractility in Fontan patients have profound effects on ventriculoarterial mechanoenergetics. This manifests in terms of mismatch between contractility and afterload, and reduces mechanical efficiency, and reduces the potential of the SV to adapt to exercise [49].

Clinical studies are ongoing to determine factors, which are detrimental to the Fontan patients. Many of these patients progress to failure, which often manifests as pleural effusions and ascites. Protein-losing enteropathy (PLE) is an uncommon (3.7%) complication of the Fontan operation occurring usually 2 or more years after surgery and has recently been a subject of review [58–60]. PLE is thought to result from bowel edema secondary to low cardiac output and elevated systemic venous and lymphatic pressures. Mesenteric vascular resistance which is generally elevated in patients with Fontan circulation is elevated more in patients with PLE. This may be due, in part, to the increased impedance to emptying of the portal venous system in patients after the Fontan operation [61, 62]. Perioperative risk factors for the development of PLE include longer cardiopulmonary bypass time and single right ventricle anatomy. Patients with PLE frequently develop peripheral edema and refractory ascites and pleural effusions. The serum albumin is low and fecal α1-antitrypsin concentration is elevated. Therapeutic options include symptomatic relief via drainage of pleural and ascitic fluid, afterload reduction, diuresis, intravenous albumin infusion, and a high protein/low fat diet. Various case reports have reported efficacy of oral steroids in the treatment of PLE [63, 64]. Other medical interventions purported in various case reports to decrease PLE via incompletely understood mechanisms include heparin, spironolactone, calcium infusion, and sildenafil [65–70]. Atrial pacing has been reported to improve PLE, likely as a result of augmented cardiac output in patients with sinus node dysfunction [71]. Surgical fenestration of the atrial septum allows some right-to-left shunting and decreases systemic venous pressure, thus reducing the risk of PLE or unremitting pleural effusions, at the expense of arterial oxygen saturation [72]. Heart transplantation is recommended for patients who have failed medical or surgical therapy due to the high mortality rate of PLE (~50%). Gamba et al. reported resolution of PLE over 18 months in six patients who underwent successful transplantation [73]. In a recent series of Fontan patients who underwent orthotopic cardiac transplantation 15 patients had PLE. Six (40%) of these patients died early after transplant (hemorrhage, RVF, multisystem organ failure, sepsis, brain death). In the nine surviving patients, signs of PLE resolved and serum albumin levels normalized within 6 weeks [74].

Pharmacology

Although drug regimen for treatment of HF in infants and children resembles that used in adults, a paucity of evidence exists regarding pharmacokinetics and treatment response. As of 2005, approximately 80% of medications given for hospitalized children with heart disease were provided off-label [75]. The most common medications are furosemide, epinephrine, dopamine, lidocaine, and milrinone. For the most part dosing and indications are extrapolated from adult studies, and do not necessarily accommodate developmental differences.

Developmental Issues with Diuretics

Diuretics have been used as a mainstay for treatment of edema and HF in infants and children. Scattered reports appeared in the 1960s and 1970, which suggested safety and efficacy for furosemide in infants and children [76]. However, these studies were retrospective reviews, and were not controlled randomized trials. Renal blood flow and glomerular filtration rate (GFR) increase substantially after 36 weeks age gestation, reaching maximal levels at 1–2 years of age. The GFR is approximately 2–4 ml/min/1.73 m^2 in term neonates, but it may be as low as 0.6–0.8 ml/min/1.73 m^2 in preterm neonates. The GFR increases rapidly during the first 2 weeks of life and then rises steadily until adult values are reached at 8–12 months of age [77]. Similarly, tubular secretion is immature at birth and reaches adult capacity during the first year of life. Immaturity of these processes partially explains the inability of neonates to excrete acid. They also exhibit higher fractional excretion of sodium. Thus, preterm infants and neonates are vulnerable to diuretic agents, agents that require mature systems for acid excretion, such as carbonic anhydrase inhibitors. Additionally, the lower GFR raises the half-life of particular drugs including diuretics. Plasma half-life of diuretics is several-fold longer in premature infants and neonates than in adults and older children. Volume of distribution is also higher in children, and albumin is lower leading to prolonged drug half-lives and increased bioavailability. These developmental differences suggest that doses should be lower, particularly in young infants. These issues are important as the premature infant in particular is vulnerable to furosemide induced ototoxicity [78].

Furosemide has been the mainstay diuretic use for pediatric HF, and is used aggressively after cardiac surgery. Pharmacodynamic studies indicate that a maximally effective dose for each patient exists, even in neonates. Therefore, a theoretical advantage exists supporting a continuous infusion strategy that avoids troughs of diuretic concentrations. However, the published studies on pediatric patients comparing intermittent with continuous infusion of furosemide have reported discrepant results regarding efficacy [79]. The most recent study reported positive results if a higher loading dose of furosemide was used prior to initiation of continuous infusion [80]. Spironolactone blocks action of excess aldosterone and provides potassium sparing during the use of loop diuretics. Considering these actions, it may be beneficial in the management of HF, particularly in infants on furosemide. There are no studies to support use of aldosterone antagonists in children with HF.

Obviously, there is a great need for controlled clinical trials to establish efficacy and safety of new diuretics in children. A recent study did evaluate torasemide, a newer loop diuretic which shows a longer elimination half-life, longer duration of action, and higher bioavailability in adults.

Torasemide did lower HF score in children. As this was not a randomized trial to compare efficacy, there is no evidence for superiority over furosemide [81].

Inotropic Agents in Pediatric Heart Failure

The therapeutic effect of inotropic agents in HF depends in part on balance between the parasympathetic and sympathetic systems. Inhibitory parasympathetic innervation is more dominant in premature infants than in term infants as exhibited by diminished heart rate variability [82]. However, the parasympathetic system matures rapidly and control function of the term neonate is similar to that in the adult. In contrast the sympathetic system matures much more slowly. Relatively low concentrations of norepinephrine occur in preterminal nerve trunks in mature animals, with higher levels in the myocardium itself. In contrast, most norepinephrine is found in nerve trunks in neonates due to the paucity of nerve terminals in the maturing myocardium [83]. Therefore, neonates rely on circulating catecholamines for circulatory support more than older children and adults. Neonates and older children also have higher levels circulating catecholamines than adults [84]. Some older studies indicate that myocardial function and cardiac output in the neonate do not respond as well to catecholamines as in the adult [85].

Use of inotropic agents for HF in adults has been reviewed in other chapters. There are a limited number of clinical studies establishing evidence for use of inotropes in pediatric HF patients. The few clinical studies that were performed collected mainly in infants and children immediately after cardiac surgery and cardiopulmonary bypass. Inotropes are used frequently in children to prevent low cardiac output syndrome after such surgery. Most of what we know regarding inotropic support evolves from animal studies. Some evidence exists supporting poor contractile response to epinephrine or norepinephrine in newborn lambs [85]. Newer studies indicate that lack of response can be overcome by increasing epinephrine dosage [33]. Maximal rates of MVO$_2$ achieved by a relatively brief course of epinephrine are similar in newborn and mature lambs, although the mitochondrial respiratory rate is driven through different mechanisms. In young sheep exposed to hypoxic stress such as frequently occurs in the newborn, endogenous circulating epinephrine and norepinephrine levels rise dramatically [37]. This dramatic response might affect cardiac function as prolonged administration of epinephrine at high dose (1.5–2 µg/kg/min over 2 h) eventually yields decreased contractility and compliance in neonatal pigs. These data provide minimal guidance for use of epinephrine in human infants. Despite lack of human data, some centers use low dose epinephrine (0.05 µg/kg/min) as a first- or second-line inotropic agent [86].

Dopamine is an endogenous precursor of norepinephrine and is used frequently in neonatal and pediatric intensive care units for circulatory support. There have been no randomized clinical trials performed to establish efficacy and safety for dopamine. Driscoll et al. showed that animals less than 7 days old displayed diminished hemodynamic responses to dopamine compared to older animals, although high doses increased systemic arterial pressure. Dopamine was noted to increase renal artery blood flow [87]. Driscoll performed retrospective reviews on the use of dopamine in children treated with a wide dosage range (0.3–25 µg kg/min) for CHD and sepsis [88]. Only 13 of 24 patients responded with increases in mean arterial pressure and urine output. Subsequently, several investigators evaluated dopamine to prevent or ameliorate low cardiac output syndrome after repair of CHD. Dopamine at doses of 5–10 µg/kg/min increased cardiac output with no change in systemic vascular resistance. It should be noted that dopamine poses significant risk for postoperative dysrhythmias in this population, and termination has been recommended if they occur. Although, the beneficial effect of dopamine for HF is not well established in children, this agent is commonly used to improve renal function after cardiopulmonary bypass or circulatory shock. The renal dose is considered as between 0.5 and 3 µg/kg/min in adults. However, studies by Girardin et al. indicate that children require somewhat higher doses (5.0 µg/kg/min) to raise glomerular filtration rate and renal plasma flow [89].

A considerable number of clinical studies have been published evaluating efficacy of dobutamine for low cardiac output syndrome in adults with severe cardiomyopathy. However, these studies show short term improvements in hemodynamics without increased long term survival. In fact there is some concern, that chronic infusion of any inotrope increases mortality. Similarly, dobutamine increases stroke volume, diastolic filling, and contractility in normal children in doses 5–20 µg/kg/min [90]. Driscoll noted increases in blood pressure and cardiac index in children with CHD undergoing catheterization [87]. Substantial evidence is lacking for supporting hemodynamic and clinical improvement by dobutamine in infants and children after cardiopulmonary bypass. A very early study by Bohn et al. showed dependent increases in cardiac output in 11 children within an extremely broad age range, 0.2–8 years [91]. Subsequently, Berner et al. published a series of papers indicating that dobutamine did not improve cardiac function in children after repair of Tetralogy of Fallot [92, 93]. Booker et al. showed that dobutamine did not elicit pulmonary vasoconstrictive effects, seen by dopamine infusion [94]. Surprisingly, literature review did not reveal a single study evaluating hemodynamic effects of dobutamine in neonates or infants, although this drug is routinely used after cardiac surgery in these groups.

Digoxin is a cardiac glycoside commonly used to treat acute and chronic CHF in infants and children. There is limited scientific basis for using digoxin in this aged group, other than combined years of experience. Berman et al. studied the effect of this drug on infants with failure secondary to unrepaired VSD [95]. Digoxin improved echocardiographic defined hemodynamic parameters in six of 11 infants. Again, no efficacy data are available.

Thyroid hormone (TH) has been considered as therapeutic and inotropic agent for treatment of low cardiac output in children after cardiopulmonary bypass. Cardiac surgery involving cardiopulmonary bypass (CPB) induces a significant and persistent reduction in circulating TH levels in the critical postoperative recovery period in all age groups [96–99]. Depressed TH levels increase post-cardiac surgery morbidity in adults [97]. Controlled, randomized studies in adults demonstrate that parenteral triiodothyronine (T_3) repletion after coronary artery bypass surgery improves postoperative ventricular function, reduces the need for inotropic support and mechanical devices, and reduces myocardial ischemia [97, 100, 101]. Postoperative depression of T_3 may contribute to hemodynamic alterations in this immature patient population [102, 103]. Triiodothyronine elicits direct "termed nongenomic"-mediated effects as well as actions through transcriptional mechanisms [104], which promote systemic vasodilation and positive inotropic effect. Several small placebo-controlled and double-blinded randomized studies have shown some positive effects on cardiac function and outcome variables in patients of children after cardiopulmonary bypass. Considering the paucity of data supporting use of other inotropic agents, these studies are quite valuable and deserve mention. Bettendorf et al. performed a randomized placebo-controlled study that examined T_3 supplementation in 40 pediatric patients after cardiac surgery [98]. Patients receiving T_3 exhibited greater increases in cardiac index during the early postoperative period and received fewer cumulative doses of the inotropic medications epinephrine and dobutamine. The subject numbers were inadequate to assess clinically important endpoints including length of intensive care unit stay and mechanical ventilation duration.

Chowdhury et al. randomized 28 patients to receive either continuous T_3 infusion at 0.05–0.15 µg/kg body weight per hour to maintain serum levels within normal levels (80–100 ng/dl) or placebo [105]. Patients with serum T_3 levels less than 40 ng/dl (or <60 ng/dl in infants) on postoperative days 0, 1, or 2 were randomized. No differences were found between groups for the degree of postoperative care, use of inotropic medications, and length of hospital stay and duration of mechanical ventilation. But this study population also had large variations in patient age and presumably diagnoses. Mackie et al. undertook a focused evaluation of T_3 supplementation on the early postoperative course of neonates undergoing aortic arch reconstruction during either the Norwood procedure (for SV anatomy) or a two-ventricle repair of interrupted aortic arch/VSD [106]. The study enrolled 42 patients in a randomized, double-blinded placebo-controlled study with patients receiving a continuous infusion of T_3 (0.05 mcg/kg/h) or placebo. Primary endpoints were a composite clinical outcome score and cardiac index at 48 h. Even though the median clinical outcome scores were the same between groups, the T_3 treated group had a statistically significantly better outcome score due to differences in the distribution of values. The T_3 group had a slightly earlier time to negative fluid balance (2.0 days in T_3 group vs. 2.5 days in the placebo group). The authors concluded that T_3 treatment in neonatal heart surgery was safe and resulted in a favorable improvement of clinical outcome scores. Portman et al. also undertook a randomized, placebo-controlled trial in children less 1-year-old undergoing surgery for repair of VSD or Tetralogy of Fallot [99]. 14 patients (seven per group) were randomized to receive either a bolus of T_3 (0.4 µg/kg) prior to CPB and after release of aortic cross-clamp or placebo. Heart rate and peak systolic pressure rate (systolic blood pressure times heart rate) were increased in T_3 treated patients at 6 h after termination of CPB. Elevation of the peak systolic pressure-rate product implies that T_3 repletion improves myocardial consumption. The Triiodothyronine for Infants and Children Undergoing Cardiopulmonary Bypass (TRICC) study was designed to overcome many of shortcomings noted in the previous studies including low patient numbers and large variation in age and diagnosis [107]. The study is a multicenter, randomized, clinical trial designed to determine the safety and efficacy of T_3 supplementation in children <2 years of age undergoing surgical procedures for CHD. The six-center study enrolled 195 patients with 99 randomized to multiple T_3 boluses over 12 h during and after surgery and 96 to placebo. Patient enrollment used a stratified design with central randomization to nine diagnostic categories in high or low risk categories based upon the commonly accepted Aristotle Score. The primary endpoint was time to extubation. Enrollment for the TRICC study was recently completed and a full evaluation of the results has yet to be published. Preliminary analyses show that T_3 treatment improved cardiac function assessed by shortening and ejection fractions, cardiac index, and/or myocardial performance index (LV Tei) at 24 h in the low and high risk patients. The primary end point, time to extubation, was not changed by T_3 treatment. However, absolute T_3 levels were associated with changes in the chance of extubation in placebo and experimental groups.

Phosphodiesterase Inhibitors

The clinical evidence supporting use of phosphodiesterase inhibitors for HF in children is sparse, yet far superior in quality to data available for diuretics or inotropic agents. Early study in a neonatal pig model showed a concentration dependent negative inotropic effect of amrinone. However, milrinone, a more selective and potent phosphodiesterase inhibitor showed positive inotropic effect [108], as well as high energy phosphate preservation in the ischemic pig myocardium [109]. Several nonrandomized studies have been performed using small series of neonates or children with low cardiac output syndrome after surgical repair of CHD [110–112]. These have shown improved cardiac index, reduced mean arterial pressure, and decreased systemic and pulmonary vascular resistance.

The Prophylatic Intravenous Use of Milrinone After Cardiac Operation in Pediatrics (PRIMACORP) study was a large double-blinded placebo-controlled trial with three parallel groups. More than 200 patients were randomized into low dose for 35 h, high dose for 35 h, or placebo. The clinical endpoint was a composite end point of death or development of low cardiac output state at 36 h. The high dose regimen, 75 µg/kg bolus followed by 0.75 µg/kg/min showed significantly lower risk of low cardiac output state compared to placebo. Accordingly, milrinone has become an essential pharmacological agent in the management of children with low cardiac output syndromes. However, no studies have substantiated the use of milrinone for chronic therapy, although some centers have reported home use as bridge to transplant [113, 114].

Vasodilator Therapy

Nitroprusside is a short acting vasodilator, sometimes used in adults with acute cardiac decompensation. Use of nitroprusside has been largely replaced by milrinone. Nitroprusside improves hemodynamic profile in patients with low cardiac output from sepsis respiratory distress. Beekman et al. noted that nitroprusside decreased right atrial and pulmonary artery wedge pressures in patients with VSD [115]. However, it also decreased systemic blood flow and increased pulmonary to systemic shunting. Another study showed that this phenomenon varied according to left ventricular loading. Artman et al. showed that the arterial vasodilator hydralazine very modestly decreased left to right shunting in six of eight patients with atrioventricular canal defects. Hydralazine failed to decrease the shunt in two patients with fairly high pulmonary vascular resistance [116]. Accordingly, nitroprusside or hydralazine should be used with great caution in patients with any shunt lesion.

ACE inhibitors are an essential pharmacological agent used for treatment of HF in adults. Similar to other drugs used for HF in children control randomized studies of ACE inhibitors are lacking. Clinical response in infants and children may relate to the etiology of HF. Captopril has been considered for use in HF caused by left to right shunts. Initially, Boucek and Chang showed that captopril increased pulmonary vascular resistance and thereby decreased left to right shunting in lambs with VSD [117]. Scammel et al. retrospectively reviewed use of captopril in 18 infants treated for severe HF. Daily weight gain was improved but patients were also on digoxin and furosemide. There was no control group for comparison [118]. Shaw et al. also retrospectively reported an increase in weight gain in infants treated with captopril for CHF [119]. However, these infants were concomitantly admitted to the hospital for intervention by skilled and persistent nursing personnel. Two studies evaluated the acute hemodynamic effects of captopril in infants with large left-to-right shunts. Captopril elicited varying hemodynamic responses, primarily dependent on baseline systemic and pulmonary vascular resistance. Although captopril decreased systemic vascular resistance (SVR) and Qp:Qs in most patients with elevated SVR, patients with normal SVR or with elevated PVR showed a significant decrease in PVR with an increase in left-to-right shunting [120, 121]. Paradoxical response with increase left to right shunt has also been noted after treatment with enalapril in children with left to right shunts [122]. Several patients in these studies demonstrated transient renal failure.

HF of alternative etiology in children may be responsive to ACE inhibitor therapy. ACE inhibitor therapy was considered beneficial for patients with Fontan type circulation due to the high SVR, ventricular hypertrophy, and associated diastolic function. One of the few randomized controlled trials showed no change in SVR, cardiac index, ventricular diastolic filling, or exercise capacity after 10 weeks of therapy. Failure of this trial to show effect may be due to the small study population and short term of therapy [123]. Bengur et al. showed some acute hemodynamic improvements in patients with primary dilated cardiomyopathy within an hour after oral administration of captopril (0.5 mg/kg). In 11 of 12 children with congestive cardiomyopathy, cardiac index and stroke volume increased and SVR increased. In contrast four children with restrictive cardiomyopathy had no change in cardiac output and showed a trend to significant hypotension [124]. The authors concluded that captopril may benefit children with congestive cardiomyopathy, but should not be used for restrictive disease. Data related to long term use with ACE inhibitors for cardiomyopathy are lacking. Chabot et al. retrospectively reviewed 27 patients treated with ACE inhibitors and compared them to 54 patients receiving conventional therapy. The authors observed better survival in the group receiving ACE inhibitors, but the study importance is limited due to the retrospective and non-randomized nature [125]. Another retrospective study showed that ten of 23 (43%) patients (age 10–20 years) treated with enalapril for cardiomyopathy secondary to Duchenne's muscular dystrophy responded with normalization of shortening fraction. Follow up time was variable [126]. Silber et al. performed the only true randomized double-blinded controlled clinical

trial comparing placebo to ACE inhibitor in a population which included children [127]. They evaluated enalapril in long-term survivors of pediatric cancer with at least one cardiac abnormality identified after anthracycline exposure. However, the ages at study enrollment ranged from 8.3 to 31.5 years and the pediatric age group was not separately evaluated. Enalapril reduced left ventricular end-systolic wall stress over the term of the study period (5 years), but did not improve exercise performance [127].

In summary, the use of ACE inhibitors for HF caused by a left to right shunt is not well supported, though is commonly used by some pediatric cardiologists. ACE inhibitors can cause increased left to right shunt and hypotension in some patients. Evidence exists that captopril acutely improves hemodynamics in children with congestive cardiomyopathy. Enalapril improved left ventricular end-systolic wall stress in a mixed population of children and adults with anthracycline cardiomyopathy, but did not improve exercise capacity. With regard to chronic use in Fontan patients and cardiomyopathy, only weak evidence stemming from a single retrospective review supports the use of chronic ACE inhibitors in children.

β-Blockers

Multiple studies in adults have demonstrated beneficial effects of β-blockers on left ventricular function, survival and symptoms. Small, nonrandomized studies suggested a possible beneficial effect of β-blockers in children with HF, but typical of most pediatric HF studies [128–131], these were limited by sample size and lack of contemporaneous control populations. Some data have indicated that although several β-blockers have been shown to be efficacious in adult HF, carvedilol may be superior [132]. Carvedilol exerts dual mechanisms of action: nonselective β-blockade and vasodilation due primarily to α1-blockade [15]. Shaddy and the Pediatric Carvedilol study group prospectively evaluated the effects of carvedilol in children and adolescents with symptomatic systemic ventricular systolic dysfunction [133]. This included patients with SV and Fontan physiology with either a morphological right or left ventricle serving as the systemic ventricle. The study represents to date the only large multi-center placebo-controlled randomized trial performed exclusively and completed in a population of children with HF. Patients included in the study were younger than 18 years with chronic symptomatic HF due to systemic ventricular systolic dysfunction. On echocardiography, patients with systemic left ventricular dysfunction were required to have an ejection fraction of less than 40%, while qualitative evidence of ventricular dilation with at least moderate systemic ventricular systolic dysfunction was required for enrollment in patients with a systemic right ventricle or SV. Patients were randomized to twice-daily dosing with placebo, low-dose carvedilol (target dose of 0.2 mg/kg per dose if weight <62.5 kg or 12.5 mg per dose if weight 62.5 kg) or high-dose carvedilol (target dose of 0.4 mg/kg per dose if weight <62.5 kg or 25 mg per dose if weight 62.5 kg). The study did not detect a treatment effect of carvedilol on the primary composite end point of clinical HF outcomes [133]. Furthermore, the study noted a high rate of improvement in both the treated and placebo populations, which has not been noted in adult populations. This was not known at the time of study design. Therefore, with the composite end-point as a primary efficacy parameter, the study was underpowered. Additionally, all patients were required to have received standard HF therapy for at least 1 month at the time of randomization, including angiotensin-converting enzyme inhibitors unless contraindicated or if patients could not tolerate it. As noted previously, the therapeutic value for these therapies remain unproven. There was a significant interaction between study drug and ventricular morphology suggesting a possible differential effect of treatment between patients with a systemic left ventricle (beneficial trend) and those whose systemic ventricle was not a left ventricle (nonbeneficial trend). The study did show that high dose carvedilol increased shortening fraction in patients with a systemic left ventricle more than low dose or placebo.

Conclusions

Congenital heart defects and associated surgery are the major causes of HF in children. Important advances have been made in surgical approaches to CHD. Similar progress in medical management, particularly related to pharmacological intervention, has been limited. Randomized placebo-controlled clinical trials have been rarely performed in this young population with the PRIMACORP trial and the Pediatric Carvedilol trial as the exceptions. Some clinical trials are currently being performed and are near completion, but more high quality evidence for drug management is necessary.

Summary

- Etiology of heart failure differs in children from adults. Congenital heart disease is a major cause of heart failure in children. Primary cardiomyopathy is a cause of heart failure, although rare.
- Quality of life measures and heart failure classifications in adults are not applicable to children. Various classifications have been developed for different age groups, though these are note validated.

- Heart failure can cause growth retardation in infants and children. Maintenance of normal growth is an important management goal for children with heart failure.
- Heart failure occurs in the fetus as a result of many different etiologies. Diagnosis depends on the presence of hydrops, and supported by echocardiography and Doppler studies.
- Fetal circulation occurs in parallel circuits, which intersect at the aortic isthmus. The right ventricle performs the most work in the fetus.
- Neonatal heart failure from left to right shunts occurs as pulmonary vascular resistance drops.
- A number of changes occur in myocardial structure and function during fetal and neonatal life, which modify the ability of the heart to deal with stress including volume and pressure overload.
- The neonatal heart undergoes transitions in ATP production and utilization, which may cause increased cardiomyocyte vulnerability to stress.
- The right ventricle fails in children, often as a result of congenital defects or surgery. Volume overloading occurs in patient with repaired Tetralogy of Fallot and pulmonary regurgitation.
- Single ventricle patients are subject to long-term volume overload. The Fontan operation relieves volume overloading but patients exhibit abnormal systolic and diastolic performance. In particular, ventricular vascular coupling is abnormal and my limit exercise performance. Protein losing enteropathy occurs in a small number of Fontan patients, but shows a poor prognosis.
- A paucity of evidence exists regarding pharmacokinetics and treatment response for heart failure in infants and children.
- Developmental changes in renal blood flow and tubular function should be considered when using diuretics.
- Although inotropic agents are frequently used in children with heart failure, limited scientific evidence exists supporting their use. Some evidence does exist supporting thyroid hormone supplementation after cardiopulmonary bypass to prevent low cardiac output syndrome.
- Use of milrinone is supported by results of the PRIMACORP study. It has become an essential pharmacological agent in the management of children with low cardiac output syndromes after heart surgery.
- The use of ACE inhibitors for heart failure caused by a left to right shunt is not well supported, though is commonly used by some pediatric cardiologists. ACE inhibitors can cause increased left to right shunt and hypotension in some patients. Evidence exists that captopril acutely improves hemodynamics in children with congestive cardiomyopathy.
- No strong evidence exists supporting the use of β-blockers in children with heart failure. Response to carvedilol may be dependent on ventricular morphology.

References

1. Ross RD, Bollinger RO, Pinsky WW (1992) Grading the severity of congestive heart failure in infants. Pediatr Cardiol 13:72–75
2. Reithmann C, Reber D, Kozlik-Feldmann R et al (1997) A post-receptor defect of adenylyl cyclase in severely failing myocardium from children with congenital heart disease. Eur J Pharmacol 330:79–86
3. Mir TS, Marohn S, Laer S, Eiselt M, Grollmus O, Weil J (2002) Plasma concentrations of N-terminal pro-brain natriuretic peptide in control children from the neonatal to adolescent period and in children with congestive heart failure. Pediatrics 110:e76
4. Tissieres P, Aggoun Y, Da Cruz E et al (2006) Comparison of classifications for heart failure in children undergoing valvular surgery. J Pediatr 149:210–215
5. Mangat J, Carter C, Riley G, Foo Y, Burch M (2009) The clinical utility of brain natriuretic peptide in paediatric left ventricular failure. Eur J Heart Fail 11:48–52
6. Farrell AG, Schamberger MS, Olson IL, Leitch CA (2001) Large left-to-right shunts and congestive heart failure increase total energy expenditure in infants with ventricular septal defect. Am J Cardiol 87:1128–1131, A10
7. Menon G, Poskitt EM (1985) Why does congenital heart disease cause failure to thrive? Arch Dis Child 60:1134–1139
8. van der Kuip M, Hoos MB, Forget PP, Westerterp KR, Gemke RJ, de Meer K (2003) Energy expenditure in infants with congenital heart disease, including a meta-analysis. Acta Paediatr 92:921–927
9. Lundell KH, Sabel KG, Eriksson BO, Mellgren G (1989) Glucose metabolism and insulin secretion in infants with symptomatic ventricular septal defect. Acta Paediatr Scand 78:620–626
10. Lundell KH, Sabel KG, Eriksson BO (1999) Plasma metabolites after a lipid load in infants with congenital heart disease. Acta Paediatr 88:718–723
11. Wilkinson JD, Sleeper LA, Alvarez JA, Bublik N, Lipshultz SE (2008) The Pediatric Cardiomyopathy Registry: 1995–2007. Prog Pediatr Cardiol 25:31–36
12. Miller TL, Neri D, Extein J, Somarriba G, Strickman-Stein N (2007) Nutrition in pediatric cardiomyopathy. Prog Pediatr Cardiol 24:59–71
13. Bellini C, Hennekam RC, Fulcheri E et al (2009) Etiology of nonimmune hydrops fetalis: a systematic review. Am J Med Genet A 149A:844–851
14. Rudolph AM (2009) The fetal circulation and congenital heart disease. Arch Dis Child Fetal Neonatal Ed. Published Online: 25 March. [Epub ahead of print]
15. Glatz JA, Tabbutt S, Gaynor JW et al (2007) Hypoplastic left heart syndrome with atrial level restriction in the era of prenatal diagnosis. Ann Thorac Surg 84:1633–1638
16. Friedman WF (1972) The intrinsic physiologic properties of the developing heart. Prog Cardiovasc Dis 15:87–111
17. Reiser PJ, Portman MA, Ning XH (2001) C. Human cardiac myosin heavy chain isoforms in fetal and failing adult atria and ventricles. Am J Physiol Heart Circ Physiol 280:H1814–H1820
18. Anderson PA, Glick KL, Killam AP, Mainwaring RD (1986) The effect of heart rate on in utero left ventricular output in the fetal sheep. J Physiol 372:557–573
19. Silverman NH, Kleinman CS, Rudolph AM et al (1985) Fetal atrioventricular valve insufficiency associated with nonimmune hydrops: a two-dimensional echocardiographic and pulsed Doppler ultrasound study. Circulation 72:825–832
20. Hofstaetter C, Hansmann M, Eik-Nes SH, Huhta JC, Luther SL (2006) A cardiovascular profile score in the surveillance of fetal hydrops. J Matern Fetal Neonatal Med 19:407–413
21. Acharya G, Archer N, Huhta JC (2007) Functional assessment of the evolution of congenital heart disease in utero. Curr Opin Pediatr 19:533–537
22. Huhta JC (2005) Fetal congestive heart failure. Semin Fetal Neonatal Med 10:542–552
23. Harada K, Suzuki T, Tamura M et al (1995) Role of age on transmitral flow velocity patterns in assessing left ventricular diastolic function in normal infants and children. Am J Cardiol 76:530–532
24. Brangenberg R, Burger A, Romer U, Kozlik-Feldmann R, Netz H (2002) Echocardiographic assessment of left ventricular size and function in normal children from infancy to adolescence: acoustic quantification in comparison with traditional echocardiographic techniques. Pediatr Cardiol 23:394–402
25. Schmitz L, Koch H, Bein G, Brockmeier K (1998) Left ventricular diastolic function in infants, children, and adolescents. Reference values and analysis of morphologic and physiologic determinants of echocardiographic Doppler flow signals during growth and maturation. J Am Coll Cardiol 32:1441–1448
26. Friedman WF, Kirkpatrick SE (1975) In situ physiological study of the developing heart. Recent Adv Stud Cardiac Struct Metab 5:497–504
27. Nassar R, Reedy MC, Anderson PA (1987) Developmental changes in the ultrastructure and sarcomere shortening of the isolated rabbit ventricular myocyte. Circ Res 61:465–483
28. Pinsky MR, Perlini S, Solda PL, Pantaleo P, Calciati A, Bernardi L (1996) Dynamic right and left ventricular interactions in the rabbit: simultaneous measurement of ventricular pressure-volume loops. J Crit Care 11:65–76
29. Satoh A, Katayama K, Hiro T et al (1996) Effect of right ventricular volume overload on left ventricular diastolic function in patients with atrial septal defect. Jpn Circ J 60:758–766
30. Walker RE, Moran AM, Gauvreau K, Colan SD (2004) Evidence of adverse ventricular interdependence in patients with atrial septal defects. Am J Cardiol 93:1374–1377, A6
31. Portman MA, Heineman FW, Balaban RS (1989) Developmental changes in the relation between phosphate metabolites and oxygen consumption in the sheep heart in vivo. J Clin Invest 83:456–464
32. Portman MA, Standaert TA, Ning X-H (1995) The relation of myocardial oxygen consumption and function to high energy phosphate utilization during graded hypoxia and reoxygenation in sheep in vivo. J Clin Invest 95:2134–2142
33. Portman MA, Xiao Y, Song Y, Ning X-H (1997) Expression of adenine nucleotide translocator parallels maturation of respiratory control in vivo. Am J Physiol Heart Circ Physiol 273: H1977–H1983
34. Murakami Y, Zhang Y, Cho YK et al (1999) Myocardial oxygenation during high work states in hearts with postinfarction remodeling. Circulation 99:942–948
35. Ochiai K, Zhang J, Gong G et al (2001) Effects of augmented delivery of pyruvate on myocardial high-energy phosphate metabolism at high workstate. Am J Physiol Heart Circ Physiol 281:H1823–H1832
36. Zhang J, Murakami Y, Zhang Y et al (1999) Oxygen delivery does not limit cardiac performance during high work states. Am J Physiol Heart Circ Physiol 277:H50–H57
37. Portman MA, Standaert TA, Ning XH (1996) Developmental changes in ATP utilization during graded hypoxia and reoxygenation in the heart in vivo. Am J Physiol Heart Circ Physiol 270:H216–H223
38. Bartelds B, Gratama JW, Knoester H et al (1998) Perinatal changes in myocardial supply and flux of fatty acids, carbohydrates, and ketone bodies in lambs. Am J Physiol 274:H1962–H1969
39. Bartelds B, Knoester H, Smid GB et al (2000) Perinatal changes in myocardial metabolism in lambs. Circulation 102:926–931
40. Bartelds B, Takens J, Smid GB et al (2004) Myocardial carnitine palmitoyltransferase I expression and long-chain fatty acid oxidation in fetal and newborn lambs. Am J Physiol Heart Circ Physiol 286:H2243–H2248
41. McGowan FX, Lee FA, CHen V, Downing SE (1992) Oxidative metabolism and mechanical function in reperfused neonatal pig heart. J Mol Cell Cardiol 24:831–840

42. Lopaschuk GD, Witters LA, Itoi T, Barr R, Barr A (1994) Acetyl-CoA carboxylase involvement in the rapid maturation of fatty acid oxidation in the newborn rabbit heart. J Biol Chem 269: 25871–25878

43. Onay-Besikci A, Campbell FM, Hopkins TA, Dyck JR, Lopaschuk GD (2003) Relative importance of malonyl CoA and carnitine in maturation of fatty acid oxidation in newborn rabbit heart. Am J Physiol Heart Circ Physiol 284:H283–H289

44. Beaufort-Krol GC, Takens J, Molenkamp MC, Smid GB, Zijlstra WG, Kuipers JR (1998) Determination of organ substrate oxidation in vivo by measurement of 13CO2 concentration in blood. J Mass Spectrom 33:328–333

45. Kantor PF, Robertson MA, Coe JY, Lopaschuk GD (1999) Volume overload hypertrophy of the newborn heart slows the maturation of enzymes involved in the regulation of fatty acid metabolism. J Am Coll Cardiol 33:1724–1734

46. Ghuysen A, Lambermont B, Kolh P et al (2008) Alteration of right ventricular-pulmonary vascular coupling in a porcine model of progressive pressure overloading. Shock 29:197–204

47. Cullen S, Shore D, Redington A (1995) Characterization of right ventricular diastolic performance after complete repair of tetralogy of Fallot. Restrictive physiology predicts slow postoperative recovery. Circulation 91:1782–1789

48. Kilner PJ, Balossino R, Dubini G et al (2009) Pulmonary regurgitation: the effects of varying pulmonary artery compliance, and of increased resistance proximal or distal to the compliance. Int J Cardiol 133:157–166

49. Szabo G, Buhmann V, Graf A et al (2003) Ventricular energetics after the Fontan operation: contractility-afterload mismatch. J Thorac Cardiovasc Surg 125:1061–1069

50. Knirsch W, Dodge-Khatami A, Kadner A et al (2008) Assessment of myocardial function in pediatric patients with operated tetralogy of Fallot: preliminary results with 2D strain echocardiography. Pediatr Cardiol 29:718–725

51. Fontan F, Baudet E (1971) Surgical repair of tricuspid atresia. Thorax 26:240–248

52. Fogel MA, Weinberg PM, Chin AJ, Fellows KE, Hoffman EA (1996) Late ventricular geometry and performance changes of functional single ventricle throughout staged Fontan reconstruction assessed by magnetic resonance imaging. J Am Coll Cardiol 28:212–221

53. Castaneda AR, Trusler GA, Paul MH, Blackstone EH, Kirklin JW (1988) The early results of treatment of simple transposition in the current era. J Thorac Cardiovasc Surg 95:14–28

54. Seliem MA, Baffa JM, Vetter JM, Chen SL, Chin AJ, Norwood WI Jr (1993) Changes in right ventricular geometry and heart rate early after hemi-Fontan procedure. Ann Thorac Surg 55:1508–1512

55. Buchhorn R, Bartmus D, Buhre W, Bursch J (2001) Pathogenetic mechanisms of venous congestion after the Fontan procedure. Cardiol Young 11:161–168

56. Akagi T, Benson LN, Green M et al (1992) Ventricular performance before and after Fontan repair for univentricular atrioventricular connection: angiographic and radionuclide assessment. J Am Coll Cardiol 20:920–926

57. Senzaki H, Masutani S, Kobayashi J et al (2002) Ventricular afterload and ventricular work in Fontan circulation: comparison with normal two-ventricle circulation and single-ventricle circulation with Blalock-Taussig shunts. Circulation 105:2885–2892

58. AboulHosn JA, Shavelle DM, Castellon Y et al (2007) Fontan operation and the single ventricle. Congenit Heart Dis 2:2–11

59. Mertens L, Hagler DJ, Sauer U, Somerville J, Gewillig M (1998) Protein-losing enteropathy after the Fontan operation: an international multicenter study. PLE study group. J Thorac Cardiovasc Surg 115:1063–1073

60. Feldt RH, Driscoll DJ, Offord KP et al (1996) Protein-losing enteropathy after the Fontan operation. J Thorac Cardiovasc Surg 112:672–680

61. Hsia TY, Khambadkone S, Deanfield JE, Taylor JF, Migliavacca F, De Leval MR (2001) Subdiaphragmatic venous hemodynamics in the Fontan circulation. J Thorac Cardiovasc Surg 121:436–447

62. Rychik J, Gui-Yang S (2002) Relation of mesenteric vascular resistance after Fontan operation and protein-losing enteropathy. Am J Cardiol 90:672–674

63. Zellers TM, Brown K (1996) Protein-losing enteropathy after the modified fontan operation: oral prednisone treatment with biopsy and laboratory proved improvement. Pediatr Cardiol 17:115–117

64. Therrien J, Webb GD, Gatzoulis MA (1999) Reversal of protein losing enteropathy with prednisone in adults with modified fontan operations: long term palliation or bridge to cardiac transplantation? Heart 82:241–243

65. Kelly AM, Feldt RH, Driscoll DJ, Danielson GK (1998) Use of heparin in the treatment of protein-losing enteropathy after Fontan operation for complex congenital heart disease. Mayo Clin Proc 73:777–779

66. Kim SJ, Park IS, Song JY, Lee JY, Shim WS (2004) Reversal of protein-losing enteropathy with calcium replacement in a patient after Fontan operation. Ann Thorac Surg 77:1456–1457

67. Kim WH, Lim HG, Lee JR et al (2005) Fontan conversion with arrhythmia surgery. Eur J Cardiothorac Surg 27:250–257

68. Ringel RE, Peddy SB (2003) Effect of high-dose spironolactone on protein-losing enteropathy in patients with Fontan palliation of complex congenital heart disease. Am J Cardiol 91:1031–1032, A9

69. Uzun O, Wong JK, Bhole V, Stumper O (2006) Resolution of protein-losing enteropathy and normalization of mesenteric Doppler flow with sildenafil after Fontan. Ann Thorac Surg 82:e39–e40

70. Zellers TM, Driscoll DJ, Mottram CD, Puga FJ, Schaff HV, Danielson GK (1989) Exercise tolerance and cardiorespiratory response to exercise before and after the Fontan operation. Mayo Clin Proc 64:1489–1497

71. Cohen MI, Rhodes LA, Wernovsky G, Gaynor JW, Spray TL, Rychik J (2001) Atrial pacing: an alternative treatment for protein-losing enteropathy after the Fontan operation. J Thorac Cardiovasc Surg 121:582–583

72. Mertens L, Dumoulin M, Gewillig M (1994) Effect of percutaneous fenestration of the atrial septum on protein-losing enteropathy after the Fontan operation. Br Heart J 72:591–592

73. Gamba A, Merlo M, Fiocchi R et al (2004) Heart transplantation in patients with previous Fontan operations. J Thorac Cardiovasc Surg 127:555–562

74. Jayakumar KA, Addonizio LJ, Kichuk-Chrisant MR et al (2004) Cardiac transplantation after the Fontan or Glenn procedure. J Am Coll Cardiol 44:2065–2072

75. Pasquali SK, Hall M, Slonim AD et al (2008) Off-label use of cardiovascular medications in children hospitalized with congenital and acquired heart disease. Circ Cardiovasc Qual Outcomes 1:74–83

76. Engle MA, Lewy JE, Lewy PR, Metcoff J (1978) The use of furosemide in the treatment of edema in infants and children. Pediatrics 62:811–818

77. Kearns GL, Abdel-Rahman SM, Alander SW, Blowey DL, Leeder JS, Kauffman RE (2003) Developmental pharmacology – drug disposition, action, and therapy in infants and children. N Engl J Med 349:1157–1167

78. Eades SK, Christensen ML (1998) The clinical pharmacology of loop diuretics in the pediatric patient. Pediatr Nephrol 12:603–616

79. Klinge J (2001) Intermittent administration of furosemide or continuous infusion in critically ill infants and children: does it make a difference? Intensive Care Med 27:623–624

80. van der Vorst MM, Ruys-Dudok van Heel I, Kist-van Holthe JE et al (2001) Continuous intravenous furosemide in haemodynamically unstable children after cardiac surgery. Intensive Care Med 27:711–715

81. Senzaki H, Kamiyama M, Masutani S et al (2008) Efficacy and safety of torasemide in children with heart failure. Arch Dis Child 93:768–771

82. Longin E, Gerstner T, Schaible T, Lenz T, Konig S (2006) Maturation of the autonomic nervous system: differences in heart rate variability in premature vs. term infants. J Perinat Med 34:303–308

83. Erath HG Jr, Boerth RC, Graham TP Jr (1982) Functional significance of reduced cardiac sympathetic innervation in the newborn dog. Am J Physiol 243:H20–H26

84. Candito M, Albertini M, Politano S, Deville A, Mariani R, Chambon P (1993) Plasma catecholamine levels in children. J Chromatogr 617:304–307

85. Teitel DF, SIdi D, CHin T, BRett C, Heymann MA, Rudolph AM (1985) Developmental changes in myocardial contractile reserve in the lamb. Pediatr Res 19:948–955

86. Bohn D (2006) Inotropic agents in heart failure. In: Chang AC, Towbin JA (eds) Heart failure in children and young adults. Saunders-Elsevier, Philadelphia, PA, pp 468–486

87. Driscoll DJ, Gillette PC, Ezrailson EG, Schwartz A (1978) Inotropic response of the neonatal canine myocardium to dopamine. Pediatr Res 12:42–45

88. Driscoll DJ, Gillette PC, Duff DF et al (1979) Hemodynamic effects of dobutamine in children. Am J Cardiol 43:581–585

89. Girardin E, Berner M, Rouge JC, Rivest RW, Friedli B, Paunier L (1989) Effect of low dose dopamine on hemodynamic and renal function in children. Pediatr Res 26:200–203

90. Harada K, Tamura M, Ito T, Suzuki T, Takada G (1996) Effects of low-dose dobutamine on left ventricular diastolic filling in children. Pediatr Cardiol 17:220–225

91. Bohn DJ, Poirier CS, Edmonds JF, Barker GA (1980) Hemodynamic effects of dobutamine after cardiopulmonary bypass in children. Crit Care Med 8:367–371

92. Berner M, Oberhansli I, Rouge JC, Jaccard C, Friedli B (1989) Chronotropic and inotropic supports are both required to increase cardiac output early after corrective operations for tetralogy of Fallot. J Thorac Cardiovasc Surg 97:297–302

93. Berner M, Rouge JC, Friedli B (1983) The hemodynamic effect of phentolamine and dobutamine after open-heart operations in children: influence of the underlying heart defect. Ann Thorac Surg 35:643–650

94. Booker PD, Evans C, Franks R (1995) Comparison of the haemodynamic effects of dopamine and dobutamine in young children undergoing cardiac surgery. Br J Anaesth 74:419–423

95. Berman W Jr, Yabek SM, Dillon T, Niland C, Corlew S, Christensen D (1983) Effects of digoxin in infants with congested circulatory state due to a ventricular septal defect. N Engl J Med 308: 363–366

96. Bennett-Guerrero E, Jimenez JL, White WD EBDA, Baldwin BI, Schwinn DA (1996) Cardiovascular effects of intravenous triiodothyronine in patients undergoing coronary artery bypass graft surgery. A randomized, double-blind, placebo- controlled trial. Duke T3 study group [see comments]. JAMA 275:687–692

97. Klemperer JD, Klein I, Gomez M et al (1995) Thyroid hormone treatment after coronary-artery bypass surgery. N Engl J Med 333:1522–1527

98. Bettendorf M, Schmidt KG, Grulich-Henn J, Ulmer HE, Heinrich UE (2000) Tri-iodothyronine treatment in children after cardiac surgery: a double-blind, randomised, placebo-controlled study. Lancet 356:529–534

99. Portman MA, Fearneyhough C, Ning X, Duncan B, Rosenthal G, Lupinetti F (2000) Triiodothyronine repletion in infants during cardiopulmonary bypass for congenital heart surgery. J Thorac Cardiovasc Surg 120:604–608

100. Dyke CM, Ding M, Abd-Elfattah AS et al (1993) Effects of triiodothyronine supplementation after myocardial ischemia. Ann Thorac Surg 56:215–222

101. Mullis-Jansson SL, Argenziano M, Corwin S et al (1999) A randomized double-blind study of the effect of triiodothyronine on cardiac function and morbidity after coronary bypass surgery. J Thorac Cardiovasc Surg 117:1128–1134

102. Bettendorf M, Schmidt KG, Tiefenbacher U, Grulich-Henn J, Heinrich UE, Schonberg DK (1997) Transient secondary hypothyroidism in children after cardiac surgery. Pediatr Res 41: 375–379

103. Dagan O, Vidne B, Josefsberg Z, Phillip M, Strich D, Erez E (2006) Relationship between changes in thyroid hormone level and severity of the postoperative course in neonates undergoing open-heart surgery. Paediatr Anaesth 16:538–542

104. Danzi S, Klein I, Portman MA (2005) Effect of triiodothyronine on gene transcription during cardiopulmonary bypass in infants with ventricular septal defect. Am J Cardiol 95:787–789

105. Chowdhury D, Ojamaa K, Parnell VA, McMahon C, Sison CP, Klein I (2001) A prospective randomized clinical study of thyroid hormone treatment after operations for complex congenital heart disease. J Thorac Cardiovasc Surg 122:1023–1025

106. Mackie AS, Booth KL, Newburger JW et al (2005) A randomized, double-blind, placebo-controlled pilot trial of triiodothyronine in neonatal heart surgery. J Thorac Cardiovasc Surg 130:810–816

107. Portman MA, Fearneyhough C, Karl TR et al (2004) The Triiodothyronine for Infants and Children Undergoing Cardiopulmonary Bypass (TRICC) study: design and rationale. Am Heart J 148:393–398

108. Ascuitto RJ, Ross-Ascuitto NT, Chen V, Downing SE (1989) Ventricular function and fatty acid metabolism in neonatal piglet heart. Am J Physiol 256:H9–H15

109. Pridjian AK, Frohlich ED, VanMeter CH, McFadden PM, Ochsner JL (1995) Pharmacologic support with high-energy phosphate preservation in the postischemic neonatal heart. Ann Thorac Surg 59:1435–1438

110. Chang AC, Atz AM, Wernovsky G, Burke RP, Wessel DL (1995) Milrinone: systemic and pulmonary hemodynamic effects in neonates after cardiac surgery. Crit Care Med 23:1907–1914

111. Bailey JM, Miller BE, Lu W, Tosone SR, Kanter KR, Tam VK (1999) The pharmacokinetics of milrinone in pediatric patients after cardiac surgery. Anesthesiology 90:1012–1018

112. Ramamoorthy C, Anderson GD, Williams GD, Lynn AM (1998) Pharmacokinetics and side effects of milrinone in infants and children after open heart surgery. Anesth Analg 86:283–289

113. Berg AM, Snell L, Mahle WT (2007) Home inotropic therapy in children. J Heart Lung Transplant 26:453–457

114. Price JF, Towbin JA, Dreyer WJ et al (2006) Outpatient continuous parenteral inotropic therapy as bridge to transplantation in children with advanced heart failure. J Card Fail 12:139–143

115. Beekman RH, Rocchini AP, Rosenthal A (1981) Hemodynamic effects of nitroprusside in infants with a large ventricular septal defect. Circulation 64:553–558

116. Artman M, Parrish MD, Boerth RC, Boucek RJ Jr, Graham TP Jr (1984) Short-term hemodynamic effects of hydralazine in infants with complete atrioventricular canal defects. Circulation 69: 949–954

117. Boucek MM, Chang RL (1988) Effects of captopril on the distribution of left ventricular output with ventricular septal defect. Pediatr Res 24:499–503

118. Scammell AM, Arnold R, Wilkinson JL (1987) Captopril in treatment of infant heart failure: a preliminary report. Int J Cardiol 16:295–301

119. Shaw NJ, Wilson N, Dickinson DF (1988) Captopril in heart failure secondary to a left to right shunt. Arch Dis Child 63: 360–363

120. Shaddy RE, Teitel DF, Brett C (1988) Short-term hemodynamic effects of captopril in infants with congestive heart failure. Am J Dis Child 142:100–105

121. Montigny M, Davignon A, Fouron JC, Biron P, Fournier A, Elie R (1989) Captopril in infants for congestive heart failure secondary to a large ventricular left-to-right shunt. Am J Cardiol 63:631–633

122. Webster MW, Neutze JM, Calder AL (1992) Acute hemodynamic effects of converting enzyme inhibition in children with intracardiac shunts. Pediatr Cardiol 13:129–135

123. Kouatli AA, Garcia JA, Zellers TM, Weinstein EM, Mahony L (1997) Enalapril does not enhance exercise capacity in patients after Fontan procedure. Circulation 96:1507–1512

124. Bengur AR, Beekman RH, Rocchini AP, Crowley DC, Schork MA, Rosenthal A (1991) Acute hemodynamic effects of captopril in children with a congestive or restrictive cardiomyopathy. Circulation 83:523–527

125. Lewis AB, Chabot M (1993) The effect of treatment with angiotensin-converting enzyme inhibitors on survival of pediatric patients with dilated cardiomyopathy. Pediatr Cardiol 14:9–12

126. Ramaciotti C, Heistein LC, Coursey M et al (2006) Left ventricular function and response to enalapril in patients with duchenne muscular dystrophy during the second decade of life. Am J Cardiol 98:825–827

127. Silber JH, Cnaan A, Clark BJ et al (2004) Enalapril to prevent cardiac function decline in long-term survivors of pediatric cancer exposed to anthracyclines. J Clin Oncol 22:820–828

128. Williams RV, Tani LY, Shaddy RE (2002) Intermediate effects of treatment with metoprolol or carvedilol in children with left ventricular systolic dysfunction. J Heart Lung Transplant 21:906–909

129. Bruns LA, Chrisant MK, Lamour JM et al (2001) Carvedilol as therapy in pediatric heart failure: an initial multicenter experience. J Pediatr 138:505–511

130. Shaddy RE, Tani LY, Gidding SS et al (1999) Beta-blocker treatment of dilated cardiomyopathy with congestive heart failure in children: a multi-institutional experience. J Heart Lung Transplant 18:269–274

131. Shaddy RE (1998) Beta-blocker therapy in young children with congestive heart failure under consideration for heart transplantation. Am Heart J 136:19–21

132. Poole-Wilson PA, Swedberg K, Cleland JG et al (2003) Comparison of carvedilol and metoprolol on clinical outcomes in patients with chronic heart failure in the Carvedilol Or Metoprolol European Trial (COMET): randomised controlled trial. Lancet 362:7–13

133. Shaddy RE, Boucek MM, Hsu DT et al (2007) Carvedilol for children and adolescents with heart failure: a randomized controlled trial. JAMA 298:1171–1179

Chapter 15
Mechanical Circulatory Support and Heart Transplantation in Children with Severe Refractory Heart Failure

Overview

Indications for mechanical circulatory support in children differ somewhat from those in adults. Extracorporeal membrane oxygenation (ECMO) provides relatively short-term life support, but newer ventricular assist devices (VAD) are now available. The primary goal of therapy is "bridge to recovery." However, transplant is now an option for patients who do not recover. Donor availability has improved through several mechanisms and decreased waiting time for recipients. The pediatric issues in mechanical circulatory support and transplant are reviewed in this chapter.

Introduction

Mechanical circulatory support is emerging as an invaluable tool in the care of children with severe refractory heart failure (HF). However, children with failing hearts often have complex issues, such as right ventricular failure, pulmonary hypertension, and anatomic variations, that challenge cannulation and support strategies. ECMO and VAD are currently available for application in neonates, infants, and smaller children. Each technique has unique advantages and disadvantages for each age group. The intraaortic balloon pump has been successfully used in bigger children, adolescents, and adults but has limited applicability in smaller children [1]. The indications for use of mechanical circulatory support have recently expanded, and outcomes have improved. As previously noted in Chap. 14, the Carvedilol trial showed that many children with HF recover. Accordingly, mechanical support in children with potentially reversible myocardial dysfunction should involve a clinical strategy to create a bridge to recovery.

Extracorporeal Membrane Oxygenation

Experience shows that in the majority of cases in children ECMO is utilized [1] for mechanical circulatory support. The summary provided as of July 2008 by the Extracorporeal Life Support (ECLS) Organization reported 3,416 cases of HF in neonates and 4,181 children [2]. The majority of runs are performed in infants and children with respiratory failure, although the cardiac cases represent a growing proportion over the past several years. For such HF in neonates and children, almost three-fifths survive to separation from extracorporeal membrane oxygenation and just over two-fifths survive to be discharged. Survival rate is highly dependent on age: 0–30 days (40%); 31 days to 1 year (49%); and 1–16 years (59%). There are multiple complications related to the use of ECLS, such as severe neurologic disorders including brain death. Myocardial stun occurs in approximately 5% of neonates on ECMO, but it can extend the run, leading to other complications. Stun has been attributed to various factors including atrophy induced by mechanical unloading of the heart.

Mechanical circulatory support is occasionally required in neonates who present with profound cyanosis and/or cardiogenic shock. Neonates with pulmonary hypertension or congenital heart defects (CHD), such as severe Ebstein's anomaly, which are refractory to conventional therapy, may require extracorporeal life support while the pulmonary vascular resistance declines. Mechanical circulatory support may be required in the postoperative period, either due to the inability to separate from cardiopulmonary bypass, or because of a progressive "late" low cardiac output syndrome. The combined experience of multiple centers demonstrates that extracorporeal membrane oxygenation can allow survival of many children with congenitally malformed hearts and refractory cardiopulmonary dysfunction. Walters et al. [3] reviewed 73 children with CHD placed on ECMO and showed superior survival for patients placed on support after weaning from cardiopulmonary bypass.

J. Marín-García, *Heart Failure*, Contemporary Cardiology,
DOI 10.1007/978-1-60761-147-9_15, © Springer Science+Business Media, LLC 2010

Survival to discharge was only 23% in patients who could not be weaned from cardiopulmonary bypass compared to 69% in patients who were cannulated postoperatively after an initial period of clinical stability. These results indicate the theory that ECMO is probably most effective if initiated after a period of stability versus immediately after cardiopulmonary bypass. Morris et al. reported on the use of ECMO in 137 children seen from January 1995 to June 2001, with an overall survival to discharge of 39% [4]. Risk factors for mortality were age below 1 month, male gender, longer duration of mechanical ventilation before support, and development of renal or hepatic dysfunction while on support. Despite early concern for the value of ECMO in patients with hypoplastic left heart syndrome (HLHS), functionally univentricular physiology and failure to separate from cardiopulmonary bypass were not associated with an increased risk of mortality. Cardiac physiology and the indications for support were not associated with the incidence of death.

Rapid resuscitation with ECMO after cardiopulmonary arrest was initially described by del Nido et al. [5]. This resuscitation requires rapid deployment and an organized effort. Extended time of cardiopulmonary resuscitation limits the effectiveness of rescue. However, prolonged effective cardiopulmonary resuscitation does not preclude survival and favorable neurologic outcomes. Some centers maintain preprimed circuits for allotted periods of time in an attempt to overcome the problem of prolonged setup. Use of these preprimed circuits accepts the added risk of infection should the circuit become contaminated, and the expense of not using the circuit during the allotted time span. Some centers have developed novel systems for cardiopulmonary support. Duncan et al. described a fully portable circuit that is maintained vacuum- and carbon dioxide-primed at all times [6].

Children with acute fulminant myocarditis can acutely decompensate and die despite conventional medical support. Therefore, mechanical circulatory support is indicated in children with acute myocarditis and persistent low cardiac output syndrome despite escalating inotropic support. The Extracorporeal Life Support Organization reports that survival with myocarditis is highest for any diagnostic group, with almost three-fifths being successfully weaned from extracorporeal membrane oxygenation [2]. ECMO is the mechanical support of choice in these patients because of the speed with which it can be instituted and its easy reversibility; in this subgroup of patients, it may be used successfully as a bridge to recovery or transplantation. Duncan et al. reviewed their experience with ECMO ($n = 12$) or Ventricular assist devices (VAD) ($n = 3$) in children with clinical, laboratory, or endomyocardial biopsy-proven myocarditis and clinical deterioration accompanied by imminently lethal cardiogenic shock or cardiac arrest [7]. Nine (60%) of the 15 patients were weaned

from support, with seven (78%) survivors; the remaining six patients were successfully bridged to transplantation, with five (83%) survivors. Deaths in this cohort of patients were secondary to post-support nosocomial infections.

Limited data exist regarding neurodevelopmental outcomes after ECMO for HF. Ibrahim et al. reported moderate to severe neurological impairment in 13 of 21 children (59%) after ECMO [8]. More recently Wagner et al. assessed 22 children who underwent ECMO for cardiac indications [9]. Moderate or severe impairment in at least two clinical assessments were found in 16 (72.7%) children. Five (22.7%) children had cerebral palsy and 15 (68.2%) had moderate or severe cognitive impairment. Eight (36%) children had pathological radiologic findings. Pathological electroencephalograms were found in 11 (50%) patients including four (18.2%) with epileptic activity. Children with radiologic findings had a slightly worse cognitive outcome. There was no association between the neurophysiologic findings and the neuropsychologic performance or the radiologic findings. Based on parental assessment, only four children had pathological scores. The authors stated that it was uncertain to which extent the impaired clinical and psychosocial functioning is caused by the primary disease or to the ECMO treatment.

ECMO use is limited to those patients who require only short-term cardiopulmonary support. Several types of mechanical support devices are available and have become standard therapy for adults with HF refractory to maximal medical management. The hemodynamic and mechanical principals and standard management of patients with these devices will not be reviewed here. There are fewer options available to children than to adults, although over the last few years, progress has been made in pediatric mechanical support. VAD are being used with increasing frequency in children with HF refractory to medical therapy for primary treatment as a long-term bridge to recovery or transplantation [1, 10, 11]. Mechanical circulatory support should be anticipated, and every attempt must be made to initiate support "urgently" rather than "emergently" before the presence of dysfunction of end organs or circulatory collapse. In an emergency, these patients can be resuscitated with ECMO and subsequently transitioned to a long-term VAD after a period of stability. Destination therapy, defined as intracorporeal insertion of a VAD with the goal of "permanent support," is currently not an option in children.

Experience in children with long-term pulsatile devices is growing [1]. These devices offer univentricular or biventricular support. Children do not require mechanical ventilation and are able to be mobilized out of the intensive care unit on relatively low levels of anticoagulation. The Berlin Heart, or EXCOR (Fig. 15.1), is a paracorporeal pneumatically driven pulsatile ventricular assist device.

The blood pumps, available in a variety of sizes, have a transparent polyurethane housing which divides an air

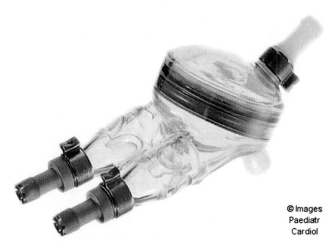

© Images
Paediatr
Cardiol

Fig. 15.1 The Berlin Heart EXCOR (Reprinted from Fuchs A, Netz H (2002) Ventricular assist devices in pediatrics. Images Paediatr Cardiol 9:24–54. With permission from © Images in Paediatric Cardiology (1999–2002))

chamber and blood chamber by a triple layer membrane. The EXCOR is offered in five different sizes providing pump capacities from 10 to 60 ml. In the United States, the Berlin Heart is not currently approved by the federal Food and Drug Administration but is available for use under a compassionate protocol as a bridge to transplantation. As of 2007, review of data from the worldwide experience using the Berlin Heart in children shows that in Europe, the United States of America, Canada, Argentina, and China, 282 children have been supported on this device [1]. Of these, about one third was supported in North America. The mean age in this population is 4.1 years. Rockett et al. have reported the largest series of patients treated with the EXCOR in the United States [11]. The Arkansas Children's Hospital placed the EXCOR in 17 children, 13 of whom received a left-sided pump and four of whom required biventricular support. Before EXCOR placement, six patients were on ECMO and one was on a centrifugal VAD. Eleven children were bridged to transplantation, one was bridged to recovery and one remains on support at the time of publication. Three children died during support and one died after explantation. There was one late death nearly 2 years after transplant. Complications included stroke in seven patients, two of which were ultimately fatal. Five patients required reoperations for bleeding or evacuation of hematoma. Despite a disappointing rate of neurologic morbidity, the authors found the results encouraging.

The MEDOS-HIA VAD, another paracorporeal, pneumatically driven blood pump, is available in Europe in three sizes for the left ventricle, providing stroke volumes of 10, 25, and 60 ml, and three sizes for the right ventricle, giving volumes of 9, 22.5, and 54 ml. This system has also

been successfully used for long-term support and bridge to transplantation. The Thoratec Ventricular Assist System, Abiomed's AB5000 Circulatory Support System, and HeartMate are pulsatile assist devices that can be used in larger children and adolescents. These systems are not practical for use in children with a body surface area smaller than 0.8 m^2 due to size limitations. Sharma et al. [12] reviewed their experience with pulsatile VAD as a bridge to heart transplantation in 18 patients over a period of 15 years. Diagnoses included dilated cardiomyopathy, myocarditis, and ventricular failure after cardiac surgery. Biventricular devices were used in just over half, with only left VAD used in the remainder. Three-quarters of the patients underwent successful transplantation. Complications included bleeding requiring reoperation, stroke, and device-related infection.

The experience with these axial flow VAD is limited in children, but they have been used successfully in those aged from 5 to 16 years with a body surface area of greater than or equal to 0.7 m^2. Advantages of axial pumps include their small size, the relatively ease of implantation and explantation, low rates of infection, and continuous flow that minimize formation of thrombus. Disadvantages include nonpulsatile flow, the limitation of size for children, and larger-sized ventricular apical cannulation. The MicroMed DeBakey VAD® is a miniaturized heart pump, which provides flow of up to 10 L of blood per minute. The implantable pump weighs less than four ounces and contains only one moving part, the impeller. The device has been used successfully to bridge several children to cardiac transplantation [61]. The Jarvik 2000 is a similar intravascular assist device. The impeller rotates at 8,000–12,000 revolutions per minute, generating a flow of 3–6 l per minute. Preliminary data in juvenile animal models in vivo experience with the pediatric Jarvik-2000 heart show that this small axial flow pump can provide partial to nearly complete circulatory support with minimal adverse effects on blood components [13].

Heart Transplantation in Pediatrics[1]

Heart transplantation is now a treatment option with good outcomes for infants and children with end-stage heart failure (HF) or inoperable CHD [14]. Over the past 15 years, approximately 400 pediatric (up to age 18 years) heart transplant procedures were performed annually [15].

---

[1]This section was authored by Robert J. Boucek Jr. M.D./M.S. Department of Pediatrics, University of Washington. Seattle, WA, USA.

Many of the advances in the science of heart transplantation in adults have formed the basis for the management of pediatric recipients. In this chapter, the substantive differences between heart transplantation in pediatrics, particularly recipients under the age of one, and adult recipients will be identified. The differences included herein are: (1) transplant indications (CHD); (2) unique opportunities for the expansion of the donor pool (ABO independent, donation after cardiac death (DCD)); (3) rejection and rejection surveillance; (4) unique long-term outcome considerations.

Recipient Age

The age of recipients at the time of transplantation is both an obvious yet profound difference between pediatric and adult cardiac transplantation. Though outcomes of heart transplantation have improved in children less than 1 year of age, defined herein as infants, the high early phase of the survival analyses demonstrate the higher early risk of the procedure in the infant recipient group compared to older children (Fig. 15.2) [15, 16] and adults [17]. Somewhat surprisingly, recipient age alone was not identified as an independent risk factor for early stage mortality [15]. Infant heart transplant recipient survival has significantly improved in the most recent era (1982–1990 vs. 2000–6/2006: p<0.0001), with the most dramatic gains in survival

achieved in the first year post-transplant (Fig. 15.3) [16]. The strong era effect offers hope that the projected half-life for infant recipients in the current era will continue to increase and decades-long survival could be a reality. In contrast, the late phase of the survival curve demonstrates a lower rate of mortality in the infant recipients (Fig. 15.3) [16]. In the interpretation of these survival results calculated using the Kaplan–Meier method, is that it incorporates information from all transplants for whom any follow-up has been provided. Since many patients are still alive and some patients have been lost to follow-up, the survival rates are estimates rather than exact rates because the time of death is not known for all patients.

Recipient age affects the indications for pediatric heart transplantation. Between 1996 and 2007, CHD was the most common (63%) indication for orthotopic transplantation in children less than 1 year of age, defined herein as infants, and overall was the most common diagnosis leading to heart transplantation in children [15]. Cardiomyopathy, on the other hand, is the most common indication in older pediatric recipients, between ages 1 and 10 years (~52%) and between ages 11 and 17 years (~61%) [15], and adult recipients (~44%) [17]. Congenital heart disease is identified as a significant risk for transplant-related deaths [15]. The most common cause of death was acute graft failure as reported in a multiinstitutional study [18]. Likely explanations for how recipient anatomy poses risks for transplantation will be discussed.

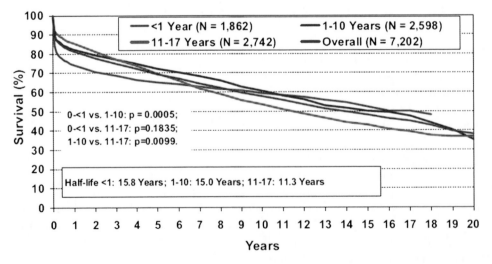

Fig. 15.2 Patient survival to 20 years stratified by age at time of transplant. Survival was calculated using the Kaplan–Meier method, which incorporates information from all transplants for whom any follow-up has been provided. Since many patients are still alive and some patients have been lost to follow-up, the survival rates are estimates rather than exact rates because the time of death is not known for all patients. The half-life is the estimated time point at which 50% of all of the recipients have died (Reprinted from Kirk et al. [16]. With kind permission from Elsevier)

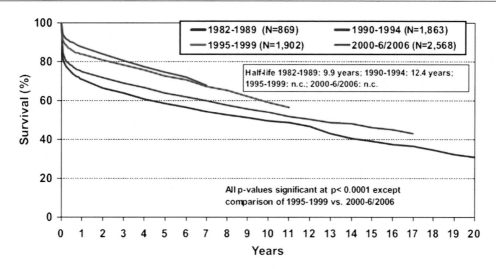

Fig. 15.3 Survival by era for recipients under 1 year of age (Reprinted from Kirk et al. [16]. With kind permission from Elsevier)

Transplant Indications: Complex Anatomy

With CHD, primary transplantation of infants with complex cardiac anatomy poses unique operative challenges compared with transplantation for cardiomyopathies. Additional surgical procedures include repositioning of transposed great arteries, reconstruction of the aortic pathway, reconstruction of the pulmonary pathway, correction of situs inversus [19] and/or visceral heterotaxy [20], and correction of anomalous pulmonary [21] or systemic venous drainage using donor and/or recipient tissue. Generally, these pose added risks but do not constitute absolute contraindications [22]. Hypoplastic pulmonary arteries or veins can constitute absolute contraindications to successful transplantation. Transplantation after palliative surgeries creates several added risk factors for transplantation [18, 22–24].

Transplant Indications: Hypoplastic Left Heart Syndrome

Primary transplantation for HLHS was pioneered by Bailey at Loma Linda and provided the first real hope for survival of infants born with congenital abnormality [25–27]. For many centers, infants with HLHS are palliated with staged surgical procedures prior to transplantation [28]. In infants where surgical palliation is not the optimal management [29], transplantation can be an excellent option [30]. In the early experience, infants with HLHS can be successfully palliated with prostaglandin E-1 while awaiting a suitable donor [26]. More recently, the PDA can be stented and the branch pulmonary arteries surgically banded (external banding) or interventionally banded [31, 32]. Transplant outcomes are good with survival ≥85% post-transplant [25, 33]. Current survival rates for initial palliative procedures such as interventional catheterization or Stage 1

surgical reconstruction, so called "Norwood," are approximately 85%. Thus, after an initial palliation, families and their physicians can elect either transplantation or three-staged surgical treatment or Norwood. Comparisons of the postoperative survival of transplantation versus Norwood favor transplantation at all ages up to 7 years [34] and differences in morbidity seem to favor transplantation. However, current limitations of donor identification and availability would not allow transplantation to be the primary option for all children born with HLHS.

Despite the demanding surgical techniques and postoperative management in very young and very sick children, 1- and 5-year actuarial survival rates are high, approximately 75 and 65%, respectively, with overall patient survival half-life greater than 10 years [15]. A number of institutional reports as well as the most recent International Society for Heart and Lung Transplantation (ISHLT) Registry data indicate 1-year survival in excess of 80% [35].

Unique Expansion of Donor Pool

As in adult heart transplantation, donor organ availability limits the number of children receiving heart transplantation and contributes to waiting time mortality. In fact, neonatal waiting time mortality and morbidity remains unacceptably high and is the highest of any solid organ, up to 30% after 90 days [33, 36, 37].

The long waiting times has been attributed to a shortage of donors. However, a past analysis of the UNOS (United Network for Organ Sharing)–ISHLT Registry database indicated that only about one-third of solid organ donors were heart donors [38] providing evidence for opportunities to improve donation rates and donor organ utilization. Distance/ischemic time has not emerged as a risk factor for pediatric transplant outcomes in the registries [15, 39], but current practice to limit ischemic time to less than 300 min may be a selection bias. More evidence is emerging to prove that expanding distance/ischemic time criteria for pediatric donor acceptance is not a risk factor for acute graft failure [40–43].

One of the most exciting opportunities to expand donor–recipient marching in pediatrics is to be able to safely transplant across ABO barriers. Infants who have not yet developed significant anti-ABO antibody have been reported to safely undergo transplantation across what had been previously thought of as ABO barriers. This was first applied in Canada [44, 45], and now the UK experience has been reported [46]. In January 1999, changes were made in the UNOS algorithm for allocation of donor hearts to permit listing across ABO barriers for infants less than a year old. DCD leading to successful heart transplantation has recently been reported for infants [47]. In the future, emphasis should be placed on optimizing donor identification, expanding the donor criteria, and better donor distribution. In addition, better identification of waiting time risks for recipients has been modeled to improve donor allocations in pediatric heart transplantation [48].

Surveillance for Rejection

Definitions

Acute rejection, as defined by the Pediatric Heart Transplant Study Group [49] and ISHLT registries [15] as well as clinical practice, is an operational definition, namely the intent to treat. Based on this definition, treated acute rejection would be more precise while in this and most discussions acute rejection is used. In clinical practice, patient symptoms and/or echocardiographic abnormalities [50, 51] alert care providers of emerging acute rejection. Severe acute rejection is often diagnosed in adult [52] and pediatric [53] recipients using clinical and echocardiographic findings while a high percentage have no, or low grades of, biopsy evidence of cellular infiltration. The diagnosis of acute *cellular* rejection can only be confirmed by histopathologic evidence for lymphocytic infiltrations and myocyte injury [54, 55]. For the most part, these definitions do not differ between adult and pediatric heart transplant communities.

Acute Rejection

Using earlier immunosuppressive regimens, pediatric heart transplant recipients experience between 1.5 and 2 acute rejection episodes/patient up to 9 years posttransplantation [49, 56]. Most acute rejection episodes in pediatric heart recipients occur in the first 3 months posttransplant [56]. Approximately, 1/3 of pediatric recipients are acute rejection-free in the first year post-transplant [56]. More recently, the ISHLT Registries report ≤20% of neonatal recipients [15] whereas between 30 and 50% of adult recipients [17] have treated acute rejection in the first year post transplant.

Acute cellular rejection is fatal in less than 10% of episodes in pediatric recipients [53]. Late acute rejection that occurs more than 1 year posttransplantation, on the other hand, has a more ominous prognosis and has been linked to poor compliance with the immunosuppressive regimen [57]. Nonischemic ventricular dysfunction that improves with augmented immunosuppression represents an additional type of rejection without biopsy evidence for cellular infiltration [58].

Echocardiographic Rejection Surveillance in Infant Recipients

As in the early days of adult heart transplantation, an objective assessment of rejection status was needed in the early days of infant heart transplantation. At the time, several investigators had identified several echocardiographic parameters relating to myocardial performance that met statistical significance but because of overlaping ranges failed to have high negative predictive value. Systematically determined quantitative 2D-guided M-mode echocardiographic parameters were found to be effective in terms of infant recipient outcomes [59]. These investigators also observed that no single echocardiographic parameter had sufficient predictive power hence the algorithm incorporated multiple echocardiographic parameters. Subsequently, an empirically derived algorithm was developed and was shown to have high predictive value for grade 3(2R) cellular rejection in prospective studies [51, 60, 61]. In this algorithm, measured patient values are compared to age-matched transplanted recipients without rejection or "normals" [51]. Most importantly, intensified immunosuppression is usually associated with a rapid improvement in the ECHO-A parameters and the derived score [51]. The positive predictive value of the algorithm was further improved when change from the patient's prerejection baseline formed the basis for scoring [61]. Of note, when this same multi-parametric algorithm was compared retrospectively in adult recipients, it retained a high level of negative predictive value for grade 3(2R) cellular rejection [60]. A similar multiparametric approach was also validated in adults as predictive of biopsy-based cellular rejection [62].

Other important observations were made in the echocardiographic assessment of infants following heart transplantation. The echocardiographic patterns of acute rejection in these younger pediatric recipients were noted to vary between patients and at different times posttransplant in the same patient. Some general trends noted were: that changes in LV posterior wall diastolic parameters often preceded changes in LV posterior wall systolic parameters; global diastolic parameters usually preceded global systolic parameters, a common finding in older children and adults [60]; new onset and significant AV valve regurgitation and/or pericardial effusion [62] were predictors independent of the function parameters; and echocardiographic changes from baseline were more predictive of acute rejection than changes from "normal" [61]. To date, single echocardiographic parameters have had limited abilities predicting cellular rejection by endomyocardial biopsy (EMB) [63–66]. Given these different patterns of rejection, it is not surprising that any single echocardiographic parameter analyzed independently [63, 67] will have sufficient predictive power.

Cardiac allograft rejection is accompanied by cellular infiltration and tissue edema resulting in myocardial relaxation abnormalities [68]. Tissue Doppler determination of posterior wall thinning has been reported to be decreased with rejection [69–72] and is independent of preloading [73], though dependent on afterload [74]. Wall thinning determined by pulse wave tissue Doppler had limited predictive value in our hands because of an apparent heart rate effect in pediatric recipients resulting in a paradoxical increase in relaxation velocities with cellular rejection [75]. Determination of LV filling characteristics using tissue Doppler assessment of mitral annulus proved to be predictive when E'/a' decreased to less than 1 [74], an abnormal LV. The mitral valve annular decent E/a ratio has been added to the current mutiparametric analysis algorithm. The tissue Doppler-derived systolic velocity, isovolumic acceleration, has the advantage of not being age-dependent or affected by regional wall motion abnormalities, common early after transplant. Compared with conventional tissue Doppler indices, isovolumic acceleration decreased with acute cellular rejection [76] and could be considered in the future as a component of a multiparametric approach to surveillance.

Despite the demonstrated predictive value of the quantitative multiparametric echocardiographic analysis algorithm ECHO-A [50], it has not been widely adopted. There are multiple reasons for this. In studies focusing on indices of systolic performance, low sensitivity has been a common finding [64], in part because systolic dysfunction is a late finding. In studies focusing on diastolic dysfunction, high sensitivity but low specificity has been a common finding, in part because diastolic parameters are load-dependent and abnormal in a significant number of recipients in the absence of rejection. The off-line use of digitized endocardial determination of the maximal velocity of posterior wall thinning, a tissue index of myocardial relaxation with high predictive value [51], has likely been a barrier. The lack of

echocardiographic standardization and institutional variations has contributed to the inability of echocardiography to compete with EMB for rejection surveillance in this country. Still, the need for noninvasive techniques has persisted in pediatrics, particularly in infants, and has been met only in certain geographical areas by standardized quantitative echocardiography. Thus, only in some centers who transplant large numbers of infants, multiparametric analysis (ECHO-A) of transthoracic echocardiograms has been used in surveillance for rejection with very high negative predictive value.

EMB-Based Surveillance Strategies

The value of routine surveillance with EMB beyond the early posttransplant period is controversial in adult recipients largely because of the very low rate of positive biopsy after 1 year posttransplant [77, 78]. In one review, the importance of even a positive biopsy is questioned in the absence of symptoms concluding that "it remains unproven whether non-treatment of moderate or greater rejection (≥3A) increases the likelihood of recurrent rejection, which if present, may increase the risk of allograft coronary disease and/or reduced long-term survival" [79]. Other limitations of the scheduled EMB in rejection surveillance are sampling error, observer variability of interpretation, quality of specimens, and limited number of opportunities for surveillance that could lead to the under recognition of late rejection.

Debate about appropriate methods for surveillance of pediatric recipients has also centered on the role of EMB. At one extreme is the position that rejection can only be detected in pediatric recipients by EMB, a statement made by respected traditional program in 2004 [55], despite the high number of negative scheduled biopsies in the absence of symptoms [80, 81]. Biopsy-based surveillance for rejection, particularly after 1 year following transplantation, is problematic in children because of risk, limited access, need for anesthesia, and costs to families. Infant heart transplantation introduced yet an additional need for less invasive surveillance for rejection than EMB as noted above. Though EMB can be performed with low risk in most pediatric recipients [82], the EMB procedure is more difficult and dangerous when performed from sites other than the internal jugular vein as in younger infants [82].

A more general question is when to perform surveillance. Should surveillance be regularly scheduled or based on some other indication such as symptoms [79]? The younger the recipient and/or the more limited the access will impose limitations on the frequency of scheduled biopsy-based surveillance. In infants, symptoms referable to left ventricular systolic and diastolic dysfunction were observed to correlate with histopathologically verified cellular rejection [83].

In older children and adults, histopathology can precede clinical symptoms of HF in the majority of patients [52]. Our center relies on clinical and echocardiographic changes to guide the decision about EMB [50]. Other centers have recommended that routine scheduled biopsy surveillance be reserved for patients at high risk of rejection [84], since significant late rejection is rare. European centers have reported that transtelephonic surveillance of ventricular-evoked responses can be used to time surveillance biopsies with high predictive value [85, 86], a strategy that would be very attractive to families of pediatric recipients.

The most compelling argument favoring continued refinement of our assessment of ventricular function and morphological changes with rejection is the observation that a significant number of children with symptomatic rejection have a biopsy score of 0 [53]. This group of patients is also at the greatest risk for death with a rejection episode. It is unclear why patients who demonstrate severe rejection clinically and by echocardiogram do not have recognized changes on EMB. While cytotoxic lymphocytes are thought to mediate myocardial damage with rejection, cytokines, such as interleukin-II or tumor necrosis factor which are released with immune activation, have been shown to have a direct myocardial depressant effect in vitro. These cytokines could cause depressed cardiac function during acute rejection, even in the absence of lymphocytes on the EMB. We speculate that the sensitivity and specificity of any one echocardiographic parameter may relate to inherent variabilities in release of these cytokine mediators with rejection.

Noninvasive Surveillance of Acute Rejection

Gene expression profiling in rejection surveillance is under review currently for pediatric heart transplant recipients [87]. The Invasive Monitoring Attenuation Through Gene Expression (IMAGE) study is a prospective, multicenter, nonblinded, randomized clinical trial designed to test the hypothesis that a primarily noninvasive rejection surveillance strategy utilizing GEP testing is not inferior to an invasive EMB-based strategy with respect to cardiac allograft dysfunction, rejection with hemodynamic compromise (HDC), and all-cause mortality in adult heart transplant recipients [88].

Late Outcomes Following Pediatric Heart Transplantation

In considering survival in pediatric heart transplantation, the current emphasis has shifted from early to late outcomes. Because the decline in survival is greatest during the first year following transplantation, the conditional survival analysis shown in Fig. 15.4 provides a more realistic expectation of survival time for recipients who survive the early posttransplant period. Younger children had a significantly improved survival over time (Fig. 15.4) [15]. In contrast to older children, the strong era effect on early mortality (see Fig. 15.3) coupled with the significant improvement in the late phase survival, particularly for neonatal recipients (see Fig. 15.4), offers hope that the projected half-life for pediatric recipients in the current era will continue to increase and decades-long survival will be a reality.

Analysis of conditional survival curves in the ISHLT registry (Figs. 15.4 and 15.5) describes the late phase survival following successful heart transplantation with a continued but low risk of mortality with time [15]. The cardiac causes of death or retransplant are the development of coronary artery disease (CAD; Fig. 15.5) [15, 89] and, to a lesser extent, rejection (Fig. 15.6) [16, 57]. The rate of late graft loss due to CAD appears to be 2–3% per year, although this rate seems to decrease over time [90].

Other risk factors for adverse late outcomes unique to pediatric heart transplantation identified in registry data include the pretransplant diagnosis of CHD (Table 15.1) and rejection posttransplant (Fig. 15.5) [15].

Late Rejection and Graft Atherosclerosis

Long-term cardiac allograft and patient survival in pediatric recipients, as in adult recipients, decreases at a low but constant rate over time [16]. The most common cause for adverse late outcomes in pediatric heart recipients, as in adult heart recipients, is reported to be accelerated CAD, or graft atherosclerosis [16]. There is a clear age at transplant dependency both on late survival and CAD (Fig. 15.7) [16]. The incidence of graft atherosclerosis varies somewhat depending on the technique used for diagnosis. Standard coronary angiography is relatively insensitive until significant coronary abnormalities are present. Using coronary angiography, the incidence of graft atherosclerosis in pediatric patients appears to be around 10–15% at 5 years. Using more sensitive techniques, such as intravascular ultrasound, the percentage increases to 15–20%. Regardless of the technique used, the incidence appears to be lower in pediatric than in adult heart transplant recipients [91]. It is not known, however, whether the difference between pediatric and adult recipients is related to diagnostic techniques, since the most sensitive measures are not applicable to the youngest recipients, and/or to immunologic immaturity of the recipients and/or perhaps even donor-specific issues.

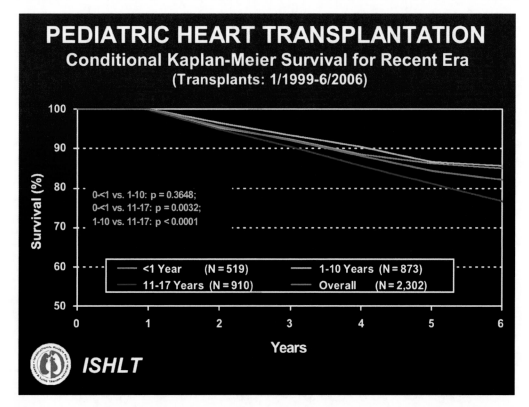

Fig. 15.4 Conditional survival by recipient age. Survival was calculated using the Kaplan–Meier method, which incorporates information from all transplants for whom any follow-up has been provided. Since many patients are still alive and some patients have been lost to follow-up, the survival rates are estimates rather than exact rates because the time of death is not known for all patients. Conditional survival is shown in this figure; this is the survival following 1 year for all patients who survived to 1 year. The conditional half-life is the estimated time point at which 50% of the recipients who survive to at least 1 year have died. Because the decline in survival is greatest during the first year following transplantation, the conditional survival provides a more realistic expectation of survival time for recipients who survive the early post-transplant period (Reproduced from Boucek et al. [15]. With kind permission from Elsevier)

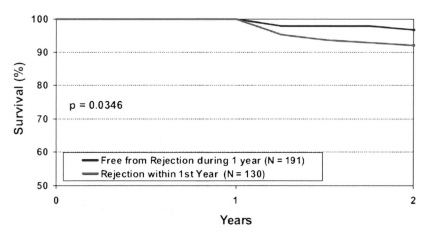

Fig. 15.5 Impact of early rejection on late outcomes in pediatric heart transplantation. Survival was calculated using the Kaplan–Meier method, which incorporates information from all transplants for whom any follow-up has been provided. Since many patients are alive and some patients have been lost to follow-up, the survival rates are estimates rather than exact rates because the time of death is not known for all patients and may never occur for some patients. Conditional survival is shown in this figure; this is the survival rate following 1 year for all patients who survived to 1 year. Survival rates were compared using the log-rank test statistic (Reprinted from Kirk et al. [16]. With kind permission from Elsevier)

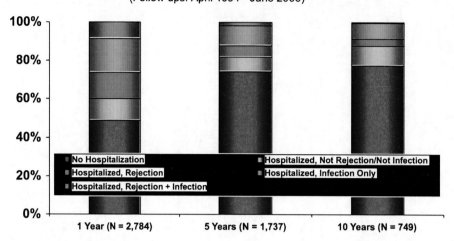

Fig. 15.6 Rehospitalization of pediatric heart recipients (Reproduced from Boucek et al. [15]. With kind permission from Elsevier)

Table 15.1 Risk factors for 5 year mortality

Variable	N	Relative risk	P value	95% confidence interval
Congenital diagnosis, age > 0, on ECMO	56	4.80	<0.0001	2.94–7.83
Congenital diagnosis, age = 0, on ECMO	63	4.74	<0.0001	2.99–7.53
Congenital diagnosis, age > 0, no EMCO	735	2.32	<0.0001	1.76–3.06
Retransplant	201	2.26	0.0001	1.52–3.36
Congenital diagnosis, age = 0, on PGE	209	1.93	0.0021	1.27–2.93
Congenital diagnosis, age = 0, no PGE or ECMO	352	1.7	0.0039	1.19–2.45
Year of transplant: 1995–1996 vs. 1999–2000	505	1.54	0.0057	1.13–2.08
On ventilator	636	1.51	0.0008	1.19–1.92
Female recipient	1,488	1.23	0.0321	1.02–1.48
Not ABO identical	759	0.77	0.0231	0.061–0.96

Reference diagnosis = Cardiomyopathy (1/1995–6/2006)

N=3,395

Multivariable analysis was performed using a proportional hazards model censoring all patients at 1 year. Continuous factors were fit using a restricted cubic spline. Analyses were limited to transplants having essentially complete information regarding risk factors (Reprinted from Kirk et al. [16]. With kind permission from Elsevier)

Late Outcomes: Quality of Life Following Pediatric Heart Transplantation

The quality of life in surviving children is excellent in the majority of recipients but will be affected by pretransplant morbidity. Most recipients do not have activity limitation and do not require frequent hospitalizations (see Fig. 15.6) [15, 92]. Somatic growth has been reported to be generally within the low normal range in infant heart transplant recipients [93]. Eighty-five percent of infant recipients who were at least 6 years old were in an appropriate grade level. However, neurodevelopmental deficits are prevalent among school-aged children with HLHS following conventional management and primary orthotopic cardiac transplant [94].

Linear growth arrest, however, has been demonstrated in the adolescent-age recipient, despite continued weight gain. Immunosuppressive medications, particularly corticosteroids and possibly calcineurin inhibitors, may affect linear growth as in adult heart transplant recipients [95].

Unique Pediatric Donor and Recipient Immunologic Variables

The ultimate goal of transplantation is donor-specific tolerance. Pediatric heart transplantation may represent a unique immunologic opportunity for organ transplantation because the development of the immune system extends not only into

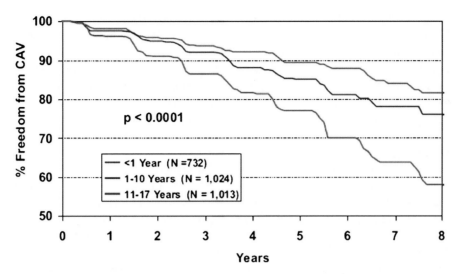

Fig. 15.7 Freedom from coronary artery disease by recipient age. Freedom from coronary artery vasculopathy (CAV) was computed using the Kaplan–Meier method. The development of CAV is reported on annual follow-ups; a date of diagnosis is not provided. For this figure the midpoint between the date of previous follow-up (when event had not occurred) and the date of follow-up when the event was reported was used as the date of occurrence. Patients were included in the analysis until an unknown response for the outcome of interest was reported. Therefore, the rates seen here may differ from those reported in the cumulative prevalence slide which is based on only those patients with known responses for each of the outcomes at all follow-up time points. Freedom from CAV rates were compared using the log-rank test statistic (Reprinted from Kirk et al. [16]. With kind permission from Elsevier)

infancy but continues throughout childhood and adolescence. Careful review of ISHLT Registry data demonstrate higher early mortality in infants with significant improvement with current era [15]. Survival is higher in many centers for recipients less than 1 year of age, predominantly due to lower early graft failure [18]. These age-related differences in early mortality for infant heart transplantation are likely due to improving skills in the management of the infant recipient. In support of a favorable immunologic opportunity for heart transplantation in childhood is the lower late phase mortality noted (see Fig. 15.4) [15]. Younger age at time of transplantation was also reported to have better early survival following polyclonal antithymocyte antibody induction [96, 97] and a lower frequency of rejection [97] compared with older children. However, in ISHLT Registry data, there was no age-related survival benefit reported with polyclonal antibody induction immunotherapy in infant heart recipients [15].

Recall that recipients less than 1 year old at transplant also have lower rates of late phase mortality and morbidity. They have a lower rate of late death/graft loss as compared to adolescents with a flattening of the late phase of the conditional survival curve (see Fig. 15.5) [15, 16]. They have higher freedom from CAD compared to adolescents (see Fig. 15.7) [16]. Though many of the late acute rejection episodes that are life threatening have been related to poor patient compliance, particularly in adolescent recipients [57], the possibility of significant age-related immunological differences should be considered further.

Favorable immune donor-specific immune responses in infant heart recipients had been anticipated since the cellular, endocrine, and humoral components of the immune system mature postnatally in humans. As noted in a prior review of this topic, cytokine production and the cytokine profile mature postnatally [98]. The absolute number of mature T-cells and killer T-cells is lower in the infant [99, 100], naive T-cells are greater than in the adult, and the lymphocyte surface receptor repertoire is age-dependent [101]. T-cell responses and phenotype are naïve, compared to adults, with decreased expression of integrins and adhesion molecules. Infants and children undergoing orthotopic cardiac transplantation typically undergo thymectomy at the time of surgery. Although absence of the thymus does not result in a detectable change in immune function in this population [102], the ability to acquire central tolerance in the absence of a thymus may be compromised and, therefore, could affect long-term graft survival [103]. Infants lack significant anti-ABO antibody and can safely undergo transplantation across ABO barriers [44]. This observation also provides compelling evidence that graft-specific tolerance, at least to B cell-mediated antibody production to blood group antigens, can be achieved in infant recipients [104].

Immunosuppression in Pediatric Heart Transplant Recipients

Maintenance immunosuppressive regimens utilized in pediatric heart transplant recipients tend to be both individual and institution-specific. The strategies take advantage of the selectivity of immunosuppressive agents for critical pathways in graft rejection. Virtually all pediatric recipients are treated with a T-cell activation inhibitor – either a calcineurin inhibitor such as cyclosporine, or tacrolimus [15]. In selected patients with significant calcineurin inhibitor-mediated toxicity, the mTOR inhibitors sirolimus or everolimus are being introduced for recipients >6 months after transplantation [105, 106]. Most patients also receive an antiproliferative agent, either mycophenolate mofetil (MMF) or azathioprine.

An early trend in infant transplantation pioneered by the Loma Linda program was to successfully wean recipients off steroids early posttransplant [107]. Similar success with steroid-free maintenance has been reported in older pediatric recipients as well [84]. Despite this lead, only 40% of pediatric recipients are not on maintenance steroids at 1 year posttransplant (08 registry), similar to that reported in the adult Registry [108]. However, about 60% of pediatric recipients report freedom from maintenance corticosteroids by 5 years [15].

Long-term corticosteroid usage in pediatric heart transplantation has been linked to several undesirable risks. For example, higher risks of opportunistic infections, diabetes, bone demineralization, and graft coronary artery disease have been linked to immunosuppressive regimens containing steroids or to their "steroid burden." Furthermore, patients who are maintained on prolonged corticosteroid therapy posttransplantation appear to be at risk for rejection when corticosteroids are later withdrawn [109]. In light of current data, many programs try to minimize the dose and duration of corticosteroid therapy after pediatric heart transplantation.

Infection/Malignancies in Pediatric Heart Transplant Recipients

Infection, due to multiple factors including immunosuppression, surgery, invasive devices, and predisposing factors, is a significant cause of morbidity and mortality after pediatric heart transplantation [110] as in adult heart transplantation. Bacteria and fungi are the major causes of infections occurring in the first month after transplantation [110]. The most common bacterial and fungal infections in heart recipients are respiratory tract or sternal wound infections [110].

Viruses play a major role in infections occurring after transplantation, particularly members of the Herpes family such as cytomegalovirus (CMV) and EBV infections. The higher the levels of immunosuppression, the greater the risk of viral infections appears to be. Therefore, prophylactic therapy against CMV infections is given in the immediate posttransplant period or with intensification of immunosuppression with rejection.

Since most infant heart recipients are serologic-negative for CMV and EBV, they will have primary infections with EBV and CMV, an important difference between adult recipients. EBV infection is related to the risk for posttransplant lymphoproliferative disorder (PTLD) in pediatric heart transplantation [111]. The proportion of malignancies that are lymphoid malignancies, due largely to PTLD, is significantly higher in pediatric [16] compared with adult recipients [17].

Minimizing the level of immunosuppression therapy following primary EBV infection should be considered to reduce the risk of PTLD. By extrapolation from other solid organ transplantation, Sirolimus could be useful to withdraw or reduce dose of the calcineurin inhibitors for toxicity or EBV-mediated PTLD [105]. The careful balance between risks of PTLD and rejection is essential but the method for assessing the level of immunosuppression is, for the most part, the drug levels. The availability of an assay to assess the responsiveness of lymphocytes could prove useful to individualize immunosuppression in primary EBV infections in pediatric heart transplant recipients [112].

The complexities and outcomes of pediatric heart transplantation are significantly different from adult heart transplantation. We have cited evidence that the youngest infant recipients have significantly lower cumulative late phase risks. We have cited evidence to suggest that infants could have significant differences in their immune responses, which may allow for reduced levels of immunosuppression. We have extensively reviewed how the need for less invasive rejection surveillance in the infant heart recipient has led to the development of an echo-based noninvasive surveillance strategy. The lessons learned that can be extrapolated to other age groups are that serial and multiparametric analyses allows for early detection of changes that relate to the onset of cellular rejection. Further refinements are still needed to survey for other forms of rejection and the development of CAD.

Survival, particularly for infants, has improved dramatically in the last decade. The most recent ISHLT Registry shows that recipients less than 1 year old at transplant and who survive the first year have greater than a 95% survival up to 4 years (see Fig. 15.3) [16]. As late outcomes continue to improve, the need for donor organs likely will increase as transplantation would provide a better quality and duration of life for children with complex CHD otherwise facing a future of multiple palliative operations, chronic congestive heart failure due to late cardiomyopathic progression. Efforts to increase potential donors and donor utilization can be supported by innovative schemes such as ABO incompatible heart transplants. Additional efforts are made more urgent when the current data indicate excellent outcomes with a large number of children in whom transplantation is deferred due to lack of donor hearts.

Conclusions

Mechanical circulatory support offers promise for patients as a bridge to recovery or transplant. However, use of these devices is associated with very serious complications and mortality. In particular, neurological abnormalities occur often as a result of thrombosis or hemorrhage. Cardiac stun still occurs in a significant number of patients, and ventricular unloading itself causes myocardial atrophy. Clinical strategies are still needed to reduce these complications. Heart transplantation is a relatively new treatment option with good outcomes for infants and children. Crossing ABO barriers has broadened the donor pool for individual recipients in the youngest age group. Newer techniques for noninvasively and accurately detect cellular rejection are described that promise to reduce the risks, costs and improve the outcomes of pediatric transplantation. This is particularly important in the young infants and children with long expected life spans and limited vascular access for performance of biopsy.

Summary

- Mechanical circulatory support is emerging as an invaluable tool in the care of children with severe refractory cardiac failure. Extracorporeal membrane oxygenation (ECMO) serves as a bridge to recovery or transplant, though many complications occur during runs.
- ECMO also provides a method of "rescue" for patients who arrest or show imminent devastating cardiac failure. This method requires organization skills.
- New ventricular assist devices are being used for infants and children including the Berlin Heart, paracorporeal pneumatically driven pulsatile ventricular assist device.
- Neurological complications occur in a large number of patients who have undergone ECMO, although the severity of these abnormalities requires further definition.
- Heart transplantation is now a treatment option with good outcomes for infants and children with end-stage heart failure or inoperable congenital cardiac defects. Recipient age affects the indications for pediatric heart transplantation. Despite the demanding surgical techniques and postoperative management in very young and very sick children, 1- and 5-year actuarial survival rates are high.
- Neonatal waiting time mortality and morbidity remains unacceptably high and is the highest of any solid organ. Several opportunities are available to expand the donor pool including transplant across ABO barriers and donation after cardiac death.
- Most acute rejection episodes in pediatric heart recipients occur in the first 3 months posttransplant. Single echocardiographic parameters have had limited abilities predicting

cellular rejection. Algorithms using multiple para-meters have been developed, which show superior predictive power.
- Infection, due to multiple factors including immunosuppression, surgery, invasive devices, and predisposing factors, is a significant cause of morbidity and mortality after pediatric heart transplantation. The most common cause for adverse late outcomes in pediatric heart recipients is reported to be accelerated coronary artery disease or graft atherosclerosis.
- The quality of life in surviving children is excellent in the majority of recipients but will be affected by pretransplant morbidity. Most recipients do not have activity limitation and do not require frequent hospitalizations. Linear growth retardation does occur in children and adolescents.

Acknowledgments Pediatric heart transplantation is successful due largely to the dedication of the parents and the programs' coordinators. The authors want to acknowledge their invaluable contributions, particularly the efforts of Judy Berger, Chris Mashburn, and Pam Hopkins. The authors acknowledge the support of the Felton Family Fund for partial support in the preparation of this chapter.

References

1. Cooper DS, Jacobs JP, Moore L et al (2007) Cardiac extracorporeal life support: state of the art in 2007. Cardiol Young 17:104–115
2. Haines NM, Rycus PT, Zwischenberger JB, Bartlett RH, Undar A (2009) Extracorporeal Life Support Registry Report 2008: neonatal and pediatric cardiac cases. ASAIO J 55:111–116
3. Walters HL 3rd, Hakimi M, Rice MD, Lyons JM, Whittlesey GC, Klein MD (1995) Pediatric cardiac surgical ECMO: multivariate analysis of risk factors for hospital death. Ann Thorac Surg 60: 329–336, discussion 36–37
4. Morris MC, Ittenbach RF, Godinez RI et al (2004) Risk factors for mortality in 137 pediatric cardiac intensive care unit patients managed with extracorporeal membrane oxygenation. Crit Care Med 32:1061–1069
5. del Nido PJ, Dalton HJ, Thompson AE, Siewers RD (1992) Extracorporeal membrane oxygenator rescue in children during cardiac arrest after cardiac surgery. Circulation 86: II300–II304
6. Duncan BW, Ibrahim AE, Hraska V et al (1998) Use of rapid-deployment extracorporeal membrane oxygenation for the resuscitation of pediatric patients with heart disease after cardiac arrest. J Thorac Cardiovasc Surg 116:305–311
7. Duncan BW, Bohn DJ, Atz AM, French JW, Laussen PC, Wessel DL (2001) Mechanical circulatory support for the treatment of children with acute fulminant myocarditis. J Thorac Cardiovasc Surg 122:440–448
8. Ibrahim AE, Duncan BW, Blume ED, Jonas RA (2000) Long-term follow-up of pediatric cardiac patients requiring mechanical circulatory support. Ann Thorac Surg 69:186–192
9. Wagner K, Risnes I, Abdelnoor M, Karlsen HM, Svennevig JL (2008) Is it possible to predict outcome in pulmonary ECMO? Analysis of pre-operative risk factors. Perfusion 23:95–99
10. Morales DL, Gunter KS, Fraser CD (2006) Pediatric mechanical circulatory support. Int J Artif Organs 29:920–937
11. Rockett SR, Bryant JC, Morrow WR et al (2008) Preliminary single center North American experience with the Berlin Heart pediatric EXCOR device. ASAIO J 54:479–482

12. Sharma MS, Webber SA, Morell VO, Gandhi SK, Wearden PD, Buchanan JR, Kormos RL (2006) Ventricular assist device support in children and adolescents as a bridge to heart transplantation. Ann Thorac Surg 82:926–932

13. Kilic A, Nolan TD, Li T et al (2007) Early in vivo experience with the pediatric Jarvik 2000 heart. ASAIO J 53:374–378

14. Canter CE, Shaddy RE, Bernstein D et al (2007) Indications for heart transplantation in pediatric heart disease: a scientific statement from the American Heart Association Council on Cardiovascular Disease in the Young; the Councils on Clinical Cardiology, Cardiovascular Nursing, and Cardiovascular Surgery and Anesthesia; and the Quality of Care and Outcomes Research Interdisciplinary Working Group. Circulation 115:658–676

15. Boucek MM, Aurora P, Edwards LB et al (2007) Registry of the International Society for Heart and Lung Transplantation: tenth official pediatric heart transplantation report. J Heart Lung Transplant 26:796–807

16. Kirk R, Edwards LB, Aurora P et al (2008) Registry of the International Society for Heart and Lung Transplantation: eleventh official pediatric heart transplantation report–2008. J Heart Lung Transplant 27:970–977

17. Taylor DO, Edwards LB, Boucek MM et al (2007) Registry of the International Society for Heart and Lung Transplantation: twenty-fourth official adult heart transplant report – 2007. J Heart Lung Transplant 26:769–781

18. Canter C, Naftel D, Caldwell R et al (1997) Survival and risk factors for death after cardiac transplantation in infants. A multi-institutional study. The Pediatric Heart Transplant Study. Circulation 96:227–231

19. Vricella LA, Razzouk AJ, Gundry SR, Larsen RL, Kuhn MA, Bailey LL (1998) Heart transplantation in infants and children with situs inversus. J Thorac Cardiovasc Surg 116:82–89

20. Larsen RL, Eguchi JH, Mulla NF et al (2002) Usefulness of cardiac transplantation in children with visceral heterotaxy (asplenic and polysplenic syndromes and single right-sided spleen with levocardia) and comparison of results with cardiac transplantation in children with dilated cardiomyopathy. Am J Cardiol 89: 1275–1279

21. Razzouk AJ, Gundry SR, Chinnock RE et al (1995) Orthotopic transplantation for total anomalous pulmonary venous connection associated with complex congenital heart disease. J Heart Lung Transplant 14:713–717

22. Chen JM, Davies RR, Mital SR et al (2004) Trends and outcomes in transplantation for complex congenital heart disease: 1984 to 2004. Ann Thorac Surg 78:1352–1361

23. Speziali G, Driscoll DJ, Danielson GK et al (1998) Cardiac transplantation for end-stage congenital heart defects: the Mayo Clinic experience. Mayo Cardiothoracic Transplant Team [see comment]. Mayo Clin Proc 73:923–928

24. Jacobs JP, Quintessenza JA, Boucek RJ et al (2005) Pediatric cardiac transplantation in children with high panel reactive antibody. Ann Thorac Surg 78:1703–1709

25. Bailey L, Nehlsen-Cannarella S, Doroshow R et al (1986) Cardiac allotransplantation in newborns as therapy for hypoplastic left heart syndrome. N Engl J Med 315:949–951

26. Bailey L, Concepcion W, Shattuck H, Huang L (1986) Method of heart transplantation for treatment of hypoplastic left heart syndrome. J Thorac Cardiovasc Surg 92:1–5

27. del Rio MJ (2000) Transplantation in complex congenital heart disease. Prog Pediatr Cardiol 11:107–113

28. Bove E, Lloyd T (1996) Staged reconstruction for hypoplastic left heart syndrome. Contemporary results. Ann Surg 224:387–394

29. Checchia PA, Larsen R, Sehra R et al (2004) Effect of a selection and postoperative care protocol on survival of infants with hypoplastic left heart syndrome. Ann Thorac Surg 77:477–483

30. Artrip JH, Campbell DN, Ivy DD et al (2006) Birth weight and complexity are significant factors for the management of hypoplastic left heart syndrome. Ann Thorac Surg 82:1252–1257, discussion 8–9

31. Chan K, Mashburn C, Boucek M (2006) Initial transcatheter palliation of hypoplastic left heart syndrome. Catheter Cardiovasc Interv 68:719–726

32. Akintuerk H, Michel-Behnke I, Valeske K et al (2002) Stenting of the arterial duct and banding of the pulmonary arteries: basis for combined Norwood stage I and II repair in hypoplastic left heart. Circulation 105:1099–1103

33. Chrisant MR, Naftel DC, Drummond-Webb J et al (2005) Fate of infants with hypoplastic left heart syndrome listed for cardiac transplantation: a multicenter study. J Heart Lung Transplant 24: 576–582

34. Jenkins PC, Flanagan MF, Jenkins KJ et al (2000) Survival analysis and risk factors for mortality in transplantation and staged surgery for hypoplastic left heart syndrome. J Am Coll Cardiol 36:1178–1185

35. Webber SA (1997) 15 years of pediatric heart transplantation at the University of Pittsburgh: lessons learned and future prospects. Pediatr Transplant 1:8–21

36. Rosenthal DN, Dubin AM, Chin C, Falco D, Gamberg P, Bernstein D (2000) Outcome while awaiting heart transplantation in children: a comparison of congenital heart disease and cardiomyopathy. J Heart Lung Transplant 19:751–755

37. Almond CSD, Thiagarajan RR, Piercey GE et al (2009) Waiting list mortality among children listed for heart transplantation in the United States. Circulation 119:717–727

38. Renlund DG, Taylor DO, Kfoury AG, Shaddy RS (1999) New UNOS rules: historical background and implications for transplantation management. United Network for Organ Sharing. J Heart Lung Transplant 18:1065–1070

39. Chin C, Naftel DC, Singh TP et al (2004) Risk factors for recurrent rejection in pediatric heart transplantation: a multicenter experience. J Heart Lung Transplant 23:178–185

40. Fukushima N, Gundry SR, Razzouk AJ et al (1995) Growth of oversized grafts in neonatal heart transplantation. Ann Thorac Surg 60:1659–1663

41. Mitropoulos FA, Odim J, Marelli D et al (2005) Outcome of hearts with cold ischemic time greater than 300 minutes. A case-matched study. Eur J Cardiothorac Surg 28:143–148

42. Scheule AM, Zimmerman GJ, Johnston JK, Razzouk AJ, Gundry SR, Bailey LL (2002) Duration of graft cold ischemia does not affect outcomes in pediatric heart transplant recipients. Circulation 106:I163–I167

43. Linam J, Law Y, Permut L et al (2009) 680: Extended donor ischemic time is not associated with poor outcome in pediatric heart transplantation. J Heart Lung Transplant 28:S301–S302

44. West LJ, Pollock-Barziv SM, Dipchand AI et al (2001) ABO-incompatible heart transplantation in infants [see comments]. N Engl J Med 344:793–800

45. West LJ, Karamlou T, Dipchand AI, Pollock-BarZiv SM, Coles JG, McCrindle BW (2006) Impact on outcomes after listing and transplantation, of a strategy to accept ABO blood group-incompatible donor hearts for neonates and infants. J Thorac Cardiovasc Surg 131:455–461

46. Roche SL, Burch M, O'Sullivan J et al (2008) Multicenter experience of ABO-incompatible pediatric cardiac transplantation [erratum appears in Am J Transplant 2008 Jun;8:1354]. Am J Transplant 8:208–215

47. Boucek MM, Mashburn C, Dunn SM et al (2008) Pediatric heart transplantation after declaration of cardiocirculatory death [see comment]. N Engl J Med 359:709–714

48. Davies RR, Russo MJ, Mital S et al (2008) Predicting survival among high-risk pediatric cardiac transplant recipients: an analysis of the United Network for Organ Sharing database. J Thorac Cardiovasc Surg 135:147–155

49. Rotando K, Naftel D, Boucek R et al (1996) Allograft rejection following cardiac transplantation in infants and children. J Heart Lung Transplant 15:S80

50. Boucek RJ Jr, Boucek MM, Asante-Korang A (2004) Advances in methods for surveillance of rejection. Cardiol Young 1:93–96

51. Boucek MM, Mathis CM, Boucek RJ Jr et al (1994) Prospective evaluation of echocardiography for primary rejection surveillance after infant heart transplantation: comparison with endomyocardial biopsy. J Heart Lung Transplant 13:66–73

52. Mills R, Naftel D, Kirklin J et al (1997) Heart transplant rejection with hemodynamic compromise: a multiinstitutional study of the role of endomyocardial cellular infiltrate. Cardiac Transplant Research Database. J Heart Lung Transplant 16:813–821

53. Pahl E, Naftel D, Canter C et al (2001) Death after rejection with severe hemodynamic compromise in pediatric heart transplant recipients: a multi-institutional study. J Heart Lung Transplant 20:279–287

54. Stewart S, Winters GL, Fishbein MC et al (2005) Revision of the 1990 working formulation for the standardization of nomenclature in the diagnosis of heart rejection [see comment]. J Heart Lung Transplant 24:1710–1720

55. Rosenthal DN, Chin C, Nishimura K et al (2004) Identifying cardiac transplant rejection in children: diagnostic utility of echocardiography, right heart catheterization and endomyocardial biopsy data. J Heart Lung Transplant 23:323–329

56. Blume ED (2003) Current status of heart transplantation in children: update 2003. Pediatr Clin North Am 50:1375–1391

57. Webber SA, Naftel DC, Parker J et al (2003) Late rejection episodes more than 1 year after pediatric heart transplantation: risk factors and outcomes. J Heart Lung Transplant 22:869–875

58. McOmber D, Ibrahim J, Lublin DM et al (2004) Non-ischemic left ventricular dysfunction after pediatric cardiac transplantation: treatment with plasmapheresis and OKT3. J Heart Lung Transplant 23:552–557

59. Boucek MM, Kanakriyeh MS, Mathis CM, Trimm RF 3rd, Bailey LL (1990) Cardiac transplantation in infancy: donors and recipients. Loma Linda University Pediatric Heart Transplant Group. J Pediatr 116:171–176

60. Tantengco MV, Dodd D, Frist WH, Boucek MM, Boucek RJ (1993) Echocardiographic abnormalities with acute cardiac allograft rejection in children: correlation with endomyocardial biopsy. J Heart Lung Transplant 12:S203–S210

61. Putzer GJ, Cooper D, Keehn C, Asante-Korang A, Boucek MM, Boucek RJ Jr (2000) An improved echocardiographic rejection-surveillance strategy following pediatric heart transplantation. J Heart Lung Transplant 19:1166–1174

62. Ciliberto GR, Mascarello M, Gronda E et al (1994) Acute rejection after heart transplantation: noninvasive echocardiographic evaluation. J Am Coll Cardiol 23:1156–1161

63. Neuberger S, Vincent R, Doelling N et al (1997) Comparison of quantitative echocardiography with endomyocardial biopsy to define myocardial rejection in pediatric patients after cardiac transplantation. Am J Cardiol 79:447–450

64. Moran AM, Lipshultz SE, Rifai NO et al (2000) Non-invasive assessment of rejection in pediatric transplant patients: serologic and echocardiographic prediction of biopsy-proven myocardial rejection. J Heart Lung Transplant 19:756–764

65. Burgess MI, Bright-Thomas RJ, Yonan N et al (2003) Can the index of myocardial performance be used to detect acute cellular rejection after heart transplantation? Am J Cardiol 92:308–311

66. Leonard GT Jr, Fricker FJ, Pruett D, Harker K, Williams B, Schowengerdt KO Jr (2006) Increased myocardial performance index correlates with biopsy-proven rejection in pediatric heart transplant recipients. J Heart Lung Transplant 25:61–66

67. Santos-Ocampo S, Sekarski T, Saffitz J et al (1996) Echocardiographic characteristics of biopsy-proven cellular rejection in infant heart transplant recipients. J Heart Lung Transplant 15:25–34

68. Puleo J, Aranda J, Weston M et al (1998) Noninvasive detection of allograft rejection in heart transplant recipients by use of Doppler tissue imaging. J Heart Lung Transplant 17:176–184

69. Puleo JA, Boucek R, Weston MW, French MF, HL F (1996) Characterization of myocardial dysfunction during heart transplant graft rejection by Doppler tissue imaging. J Heart Lung Transplant 15:S58

70. Mankad S, Murali S, Mandarino WA, Kormas RL, Gorcsan J (1997) Assessment of acute cardiac allograft rejection by quantitative tissue Doppler echocardiography. Circulation 96:I-342

71. Dandel M, Hummel M, Muller J, Meyer R, Ewert R, Hetzer R (2001) Wall motion assessment by tissue Doppler imaging after heart transplantation: timing of endomyocardial biopsies and facilitation of therapeutic decisions during acute cardiac rejection. J Heart Lung Transplant 20:213

72. Dandel M, Hummel M, Muller J et al (2001) Reliability of tissue Doppler wall motion monitoring after heart transplantation for replacement of invasive routine screenings by optimally timed cardiac biopsies and catheterizations. Circulation 104:I184–I191

73. Garcia M, Thomas J, Klein A (1998) New Doppler echocardiographic applications for the study of diastolic function [Review] [68 refs]. J Am Coll Cardiol 32:865–875

74. Oki T, Tabata T, Mishiro Y et al (1999) Pulsed tissue Doppler imaging of left ventricular systolic and diastolic wall motion velocities to evaluate differences between long and short axes in healthy subjects. J Am Soc Echocardiogr 12:308–313

75. Asante-Korang A, Fickey M, Boucek MM, Boucek RJ Jr (2004) Diastolic performance assessed by tissue Doppler after pediatric heart transplantation. J Heart Lung Transplant 23:865–872

76. Pauliks LB, Pietra BA, DeGroff CG, Kirby KS, Knudson OA, Logan L, Boucek MM, Valdes-Cruz LM (2005) Non-invasive detection of acute allograft rejection in children by tissue Doppler imaging: myocardial velocities and myocardial acceleration during isovolumic contraction. J Heart Lung Transplant 24:S239–S248

77. Stehlik J, Starling RC, Movsesian MA et al (2006) Utility of long-term surveillance endomyocardial biopsy: a multi-institutional analysis. J Heart Lung Transplant 25:1402–1409

78. Levi DS, DeConde AS, Fishbein MC, Burch C, Alejos JC, Wetzel GT (2004) The yield of surveillance endomyocardial biopsies as a screen for cellular rejection in pediatric heart transplant patients [see comment]. Pediatr Transplant 8:22–28

79. Kirklin JK (2005) Is biopsy-proven cellular rejection an important clinical consideration in heart transplantation? Curr Opin Cardiol 20:127–131

80. Chin C, Akhta MJ, Rosenthal D, Bernstein D (2000) Safety and utility of the routine surveillance biopsy in pediatric patients 2 years after heart transplantation. J Pediatr 136:238–242

81. Wagner K, Oliver MC, Boyle GJ et al (2000) Endomyocardial biopsy in pediatric heart transplant recipients: a useful exercise? (Analysis of 1, 169 biopsies). Pediatr Transplant 4:186–192

82. Pophal SG, Gunnlaugur S, Booth KL et al (1999) Complications of endomyocardial biopsy in children. J Am Coll Cardiol 34:2105–2110

83. Boucek MM, Mathis CM, Kanakriyeh MS, Hodgkin DD, Boucek RJ Jr, Bailey LL (1993) Serial echocardiographic evaluation of cardiac graft rejection after infant heart transplantation. J Heart Lung Transplant 12:824–831

84. Leonard HCO, Sullivan JJ, Dark JH (2000) Long-term follow-up of pediatric cardiac transplant recipients on a steroid-free regime: the role of endomyocardial biopsy. J Heart Lung Transplant 19:469–472

85. Grasser B, Iberer F, Schreier G et al (2000) Non-invasive cardiac allograft monitoring: the graz experience. J Heart Lung Transplant 19:653–659

86. Kniepeiss D, Iberer F, Grasser B, Schaffellner S, Schreier G, Tscheliessnigg KH (2001) Noninvasive cardiac allograft monitoring. Transplant Proc 33:2456–2457

87. Bernstein D, Williams GE, Eisen H et al (2007) Gene expression profiling distinguishes a molecular signature for grade 1B mild acute cellular rejection in cardiac allograft recipients. J Heart Lung Transplant 26:1270–1280

88. Pham MX, Deng MC, Kfoury AG, Teuteberg JJ, Starling RC, Valantine H (2007) Molecular testing for long-term rejection surveillance in heart transplant recipients: design of the Invasive Monitoring Attenuation Through Gene Expression (IMAGE) trial. J Heart Lung Transplant 26:808–814

89. Sigfusson G, Fricker FJ, Bernstein D et al (1997) Long-term survivors of pediatric heart transplantation: a multicenter report of sixty-eight children who have survived longer than five years [see comments]. J Pediatr 130:862–871

90. Pahl E, Naftel DC, Kuhn MA et al (2005) The impact and outcome of transplant coronary artery disease in a pediatric population: a 9-year multi-institutional study. J Heart Lung Transplant 24:645–651

91. Pietra B, Boucek M (2000) Immunosuppression for pediatric cardiac transplantation in the modern era. Prog Pediatr Cardiol 11:115–129

92. Chinnock R, Sherwin T, Robie S, Baum M, Janner D, Mellick L (1995) Emergency department presentation and management of pediatric heart transplant recipients. Pediatr Emerg Care 11: 355–360

93. Chinnock R, Baum M (1998) Somatic growth in infant heart transplant recipients. Pediatr Transplant 2:30–34

94. Mahle WT, Visconti KJ, Freier MC et al (2006) Relationship of surgical approach to neurodevelopmental outcomes in hypoplastic left heart syndrome. Pediatrics 117:e90–e97

95. Guo CY, Johnson A, Locke TJ, Eastell R (1998) Mechanisms of bone loss after cardiac transplantation. Bone 22:267–271

96. Boucek RJ Jr, Naftel D, Boucek MM et al (1999) Induction immunotherapy in pediatric heart transplant recipients: a multicenter study. J Heart Lung Transplant 18:460–469

97. Ibrahim J (2002) Rejection is reduced in thoracic organ recipients when transplanted in the first year of life. J Heart Lung Transplant 21:311–318

98. Vigano A, Esposito S, Arienti D, Zagliani A, Massironi E, Principi N, Clerici M (1999) Differential development of type 1 and type 2 cytokines and beta-chemokines in the ontogeny of healthy newborns. Biol Neonate 75:1–8

99. Schelonka RL, Raaphorst FM, Infante D, Kraig E, Teale JM, Infante AJ (1998) T cell receptor repertoire diversity and clonal expansion in human neonates. Pediatr Res 43:396–402

100. Schelonka RL, Infante AJ (1998) Neonatal immunology [Review] [65 refs]. Semin Perinatol 22:2–14

101. Neubert R, Delgado I, Abraham K, Schuster C, Helge H (1998) Evaluation of the age-dependent development of lymphocyte surface receptors in children. Life Sci 62:1099–1110

102. Wells WJ, Parkman R, Smogorzewska E, Barr M (1998) Neonatal thymectomy: does it affect immune function? J Thorac Cardiovasc Surg 115:1041–1046

103. Ogle BM, West LJ, Driscoll DJ et al (2006) Effacing of the T cell compartment by cardiac transplantation in infancy. J Immunol 176:1962–1967

104. Fan X, Ang A, Pollock-Barziv SM et al (2004) Donor-specific B-cell tolerance after ABO-incompatible infant heart transplantation [see comment]. Nat Med 10:1227–1233

105. Sindhi R, Webber S, Venkataramanan R, McGhee W, Phillips S, Smith A, Baird C, Iurlano K, Mazariegos G, Cooperstone B, Holt DW, Zeevi A, Fung JJ, Reyes J (2001) Sirolimus for rescue and primary immunosuppression in transplanted children receiving tacrolimus. Transplantation 72:851–855

106. Lobach NE, Pollock-Barziv SM, West LJ, Dipchand AI (2005) Sirolimus immunosuppression in pediatric heart transplant recipients: a single-center experience. J Heart Lung Transplant 24: 184–189

107. Bailey L, Assaad A, Trimm R et al (1988) Orthotopic transplantation during early infancy as therapy for incurable congenital heart disease. Ann Surg 208:279–286

108. Aurora P, Boucek MM, Christie J et al (2007) Registry of the International Society for Heart and Lung Transplantation: tenth official pediatric lung and heart/lung transplantation report – 2007. J Heart Lung Transplant 26:1223–1228

109. Canter CE, Moorhead S, Saffitz JE, Huddleston CB, Spray TL (1994) Steroid withdrawal in the pediatric heart transplant recipient initially treated with triple immunosuppression. J Heart Lung Transplant 13:74–79

110. Schowengerdt KO, Naftel DC, Seib PM et al (1997) Infection after pediatric heart transplantation: results of a multiinstitutional study. The Pediatric Heart Transplant Study Group. J Heart Lung Transplant 16:1207–1216

111. Boyle GJ, Michaels MG, Webber SA et al (1997) Posttransplantation lymphoproliferative disorders in pediatric thoracic organ recipients. J Pediatr 131:309–313

112. Barnes AP, Daneman SM, Guleserian KJ, Ring WS, Fixler DE (2008) Low Cylex(TM) immune response associated with increased risk of infection in pediatric heart transplants. J Heart Lung Transplant 27:S242

Section VIII
Aging and the Failing Heart

Chapter 16
Basic Mechanisms Mediating Cardiomyopathy and Heart Failure in Aging

Overview

Biological aging represents the major risk factor for the development of heart failure (HF), malignancies, and neuro-degenerative diseases. While risk factors such as lifestyle patterns, genetic traits, blood lipid levels, and diabetes can contribute to its development, advancing age remains the most determinant predictor of cardiac disease. Several parameters of left ventricular function may be affected with aging, including increased duration of systole, decreased sympathetic stimulation, and increased left ventricle ejection time, while compliance decreases. In addition, changes in cardiac phenotype with diastolic dysfunction, reduced contractility, left ventricular hypertrophy, and HF, all increase in incidence with age. Given the limited capacity that the heart has for regeneration, reversing or slowing the progression of these abnormalities poses a major challenge. In this chapter, we present a discussion on the molecular and cellular mechanisms involved in the pathogenesis of cardiomyopathies and HF in aging and the potential involvement of specific genes identified as primary mediators of these diseases.

Introduction

Although our current knowledge of age-associated cardiac pathologies has outpaced our understanding of the basic mechanisms underlying these processes, with the availability of the Human Genome Project (HGP) and an increasing number of animal models, as well as new and exciting molecular technologies, the unraveling of the underlying basic mechanisms of the failing aging heart has already begun.

Changes occurring in the aging heart include decreased β-adrenergic sympathetic responsiveness [1, 2], slowed and delayed early diastolic filling [3, 4], increased vascular stiffness [5, 6], and endothelial dysfunction [7, 8]. Of significance is the fact that the cellular changes of aging are most pronounced in postmitotic organs (e.g., brain and heart) and defects in the structure and function of cardiomyocytes may

be the determinant factors in the overall cardiac aging process, particularly in HF.

With aging, myocytes undergo hypertrophy, and this may be accompanied by intracellular changes, including mito-chondrial-derived oxidative stress (OS) that will contribute to the overall cellular aging as well as to ischemia-induced myocardial damage. Following an episode of ischemia and reperfusion (I/R), the aging heart suffers greater damage than the adult heart; however, the occurrence and degree of aging-related defects remain uncertain. Basic mechanisms that have been proposed for cardiac aging are discussed in this chapter including cell senescent, accumulation of reactive oxygen species (ROS), inflammatory changes, decreased α and β-adrenoreceptors (AR) mediated contractility, increased levels of G-proteins-coupled receptors, impaired intracellular Ca^{2+} homeostasis, decreased IGF-1 levels, cellular damage/cell loss, telomerase inactivation, abnormal autophagy, and altered membrane structure and permeability, all of which may lead to abnormal cardiac contractile function and contribute to the development of HF [9, 10].

Accumulation of Reactive Oxygen Species

The "free radical theory of aging" has drawn great attention in the assessment of cardiac aging. This theory presupposes that in biological systems, reactive oxidatives species (ROS) attack molecules and cause a decline in the function of organ systems, eventually leading to failure and death. All cell types including cardiomyocytes are capable of generating ROS, and the major sources of their production include mitochondria, xanthine oxidases and the NADPH oxidases. Under pathophysiological conditions, ROS levels can increase and cause cellular damage and dysfunction targeting primarily the mitochondria.

Interestingly, in addition to its damaging effect, ROS play an important role in a number of signal transduction pathways in the cardiomyocyte. Whether the effects of this signaling role are beneficial or harmful may depend upon

J. Marín-García, *Heart Failure*, Contemporary Cardiology,
DOI 10.1007/978-1-60761-147-9_16, © Springer Science+Business Media, LLC 2010

the site, source and amount of ROS produced, as well as the overall redox status of the cell. ROS have been implicated in the development of cardiac hypertrophy, cardiomyocyte death by apoptosis, and remodeling of the heart, largely by upregulating proapoptotic proteins and the mitochondrial-dependent pathways. Cardiomyocyte apoptosis has been reported in a variety of cardiovascular diseases, including myocardial infarction, ischemia/reperfusion and HF.

ROS mediates oxidative damage to lipids and proteins in the aging heart, and both myocardial mtDNA and nuclear DNA damage will result in further accumulation of oxidative species and, in particular, mitochondrial DNA damage will accumulate because of its inefficient repair machinery and its close proximity to the sources of ROS (Fig. 16.1). Thus, in the aging failing heart, neutralization of ROS by mitochondrial antioxidants such as superoxide dismutase (SOD), catalase

(CA), glutathione peroxidase (GPx), and glutathione becomes critically important. During aging, mitochondrial dysfunction and ROS generation may also trigger increased apoptosis, with resultant cell loss. This loss in cardiomyocytes may be secondary to mitochondrial dysfunction caused by chronic exposure to ROS, damage to mtDNA (mutations and deletions) and to mitochondrial membranes. While mtDNA damage occurs with aging, mtDNA levels, although decreased in liver and skeletal muscle, are for the most part preserved in the aging heart.

Data from in vitro studies indicate that mitochondrial OS and declining mitochondrial energy production can lead to the activation of apoptotic pathways, but whether this also occurs in the in vivo aging heart is not clear. While the role and extent of apoptosis in normal myocardial aging is presently unknown, ample evidence of cardiomyocyte apoptosis

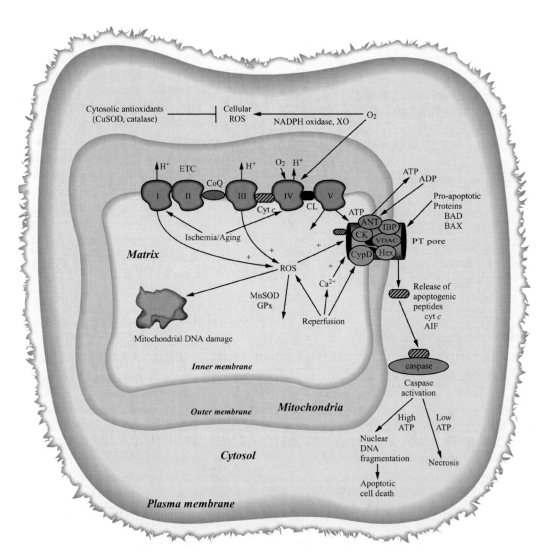

Fig. 16.1 ROS generation and antioxidant enzymes in the aging heart. Cytosolic pathways of ROS generation involving NADPH oxidase and xanthine oxidase (XO), the cytosolic antioxidant enzymes copper SOD (CuSOD) and catalase are shown, as well as the mitochondrial pathway of ROS generation (primarily through complex I and III) and mitochondrial antioxidant response featuring MnSOD, GPx and glutathione peroxidase (GPx). Primary mitochondrial targets of ROS including the PT pore, mitochondrial apoptotic pathway and mtDNA are also represented

is supported by studies in the aging rat heart showing the release of cytochrome *c* from mitochondria and decreased levels of Bcl-2 (an antiapoptotic protein), while Bax, a proapoptotic protein, remained unchanged [11, 12].

The occurrence and degree of aging-related defects in mitochondrial OXPHOS remain questionable. Interestingly, aging-related defects have been found in the interfibrillar mitochondria (IFM), in which complex III and IV activity and rate of OXPHOS were decreased, while the subsarcolemmal mitochondrial (SSM) electron transport chain (ETC) activity remained normal [13–15]. The selective alteration of IFM during aging suggests that the consequences of aging-induced mitochondrial dysfunction may be enhanced in specific subcellular regions of the senescent cardiomyocyte. Recent observations suggested that mitochondrial ROS cause OS and impaired mitochondrial function in IFM to a greater degree than in SSM with age, and because of their proximity to myofibrils, IFM are probably the primary source of ATP for myosin ATPases, and therefore OS in IFM may be the culprit for the myocardial dysfunction occurring with aging [16]. It is important to keep in mind that the subfractionation of mitochondria may provide a mixture of organelles of SSM and IFM that may complicate the assessment of the age-related changes in mitochondrial oxidant production and OS. Therefore, further studies in this area are needed.

In early myocardial reperfusion, a burst of ROS occurs in association with changes in mitochondria (e.g., PT pore opening) and myocardial injury. The source of this ROS generation may be of either mitochondrial or cytoplasmic origin. On the other hand, the source of ROS generated during ischemia (and likely in the early/acute pathway of ischemic preconditioning) involves more distinctively the mitochondrial ETC and may be different than the source of ROS generated in early reperfusion [17, 18]. OS also appears to participate in the generation of large-scale myocardial mtDNA deletions as demonstrated in pacing-induced cardiac failure [19], as well as in studies of ameroid constriction-mediated myocardial ischemia in the dog [20]. Moreover, neonatal cardiac myocytes treated with tumor necrosis factor-α (TNF-α) showed a significant increase in ROS levels, and this is accompanied by an overall decline in mtDNA copy number and decreased complex III activity [21]. These findings suggest that the TNF-α-mediated decline in mtDNA copy number might result from an increase in mtDNA deletions. Thus, in aging and in the aging failing heart, accumulation of ROS initiates a vicious circle following somatic mtDNA damage as shown in Fig. 16.2. During aging and after myocardial infarction, ROS-induced mtDNA damage, resulting in respiratory complex enzyme dysfunction, contributes to the progression of left ventricular (LV) remodeling. In a murine model of MI and remodeling created by ligation of the left anterior descending coronary artery, increased ROS production (e.g., OH$^{\cdot}$ level) was shown in association with decreased levels of mtDNA and

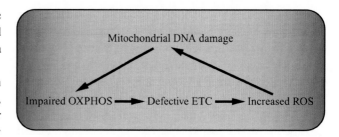

Fig. 16.2 Increased accumulation of ROS initiates a vicious circle following somatic mtDNA damage

ETC activities, suggesting mitochondrial dysfunction [22]. Significantly, the chronic release of ROS has been linked to the development of left ventricular hypertrophy and advanced HF. As noted in previous chapters, chronic ROS generation can derive both from mitochondria and from nonmitochondrial NADPH oxidase that in endothelial cells is activated by cytokines, neurohormones, and growth factors (e.g., angiotensin II, norepinephrine, TNF-α) [23, 24]. Furthermore, changes in the cardiac phenotype can be driven by redox-sensitive gene expression, in this way ROS may act as potent intracellular second messengers.

NADPH oxidase plays a prominent role in the hypertrophic signaling pathway [25–27] in cardiac myocytes, and NADPH oxidase activity is significantly increased in the failing myocardium [28]. Interestingly, statins (i.e., 3-hydroxyl-3-methylglutaryl coenzyme A (HMG-CoA) reductase inhibitors) by modulating the ROS-generating activity of NADPH oxidase can inhibit cardiac hypertrophy by cholesterol-independent mechanisms [29, 30]. Also, statins block the isoprenylation and activation of members of the Rho guanosine triphosphatase (GTPase) family such as Rac1, an essential component of NADPH oxidase. Thus, blocking the ROS production with statins may be beneficial to the aging patients with myocardial hypertrophy and chronic HF.

Cardiac overexpression of heavy metal-scavenging antioxidant metallothionein prolongs life span, alleviates aging-associated cardiac contractile dysfunction, insulin insensitivity, and mitochondrial damage [31]. A recent study tested the hypothesis that catalase, an enzyme which detoxifies H_2O_2, might interfere with cardiac aging [32]. Contractile and intracellular Ca^{2+} properties were evaluated in cardiomyocytes from young and old FVB (inbred strains of mice that carry the Fv1b allele for sensitivity to the B strain of Friend leukaemia virus) and transgenic mice with cardiac overexpression of catalase. Contractile indices analyzed included peak shortening (PS), time-to-90% PS (TPS90), time-to-90% relengthening (TR90), half-width duration (HWD), maximal velocity of shortening/relengthening ($\pm$dL/dt), and intracellular Ca^{2+} levels or decay rate. Levels of advanced glycation endproduct (AGE), Na^+/Ca^{2+} exchanger (NCX), sarco(endo)plasmic reticulum Ca^{2+}-ATPase (SERCA2a), phospholamban (PLB), myosin heavy chain (MHC), membrane Ca^{2+} and K^+ channels were measured by Western blotting Catalase transgene prolonged survival while did not alter myocyte function by itself. Aging depressed $\pm dL/dt$, prolonged HWD, TR90 and intracellular Ca^{2+} decay without affecting other indices in FVB myocytes. Aged FVB myocytes exhibited a stepper decline in PS in response to elevated stimulus or a dampened rise in PS in response to elevated extracellular Ca^{2+} levels. Aging-induced defects were attenuated by catalase. AGE level was elevated in aged FVB compared with young FVB mice, which was reduced by catalase. Expression of SERCA2a, NCX and Kv1.2 K^+ channel was significantly reduced although levels of PLB, L-type Ca^{2+} channel dihydropyridine receptor and β-MHC isozyme remained unchanged in aged FVB hearts. Catalase restored NCX and Kv1.2 K^+ channel but not SERCA2a level in the aged mice. These data suggest that catalase protects the cardiomyocytes from aging-induced contractile dysfunction possibly via improved intracellular Ca^{2+} handling. By catalyzing conversion of H_2O_2 to oxygen and water, catalase would shift redox balance toward antioxidant end, leading to increased myocardial antioxidant capacity, which may offset the detrimental effect of H_2O_2 (a model illustrating the triggering stimuli and cellular pathways involved in the onset and progression of HF is shown in Chap. 5) (see Fig. 5.1).

NO also plays a significant role in myocardial OS as demonstrated by Li and associates. Upon examining the role of inducible nitric oxide synthase (iNOS) in aging-related myocardial ischemic injury, as well as its relation to β-AR stimulation, they found that iNOS is upregulated in the aging rat heart [33]. Isolated perfused hearts from young (3–5 months) and aging (24–25 months) rats subjected to 30 min of myocardial ischemia resulted in cardiac dysfunction. Infusion of isoproterenol for 30 min caused a partial recovery of cardiac function in hearts from young rats, receiving either vehicle or 1,400 W (a nonselective iNOS inhibitor). In striking contrast, isoproterenol infusion to hearts from aging animals receiving vehicle failed to improve ischemia-induced cardiodepression and worsened cardiac function, with a significant increase in myocardial NO production, peroxynitrite formation, caspase-3 activation, and creatine kinase release. Therefore, β-AR stimulation interacts with ischemia and triggers a significant increase in myocardial NO production, creates a nitrosative stress, generates toxic peroxynitrite, activates apoptosis, and eventually causes cardiac dysfunction and myocardial injury in the aging heart. Moreover, myocardial NO production, peroxynitrite formation, and caspase-3 activation were attenuated and LV function significantly improved in aging heart treated with the iNOS inhibitor, 1,400 W. Compared to young rat hearts, significant increases in iNOS protein expression, activity, and immunoreactivity were found in the aging heart, confirming that aging induces a phenotypic upregulation of myocardial iNOS and that there is a critical link between iNOS-generated NO production and aging-associated myocardial ischemia.

Inflammatory Mechanisms/Signaling

Besides ROS, NO and iNOS other molecules and signaling pathways such as inflammatory signaling are actively involved in the aging process. Gathered observations have shown the fundamental role that immunity has in mediating artherosclerosis from initiation through progression and, ultimately, the thrombotic complications of atherosclerosis [34–36]. Increase in markers of inflammation may predict outcomes of patients with acute coronary syndromes, independently of myocardial damage.

Inflammatory markers have been identified as significant independent risk indicators for cardiovascular events including HF. Kritchevsky et al. [37] have examined the role that inflammatory markers play in predicting the incidence of CVD, specifically in older adults. Interestingly, IL-6, TNF-α, and IL-10 levels appear to predict cardiovascular outcomes in adults <65 years. Data on C-reactive protein (CRP) levels were rather inconsistent and appeared to be less reliable in old age than in middle age. In addition, fibrinogen levels have some value in predicting mortality but in a nonspecific manner. The authors indicated that in the elderly, inflammatory markers are nonspecific measures of health and may predict both disability and mortality, even in the absence of clinical CVD.

Interventions designed to prevent CVD through the modulation of inflammation may be helpful in reducing disability and mortality. The role of increased inflammatory markers such as IL-6 and IL-1β as a risk factor in aging, and in the development of MI has also been reported [38]. Analysis of polymorphisms in *IL-6* gene promoter (−174 G>C) revealed that elderly patients with acute coronary syndrome (ACS) carrying *IL-6* −174 GG genotypes exhibited a marked increase in 1 year follow-up mortality rate, suggesting that *IL-6* −174 G → C polymorphisms can be added to the other clinical markers such as CRP serum levels and a history of CAD, useful in identifying elderly male patients at higher risk of death after ACS [39]. In addition, data from the InCHIANTI study suggest that increased levels of serum IL-1β are associated with high risk of congestive HF and angina pectoris [40].

Adrenergic Receptors in the Aging Heart

The decline in cardiac performance that occurs with aging is in part due to a decrease in α- and β-AR-mediated contractility. While impairment in β-AR signaling is known to occur in the aging heart, the components of the α1-AR signaling cascade that are responsible for the aging-associated deficit in α1-AR contractile function have just begun to be identified. To determine that the aged heart has an impaired response to α1-adrenergic stimulation, Montagne et al. [41] measured both cardiomyocyte Ca^{2+}-transient and cardiac protein kinase C (PKC) activity in young (3 months) and old

Wistar rats (24 months). Ca^{2+} transients were obtained under 1 Hz pacing by microfluorimetry of cardiomyocyte loaded with indo-1 and compared during control conditions and after α1-adrenergic stimulation (phenylephrine or cirazoline, an α1-specific agonist). In addition, the activity of PKC and PKC translocation index were assayed before and after α1-adrenergic stimulation. In the young animals, cirazoline induced a significant increase in Ca^{2+} transient for up to 10^{-9}M concentration which returned to control values for larger concentrations. In contrast, in the old animals, there was a constant negative effect of cirazoline on the Ca^{2+} transient with a significant decrease at 10^{-6}M compared with both baseline and Kreb's solution. In a dose–response curve to phenylephrine, prior experiments showed that the response of Ca^{2+} transient was maximal at 10^{-7}M. This concentration induced a significant increase in Ca^{2+} transient in the young and a significant decrease in old rats. The same concentration was chosen to perform PKC activity measurements under α1-adrenergic stimulation. In the basal state, PKC activity was higher in the older than in the younger animals but was not different in cytosolic fractions; thus, the translocation index was higher in the old group. Following the administration of phenylephrine, translocation of PKC toward the particulate fraction was observed in the young but not in old rats. Taken together, the data showed that cardiac α1-adrenoceptor response was impaired in aged hearts and that the negative effect of α1-adrenergic stimulation on Ca^{2+} transient in cardiomyocytes in the old rats can be related to an absence of α1-adrenergic-induced PKC translocation.

Korzick et al. [42] have also measured α1-adrenergic stimulation in the senescent rat heart. Cardiac contractility (dP/dt) was analyzed using the Langendorff-perfused hearts isolated from 5 month adult and 24 month old aging Wistar rats, following maximal α1-AR stimulation with phenylephrine. Upon assessing the subcellular distribution of PKCα and PKCϵ, and their respective anchoring proteins RACK1 and RACK2 by Western blotting, they found that the subcellular translocation of PKCα and PKCϵ, in response to α1-AR stimulation, is disrupted in the aging myocardium. Age-related reductions in RACK1 and RACK2 levels were also observed, suggesting that alterations in PKC-anchoring proteins may contribute to impaired PKC translocation and defective α1-AR contraction in the aged rat heart. Interestingly, the investigators also sought to determine whether age-related defects in α1-AR contraction could be reversed by chronic exercise training (treadmill) in adult and aged rat [43]. The data revealed that age-related decrease in α1-AR contractility in the rat heart can be partially reversed by exercise suggesting that alterations in PKC levels underlie, at least in part, exercise training-induced improvements in α1-AR contraction.

Reperfusion of an isolated mammalian heart with a calcium-containing solution after a brief calcium-free perfusion results in irreversible cell damage (the calcium paradox). Activation of the α1-AR pathway confers protection against the lethal injury of the Ca^{2+} paradox via PKC-mediated signaling pathways, and this protection is shared by stimuli common with calcium preconditioning [44]. Notwithstanding these findings, the effect of aging on the human sympathetic nervous system remains a controversial issue. At present, interest in this subject has significantly increased, mainly because diverse cardiac pathologies, including essential hypertension, CAD, HF, and dysrhythmias increase with age, and the sympathetic nervous system may be an important pathophysiological component [45]. However, aging does not have an additive effect in the activation of the sympathetic nervous system that occurs in HF; suggesting that other factors such as CAD and MI may impact the increased incidence of HF with aging [46].

Cardiac G-Protein-Coupled Receptors

Cardiac G-protein-coupled receptors (GPCRs) that function through stimulatory G-protein $G\alpha_s$, such as β1- and β2-ARs, play a key role in cardiac contractility (see Chap. 8). Several $G\alpha_s$-coupled receptors in the heart also activate $G\alpha_i$, including β2-ARs (but not β1-ARs); PKA-dependent phosphorylation of β2-AR can shift its coupling preference from $G\alpha_s$ to $G\alpha_i$ [47]. Coupling of cardiac β2-ARs to $G\alpha_i$ inhibits adenylyl cyclase (AC) and opposes β1-AR-mediated apoptosis [48]. Studies on advanced HF have shown that $G\alpha_{i2}$ levels increase with age in both human atria [49], and in ventricles of old (24 months) Fischer 344 rats resulting in diminished AC activity [48]. These levels may subsequently increase the receptor-mediated activation of G_i through multiple GPCRs. Furthermore, increased G_i activity is likely to have an adverse effect on heart function since G_i-coupled signaling pathways in the heart reduce both the rate and force of contraction [50].

Investigation of the effects of age on GPCR signaling in human atrial tissue showed that the density of atrial muscarinic acetylcholine receptor (mAChR) increases with age but reaches statistical significance only in patients with diabetes [51]. Interestingly, in elderly subjects of similar ages, those with diabetes have 1.7-fold higher levels of $G\alpha_{i2}$ and twofold higher levels of $G\beta_1$. On the other hand, it has been reported that right atrial mAChR density significantly decreased in advanced age [52]. The disparity between these findings could be explained by differences in age between patient groups; one study examined only adults with an age range from 41 to 85 years [51], while the other study group's age ranged from 5 days to 76 years [52]. Analysis of G-protein-coupled receptor kinase (GRK) activity (by in vitro rhodopsin phosphorylation) in the right atria from 16 children (mean age 9 ± 2 years) and 17 elderly patients (mean age 67 ± 2 years) without apparent HF and the RA from four patients with end-stage HF showed that in contrast to the failing human heart, in the aging human heart, GRK activity was not increased [54]. These observations suggest that GRK activity may not have an important role in β-AR desensitization in the aging human heart, but why GRK's regulation is different in the human aging heart than in the failing human heart is not yet completely understood. Leineweber et al. [53] have found that with aging increase in sympathetic activity develops slowly and moderately, since plasma noradrenaline levels (often taken as an indirect index of sympathetic activity) [54] increase continuously at a 10–15% rate per decade due to enhanced spillover of noradrenaline into the circulation [55, 56]. In contrast, in HF, increases in sympathetic activity occur much more rapidly and are more pronounced than in the aging heart [57]. Thus, the time course and intensity of increases in sympathetic activity in the aging and the failing human heart are dissimilar, and this may explain differences in regulation of GRKs in the aging compared to the failing human heart.

To determine whether changes in GRK activity are an early or late occurrence in human HF, and whether β-adrenoceptor blocker treatment is able to influence myocardial GRK activity, Leineweber et al. [58] have measured β-AR density (by (−)-[(118)I]-iodocyanopindolol binding) and GRK activity (by an in vitro rhodopsin phosphorylation assay) in the right atria from patients at different stages of HF treated with and without β-adrenoceptor blockers, as well as in the four chambers of explanted hearts from patients with end-stage HF. Increase in GRK activity was an early and transient event in the course of HF that may be prevented by β-adrenoceptor blocker treatment. It has been reported that in humans, after 50 years of age, atrial mAChR density exhibits an upward trend with age [51] which differs from most animal studies data, which have been less conclusive by either showing unchanged muscarinic receptor levels [59–62], or by indicating decreased mAChR density with age [63].

SERCA and Thyroid Hormone in the Aging Heart

Myocardial contraction and relaxation are regulated by the concentration of Ca^{2+} around the contractile elements in cardiomyocytes. After contraction, relaxation is brought about by lowering Ca^{2+} levels. A major contribution to this process is made by the sarcoplasmic reticulum Ca^{2+} ATPase (SERCA), a 110-kD transmembrane protein, which pumps cytoplasmic Ca^{2+} into the sarcoplasmic reticulum (SR) [64]. Three SERCA genes have been identified so far as SERCA1, SERCA2, and SERCA3 encoding six distinct proteins isoforms by alternative explicing [65, 66] with the SERCA2a being the predominant isoform expressed in the heart. Since SERCA2a plays an important role in intracellular Ca^{2+} hemostasis and cardiac contractility, the abnormal expression of SERCA2a in the senescent heart is likely to have major biochemical and pathophysiological effects. As a matter of fact, senescent is characterized by reduced myocardial contractility velocity and prolonged relaxation time. These changes might be related to decreased expression and activity of SERCA, which controls the rate of SR calcium uptake during relaxation. The cardiac SERCA pumps Ca^{2+} from the cytosol back to the SR and is considered an important determinant of intracellular Ca^{2+} signaling and cardiac contractility. At least in part, the increased susceptibility to HF of the aging heart may be mediated by abnormal Ca^{2+} handling and decreased expression of the SERCA gene [67]. The molecular mechanisms that regulate cardiac SERCA expression in aging are still unclear; however, new studies implicated a decreased thyroid hormone (TH) responsiveness in the aging rat heart; in large part, this decrease involves binding of the TH receptor (TR) and retinoid X receptor (RXR) heterodimer to TH-responsive elements (TREs) located in the SERCA and cardiac myosin heavy chain (MHC) gene promoters. Age-associated changes in the TR and RXR could explain the age-associated changes in SERCA and MHC expression. Long et al. found no significant myocardial changes in RXRα or RXRβ mRNA levels in the aging rat heart, although both α1 and α2 TR mRNA levels decreased significantly between 2 and 6 months of age [68]. During this time period, the mRNA levels for α-MHC declined by more than half, whereas β-MHC mRNA levels remained unchangingly low. In contrast, between 6 and 24 months, when mRNA levels for β-MHC increased and α-MHC continued to decrease, there was a significant decline in TRβ1 and RXRγ mRNA levels accompanied by a reduction in the TRβ1 and RXRγ protein levels. Taken together, these findings suggest that decline in α-MHC gene expression may be biphasic and in part due to a decline in α1 (and possibly α2) TR levels between 2 and 6 months of age, and a decline in TRβ1 and RXRγ levels at later age.

Aging-mediated down-regulation of MHC and SERCA mediated by myocardial TH/TR signaling-mediated transcriptional control can be reversed with exercise [69]. While the expression of myocardial TRα1 and TRβ1 proteins is significantly lower in sedentary aged rats than in sedentary young rats, their expression is significantly higher in exercise-trained than in sedentary aged rats. Furthermore, the activity of TR DNA binding to the TRE transcriptional regulatory region in the α-MHC and SERCA genes and the myocardial expression of α-MHC and SERCA (both mRNA and protein) were upregulated with exercise training in the aging heart, in association with changes in the myocardial TR protein levels. In addition, plasma 3,3′-triiodothyronine (T3) and TH levels, which decrease with aging [70, 71], are increased after exercise training. The reversal of aging-induced down-regulation of myocardial TR signaling-mediated transcription of MHC and SERCA genes by exercise training appears to be related to the cardiac functional improvement observed in trained aged hearts.

Identification of the specific mechanisms contributing to decreased TH signaling in the aging heart may provide novel insights into potential therapies, keeping in mind that in the aging heart decreased TH activity may be a physiological adaptation. In the aging heart, therapies that increase SERCA activity might improve cardiac performance, and Ca^{2+} cycling proteins can be targeted to improve cardiac function [72]. Decline in myocardial SERCA content with age may also contribute to the development of impaired function after I/R. Moreover, the ratio of SERCA to either phospholamban or calsequestrin decreased in the senescent human myocardium [73]. Decreased rates of Ca^{2+} transport mediated by the SERCA isoform are responsible for the slower sequestration of cytosolic Ca^{2+} and consequently prolonged muscle relaxation times in the aging heart. Knyushko et al. [74] found that senescent Fischer 344 rat heart had a 60% decrease in SERCA activity in comparison to that of young adult hearts, and this functional reduction in activity could be attributed in part to both lower abundance of SERCA protein and increased 3-nitrotyrosine modifications of multiple tyrosines within the cardiac SERCA protein. Nitration in the senescent heart was found to increase by more than two nitrotyrosines per Ca^{2+}-ATPase, coinciding with the appearance of partially nitrated Tyr(294), Tyr(295), and Tyr(753) residues. In contrast, skeletal muscle SERCA exhibited a homogeneous pattern of nitration, with full site nitration of Tyr(753) in the young, with additional nitration of Tyr(294) and Tyr(295) in the senescent muscle. The nitration of these latter sites correlates with diminished transport function in both types of muscle, suggesting that these sites have a potential role in the down-regulation of ATP utilization by the Ca^{2+}-ATPase under conditions of nitrosative stress.

Growth Hormone and IGF-I

IGF-1/GH/IGF-1 receptor system not only plays an important role in determining organism development and lifespan but is in itself affected by age. IGF-1 decreased linearly with age in both sexes, with significantly higher levels in men than women [75]. The decrease in GH-induced IGF-1 secretion in the elderly suggests that resistance to the action of GH may be a secondary contributing factor in the low plasma IGF-1 concentrations [76]. Decreased IGF-1 levels with age may contribute to the increase in cardiac disease found in the elderly, including HF [77]. Findings from the Framingham Heart Study in a prospective, community-based investigation indicated that serum IGF-1 level was inversely related to the risk for HF in the elderly without a previous MI, suggesting that the maintenance of an optimal IGF-1 levels in aged individuals may reduce the risk for HF [78]. In addition, this study revealed that greater levels or production of the catabolic cytokines TNF-α and interleukin 6 were associated with

increased mortality in community-dwelling elderly adults, whereas IGF-1 levels had the opposite effect [79]. In aged animals and humans, the secretion of GH and the response of GH to the administration of GH-releasing hormone (GHRH) are lower than in young adults [80]. In rodents, a twofold increase in GH receptors has been observed with age but this increase fails to compensate for the reduction in GH secretion [81, 82]. Further studies revealed that the apparent size of the GH receptor was not altered with age, whereas the capacity of GH to induce *IGF-1* gene expression and secretion was 40–50% less in old than in young animal [77].

There is considerable literature indicating that GH administration to old animals and humans raises plasma IGF-1 levels and results in increases in skeletal muscle and lean body mass, a decrease in adiposity, increased immune function, improvements in learning and memory, and increases in cardiovascular function. Interestingly, GH can induce improvement in hemodynamic and clinical status in some patients with chronic HF, largely resulting from the ability of GH to increase cardiac mass [83]. However, disappointing results have been reported in patients with DCM undergoing infusion of GH [84]; this could be related to the choice of an incorrect agent (GH instead of IGF-1) and/or failure to selectively target patients with low IGF-1 levels [85]. Recently, in a meta-analysis of clinical studies, Tritos and Danias [86] evaluated the efficacy and safety of recombinant human growth hormone (rhGH) therapy in severe HF. Therapy with rhGH appears to have beneficial clinical effects in HF including improved exercise duration, maximum oxygen consumption, and New York Heart Association class. Also, there was hemodynamic improvement, including increased cardiac output, decreased systemic vascular resistance and improved left ventricular (LV) ejection fraction, with no adverse effects on diastolic function. Most of the beneficial effects were driven by either uncontrolled or longer duration studies. Interestingly, rhGH therapy slightly increased the risk for ventricular dysrhythmias; although this finding was driven by a single small study. This meta-analysis suggests that rhGH therapy may have beneficial effects in cases of HF secondary to LV systolic dysfunction and that the possibility of prodysrhythmia associated with rhGH therapy merits further assessment. Furthermore, larger randomized trials with longer treatment duration are needed to fully elucidate the efficacy and safety of rhGH therapy in human HF.

Pharmacological administration of GH to adults may pose some risks; mice transgenic for GH and acromegalic patients secreting high amounts of GH have premature death [87]. Thus, caution must be used in the use of IGF-1 for treatment of cardiac diseases. Given its potent antiapoptotic role in proliferation, several studies reported the association of high dosage IGF-1 with human cancers [88, 89], in contrast another study found that overexpression of *IGF-1* in animals or the administration of rhIGF-1 does not have a carcinogenic effect [90].

Interestingly, the Klotho protein which functions as a circulating hormone binds to a cell-surface receptor and represses intracellular signals of insulin and IGF-1, stops aging in mice (a subject that will be further discussed later in this chapter). Amelioration of the aging-like phenotypes in Klotho-deficient mice has been observed by disturbing insulin and IGF-1 signaling, suggesting that Klotho-mediated inhibition of insulin and IGF-1 signaling contributes to its antiaging properties [91].

Cellular Damage/Cell Loss

Since cell damage occurs at random in any organ or tissue, including the heart, a population of damaged cells will always coexist with normal cells at any time in the process of aging; an important unknown relates to the number of damaged cells required to impair organ/tissue function. Kirkwood [92] pointed out that there is a significant difference in assessing cell damage in vitro versus in vivo, with cells in culture reaching a limit in their potential for cell division/differentiation, which may not occur in vivo. Therefore, caution is called for regarding the interpretation of data using different methodologies. During aging, there is a significant loss of postmitotic cells, such as cardiac myocytes, potentially triggered by the onset of mitochondrial dysfunction and ROS generation. For instance, in vitro studies of H_2O_2-treated cardiomyocytes showed that increased mitochondrial OS and declining mitochondrial energy production lead to the activation of apoptotic pathways [93, 94], but whether this also occurs in the aging heart in vivo is not known. While the role and extent of apoptosis in normal myocardial aging is under considerable debate, evidence of cardiomyocyte apoptosis has been confirmed by data showing that the aging rat heart had significantly elevated levels of cytochrome c release from mitochondria, as well as decreased levels of the anti-apoptotic protein Bcl-2, whereas levels of the proapoptotic protein Bax were unchanged [12]. Furthermore, myocytes derived from hearts of old mice displayed increased levels of markers of cell death and senescence, compared to myocytes from younger animals [95]. It is possible that apoptosis, at least to a certain degree in cardiac aging, may be a protective mechanism to get rid of damaged, potentially dangerous cells in a mechanistic effort to tilt the balance toward healthy cells, although, we do not know where this balance is.

According to Uhrborn et al. [96], glioma cells stained for senescence-associated β-galactosidase activity, apparently specific for senescent cells, showed that enlarged cells gave a distinctive positive staining reaction. This senescence phenotype appears to be dependent on the continuous expression of p16INK4A. Thus, induced expression of p16INK4A in these cells reverted their immortal phenotype and caused immediate cellular senescence. Increased expression of p16INK4A also occurred in aging cardiomyocytes [95]. Proteins implicated in growth arrest and senescence, such as p27Kip1, p53, p16INK4a, and p19ARF, were also present in myocytes of young mice, and their expression increased with age. In addition, DNA damage and myocyte death were found to exceed cell formation in older mice, leading to a decline in the number of myocytes and to HF. This effect did not occur in transgenic mice, in which cardiac stem cells-mediated myocyte regeneration compensated for the extent of cell death and prevented ventricular dysfunction.

Telomeres and Telomere-Related Proteins

In human, there is a remarkable variability in the age of onset and the severity of the manifestations of cardiovascular diseases. Although this cannot be explained by established risk factors, it may be explained by variation in biological age. During aging, telomeres length is progressively reduced in most somatic cells, and after a number of cell cycles, telomere length reaches a critical size, cellular replication stops and the cell becomes senescent (Fig. 16.3). Age-dependent telomere shortening in most somatic cells, including vascular endothelial cells, SMCs, and cardiomyocytes, appears to impair cellular function and the viability of the aged organism. While the association of telomere length and CVD appears likely, whether telomere shortening is a direct cause of the vascular pathology of aging or a consequence is not known [97]. Recently, telomere length has been reported to be shorter in circulating leukocytes of patients with HF compared with age-balanced and gender-balanced control patients, and appears to be related to the severity of disease. Furthermore, telomere length has been found to be incrementally shorter in relation to the presence and extent of atherosclerotic disease manifestations [98]. Notwithstanding, telomere dysfunction and reduction in telomere length has been observed with age in SMCs, endothelial, and white blood cells, and they may be the primary factor in predisposing vascular tissues to atherosclerosis, and also to a decreasing capacity for neovascularization [97]. This attrition of telomere length is most prominent under conditions of high OS, but particularly prevalent in hypertensives, diabetics, and individuals with CAD.

In endothelial cells, glutathione-dependent redox homeostasis plays a central role in the preservation of telomere function [99]. Under conditions of mild chronic OS, the loss of telomere integrity is a major trigger for the onset of premature senescence. Interestingly, antioxidants and statins can delay the replicative senescence of endothelial cells by inhibition of the nuclear export of telomerase reverse transcriptase into the cytosol [100]. Further studies

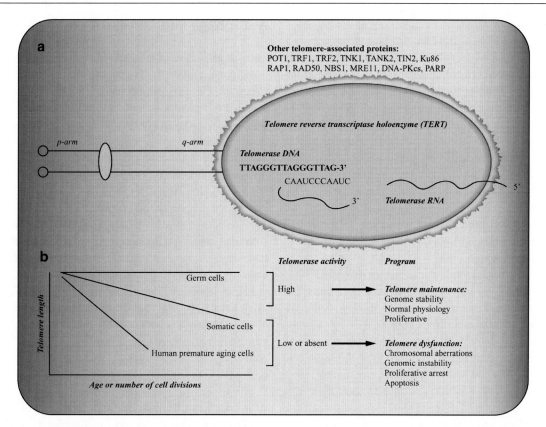

Fig. 16.3 Telomeres, telomerase and cell proliferation. (**a**) Telomeres present at the ends of the chromosomes (one end at the Q arm is shown here) are composed of a tandem repeated sequence in telomeric DNA, a telomerase ribonucleoprotein complex including a catalytic telomerase reverse transcriptase holoenzyme (TERT), an RNA component and additional telomeric proteins (listed on top). (**b**) Telomere length decreases in aging in somatic cells but not in germ cells. As telomerase activity is low or absent in most somatic cells, progressive telomere erosion occurs with each mitotic division during normal aging. In germ cells (and tumor cells) containing high telomerase activity, no change in telomere length is seen with aging or progressive divisions. Accelerated telomere attrition is associated with human premature aging. Some of the phenotypic changes associated with telomere length are shown on the *bottom right*

have shown that telomere biology plays a significant role in the functional augmentation of endothelial progenitor cells (EPCs) by statins [101]. These studies found that the *ex vivo* culturing of EPCs leads to premature replicative senescence associated with the "uncapping" and dysfunction of telomeres, and loss of telomere repeat-binding factor (TRF2). In addition, cotreatment of the cultured EPCs with statins delayed their premature senescence, in part by enhancing TRF2 expression at the posttranslational level.

While the ability of EPCs to sustain ischemic tissue and repair may be limited in the aging/senescence heart, estrogens have been shown to accelerate the recovery of the endothelium after vascular injury, significantly increasing telomerase activity [102]. RT-PCR analysis showed that 17β-estradiol administered in a dose-dependent fashion increased levels of the telomerase catalytic subunit (TERT), an effect that was significantly inhibited by pharmacological PI3K blockers (either wortmannin or LY294002). In addition, EPCs treated with 17β-estradiol had significantly enhanced mitogenic potential and release of VEGF protein;

also, EPCs treated with both 17β-estradiol and VEGF were more likely to integrate into the network formation than those treated with VEGF alone. Telomerase inactivation during aging may also be related to the oxidized low-density lipoprotein-accelerated onset of EPC senescence, which leads to the impairment of proliferative capacity and network formation [103].

Estrogen also stimulates NO production in vascular endothelial cells [104], which in turn induces telomerase in these cells [105]. The cardioprotective effects of estrogens via indirect actions on lipoprotein metabolism, and through direct effects on vascular endothelial cells and SMCs are likely to contribute to the lower incidence of CVD observed in premenopausal women compared with men; significantly, women have a decelerated rate of age-dependent telomere attrition over men [106].

In a paper on the relation of telomere biology and cardiovascular disease, Fuster and Andrés [107] reviewed experimental and human studies that linked telomeres and associated proteins to several factors that influence cardiovascular risk (e.g., estrogens, OS, hypertension, diabetes, and psychological stress), as well as to neovascularization and the pathogenesis of atherosclerosis and heart disease. They identify two still unanswered critical questions: (1) Whether telomere shortening is cause or consequence of cardiovascular disease, and (2) if therapies targeting the telomere may be applicable in treating these disorders (e.g., cell "telomerization" to engineer blood vessels of clinical value for bypass surgery, and to facilitate cell-based myocardial regeneration strategies). Since current research has been mainly focused on the role of telomerase, a suggestion is made that it is of up most importance to investigate whether defects in additional telomere-associated proteins may contribute to the pathogenesis of cardiovascular disease.

Most human somatic cells can undergo only limited replication in vitro, and senescence can be triggered when telomeres cannot carry out their normal protective functions. Moreover, senescent human fibroblasts display molecular markers characteristic of cells bearing DNA double-strand breaks and inactivation of DNA damage checkpoint kinases in senescent cells may restore the cell-cycle progression into S phase [108]. This telomere-initiated senescence may reflect a DNA damage checkpoint response that is activated with a direct contribution from dysfunctional telomeres. A high rate of age-dependent telomere attrition has been noted in the human distal abdominal aorta, probably reflecting enhanced cellular turnover rate due to local factors, such as increase in shear wall stress in this vascular segment [109]. These data appear to contradict findings in mice that short telomeres provide a protective effect from diet-induced atherosclerosis [110]. These apparently conflicting findings might be reconciled if cellular damage accumulation imposed by prolonged exposure to cardiovascular risk factors ultimately prevails over protective mechanisms, including telomere shortening [106].

Several observations support the concept that the average telomere length is better maintained in conditions of low OS [111], and selective targeting of antioxidants, directly into the mitochondria, can counteract telomere shortening and increase lifespan in fibroblasts under mild OS [112]. Mitochondrial dysfunction can lead to a loss of cellular proliferative capacity through telomere shortening (Fig. 16.4), and the generation of ROS may signal the nucleus to limit cell proliferation through telomere shortening and telomeres as sensors to damaged mitochondria [113].

There is increasing evidence that telomere dysfunction is emerging as an important factor in the pathogenesis of human CVDs associated with aging, including hypertension, atherosclerosis, and HF (Fig. 16.5). In the future, further research should also be oriented toward finding the potential role that additional telomere-associated proteins, other than telomerase, play in aging and in HF, and to use these discoveries to develop novel and more effective cardiovascular therapies.

Autophagy and Cardiac Aging

The process where cells faced with a short supply of nutrients in their extracellular fluid begin to engulf specific, often defective, organelles (e.g., mitochondria) to reuse their components is called autophagy. This process is well conserved in nature from lower eukaryotes to mammals and has been attributed to disparate physiological events including cell death, which mechanism is different from apoptosis. A number of steps are involved in autophagy: (1) formation of a double membrane within the cell; (2) confinement of the material to be degraded into an autophagosome; (3) fusion of the autophagosome with a lysosome, and (4) the enzymatic degradation of the materials. Activated class I phosphatidylinositol 3-kinase and mammalian target of rapamycin (mTOR) inhibit autophagy, while class III phosphatidylinositol 3-kinase acts as a facilitator [114]. Autophagy decreases during the development of myocardial hypertrophy and is enhanced during the regression of hypertrophy. It occurs in many types of cells during development including cardiomyocytes, and in pressure-overloaded animal models cardiomyocyte loss due to autophagy which occurs during the progression from compensated hypertrophy to HF. Moreover, in cardiac diseases associated with aging such as ischemic heart disease and cardiomyopathy, intralysosomal degradation of cells plays an essential role in the renewal of cardiac myocytes; being the interaction of mitochondria and lysosomes in cellular homeostasis of great significance, since both organelles suffer significant age-related alterations in postmitotic cells [115]. Many mitochondria undergo enlargement and structural disorganization, and since lysosomes responsible for mitochondrial turnover experience a loss of function, the rate of total mitochondrial protein turnover declines with age [116]. Coupled mitochondrial and lysosomal defects contribute to irreversible functional impairment and cell death, and similarly mitochondrial interaction with other functional compartments of the cardiac cell (e.g., the ER for Ca^{2+} metabolism, peroxisomes for the interchange of antioxidant enzymes essential in the production and decomposition of H_2O_2) must be kept in check since defects in communication between these organelles may accelerate the aging process.

Several mechanisms may potentially contribute to the age-related accumulation of damaged mitochondria following initial oxidative injury, including clonal expansion of defective mitochondria, reduction in the number of mitochondria targeted for autophagocytosis (secondary to mitochondrionmegaly or decreased membrane damage associated with decrease mitochondrial respiration), suppressed autophagy because of heavy lipofuscin loading of lysosomes, and decreased efficiency of Lon protease [117].

Abnormal autophagic degradation of damaged macromolecules and organelles, known as biological "garbage," is also

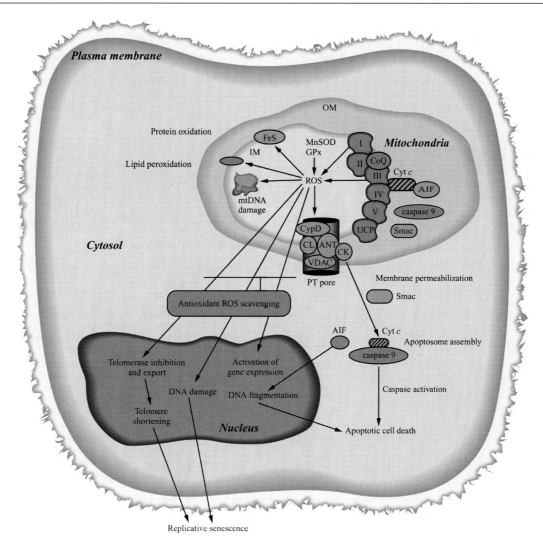

Fig. 16.4 Mitochondrial ROS production contributes to telomere-dependent replicative senscence. Production of ROS by aberrant mitochondrial respiratory complexes thought to occur in aging leads to mtDNA and protein damage and lipid peroxidation, PT pore and apoptotic progression (via cytochrome c release, membrane permeabilization, apoptosome formation and nuclear DNA fragmentation). ROS also affects the nucleus by reducing telomerase activity and increasing its export from the nucleus, causing direct DNA damage and activating specific gene expression – all of which contribute to the signaling of replicative senescence. Also shown is the involvement of antioxidant response both in the mitochondria (e.g., MnSOD and GpX) and in the cytosol which can remove ROS by scavenging free radicals

considered an important contributor to aging and the death of postmitotic cells, including cardiomyocytes. Stroikin et al. compared the survival of density-dependent growth-arrested and proliferating human fibroblasts and astrocytes following inhibition of autophagic sequestration with 3-methyladenine (3MA) [118]. Exposure of confluent fibroblast cultures to 3MA for 2 weeks resulted in an increased number of dying cells compared to both untreated confluent cultures and dividing cells with 3MA-inhibited autophagy. Similarly, autophagic degradation was suppressed by the protease inhibitor leupeptin. These findings suggest that lysosomal "garbage" accumulation plays an important role in the aging and death of postmitotic cells, and also support the antiaging role of cell division. Thus, autophagy can be considered an important participant

in the regulation of cellular metabolism, organelle homeostasis and redox equilibrium playing a paramount role in maintaining a normal myocardium.

Myocardial Remodeling and Aging

To determine the effects of aging on the human myocardium, hearts from individuals (aged 17–90 years) who died from causes other than cardiovascular disease have been studied [119]. The aging process was characterized by a loss of 38 million and 14 million nuclei/year in the left and right ventricles, respectively. This loss in muscle mass was accompanied

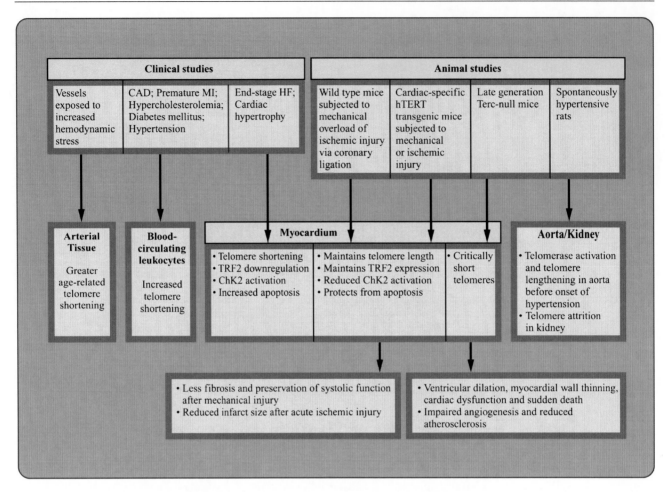

Fig. 16.5 Telomeres and telomerase in both human and animal CVD. Telomere and telomerase phenotype in different tissues of patients with indicated CVD disorders, and of selected animal models of CVD including both wild-type and genetically modified mice (e.g., cardiac-specific hTERT and Terc-null strains) and in spontaneously hypertensive rats

by a progressive increase in myocyte cell volume per nucleus, resulting in the preservation of ventricular wall thickness. However, the cellular hypertrophic response was unable to maintain normal cardiac mass. Left and right ventricular weights decreased by 0.70 and 0.21 g/year, respectively. Therefore, it was proposed that about one third of the cardiomyocytes are lost from the human heart between the ages of 17 and 90 years [119]. Several studies, however, have challenged the widely held, but unproven paradigm that describes the heart as a postmitotic organ [120]. Recent developments in the field of stem cell biology have led to the recognition that the possibility exists for extrinsic and intrinsic regeneration of myocytes and coronary vessels, leading to the reevaluation of cardiac homeostasis and myocardial aging [121]. A newer paradigm views the adult mammalian heart as composed of nondividing myocytes (primarily terminally differentiated), and a small and continuously renewed subpopulation of cycling myocytes produced by the differentiation of cardiac stem cells. A dynamic balance between myocyte death and the formation of new myocytes by cardiac stem cells is an important regulator of myocardial maintenance of function and mass from birth to adulthood and very critical in old age. Increasing evidence suggests that numerous pathological or physiological stimuli can activate stem cells to enter the cell cycle and differentiate into new myocytes, and in some cases vasculature which significantly contribute to changes in cardiac output and myocardial mass [122].

Telomere length is a useful marker of these processes. Studies in fetal, neonatal, and senescent (27 month-old) Fischer 344 rats found that while the loss of telomeric DNA was minimal in fetal and neonatal myocytes, telomeric shortening increased with age in a subgroup of myocytes that constituted nearly 20% of the myocyte population, suggesting that this population reflects the most actively dividing myocyte class in the organ. Early studies found in the remaining nondividing rat myocytes, the progressive accumulation of another marker of cellular senescence, senescent associated nuclear protein, p16(INK4) [123].

When cardiomyocytes from aging individuals with age-related HF were compared to myocytes from individuals with idiopathic DCM, several differences in heart and myocyte phenotype were observed [124]. While aged diseased hearts exhibited moderate hypertrophy and dilation, they also displayed an accumulation of p16INK4a positive primitive stem cells and myocytes. A marked increase in cell death was primarily limited to cells expressing p16INK4a with significant telomeric shortening. Importantly, this finding suggested that stem cells could also be targeted by senescence. While cell multiplication, mitotic index, and telomerase increased in the aging heart, new evidence suggested that regenerative events could not compensate for cell death or prevent telomeric shortening. This study [124] also demonstrated that hearts from subjects with idiopathic DCM had more severe hypertrophy and dilation, more extensive cardiac interstitial fibrosis and tissue inflammatory injury, increased necrosis, and a reduced level of myocytes with p16INK4a labeling. This is consistent with the involvement of p16INK4a with death signals linked to apoptosis in senescent myocardium in contrast to idiopathic DCM, in which myocyte necrosis predominates and myocyte death is largely independent from the expression of the kinase inhibitor p16INK4a. Nonetheless, some important commonalities were also found: while idiopathic DCM had increased necrosis compared to aging tissues, aged diseased hearts and idiopathic DCM subjects had similar levels of myocyte apoptosis. In addition, extensive stem cell death was found in both cases and not in healthy controls, suggesting that mechanisms (e.g., OS) that target stem cells may contribute to the phenotype of cardiac dysfunction in both the aging and cardiomyopathic heart. Torella et al. have identified a population of cardiac stem cells in young and senescent mice that with aging display increased evidence of senescence, i.e., p16ink4a expression, telomere shortening (indicative of reduced telomerase activity), and apoptosis [95]. Interestingly, the effect of murine aging on cardiac stem cells (including the expression of gene products implicated in growth arrest and senescence, such as p27Kip1, p53, p16INK4a, and p19ARF), and on the resulting cardiac dysfunction was remarkably attenuated in aged transgenic mice containing overexpressed IGF-1. It remains to be seen whether similar effects of IGF-1 on preserving stem cell regenerative function would be found in strains with idiopathic DCM.

Recently, Gonzalez et al. [125] reported that chronological age leads to telomeric shortening in cardiac progenitor cell (CPCs), which generate a differentiated progeny that rapidly acquires the senescent phenotype, conditioning organ aging. Attenuation of the IGF-1/IGF-1 receptor and hepatocyte growth factor/c-Met systems mediate the CPC aging, which does not counteract any longer the CPC renin–angiotensin system, resulting in cellular senescence, growth arrest, and apoptosis. However, the senescent heart contains functionally competent CPCs with the properties of stem cells as demonstrated by pulse-chase 5-bromodeoxyuridine-labeling assay. This subset of telomerase-competent CPCs have long telomeres and, following activation, migrate to the regions of damage, where they generate a population of young cardiomyocytes reversing partly the aging myopathy. Thus, a senescent heart phenotype and HF may be corrected, and this may lead to prolongation of maximum lifespan.

p66(Shc) longevity gene regulates both steady-state and environmental stress-dependent ROS generation and its deletion in mice protects against experimental diabetic glomerulopathy by preventing diabetes-induced OS [126]. The increasing oxygen toxicity that occurs in diabetes mellitus may affect CPCs function resulting in abnormal CPC growth and myocyte formation, which may favor premature myocardial aging and HF. Using a model of insulin-dependent diabetes mellitus, Rota et al. [127] reported that generation ROS leads to telomeric shortening, expression of the senescent associated proteins p53 and p16INK4a, and apoptosis of CPCs, impairing the growth reserve of the heart. Ablation of the p66shc gene prevents these CPCs negative adaptations, interfering with the acquisition of the heart senescent phenotype and the development of HF with diabetes. Low ROS levels activate cell growth, intermediate ROS levels trigger cell apoptosis, and high levels initiate cell necrosis. CPCs replication predominates in diabetic p66shc−/−, whereas CPC apoptosis, and myocyte apoptosis and necrosis prevail in diabetic wild type. Expansion of CPCs and developing myocytes preserves cardiac function in diabetic p66shc−/−, suggesting that intact CPCs can effectively counteract the impact of uncontrolled diabetes on the heart. The recognition that p66shc conditions the destiny of CPCs raises the possibility that diabetic cardiomyopathy is a stem cell disease, in which abnormalities in CPCs define the life and death of the heart. These data suggest a genetic link between diabetes and ROS and between CPC survival and growth.

Since aging and a number of potential risk factors for coronary artery disease affect the functional activity of the endogenous stem/CPCs, their therapeutic potential application seems rather limited. Furthermore, the aging failing heart may not offer an adequate tissue environment in which cells are infused or injected. To ameliorate this Dimmeler and Leri suggested that pretreatment of cells or the target tissue by small molecules, polymers, growth factors, or a combination thereof may enhance the effect of cell therapy for cardiovascular diseases [128]. However, further research in animal models is necessary before clinical application to aging individual in HF can be carried out.

Besides stem cells and myocytes, another critical component of the aging heart milieu is the cardiac fibroblasts, the predominant cell type in the heart. Fibroblasts activated by various autocrine and paracrine factors, such as angiotensin II (ANGII), aldosterone, endothelins, cytokines, and growth factors likely play a key role in the formation and maintenance of fibrous tissue by the production of various extracellular-matrix (ECM) proteins, such as collagen, fibronectin, and integrin [129]. Cardiac fibrosis is characterized by excessive accumulation of fibrillar collagen in the extracellular space, in part arising as a loss of cardiomyocytes (replacement fibrosis) and as an interstitial response to various chronic cardiovascular diseases such as hypertension, myocarditis, and severe HF (reactive fibrosis), and is generally considered to be elevated in the aging human heart [1, 130]. Collagen concentration (primarily collagen type 1) and the intermolecular cross-linking of collagen increase with age [131]; however, being a rather complex process, the mechanisms of fibroblast involvement in aging-associated myocardial fibrosis remain undetermined. Surprisingly, both ANGII stimulation of collagen synthesis and fibroblast proliferation are diminished in aging compared to young cardiac fibroblasts [132]. Also, enzymes involved in the degradation of ECM components including the matrix metalloproteinases (MMPs) such as MMP-3, MMP-8, MMP-9, MMP-12, and MMP-14 increased in concert with decreased insoluble collagen in aging mice, suggesting that the accumulated collagen and fibronectin are not attributable to aging-mediated decline in degradation [133, 134]. This suggests that the increased fibrosis and stiffness found in the aging heart must have another mechanism. For example, age-mediated changes in glycation and integrin kinase signaling may contribute to the accumulation of collagen cross-interactions and fiber bundling, which can lead to fibrosis [135, 136]. Increased fibrosis with age leads to increased diastolic stiffness and contractile dysfunction in the heart and its larger vessels, and can reduce the electrical coupling between cardiac myocytes resulting in nonuniform depolarization, conduction delays, and dysrhythmias. It is evident that excessive collagen deposition or pathological fibrosis is an important contributor to LV dysfunction and poor outcome in patients with hypertension, myocardial infarction, and HF.

As previously discussed, HF with preserved LV ejection fraction frequently occurs in the elderly, and this type of HF is known as diastolic heart failure (DHF). Observations on the structural changes of DHF have shown that DHF patients had stiffer cardiomyocytes, as suggested by a higher resting tension (F(passive)) at the same sarcomere length. Collagen volume fraction and F(passive) determined in vivo diastolic LV dysfunction. Correction of this high F(passive) by protein kinase A (PKA) suggests that reduced phosphorylation of sarcomeric proteins is involved in DHF [137]. Cardiomyocytes of DHF patients had higher F(passive), but their total force is comparable to systolic heart failure (SHF). Cardiomyocyte diameter has been found to be higher in DHF [138], but collagen volume fraction was equally elevated in both types of HF, with myofibrillar density lower in SHF. Cardiomyocytes in DHF patients had higher F(passive), but their total force was comparable to SHF. After administration of PKA to cardiomyocytes, the drop in F(passive) was larger in DHF than in SHF [138]. The data suggest that LV myocardial structure and function differ in SHF and DHF because of distinct cardiomyocyte abnormalities, and underline the separation of HF into two different phenotypes of SHF and DHF.

Hypertrophic Cardiomyopathy

A number of hypertrophic cardiomyopathy (HCM)-associated alleles have been primarily described in very young individuals showing what is termed early-onset presentation; these phenotypes are often associated with sudden cardiac death and are of significant concern mainly in neonates and young athletes (including specific mutations in β-MHC and cardiac troponin T). Several mutations in fatty acid metabolism (e.g., ACADVL, carnitine transport), and in bioenergetic metabolism (e.g., NDUFV2, COX 15) and a number of mtDNA mutations have also been primarily identified in neonates and children. Interestingly, while the relationship between genotype and phenotype with HCM mutations is often not clear-cut, the distribution of specific mutations in elderly onset disease is often markedly different from specific mutations found in familial early onset HCM [139]. For instance, mutations in *MYBPC3* encoding cardiac myosin binding protein-C, show delayed onset of HCM and induce the disease predominantly in the fifth or sixth decade of life and along with specific troponin I, and α-myosin heavy chain alleles are more prevalent in elderly onset HCM [140, 141]. Mutations which alter the charge of the encoded amino acid tend to affect patient survival more significantly than those that produce a conservative amino acid change [142]. The milder cardiac phenotype in many of the patients with elderly onset HCM genes is also consistent with the observation that HCM is frequently well tolerated and compatible with normal life expectancy, and it may remain clinically dormant for long periods of time with symptoms and initial diagnosis deferred until late in life [143].

Mutations in the X-linked GLA gene encoding the lysosomal enzyme α-galactosidase A, causing α-galactosidase A deficiency, is a genetic defect with significant association to late-onset HCM, and leads to an inborn lysosomal storage disorder characterized by pathological intracellular glycosphingolipids deposition. Cardiac involvement consisting of progressive left ventricular hypertrophy is very common and constitutes the most frequent cause of death. Mutations in this gene have been found in up to 6% of men with late-onset HCM, and in 12% of women with late-onset HCM [144, 145].

Of the HCM-causing genes thus far identified (Table 16.1), a large proportion encode protein components of the cardiac sarcomere, which were the first class of HCM genes to be

Table 16.1 Genes implicated in clinical HCM

Gene	Protein	Function
TNNT2	Cardiac troponin T	Sarcomeric
TTN	Titin	Z disc
MYL3	Essential myosin light chain	Sarcomeric
TNNC1	Cardiac troponin C	Sarcomeric
MYBPC3	Cardiac myosin binding protein C	Sarcomeric
CSRP3	Cardiac muscle LIM protein	Cytoskeletal/Z disc
MYL2	Regulatory myosin light chain	Sarcomeric
MYH7	β-Myosin heavy chain	Sarcomeric
ACTC	Cardiac actin	Sarcomeric
TPM1	α-Tropomyosin	Sarcomeric
TNNI3	Cardiac troponin I	Sarcomeric
CAV3	Caveolin-3	Signaling
LAMP2	Lysosome associated membrane protein 2	Lysosome
TCAP	T-Cap (telethonin)	Cytoskeletal/Z disc
MYOZ2	Myozenin 2	Cytoskeletal/Z disc
PRKAG2	AMP-activated protein kinase (regulatory subunit)	Energy sensor
SCO2	COX assembly	Energy metabolism
NDUFV2	Respiratory complex I subunit	Energy metabolism
NDUFS2	Respiratory complex I subunit	Energy metabolism
ANT	Adenine nucleotide transporter/ mtDNA maintenance	Energy metabolism
ACADVL	VLCAD activity (Fatty acid oxidation)	Energy metabolism
FRDA	Mitochondrial iron import	Energy metabolism
COX10	COX assembly	Energy metabolism
SLC22A4	Carnitine transporter (OCTN2)	Energy metabolism
COX15	COX assembly	Energy metabolism
GLA	α-Galactosidase	Lysosomal storage

identified, and still remain the most prevalent [146]. Mutations have been found in genes that encode components of the thick filament proteins (i.e., β-MHC, essential MLC, regulatory MLC, and cMyBP-C), genes that encode thin filament proteins (i.e., cardiac actin, cardiac troponin T, cardiac troponin I, cardiac troponin C, and α-tropomyosin). HCM mutations have also been found in genes involved in the cytoskeleton including titin, telethonin, myozenin, and cardiac muscle LIM protein. In addition, mutations resulting in HCM have also been reported in genes encoding nonsarcomeric/noncytoskeletal proteins including the γ2-regulatory subunit of an AMP-activated protein kinase (AMPK) [147], LAMP-2, a lysosome-associated membrane glycoprotein, and caveolin-3, a contributor to the caveolae micro-domains involved in cellular signaling [148]. Another significant subgroup of mutant genes identified in patients with HCM are comprised of genes encoding proteins involved in mitochondrial bioenergetic metabolism. These include subunits of the mitochondrial respiratory chain (NDUFV2, NDUFS2), SCO2 encoding a copper metallochaperone, COX10, and COX15 involved in the assembly of the multisubunit mitochondrial respiratory complex IV enzyme also known as cytochrome *c* oxidase;

genes involved in fatty acid transport and oxidation (SLC22A4, ACADVL) and iron import (FRDA/frataxin); mutations in ANT encoding the adenine nucleotide translocator which also has been recently found to play a role in mtDNA maintenance. Moreover, numerous mutations in mtDNA have also been reported associated with the development of HCM often in conjunction with multisystemic disorders including hypotonia, myopathies, muscle-weakness, lactic acidosis, deafness, ophthalmic disease, and diabetes.

Dilated Cardiomyopathy

Dilated cardiomyopathy (DCM) is a heterogeneous disease that often overlaps with inflammatory heart disease. Although in the majority of cases the etiology of DCM is unknown, microarray techniques, performed using endomyocardial biopsy specimens, may allow novel insights into the unique disease-specific gene expression that exists in end-stage cardiomyopathy of different etiologies presenting with HF. Importantly, expression profile analysis of DCM may facilitate its early detection and prognostic assessment. Recently, Ruppert et al. [149] characterized different types of DCM employing gene expression profiling of biopsied cardiac tissue with microarrays performed by hybridization of synthesized complementary DNA against a Lab-Arraytor60-combi microarray. One pattern of gene expression was consistent with DCM and inflammatory cardiomyopathy, and another with inflammatory heart disease. Additionally, the microarray data were confirmed by showing that DCM is associated with a reduced myocardial toll-like receptor 9 expression resulting from progressive loss of functional cardiomyocytes. Collectively, these findings demonstrated the utility and validity of microarrays from endomyocardial biopsy specimens to detect subclasses of DCM that do not differ histopathologically, but transcriptionally, from each other. Furthermore, the gene expression profile observed in these patients with DCM suggested ongoing immune activation. Haeidecker et al. have assessed individual risk of new-onset HF by analysis of transcriptome biomarkers using microarrays techniques [150]. From a total of 350 endomyocardial biopsy samples, they were able to identify 180 with idiopathic DCM. Patients with phenotypic extremes in survival were selected: 25 considered to have good prognosis (event-free survival for at least 5 years) and 18 with poor prognosis (events (death, requirement for LVAD, or cardiac transplant) and showing within the first 2 years of presentation clinical HF). Forty-six overexpressed genes were identified in patients with good versus poor prognosis, of which 45 genes were selected by prediction analysis of microarrays for prognosis in a train set ($n = 29$) with subsequent validation in test sets ($n = 14$ each). Interestingly, the biomarker performed with 74% sensitivity and 90% specificity after 50 random partitions. These findings suggest that transcriptomic biomarkers may predict prognosis in patients with new-onset HF from a single endomyocardial biopsy sample. Moreover, and based on these findings, novel therapeutic targets for HF and cardiomyopathy might become possible.

Kittleson et al. [151], also using gene expression analysis of microarrays, have tested the hypothesis that nonischemic (NICM) and ischemic cardiomyopathy (ICM) would have both shared and have distinct differentially expressed genes relative to normal hearts. Comparison of gene expression of 21 NICM and 10 ICM samples with that of six nonfailing (NF) hearts was carried out using Affymetrix U133A Gene Chips and significance analysis of microarrays. Compared with NF, 257 genes were differentially expressed in NICM and 72 genes in ICM. Only 41 genes were shared between the two comparisons, mainly involved in cell growth and signal transduction. Those uniquely expressed in NICM were frequently involved in metabolism, and those in ICM more often had catalytic activity. Novel genes, which were upregulated in NICM but not ICM included angiotensin-converting enzyme-2 (ACE2) suggesting that ACE2 may offer differential therapeutic efficacy in NICM and ICM. In addition, a tumor necrosis factor receptor was downregulated in both NICM and ICM, demonstrating the different signaling pathways involved in the pathophysiology of HF. Thus, transcriptome analysis offers novel insights into the pathogenesis-based therapies in HF management and complements studies using expression-based profiling to diagnose HF of different etiologies. In contrast, Kuner et al. [152] have reported poor separation of ischemic and nonischemic cardiomyopathies by genomic analysis. They analyzed one cDNA and two publicly available high-density oligonucleotide microarray studies comprising a total of 279 end-stage human HF samples. When classifiers identified in a single study were applied to the remaining studies, misclassification rates >25% for ICM and NICM specimens were noted, indicating poor separation of both etiologies. However, data mining of 458 classifier genes that were concordantly identified in at least two of the three data sets points to different biological processes in ICM vs. NICM. Consistent with the underlying ischemia, cytokine signaling pathways and immediate-early response genes were overrepresented in ICM samples, whereas NICM samples displayed a deregulation of cytoskeletal transcripts, genes encoding for the major histocompatibility complex, and antigen processing and presentation pathways, potentially pointing to immunologic processes in NICM. These data suggest that ICM and NICM exhibit substantial heterogeneity at the transcriptomic level. However, prospective studies will be necessary to test whether etiology-specific gene expression patterns are present at earlier disease stages or in subsets of both etiologies.

Other than immune-inflammatory and ischemic etiologies, most often than not, the cause of DCM is unknown and fre-

quently appears to be secondary to mutations in a large number of genes with diverse functions, with a familial inheritance [146]. These mutations may be present at a wide variety of genetic loci that confirm its genetic heterogeneity (Table 16.2). A compounding factor in the development of DCM is age. With aging the incidence of idiopathic DCM increases, males are afflicted at a higher rate than females and elderly patients have a worse prognosis than their younger counterparts with this disease. Moreover, age-related penetrance, i.e., absence of disease manifestations in genotype-positive individuals until after a particular age, and nonpenetrance, has contributed to the underestimation of the prevalence of familial type of this disease [153, 154].

The first gene identified by candidate gene analysis in DCM was cardiac actin. Mutations in five other genes encoding sarcomere proteins have been implicated in DCM (all of which can also cause HCM) including β-MHC, cMyBP-C, cardiac troponin T, α-tropomyosin, and titin. While a subset of HCM patients develop a dilated phenotype, DCM resulting from sarcomeric gene mutations often arises without previous HCM. Mutations were subsequently described in genes encoding cytoskeletal proteins including desmin, δ-sarcoglycan, muscle LIM protein, α-actinin-2, Cypher/Zasp, Tcap/telethonin and metavinculin, which stabilize the myofibrillar apparatus and link the cytoskeleton to the contractile apparatus. Dystrophin is another critical gene involved in the intracellular cytoskeleton (linking it to the ECM and contributing to intracellular organization, force transduction, and membrane stability), whose mutation can lead to DCM either in association with Duchenne muscular dystrophy or result in an adult-onset X-linked DCM without skeletal myopathy. Furthermore, mutations in gene-products serving critical electrophysiological function in the heart have been associated with DCM in a limited number of cases, including the ABCC9 gene encoding SUR2A, the regulatory subunit of the cardiac K_{ATP} channel, and the SCN5A gene encoding the cardiac sodium channel, involved in the generation of the action potential. Mutations in the phospholamban (PLN) gene encoding a transmembrane phosphoprotein which by inhibiting the cardiac sarcoplasmic reticular Ca^{2+}-adenosine triphosphatase (SERCA2a) pump is a critical regulator of calcium cycling, have also been found in individuals with DCM [155–157]. A T116G point mutation, substituting a termination codon for Leu-39 (L39stop), and resulting in loss-of-function mutation (PLN null allele) was identified in two families with hereditary HF; subjects homozygous for L39stop developed DCM and HF, requiring cardiac transplantation [156].

DCM-causing mutations have also been found in proteins which appear to be involved in the maintenance of nuclear integrity as well as playing roles in other nuclear processes including gene transcription, cell cycle regulation, and chromatin remodeling. For example, mutations in the LMNA

Table 16.2 Genes implicated in familial human dilated cardiomyopathy (DCM)

Gene	Protein	Function	Chromosomal locus	Inher.
ABCC9	SUR2A, regulatory subunit of cardiac K_{ATP} channel	Membrane channel	12p12.1	AD
ACTC	Cardiac α-actin	Sarcomeric	15q14	AD
ACTN2	α-actinin-2	Cytoskeletal	1q43	AD
DES	Desmin	Cytoskeletal	2q35	AD
DMD	Dystrophin	Cytoskeletal	Xp21	X-R
FOXD4	Forkhead Box D4	Transcription factor	9p11–q11	Nd
TAZ (G4.5)	Tafazzin	Metabolic	Xq28	X-R
LMNA	Lamins A and C	Nuclear membrane	1p1–q21	AD
CSRP3	muscle LIM protein	Cytoskeletal	11p15	AD
MYBPC3	Cardiac myosin binding protein C	Sarcomeric	11p11	AD
MYH6	α-myosin heavy chain	Sarcomeric	14q12	AD
MYH7	β-myosin heavy chain	Sarcomeric	14q12	AD
PLN	Phospholamban	Calcium cycling	6q22.1	AD
SCN5A	Cardiac sodium channel	Membrane channel	3p22–25	AD
SGCD	δ-sarcoglycan	Cytoskeletal	5q33	AD
STA	Emerin	Nuclear membrane	Xq28	X-R
TCAP	Tcap/telethonin	Cytoskeletal	17q12	AD
TNNC1	Cardiac troponin C	Sarcomeric	3p21.3–3p14.3	AD
TNNI3	Cardiac troponin I	Sarcomeric	19q13.4	AR
TNNT2	Cardiac troponin T	Sarcomeric	1q32	AD
TPM1	α-Tropomyosin	Sarcomeric	15q22	AD
TTN	Titin	Cytoskeletal	2q31	AD
VCL	Metavinculin	Cytoskeletal	10q22–q23	AD
ZASP	Cypher/Zasp	Cytoskeletal	10q22.3–q23.2	AD

AD autosomal dominant; *AR* autosomal recessive; *X-R* X-linked recessive; *Nd* not determined

gene encoding lamin A and the STA gene encoding emerin, both multifunctional nuclear membrane proteins, have been found to lead to DCM, the latter most commonly in association with Emery–Dreifuss muscular dystrophy. A mutation disrupting an extremely highly conserved tryptophan residue in the forkhead domain of FOXD4, a nuclear transcription factor of the forkhead/winged helix box (FOX) gene family has been identified in a pedigree presenting with a complex phenotype including DCM [158].

DCM may be also associated to mutations in proteins involved in energy metabolism, and to specific pathogenic mutations in mtDNA (often in conjunction with multisystemic disorders). Clearly, the wide spectrum of defective intracellular functions that can lead to DCM suggests that multiple pathophysiological mechanisms are likely involved in triggering this disorder, consistent with its frequently heterogeneous presentation. A number of the aforementioned genetic defects are associated with late-onset DCM with higher incidence of presentation in the elderly. In a large-scale mutation analysis of European patients with DCM, carriers of mutations in the β myosin heavy chain (MYH7) gene were significantly older (mean age at diagnosis was 48 years) compared to carriers of mutations in the cardiac T troponin (TNNT2) gene (mean age at diagnosis was 23 years) [159]. Also, several specific DCM-associated mutations are associated with a milder presentation and increased disease presen-

tation with age. While mutations in the MyBP-C have been previously described in association with a favorable clinical course and with late onset HCM, late-onset DCM has been reported in association with an Arg820Gln mutation in the MyBP-C gene [160]. Similarly, carriers of the Arg71Thr mutation in the SGCD gene encoding the cytoskeletal δ-sarcoglycan had a relatively mild phenotype and a late onset of DCM [161].

Mutations in the DMD gene have been reported in both familial and sporadic cases of Duchenne (DMD) and Becker (BMD) muscular dystrophies [162, 163]. DMD usually presents in early childhood with progressive skeletal muscle weakness, mainly of the large proximal muscle groups, and loss of ambulation generally by early adolescence; DCM and conduction defects present late in the disease and the majority of patients die in their twenties, most commonly as a result of respiratory failure. Individuals with DMD usually have frameshift or nonsense DMD mutations that result in premature termination of translation, and a reduction or absence of dystrophin; typically, patients with DMD lack any detectable dystrophin expression in their skeletal muscles. In contrast, BMD is a milder, allelic form of DMD with affected males presenting later in life, exhibiting a milder course and displaying a high incidence of cardiac involvement, despite their milder skeletal muscle disease; the most common cause of death in BMD is HF. While clinical expression occurs primarily in the young adult, expression including severe DCM has also been reported in the older adult (>50 years old) [164, 165]. Subjects with BMD usually have DMD deletions that result in truncation or reduced levels of expression of dystrophin. Skeletal muscle from patients with BMD contains dystrophin of altered size and/ or reduced abundance. Interestingly, female carriers of DMD and BMD experience a high incidence of cardiac involvement that progresses with age and manifests primarily as cardiomyopathy.

A D626N mutation in the Cypher/ZASP encoding the Z-disc associated protein was found in all affected individuals in a family and was associated with late-onset DCM [166]. This mutation also proved interesting in that it alters the binding function of the Cypher/ZASP LIM domain and increased its interaction with protein kinase C (PKC), suggesting an association between DCM and the inherited abnormality involved in signal transduction.

Mutations in other signal transduction proteins appear to play a role in late-onset DCM. For instance, in a family with deletion of arginine 14 in the PLN gene, members did not present with DCM until their seventh decade with mildly symptomatic HF [155]. While this finding suggests that PLN mutations should be considered a contributory factor in the development of late onset cardiomyopathy, the finding that other heterozygous individuals with the identical PLN Arg 14 mutation have been reported to exhibit more severe disease at an earlier age (i.e., left ventricular dilation, contractile dysfunction, and episodic ventricular dysrhythmias, with overt HF by middle-age) suggests that other modulatory factors are likely involved in the expression of the DCM phenotype [167].

Another connection between genes involved in DCM and aging phenotypes has emerged with the characterization of LMNA mutations affecting lamin A/C. In addition to a variety of laminopathies including DCM along with neuropathy, lipodystrophy, limb girdle muscular dystrophy (LGMD), and autosomal dominant Emery–Dreifuss muscular dystrophy (EDMD), mutations in LMNA can result in premature aging syndromes or progeria. LMNA mutations have been reported in segmental progerias: Hutchinson–Gilford Progeria Syndrome (HGPS) [168], and Atypical Werner Syndrome [169]. In these aging diseases, the age of onset is quite different. In sharp contrast to Werner Syndrome, which becomes apparent at or shortly after puberty and early adulthood, HGPS manifests early in childhood. Growth retardation can be observed by 3–6 months of age, with degenerative changes in cutaneous, musculoskeletal, and cardiovascular systems showing shortly thereafter; baldness occurs by age 2 and median age of death is 13.5 years with mortality primarily attributable to myocardial infarction or severe HF. While many of the diseases secondary to LMNA mutations arise from dominant missense mutations (e.g., DCM type 1A, LGMD) some are autosomal recessive

(e.g., Charcot–Marie–Tooth disease) and others sporadic (e.g., HGPS, EDMD). It is clear, although largely unexplained, that different mutations in the same gene can lead to diverse dysfunctions and limited phenotypic overlap, with specific tissues targeted in each pathology [170]. An important unanswered question is why defects in nuclear envelope proteins that are found in most adult cell types should give rise to pathologies associated predominantly with skeletal and cardiac muscle and adipocytes. Among three different LMNA-mediated myopathies (i.e., EDMD, DCM and LGMD), cardiomyopathy occurs with the underlying potential of sudden death because of cardiac dysrhythmia. Moreover, the cardiac disease of mutated LMNA is often defined by conduction system and rhythm disturbances occurring early in the course of the disease, followed by DCM and HF. Affected individuals of a family comprised of members heterozygous for the same single nucleotide deletion in exon 6 of the LMNA gene showed different presentations, one with LGMD, one with EDMD, and another with DCM. The intrafamilial variability and mutational pleiotrophy observed in this and other studies suggests that other modifying factors (genetic, environmental or epigenetic) likely influence phenotypic expression [171].

While over 20 LMNA mutations (primarily missense defects localized in exons 1 and 3) have been reported to lead to autosomal dominant DCM (type 1A), evidence has been presented that different LMNA mutations can have significant different age-expression. Molecular analysis of two 4-generation white families with autosomal dominant familial DCM and conduction system disease revealed novel mutations in the rod segment of LMNA [172]. A missense mutation (nucleotide G607A, amino acid E203K) was identified in 14 adult subjects of family A with a cardiac phenotype primarily manifested as progressive conduction disease, occurring in the fourth and fifth decades with ensuing death due to HF. In contrast, a nonsense mutation (nucleotide C673T, amino acid R225X) was identified in ten adult subjects of family B with progressive conduction disease occurring with an earlier onset (third and fourth decades), accompanied by ventricular dysrhythmias, left ventricular enlargement, and systolic dysfunction and death caused by HF or sudden cardiac death.

Given the multiplicity of lamin A/C intracellular functions, a clear picture of the pathogenic mechanism by which LMNA mutations causes DCM (and conduction defects) is not yet evident [170–173]. One attractive hypothesis suggests that defective lamin A/C undermines the structural integrity of the nuclear envelope, promoting a mechanical nuclear fragility, and by its interactions with the cytoskeletal desmin results in a whole cell-mechanical vulnerability particularly notable under conditions of constant mechanical stress typical of cardiac and skeletal muscle cells, with resultant impairment of force transmission and contractile function. Other potential pathogenic mechanisms include loss or rearrangement of other LMNA-associated protein (e.g., emerin) and nuclear pore modification, changes in heterochromatin relative to the nuclear lamina, and altered gene expression due to disrupted interaction with RNA polymerases and transcription factors (this is further discussed in Chap. 6).

Restrictive Cardiomyopathy

Restrictive cardiomyopathy (RCM), the rarest form of cardiomyopathy, involves impaired ventricular filling and reduced diastolic volume in the presence of normal systolic function, and normal or near normal myocardial thickness. RCM is most frequently caused by pathological conditions that stiffen the myocardium by promoting infiltration or fibrosis, including endomyocardial disease, amyloidosis, sarcoidosis, scleroderma, storage diseases (e.g., hemochromatosis, Gaucher's disease, Fabry disease, glycogen storage disease), metastatic malignancy, anthracycline toxicity, or radiation damage. Several of the infiltrative diseases resulting in RCM can be inherited, including familial amyloidosis, hemochromatosis, Gaucher's disease, and glycogen storage disease. Most of the congestive HF in the elderly is due to diastolic dysfunction with preserved systolic function suggesting that RCM is an important entity [174]. Amyloidosis is the most prevalent underlying cause of RCM [175], and results from replacement of normal myocardial contractile elements by infiltration and interstitial deposits of amyloid, leading to alterations in cellular metabolism, Ca^{2+} transport, receptor regulation, and cellular edema. Amyloid myocardium becomes firm, rubbery, and noncompliant, and can also involve the cardiac conduction system presenting with different types of conduction defects and dysrhythmias.

Familial amyloidosis, or hereditary amyloidosis, while overall less common than immunoglobin amyloidosis (AL), is more frequently associated with RCM, and is most often caused by an autosomal-dominant mutation in the serum protein transthyretin encoded by the TTR gene. This gene encodes a protein containing 127-amino acid residues of four identical, noncovalently linked subunits that dimerize in the plasma protein complex. Over 60 distinct amino acid substitutions distributed throughout the TTR sequence have been correlated with increased amyloidogenicity of TTR [175]. The pattern of myocardial involvement varies according to the specific mutation and has distinct age-expression. A large number of these mutations have been associated with late-onset amyloid cardiomyopathy, as well as with polyneuropathy.

Patients with the Met 30 transthyretin variant, the most prevalent *TTR* mutation, primarily display conduction defects and often require pacemaker implantation [176]. In early-onset cases (i.e., patients younger than 50 years old), cardiac amyloid deposition was most prominent in the atrium and subendocardium but became evident throughout the myocar-

dium in late-onset cases. The Tyr77 mutation, the second most prevalent TTR mutation was studied in a large family with 12 affected individuals over four generations; the clinical phenotype is characterized by (sometimes prolonged) carpal tunnel syndrome, beginning between the sixth and seventh decade, with subsequent RCM [177]. Moreover, different ethnic groups have been shown to have varying degrees of susceptibility to cardiac amyloid deposition, while other groups do not have cardiac involvement. Substitution of isoleucine for valine at position 122 of the TTR gene has been reported to be more prevalent in African-Americans (estimated to be present in approximately 4% of the black population) [178], and is also associated with the occurrence of late-onset RCM [179]. Molecular analysis revealed that the substitution of isoleucine for valine shifts the equilibrium toward monomer (indicating lower tetramer stability), and favors tetramer dissociation required for amyloid fibril formation and resulting in accelerated amyloidosis [180].

RCM can also be associated with an iron-overload cardiomyopathy that manifests systolic or diastolic dysfunction primarily attributable to increased cardiac of iron deposition, and occurs with common genetic disorders such as hemochromatosis [181]. While the precise mechanism of iron-induced HF is not clear, the toxicity of iron in biological systems has largely been attributed to its ability to catalyze ROS generation. Hereditary hemochromatosis is a common autosomal recessive disorder among Caucasians with the genotype at risk accounting for 1:200–400 individuals of Northern European ancestry. Clinical complications appear late in life and often include cardiomyopathy (primarily but not necessarily restrictive) with subsequent development of congestive HF limited to homozygotes. As with many cardiomyopathies, phenotypic expression of the disease shows intrafamilial variability, likely as a result of the effects of modifier genes or to environmental factors. Hereditary hemochromatosis has been linked to pathogenic mutations in the gene coding for HFE, an atypical HLA class I molecule on chromosome 6 (6p21.3), hemojuvelin (HJV or HFE2) on chromosome 1 (most often associated with the juvenile form of hemochromatosis) and more rarely the gene coding for hepcidin (HAMP) on chromosome 19, and the gene encoding serum transferrin receptor 2 [181–183]. Two missense mutations in HFE have been found to be responsible for the majority of cases, C282Y and H63D; the C282Y mutation has a higher penetrance than the H63D mutation, and appears to result in a greater loss of HFE protein function [181]. Iron-overload in the heart resulting from HFE knockout in mice can also lead to increased susceptibility to myocardial ischemia/reperfusion injury as indicated by increased postischemic ventricular dysfunction, increased myocardial infarct size and myocyte apoptosis, with the degree of injury significantly elevated by high-iron diet [184]. While HFE mutations have been reported to be involved in several age-related chronic diseases such as Alzheimer's disease and CAD, one study suggested that in some populations the same HFE mutations associated with cardiomyopathy and CVDs paradoxically have also shown an increased prevalence (in the heterozygous state) in centenarians (primarily women), suggesting a beneficial role with respect to longevity [185]. This may be because individuals heterozygous for the C282Y mutation tend to have slightly but significantly higher values for serum iron and transferrin saturation and are therefore less likely to exhibit anemia secondary to iron deficiency; however, other studies have failed to replicate this relationship in different ethnic groups [186, 187].

Conclusion

The increased use of gene profiling in hearts from subjects with age-associated diseases such as cardiomyopathy and HF has begun to define a molecular signature of cardiac dysfunction whose component elements can be informatively compared between diseases, various populations (e.g., ethnic/racial, gender), a variety of treatment regimens (e.g., LV assist devices, pharmacological treatments) and of course, age. Efforts are also being undertaken to define a proteomic profile of age-associated cardiac disease, albeit as we have previously noted, for numerous pragmatic reasons most studies have chosen to target and define limited proteomes (e.g., mitochondrial/organelle-specific, specific classes of protein-modification).

While a number of polymorphic gene variants of candidate-genes in association with age-mediated cardiac diseases have been identified, in general these findings have been extraordinarily difficult to replicate and there are indications that modifying genes and/or environmental and epigenetic factors markedly influence the effects of these genes on the expression of cardiac disease and cardiac phenotype. Newer techniques of gene mapping, including very powerful haplotype mapping, may be applied in defining the genes involved in susceptibility and progression of these diseases in the elderly. Similarly, new techniques are urgently needed and will undoubtedly be developed to elucidate gene–environmental interactions.

In the dawning era of genomic- and post-genomic medicine, although there has not been widespread practical use of genomic information in everyday practice, there are many examples of how this information is beginning to transform the way we look at disease states in terms of diagnosis, prognosis and treatment. The gathered experience with molecular analysis of other non-cardiac diseases will be helpful in developing information to be applied to the management of HF including diagnosis, prognosis, and treatment response. We concur with others [188] that this information may not only be clinically useful but also helpful in advancing research and discovery of new drugs and translational medicine. Therefore, new genomic technologies and information should enhance our understanding of HF and cardiomyopathies, and in particular the cardiomyopathy of aging.

Although many pharmacodynamic studies have focused primarily on healthy older people, the pathophysiology of CVDs, including HF in the elderly is different than in younger individuals, and this may change the pharmacodynamic response and therapeutic outcome. In spite of the fact that most of the clinical trials on HF have recruited younger men (younger than 65 years old) with systolic dysfunction secondary to ischemic heart disease, in clinical practice, HF is often a syndrome of older women with diastolic dysfunction, perhaps secondary to systemic hypertension. This difference in the pathophysiology of the disease in aging may explain why the survival benefits seen with angiotensin-converting enzyme inhibitors and β-blockers in younger adult are reduced in older people, particularly older women [189, 190]. Finally, the primary goal of the pharmacogenomics of HF, should be to increasingly effectuate a personalized medicine defining the most effective treatment plan (e.g., drug regimens and dosage) to treat disease in patients of specific genetic backgrounds, and ages. Lately, great progress is being made in that direction.

Summary

- During aging, a significant loss of cardiac myocytes occurs, probably related to programmed cell death (apoptosis). The cumulative effect of this loss may result in significant physiological decline.
- Loss in cardiomyocytes may be secondary to mitochondrial dysfunction, likely caused by chronic exposure to oxidative free radicals, damage to mtDNA (mutations and deletions) and mitochondrial membranes.
- Besides cells loss, other mechanisms involved in cardiac aging are: ROS and oxidative stress, inflammatory mechanisms/signaling, adrenergic, muscarinics, and other cardiac G-protein-coupled receptors, SERCA, thyroid hormone, growth hormone and IGF-1, telomeres and telomere-related proteins, autophagy and cardiac aging, gender, genetic make-up, susceptibiliy genes, and epigenetic/environmental factors.
- Numerous genes mutations have been identified as a common etiological factor in the more prevalent varieties of cardiomyopathy, HCM and DCM, and also in the more rarely found phenotypes such as RCM.
- Numerous genetic defects have also been implicated in the pathogenesis of metabolic cardiomyopathies (often associated with extra-cardiac presentations) including mitochondrial cardiomyopathies and the cardiomyopathy associated with diabetes.
- Defects in genes encoding sarcomeric and cytoskeletal proteins have been linked to the progression of HCM, a number of which display age-mediated expression.

- Defects in non-sarcomeric/non-cytoskeletal genes have also been associated with familial and sporadic HCM includes defects in metabolic regulatory genes (PRAKG2), signaling proteins (caveolin) and nuclear membrane proteins (Lamin A/C).
- Defects in genes encompassing a wide range of functions have been identified in association with dilated cardiomyopathy (DCM); a number of the associated defects show increased expression in the elderly.
- Research in transgenic animals (primarily mice) models as well as rat and hamster have resulted in informative models of cardiomyopathy and HF which recapitulate clinical phenotypes. Both loss-of-function and gain-of-function models have been used to examine the role of defective metabolic, intracellular signaling and cardiomyocyte contractile and structural components and pathways that can lead to cardiac dysfunction, several with specific aging-related phenotypic expression.
- In addition to providing information concerning pathogenesis, these animal models have often proved useful for testing new treatments of HF.
- Although, most of the clinical trials of HF have recruited younger men (younger than 65 years) with systolic dysfunction secondary to ischemic heart disease, in clinical practice HF is often a syndrome of older women with diastolic dysfunction, perhaps secondary to systemic hypertension.
- The increased use of gene profiling in hearts from subjects with age-associated diseases such as cardiomyopathy and HF has begun to define a molecular signature of cardiac dysfunction whose component elements can be informatively compared between diseases, various populations and of course, age.
- Better understanding of the causes of aging-related diseases including HF, is essential before we can even think if the abolition of human senescence is possible.

References

1. Lakatta EG (1993) Cardiovascular regulatory mechanisms in advanced age. Physiol Rev 73:413–467
2. Lakatta EG, Gerstenblith G, Angell CS, Shock NW, Weisfeldt ML (1975) Diminished inotropic response of aged myocardium to catecholamines. Circ Res 36:262–269
3. Lakatta EG, Gerstenblith G, Angell CS, Shock NW, Weisfeldt ML (1975) Prolonged contraction duration in aged myocardium. J Clin Invest 55:61–68
4. Schulman SP, Lakatta EG, Fleg JL, Lakatta L, Becker LC, Gerstenblith G (1992) Age-related decline in left ventricular filling at rest and exercise. Am J Physiol 263:H1932–H1938
5. Merillon JP, Motte G, Masquet C, Azancot I, Aumont MC, Guiomard A, Gourgon R (1982) Changes in the physical properties of the arterial system and left ventricular performance with age and in permanent arterial hypertension: their interrelation. Arch Mal Coeur Vaiss 75:127–132
6. Roman MJ, Ganau A, Saba PS, Pini R, Pickering TG, Devereux RB (2000) Impact of arterial stiffening on left ventricular structure. Hypertension 36:489–494
7. Taddei S, Virdis A, Mattei P, Ghiadoni L, Fasolo CB, Sudano I, Salvetti A (1997) Hypertension causes premature aging of endothelial function in humans. Hypertension 29:736–743
8. Taddei S, Virdis A, Mattei P, Ghiadoni L, Gennari A, Fasolo CB, Sudano I, Salvetti A (1995) Aging and endothelial function in normotensive subjects and patients with essential hypertension. Circulation 91:1981–1987
9. Lakatta EG (2000) Cardiovascular aging in health. Clin Geriatr Med 16:419–444
10. Kass DA, Shapiro EP, Kawaguchi M, Capriotti AR, Scuteri A, deGroof RC, Lakatta EC (2001) Improved arterial compliance by a novel advanced glycation end-product crosslink breaker. Circulation 104:1464–1470
11. Phaneuf S, Leeuwenburgh C (2002) Cytochrome c release from mitochondria in the aging heart: a possible mechanism for apoptosis with age. Am J Physiol Integr Comp Physiol 282:R423–R430
12. Pollack M, Phaneuf S, Dirks A, Leeuwenburgh C (2002) The role of apoptosis in the normal aging brain, skeletal muscle, and heart. Ann N Y Acad Sci 959:93–107
13. Fannin SW, Lesnefsky EJ, Slabe TJ, Hassan MO, Hoppel CL (1999) Aging selectively decreases oxidative capacity in rat heart interfibrillar mitochondria. Arch Biochem Biophys 372:399–407
14. Hoppel CL, Moghaddas S, Lesnefsky EJ (2002) Interfibrillar cardiac mitochondrial comples III defects in the aging rat heart. Biogerontology 3:41–44
15. Suh JH, Heath SH, Hagen TM (2003) Two subpopulations of mitochondria in the aging rat heart display heterogenous levels of oxidative stress. Free Radic Biol Med 35:1064–1072
16. Judge S, Jang YM, Smith A, Hagen T, Leeuwenburgh C (2005) Age-associated increases in oxidative stress and antioxidant enzyme activities in cardiac interfibrillar mitochondria: implications for the mitochondrial theory of aging. FASEB J 19:419–421
17. Becker LB (2004) New concepts in reactive oxygen species and cardiovascular reperfusion physiology. Cardiovasc Res 61:461–470
18. Becker LB, vanden Hoek TL, Shao ZH, Li CQ, Schumacker PT (1999) Generation of superoxide in cardiomyocytes during ischemia before reperfusion. Am J Physiol 277:H2240–H2246
19. Marin-Garcia J, Goldenthal MJ, Moe GW (2001) Abnormal cardiac and skeletal muscle mitochondrial function in pacing-induced cardiac failure. Cardiovasc Res 52:103–110
20. Marin-Garcia J, Goldenthal MJ, Ananthakrishnan R, Mirvis D (1996) Specific mitochondrial DNA deletions in canine myocardial ischemia. Biochem Mol Biol Int 40:1057–1065
21. Suematsu N, Tsutsui H, Wen J, Kang D, Ikeuchi M, Ide T, Hayashidani S, Shiomi T, Kubota T, Hamasaki N, Takeshita A (2003) Oxidative stress mediates tumor necrosis factor-alpha-induced mitochondrial DNA damage and dysfunction in cardiac myocytes. Circulation 107:1418–1423
22. Ide T, Tsutsui H, Hayashidani S, Kang D, Suematsu N, Nakamura K, Utsumi H, Hamasaki N, Takeshita A (2001) Mitochondrial DNA damage and dysfunction associated with oxidative stress in failing hearts after myocardial infarction. Circ Res 88:529–535
23. Sorescu D, Griendling K (2002) Reactive oxygen species, mitochondria, and NAD(P)H oxidases in the development and progression of heart failure. Congest Heart Fail 8:132–140
24. Griendling KK, Sorescu D, Ushio-Fukai M (2000) NAD(P)H oxidase: role in cardiovascular biology and disease. Circ Res 86:494–501
25. Sabri A, Hughie HH, Lucchesi PA (2003) Regulation of hypertrophic and apoptotic signaling pathways by reactive oxygen species in cardiac myocytes. Antioxid Redox Signal 5:731–740
26. Li JM, Gall NP, Grieve DJ, Chen M, Shah AM (2002) Activation of NADPH oxidase during progression of cardiac hypertrophy to failure. Hypertension 40:477–484

27. Xiao L, Pimentel DR, Wang J, Singh K, Colucci WS, Sawyer DB (2002) Role of reactive oxygen species and NAD(P)H oxidase in alpha(1)-adrenoceptor signaling in adult rat cardiac myocytes. Am J Physiol Cell Physiol 282:C926–C934

28. Heymes C, Bendall JK, Ratajczak P, Cave AC, Samuel JL, Hasenfuss G, Shah AM (2003) Increased myocardial NADPH oxidase activity in human heart failure. J Am Coll Cardiol 41:2164–2171

29. Nakagami H, Liao JK (2004) Statins and myocardial hypertrophy. Coron Artery Dis 15:247–250

30. Maack C, Kartes T, Kilter H, Schafers HJ, Nickenig G, Bohm M, Laufs U (2003) Oxygen free radical release in human failing myocardium is associated with increased activity of rac1-GTPase and represents a target for statin treatment. Circulation 108:1567–1574

31. Fang CX, Doser TA, Yang X, Sreejayan N, Ren J (2006) Metallothionein antagonizes aging induced cardiac contractile dysfunction: role of PTP1B, insulin receptor tyrosine phosphorylation and Akt. Aging Cell 5:177–185

32. Ren J, Li Q, Wu S, Li SY, Babcock SA (2007) Cardiac overexpression of antioxidant catalase attenuates aging-induced cardiomyocyte relaxation dysfunction. Mech Ageing Dev 128:276–285

33. Li D, Qu Y, Tao L, Liu H, Hu A, Gao F, Sharifi-Azad S, Grunwald Z, Ma XL, Sun JZ (2005) Inhibition of iNOS protects the aging heart against beta-adrenergic receptor stimulation-induced cardiac dysfunction and myocardial ischemic injury. J Surg Res 131:64–72

34. Ross R (1999) Atherosclerosis: an inflammatory disease. N Engl J Med 340:115–126

35. Lusis AJ (2000) Atherosclerosis. Nature 407:233–241

36. Libby P (2002) Inflammation in atherosclerosis. Nature 420:868–874

37. Kritchevsky SB, Cesari M, Pahor M (2005) Inflammatory markers and cardiovascular health in older adults. Cardiovasc Res 66: 265–275

38. Deten A, Marx G, Briest W, Volz HC, Zimmer H-G (2005) Heart function and molecular biological parameters are comparable in young adult and aged rats after chronic myocardial infarction. Cardiovasc Res 66:364–373

39. Antonicelli R, Olivieri F, Bonafe M, Cavallone L, Spazzafumo L, Marchegiani F, Cardelli M, Recanatini A, Testarmata P, Boemi M, Parati G, Franceschi C (2005) The interleukin-6 -174 G>C promoter polymorphism is associated with a higher risk of death after an acute coronary syndrome in male elderly patients. Int J Cardiol 103:266–271

40. Di Iorio A, Ferrucci L, Sparvieri E, Cherubini A, Volpato S, Corsi A, Bonafe M, Franceschi C, Abate G, Paganelli R (2003) Serum IL-1beta levels in health and disease: a population-based study. 'The InCHIANTI study'. Cytokine 22:198–205

41. Montagne O, Le Corvoisier P, Guenoun T, Laplace M, Crozatier B (2005) Impaired alpha1-adrenergic responses in aged rat hearts. Fundam Clin Pharmacol 19:331–339

42. Korzick DH, Holiman DA, Boluyt MO, Laughlin MH, Lakatta EG (2001) Diminished alpha1-adrenergic-mediated contraction and translocation of PKC in senescent rat heart. Am J Physiol Heart Circ Physiol 281:H581–H589

43. Korzick DH, Hunter JC, McDowell MK, Delp MD, Tickerhoof MM, Carson LD (2004) Chronic exercise improves myocardial inotropic reserve capacity through alpha1-adrenergic and protein kinase C-dependent effects in senescent rats. J Gerontol A Biol Sci Med Sci 59:1089–1098

44. Wang Y, Ashraf M (1998) Activation of alpha1-adrenergic receptor during Ca2+ pre-conditioning elicits strong protection against Ca2+ overload injury via protein kinase C signaling pathway. J Mol Cell Cardiol 30:2423–2435

45. Esler M, Kaye D (2000) Sympathetic nervous system activation in essential hypertension, cardiac failure and psychosomatic heart disease. J Cardiovasc Pharmacol 35:S1–S7

46. Kaye D, Esler M (2005) Sympathetic neuronal regulation of the heart in aging and heart failure. Cardiovasc Res 66:256–264

47. Daaka Y, Luttrell LM, Lefkowitz RJ (1997) Switching of the coupling of the beta2-adrenergic receptor to different G proteins by protein kinase A. Nature 390:88–91

48. Kilts JD, Akazawa T, Richardson MD, Kwatra MM (2002) Age increases cardiac Galpha (i2) expression, resulting in enhanced coupling to G protein-coupled receptors. J Biol Chem 277:31257–31262

49. Kilts JD, Akazawa T, El-Moalem HE, Mathew JP, Newman MF, Kwatra MM (2003) Age Increases Expression and receptor-mediated activation of Galpha i in human atria. J Cardiovasc Pharmacol 42:662–670

50. Brodde O-E, Michel MC (1999) Adrenergic and muscarinic receptors in the human heart. Pharmacol Rev 51:651–689

51. Richardson MD, Kilts JD, Kwatra MM (2004) Increased expression of Gi-coupled muscarinic acetylcholine receptor and Gi in atrium of elderly diabetic subjects. Diabetes 53:2392–2396

52. Brodde O-E, Konschack U, Becker K, Rüter F, Poller U, Jakubetz J, Radke J, Zerkowski H-R (1998) Cardiac muscarinic receptors decrease with age: in vitro and in vivo studies. J Clin Invest 101: 471–478

53. Leineweber K, Klapproth S, Beilfuss A, Silber RE, Heusch G, Philipp T, Brodde OE (2003) Unchanged G-protein-coupled receptor kinase activity in the aging human heart. J Am Coll Cardiol 42:1487–1492

54. Goldstein DS (1988) Plasma catecholamines and essential hypertension: an analytical review. Hypertension 5:86–99

55. Folkow B, DiBona GF, Hjemdahl P, Toren PH, Wallin BG (1983) Measurements of plasma norepinephrine concentrations in human primary hypertension. Hypertension 5:399–403

56. Esler MD, Turner AG, Kaye DM et al (1995) Aging effects on human sympathetic neuronal function. Am J Physiol 268:R278–R285

57. Francis GS, Goldsmith SR, Cohn JN (1982) Relationship of exercise capacity to resting left ventricular performance and basal plasma norepinephrine levels in patients with congestive heart failure. Am Heart J 104:725–731

58. Leineweber K, Rohe P, Beilfuss A, Wolf C, Sporkmann H, Bruck H, Jakob HG, Heusch G, Philipp T, Brodde OE (2005) G-protein-coupled receptor kinase activity in human heart failure: effects of beta-adrenoceptor blockade. Cardiovasc Res 66:512–590

59. Su N, Duan J, Moffat MP, Narayanan N (1995) Age-related changes in electrophys-iological responses to muscarinic receptor stimulation in rat myocardium. Can J Physiol Pharmacol 73:1430–1436

60. Narayanan N, Derby JA (1983) Effects of age on muscarinic cholinergic receptors in rat myocardium. Can J Physiol Pharmacol 61:822–829

61. Hardouin S, Mansier P, Bertin B, Dakhly T, Swynghedauw B, Moalic JM (1997) β-Adrenergic and muscarinic receptor expression are regulated in opposite ways during senescence in rat left ventricle. J Mol Cell Cardiol 29:309–319

62. Elfellah MS, Johns A, Shepherd AMM (1986) Effect of age on responsiveness of isolated rat atria to carbachol and on binding characteristics of atrial muscarinic receptors. J Cardiovasc Pharmacol 8:873–877

63. Lo S-H, Liu I-M, Huang LW, Cheng J-T (2001) Decrease of muscarinic M2 cholinoceptor gene expression in the heart of aged rat. Neurosci Lett 300:185–187

64. Periasamy M, Huke S (2001) SERCA pump level is a critical determinant of Ca2+homeostasis and cardiac contractility. J Mol Cell Cardiol 33:1053–1063

65. Brandl CJ, Green NM, Korczak B, MacLennan DH (1986) Two Ca2+ ATPase genes: homologies and mechanistic implications of deduced amino acid sequences. Cell 44:597–607

66. Anger M, Samuel JL, Marotte F, Wuytack F, Rappaport L, Lompré AM (1993) The sarco(endo)plasmic reticulum Ca(2+)-ATPase mRNA isoform, SERCA 3, is expressed in endothelial and epithelial cells in various organs. FEBS Lett 334:45–48

67. Maciel LM, Polikar R, Rohrer D, Popovich BK (1990) Dillmann WH Age-induced decreases in the messenger RNA coding for the

sarcoplasmic reticulum (Ca2+)-ATPase of the rat heart. Circ Res 67:230–234

68. Long X, Boluyt MO, O'Neill L, Zheng JS, Wu G, Nitta YK, Crow MT, Lakatta EG (1999) Myocardial retinoid X receptor, thyroid hormone receptor, and myosin heavy chain gene expression in the rat during adult aging. J Gerontol A Biol Sci Med Sci 54:B23–B27

69. Iemitsu M, Miyauchi T, Maeda S, Tanabe T, Takanashi M, Matsuda M, Yamaguchi I (2004) Exercise training improves cardiac function-related gene levels through thyroid hormone receptor signaling in aged rats. Am J Physiol Heart Circ Physiol 286:H1696–H1705

70. Tang F (1985) Effect of sex and age on serum aldosterone and thyroid hormones in the laboratory rat. Horm Metab Res 17:507–509

71. Buttrick P, Malhotra A, Factor S, Greenen D, Leinwand L, Scheuer J (1991) Effect of aging and hypertension on myosin biochemistry and gene expression in the rat heart. Circ Res 68:645–652

72. Schmidt U, del Monte F, Miyamoto MI, Matsui T, Gwathmey JK, Rosenzweig A, Hajjar RJ (2000) Restoration of diastolic function in senescent rat hearts through adenoviral gene transfer of sarcoplasmic reticulum Ca(2+)-ATPase. Circulation 101: 790–796

73. Cain BS, Meldrum DR, Joo KS, Wang JF, Meng X, Cleveland JC Jr, Banerjee A, Harken AH (1998) Human SERCA2a levels correlate inversely with age in senescent human myocardium. J Am Coll Cardiol 32:458–467

74. Knyushko TV, Sharov VS, Williams TD, Schoneich C, Bigelow DJ (2005) 3-Nitro-tyrosine modification of SERCA2a in the aging heart: a distinct signature of the cellular redox environment. Biochemistry 44:13071–13081

75. Goodman-Gruen D, Barrett-Connor E (1997) Epidemiology of insulin-like growth factor-I in elderly men and women. The Rancho Bernardo Study. Am J Epidemiol 145:970–976

76. Lieberman SA, Mitchell AM, Marcus R, Hintz RL, Hoffman AR (1994) The insulin-like growth factor I generation test: resistance to growth hormone with aging and estrogen replacement therapy. Horm Metab Res 26:229–233

77. Khan AS, Sane DC, Wannenburg T, Sonntag WE (2002) Growth hormone, insulin-like growth factor-1 and the aging cardiovascular system. Cardiovasc Res 54:25–35

78. Vasan RS, Sullivan LM, D'Agostino RB, Roubenoff R, Harris T, Sawyer DB, Levy D, Wilson PW (2003) Serum insulin-like growth factor I and risk for heart failure in elderly individuals without a previous myocardial infarction: the Framingham Heart Study. Ann Intern Med 139:642–648

79. Roubenoff R, Parise H, Payette HA, Abad LW, D'Agostino R, Jacques PF, Wilson PW, Dinarello CA, Harris TB (2003) Cytokines, insulin-like growth factor 1, sarcopenia, and mortality in very old community-dwelling men and women: the Framingham Heart Study. Am J Med 115:429–435

80. Ghigo E, Arvat E, Gianotti L, Ramunni J, DiVito L, Maccagno B, Grottoli S, Camanni F (1996) Human aging and the GH-IGF-I axis. J Pediatr Endocrinol Metab 9:271–278

81. Takahashi S, Meites J (1987) GH binding to liver in young and old female rats: relation to somatomedin-C secretion. Proc Soc Exp Biol Med 186:229–233

82. Xu X, Bennett SA, Ingram RL, Sonntag WE (1995) Decreases in growth hormone receptor signal transduction contribute to the decline in insulin-like growth factor I gene expression with age. Endocrinology 136:4551–4557

83. Colao A, Marzullo P, Di Somma C, Lombardi G (2001) Growth hormone and the heart. Clin Endocrinol 54:137–154

84. Osterziel KJ, Strohm O, Schuler J, Friedrich M, Hänlein D, Willenbrock R, Anker SD, Poole-Wilson PA, Ranke MB, Dietz R (1998) Randomised, double-blind, placebo-controlled trial of human recombinant growth hormone in patients with chronic heart failure due to dilated cardiomyopathy. Lancet 351:1233–1237

85. Wang PH (2001) Roads to survival: insulin-like growth factor-1 signaling pathways in cardiac muscle. Circ Res 88:552–554

86. Tritos NA, Danias PG (2008) Growth hormone therapy in congestive heart failure due to left ventricular systolic dysfunction: a meta-analysis. Endocr Pract 14:40–49

87. Laron Z (2005) Do deficiencies in growth hormone and insulin-like growth factor-1 (IGF-1) shorten or prolong longevity? Mech Ageing Dev 126:305–307

88. Chan JM, Stampfer MJ, Giovannucci E, Gann PH, Ma J, Wilkinson P, Hennekens CH, Pollak M (1998) Plasma insulin-like growth factor-I and prostate cancer risk: a prospective study. Science 279:563–566

89. Hankinson SE, Willett WC, Colditz GA, Hunter DJ, Michaud DS, Deroo B, Rosner B, Speizer FE, Pollak M (1998) Circulating concentrations of insulin-like growth factor-I and risk of breast cancer. Lancet 351:1393–1396

90. Clark RG (2004) Recombinant human insulin-like growth factor I (IGF-I): risks and benefits of normalizing blood IGF-I concentrations. Horm Res 62:93–100

91. Kurosu H, Yamamoto M, Clark JD, Pastor JV, Nandi A, Gurnani P, McGuinness OP, Chikuda H, Yamaguchi M, Kawaguchi H, Shimomura I, Takayama Y, Herz J, Kahn CR, Rosenblatt KP, Kuro-o M (2005) Suppression of aging in mice by the hormone Klotho. Science 309:1829–1833

92. Kirkwood TB (2005) Understanding the odd science of aging. Cell 120:437–447

93. Cook SA, Sugden PH, Clerk A (1999) Regulation of Bcl-2 family proteins during development and in response to oxidative stress in cardiac myocytes: association with changes in mitochondrial membrane potential. Circ Res 85:940–949

94. Long X, Goldenthal MJ, Wu GM, Marín-García J (2004) Mitochondrial Ca2+ flux and respiratory enzyme activity decline are early events in cardiomyocyte response to H2O2. J Mol Cell Cardiol 37:63–70

95. Torella D, Rota M, Nurzynska D, Musso E, Monsen A, Shiraishi I, Zias E, Walsh K, Rosenzweig A, Sussman MA, Urbanek K, Nadal-Ginard B, Kajstura J, Anversa P, Leri A (2004) Cardiac stem cell and myocyte aging, heart failure, and insulin-like growth factor-1 overexpression. Circ Res 94:514–524

96. Uhrbom L, Nister M, Westermark B (1997) Induction of senescence in human malignant glioma cells by p16INK4A. Oncogene 15:505–514

97. Edo MD, Andrés V (2005) Aging, telomeres, and atherosclerosis. Cardiovasc Res 66:213–221

98. van der Harst P, van der Steege G, de Boer RA, Voors AA, Hall AS, Mulder MJ, van Gilst WH, van Veldhuisen DJ; MERIT-HF Study Group (2007) Telomere length of circulating leukocytes is decreased in patients with chronic heart failure. J Am Coll Cardiol 49:1459–1464

99. Kurz DJ, Decary S, Hong Y, Trivier E, Akhmedov A, Erusalimsky JD (2004) Chronic oxidative stress compromises telomere integrity and accelerates the onset of senescence in human endothelial cells. J Cell Sci 117:2417–2426

100. Haendeler J, Hoffmann J, Diehl JF, Vasa M, Spyridopoulos I, Zeiher AM, Dimmeler S (2004) Antioxidants inhibit nuclear export of telomerase reverse transcriptase and delay replicative senescence of endothelial cells. Circ Res 94:768–775

101. Spyridopoulos I, Haendeler J, Urbich C, Brummendorf TH, Oh H, Schneider MD, Zeiher AM, Dimmeler S (2004) Statins enhance migratory capacity by upregulation of the telomere repeat-binding factor TRF2 in endothelial progenitor cells. Circulation 110:3136–3142

102. Imanishi T, Hano T, Nishio I (2005) Estrogen reduces endothelial progenitor cell senescence through augmentation of telomerase activity. J Hypertens 23:1699–1706

103. Imanishi T, Hano T, Sawamura T, Nishio I (2004) Oxidized low-density lipoprotein induces endothelial progenitor cell senescence, leading to cellular dysfunction. Clin Exp Pharmacol Physiol 31:407–413

104. Simoncini T, Hafezi-Moghadam A, Brazil DP, Ley K, Chin WW, Liao JK (2000) Interaction of oestrogen receptor with the regulatory subunit of phosphatidylinositol-3-OH kinase. Nature 407:538–541

105. Vasa M, Breitschopf K, Zeiher AM, Dimmeler S (2000) Nitric oxide activates telomerase and delays endothelial cell senescence. Circ Res 87:540–542

106. Serrano AL, Andres V (2004) Telomeres and cardiovascular disease: does size matter? Circ Res 94:575–584

107. Fuster JJ, Andrés V (2006) Telomere biology and cardiovascular disease. Circ Res 99:1167–1168

108. d'Adda di Fagagna F, Reaper PM, Clay-Farrace L, Fiegler H, Carr P, Von Zglinicki T, Saretzki G, Carter NP, Jackson SP (2003) A DNA damage checkpoint response in telomere-initiated senescence. Nature 426:194–198

109. Okuda K, Khan MY, Skurnick J, Kimura M, Aviv H, Aviv A (2000) Telomere attrition of the human abdominal aorta: relationships with age and atherosclerosis. Atherosclerosis 152:391–398

110. Poch E, Carbonell P, Franco S, Díez-Juan A, Blasco MA, Andrés V (2004) Short telomeres protect from diet-induced atherosclerosis in apolipoprotein E-null mice. FASEB J 18:418–420

111. von Zglinicki T, Pilger R, Sitte N (2000) Accumulation of single-strand breaks is the major cause of telomere shortening in human fibroblasts. Free Radic Biol Med 28:64–74

112. Saretzki G, Murphy MP, von Zglinicki T (2003) MitoQ counteracts telomere shortening and elongates lifespan of fibroblasts under mild oxidative stress. Aging Cell 2:141–143

113. Passos JF, von Zglinicki T (2005) Mitochondria, telomeres and cell senescence. Exp Gerontol 40:466–472

114. Goswami SK, Das DK (2006) Autophagy in the myocardium: dying for survival? Exp Clin Cardol 11:183–188

115. Brunt UT, Terman A (2002) The mitochondrial-lysosomal axis theory of aging: accumulation of damaged mitochondria as a result of imperfect autophago-cytosis. Eur J Biochem 269:1996–2002

116. Rooyackers OE, Adey DB, Ades PA, Nair KS (1996) Effect of age on in vivo rates of mitochondrial protein synthesis in human skeletal muscle. Proc Natl Acad Sci USA 93:15364–15369

117. Terman A, Brunk UT (2004) Myocyte aging and mitochondrial turnover. Exp Gerontol 39:701–705

118. Stroikin Y, Dalen H, Brunk UT, Terman A (2005) Testing the "garbage" accumulation theory of ageing: mitotic activity protects cells from death induced by inhibition of autophagy. Biogerontology 6:39–47

119. Olivetti G, Melissari M, Capasso JM, Anversa P (1991) Cardiomyopathy of the aging human heart. Myocyte loss and reactive cellular hypertrophy. Circ Res 68:1560–1568

120. Anversa P, Rota M, Urbanek K, Hosoda T, Sonnenblick EH, Leri A, Kajstura J, Bolli R (2005) Myocardial aging – a stem cell problem. Basic Res Cardiol 100:482–493

121. Nadal-Ginard B, Kajstura J, Leri A, Anversa P (2003) Myocyte death, growth, and regeneration in cardiac hypertrophy and failure. Circ Res 92:139–150

122. Ellison GM, Torella D, Karakikes I, Nadal-Ginard B (2007) Myocyte death and renewal: modern concepts of cardiac cellular homeostasis. Nat Clin Pract Cardiovasc Med 4:S52–S59

123. Kajstura J, Pertoldi B, Leri A, Beltrami CA, Deptala A, Darzynkiewicz Z, Anversa P (2000) Telomere shortening is an in vivo marker of myocyte replication and aging. Am J Pathol 156:813–819

124. Chimenti C, Kajstura J, Torella D, Urbanek K, Heleniak H, Colussi C, Di Meglio F, Nadal-Ginard B, Frustaci A, Leri A, Maseri A, Anversa P (2003) Senescence and death of primitive cells and myocytes lead to premature cardiac aging and heart failure. Circ Res 93:604–613

125. Gonzalez A, Rota M, Nurzynska D, Misao Y et al (2008) Activation of cardiac progenitor cells reverses the failing heart senescent phenotype and prolongs lifespan. Circ Res 102:597–606

126. Menini S, Amadio L, Oddi G, Ricci C et al (2006) Deletion of p66Shc longevity gene protects against experimental diabetic glomerulopathy by preventing diabetes-induced oxidative stress. Diabetes 55:1642–1650

127. Rota M, LeCapitaine N, Hosoda T et al (2006) Diabetes promotes cardiac stem cell aging and heart failure, which are prevented by deletion of the p66shc gene. Circ Res 99:42–52

128. Dimmeler S, Leri A (2008) Aging and disease as modifiers of efficacy of cell therapy. Circ Res 102:1319–1330

129. Jugdutt BI (2003) Remodeling of the myocardium and potential targets in the collagen degradation and synthesis pathways. Curr Drug Targets Cardiovasc Haematol Disord 3:1–30

130. Allessie M, Schotten U, Verheule S, Harks E (2005) Gene therapy for repair of cardiac fibrosis: a long way to Tipperary. Circulation 111:391–393

131. de Souza RR (2002) Aging of myocardial collagen. Biogerontology 3:325–335

132. Shivakumar K, Dostal DE, Boheler K, Baker KM, Lakatta EG (2003) Differential response of cardiac fibroblasts from young adult and senescent rats to ANG II. Am J Physiol Heart Circ Physiol 284:H1454–H1459

133. Lindsey ML, Goshorn DK, Squires CE, Escobar GP, Hendrick JW, Mingoia JT, Sweterlitsch SE, Spinale FG (2005) Age-dependent changes in myocardial matrix metalloproteinase/tissue inhibitor of metalloproteinase profiles and fibroblast function. Cardiovasc Res 66:410–419

134. Li YY, McTiernan CF, Feldman AM (2000) Interplay of matrix metalloproteinases, tissue inhibitors of metalloproteinases and their regulators in cardiac matrix remodeling. Cardiovasc Res 46:214–224

135. Chen X, Li Z, Feng Z, Wang J, Ouyang C, Liu W, Fu B, Cai G, Wu C, Wei R, Wu D, Hong Q (2006) Integrin-linked kinase induces both senescence-associated alterations and extracellular fibronectin assembly in aging cardiac fibroblasts. J Gerontol A Biol Sci Med Sci 61:1232–1245

136. Brown RD, Ambler SK, Mitchell MD, Long CS (2005) The cardiac fibroblast: therapeutic target in myocardial remodeling and failure. Annu Rev Pharmacol Toxicol 45:657–687

137. Borbély A, van der Velden J, Papp Z, Bronzwaer JG, Edes I, Stienen GJ, Paulus WJ (2005) Cardiomyocyte stiffness in diastolic heart failure. Circulation 111:774–781

138. van Heerebeek L, Borbély A, Niessen HW, Bronzwaer JG, van der Velden J, Stienen GJ, Linke WA, Laarman GJ, Paulus WJ (2006) Myocardial structure and function differ in systolic and diastolic heart failure. Circulation 113:1966–1973

139. Richard P, Villard E, Charron P, Isnard R (2006) The genetic bases of cardiomyopathies. J Am Coll Cardiol 48:A79–A89

140. Niimura H, Patton KK, McKenna WJ, Soults J, Maron BJ, Seidman JG, Seidman CE (2002) Sarcomere protein gene mutations in hypertrophic cardiomyopathy of the elderly. Circulation 105:446–451

141. Charron P, Dubourg O, Desnos M, Bennaceur M, Carrier L, Camproux AC, Isnard R, Hagege A, Langland JM, Bonne G, Richard P, Hainque B, Bouhour JB, Schwartz K, Komajda M (1998) Clinical features and prognostic implications of familial hypertrophic cardiomyopathy related to the cardiac myosin-binding protein C gene. Circulation 97:2230–2236

142. Anan R, Greve G, Thierfelder L, Watkins H et al (1994) Prognostic implications of novel beta cardiac myosin heavy chain gene mutations that cause familial hypertrophic cardiomyopathy. J Clin Invest 93:280–285

143. Maron BJ, Casey SA, Hauser RG, Aeppli DM (2003) Clinical course of hypertrophic cardiomyopathy with survival to advanced age. J Am Coll Cardiol 42:882–888

144. Chimenti C, Pieroni M, Morgante E, Antuzzi D, Russo A, Russo MA, Maseri A, Frustaci A (2004) Prevalence of Fabry disease in female patients with late-onset hypertrophic cardiomyopathy. Circulation 110:1047–1053

145. Sachdev B, Takenaka T, Teraguchi H, Tei C, Lee P, McKenna WJ, Elliott PM (2002) Prevalence of Anderson-Fabry disease in male patients with late onset hypertrophic cardiomyopathy. Circulation 105:1407–1411

146. Fatkin D, Graham RM (2002) Molecular mechanisms of inherited cardiomyopathies. Physiol Rev 82:945–980

147. Taylor MR, Carniel E, Mestroni L (2004) Familial hypertrophic cardiomyopathy: clinical features, molecular genetics and molecular genetic testing. Expert Rev Mol Diagn 4:99–113

148. Roberts R, Sidhu J (2003) Genetic basis for hypertrophic cardiomyopathy: implications for diagnosis and treatment. Am Heart Hosp J 1:128–134

149. Ruppert V, Meyer T, Pankuweit S, Möller E, Funck RC, Grimm W, Maisch B (2008) German Heart Failure Network. Gene expression profiling from endomyocardial biopsy tissue allows distinction between subentities of dilated cardiomyopathy. J Thorac Cardiovasc Surg 136:360–369

150. Heidecker B, Kasper EK, Wittstein IS, Champion HC, Breton E, Russell SD, Kittleson MM, Baughman KL, Hare JM (2008) Transcriptomic biomarkers for individual risk assessment in new-onset heart failure. Circulation 118:238–246

151. Kittleson MM, Minhas KM, Irizarry RA, Ye SQ, Edness G, Breton E, Conte JV, Tomaselli G, Garcia JG, Hare JM (2005) Gene expression analysis of ischemic and nonischemic cardiomyopathy: shared and distinct genes in the development of heart failure. Physiol Genomics 21:299–307

152. Kuner R, Barth AS, Ruschhaupt M, Buness A, Zwermann L, Kreuzer E, Steinbeck G, Poustka A, Sültmann H, Nabauer M (2008) Genomic analysis reveals poor separation of human cardiomyopathies of ischemic and nonischemic etiologies. Physiol Genomics 34:88–94

153. Burkett EL, Hershberger RE (2005) Clinical and genetic issues in familial dilated cardiomyopathy. J Am Coll Cardiol 45: 969–981

154. Mestroni L, Rocco C, Gregori D, Sinagra G, Di Lenarda A, Miocic S, Vatta M, Pinamonti B, Muntoni F, Caforio ALP, McKenna WJ, Falaschi A, Giacca M, Camerini F (1000) Familial dilated cardiomyopathy: evidence for genetic and phenotypic heterogeneity. J Am Coll Cardiol 34:181–190

155. DeWitt MM, MacLeod HM, Soliven B, McNally EM (2006) Phospholamban R14 deletion results in late-onset, mild, hereditary dilated cardiomyopathy. J Am Coll Cardiol 48:1396–1398

156. Haghighi K, Kolokathis F, Pater L, Lynch RA et al (2003) Human phospholamban null results in lethal dilated cardiomyopathy revealing a critical difference between mouse and human. J Clin Invest 111:869–876

157. Schmitt JP, Kamisago M, Asahi M, Li GH, Ahmad F, Mende U, Kranias EG, MacLennan DH, Seidman JG, Seidman CE (2003) Dilated cardiomyopathy and heart failure caused by a mutation in phospholamban. Science 299:1410–1413

158. Minoretti P, Arra M, Emanuele E, Olivieri V, Aldeghi A, Politi P, Martinelli V, Pesenti S, Falcone C (2007) A W148R mutation in the human FOXD4 gene segregating with dilated cardiomyopathy, obsessive-compulsive disorder, and suicidality. Int J Mol Med 19:369–372

159. Villard E, Duboscq-Bidot L, Charron P, Benaiche A, Conraads V, Sylvius N, Komajda M (2005) Mutation screening in dilated cardiomyopathy: prominent role of the beta myosin heavy chain gene. Eur Heart J 26:794–803

160. Konno T, Shimizu M, Ino H, Matsuyama T, Yamaguchi M, Terai H, Hayashi K, Mabuchi T, Kiyama M, Sakata K, Hayashi T, Inoue M, Kaneda T, Mabuchi H (2003) A novel missense mutation in the myosin binding protein-C gene is responsible for hypertrophic cardiomyopathy with left ventricular dysfunction and dilation in elderly patients. J Am Coll Cardiol 41:781–786

161. Karkkainen S, Miettinen R, Tuomainen P, Karkkainen P, Helio T, Reissell E, Kaartinen M, Toivonen L, Nieminen MS, Kuusisto J, Laakso M, Peuhkurinen K (2003) A novel mutation, Arg71Thr, in the delta-sarcoglycan gene is associated with dilated cardiomyopathy. J Mol Med 81:795–800

162. Bonne G, Mercuri E, Muchir A, Urtizberea A et al (2000) Clinical and molecular genetic spectrum of autosomal dominant Emery-Dreifuss muscular dystrophy due to mutations of the lamin A/C gene. Ann Neurol 48:170–180

163. Wehnert MS, Bonne G (2002) The nuclear muscular dystrophies. Semin Pediatr Neurol 9:100–107

164. Vandenhende MA, Bonnet F, Sailler L, Bouillot S, Morlat P, Beylot J (2005) [Dilated cardiomyopathy and lipid-lowering drug muscle toxicity revealing late-onset Becker's disease]. Rev Med Interne 26:977–979

165. Yazaki M, Yoshida K, Nakamura A, Koyama J, Nanba T, Ohori N, Ikeda S (1999) Clinical characteristics of aged Becker muscular dystrophy patients with onset after 30 years. Eur Neurol 42: 145–149

166. Arimura T, Hayashi T, Terada H, Lee SY, Zhou Q, Takahashi M, Ueda K, Nouchi T, Hohda S, Shibutani M, Hirose M, Chen J, Park JE, Yasunami M, Hayashi H, Kimura A (2004) A Cypher/ZASP mutation associated with dilated cardiomyopathy alters the binding affinity to protein kinase C. J Biol Chem 279:6746–6752

167. Haghighi K, Kolokathis F, Gramolini AO, Waggoner JR et al (2006) A mutation in the human phospholamban gene, deleting arginine 14, results in lethal, hereditary cardiomyopathy. Proc Natl Acad Sci USA 103:1388–1393

168. De Sandre-Giovannoli A, Bernard R, Cau P, Navarro C, Amiel J, Boccaccio I, Lyonnet S, Stewart CL, Munnich A, Le Merrer M, Levy N (2003) Lamin a truncation in Hutchinson-Gilford progeria. Science 300:2055

169. Chen L, Lee L, Kudlow BA, Dos Santos HG et al (2003) LMNA mutations in atypical Werner's syndrome. Lancet 362:440–445

170. Capell BC, Collins FS (2006) Human laminopathies: nuclei gone genetically awry. Nat Rev Genet 7:940–952

171. Brodsky GL, Muntoni F, Miocic S, Sinagra G, Sewry C, Mestroni L (2000) Lamin A/C gene mutation associated with dilated cardiomyopathy with variable skeletal muscle involvement. Circulation 101:473–476

172. Jakobs PM, Hanson EL, Crispell KA, Toy W, Keegan H, Schilling K, Icenogle TB, Litt M, Hershberger RE (2001) Novel lamin A/C mutations in two families with dilated cardiomyopathy and conduction system disease. J Card Fail 7:249–256

173. Fatkin D, MacRae C, Sasaki T, Wolff MR, Porcu M, Frenneaux M, Atherton J, Vidaillet HJ Jr, Spudich S, De Girolami U, Seidman JG, Seidman C, Muntoni F, Muehle G, Johnson W, McDonough B (1999) Missense mutations in the rod domain of the lamin A/C gene as causes of dilated cardiomyopathy and conduction-system disease. N Engl J Med 341:1715–1724

174. Tresch DD, McGough MF (1995) Heart failure with normal systolic function: a common disorder older people. J Am Geriatr Soc 43:1035–1042

175. Hassan W, Al-Sergani H, Mourad W, Tabbaa R (2005) Amyloid heart disease. New frontiers and insights in pathophysiology, diagnosis, and management. Tex Heart Inst J 32:178–184

176. Koike H, Misu K, Sugiura M, Iijima M, Mori K, Yamamoto M, Hattori N, Mukai E, Ando Y, Ikeda S, Sobue G (2004) Pathology of early- vs late-onset TTR Met30 familial amyloid polyneuropathy. Neurology 63:129–138

177. Blanco-Jerez CR, Jimenez-Escrig A, Gobernado JM, Lopez-Calvo S, de Blas G, Redondo C, Garcia Villanueva M, Orensanz L (1998) Transthyretin Tyr77 familial amyloid polyneuropathy: a clinicopathological study of a large kindred. Muscle Nerve 21:1478–1485

178. Hamidi Asl K, Nakamura M, Yamashita T, Benson MD (2001) Cardiac amyloidosis associated with the transthyretin Ile122 mutation in a Caucasian family. Amyloid 8:263–269

179. Yamashita T, Asl KH, Yazaki M, Benson MD (2005) A prospective evaluation of the transthyretin Ile122 allele frequency in an African-American population. Amyloid 12:127–130

180. Jiang X, Buxbaum JN, Kelly JW (2001) The V122I cardiomyopathy variant of transthyretin increases the velocity of rate-limiting tetramer dissociation, resulting in accelerated amyloidosis. Proc Natl Acad Sci USA 98:14943–14948

181. Burke W, Press N, McDonnell SM (1998) Hemochromatosis: genetics helps to define a multifactorial disease. Clin Genet 54:1–9

182. Hanson EH, Imperatore G, Burke W (2001) HFE gene and hereditary hemochromatosis: a HuGE review. Human Genome Epidemiology. Am J Epidemiol 154:193–206

183. Papanikolaou G, Samuels ME, Ludwig EH, MacDonald ML (2004) et al.Mutations in HFE2 cause iron overload in chromosome 1q-linked juvenile hemochromatosis. Nat Genet 36:77–82

184. Turoczi T, Jun L, Cordis G, Morris JE, Maulik N, Stevens RG, Das DK (2003) HFE mutation and dietary iron content interact to increase ischemia/reperfusion injury of the heart in mice. Circ Res 92:1240–1246

185. Lio D, Balistreri CR, Colonna-Romano G, Motta M, Franceschi C, Malaguarnera M, Candore G, Caruso C (2002) Association between the MHC class I gene HFE polymorphisms and longevity: a study in Sicilian population. Genes Immun 3:20–24

186. Coppin H, Bensaid M, Fruchon S, Borot N, Blanche H, Roth MP (2003) Longevity and carrying the C282Y mutation for haemochromatosis on the HFE gene: case control study of 492 French centenarians. BMJ 327:132–133

187. Lio D, Pes GM, Carru C, Listi F, Ferlazzo V, Candore G, Colonna-Romano G, Ferrucci L, Deiana L, Baggio G, Franceschi C, Caruso C (2003) Association between the HLA-DR alleles and longevity: a study in Sardinian population. Exp Gerontol 38: 313–317

188. McLean AJ (2004) DG.Aging biology and geriatric clinical pharmacology. Pharmacol Rev 56:163–184

189. Flather MD, Yusuf S, Kober L, Pfeffer M, Hall A, Murray G, Torp-Pedersen C, Ball S, Pogue J, Moye L, Braunwald E (2000) Long-term ACE-inhibitor therapy in patients with heart failure or left-ventricular dysfunction: a systematic overview of data from individual patients. ACE-Inhibitor Myocardial Infarction Collaborative Group. Lancet 355:1575–1581

190. Richardson LG, Rocks M (2001) Women and heart failure. Heart Lung 30:87–97

Chapter 17
Heart Failure of Aging: Clinical Considerations

Overview

Although the physiological decline occurring during aging is much more subtle than that observed in young people and adults with cardiac disease, heart failure (HF) is a disease of the elderly. This may be related to a significant loss of cardiac myocytes occurring through apoptosis; this loss may be secondary to mitochondrial dysfunction, probably caused by chronic exposure to ROS, which will result in damaged mtDNA (mutations and deletions) and mitochondrial membranes. In this chapter, we will discuss clinical aspects of HF in the elderly and define their etiology, pathophysiology, clinical presentation, diagnosis and common approaches to therapeutic interventions, including pharmacotherapy, and device and replacement therapies.

Introduction

HF is predominantly a disease of the elderly, with prevalence increasing from <1% in the population aged <50 to 10% in persons over the age of 80 [1], and 80% of hospitalizations for HF occurs in patients over 65 years [2]. In the aging heart, significant alterations in cardiac structure and function occur, and some of these changes may predispose an individual to the development of HF [2]. The functional reserve of the heart decreases with aging, and the loss of myocytes contributes to the attenuation of the response of the aging heart to sudden changes in ventricular loading [3]. Diastolic HF is more common in the elderly: at the age of 70 years, almost half of all patients with HF have diastolic HF. Indeed, HF with preserved systolic function accounts for less than 10% of all HF cases in persons under the age of 65 but more than 50% of cases over the age of 75 [4, 5]. Common underlying disorders in patients with diastolic HF are hypertension and obesity. A distinctive feature distinguishing HF that occurs in the elderly from the younger individuals is the much higher frequency of HF occurring in the absence of systolic dysfunction, i.e., diastolic HF or HF with preserved systolic function.

Pathophysiologic Considerations

The association of age and decreasing heart function has been amply documented. Aging is associated with significant alterations in cardiac structure and function, and some of these changes may predispose an individual to the development of HF [3]. The changes at a whole-organ level include reduced vascular compliance, which increases the impedance to left ventricular ejection and impairs ventricular diastolic performance [6]; about one third of the cardiomyocytes are lost from the human heart between the ages of 17 and 90 years [7]. Attenuated β-adrenergic responsiveness to inotropic stimulation and degenerative changes in the sinoatrial node limit the functional reserve and, in particular, its response to stress. The latter impairment is exacerbated by mitochondrial dysfunction with reduced capacity to generate high-energy phosphates [6, 8]. Nevertheless, mitochondrial enzymatic dysfunction is unlikely to result from an aging-induced decline in mitochondrial transcription, mtDNA depletion, or defective mitochondrial biogenesis. The search for the mechanism of mitochondrial enzyme dysfunction may focus on the posttranslational modification of the proteins, mainly in mtDNA-encoded enzyme-subunits. It is worth noting that examination of all of the components involved in each aging-affected respiratory enzyme using blue native polyacrylamide gel electrophoresis (BN-PAGE) analysis (in which catalytic activities can be maintained) may distinguish amongst the possible mechanisms of enzymatic dysfunction [9].

In addition, mitochondrial stress response with increased expression of heat shock protein 60 (HSP60) and glutathione peroxidase (GPx), probably related to elevated ROS production, occurs in the senescent heart and may be mediated by the increased transcription of NF-κB. The roles of both aging-dependent mtDNA damage and the increased sensitivity of the PT pore need to be further delineated, both as indicators of oxidative damage and as potential stimuli or signaling events of downstream cellular transcriptional and apoptotic events in myocardial aging. Importantly, the larger context of myocardial nuclear gene expression governing mitochondrial function needs to be considered and fully examined, given the relative scarcity of aging-regulation data presently available. A comprehensive analysis of mitochondrial events may be extremely useful in assessing both the individual pathway responses and the overall cardiac phenotype in the aging process in general and in HF in particular.

The cellular changes of aging are most pronounced in postmitotic organs (e.g., brain and heart), and abnormalities in the structure and function of cardiac myocytes may be the definitive factors in the overall cardiac aging process. As the heart ages, myocytes undergo hypertrophy that may be accompanied by intracellular changes, including mitochondrial-derived oxidative injury that will contribute to the overall cellular aging as well as to ischemia-induced tissue damage. Increasingly, the interaction of the cellular organelles, i.e., mitochondria, endoplasmic reticulum (ER), peroxisomes, and lysosomes, in cellular homeostasis is considered to be of significance, lysosomes and mitochondria being the organelles that suffer the most remarkable age-related alterations in postmitotic cells [10]. Linked mitochondrial and lysosomal defects contribute to irreversible myocyte functional impairment and cell death. Therefore, interactions among the different components of the cardiac cells must be regulated (e.g., mitochondria–nucleus for adequate expression of a number of genes, the ER–mitochondria for Ca^{2+} metabolism and peroxisomes–mitochondria for the interchange of antioxidant enzymes essential in the production and decomposition of H_2O_2), since defects in communication between these organelles will accelerate the aging process.

Clinical Considerations

Etiologies and Precipitating Factors

Systemic hypertension and coronary heart disease (CHD) account for 70–80% of HF cases at older age in the USA [11]. Hypertension is the most common etiology in older women, particularly in those subjects with preserved systolic function. In older men, HF can often be attributable to CHD. Other causes include valvular heart disease and cardiomyopathy. The most common etiologies are summarized in Table 17.1. Furthermore, worsening of HF may be precipitated by factors such as dysrhythmias, renal failure, anemia (see Chap. 12), infection, drugs side-effect, and by lack of compliance with medication and/or diet. Most importantly, HF in the elderly is frequently multifactorial in etiologies, and this fact needs to be recognized in the management of these patients. In addition to determining the etiologies, it is important to identify factors that commonly precipitate or contribute to HF exacerbation (Table 17.2). As discussed below, noncompliance with medications and diet is the most

Table 17.1 Etiologies of heart failure in the aged population

1. Hypertensive heart disease
2. Coronary heart disease: (a) acute myocardial infarction, (b) chronic ischemic cardiomyopathy
3. Age-related diastolic dysfunction
4. Valvular heart disease: (a) aortic stenosis or insufficiency, (b) mitral valve regurgitation, (c) prosthetic valve malfunction
5. Cardiomyopathy: (a) HCM, (b) DCM/ischemic, (c) nonischemic (dilated), (d) restrictive

Table 17.2 Precipitants of heart failure exacerbations in the aged population

1. Myocardial ischemia or infarction
2. Uncontrolled hypertension
3. Dietary sodium excess
4. Noncompliance with medications/inappropriate reductions of HF drugs
5. Dysrhythmias: atrial fibrillation, ventricular tachy/bradydysrhythmias
6. Pulmonary embolism
7. Intercurrent illness: fever, pneumonia/respiratory process, anemia, worsening renal function
8. Drugs and toxins: alcohol, antidysrhythmic agents/digitalis intoxication, calcium channel blockers, nonsteroidal antiinflammatory agents

common cause of HF exacerbation [12]. Other contributory factors include myocardial ischemia, volume overload owing to excess fluid intake, dysrhythmias (especially atrial fibrillation), intercurrent infections, anemia, and various toxins including alcohol.

Clinical Presentation and Diagnostic Challenges

An accurate diagnosis of the HF syndrome at older age is complicated by the atypical symptoms and signs frequently displayed by older subjects. Exertional dyspnea, orthopnea, lower extremity edema, and impaired exercise tolerance are the cardinal symptoms of HF. However, with increasing age, often accompanied by reduced physical activity, exertional symptoms become less prominent [13]. Although most clinical trials of therapy have studied patients with an average age in the mid-sixties, HF is more prevalent in the elderly, who bear a greater burden of co-morbidity and polypharmacy [14] as well as psychogeriatric comorbidities (further discussion is presented in Chap. 13), health service utilization, functional decline, and frailty [15]. Frailty characterizes elderly persons in whom the ability to independently perform activities of daily living, such as bathing, toileting, dressing, grooming, and feeding, is progressively eroded, and these associations have ramifications on the diagnosis and prognosis of HF [13, 16].

Elderly patients with HF often have a clinical presentation, which is not commonly encountered in younger patients, and that may confound the diagnosis [16]. HF and cognitive impairment is becoming more prevalent in the aging individual and is associated with defects in the domains of attention, short-term memory, and executive function (insight, judgment, problem solving, and decision-making), and these attributes have been closely related with nonadherence to treatment, accelerated functional decline, and even mortality [17]. Acute and fluctuating cognitive impairment, or delirium, can be precipitated by decompensated HF. Generally underrecognized by health care providers, delirium is usually reversible, though it may persist well beyond hospital discharge [18]. Cognitive impairment can occur in patients with stable HF, and this is called dementia if it impinges upon independent function such as adherence to prescribed therapy. Also, symptoms of depression are common in HF patients [19]. Depression reduces quality of life, increases the risk of functional impairment, rehospitalization, and mortality, and may reduce adherence to prescribed therapy. Depression and HF share common clinical features in elderly patients, including weight gain, sleep disturbances, fatigue, poor energy, and cognitive disturbances [20]. Pooled analysis has shown diminished neuropsychological performance in HF patients in comparison to controls. In a pooled sample of 2,937 HF patients and 14,848 control subjects, the odds ratio for cognitive impairment was 1.62 (95% confidence interval: 1.48–1.79, $p < 0.0001$) among subjects with HF. These findings underline the need for additional systematic neuropsychological data and adequate neuroimaging from representative populations of HF patients [21].

Vogels et al. have evaluated magnetic resonance imaging (MRI) and cognitive performance in nondemented outpatients with HF and found that medial temporal lobe atrophy was related to cognitive dysfunction, involving memory impairment and executive dysfunction, whereas white matter hyperintensities were related to depression and anxiety. In addition, disease severity and ApoE genotype were considered important determinants for cognitive impairment in patients with chronic HF [22, 23].

Biomarkers in the Diagnosis of Heart Failure in the Elderly

Because of the atypical presentations, the use of biomarkers such as B-type natriuretic peptide (BNP) in the diagnosis of HF in the elderly may be particularly useful. In a prospective study, Cournot et al. [24] evaluated 61 HF patients older than

70 years (mean age, 82.7 years). Patients' workup on admission and at discharge included clinical, radiologic, biologic, and echocardiographic evaluation. The median BNP level at admission was 1,136 pg/mL and the mean change during the hospitalization was −32%. Cardiac death or readmissions were best predicted by the change in BNP levels, with the poorest prognosis in patients who did not achieve a decrease of at least 40%. As hospitalization of elderly patients with decompensated HF is a common event, it appears that measurements of BNP on admission and discharge provide reliable information on the long-term prognosis on these patients. Cournot et al. [25] have also evaluated whether accurate risk stratification can be obtained using BNP level after stabilization on treatment, the change in BNP under optimal treatment, or a combination of both. They studied 157 consecutive patients aged ≥70 (mean 83 years) hospitalized for decompensated HF. As in previous studies, these investigators collected clinical, radiologic, biologic, and ultrasonography data on admission and at discharge. The median BNP level on admission was 1,057 pg/mL, and the mean change during hospitalization was −42%. Cardiac death or readmissions were independently predicted by both predischarge BNP and the change in BNP levels. The highest event rate was observed in patients with both a predischarge BNP ≥ 360 pg/mL and a decrease < 50% during hospitalization compared with patients with a predischarge BNP < 360 pg/mL and a decrease ≥50. The remaining patients constituted an intermediate risk group. Taken together, these findings suggest that predischarge BNP and inhospital BNP change should not be interpreted independently from each other. The highest risk group includes patients with a high predischarge BNP level corresponding to more than half of the BNP on admission. Evidently, these patients may benefit from close monitoring for potential signs of cardiac decompensation.

Interleukin-6 (IL-6) is another prognostic marker that may be useful in the assessment of HF in the elderly. Previously, increased proinflammatory cytokines have mainly been studied in younger patients with HF. Haugen et al. [26] have evaluated if inflammation was equally important in the progression of HF in the elderly, as it has been previously reported in younger patients, and also if cytokine level can predict mortality in elderly HF patients. Cytokine profile in an elderly patient group with severe HF ($n = 54$, age of 80.1 ± 5.0 years, New York Heart Association (NYHA) class III or IV) was compared with that of age-matched healthy individuals ($n = 70$). Of the 54 study patients, 46% were hypertensive, 54% had CAD, 43% had atrial fibrillation (AF), and 24% had a previous stroke. One-year mortality was 24%. Their results revealed increased levels of IL-6, tumor necrosis factor-α (TNF-α) and epidermal growth factor in the HF patients compared with those in the control group. IL-6, TNF-α and vascular endothelial growth factor were significantly increased in those who died within 1 year.

Further logistic regression analyses showed that IL-6 was the only significant predictor of 1-year mortality. While in a subgroup of HF patients with AF, there were also significant cytokine activations; in patients with associated ischemia or diabetes, cytokines were less activated. This study revealed that in octogenarian HF patients there were significant increases of inflammatory cytokines that were associated with mortality, and IL-6 was the only cytokine able to predict 1-year mortality. In addition, cytokine activation was more pronounced in the subgroup of patients with HF and associated AF.

Pharmacological Therapy

In contrast to HF with a low ejection fraction, there is no definitive evidence-based treatment for HF with preserved ejection fraction. The overall survival of patients with HF and reduced ejection fraction (EF) seems to significantly improve over time; in contrast, no such improvement has been seen among patients with HF-preserved ejection fraction (PEF). Das et al. [27] recently evaluated two large randomized clinical trials completed in HF-PEF patients that did not achieve a statistical significance in benefit of renin–angiotensin system blockade on their primary combined endpoints of morbidity and mortality. Both trials, however, suggested a benefit of the angiotensin receptor and angiotensin-converting enzyme (ACE) blockade on HF hospitalization. Furthermore, no clear benefit of β-blockers was demonstrated specifically in patients with HF-PEF. Thus, current therapeutic recommendations for HF-PEF are mostly aimed at symptomatic management and treatment of concomitant comorbidities. On the other hand, in their evaluation of a nationwide sample of 13,533 eligible Medicare beneficiaries aged ≥65 years who were hospitalized with a primary discharge diagnosis of HF and had chart documentation of preserved left ventricular ejection fraction between April 1998 and March 1999 or between July 2000 and June 2001, Shah et al. [28] found that irrespective of total cholesterol level or CAD status, diabetes, hypertension, and age, statin therapy was associated with significant differences in mortality rates. Similarly, angiotensin-converting enzyme inhibitors were associated with better survival at 1 year and 3 years, and β-blocker therapy was associated with a nonsignificant trend at 1 year and significant survival benefits at 3 years. Altogether, their data demonstrated that statins, angiotensin-converting enzyme inhibitors, and β-blockers are associated with better short- and long-term survival in patients ≥65 years with HF-PEF. To ascertain if above therapies are beneficial to aging patients in HF-PEF, we are looking for the results of ongoing, and new, clinical trials assessing the inhibition of the angiotensin and the aldosterone receptors (Table 17.3).

Besides the ongoing general clinical trials on inhibition of the angiotensin and the aldosterone receptors in HF-PEF

Table 17.3 Outcome trials in patients with heart failure and preserved systolic function

Name	Agent	Outcome
PEP-CHF [29]	Perindopril	Neutral
CHARM-preserved [30]	Candesartan	Neutral
I-PRESERVE [31]	Irbesartan	Neutral
SENIORS [32]	Nebivolol	Positive
TOPCAT	Spironolactone	Ongoing

PEP-CHF the perindopril in elderly people with chronic heart failure; *CHARM-Preserved* candesartan in heart failure assessment of reduction in mortality and morbidity-preserved systolic function arm; *I-PRESERVE* irbesartan in patients with heart failure and preserved ejection fraction; *SENIORS* study of the effects of nebivolol intervention on outcomes and rehospitalization in seniors with heart failure; *TOPCAT* treatment of preserved cardiac function heart failure with an aldosterone antagonist

mentioned earlier, a small number of randomized trials of therapies have been conducted specifically in the elderly populations. This, together with a multitude of data from observational data sets, suggests that most recommendations on HF therapies are applicable to elderly patients. Observational data suggest that ACE inhibitor use in elderly HF patients may preserve cognition, slow functional decline, and reduce hospitalizations and perhaps mortality, even in patients with relative contraindications such as mild to moderate renal impairment [33]. The β-blocker nebivolol has been studied in over 2,000 patients ≥70 years with clinical evidence of HF, regardless of ejection fraction (EF) [34]. After follow-up of less than 2 years, a significant benefit for nebivolol was seen with reduction of the combined primary endpoint of mortality and cardiovascular hospitalization. The Japanese Diastolic Heart Failure Study assessed the effects of the β-blocker carvedilol in 800 elderly Japanese patients with HF and documented EF>40% [35].

Therapies at correcting mitochondrial defects, including ROS and FAO metabolism present in the aging and in the failing heart, have also been suggested. For example, supplements of acetyl-L-carnitine (ALCAR) and (R)-alpha-lipoic acid may improve myocardial bioenergetics and decrease the oxidative stress (OS) associated with aging [36]. Old rats fed with ALCAR have shown a reversal of the age-related decline in carnitine levels and improved mitochondrial fatty acid β-oxidation in a number of tissues studied. However, ALCAR supplementation does not appear to reverse the age-related decline in the cardiac antioxidant status and may not improve the indices of OS. Lipoic acid, a potent thiol antioxidant and mitochondrial metabolite, appears to increase low molecular weight antioxidants, decreasing the age-associated oxidative insult. Seemingly, ALCAR along with lipoic acid may be effective supplemental regimens to maintain myocardial function in aging. Moreover, the lipophilic antioxidant and mitochondrial redox coupler coenzyme Q_{10} may have the potential to improve energy production in the aging and

Table 17.4 Atypical clinical features of heart failure in the frail elderly

Symptoms	Signs
Delirium	Ankle edema: may reflect venous insufficiency, drug effects and malnutrition
Falls	Sacral edema
Sudden functional decline	Rales/crackles are nonspecific
Sleep disturbances	
Nocturia	

failing heart mitochondria by bypassing defective components in the respiratory chain, as well as by reducing the effects of OS. Studies in rats and human have suggested that coenzyme Q_{10} protects the aging heart against stress [37].

Elderly patients are vulnerable to adverse drug events (ADE), due to the growing complexity of medication regimens, age-related physiologic changes, and a higher burden of co-morbid illnesses. Cardiovascular medications are frequently associated with ADE in the elderly [38]. Digitalis toxicity can occur at therapeutic serum levels [39]. Falls constitute common clinical presentations of ADE in the elderly, often from postural hypotension (Table 17.4). In randomized trials of drug treatment for HF, titration to target doses is less frequently successful in older patients due to higher side-effect rates. As such, care must be taken with titration of medications to target doses in order to avoid ADE. In particular, orthostatic hypotension is a frequent side-effect in elderly patients, but if recognized, and managed, can be controlled in order to allow for use of evidence-based therapies. Cardiovascular medications in general, and HF medications specifically, are underprescribed in the elderly patients, despite the observation that because of higher event rate, the absolute benefit of evidence-based therapies may be greatest in the elderly [40].

Disease Management Programs for Heart Failure in the Elderly

Several systematic reviews support the role of HF management programs in elderly HF patient populations [41]. While active involvement of caregivers in patient monitoring and medication adjustment is common to studies showing benefit, the optimal way of providing HF management remains controversial. The precise design of such care delivery systems depends in part upon local resources and infrastructure. Comprehensive geriatric assessment, shown to improve function, prevent hospitalization and institutionalization, reduce the risk of adverse drug reactions, and improve suboptimal prescribing, may have a role to play in the management of frail elderly patients with HF.

The occurrence of diabetes mellitus and renal insufficiency in older HF patients portends a significantly worse prognosis and a greater likelihood of adverse drug events. There exists a potential for contradictory recommendations when these comorbidities are managed in separate settings. Conflicting advice from multiple care providers can result in patient confusion, nonadherence, and adverse outcomes. For example, recommendations to limit diuretic use in order to maintain renal function, or dietary advice for controlling blood glucose that results in increased sodium intake, may lead to worsening HF symptoms. An integrative approach to care is required, based on shared therapeutic goals and involving all care providers, and including the primary care physician and the patient.

Recently, it had been noted that the process of assessing health-related quality of life (HRQoL) in elderly patients with HF and quality-adjusted life year (QALY) weights is complicated and time-consuming. Alehagen et al. have [42] evaluated NYHA functional status of 323 elderly HF patients independently, both by the patients themselves and by the examining cardiologist. HRQoL was assessed using the Short Form (SF)-36 questionnaire and a time trade-off (TTO) scenario. The TTO technique generates direct QALY weights. Both the TTO technique and SF-36 values demonstrated a statistically significant correlation with NYHA functional status. The TTO values also correlated with all SF-36 dimensions. Increasing deterioration was associated with statistically significant drops in both SF-36 values and TTO-based QALY weights. From NYHA class I–IV symptom the QALY weights were 0.77, 0.68, 0.61, and 0.50, respectively. In sum, in elderly patients, symptoms of HF have a significant impact on perceived quality of life.

Device and Cardiac Replacement Therapy in the Elderly

Cardiac resynchronization therapy (CRT) with or without concurrent use of implantable cardioverter defibrillator (ICD) is now a widely used treatment modality both for primary and secondary prevention in HF patients. There are still limited data on the impact of this type of device therapy in the elderly as most large-scale efficacy trials either excluded the very elderly patients, or the number of elderly patients studied was small. Bleeker et al. have studied the effects of CRT in elderly patients [43]. This study included 170 consecutive patients whose clinical and echocardiographic changes were evaluated after 6 months of follow-up. Survival was evaluated up to 2 years. The effects of CRT in elderly patients (age >70 years) were compared with those in younger patients (age <70 years). After 6 months of follow-up, CRT was beneficial in both groups, as reflected by improvements in clinical and echocardiographic parameters. Moreover, the magnitude of improvement was comparable between the two groups in clinical (NYHA class, quality-of-life score, and 6-min walking distance) and echocardiographic parameters (improvement in LV ejection fraction and extent of LV reverse remodeling). In addition, the number of nonresponders was comparable between the patients aged <70 years (25%) and those aged ≥70 years (22%), and survival was not different between the two groups.

More recently, in a prospective observational study, Delnoy at al. [44] evaluated the clinical and echocardiographic response to CRT in a group of 107 elderly (age >75 years) patients. Echocardiographic and clinical parameters were assessed at baseline and at 3, 12, and 24 months. Data were compared with a group of patients ≤75 years of age (mean 67 years). Clinical baseline characteristics between the two groups were comparable. At follow-up, similar and sustained improvement were observed in both groups based on NYHA class, quality of life score, and left ventricular (LV) ejection fraction. Clinical response, defined as survival with improvement (≥1 score) of NYHA class without hospital admission for HF, was seen in 67% and 69% (group aged ≤75 years) versus 65 and 60% (group aged >75 years) after 3 months and 1 year, respectively. Reverse LV remodeling was observed in 79 and 87% (group aged ≤75 years) versus 71 and 79% (group aged >75 years) after 3 months and 1 year, respectively. Hospitalization for HF decreased significantly in both groups in the year after CRT. Significant improvement in NYHA class and LV ejection fraction was also observed in a subgroup of 39 octogenarians (>80 years) with similar LV reverse remodeling (75 and 84%) after 3 months and 1 year, respectively. Thus, this study showed that clinical and echocardiographic improvement of CRT occurred in patients aged >75 years and even in octogenarians. Moreover, as ventricular assist device technology improves, it may be used to complement heart transplantation to avoid immunosuppression and its side-effect of malignancy in older patients with advanced HF.

To address the use of CRT outside clinical trials, Piccini et al. ("Get With The Guidelines-Heart Failure" program) [45] evaluated the use of CRT in patients admitted to a hospital with HF. From a group of 33,898 patients admitted to one of the 228 participant hospital between January 2005 and September 2007, 4201 patients (12.4%) were discharged alive with CRT, including 811 new implants. Patients discharged with CRT were older (median age, 75 versus 72 years), sicker, had lower median LVEF, had more frequent ischemic cardiomyopathy, dysrhythmias, and higher use of β-blocker and aldosterone antagonist than those without CRT. The conclusion was that although CRT is a class I recommendation for patients with LV dysfunction, QRS prolongation, and class III to IV HF, significant variations exist for CRT therapy by hospital and region of the country and appear to be influenced by patient age and race. Interestingly, 10% of patients with a new CRT had a LVEF >35% before implan-

tation (6% had a LVEF of 40%) suggesting a potential overuse of CRT in some patient groups since this therapy is currently recommended only for patients with LVEF ≤ 35%, as a result of a lack of randomized trial data in patients with preserved systolic function. As pointed out by McAllister in his recent editorial [46], although it is possible that some CRT implants in cases with less severe systolic dysfunction were done prophylactically (to prevent worsening systolic function in patients who required a right ventricular pacemaker for bradydysrhythmias), the 10% proportion raised the suspicion of CRT overuse. Clearly, to understand the reasons for the variations in CRT use at the patient, physician, and hospital levels and being able to implement programs to improve the awareness and promotion of evidence-based use of medical devices in HF further research is warranted.

Since heart transplantation has become a highly successful therapeutic option for patients with end-stage HF, the criteria for patient selection, including recipients' upper age limits have been expanded, with an increasing number of people older than 60 years of age now undergoing transplantation. Several studies have now reported similar long-term survival rate in patients transplanted at age >60 versus patients transplanted at younger age [47–49]. Older transplant recipients have equal or less rejection episodes [50] but may have equal or higher rate of infection and transplant CAD [51].

The long-term outcomes of heart transplantation in older recipients have been recently evaluated by Marelli et al. [52] in a cohort of 182 patients aged 62–75 years (mean ± SD: 66.3 ± 11.4 years) operated at a single institution. They were compared with a control group of 348 adult recipients aged 18–62 years (mean ± SD: 48.2 ± 11.4 years). All recipients in this consecutive cohort had a follow-up of at least 5 years. End-points studied were Kaplan–Meier survival, freedom from dialysis, and freedom from malignancy at 100 months. Follow-up was 100% at 100 months. At 100 months, survival for the elderly was 55% (46 remaining at risk) and 63% (102 remaining at risk) for controls ($p = 0.051$, log-rank test). Retransplant and dialysis, but not recipient age or malignancy, were predictive of survival by regression analysis. Freedom from malignancy at 100 months was 68% for the elderly and 95% for controls. Age predicted malignancy by regression analysis. At 100 months, freedom from dialysis was 81% for the elderly and 87% for controls with preoperative creatinine, but not age, predicting the need for dialysis. Taken together, these data showed that the long-term survival of older heart transplant recipients although acceptable is significantly lower than in young recipients. Furthermore, the increased risk of renal failure and malignancy among elderly patients likely influences the difference in survival observed between the two groups.

Recently, the United Network for Organ Sharing (UNOS) database has been retrospectively reviewed by Weiss et al.

[53]. They identified 14,401 first-time orthotopic heart transplantation (OHT) recipients between the years 1999 and 2006. Stratification was carried out by age into those ≥60 years (30%) and younger patients aged 18–59 years. The primary end-point was all-cause mortality during the study period. Secondary outcomes included length of hospital stay (LOS), postoperative stroke, postoperative infections, acute renal failure and rejection within 1 year of transplant. The elderly group had higher serum creatinine levels, longer wait list time, and were more likely to have hypertension (HTN) or diabetes mellitus (DM). Survival at 30 days, 1 year, and 5 years was 94, 87, and 75%, respectively, for the young group, and 93, 84, and 69%, respectively, for the older group. Multivariate analysis revealed age ≥60 years, donor age, ischemic time, creatinine, HTN, and DM to be independent predictors of mortality. Older patients had more infections and longer LOS but had lower rates of rejection as compared to younger recipients. As observed by these investigators, the UNOS database has provided a large multiinstitutional sample examining OHT in the elderly and while the survival in patients ≥60 years of age is lower than in younger one, the cumulative 5-year survival in the older group close to 70% is acceptable. Thus, OHT should not be restricted on the basis of age.

Conclusions and Future Directions

The increased use of gene profiling in hearts from subjects with age-associated diseases such as cardiomyopathy and HF has begun to define a molecular signature of cardiac dysfunction whose component elements can be informatively compared between diseases, various populations (e.g., ethnic/racial, gender), a variety of treatment regimens (e.g., LV assist devices, pharmacological treatments), and of course age. Efforts are also being undertaken to define a proteomic profile of age-associated cardiac disease; albeit for numerous pragmatic reasons, most studies have chosen to target and define limited proteomes (e.g., mitochondrial/organelle-specific, specific classes of protein modification).

Many pharmacodynamic studies have focused primarily on healthy older people; however, the pathophysiology of CVDs, including HF in the elderly, is different than in younger people, and this may change the pharmacodynamic response and therapeutic outcome. Although, most of the clinical trials of HF have recruited younger men (younger than 65 years old) with systolic dysfunction secondary to ischemic heart disease, in clinical practice, HF is often a syndrome of older women with diastolic dysfunction, perhaps secondary to systemic hypertension. This difference in the pathophysiology of the disease in aging may explain why the survival benefits seen with angiotensin-converting enzyme inhibitors and β-blockers in younger adults are reduced in older people, particularly

older women [54, 55]. Importantly, the primary goal of pharmacogenomics of HF should be to develop a personalized medicine that could define the most effective treatment plan (e.g., drug regimens and dosage) to treat disease in patients of specific genetic backgrounds and age.

Looking forward, it is noteworthy that studies with transgenic animals (primarily mice) and genetic models in the rat and hamster have provided invaluable models of cardiomyopathy and HF, which recapitulate the clinical phenotypes. Both loss-of-function and gain-of-function models have been used to examine the role of defective metabolic, intracellular signaling and cardiomyocyte contractile, and structural components and pathways that can lead to cardiac dysfunction, a number with specific aging-related phenotypic expression. Furthermore, besides providing information concerning the pathogenesis, these animal models have often proved useful as substrates for testing new therapies of HF. Finally, increasing experience with molecular analysis of other noncardiac diseases will be helpful in developing information to be applied to the management of HF, including diagnosis, prognosis, and treatment response. This information may not only be clinically useful but also helpful in advancing the research and discovery of new drugs and translational medicine [56]. Therefore, new genomic technologies and information should enhance our understanding of HF and cardiomyopathies, particularly the cardiomyopathy and HF occurring with aging.

Summary

- Heart failure (HF) is predominantly a clinical syndrome of aging, with prevalence increasing from nearly 1% in the population age <50 to over 10% in persons over the age of 80, with 80% of hospitalizations for HF found in patients over age 65.
- HF in the elderly is frequently multifactorial in etiologies with common etiologies including hypertensive heart disease, coronary artery disease (CAD), age-related diastolic dysfunction, valvular heart disease, and cardiomyopathy.
- Factors that commonly precipitate or contribute to exacerbation of HF in the elderly include myocardial ischemia, dietary sodium excess, noncompliance with medications, volume overload owing to excess fluid intake, arrhythmias (especially atrial fibrillation), intercurrent infections and fever, anemia and various drugs, and toxins including alcohol and antiarrhythmic agents.
- While exertional dyspnea, orthopnea, lower extremity edema, and impaired exercise tolerance are cardinal symptoms of HF, with reduced physical activity often found in increasing age, exertional symptoms become less prominent.

- A prominent feature that distinguishes HF in the elderly from the younger individuals is a much higher frequency of HF occurring in the absence of systolic dysfunction, i.e., diastolic HF or HF with preserved systolic function.

- Elderly patients with HF often have atypical clinical presentation, not found in younger patients, with cognitive impairment, defective short-term memory, and executive dysfunction, and these features have been associated with nonadherence to treatment, accelerated functional decline, and mortality.

- Approaches to HF treatment in the elderly include pharmacotherapy, cardiac resynchronization therapy (CRT) with or without concurrent use of implantable cardioverter defibrillator (ICD), and heart transplantation for end-stage disease.

- Some CRT implants in cases with less severe systolic dysfunction may have been done prophylactically.

- Besides providing information concerning the pathogenesis, animal models have often proved useful as substrates for testing new therapies of HF.

- New genomic technologies and information should enhance our understanding of HF and cardiomyopathies, particularly the cardiomyopathy and HF occurring with aging.

References

1. O'Connell J (2000) The economic burden of heart failure. Clin Cardiol 23:III6–III10
2. Kannel WB, Belanger AJ (1991) Epidemiology of heart failure. Am Heart J 121:951–957
3. Anversa P, Rota M, Urbanek K, Hosoda T, Sonnenblick EH, Leri A, Kajstura J, Bolli R (2005) Myocardial aging – a stem cell problem. Basic Res Cardiol 100:482–493
4. Vasan RS, Larson MG, Benjamin EJ, Evans JC, Reiss CK, Levy D (1999) Congestive heart failure in subjects with normal versus reduced left ventricular ejection fraction: prevalence and mortality in a population-based cohort. J Am Coll Cardiol 33:1948–1955
5. Kitzman DW (2000) Heart failure with normal systolic function. Clin Geriatr Med 16:489–512
6. Wei JY (1992) Age and the cardiovascular system. N Engl J Med 327:1735–1739
7. Olivetti G, Melissari M, Capasso JM, Anversa P (1991) Cardiomyopathy of the aging human heart. Myocyte loss and reactive cellular hypertrophy. Circ Res 68:1560–1568
8. Lakatta EG (2000) Cardiovascular aging in health. Clin Geriatr Med 16:419–444
9. Van Coster R, Smet J, George E, De Meirleir L et al (2001) Blue native polyacrylamide gel electrophoresis: a powerful tool in diagnosis of oxidative phosphorylation defects. Pediatr Res 50:658–665
10. Brunt UT, Terman A (2002) The mitochondrial-lysosomal axis theory of aging: accumulation of damaged mitochondria as a result of imperfect autophagocytosis. Eur J Biochem 269:1996–2002
11. Gottdiener JS, Arnold AM, Aurigemma GP, Polak JF et al (2000) Predictors of congestive heart failure in the elderly: the Cardiovascular Health Study. J Am Coll Cardiol 35:1628–1637
12. Ghali JK, Kadakia S, Cooper R, Ferlinz J (1988) Precipitating factors leading to decompensation of heart failure. Traits among urban blacks. Arch Intern Med 148:2013–2016
13. Tresch DD (2000) Clinical manifestations, diagnostic assessment, and etiology of heart failure in elderly patients. Clin Geriatr Med 16:445–456
14. Heiat A, Gross CP, Krumholz HM (2002) Representation of the elderly, women, and minorities in heart failure clinical trials. Arch Intern Med 162:1682–1688
15. Incalzi AR, Capparella O, Gemma A, Porcedda P, Raccis G, Sommella L, Carbonin PU (1992) A simple method of recognizing geriatric patients at risk for death and disability. J Am Geriatr Soc 40:34–38
16. Arnold JM, Liu P, Demers C, Dorian P et al (2006) Canadian Cardiovascular Society consensus conference recommendations on heart failure 2006: diagnosis and management. Can J Cardiol 22:23–45
17. Zuccala G, Pedone C, Cesari M, Onder G, Pahor M, Marzetti E, Lo Monaco MR, Cocchi A, Carbonin P, Bernabei R (2003) The effects of cognitive impairment on mortality among hospitalized patients with heart failure. Am J Med 115:97–103
18. Kelly KG, Zisselman M, Cutillo-Schmitter T, Reichard R, Payne D, Denman SJ (2001) Severity and course of delirium in medically hospitalized nursing facility residents. Am J Geriatr Psychiatry 9:72–77
19. Gottlieb SS, Khatta M, Friedmann E, Einbinder L et al (2004) The influence of age, gender, and race on the prevalence of depression in heart failure patients. J Am Coll Cardiol 43:1542–1549
20. Joynt KE, Whellan DJ, O'Connor CM (2004) Why is depression bad for the failing heart? A review of the mechanistic relationship between depression and heart failure. J Card Fail 10:258–271
21. Vogels RL, Scheltens P, Schroeder-Tanka JM, Weinstein HC (2007) Cognitive impairment in heart failure: a systematic review of the literature. Eur J Heart Fail 9:440–449
22. Vogels RL, Oosterman JM, van Harten B, Gouw AA, Schroeder-Tanka JM, Scheltens P, van der Flier WM, Weinstein HC (2007) Neuroimaging and correlates of cognitive function among patients with heart failure. Dement Geriatr Cogn Disord 24:418–423
23. Vogels RL, Oosterman JM, van Harten B, Scheltens P, van der Flier WM, Schroeder-Tanka JM, Weinstein HC (2007) Profile of cognitive impairment in chronic heart failure. J Am Geriatr Soc 55:1764–1770
24. Cournot M, Leprince P, Destrac S, Ferrieres J (2007) Usefulness of in-hospital change in B-type natriuretic peptide levels in predicting long-term outcome in elderly patients admitted for decompensated heart failure. Am J Geriatr Cardiol 16:8–14
25. Cournot M, Mourre F, Castel F, Ferrières J, Destrac S (2008) Optimization of the use of B-type natriuretic peptide levels for risk stratification at discharge in elderly patients with decompensated heart failure. Am Heart J 155:986–989
26. Haugen E, Gan LM, Isic A, Skommevik T, Fu M (2008) Increased interleukin-6 but not tumour necrosis factor-alpha predicts mortality in the population of elderly heart failure patients. Exp Clin Cardiol 13:19–24
27. Das A, Abraham S, Deswal A (2008) Advances in the treatment of heart failure with a preserved ejection fraction. Curr Opin Cardiol 23:233–240
28. Shah R, Wang Y, Foody JM (2008) Effect of statins, angiotensin-converting enzyme inhibitors, and beta blockers on survival in patients > or =65 years of age with heart failure and preserved left ventricular systolic function. Am J Cardiol 101:217–222
29. Cleland JG, Tendera M, Adamus J, Freemantle N, Polonski L, Taylor J (2006) The perindopril in elderly people with chronic heart failure (PEP-CHF) study. Eur Heart J 27:2338–2345
30. Yusuf S, Pfeffer MA, Swedberg K, Granger CB, Held P, McMurray JJ, Michelson EL, Olofsson B, Ostergren J (2003) Effects of candesartan in patients with chronic heart failure and preserved left-ventricular ejection fraction: the CHARM-Preserved Trial. Lancet 362:777–781

31. Massie BM, Carson PE, McMurray JJ, Komajda M, McKelvie R, Zile MR, Anderson S, Donovan M, Iverson E, Staiger C, Ptaszynska A (2008) Irbesartan in patients with heart failure and preserved ejection fraction. N Engl J Med 359:2456–2467

32. van Veldhuisen DJ, Cohen-Solal A, Bohm M, Anker SD, Babalis D, Roughton M, Coats AJ, Poole-Wilson PA, Flather MD (2009) Beta-blockade with nebivolol in elderly heart failure patients with impaired and preserved left ventricular ejection fraction: data from SENIORS (Study of Effects of Nebivolol Intervention on Outcomes and Rehospitalization in Seniors With Heart Failure). J Am Coll Cardiol 53:2150–2158

33. Ahmed A, Kiefe CI, Allman RM, Sims RV, DeLong JF (2002) Survival benefits of angiotensin-converting enzyme inhibitors in older heart failure patients with perceived contraindications. J Am Geriatr Soc 50:1659–1666

34. Flather MD, Shibata MC, Coats AJ, Van Veldhuisen DJ et al (2005) Randomized trial to determine the effect of nebivolol on mortality and cardiovascular hospital admission in elderly patients with heart failure (SENIORS). Eur Heart J 26:215–225

35. Hori M, Kitabatake A, Tsutsui H, Okamoto H, Shirato K, Nagai R, Izumi T, Yokoyama H, Yasumura Y, Ishida Y, Matsuzaki M, Oki T, Sekiya M (2005) Rationale and design of a randomized trial to assess the effects of beta-blocker in diastolic heart failure; Japanese Diastolic Heart Failure Study (J-DHF). J Card Fail 11:542–547

36. Hagen TM, Moreau R, Suh JH, Visioli F (2002) Mitochondrial decay in the aging rat heart: evidence for improvement by dietary supplementation with acetyl-L-carnitine and/or lipoic acid. Ann NY Acad Sci 959:491–507

37. Tiano L, Fedeli D, Santoni G, Davies I, Wakabayashi T, Falcioni G (2003) Ebselen prevents mitochondrial ageing due to oxidative stress: in vitro study of fish erythrocytes. Mitochondrion 2:428–436

38. Gurwitz JH, Field TS, Harrold LR, Rothschild J, Debellis K, Seger AC, Cadoret C, Fish LS, Garber L, Kelleher M, Bates DW (2003) Incidence and preventability of adverse drug events among older persons in the ambulatory setting. JAMA 289:1107–1116

39. Miura T, Kojima R, Sugiura Y, Mizutani M, Takatsu F, Suzuki Y (2000) Effect of aging on the incidence of digoxin toxicity. Ann Pharmacother 34:427–432

40. Cleland JG, Cohen-Solal A, Aguilar JC, Dietz R et al (2002) Management of heart failure in primary care (the IMPROVEMENT of Heart Failure Programme): an international survey. Lancet 360:1631–1639

41. Gonseth J, Guallar-Castillon P, Banegas JR, Rodriguez-Artalejo F (2004) The effectiveness of disease management programmes in reducing hospital re-admission in older patients with heart failure: a systematic review and meta-analysis of published reports. Eur Heart J 25:1570–1595

42. Alehagen U, Rahmqvist M, Paulsson T (2008) Levin LA.Quality-adjusted life year weights among elderly patients with heart failure. Eur J Heart Fail 10:1033–1039

43. Bleeker GB, Schalij MJ, Molhoek SG, Boersma E, Steendijk P, van der Wall EE, Bax JJ (2005) Comparison of effectiveness of cardiac resynchronization therapy in patients <70 versus > or =70 years of age. Am J Cardiol 96:420–422

44. Delnoy PP, Ottervanger JP, Luttikhuis HO, Elvan A, Misier AR, Beukema WP, van Hemel NM (2008) Clinical response of cardiac resynchronization therapy in the elderly. Am Heart J 155: 746–751

45. Piccini JP, Hernandez AF, Dai D, Thomas KL, Lewis WR, Yancy CW, Peterson ED, Fonarow GC; Get With the Guidelines Steering Committee and Hospitals (2008) Use of cardiac resynchronization therapy in patients hospitalized with heart failure. Circulation 118:926–933

46. McAlister FA (2008) Cardiac resynchronization therapy for heart failure: a hammer in search of nails. Circulation 118:901–903

47. Morgan JA, John R, Weinberg AD, Remoli R et al (2003) Long-term results of cardiac transplantation in patients 65 years of age and older: a comparative analysis. Ann Thorac Surg 76:1982–1987

48. Zuckermann A, Dunkler D, Deviatko E, Bodhjalian A, Czerny M, Ankersmit J, Wolner E, Grimm M (2003) Long-term survival (>10 years) of patients >60 years with induction therapy after cardiac transplantation. Eur J Cardiothorac Surg 24:283–291

49. Potapov EV, Loebe M, Hubler M, Musci M, Hummel M, Weng Y, Hetzer R (1999) Medium-term results of heart transplantation using donors over 63 years of age. Transplantation 68:1834–1838

50. Blanche C, Kamlot A, Blanche DA, Kearney B, Magliato KE, Czer LS, Trento A (2002) Heart transplantation with donors fifty years of age and older. J Thorac Cardiovasc Surg 123:810–815

51. Morgan JA, John R, Weinberg AD, Remoli R, Kherani AR, Vigilance DW, Schanzer BM, Bisleri G, Mancini DM, Oz MC, Edwards NM (2003) Long-term results of cardiac transplantation in patients 65 years of age and older: a comparative analysis. Ann Thorac Surg 76:1982–1987

52. Marelli D, Kobashigawa J, Hamilton MA, Moriguchi JD, Kermani R, Ardehali A, Patel J, Noguchi E, Beygui R, Laks H, Plunkett M, Shemin R, Esmailian F (2008) Long-term outcomes of heart transplantation in older recipients. J Heart Lung Transplant 27:830–834

53. Weiss ES, Nwakanma LU, Patel ND, Yuh DD (2008) Outcomes in patients older than 60 years of age undergoing orthotopic heart transplantation: an analysis of the UNOS database. J Heart Lung Transplant 27:184–191

54. Flather MD, Yusuf S, Kober L, Pfeffer M, Hall A et al (2000) Long-term ACE-inhibitor therapy in patients with heart failure or left-ventricular dysfunction: a systematic overview of data from individual patients. ACE-Inhibitor Myocardial Infarction Collaborative Group. Lancet 355:1575–1581

55. Richardson LG, Rocks M (2001) Women and heart failure. Heart Lung 30:87–97

56. McLean AJ, Le Couteur DG (2004) Aging biology and geriatric clinical pharmacology. Pharmacol Rev 56:163–184

Chapter 18
Diagnosis of Heart Failure: Evidence-Based Perspective

Overview

The evaluation of symptomatic patients with suspected heart failure (HF) is directed at confirming the diagnosis, determining the cause, identifying concomitant illnesses, establishing the severity of HF, and guiding therapy. However, HF is a clinical diagnosis, and no single test can establish its presence or absence. The diagnosis of HF is therefore made when symptoms and signs of impaired cardiac output and/or volume overload are documented in the setting of abnormal systolic and/or diastolic cardiac function. The cardinal triad of edema, fatigue, and dyspnea are neither sensitive nor specific manifestations of HF, and atypical presentations of HF should always be recognized, particularly when evaluating women, obese patients, and the elderly. A focused clinical history and physical examination should be performed in all patients and initial investigations should be targeted to confirm or exclude HF as the diagnosis and to identify systemic disorders (e.g., thyroid dysfunction) that may impact on its development or progression. Measurement of plasma biomarkers including natriuretic peptides, such as B-type natriuretic peptide (BNP), is likely to become more widely available and is helpful as low levels are useful in excluding HF and high levels can confirm HF in patients presenting with dyspnea, when the clinical diagnosis remains uncertain. Two-dimensional and Doppler echocardiography are the initial imaging modalities of choice in patients suspected to have HF as they assess systolic and diastolic ventricular function, wall thickness, chamber sizes, valvular function, and pericardial disease. Radionuclide angiography is useful in patients whose echocardiographic images may be poor (e.g., obese patients, patients with emphysema).

Cardiac catheterization with hemodynamic measurements and contrast ventriculography, or magnetic resonance imaging when available, may be used in specific cases where initial non-invasive tests are inconclusive. When coronary artery disease (CAD) is suspected, non-invasive testing, such as radionuclide perfusion imaging or stress echocardiography, is useful to ascertain the presence or extent of myocardial infarction, ischemia, or viability that may warrant further evaluation. Coronary angiography should also be considered, especially in those who have angina or positive non-invasive tests and are candidates for revascularization. Endomyocardial biopsy is not recommended in the routine evaluation of HF; it has limited diagnostic value except in suspected rare disorders such as infiltrative or inflammatory myocardial diseases. Patients with CAD, hypertension, diabetes mellitus, exposures to cardiotoxic drugs, alcohol abuse, or family history of cardiomyopathy are at high risk for HF and may benefit from primary screening.

Introduction

HF can be defined as an inability of the myocardium to deliver sufficient oxygenated blood to meet the needs of tissues and organs during exercise or at rest. Because diagnostic criteria for this clinical syndrome remain ill defined, the actual prevalence is difficult to determine. The spectrum of patients who may be suspected of having HF ranges from those who are asymptomatic but at high risk for HF (i.e., patients who have CAD, hypertension, diabetes mellitus, obesity, exposure to cardiotoxic drugs, or familial history of cardiomyopathy) to those with overt signs and symptoms of HF. The American College of Cardiology and the American Heart Association identify four stages in the progression of HF [1]. Patients in stage A have no structural abnormalities but are at high risk for HF. In stage B, patients are asymptomatic but have structural heart disease. Patients in stage C have structural abnormalities and past or present HF. In stage D, patients have end-stage HF and require mechanical circulatory support, infusion of inotropic agents, cardiac transplantation, or hospice care. The fact that patients can progress from asymptomatic left ventricular dysfunction, i.e., stage B, to progressive HF, i.e., stages C and D; the high morbidity and mortality rates associated with the condition; and the fact that early treatment can delay the onset of overt HF have raised questions about the need to screen patients for HF [2]. General screening of the general population cannot

J. Marín-García, *Heart Failure*, Contemporary Cardiology,
DOI 10.1007/978-1-60761-147-9_18, © Springer Science+Business Media, LLC 2010

be recommended at present [3]. However, screening echocardiography may be appropriate in selected patients who are at high risk for developing systolic dysfunction, such as patients with a strong family history of cardiomyopathy and patients with exposure to cardiotoxic drugs, although the prevalence of these patients is unclear at this point [1]. This chapter will focus on the diagnosis of HF from an evidence-based perspective.

General Considerations Relevant to the Diagnosis of Heart Failure

Confirming the diagnosis of HF may also involve determining the cause, identifying concomitant illnesses, establishing the severity of disease, and guiding subsequent therapy, which requires an understanding of the etiologies and forms of HF. The pathophysiology of HF has been discussed in other chapters. In brief, normal myocardial function requires sufficient nutrient-rich, toxin-free blood at rest and during exercise; sequential depolarization of the myocardium; normal myocardial contractility during systole and relaxation during diastole; normal intracardiac volume before contraction (preload); and limited impedance to the flow of blood out of the heart (afterload). The capacity of the heart to adapt to short-term changes in preload or afterload is substantial, but sudden or sustained changes in preload (e.g., acute valvular regurgitation, excessive intravenous hydration), afterload (e.g., aortic stenosis, severe uncontrolled hypertension), or demand (e.g., severe anemia or hyperthyroidism) may lead to progressive failure of myocardial function. Asymptomatic cardiac dysfunction can progress steadily to overt HF.

The list of etiologies of HF that are commonly encountered in clinical practice is shown in Table 18.1. CAD accounts for nearly 75% of all cases of HF [4], followed by diabetes mellitus and valvular heart disease. HF can also be multifactorial, i.e., the syndrome can result from acute myocardial infarction (loss of myocardial contractility) with papillary muscle dysfunction (increased preload) and acute pulmonary edema (hypoxemia). HF phenotypes may be classified based on the role of diastolic or systolic dysfunction and based on the anatomic area of involvement (Table 18.2). The types of HF resulting from systolic dysfunction include high output HF, low cardiac output syndrome, right HF, left HF, and biventricular failure. High output HF occurs when the demand for blood exceeds the capacity of an otherwise normal heart to meet the demand. This type of HF may occur in patients with severe anemia, arteriovenous malformations with shunting of blood, or hyperthyroidism. Patients with low cardiac output syndrome have fatigue and loss of lean muscle mass as their most prominent symptoms, but they also may have dyspnea, impaired renal function, or altered

mental status. Right heart failure (RHF) is characterized by peripheral edema, whereas left heart failure is characterized by pulmonary congestion; both systemic and pulmonary congestion are present in patients with biventricular HF. RHF is a more specific form of HF as it relates to diagnosis and management and is therefore considered in more detail in this chapter.

Table 18.1 Etiologies of heart failure

Common
Coronary heart disease
Hypertension
Idiopathic
Diabetes mellitus
Valvular disease
Less common
Anemia
Connective tissue disease
Viral myocarditis
Hemochromatosis
Human immunodeficiency virus infection
Hyperthyroidism, hypothyroidism
Hypertrophic cardiomyopathy
Infiltrative disease (including amyloidosis and sarcoidosis)
Mediastinal radiation
Peripartum cardiomyopathy
Restrictive pericardial disease
Tachyarrhythmia
Toxins (including drugs and alcohol)
Trypanosomiasis (Chagas' disease)

Table 18.2 Classification of heart failure phenotypes

Diastolic dysfunction/ preserved systolic function	Normal myocardial contractility, left ventricular volume and ejection fraction; impaired relaxation; diminished early diastolic filling
Systolic dysfunction	Absolute or relative impairment of myocardial contractility, low ejection fraction
High output heart failure	Bounding pulses, wide pulse pressure, accentuated heart sounds, peripheral vasodilatation, increased cardiac output and ejection fraction, moderate four-chamber enlargement
Low output syndrome	Fatigue, loss of lean body mass, prerenal azotemia, peripheral vasoconstriction, reduced left or right contractility
Right heart failure	Dependent edema, jugular venous distention, right atrial and ventricular dilatation, reduced right-sided contractility
Left heart failure	Dyspnea, pulmonary vascular congestion reduced left-sided contractility
Biventricular failure	Dyspnea, dependent edema, jugular venous distention, pulmonary vascular congestion, bilateral reduced contractility

RHF is a clinical syndrome that occurs when the right ventricle (RV), due to systolic and/or diastolic dysfunction, is unable to produce adequate cardiac output for the needs of the individual, or is unable to do so with normal filling pressures. RHF may occur as pure right-sided failure (uncommon), or in association with left-sided failure (less common). Recent reviews and working groups have described in detail normal and abnormal function and disease states of the right ventricle [5]. In order for diagnosis of RHF to be made, at least two features should be present:

1. Signs and symptoms consistent with RHF
2. Objective evidence of abnormal right-sided cardiac structure or function or elevated filling pressure

The etiology of RHF is shown in Table 18.3. The clinical presentation of RHF is variable but typically involves exercise limitation, fatigue, and evidence of systemic venous congestion. This falls into three general categories:

1. Fluid retention (ascites, peripheral edema)
2. Exercise intolerance and fatigue (low cardiac output, diastolic and systolic dysfunction)
3. Hypotension (especially with atrial and ventricular dysrhythmias, low cardiac output).

In addition, gastrointestinal symptoms, including anorexia, bloating, nausea, and constipation, may be present and are common in the advanced stages. There are also several conditions, which may give rise to suspicion of RHF, including liver cirrhosis, nephrotic syndrome, and renal failure with significant volume overload. These conditions should be excluded before ascribing the clinical presentation as primarily due to RHF.

The underlying pathophysiology in RHF may include venous congestion, RV enlargement, increased pulmonary artery pressures, and tricuspid or pulmonary valvular dysfunction. These are in turn suggested by several physical examination findings. Most often an abnormal jugular venous pressure is seen, which may represent reduced RV compliance and/or venous hypertension. In more severe cases, pitting sacral or peripheral edema will be present, as may liver enlargement, tenderness and ascites. RV enlargement is manifested through a palpable impulse (lift or heave) present along the left sternal border while a palpable

Table 18.3 Causes of Right Heart Failure

1. As a consequence of increased afterload, including left HF and pulmonary arterial hypertension
2. RV myopathic process, RV infarction and restrictive heart disease
3. Right-sided valvular heart disease
4. Congenital heart disease and surgical residua
5. Pericardial disease[a]

RV right ventricle; *RHF* right heart failure
[a]Mimic of RHF

pulmonary artery pulsation at the left upper sternal border may be present in the setting of significant pulmonary artery dilatation. With pulmonary arterial hypertension, the pulmonary valvular closure sound may be delayed, resulting in increase splitting of the second heart sound, or increased in intensity or even palpable. If pulmonary regurgitation is present with normal pulmonary pressure, a low-pitched and variable length pulmonary decrescendo murmur may be present at the left sternal border. In the setting of pulmonary hypertension a high-pitched Graham-Steele murmur is heard. Tricuspid regurgitation, when audible, is usually heard as a regurgitant type murmur heard at the left lower sternal border. A right-sided S3 may be present and increases with inspiration, as do nearly all right-sided heart sounds, extracardiac sounds, and murmurs. Table 18.4 includes several clinical and diagnostic abnormalities associated with RHF with or without pulmonary hypertension.

Clinical Evaluation of Patients with Heart Failure

HF is a clinical syndrome, no single test can establish its presence or absence, and clinical evaluation remains the most important initial step in the diagnosis of HF. In patients with this condition, the most frequent clinical findings are related to decreased exercise tolerance or fluid retention [6, 7]. Decreased exercise tolerance typically presents as dyspnea or, much less commonly, fatigue on exertion. Fluid retention results in orthopnea, rales, elevated jugular venous pressure, dependent edema, and the typical radiographic findings of cardiomegaly, pulmonary edema, and pleural effusion. There currently are no validated clinical decision rules to estimate the contribution of each of these findings to HF. Nearly all patients with HF present with dyspnea. Thus, the absence of dyspnea makes HF highly unlikely (sensitivity > 95%), and alternative explanations for the patient's symptoms should be sought first. It is important to note that HF is present in only about 30% of patients who present with dyspnea in the primary care setting. Other common causes of dyspnea in adult primary care patients include asthma (33%), chronic obstructive pulmonary disease (9%), dysrhythmia (7%), infection (5%), interstitial lung disease (4%), anemia (2%), and pulmonary embolism (<2%) [8]. Accordingly, 30% is a reasonable pretest estimate of the probability of HF with or without systolic dysfunction in patients presenting with dyspnea in the primary care setting. In patients with dyspnea, a focused history and physical examination, combined with selected diagnostic testing, can identify HF [1, 6, 7, 9]. This diagnostic approach, which avoids unnecessary

Table 18.4 Diagnosis of Right Heart Failure

Common features	Right heart failure without pulmonary hypertension	Cor pulmonale
Symptoms	Fatigue	Fatigue
	Hepatic congestion	Hemoptysis
	Right upper quadrant discomfort	*Hoarseness*
	Anorexia/early satiety	Hepatic congestion
	Peripheral edema	Right upper quadrant discomfort
	Cough	Anorexia/early satiety
	Dyspnea/orthopnea[a]	Peripheral edema
		Cough
		Shortness of breath/orthopnea[a]
Physical signs	Elevated jugular venous pulsation, positive hepatojugular reflux or Kussmaul sign	Elevated jugular venous pulsation, positive hepatojugular reflux or Kussmaul sign
	Peripheral or sacral edema	Peripheral or sacral edema
	Ascites	Ascites
	Hepatomegaly or liver tenderness	Hepatomegaly or liver tenderness
	Right-sided third heart sound	Right-sided third heart sound, *increased pulmonary closure sound, pulmonary ejection* click
	Murmur of tricuspid regurgitation	Murmur of tricuspid regurgitation
	Signs of right ventricular enlargement	Signs of right ventricular enlargement
		Evidence of co-existent underlying pulmonary cause of cor pulmonale
Diagnostic testing	EKG: Right axis deviation, right ventricular hypertrophy, p pulmonale pattern low-voltage QRS, incomplete or complete right bundle branch block	EKG: Right axis deviation, right ventricular hypertrophy, p pulmonale pattern low-voltage QRS, incomplete or complete right bundle branch block
	Chest X-ray: right sided cardiac enlargement, enlargement of pulmonary arteries (uncommon), oligemic peripheral lung fields (rare), right sided pleural effusion[a]	Chest X-ray: right sided cardiac enlargement, enlargement of pulmonary arteries, oligemic peripheral lung fields, right sided pleural effusion[a]
	Echocardiogram: evidence of abnormal right ventricular structure and/or function. No evidence of increased pulmonary pressure. Septal flattening during diastole but not systole	Echocardiogram: evidence of abnormal right ventricular structure and/or function. *Evidence of increased pulmonary pressure. Septal flattening during* systole

[a]Less commonly found but may occur; *COPD* chronic obstructive pulmonary disease; *ILD* interstitial lung disease. Items appearing in italics occur in the setting of Cor pulmonale but are uncommon in its absence

testing and expense, is guided by the sensitivity and specificity of various clinical findings (see Table 18.5) [6, 7, 9, 10]. Thus, a history of myocardial infarction (MI) is of limited value in advancing the diagnosis of HF where a positive history only slightly increases the probability of HF and a negative history is associated with only a small decrease in probability. Likewise, dependent edema provides minimal help in diagnosing HF. If present, hepatojugular reflux increases the likelihood of HF moderately; absence of this finding does little to reduce the likelihood of HF [7, 10]. HF can be ruled in if jugular venous distention, displacement of cardiac apical pulsation, or a gallop rhythm is present (specificity ≥95%); however, absence of these findings is of limited help in ruling out HF. It is important to note that the ability to detect physical findings of HF depends on proper technique and the skill of the examiner [10]. Chest roentgenogram (CR) and electrocardiogram (EKG) should be obtained in patients with dyspnea and suspected HF. A normal CR marginally decreases the probability of HF and helps identify pulmonary causes of dyspnea. A normal EKG makes HF

unlikely (sensitivity 94%). If both the EKG and CR are normal, HF is highly unlikely (sensitivity 90%), and other etiologies should be entertained [6, 9]. With regard to the EKG, the probability of HF is increased by anterior Q waves or left bundle branch block on the EKG. Therefore, patients with dyspnea and suggestive abnormalities on the EKG or CR should undergo natriuretic peptide testing, if available and/or two-dimensional echocardiography with Doppler flow studies. The echocardiogram is the diagnostic standard for identifying both systolic and diastolic dysfunction. Radionuclide angiography or contrast cineangiography may be helpful if the echocardiogram is equivocal or technically inadequate but will not give detailed information on cardiac structures and flow [11].

Standard laboratory testing may reveal the presence of disorders or conditions that can lead to or exacerbate HF. The initial evaluation of patients with HF should include a complete blood count, urinalysis, serum electrolytes (including calcium and magnesium), glycohemoglobin, and blood lipids, as well as tests of both renal and hepatic function, a CR,

Table 18.5 Sensitivity of clinical findings in the diagnosis of heart failure

Clinical findings [6, 7, 9, 10]	Reference standard	Sensitivity (%)	Specificity (%)
History			
Dyspnea on exertion	LV dysfunction on echocardiogram	100	17
Paroxysmal nocturnal dyspnea	LV dysfunction on echocardiogram	39	80
Previous myocardial infarction	LV dysfunction on echocardiogram	59	86
Physical examination			
Displaced cardiac apex	LV dysfunction on echocardiogram	66	95
Dependent edema	LV dysfunction on echocardiogram	20	86
Gallop rhythm	LV dysfunction on echocardiogram	24	99
Hepatojugular reflux	Clinicoradiographic score	33	94
Jugular venous distention	LV dysfunction on echocardiogram	17	98
Pulmonary rales	LV dysfunction on echocardiogram	29	77
Tests			
Chest roentgenogram: cardiomegaly, pulmonary edema, or both	LV dysfunction on echocardiogram	71	92
EKG: anterior Q waves or LBBB	LV dysfunction on echocardiogram	94	61

and a 12-lead EKG. Thyroid function tests (especially) should be measured, because both hyperthyroidism and hypothyroidism can be a primary or contributory cause of HF. A fasting transferrin saturation is useful to screen for hemochromatosis; several mutated alleles for this disorder are common in individuals of Northern European descent, and affected patients may show improvement in LV function after treatment with phlebotomy and chelating agents. Screening for human immunodeficiency virus (HIV) is reasonable and should be considered for all high-risk patients. However, other clinical signs of HIV infection typically precede any HF symptoms in those patients who develop HIV cardiomyopathy. Serum titers of antibodies developed in response to infectious organisms are occasionally measured in patients with a recent onset of HF (especially in those with a recent viral syndrome), but the yield of such testing is low, and the therapeutic implications of a positive result are uncertain.

Assays for connective tissue diseases and for pheochromocytoma should be performed if these diagnoses are suspected, and serum titers of Chagas disease antibodies should be checked in patients with nonischemic cardiomyopathy who have traveled in or emigrated from an endemic region.

Role of Echocardiography in the Diagnosis of Heart Failure

Two-dimensional echocardiography can detect structural abnormality, systolic dysfunction, diastolic dysfunction, or a combination of these abnormalities that need to be documented in patients who present with resting and/or exertional symptoms suggestive of HF to establish the diagnosis. Indeed, both the ACC/AHA guidelines as well as the European

Society of Cardiology (ESC) guidelines strongly recommend the use of echocardiography in the diagnosis of HF [12, 13].

Heart Failure with Systolic Dysfunction

HF due to systolic dysfunction is relatively easy to diagnose by echocardiography. This demonstrates a dilated left ventricle with a reduced ejection fraction. In systolic HF, however, echocardiography has other roles beyond the recognition of systolic HF since dilatation of the LV results in alteration of intracardiac geometry and hemodynamics and these abnormalities are associated with increased morbidity and mortality [14]. LV dimensions, volumes, and wall thicknesses are echocardiographic measurements widely used in both clinical practice and research. If acceptable parasternal views can be obtained, it is useful to record LV chamber dimensions routinely and to measure wall thickness. In patients with CAD, where segmental wall motion abnormalities may be present, it is not satisfactory to use M mode estimations of ejection fraction. Major wall motion abnormalities should be noted. Provided good visualization of endocardium from apical views is recommended, and it is useful to calculate ejection fraction (EF) using any of the well established methods [15]. If there are major wall motion abnormalities, measurements of EF should be made in both four-chamber and two-chamber views. There is disagreement as to whether measurements of EF should be made, or whether rough "eyeball" estimates of LV global systolic function should be reported instead. Clinicians want this information on which to base treatment decisions but need to realize the limitations of EF measurement, by whatever method, and not base treatment decisions purely on numbers. Echocardiographers need to be aware of clinician's needs for information, and to be as accurate as possible.

Valvular Regurgitation

Cardiac valvular regurgitation, particularly mitral valve regurgitation (MVR), is a common finding in patients with HF. In patients with dilated LV and ischemic cardiomyopathy, the MVR is typically functional and reflects geometric distortions of LV chamber, which displaces the normal valve and subvalvar closing mechanisms [16]. This functional mitral regurgitation is a consequence of adverse LV remodeling and increased sphericity of the chamber. Functional MVR is typically dynamic, occurs with a structurally normal valve, and is a marker of adverse prognosis [17]. MVR increases the propensity for progression of HF. In fact, LV dilatation begets MVR and MVR begets further LV dilatation, progressive remodeling, and contractile dysfunction [18]. The presence and degree of MVR complicating HF are unrelated to the severity of systolic dysfunction. Local LV remodeling (apical and posterior displacement of papillary muscles) leads to excess valvular tenting independent of global LV remodeling. In turn, excess tenting and loss of systolic annular contraction are associated with larger MVR. Tenting is characterized by insufficient systolic leaflet body displacement toward the annulus, with coaptation limited to leaflet tips. Valvular tenting area was measured by the area enclosed between the annular plane and mitral leaflets from the parasternal long-axis view at early and late systole. The distance between leaflet coaptation and the mitral annulus plane at early and end systole measured displacement of mitral coaptation toward the LV apex [16, 18].

Heart Failure with Preserved Systolic Function

As discussed in previous chapters, a large number of patients who suffer from the HF syndrome have preserved systolic function, although there is no universal agreement as to the frequency of this finding [19]. It is assumed that some of these patients have HF because of diastolic dysfunction. The diagnosis of diastolic dysfunction may be problematic. Diagnostic criteria for this type of HF are poorly defined, diastolic dysfunction often is present in patients who also have left ventricular systolic dysfunction, and most patients with diastolic dysfunction have other conditions that could explain their symptoms [20].

Diastolic dysfunction refers to the presence of abnormalities in filling of the ventricle. LV filling consists of a series of hemodynamic events that are affected by multiple intrinsic and extrinsic factors. The initial diastolic event is myocardial relaxation, an active energy-dependent process that causes a decrease rapidly in the pressure of left ventricle after the end of contraction and during early diastole. Doppler echocardio-

graphy is an extremely sensitive tool for the detection and measurement of pressure gradient (driving force) from the left atrium to the LV during diastole. Mitral flow velocities are obtained by pulsed-wave Doppler echocardiography with the sample volume located between the tips of mitral leaflets during diastole. Initial classification of diastolic filling is made from peak velocity of early rapid filling wave (E), peak velocity of late filling wave caused by atrial contraction (A), and E/A ratio. Diastolic filling pattern is characterized further by measuring deceleration time, which is the interval from the peak of E velocity to its extrapolation to the baseline [21]. In the early stages of diastolic dysfunction, impaired (delayed) relaxation of the left ventricle predominates, and this decreases early diastolic filling. An abnormal relaxation pattern is seen on the mitral flow velocity curve and consists of a low E velocity, prolongation of the deceleration time, and increased filling at atrial contraction. The deceleration time is characteristically prolonged because it takes longer for left atrial and LV pressures to be equilibrated with a slower and continued fall in LV pressure until mid to late diastole and a reduced rate of filling during early diastole (E). At this stage, there is little if any increase in rest left ventricular diastolic filling pressure [22]. With disease progression, left atrial pressure increases, thus increasing the driving pressure across the mitral valve. There is a gradual increase in the E velocity on the mitral flow velocity curve. As effective operative compliance decreases, the deceleration time shortens, and a pseudonormal pattern appears. In more advanced disease, the left atrial pressure is higher and ventricular compliance is poor, producing a restriction to filling pattern. Using Doppler technique, pulmonary artery pressure can also often be estimated, if patients have enough tricuspid regurgitation to provide a complete flow/velocity "envelope" [23].

Tissue Doppler imaging (TDI) is an echocardiographic technique with the capacity to quantify systolic and diastolic functions both globally and regionally [24]. TDI is useful for the detection of left ventricular systolic and diastolic dysfunction, because it integrates detailed information of regional function to estimate global cardiac function. Systolic function is one of the most important determinants of diastolic function: in fact systolic and diastolic functions are closely coupled in the cardiac cycle and both are energy-dependent processes. Yu et al. demonstrated that, in patients with diastolic heart failure, there is objective evidence of impaired left ventricular systolic function as demonstrated by TDI [25]. In these patients, the regional function, assessed by mitral annulus peak systolic velocity, was decreased. The mitral annulus peak systolic velocity appears to be a more sensitive index of early systolic dysfunction than ejection fraction and, hence, in a proportion of these patients the systolic function was labeled as "normal" by conventional methods. This indicates the coexistence of systolic and diastolic dysfunction in a spectrum of different severity in the pathophysiological process of HF. The velocity of annular motion reflects shortening and lengthening of the myocardial fibers along a longitudinal plane. The mitral annulus early diastolic velocity (Ea) is an index of LV relaxation that may not be influenced by left atrial pressure. Ea is lower at the septal annulus (normal >10 cm/s) compared to the lateral annulus (normal >15 cm/s). Using early diastolic velocity of mitral annulus, Nagueh et al. identified patients with relaxation abnormalities independent of the filling pressures and, consequently, differentiated the pseudonormal from the normal LV filling pattern [26]. Furthermore, the ratio of the transmitral E velocity of mitral flow and early diastolic velocity of mitral annulus is related significantly with pulmonary capillary wedge pressure, suggesting that this measurement can be used as an index of filling pressures.

Other Diagnostic Tests

Other tests may be used to provide information regarding the nature and severity of the cardiac abnormality. Radionuclide ventriculography (RVG) can provide highly accurate measurements of LV function and RVEF, but it is unable to directly assess valvular abnormalities or cardiac hypertrophy as in echocardiography. Magnetic resonance imaging (MRI) or computed tomography (CT) may be useful in evaluating chamber size and ventricular mass, detecting RV dysplasia, or recognizing the presence of pericardial disease, as well as in assessing cardiac function and wall motion [27]. Magnetic resonance imaging is also used to identify myocarditis, myocardial viability and scar tissue [28].

Biomarkers in the Diagnosis of Heart Failure

The diagnosis of HF is usually based on history, physical examination, CR and if available, LV function assessment. However, diagnosing HF based on conventional measures may be exceedingly difficult. LV function assessment may not be available and patients with preserved systolic LV function may have unremarkable echocardiographic findings [20, 29]. Indeed, many studies have demonstrated that making a diagnosis of HF based on clinical assessment and standard testing may be inadequate [30–33]. Therefore, there has been great effort to develop biomarkers that would offer incremental value to conventional tools to establish rapid and accurate diagnosis and risk stratification of patients with HF.

The term "biomarker" was first introduced in the late 1980s as a subject heading term: "measurable and quantifiable biological parameters … which serve as indices for health- and physiology-related assessments" [34]. In 2001, a National Institute of Health working group standardized the definition as "a characteristic that is objectively measured and evaluated as an indicator of normal biological processes, pathogenic processes, or pharmacologic responses to a therapeutic intervention" [35]. Indeed, one application of biomarkers is in the management of HF. To date, the only biomarkers that have been developed for clinical use in HF are the natriuretic peptides (NP). The NP family consists of the atrial natriuretic peptide (ANP), B-type or brain natriuretic peptide (BNP), and three other structurally similar peptides: C-type natriuretic peptide mostly of central nervous system and endothelial origin, urodilatin from the kidney and dendroaspis NP which is of unknown significance [36–38]. BNP and the amino-terminal fragment of the prohormone, NT-proBNP, have evolved to be useful biomarkers of cardiac function as well as prognosis in HF and other cardiovascular (CV) disorders. Studies have established a close association between the blood level of BNP and NT-proBNP, and the diagnosis of HF [32, 39–42] as well as an independent prediction of mortality and subsequent HF events [43–47]. Use of BNP/NT-proBNP as an adjunct to clinical evaluation in diagnosis of HF particularly in the acute setting has been recommended in the HF management guidelines of several countries [48–53]. Cumulative evidence to date attesting to the utility of BNP and NT-proBNP as a diagnostic and prognostic marker in acute HF have been summarized in recent reviews and consensus recommendations[38, 53–55]. In practice, measurements of BNP and NT-proBNP essentially offer the same performance with optimal values typically providing 98% or better negative predictive value, sensitivities of 90%, specificity and positive predictive values of about 80%, and areas under receiver-operator curves (ROC) of >0.85 [41, 56–59]. A recent study that took combined measurements of BNP and NT-proBNP levels in the renal arteries and veins of hypertensive subjects undergoing renal arteriography has suggested that both BNP and NT-proBNP are equally dependent on renal function and clearance [60].

Accompanying the observational data is increasing evidence from randomized controlled trial (RCT) supporting a concept that the provision of knowledge of plasma BNP/NT-proBNP levels may be translated to improved overall management of patients with acute HF. The Acute Shortness of Breath Evaluation (BASEL) study was a single centre prospective, RCT of 452 patients presenting to an emergency department (ED) in Basel, Switzerland, with acute dyspnea [61, 62]. Two hundred twenty-five patients were randomized to a strategy with measurement of BNP levels and 227 were assessed in a standard manner. The use of BNP levels reduced the need for hospitalization. The median time to discharge was 8.0 days in the BNP group and 11.0 days in the control group. The mean total cost was US$5,410 in the BNP group versus $7,264 in the control group. Up until recently, studies, particularly those that studied NT-proBNP had either involved small

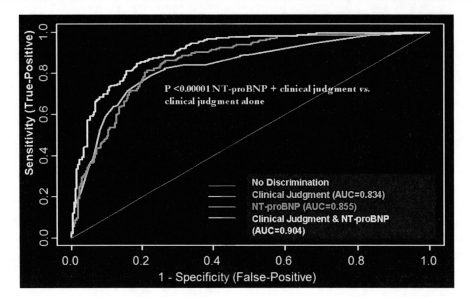

Fig. 18.1 Natriuretic peptide testing enhances the diagnostic performance of clinical evaluation. Receiver-operating characteristics (ROC) curves comparing the sensitivity and specificity of clinical judgment alone, NT-proBNP testing and the two combined are shown in this slide. Clinical judgment alone using different level of certainty generated an AUC of 0.834, 95% CI 0.80–0.84, $P<0.001$ (Clinician assessment of acute HF could also be expressed as a binary outcome. The sensitivity in this case was 78% whereas the specificity was 81%). Adding NT-proBNP results to those of clinical judgment alone significantly improved the performance, increasing the AUC to 0.904, 95% CI 0.90–0.93, $P<0.0001$ ($P=0.00001$ versus clinical judgment). Although not a pre-specified analysis, when compared to clinical judgment alone, NT-proBNP results (AUC 0.855, 95% CI 0.84–0.89, $P<0.001$) was numerically superior to ED physician estimated likelihood of acute HF, the difference was not statistically significant

number of patients [63, 64], were conducted in single centers [39, 64, 65], or were not randomized in design [41]. The larger scale studies of BNP and NT-proBNP were conducted mostly in the US [39, 41] where per capita health care spending is higher than other countries [64]. These data, while important, were not necessarily applicable to countries with publicly funded universal healthcare coverage systems [65]. These concerns prompted the design of the multicenter Improved Management of Patient with Congestive Heart Failure (IMPROVE-CHF) study. This prospective RCT was designed to test the hypothesis that a strategy that included knowledge of NT-proBNP results would improve the management of patients with suspected acute HF [42]. The specific aims were to evaluate: (1) whether NT-proBNP added incremental value to clinical judgment in diagnosing acute HF; and (2) whether a management strategy that incorporated knowledge of NT-proBNP results would lead to cost-savings without compromising clinical outcomes. Five hundred patients presenting with dyspnea to seven emergency departments were studied. For the diagnosis of acute HF, adding NT-proBNP to clinical judgment enhanced accuracy, the area under the ROC curve increased from 0.83 to 0.90 ($P<0.00001$) (Fig. 18.1). Knowledge of NT-proBNP values reduced the duration of ED visit by 21% (6.3–5.6 h, $P=0.031$), number of patients readmitted over 60 days by 35% (51 to 33, $P=0.046$) and direct medical cost of ED visits, hospitalizations, and outpatient services (US$6,129 to $5,180 per patient, $P=0.023$). The recommended cut points for ruling in and ruling out a diagnosis of HF in patients presenting with dyspnea and based on the results of some of the above studies are shown in Fig. 18.2.

Conclusions

Heart failure is a complex clinical syndrome that can result from any structural or functional cardiac disorder that impairs the ability of the ventricle to fill with or eject blood. The cardinal manifestations of HF are dyspnea and fatigue, which may limit exercise tolerance, and fluid retention, which may lead to pulmonary congestion and peripheral edema. Both abnormalities can impair the functional capacity and quality of life of affected individuals, but they do not necessarily dominate the clinical picture at the same time. Although HF is a clinical diagnosis, there may be widespread inaccuracies in diagnosis when clinical methods alone are used. Many patients in whom the diagnosis is made, particularly in the primary care setting, may turn out not to have the condition upon further investigation. More advanced and newer diagnostic modalities such as echocardiography and natriuretic peptides testing may be extremely useful and complimentary to clinical evaluation. These tests yield the best results when used in the appropriate patient groups. Radionuclide angiography or contrast cineangiography may be necessary when clinical suspicion for heart failure is high and the echocardiogram is equivocal.

	Age (years)	HF is unlikely	HF is possible but other diagnoses need to be considered	HF is highly likely
BNP	All	< 100 pg/ml	100-500 pg/ml	> 500 pg/ml
NT-proBNP	< 50	< 300 pg/ml	300-450 pg/ml	> 450 pg/ml
	50 - 75	< 300 pg/ml	450-900 pg/ml	> 900 pg/ml
	> 75	< 300 pg/ml	900-1800 pg/ml	> 1800 pg/ml

Fig. 18.2 BNP and NT-proBNP assay cut points for the diagnosis of acute heart failure. *HF* heart failure

Summary

- Heart failure is defined by an inability of the myocardium to deliver sufficient oxygenated blood to meet the needs of tissues and organs during exercise or at rest.
- Evaluation of patients with suspected HF is directed at confirming the diagnosis, determining the cause, identifying concomitant illnesses, establishing the severity of HF, and ultimately guiding therapy. Heart failure is a clinical diagnosis, and no single test can establish its presence or absence.
- Coronary heart disease accounts for most cases of HF, followed by diabetes mellitus and valvular heart disease.
- Heart failure also can be multifactorial i.e., the syndrome can result from MI (loss of myocardial contractility) with papillary muscle dysfunction (increased preload) and acute pulmonary edema (hypoxemia).
- Heart failure may also be classified into several types based on the role of diastolic or systolic dysfunction and based on the anatomic area of involvement.
- In patients with HF, the most frequent clinical findings are related to decreased exercise tolerance or fluid retention. Fluid retention results in orthopnea, rales, elevated jugular venous pressure, dependent edema, and the typical radiographic findings of cardiomegaly, pulmonary edema, and pleural effusion. There currently are no validated clinical decision rules to estimate the contribution of each of these findings to HF.
- Nearly all patients with HF present with dyspnea. Thus, the absence of dyspnea makes HF highly unlikely. A focused history and physical examination, combined with selected diagnostic testing, therefore can identify HF in most instances.
- Two dimensional echocardiography can detect structural abnormality, systolic dysfunction, diastolic dysfunction, regurgitant flow, or a combination of these abnormalities that need to be documented in patients who present with resting and/or exertional symptoms suggestive of HF to establish the diagnosis.
- Tissue Doppler imaging has the capacity to quantify systolic and diastolic functions both globally and regionally. It is particularly useful for the detection of left ventricular systolic and diastolic dysfunction, because it integrates detailed information of regional function to estimate global cardiac function.
- In spite of the rapid development of new techniques, due to high cost and the need for skilled technicians, in the absence of some other clinical indication, such as a prior myocardial infarction, abnormality of electrocardiogram, family history of cardiomyopathy, or HF symptoms, routine comprehensive echocardiography cannot be recommended at present.
- Diagnosing HF based on conventional measures may at times be quite difficult. LV function assessment may not be available and patients with preserved systolic LV function may have unremarkable echocardiographic findings.
- There has been great effort to develop biomarkers that would offer incremental value to conventional tools to establish rapid and accurate diagnosis and risk stratification of patients with HF. To date, the only biomarkers that have been developed for clinical use in HF are the natriuretic peptides (NP).
- BNP and the amino-terminal fragment of the prohormone, NT-proBNP, have evolved to be useful biomarkers of cardiac function as well as prognosis in HF and other cardiovascular disorders. Studies have established a close association between the blood level of BNP and NT-proBNP, and the diagnosis of HF as well as an independent prediction of mortality and subsequent HF events.
- Use of BNP/NT-proBNP as an adjunct to clinical evaluation in diagnosis of HF particularly in the acute setting has been recommended in the HF management guidelines.

References

1. Hunt SA, Baker DW, Chin MH et al (2001) ACC/AHA guidelines for the evaluation and management of chronic heart failure in the adult: executive summary. A report of the American College of Cardiology/American Heart Association Task Force on Practice Guidelines (Committee to revise the 1995 Guidelines for the Evaluation and Management of Heart Failure). J Am Coll Cardiol 38:2101–2113
2. Pfeffer MA, Braunwald E, Moye LA et al (1992) Effect of captopril on mortality and morbidity in patients with left ventricular dysfunction after myocardial infarction. Results of the survival and ventricular enlargement trial. The SAVE Investigators. N Engl J Med 327:669–677
3. Wang TJ, Levy D, Benjamin EJ, Vasan RS (2003) The epidemiology of "asymptomatic" left ventricular systolic dysfunction: implications for screening. Ann Intern Med 138:907–916
4. Gheorghiade M, Bonow RO (1998) Chronic heart failure in the United States: a manifestation of coronary artery disease. Circulation 97:282–289

5. Haddad F, Hunt SA, Rosenthal DN, Murphy DJ (2008) Right ventricular function in cardiovascular disease, part I: anatomy, physiology, aging, and functional assessment of the right ventricle. Circulation 117:1436–1448

6. Davie AP, Francis CM, Love MP, Caruana L, Starkey IR, Shaw TR, Sutherland GR, McMurray JJ (1996) Value of the electrocardiogram in identifying heart failure due to left ventricular systolic dysfunction. BMJ 312:222

7. Davie AP, Francis CM, Caruana L, Sutherland GR, McMurray JJ (1997) Assessing diagnosis in heart failure: which features are any use? QJM 90:335–339

8. Mulrow CD, Lucey CR, Farnett LE (1993) Discriminating causes of dyspnea through clinical examination. J Gen Intern Med 8: 383–392

9. Gillespie ND, McNeill G, Pringle T, Ogston S, Struthers AD, Pringle SD (1997) Cross sectional study of contribution of clinical assessment and simple cardiac investigations to diagnosis of left ventricular systolic dysfunction in patients admitted with acute dyspnoea. BMJ 314:936–940

10. Cook DJ, Simel DL (1996) The Rational Clinical Examination. Does this patient have abnormal central venous pressure? JAMA 275:630–634

11. Naik MM, Diamond GA, Pai T, Soffer A, Siegel RJ (1995) Correspondence of left ventricular ejection fraction determinations from two-dimensional echocardiography, radionuclide angiography and contrast cineangiography. J Am Coll Cardiol 25:937–942

12. Dickstein K, Cohen-Solal A, Filippatos G et al (2008) ESC Guidelines for the diagnosis and treatment of acute and chronic heart failure 2008: the Task Force for the Diagnosis and Treatment of Acute and Chronic Heart Failure 2008 of the European Society of Cardiology. Developed in collaboration with the Heart Failure Association of the ESC (HFA) and endorsed by the European Society of Intensive Care Medicine (ESICM). Eur Heart J 29: 2388–2442

13. Hunt SA, Abraham WT, Chin MH et al (2009) 2009 Focused update incorporated into the ACC/AHA 2005 Guidelines for the Diagnosis and Management of Heart Failure in Adults A Report of the American College of Cardiology Foundation/American Heart Association Task Force on Practice Guidelines Developed in Collaboration With the International Society for Heart and Lung Transplantation. J Am Coll Cardiol 53:e1–e90

14. St John SM, Pfeffer MA, Plappert T et al (1994) Quantitative two-dimensional echocardiographic measurements are major predictors of adverse cardiovascular events after acute myocardial infarction. The protective effects of captopril. Circulation 89:68–75

15. Schiller NB, Shah PM, Crawford M et al (1989) Recommendations for quantitation of the left ventricle by two-dimensional echocardiography. American Society of Echocardiography Committee on Standards, Subcommittee on Quantitation of Two-Dimensional Echocardiograms. J Am Soc Echocardiogr 2:358–367

16. Yiu SF, Enriquez-Sarano M, Tribouilloy C, Seward JB, Tajik AJ (2000) Determinants of the degree of functional mitral regurgitation in patients with systolic left ventricular dysfunction: a quantitative clinical study. Circulation 102:1400–1406

17. Lancellotti P, Gerard PL, Pierard LA (2005) Long-term outcome of patients with heart failure and dynamic functional mitral regurgitation. Eur Heart J 26:1528–1532

18. Trichon BH, Felker GM, Shaw LK, Cabell CH, O'Connor CM (2003) Relation of frequency and severity of mitral regurgitation to survival among patients with left ventricular systolic dysfunction and heart failure. Am J Cardiol 91:538–543

19. Aguirre FV, Pearson AC, Lewen MK, McCluskey M, Labovitz AJ (1989) Usefulness of Doppler echocardiography in the diagnosis of congestive heart failure. Am J Cardiol 63:1098–1102

20. Caruana L, Petrie MC, Davie AP, McMurray JJ (2000) Do patients with suspected heart failure and preserved left ventricular systolic function suffer from "diastolic heart failure" or from misdiagnosis? A prospective descriptive study. BMJ 321: 215–218

21. Garcia MJ, Thomas JD, Klein AL (1998) New Doppler echocardiographic applications for the study of diastolic function. J Am Coll Cardiol 32:865–875

22. Nishimura RA, Appleton CP, Redfield MM, Ilstrup DM, Holmes DR Jr, Tajik AJ (1996) Noninvasive Doppler echocardiographic evaluation of left ventricular filling pressures in patients with cardiomyopathies: a simultaneous Doppler echocardiographic and cardiac catheterization study. J Am Coll Cardiol 28:1226–1233

23. Yock PG, Popp RL (1984) Noninvasive estimation of right ventricular systolic pressure by Doppler ultrasound in patients with tricuspid regurgitation. Circulation 70:657–662

24. Yu CM, Sanderson JE, Marwick TH, Oh JK (2007) Tissue Doppler imaging a new prognosticator for cardiovascular diseases. J Am Coll Cardiol 49:1903–1914

25. Yu CM, Lin H, Yang H, Kong SL, Zhang Q, Lee SW (2002) Progression of systolic abnormalities in patients with "isolated" diastolic heart failure and diastolic dysfunction. Circulation 105:1195–1201

26. Nagueh SF, Middleton KJ, Kopelen HA, Zoghbi WA, Quinones MA (1997) Doppler tissue imaging: a noninvasive technique for evaluation of left ventricular relaxation and estimation of filling pressures. J Am Coll Cardiol 30:1527–1533

27. Ritchie JL, Bateman TM, Bonow RO et al (1995) Guidelines for clinical use of cardiac radionuclide imaging. Report of the American College of Cardiology/American Heart Association Task Force on Assessment of Diagnostic and Therapeutic Cardiovascular Procedures (Committee on Radionuclide Imaging), developed in collaboration with the American Society of Nuclear Cardiology. J Am Coll Cardiol 25:521–547

28. Bello D, Shah DJ, Farah GM et al (2003) Gadolinium cardiovascular magnetic resonance predicts reversible myocardial dysfunction and remodeling in patients with heart failure undergoing beta-blocker therapy. Circulation 108:1945–1953

29. Cabanes L, Richaud-Thiriez B, Fulla Y, Heloire F, Vuillemard C, Weber S, Dusser D (2001) Brain natriuretic peptide blood levels in the differential diagnosis of dyspnea. Chest 120: 2047–2050

30. Remes J, Miettinen H, Reunanen A, Pyorala K (1991) Validity of clinical diagnosis of heart failure in primary health care. Eur Heart J 12:315–321

31. Stevenson LW, Perloff JK (1989) The limited reliability of physical signs for estimating hemodynamics in chronic heart failure. JAMA 261:884–888

32. McCullough PA, Nowak RM, McCord J et al (2002) B-type natriuretic peptide and clinical judgment in emergency diagnosis of heart failure: analysis from Breathing Not Properly (BNP) Multinational Study. Circulation 106:416–422

33. Thomas JT, Kelly RF, Thomas SJ, Stamos TD, Albasha K, Parrillo JE, Calvin JE (2002) Utility of history, physical examination, electrocardiogram, and chest radiograph for differentiating normal from decreased systolic function in patients with heart failure. Am J Med 112:437–445

34. Vasan RS (2006) Biomarkers of cardiovascular disease: molecular basis and practical considerations. Circulation 113:2335–2362

35. (2001) Biomarkers and surrogate endpoints: preferred definitions and conceptual framework. Clin Pharmacol Ther 69:89–95

36. Clerico A, Emdin M (2004) Diagnostic accuracy and prognostic relevance of the measurement of cardiac natriuretic peptides: a review. Clin Chem 50:33–50

37. Levin ER, Gardner DG, Samson WK (1998) Natriuretic peptides. N Engl J Med 339:321–328

38. Moe GW (2005) BNP in the Diagnosis and Risk Stratification of Heart Failure. Heart Fail Monit 4:116–122

39. Januzzi JL Jr, Camargo CA, Anwaruddin S et al (2005) The N-terminal Pro-BNP investigation of dyspnea in the emergency department (PRIDE) study. Am J Cardiol 95:948–954

40. Maisel A, Hollander JE, Guss D et al (2004) Primary results of the Rapid Emergency Department Heart Failure Outpatient Trial (REDHOT). A multicenter study of B-type natriuretic peptide levels, emergency department decision making, and outcomes in patients presenting with shortness of breath. J Am Coll Cardiol 44:1328–1333

41. Maisel AS, Krishnaswamy P, Nowak RM et al (2002) Rapid measurement of B-type natriuretic peptide in the emergency diagnosis of heart failure. N Engl J Med 347:161–167

42. Moe GW, Howlett J, Januzzi JL, Zowall H (2007) N-terminal pro-B-type natriuretic peptide testing improves the management of patients with suspected acute heart failure: primary results of the Canadian prospective randomized multicenter IMPROVE-CHF study. Circulation 115:3103–3110

43. Januzzi JL (2006) van KR, Lainchbury J, Bayes-Genis A, Ordonez-Llanos J, Santalo-Bel M, Pinto YM, Richards M. NT-proBNP testing for diagnosis and short-term prognosis in acute destabilized heart failure: an international pooled analysis of 1256 patients: the International Collaborative of NT-proBNP Study. Eur Heart J 27:330–337

44. Januzzi JL Jr, Sakhuja R, O'Donoghue M et al (2006) Utility of amino-terminal pro-brain natriuretic peptide testing for prediction of 1-year mortality in patients with dyspnea treated in the emergency department. Arch Intern Med 166:315–320

45. Anand IS, Fisher LD, Chiang YT et al (2003) Changes in brain natriuretic peptide and norepinephrine over time and mortality and morbidity in the Valsartan Heart Failure Trial (Val-HeFT). Circulation 107:1278–1283

46. Fisher C, Berry C, Blue L, Morton JJ, McMurray J (2003) N-terminal pro B type natriuretic peptide, but not the new putative cardiac hormone relaxin, predicts prognosis in patients with chronic heart failure. Heart 89:879–881

47. Harrison A, Morrison LK, Krishnaswamy P et al (2002) B-type natriuretic peptide predicts future cardiac events in patients presenting to the emergency department with dyspnea. Ann Emerg Med 39:131–138

48. (2006) Executive summary: HFSA 2006 Comprehensive Heart Failure Practice Guideline. J Card Fail 12:10–38

49. Hunt SA, Abraham WT, Chin MH et al (2005) ACC/AHA 2005 Guideline Update for the Diagnosis and Management of Chronic Heart Failure in the Adult – Summary Article: A Report of the American College of Cardiology/American Heart Association Task Force on Practice Guidelines (Writing Committee to Update the 2001 Guidelines for the Evaluation and Management of Heart Failure): Developed in Collaboration With the American College of Chest Physicians and the International Society for Heart and Lung Transplantation: Endorsed by the Heart Rhythm Society. Circulation 112:1825–1852

50. Nieminen MS, Bohm M, Cowie MR et al (2005) Executive summary of the guidelines on the diagnosis and treatment of acute heart failure: the Task Force on Acute Heart Failure of the European Society of Cardiology. Eur Heart J 26:384–416

51. Remme WJ, Swedberg K (2001) Guidelines for the diagnosis and treatment of chronic heart failure. Eur Heart J 22:1527–1560

52. Arnold JM, Liu P, Demers C et al (2006) Canadian Cardiovascular Society consensus conference recommendations on heart failure 2006: diagnosis and management. Can J Cardiol 22:23–45

53. Arnold JM, Howlett JG, Dorian P et al (2007) Canadian Cardiovascular Society Consensus Conference recommendations on heart failure update 2007: prevention, management during intercurrent illness or acute decompensation, and use of biomarkers. Can J Cardiol 23:21–45

54. Moe GW (2002) Natriuretic peptide in heart failure. In: Braunwald E, Fauci AS, Isselbacher KJ et al (eds) Harrison's online. McGraw-Hill, New York

55. Januzzi JL Jr, Chen-Tournoux AA, Moe G (2008) Amino-terminal pro-B-type natriuretic peptide testing for the diagnosis or exclusion of heart failure in patients with acute symptoms. Am J Cardiol 101:29–38

56. Cowie MR, Struthers AD, Wood DA, Coats AJ, Thompson SG, Poole-Wilson PA, Sutton GC (1997) Value of natriuretic peptides in assessment of patients with possible new heart failure in primary care. Lancet 350:1349–1353

57. Dao Q, Krishnaswamy P, Kazanegra R et al (2001) Utility of B-type natriuretic peptide in the diagnosis of congestive heart failure in an urgent-care setting. J Am Coll Cardiol 37:379–385

58. Davis M, Espiner E, Richards G et al (1994) Plasma brain natriuretic peptide in assessment of acute dyspnoea. Lancet 343:440–444

59. Lainchbury JG, Campbell E, Frampton CM, Yandle TG, Nicholls MG, Richards AM (2003) Brain natriuretic peptide and n-terminal brain natriuretic peptide in the diagnosis of heart failure in patients with acute shortness of breath. J Am Coll Cardiol 42:728–735

60. van Kimmenade RR, Januzzi JL Jr, Bakker JA et al (2009) Renal clearance of B-type natriuretic peptide and amino terminal pro-B-type natriuretic peptide a mechanistic study in hypertensive subjects. J Am Coll Cardiol 53:884–890

61. Mueller C, Scholer A, Laule-Kilian K et al (2004) Use of B-type natriuretic peptide in the evaluation and management of acute dyspnea. N Engl J Med 350:647–654

62. Mueller C, Laule-Kilian K, Schindler C et al (2006) Cost-effectiveness of B-type natriuretic peptide testing in patients with acute dyspnea. Arch Intern Med 166:1081–1087

63. Bayes-Genis A, Santalo-Bel M, Zapico-Muniz E et al (2004) N-terminal probrain natriuretic peptide (NT-proBNP) in the emergency diagnosis and in-hospital monitoring of patients with dyspnoea and ventricular dysfunction. Eur J Heart Fail 6:301–308

64. Lainchbury JG, Yandle TG, Campbell E, Richards M (2003) Brain natriuretic peptide and N-terminal brain natriuretic peptide in the diagnosis of heart failure in patients with acute shortness of breath (abstract). J Am Coll Cardiol 41:184A

65. Lasser KE, Himmelstein DU, Woolhandler S (2006) Access to care, health status, and health disparities in the United States and Canada: results of a cross-national population-based survey. Am J Public Health 96:1300–1307

Chapter 19

"Omics" Application in Heart Failure: Novel Diagnostic and Prognostic Markers to Understand Pathophysiology and Find New Therapies

Overview

Using conventional tools such as history, physical examination, and radiographic and echocardiographic evaluations, a diagnosis of the HF syndrome is usually not difficult [Chap. 18]. However, because of low specificity, the value of these conventional tools to identify etiologies and prognosis, is in general relatively limited. Thus, there is a need for new methods that together with establishing the genetic makeup of the individual can also provide information about potential changes in protein and transcript expression related to the interaction of genes and their environment. The term "-omics" is employed to describe a field of study in biology such as genomics or proteomics. The related neologism "ome" addresses the objects of study of such fields, such as the genome, transcriptome, or proteome, or other molecular components of cells, tissues, or organisms. In this chapter, we discuss the use of these technologies and others that are either presently at our disposal or in the developmental phase.

Introduction

The diagnosis of HF may be rather difficult using only conventional tools (i.e., history, physical examination, chest radiogram, and echocardiogram). As previously discussed in Chap. 18, the availability of cardiac biomarkers, most notably B-type or brain natriuretic peptide (BNP), had proved to be extremely helpful in HF diagnosis. Indeed, the cardiac natriuretic peptides, particularly BNP, are useful biomarkers not only in the assessment of cardiac function but also in the prognostication of HF as well as in other cardiovascular diseases (CVDs). Several observations have shown the close relationship between plasma BNP and the N-terminal fragment of the BNP prohormone (NT-proBNP) with the diagnosis of HF, and as an independent prediction of short-term mortality and HF events [1–5]. Preliminary data from randomized controlled trials suggest that the knowledge of BNP and/or NT-proBNP level can improve the management of patients with HF, and large-scale randomized controlled tri-

als that evaluate BNP/NT-proBNP-guided therapy are currently underway.

In HF, there is activation of neurohormones and proinflammatory cytokines, which likely mediate its progression (i.e., the neurohormone and cytokine hypotheses) [6, 7]. The number of circulating biomarkers of neurohormone and cytokine activation is increasing and some of these biomarkers are known to be prognostic in patients with HF [6, 8], but none of these biomarkers, except for BNP and NT-proBNP, have been used extensively in clinical practice, particularly as they relate to clinical decision-making. Notwithstanding, besides BNP and TNF-α, more specific genetic markers are required, not only for the diagnosis of specific cardiomyopathy (as opposed to HF in general) or specific etiologies of HF but also to establish a more accurate prognosis since traditional risk assessments tools are rather limited. Previously, in Chap. 3, we have examined the current use of microarrays for gene/transcriptome profiling and protein biomarkers in HF. In this chapter, we have further discussed these and other emergent technologies, which can be complementary to techniques such as genomics and proteomics and aimed at improving the identification of the etiology, diagnosis, and prognosis of HF.

Use of Gene Profiling and Proteomics in HF

At the outset, it suffices to say that while not as easy or convenient to perform as the screening of circulating biomarkers, the use of gene/transcriptome profiling in HF patients with or without dysrhythmias may provide important information that is unavailable with other approaches and may augment the growing list of important (and novel) biomarkers. For example, using micoarray technology for transcriptional profiling of genes modulated in patients with atrial fibrillation (AF), a group of 33 AF-specific genes that were significantly activated were identified in comparison to patients in sinus rhythm used as controls [9]. These genes encode proteins with multiple functions such as ion channel, antioxidant, inflammatory, cell growth/cell cycle, transcription factors (e.g., NF-κB), and cell signaling. On the other hand, 63 sinus rhythm-specific genes were identified, including several genes with cell signaling function (such as SERCA 2), cellular respiration, energy production, and antiproliferative or negative regulator of cell growth. This gene profiling will allow further inroads in understanding the role that modulated the expression of these genes plays in the initiation or perpetuation of AF either isolated or in association to HF. In addition, gene profiling may allow the assessment of the gene-specific contribution to the pathophysiological mechanism of atrial remodeling as well as furnishing potential biomarkers that could be useful in the prediction of AF.

As previously mentioned, a large number of inflammatory mediators including circulating inflammatory cytokines (e.g., IL-6 and TNF-α) or the hepatic product C-reactive protein are useful biomarkers of long-term cardiovascular risk in apparently healthy populations and in those with already established CVD. Previously, it has been shown that T cells from HF patients exhibit enhanced gene expression of chemokines, ligands for the tumor necrosis factor superfamily, as well as inflammatory cytokines, interferon-γ and interleukin-18, with a pattern that appears similar in ischemic and DCM of unknown etiology. On the other hand, no differences in cytokine gene expression were found in monocytes from HF patients compared to controls [10]. Interestingly, T-cells from HF patients had enhanced surface expression of the activation markers CD69 and CD25, while there was no upregulation of the monocyte activation marker CD32. These observations suggest that T cells may be part of the inflammatory response during HF but they are independent of its etiology. Thus, chemokines gene expression can be useful to establish the etiology of HF, and the blocking of the activation of unwanted T cells might also be a new target for the treatment of HF.

Experimentally, it has been demonstrated that cardiac cytokine gene expression profiling by microarray technology can be very helpful in the evaluation and diagnosis of HF pathogenesis. Using microarray technology, Husberg et al. have recently reported alterations in gene expression during HF progression in noninfarcted left ventricular (LV) murine tissue at various time points after myocardial infarction (MI) [11]. The highest number of regulated genes was found 5 days after MI. They identified 14 regulated genes encoding cytokines with no previous association to HF. The strongest upregulation was found for the chemokine fractalkine (CX3CL1). Screening human failing hearts, they detected a threefold increase in CX3CL1 protein production, and both cardiomyocytes and fibrous tissue showed immunoreactivity for CX3CL1 and its specific receptor CX3CR1. The circulating level of CX3CL1 was also increased in patients with HF and was related to its severity (1.6-fold in New York Heart Association (NYHA) II, 2.2-fold in NYHA III and 2.9-fold in NYHA IV). CX3CL1 production could be induced in in vitro experiments by inflammatory cytokines known to be highly

expressed in HF. CX3CL1 itself induced the expression of markers of cardiac hypertrophy and protein phosphatases in neonatal cardiomyocytes. Taken together, the findings of increased CX3CL1 production in both experimental animal model and in patients with HF, plus its direct effects on cardiomyocytes suggest that CX3CL1 and its receptor CX3CR1 have a role in the pathogenesis of HF and may potentially serve as biomarkers.

While circulating biomarkers are generally produced from blood–borne cells (e.g., macrophages and T cells), retained in the intima layer and activated resident cells of vascular origin (e.g., endothelial cells), inflammatory mediators originating outside the coronary artery are capable of inducing compositional changes in the intima layer. Such inflammatory mediators originating from remote extravascular sources can provide an explanation for the increased cardiovascular risk in certain patient populations, including not only patients with chronic infections or chronic inflammation (e.g., rheumatoid arthritis) but also insulin-resistant individuals who exhibit increased release of cytokines from adipose tissue. In fact, gene profiling has demonstrated increased expression of a panel of inflammatory genes (e.g., MCP-1, IL-6, IL-1β and TNF-α) in epicardial adipose tissue in patients with established coronary artery disease (CAD). Importantly, these inflammatory signals present in epicardial adipose tissue were neither strongly correlated with plasma inflammatory biomarkers nor attenuated by chronic treatment with conventional cardiovascular therapies, including statins or ACE inhibitors/angiotensin II receptor blockers [12]. While these findings are suggestive that the presence of inflammatory mediators, and bioactive molecules, in the localized tissues surrounding epicardial coronary arteries may profoundly alter arterial homeostasis (e.g., leading to amplification of vascular inflammation or plaque instability) in a manner not revealed by plasma biomarkers and refractory to some treatment options, they also suggest a fundamental limitation with biomarkers as presently configured. Studies with epicardial fat biopsies from patients undergoing coronary artery bypass grafting (CABG) have extended the genes profiled to include other inflammatory markers such as resistin (a recently identified adipocytokine), CRP, adiponectin, leptin, and the macrophage marker CD45, compared to both plasma levels and other fat depots [12]. These findings revealed increased macrophage infiltration (e.g., increased CD45) into epicardial fat in CABG patients, and they are indicative of significant local inflammation and evidence of a pathogenic gene profile in these tissues, including markedly decreased levels of adiponectin. Adiponectin exhibits both insulin sensitivity and anti-inflammatory and antiatherogenic properties, and its serum levels have been reported to be reduced in both type 2 diabetes mellitus and CAD [13]. Interestingly, the serum profile of CABG patients showed significantly higher levels of both CRP and resistin and significantly lower levels of adiponectin when compared to matched controls.

Delineation of both plasma and genetic biomarkers should prove informative in the clinical setting of stent therapy for the treatment of atherosclerotic CAD, in particular to risk-stratify patients prior to therapy [14]. Prospective risk stratification may allow the rational selection of specialized treatments against the development of in-stent restenosis (ISR), as might be promoted in some individuals by drug-eluting stents. A large scale trial study is presently underway to both understand the molecular mechanisms of restenosis and to identify genetic biomarkers predictive of restenosis. A combined proteomic analysis of plasma and microarray profiling are being used to identify candidate genes that show differential expression. Moreover, the screening of candidate genes to identify variants (e.g., in promoter regions, SNPs, etc.) by genotype analysis can be carried out as well as a genome-wide scan to identify genetic loci that are associated with ISR.

Proteome Analysis in HF

In proteome research, two major approaches have been employed, the complete proteomic approach, in which the entire proteome-(all proteins) are characterized, and a more limited proteomic analysis, which is either targeted to specific candidate proteins or limited to specific classes of proteins or subproteomes [15]. A complete proteomic analysis of plasma proteins while extremely desirable in the long-run is likely unattainable with the presently available proteomic technology. This is largely due to the high sensitivity required to evaluate in depth the plasma proteome, reflecting both the dynamic range of its constituent specific protein levels, such as regulatory factors and cytokines simply undetectable by present proteomic technology, as well as the astonishing level of posttranslational modifications that most proteins undergo. In strong advocacy of a targeted approach, particularly in regard to cardiovascular biomarkers, Anderson has presented a list of 177 candidate proteins, many of which can be simultaneously analyzed using available mass spectrometry (MS) technology (specifically SPE-LC-MS/MS) [16]. This is a widely used methodology for the precise quantitative determination of small molecules such as drugs, drug metabolites, and hormones. It might also be achieved by using multiplex assessment with immunoblot microarrays; however, at present, the use of antibody arrays, which could provide the high sensitivity and specificity required, are limited by the availability (and expense) of suitable antibodies. Analysis by MS/MS techniques focused on examining multiple small peptides generated (by proteolytic digestion) from the larger plasma proteins, would have a high sensitivity, and also it would be extremely rapid and quantitative (compared to other proteomic techniques such as electrophoresis which tend to show great variability in quantitative assessment). Furthermore, the

preselection or prefractionation of a group of candidate proteins may allow the use of assay technologies with higher sensitivity and a greater dynamic range than what is available with current proteomics. The simultaneous profiling analysis of multiple independent disease-related circulating marker proteins and their peptides, considered in the aggregate, would also be less prone to the influence of heterogenous genetic factors and disease processes, as well as environmental "noise" that might impact on the level of a single marker protein, giving a better fingerprint for a disease state.

It has been noted that multiple biomarkers, considered as a composite, may provide better prediction of disease state than single markers (e.g., in the assessment of inflammation with a panel of weak acute phase reactants compared to a single marker such as CRP or serum amyloid A) [17]. Similarly, the relative risk of CAD is better predicted by CRP and LDL-cholesterol together than by either marker alone [18].

Interestingly, a novel cardiac multimarker approach has been used based on protein biochip array technology simultaneously assessing cTnI, CK-MB, myoglobin, carbonic anhydrase III (CAIII), and fatty acid-binding protein (FABP) in a single chip [19]. This methodology has been applied to the clinical diagnosis of acute coronary syndrome (ACS), and the data obtained have showed that FABP had a better diagnostic profile than myoglobin in the detection of acute myocardial infarct (MI) during the first hours after the onset of the chest pain. Furthermore, myoglobin/CAIII ratio, previously noted to be a sensitive and specific marker for perioperative MI [20], significantly improved the myoglobin specificity.

The HUPO Plasma Proteome Project pilot phase has been initiated to accelerate the identification and development of novel cardiovascular biomarkers provided by proteomic profiling of accessible body fluids, such as plasma. Launched from multiple laboratories worldwide, this project incorporates data derived from the analyses of human plasma using a myriad of distinct proteomic approaches. A subset of the 3,020 proteins thus far identified (by MS/MS spectra) are related to cardiovascular function and have been organized into eight groups: markers of inflammation and/or CVD, vascular and coagulation, signaling, growth and differentiation, cytoskeletal, transcription factors, channels/receptors and HF, and remodeling [21]. The functional annotation of these proteins and structural analyses are available as a shared database and constitute a significant resource for further development of molecular biosignatures for diseases such as myocardial ischemia and atherosclerosis [22]. This type of analysis has emerged in several areas of cardiovascular medicine/biology. For example, Serum Proteomic Pattern Diagnostics is a new type of proteomic platform in which patterns of proteomic signatures from MS data are used as a diagnostic classifier [23]. This approach has shown promise in early detection of cancers and recently has also been applied in the detection of anthracycline-induced cardiotoxicity using analysis of serum proteins from rats. This new technology emphasized the clinical utility of diagnostic proteomic patterns in which low molecular weight peptides and protein fragments may have higher accuracy than traditional biomarkers of cardiotoxicity such as troponin.

The use of proteome analysis has been expanded to include the assessment of HF prognosis. For example, to predict clinical deterioration of HF patients, Sugiura et al. measured circulating levels of myocardium-specific proteins [24]. Seventy-eight patients with advanced HF from DCM in stable conditions were enrolled, and blood levels of myosin light chain-I (MLC-I), troponin T (TnT), heart fatty acid-binding protein (H-FABP), and creatine kinase isoenzyme MB (CK-MB) were measured. Patients were followed up for 951 ± 68 days, with the endpoint being acute deterioration. Univariate analysis revealed that MLC-I, TnT, H-FABP, and CK-MB were significant predictors for acute deterioration of HF. Application of the Kaplan–Meier method using cutoff values determined by analysis of receiver operating characteristics curves demonstrated that the incidence of acute deterioration was significantly higher in patients with higher values of MLC-I (61.9%), TnT (52.4%), H-FABP (50.0%), or CK-MB (38.6%) than in those with lower values of these markers (15.8, 20.4, 13.6, and 16.1%, respectively). These data suggest that increased circulating levels of the specific myocardial proteins are related to a higher probability of future acute deterioration in HF patients in a stable condition associated with DCM.

It has been proposed that cytosolic marker H-FABP is more sensitive than TnT in the detection of ongoing myocardial damage (OMD) in HF patients. Niizeki et al. have measured serum H-FABP and TnT levels in 126 consecutive HF patients at admission and were followed-up with a mean period of 474 ± 328 days [25]. Cutoff values for H-FABP (4.3 ng/mL) and TnT (0.01 ng/mL) were determined from previous studies. Positive rate of H-FABP was higher than that of TnT in all HF patients (46% (58/126) versus 26% (33/126), $P < 0.0001$), and in severe HF (New York Heart Association III/IV) patients (69% (34/49) versus 47% (23/49), $P = 0.0121$). There were 27 cardiac events during the follow-up period. In patients with cardiac events, H-FABP was more frequently detected than TnT (88% (24/27) versus 44% (12/27), $P = 0.0103$). There were 33 patients with positive H-FABP among 93 patients with negative TnT. These patients had greater NYHA functional class, higher levels of BNP, and higher rates of cardiac events (36% versus 5%, $P < 0.0001$) compared with those in whom both H-FABP and TnT were negative. Kaplan–Meier analysis demonstrated that in patients with negative TnT, positive H-FABP group had higher risk for cardiac events than negative H-FABP group. A multivariate analysis with Cox proportional hazard model showed that H-FABP was the only independent predictor of cardiac events. The area under the receiver operating characteristic curve was greater for H-FABP than for

TnT (0.779 versus 0.581; $P = 0.009$), suggesting that H-FABP had greater predictive capacity for cardiac events than TnT. These findings showed that H-FABP appears to be more sensitive to detect OMD and could identify patients at high risk more effectively than TnT. On the other hand, to predict potential adverse outcomes in patients with HF (death or rehospitalization), levels of both cardiomyocyte membrane and myofibril damage markers T and H-FABP were recently measured by Setsuta et al. [26]. TnT and H-FABP were measured in 103 HF patients and in 31 controls. Patients were classified into four groups based on detectable (≥ 0.01 ng/mL) or undetectable TnT (TnT+ or TnT−) and H-FABP $\geq$ or <4.5 ng/mL (high-H-FABP or low-H-FABP). Kaplan-Meier analysis showed that the CE-free rate ($n = 43$) was significantly lower in patients with TnT+ and high-H-FABP than in patients in the other three groups (patients with TnT+ and low-H-FABP, TnT− and high-H-FABP, and TnT− and low-H-FABP). In stepwise multivariate Cox proportional hazard analysis, TnT+ and high-H-FABP were independent predictors of future CE. Thus, elevated levels of both TnT and H-FABP predict adverse outcomes in HF patients.

Endomyocardial biopsy, although the most reliable method to detect rejection following cardiac transplantation in HF patients, is nonetheless an invasive procedure. To detect rejection noninvasively, other methods are desirable but they are not currently available; it is possible that proteomics may be the needed method to identify novel blood markers of rejection. Sequential cardiac biopsies have been analyzed by 2-D gel electrophoresis and classified according to whether they showed rejection ($n = 16$) or no rejection ($n = 17$) [27]. In this analysis, over 100 proteins were found to be upregulated by between 2- and 50-fold during rejection; 13 of these were identified and found to be cardiac specific or HSPs. Levels of two of these proteins (i.e., alphaβ-crystallin, tropomyosin) were measured by ELISA in the sera of 17 patients and followed for 3 months after their transplants. These proteins were significantly higher in the sera of patients whose cardiac biopsies showed rejection compared to those with no rejection. These findings suggest that proteomic analysis can be used in the identification of novel serum markers of human cardiac allograft rejection. Thus, current advances in translational protein-based diagnostics are making biomarkers testing readily available from the bench to both the clinic and at the bedside.

Metabolome in HF

Metabolomics represents the global analysis of metabolites (i.e., small molecules products of metabolism), and the metabolome represents the collection of all metabolites in a biological organism that are the end products of its gene expression.

While mRNA gene expression data and proteomic analyses do not tell the whole story of what might be happening at the level of cardiomyocytes, metabolic profiling can give an instantaneous snapshot of the physiology of that cell. First described by Oliver et al., the metabolome [28] refers to the complete set of small molecules such as metabolic intermediates, hormones and other signaling molecules, and secondary metabolites to be found within a biological sample, such as a single organism. The word metabolomics was coined in analogy with transcriptomics and proteomics; like the transcriptome and the proteome, the metabolome is dynamic, changing from second to second. Notwithstanding, while the metabolome can be defined readily enough, it is not currently possible to analyze the entire range of metabolites by a single analytical method. In January 2007, scientists at the University of Alberta and the University of Calgary in Canada completed the first draft of the human metabolome. They catalogued approximately 2,500 metabolites, 1,200 drugs, and 3,500 food components that can be found in the human body [29–31].

While metabolimics are relatively new to organ transplantation, the appraisal of metabolites as a quick, noninvasive method of organ function is not that new [32]. Measurements of serum creatinine have been previously used to assess pre- and postoperative organ function, and during the last decade, a number of lesser-known, organ-specific metabolites have also been shown to be good diagnostic indicators of both organ function and viability. While expression of a number of transcripts, protein abundance and/or tissue changes may take days or weeks to occur, metabolic changes happened rapidly after an "event" (i.e., HF/ischemia). Therefore, metabolomic measurements may offer a particularly useful and inexpensive diagnostic tool to monitor HF as well as heart viability before or after transplantation. Nonetheless, more experience is necessary since this is a new method for rapid metabolite identification, and metabolites are only one part of a very complex picture as HF is. Besides creatinine, serum metabolomics have shown many novel metabolic markers of HF, including pseudouridine and 2-oxoglutarate. Dunn et al. have evaluated 52 patients with systolic HF (EF < 40% plus signs and symptoms of failure) and 57 controls [33]. Serum samples were analyzed by gas chromatography-time of flight – mass spectrometry and the raw data reduced to 272 statistically robust metabolite peaks. 38 peaks showed a significant difference between case and control ($P < 5 \times 10^{-5}$). Pseudouridine, a modified nucleotide present in t- and rRNA and a marker of cell turnover, as well as the tricarboxylic acid cycle intermediate 2-oxoglutarate were two of such metabolites. In addition, three new compounds were also excellent discriminators between patients and controls: 2-hydroxy, 2-methylpropanoic acid, erythritol, and 2,4,6-trihydroxypyrimidine. Although renal disease may be associated with HF, and metabolites associated with renal disease and other markers were also elevated (e.g., urea, creatinine and uric acid), no correlation was found within the patients group between these metabolites and their HF biomarkers, indicating that these were indeed biomarkers of HF and not renal disease per se. Taken together, these findings demonstrated the power of data-driven metabolomics approaches to identify such markers of disease.

Metabolic Imaging

The heart is a high energy-demand organ that consumes more energy per gram of weight than any other organ, and its principal enzyme responsible for energy reserve is creatine kinase (CK). However, direct measures of CK flux in the beating human heart has not been possible so far. Weiss et al. using an image-guided molecular assessment of endogenous ATP turnover have measured ATP flux through CK in normal, stressed, and failing human hearts [34]. They found that cardiac CK flux in healthy humans is faster than that estimated through OXPHOS, and CK flux does not increase during a doubling of the heart rate–blood pressure product by dobutamine. Also, the cardiac ATP flux through CK is reduced by 50% in mild-to-moderate human HF. Thus, magnetic resonance strategies can now directly assess human myocardial CK energy flux, and the deficit in ATP supplied by CK in HF appears to be cardiac-specific and potentially of sufficient magnitude, even in the absence of a significant reduction in ATP stores, to contribute to the pathophysiology of human HF. These observations support the search for new therapies to reduce energy demand and/or augment energy transfer in HF and suggest that treatment effectiveness can be assessed by cardiac magnetic resonance.

To test the hypothesis that ATP flux through CK is impaired in the hypertrophied failing human heart, Smith et al. have measured myocardial CK metabolite concentrations and ATP synthesis through CK [35]. Myocardial ATP levels were normal, but creatine phosphate levels were 35% lower in left ventricular hypertrophy (LVH) patients than in normal subjects. LV mass and CK metabolite levels in LVH were not different from those in patients with LVH and HF; while myocardial CK pseudo first-order rate constant was normal in LVH, it was one half in LVH + HF. The net ATP flux through CK was significantly reduced by 30% in LVH and by a dramatic 65% in LVH + HF. Based on these observations in human LVH, it is evident that it is not the relative or absolute CK metabolite pool sizes but rather the kinetics of ATP turnover through CK that discern failing from nonfailing hypertrophic hearts. Interestingly, the deficit in ATP kinetics was similar in systolic and nonsystolic HF and was not related to the severity of hypertrophy but to the presence of HF. Because CK temporally buffers ATP, these findings support the concept that decreased myofibrillar energy delivery contributes to HF pathophysiology in human LVH.

It has been established that magnetic resonance spectroscopy (MRS) allows for the noninvasive detection of a wide variety of metabolites in the heart. Ten Hove et al. [36] have studied the metabolic changes that occur in HF using ^{31}P and ^{1}H-MRS in both patients and experimental animal studies. (31)P-MRS allows for the detection of phosphocreatine (PCr), ATP, inorganic phosphate (Pi), and intracellular pH, while ^{1}H-MRS allows for the detection of total creatine. Using cardiac MRS, the PCr/CK system was found to be impaired in the failing heart. In both patients and experimental models, PCr levels as well as total creatine levels are reduced, and in severe HF, ATP is also reduced. PCr/ATP ratios correlate with the clinical severity of HF and are a prognostic indicator of mortality. Furthermore, chemical flux through the CK reaction, measured with ^{31}P saturation transfer MRS, is reduced more than the steady-state levels of high-energy phosphates in failing myocardium in both experimental models and in patients. Experimental studies suggest that these changes can result in increased free ADP levels when the failing heart is stressed. Increased free ADP levels, in turn, result in a reduction in the available free energy of ATP hydrolysis, which may directly contribute to contractile dysfunction. Furthermore, observations from transgenic mouse models also suggest that an intact creatine/CK system is critical in situations of cardiac stress and also underlie the vital role that energy metabolism plays in HF.

Assessment of Genetic Influences on Drug Targets and Drug Metabolism in HF

Evaluation of genes influence on drugs response and metabolism is an important goal in the care of HF patients. A number of drug-metabolizing enzymes have inactivating mutations, leading to absent or nonfunctional proteins. For drugs with a high dependence on a particular enzyme for their elimination, these polymorphisms may have clinical consequences. In the case of drugs used in the treatment of HF, there are a few substrates for enzymes that exhibit genetic variability, but most do not have important clinical significance. For example, about 70% of the metabolism of the β-blocker metoprolol, a drug used widely in the treatment of HF associated with systolic dysfunction, is controlled by the polymorphic cytochrome P450 2D6 (CYP2D6) enzyme, and patients with inactivating mutations on both alleles have no functional protein. The "poor metabolizers" have up to five times higher drug concentrations and yet nei-

ther drug plasma concentration nor CYP2D6 genotype are determinants of tolerability or adverse effects in patients with HF [37, 38].

Genetic variability in the proteins involved in drug pharmacodynamics is likely to be more informative than in drug metabolism for pharmacogenomics studies. At present, there are data supporting genetic associations between drug targets and response for β-blockers, ACE inhibitors, and angiotensin receptor blockers [39, 40]. Of most relevance to the treatment of HF is the emerging data on the genetic determinants of response to β-blockers. Several studies have now reported that Arg389Arg genotype of the β1-adrenergic receptor is associated with the greatest response, both in terms of LV systolic function as well as improvement in survival [38, 41, 42]. On the other hand, there are now genetic markers that can potentially predict cardiac toxicity of drugs. A recent study of genotyped patients with non-Hodgkin lymphoma treated with doxorubicin was undertaken and followed for the development of HF [43]. Single-nucleotide polymorphisms were selected from 82 genes with conceivable relevance to anthracycline-induced cardiotoxicity. Of 1697 patients, 55 developed acute and 54 developed chronic toxicity. Five significant associations with polymorphisms of the NAD(P)H oxidase and doxorubicin efflux transporters were detected. Chronic toxicity was associated with a variant of the NAD(P)H oxidase subunit NCF4 (-212AG). Acute toxicity was associated with the His72Tyr polymorphism in the p22phox subunit and with the variant 7508TA of the RAC2 subunit of the same enzyme. Mice deficient in NAD(P)H oxidase activity, unlike wild-type mice, were resistant to chronic doxorubicin treatment. In addition, acute toxicity was associated with the Gly671Val variant of the doxorubicin efflux transporter multidrug resistance protein 1 (MRP1) and with the Val1188Glu and Cys1515Tyr haplotype of the functionally similar MRP2, a drug transporter gene. Polymorphisms in adrenergic receptors, previously found to be predictive of HF, were not associated with anthracycline cardiac toxicity. Thus, genetic variants in doxorubicin transport and free radical metabolism may modulate the individual risk to develop doxorubicin-induced cardiotoxicity.

Pharmacogenetics/Pharmacogenomics

To improve the efficacy and safety and to understand the disposition and clinical consequences of drugs in HF, two rapidly developing fields – pharmacogenetics (focusing on single genes) and pharmacogenomics (focusing on many genes) – could be used for the genetic personalization of drug response. This is so because many drug responses appear to be genetically determined, and the relationship between genotype and drug response may have an important diagnostic value. Identification and characterization of a large number of genetic polymorphisms (biomarkers) in drug metabolizing enzymes and drug transporters in an ethnically diverse group of individuals in HF may provide substantial knowledge about the mechanisms of interindividual differences in drug response.

Recent clinical trials have clearly demonstrated that the administration of β-blockers decreases mortality in patients with HF; however, significant heterogeneity exists in the effectiveness of β-blockers among individual cases. Recently, 39 polymorphisms in 16 genes related to the adrenergic system, and their association with the response to β-blockers, have been assessed in 80 patients with HF secondary to DCM [44]. Polymorphisms of NET T 182C ($P = 0.019$), ADRA1D T1848A ($P = 0.023$), and ADRA1D A1905G ($P = 0.029$) were associated with improvement on left ventricular fractional shortening (LVFS) by β-blockers, and a combined genotype analysis of NET T 182C and ADRA1D T1848A among genotype groups demonstrated a significant difference in LVFS improvement. In addition, it seems that NET (T 182C) and ADRA1D (T1848A and A1905G) polymorphisms may be predictive markers of the response to β-blockers, and the genotyping of these polymorphisms in HF patients may provide clinical insights into individual differences in the response to β-blockers.

Increasing understanding of the human genome and the development of a wide assortment of pharmacologic and mechanical therapies in HF, a potentially realizable goal, will integrate pharmacogenetics, pharmacogenomics, and therapy so that more tailored treatment can be delivered [39]. A list of specific drugs widely used in the treatment of HF is shown in Table 19.1.

Table 19.1 Examples of pharmacological agents used in the treatment of HF with evidence of association between genetic, and efficacy or adverse effects

Drug class	Genes associated with efficacy or toxicity
β-agonists	β$_2$-adrenergic receptors
β-blockers	β$_1$-adrenergic receptors
	ACE
	G$_s$ protein α subunit
	CYP2D6
ACE inhibitors	ACE
	Angiotensinogen
	AT$_1$ receptor subtype
	Bradykinin B$_2$
AT$_1$ receptor blockers	AT$_1$ receptor subtype
Digoxin	P-glycoprotein drug transporter MDR1
Anti-hypertensives	Adducin (ADD 1-3),
Diuretics	G protein β$_3$-subunit (GNβ3)
Hydralazine	N-acetyltransferase (NAT2)

Use of Cardiac Expression Modules/ Integrative Bioinformatics in HF

Cardiac expression modules/Module Map algorithm is being used to uncover groups of genes that have a similar pattern of expression under various conditions of stress, including HF. These groups of genes are called modules and may serve as computational predictions of biological pathways for the various clinical situations. The Module Map algorithm allows a large-scale analysis of genes expressed. Akavia et al. [45] have applied this algorithm to 700 different mouse experiments downloaded from the Gene Expression Omnibus (GEO) database, which identified 884 modules. They have shown a role for genes related to the immune system in conditions of heart remodeling and failure, and changes in the expression of genes involved in energy metabolism and expression of cardiac contractile proteins following MI. Whereas focusing on another module they noted a novel correlation between genes related to osteogenesis and HF, including Runx2 and Ahsg, whose role in HF was unknown. Despite a lack of prior biological knowledge, the Module Map algorithm reconstructed known pathways, confirming the strength of this new method for analyzing gene profiles related to clinical phenomenon, and therefore uncovering the correlation of clinical conditions to the molecular level.

Recently, Camargo and Azuaje have reported on linking gene expression and functional network data (i.e., integrative bioinformatics) in human HF [46]. Global protein–protein interaction (PPI) network in HF, which by itself represents a useful compendium of the current status of human HF-relevant interactions, was assembled. This provided the basis for analysis of interaction connectivity patterns in relation to a HF gene expression data set. They established the relationships between significance of the differentiation of gene expression and connectivity degrees in the PPI network, and analyzed the relationships between gene coexpression and PPI network connectivity. Genes that are not significantly differentially expressed may encode proteins that exhibit diverse network connectivity patterns. Furthermore, genes that were not defined as significantly differentially expressed may encode proteins with many interacting partners; also, genes encoding network hubs may exhibit weak coexpression with the genes encoding their interacting protein partners. These investigators also found that hubs and superhubs display a significant diversity of coexpression patterns in comparison to peripheral nodes. Evaluation of Gene Ontology (GO) demonstrated that highly connected proteins are likely to be engaged in higher level GO biological process terms, while low-connectivity proteins tend to be engaged in more specific disease-related processes. Taken together, these data support the hypothesis that integrative analysis of differential gene expression and PPI network analysis may be useful in determining the functional roles and identification of potential drug targets in human HF.

Systems Biology: An Integrated Approach to HF

Systems Biology represents a combination of concepts from different scientific disciplines in the search for an integral understanding of complex biological systems, based on their components and interactions. Moving away from the reductionistic approaches, there is increasing interest in integrating transcriptome, proteome, and physiome data, as well as from mutant gene to dysfunctional cell, organ, phenotype, and disease. A major challenge facing cardiovascular medicine in general, and HF in particular is how to translate the wealth of data on molecules, cells, and tissues into a clear understanding of how these systems function and how they are perturbed in the disease processes. The huge and ever-growing databases containing genomic, proteomic, biochemical, anatomical, and physiological information that can be searched and retrieved via the Internet may help further to understand the functioning of the healthy heart in general, and the complexity of the HF syndrome in particular. Eventually, databases may lead to a model of cardiac function at the genetic, molecular, and physiological levels that can predict which interventions are to be made. Furthermore, such simulated modeling might highlight the existing gaps in our knowledge and elicit new perspectives in how to fill them [47].

Early work on this type of integrative biology approach (prior to the acquisition of much of the proteomic/genomic/molecular data) has employed data on ion concentration and metabolite levels during cardiac ischemia to construct a simulated computer model that integrates cardiac energetics with electrophysiological changes, which proved informative in predicting the effects of specific therapeutic interventions [48]. Besides the identification of the electrophysiological effects of therapeutic interventions such as Na^+–H^+ exchange block, this model suggested an effective strategy to control cardiac dysrhythmias during calcium overload by regulating sodium–calcium exchange. In addition to myocardial ischemia, other types of cardiovascular disorders that have been "modeled" using this approach include cardiac dysrhythmias and contractile disorders [49–51].

A clear understanding of the HF syndrome's overall mechanisms and the role that genes play in fostering its complex phenotypes will require integrating the large comprehensive and ever-growing information concerning genomic, proteomic, biochemical, anatomical, and physiological data from HF patients. Since HF tends to progress in a system-wide fashion, increased emphasis should be placed on the overall cellular networks involved in gene regulation, metabolic and

growth pathways, and protein–protein interaction rather than focusing on single genes and proteins (i.e., microscopic/reductionist approach). An attractive feature of systems biology is its model-building integrating data, incorporating unconnected observations and theories to test *via* simulation, and allowing the generation and refinement of hypothesis concerning HF. Interestingly, much of this information is already broadly available both in the published literature and in online databases that can be searched and retrieved. Eventually, this approach could lead to simulated modeling of cardiac function (or dysfunction) at the genetic, molecular, and physiological levels and could allow predictions about potential interventions to be made. The construction of these models, in addition to the array of data discussed above, requires extensive and sophisticated mathematical and computer algorithmic treatment [52], and, obviously, a multidisciplinary approach involving mathematics, computer knowledge, molecular and cell biology, genetics, physiology, and anatomy. Parenthetically, system-modeling approaches can be divided into bottom-up and top-down. In top-down mode, the system as a whole is deconstructed into its component parts (i.e., functional groups such as a tissues and cells) and links. The bottom-up approach tends to be more reductionist, focusing on the gene and proteins and the pathways they define. As pointed out by Kriete et al. [53], presently, there are limited quantitative data regarding higher levels of biological organization depicting cells, their arrangements in tissues and supply networks to optimize nutrient distribution and thereby regulate metabolism, in contrast to the expanding wealth of information relating to bottom-up modeling (i.e., derived from molecular studies). However, defining and integrating both approaches appears to be of significance for successful modeling since models built from bottom-up data alone appear to have limited capacity for examining the effect of perturbations on cells as a whole, and even more so, on modeling multicellular entities or organisms. Moreover, a top-down model of HF can predict turnover rates in mitochondrial respiratory enzymes, which in turn can lead to ROS and OS generation linked to HF, as well as to aging. The bottom-up model in aging has tended to concentrate on the identification of gene regulation, chromatin functional remodeling (e.g., telomere function), intracellular signaling, protein and DNA repair networks. These models applied to HF as well as to aging will recognize and address the dual-sided features of ROS, both as a participant in the stochastic mechanisms involved in the cell (and DNA) and as a critical signaling molecule in executing programmed transcriptional responses dealing with cardiomyocyte survival and cytoprotection.

From a physiome perspective, it is apparent that HF could affect all levels of the system network in an interconnected and multidirectional fashion as well as several feedback loops between the genomic, organelle, cellular and organ level (Fig. 19.1). Importantly, the models discussed above

Fig. 19.1 Systems biology. Top-down and bottom-up analysis of the phenome

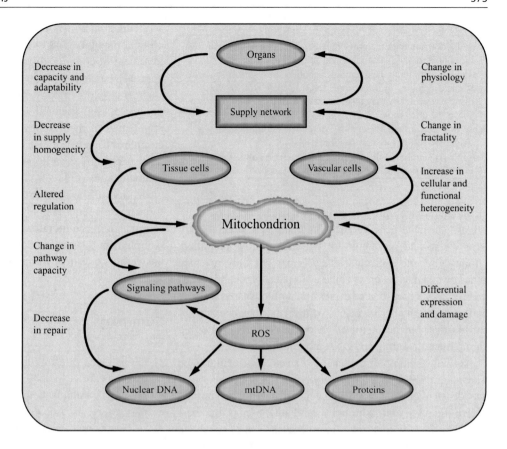

underscore the fact that much critical postgenomic data remain to be obtained including the identification of gene–environmental factor and protein–protein interactions, which appear to underlie many phenotypic changes in HF and signaling events in the cardiomyocyte.

Biomolecular interactions revealed by proteomic information will be important for unraveling metabolic and signaling pathways operating in the cell, and, in particular, in response to heart disease and injury. The identification of functional interactions between signaling pathways and genetic networks can be of great significance in providing a window into regulation of the coordinate expression of functional groups of genes, with a few key pathways switching between alternative cell fates. Underlying these models is the important recognition that the heart and vascular system are dynamic and more than just electrical circuitry or mechanical pumps, and they have the ability to grow and remodel in response to changing environments partly determined by genes and partly by their physical environment [54].

Conclusions and Future Directions

Novel diagnostics techniques that actually are being used, and techniques that have the promise of being potentially helpful

for evaluation of the etiology, diagnostics, and prognostication of HF have been discussed in this chapter. Studies involving transcriptome analysis of endomyocardial biopsies from HF patients have begun to provide an overall picture of which genes are upregulated and which are downregulated. This can provide a "snapshot" or molecular signature of HF that depicts some general programming changes in overall gene expression, dependent on sampling time and tissue. This type of analysis has begun to facilitate the identification of biomarkers that are not only reflective of phenotypic changes but are also responsive to treatment interventions. These observations have also unveiled a classical pattern of heterogeneity in genotypic expression that seems to characterize postmitotic tissues such as the heart. This heterogeneity arising from the multiple cell types that comprise these tissues is even more evident in cell-to-cell studies of single cardiomyocytes.

So far, the use of proteomic analysis in HF studies has been rather limited. The most informative proteomic studies of HF have targeted either specific groups of proteins, either organelle-specific (e.g., mitochondrial), functional (e.g., metabolic), or modified (e.g., nitrated proteins) rather than using global snapshots of the whole proteome. On the other hand, and in reference to the genetic analysis of HF, despite the problems posed by the pronounced heterogeneity in genotypes, difficult-to-control environmental factors, practical problems in conducting longitudinal studies, and frequent methodological

Table 19.2 Four phases in architecture of diagnostic research [55]

Phase I – determining the normal range of values for a diagnostic test through observational studies in healthy people

Phase II – determining the diagnostic accuracy through case–control studies, including healthy people and (a) people with known disease assessed by diagnostic standard and (b) people with suspected disease

Phase III – determining the clinical consequences of introducing a diagnostic test through randomized trials

Phase IV – determining the effects of introducing a new diagnostic test into clinical practice by surveillance in large cohort studies

inconsistencies in sampling and assessing phenotypes, a number of genes and gene variants that contribute to human HF have been and continue to be successfully identified. Furthermore, the molecular analysis has not only revealed genes involved in the onset of these HF phenotypes and identified commonalities of gene expression profiles shared with the normal heart but also has begun to unveil the epigenetic mechanisms that can be disrupted in progressive HF, including chromatin remodeling and DNA modifications.

Notwithstanding all evidence obtained from randomized trials, definitive proof is necessary before the introduction of new drugs in clinical practice in general and in the treatment of HF in particular. Similarly, randomization is the best method for comparing interventions that evaluate the potential effects of a new diagnostic test since methodologic shortcomings can overestimate the accuracy of the test. We agree with Gluud and Gluud that so far only limited randomized trials have dealt with diagnostic tests [55]. As noted when looking at the four phases in the architecture of diagnostic research, the demand for diagnostic phase III and phase IV studies is and will be increasing with the continuous development of new diagnostic methods as discussed above. During the development of new diagnostic methods, the so called four temporal phases (Table 19.2) of research provide a logical, stepwise procedure for their development. However, these phases do not apply to all diagnostic tests or provide an adequate basis for all types of diagnostic studies. Nevertheless, the phase concept as a guide may be adjusted according to individual circumstances.

Finally, the use of systems biology, which blends stochastic and deterministic features might have a relevant impact on current cardiovascular biology. As the methodology progresses, complex, multifactorial diseases including HF, diabetes, arthritis, and cancer might be understood in terms of failure of molecular components to cooperate properly. Consequently, these diseases may be studied and treated in a rational and successful way. Example of this concept is the model of the human heart that blends at the molecular, cellular, and organ levels in a quantitative and predictable manner [49]. Thus, the ultimate goal of systems biology is to tailor drugs and therapies to the needs of individual patients, improving the safety and efficacy of HF treatment.

Reductionism has been so far the prevalent approach in clinical medicine and employed in clinical diagnostics and treatment of complex diseases, including HF; however, this approach has serious limitations, and an alternative approach, such as systems biology, maybe at least complement it. As pointed out by Ahn et al. [56] in their review on the clinical application of the systems approach, rather than dividing a complex problem (i.e., HF) into its component parts, the systems perspective can appreciate the holistic and composite characteristics of the disease with the perspective that in the evaluation of the problem computational and mathematical tools may be required. Nevertheless, there is still significant skepticism in the literature about how systems biology will complement classic reductionist approaches. In order to answer this question, further research is needed.

Summary

- Global gene profiling analysis has proven informative in diverse cardiac pathologies including cardiac hypertrophy, myocardial ischemia, dilated cardiomyopathy, coronary artery disease, atrial fibrillation, and heart failure.
- In tissues and cells of both animal models and human subjects of HF, gene profiling has shown genes involved (or altered) in HF, apoptotic progression, and proinflammatory events in vascular cells.
- Proteomic analysis allows the assessment of gene expression at the protein level as well as the identification of novel vascular and cardiac-specific biomarkers of HF.
- Most informative proteomic studies have eschewed a complete proteomic approach in which the entire proteome is characterized and rather have utilized a more focused proteomic analysis targeted to specific candidate proteins by function, or limited to specific classes of proteins, or subproteomes of specific organelles (e.g., mitochondria or lysosomes) or containing specific protein modifications (e.g., nitration).
- Genome-wide screening in some defined populations (e.g., centenarians and their families) and SNP polymorphic variant analysis in case–association studies have allowed the identification of several genes associated with human aging.
- Genes involved in lipoprotein metabolisms (APOE), signaling, inflammation, and immune-regulation have been clearly associated with differences in cardiac diseases in general and HF in particular, as well as in the susceptibility to aging-associated diseases.
- Molecular genetic analysis has begun to reveal the mechanism of significant epigenetic contributions to the expression of HF phenotype, including DNA methylation and chromatin remodeling, primarily through modifications of chromatin proteins including histones.

- The ultimate goal of systems biology is to tailor drugs and therapies to the needs of individual patients improving the safety and efficacy of HF treatment.
- There is still significant skepticism about how systems biology will complement classic reductionist approaches. To answer this question, further research is needed.

References

1. Moe GW (2005) BNP in the diagnosis and risk stratification of heart failure. Heart Fail Monit 4:116–122
2. Januzzi JL, van Kimmenade R, Lainchbury J, Bayes-Genis A et al (2006) NT-proBNP testing for diagnosis and short-term prognosis in acute destabilized heart failure: an international pooled analysis of 1256 patients The International Collaborative of NT-proBNP Study. Eur Heart J 27:330–337
3. Januzzi JL Jr, Camargo CA, Anwaruddin S, Baggish AL et al (2005) The N-terminal Pro-BNP investigation of dyspnea in the emergency department (PRIDE) study. Am J Cardiol 95:948–954
4. Maisel AS, Krishnaswamy P, Nowak RM, McCord J et al (2002) Rapid measurement of B-type natriuretic peptide in the emergency diagnosis of heart failure. N Engl J Med 347:161–167
5. McDonagh TA, Robb SD, Murdoch DR, Morton JJ, Ford I, Morrison CE, Tunstall-Pedoe H, McMurray JJ, Dargie HJ (1998) Biochemical detection of left-ventricular systolic dysfunction. Lancet 351:9–13
6. Armstrong PW, Moe GW (1993) Medical advances in the treatment of congestive heart failure. Circulation 88:2941–2952
7. Seta Y, Shan K, Bozkurt B, Oral H, Mann DL (1996) Basic mechanisms in heart failure: the cytokine hypothesis. J Card Fail 2:243–249
8. Vidal B, Roig E, Perez-Villa F, Orus J, Perez J, Jimenez V, Leivas A, Cuppoletti A, Roque M, Sanz G (2002) Prognostic value of cytokines and neurohormones in severe heart failure. Rev Esp Cardiol 55:481–486
9. Ohki R, Yamamoto K, Ueno S, Mano H, Misawa Y, Fuse K, Ikeda U, Shimada K (2005) Gene expression profiling of human atrial myocardium with atrial fibrillation by DNA microarray analysis. Int J Cardiol 102:233–238
10. Yndestad A, Holm AM, Müller F, Simonsen S, Frøland SS, Gullestad L, Aukrust P (2003) Enhanced expression of inflammatory cytokines and activation markers in T-cells from patients with chronic heart failure. Cardiovasc Res 60:141–146
11. Husberg C, Nygård S, Finsen AV, Damås JK, Frigessi A, Oie E, Waehre A, Gullestad L, Aukrust P, Yndestad A, Christensen G (2008) Cytokine expression profiling of the myocardium reveals a role for CX3CL1 (fractalkine) in heart failure. J Mol Cell Cardiol 45:261–269
12. Mazurek T, Zhang L, Zalewski A, Mannion JD et al (2003) Human epicardial adipose tissue is a source of inflammatory mediators. Circulation 108:2460–2466
13. Baker AR, Silva NF, Quinn DW, Harte AL, Pagano D, Bonser RS, Kumar S, McTernan PG (2006) Human epicardial adipose tissue expresses a pathogenic profile of adipocytokines in patients with cardiovascular disease. Cardiovasc Diabetol 5:1–7
14. Ganesh SK, Skelding KA, Mehta L, O'Neill K, Joo J, Zheng G, Goldstein J, Simari R, Billings E, Geller NL, Holmes D, O'Neill WW, Nabel EG (2004) Rationale and study design of the CardioGene Study: genomics of in-stent restenosis. Pharmacogenomics 5:952–1004
15. Stanley BA, Gundry RL, Cotter RJ, Van Eyk JE (2004) Heart disease, clinical proteomics and mass spectrometry. Dis Markers 20:167–178
16. Anderson L (2005) Candidate-based proteomics in the search for biomarkers of cardiovascular disease. J Physiol 563:23–60
17. Doherty NS, Littman BH, Reilly K, Swindell AC, Buss JM, Anderson NL (1998) Analysis of changes in acute-phase plasma proteins in an acute inflammatory response and in rheumatoid arthritis using two-dimensional gel electrophoresis. Electrophoresis 19:355–363
18. Ridker PM, Rifai N, Rose L, Buring JE, Cook NR (2002) Comparison of C-reactive protein and low-density lipoprotein cholesterol levels in the prediction of first cardiovascular events. N Engl J Med 347:1557–1565
19. Di Serio F, Amodio G, Ruggieri E, De Sario R, Varraso L, Antonelli G, Pansini N (2005) Proteomic approach to the diagnosis of acute coronary syndrome: preliminary results. Clin Chim Acta 357:226–235
20. Vuotikka P, Ylitalo K, Vuori J, Vaananen K, Kaukoranta P, Lepojarvi M, Peuhkurinen K (2003) Serum myoglobin/carbonic anhydrase III ratio in the diagnosis of perioperative myocardial infarction during coronary bypass surgery. Scand Cardiovasc J 37:23–29
21. Berhane BT, Zong C, Liem DA et al (2005) Cardiovascular-related proteins identified in human plasma by the HUPO Plasma Proteome Project pilot phase. Proteomics 5:3520–3530
22. Gallego-Delgado J, Lazaro A, Osende JI et al (2005) Proteomic approach in the search of new cardiovascular biomarkers. Kidney Int Suppl S103–S107
23. Petricoin EF, Rajapaske V, Herman EH et al (2004) Toxicoproteomics: serum proteomic pattern diagnostics for early detection of drug induced cardiac toxicities and cardioprotection. Toxicol Pathol 32:122–130
24. Sugiura T, Takase H, Toriyama T, Goto T, Ueda R, Dohi Y (2005) Circulating levels of myocardial proteins predict future deterioration of congestive heart failure. J Card Fail 11:504–509
25. Niizeki T, Takeishi Y, Arimoto T et al (2007) Heart-type fatty acid-binding protein is more sensitive than troponin T to detect the ongoing myocardial damage in chronic heart failure patients. J Card Fail 13:120–127
26. Setsuta K, Seino Y, Kitahara Y, Arau M, Ohbayashi T, Takano T, Mizuno K (2008) Elevated levels of both cardiomyocyte membrane and myofibril damage markers predict adverse outcomes in patients with chronic heart failure. Circ J 72:569–574
27. Borozdenkova S, Westbrook JA, Patel V et al (2004) Use of proteomics to discover novel markers of cardiac allograft rejection. J Proteome Res 3:282–288
28. Oliver SG, Winson MK, Kell DB, Baganz F (1998) Systematic functional analysis of the yeast genome. Trends Biotechnol 16:373–378
29. Dunn WB, Ellis DI (2005) Metabolomics: current analytical platforms and methodologies. Trends Anal Chem 24:285–294
30. Ellis DI, Goodacre R (2006) Metabolic fingerprinting in disease diagnosis: biomedical applications of infrared and Raman spectroscopy. Analyst 131:875–885
31. Wishart DS, Tzur D, Knox C et al (2007) HMDB: the Human Metabolome Database. Nucleic Acids Res 35: D521–D526
32. Wishart DS (2005) Metabolomics: the principles and potential applications to transplantation. Am J Transplant 5:2814–2820
33. Dunn WB, Broadhurst DI, Deepak SM, Buch MH et al (2007) Serum metabolomics reveals many novel metabolic markers of heart failure, including pseudouridine and 2-oxoglutarate. Metabolomics 3:413–426
34. Weiss RG, Gerstenblith G, Bottomley PA (2005) ATP flux through creatine kinase in the normal, stressed, and failing human heart. Proc Natl Acad Sci USA 102:808–813
35. Smith CS, Bottomley PA, Schulman SP, Gerstenblith G, Weiss RG (2006) Altered creatine kinase adenosine triphosphate kinetics in failing hypertrophied human myocardium. Circulation 114:1151–1158
36. Ten Hove M, Neubauer S (2007) MR spectroscopy in heart failure – clinical and experimental findings. Heart Fail Rev 12:48–57

37. McGourty JC, Silas JH, Lennard MS, Tucker GT, Woods HF (1985) Metoprolol metabolism and debrisoquine oxidation polymorphism – population and family studies. Br J Clin Pharmacol 20:555–566

38. Terra SG, Pauly DF, Lee CR et al (2005) Beta-Adrenergic receptor polymorphisms and responses during titration of metoprolol controlled release/extended release in heart failure. Clin Pharmacol Ther 77:127–137

39. Johnson JA, Cavallari LH (2005) Cardiovascular pharmacogenomics. Exp Physiol 90:283–289

40. Roden DM (2003) Cardiovascular pharmacogenomics. Circulation 108:3071–3074

41. Mialet PJ, Rathz DA, Petrashevskaya NN et al (2003) Beta 1-adrenergic receptor polymorphisms confer differential function and predisposition to heart failure. Nat Med 9:1300–1305

42. Terra SG, Hamilton KK, Pauly DF et al (2005) Beta1-adrenergic receptor polymorphisms and left ventricular remodeling changes in response to beta-blocker therapy. Pharmacogenet Genomics 15:227–234

43. Wojnowski L, Kulle B, Schirmer M et al (2005) NAD(P)H oxidase and multidrug resistance protein genetic polymorphisms are associated with doxorubicin-induced cardiotoxicity. Circulation 112:3754–3762

44. Nonen S, Okamoto H, Fujio Y et al (2008) Polymorphisms of norepinephrine transporter and adrenergic receptor alpha1D are associated with the response to bold italic beta-blockers in dilated cardiomyopathy. Pharmacogenomics J 8:78–84

45. Akavia UD, Benayahu D (2008) Meta-analysis and profiling of cardiac expression modules. Physiol Genomics 35:305–315

46. Camargo A, Azuaje F (2007) Linking gene expression and functional network data in human heart failure. PLoS One 2:e1347

47. Bassingthwaighte JB, Qian H, Li Z (1999) The Cardiome Project. An integrated view of cardiac metabolism and regional mechanical function. Adv Exp Med Biol 471:541–553

48. Ch'en F, Clarke K, Vaughan-Jones R, Noble D (1997) Modeling of internal pH, ion concentration, and bioenergetic changes during myocardial ischemia. Adv Exp Med Biol 430:281–290

49. Noble D (2002) Modeling the heart – from genes to cells to the whole organ. Science 295:1678–1682

50. Rudy Y (2000) From genome to physiome: integrative models of cardiac excitation. Ann Biomed Eng 28:945–950

51. Hunter P, Smith N, Fernandez J, Tawhai M (2005) Integration from proteins to organs: the IUPS Physiome Project. Mech Ageing Dev 126:187–192

52. Crampin EJ, Halstead M, Hunter P et al (2004) Computational physiology and the Physiome Project. Exp Physiol 89:1–26

53. Kriete A, Sokhansanj BA, Coppock DL, West GB (2006) Systems approaches to the networks of aging. Ageing Res Rev 5: 434–448

54. Noble D (2002) Modelling the heart: insights, failures and progress. Bioessays 24:1155–1163

55. Gluud C, Gluud LL (2005) Evidence based diagnostics. BMJ 330:724–726

56. Ahn AC, Tewari M, Poon CS, Phillips RS (2006) The clinical applications of a systems approach. PLoS Med 3:e209

Section X
Available and Forthcoming Therapies for Heart Failure

Chapter 20
Treatment of Chronic Heart Failure

Overview

Over the past two decades, enormous progress has been made in the pharmacotherapy of heart failure (HF). Large randomized controlled trials involving the inhibition of the renin–angiotensin–aldosterone system and sympathetic nervous system have led to substantial improvements in both morbidity and mortality [1–3]. Indeed, with optimal pharmacologic therapy, the annual mortality rate for those with New York Heart Association (NYHA) Class II symptoms of HF has declined to less than 10% per annum [4]. Furthermore, advances in device therapy including cardiac resynchronization therapy (CRT) with or without implantable defibrillators (CRT-D), in addition to medical treatment, for more severe HF have brought down the annual mortality rate for those with NYHA Class III HF to about 11% at 1 year [5, 6]. Cardiac transplantation is now a valuable option for selected patients with end-stage HF despite optimal medical therapy, with a 1-year survival approaching 90%, a 5-year survival rate of approximately 70%, and a median survival in excess of 10 years [7]. In this chapter, all aspects of available therapy of HF will be reviewed followed by a brief glimpse into the future.

Introduction

The aim of treating HF is not different from any other medical condition, namely to bring about a reduction of mortality and morbidity. Since the mortality of HF is so high, particular emphasis has been put on this end-point in clinical trials. However, for many patients, and notably the elderly, the ability to lead an independent life, freedom from excessively unpleasant symptoms, and reduction of admission to hospital, constitutes treatment goals, which, on occasions, may be as important as the prolongation of life. Prevention of heart disease or its progression remains an essential part of management. Many of the randomized clinical trials in HF have evaluated patients with systolic dysfunction based on an ejection frac-

tion of 35–40%. This is admittedly a relatively arbitrary cutoff level, and there is limited trial evidence in the large population with symptomatic HF and an EF between 40 and 50%.

Because treatment of HF has improved over the past decade, the older prognostic models need to be revalidated [8], and newer prognostic models may have to be developed. Outcomes have been improved for most high-risk patients, which has resulted in a shift in the selection process for patients referred for heart transplantation [8]. Routine use of ambulatory electrocardiographic monitoring, T-wave alternans analysis, heart rate variability measurement, and signal-averaged electrocardiography have not been shown to provide incremental value in assessing overall prognosis, although ambulatory electrocardiographic monitoring can be useful in decision making regarding placement of implantable cardioverter-defibrillators (ICDs) [9]. Likewise, although the natriuretic peptides are strong predictors of prognosis in patients HF, a natriuretic peptide-targeted treatment approach has not been proven convincingly to be of value in following patients with chronic HF [10, 11].

General Measures

Nonpharmacologic strategies represent an important contribution to HF therapy, and they can significantly impact patient stability, functional capacity, mortality, and quality of life. Dietary instruction regarding sodium intake is recommended for all patients with HF. Patients with HF and diabetes, dyslipidemia, or obesity should be given specific instructions regarding carbohydrate or caloric constraints as per disease-specific guidelines. Dietary sodium restriction (2–3 g everyday) is recommended for patients with the clinical syndrome of HF. Further restriction (<2 g daily) may be considered in moderate to severe HF. Restriction of daily fluid intake to <2 l is recommended in patients with severe hyponatremia (serum sodium <130 mEq/l) and should be considered for all patients with signs of fluid retention that are difficult to control despite high doses of diuretic and sodium restriction. The identification of concurrent treatable conditions as discussed in Chap. 12,

J. Marín-García, *Heart Failure*, Contemporary Cardiology,
DOI 10.1007/978-1-60761-147-9_20, © Springer Science+Business Media, LLC 2010

such as sleep-disordered breathing, urologic abnormalities, restless leg syndrome, and depression should be considered in patients with HF and chronic insomnia. Pharmacologic aids to sleep induction may be necessary. Agents that do not risk physical dependence are preferred.

HF is a syndrome with an enormous impact on the quality of life of patients and families. HF can affect employment, relationships, leisure activities, eating, sleeping, and sexual activity. Physicians have a significant opportunity to improve their patients' quality of life by initiating discussion regarding these issues and providing education, feedback, and support. Patients with HF should be advised to stop smoking and to limit alcohol consumption to <2 standard drinks per day in men, or <1 standard drink per day in women. Patients suspected of a diagnosis of alcohol-induced cardiomyopathy should be advised to abstain from alcohol consumption. Patients suspected of using illicit drugs should be counseled to discontinue such use. Pneumococcal and annual influenza vaccines are recommended in all patients with HF in the absence of contraindications. Nonsteroidal antiinflammatory drugs, including cyclooxygenase-2 inhibitors, are not recommended in patients with chronic HF. The risk of renal failure and fluid retention is markedly increased in the setting of reduced renal function or angiotensin-converting enzyme (ACE) inhibitor therapy.

Exercise intolerance is recognized as a hallmark of HF. Until the late 1980s, HF patients were advised to avoid physical activity in the hope that it might minimize symptoms and protect the already damaged heart. It is now understood that exercise intolerance in HF has a multifactorial etiology and that parameters such as intracardiac filling pressures and left ventricular ejection fraction may not be reliable predictors of exercise capacity. Changes in the periphery and left ventricular function are both important determinants of exercise capacity. Exercise training programs in selected patients have been shown to be not only safe but also can reverse many of these peripheral abnormalities felt to play a role in exercise intolerance and improve overall exercise capacity [12]. As a result, there has been a gradual move from reluctance to consider exercise programs for patients with HF and left ventricular dysfunction toward referral of selected patients.

Numerous clinical and mechanistic studies and some randomized studies have shown that regular exercise performed by either interval training (e.g., biking and treadmill) or steady-state exercise can safely increase physical capacity by 15–25% and improve symptoms and quality of life in patients with NYHA II–III HF [12, 13]. However, these studies have been small and have used mainly physiological end points. The ExTraMATCH Collaborative Trial [13] addressed the question as to whether exercise training reduces morbidity and mortality in HF patients by using individual patient data from nine relatively small studies published since 1990

involving 801 patients. The ExTraMATCH review provided further support for the safety of exercise training in stabilized NYHA I–III HF patients and reported relative risk reductions of 32% for death and 23% for the combined endpoint of death and hospital admission, respectively, for exercise training versus usual care. Several detailed discussions have been provided on exercise and HF [14, 15].

Results of the National Institute of Health-sponsored A Controlled Trial Investigating Outcomes of Exercise Training (HF-ACTION) trial have been published recently [16]. In this multicenter trial, 2,331 stable outpatients with HF and reduced ejection fraction were assigned to usual care plus aerobic exercise training, consisting of 36 supervised sessions followed by home-based training or usual care alone. Median LV ejection fraction was 25%. Exercise adherence decreased from a median of 95 min per week during months 4–6 of follow-up to 74 min per week during months 10–12. A total of 759 patients (65%) in the exercise training group died or were hospitalized compared with 796 patients (68%) in the usual care group (hazard ratio (HR), 0.93 (95% confidence interval (CI), 0.84–1.02); $P=0.13$). There were nonsignificant reductions in the exercise training group for mortality (189 patients (16%) in the exercise training group vs. 198 patients (17%) in the usual care group; HR, 0.96 (95% CI, 0.79–1.17); $P=0.70$), cardiovascular (CV) mortality or CV hospitalization (632 (55%) in the exercise training group vs. 677 (58%) in the usual care group; HR, 0.92 (95% CI, 0.83–1.03); $P=0.14$), and CV mortality or HF hospitalization (344 (30%) in the exercise training group vs. 393 (34%) in the usual care group; HR, 0.87 (95% CI, 0.75–1.00); $P=0.06$). In prespecified supplementary analyses adjusting for highly prognostic baseline characteristics, the HR were 0.89 (95% CI, 0.81–0.99; $P=0.03$) for all-cause mortality or hospitalization, 0.91 (95% CI, 0.82–1.01; $P=0.09$) for cardiovascular mortality or CV hospitalization, and 0.85 (95% CI, 0.74–0.99; $P=0.03$) for cardiovascular mortality or HF hospitalization. Therefore, in the protocol-specified primary analysis, exercise training resulted in nonsignificant reductions in the primary end-point of all-cause mortality or hospitalization and in key secondary clinical end-points. After adjustment for prognostic predictors of the primary end-point, exercise training was associated with modest significant reductions for both all-cause mortality or hospitalization and cardiovascular mortality or HF hospitalization.

Based on available data to date, one can recommend regular physical activity for all patients with stable HF symptoms and impaired LV systolic function. Exercise training three to five times a week for 30–45 min per session (to include warm up and cool down) should be considered. Prior to starting an exercise program, all patients should have a graded exercise stress test to assess functional capacity, identify angina or ischemia, and determine an optimal target heart rate for training. Training for both aerobic activity and resistance training should be at a moderate intensity. Individualized exercise training may initially be performed in a supervised setting with trained personnel and external defibrillators when resources are available and accessible.

Pharmacologic Therapy

There have now been many landmark clinical trials on the use of ACE inhibitors [1, 17–21] and β-blockers (Fig. 20.1) [2, 22–24] as well as meta-analyses [25, 26] in HF such that these agents have become standard therapy and should be considered in all patients diagnosed with HF in the presence of systolic dysfunction. The timing of the introduction should be individualized to maximize tolerability and long-term persistence with therapy. In general, acute symptoms should be relieved first, such as with the use of diuretics, but an ACE inhibitor or a β-blocker should be introduced as early as the

patient's condition allows. Heart rate and blood pressure abnormalities may dictate which drug class should be used first or preferentially uptitrated. As most of the clinical trials administered ACE inhibitors first, most physicians would start with an ACE inhibitor and add a β-blocker but not necessarily delay introduction until target ACE inhibitor dose was reached. A recent open-label trial of 1,010 patients with mild to moderate HF and LV ejection fraction ≤35%, CIBIS III [27], showed either strategy of ACE inhibitor or β-blocker for the first 6 months, followed by the combination for 6–24 months, to be similar with some small nonsignificant differences in tolerability and outcomes. Heart rate, blood pressure, and comorbidities may dictate which drug class should be used first or preferentially uptitrated. If an ACE inhibitor is not tolerated, there is now good evidence that an angiotensin receptor blocker (ARB) can be substituted [28, 29] and this may also apply if a β-blocker is not tolerated, although those data are not as robust. In patients who are already on combination ACE inhibitor plus β-blocker, but

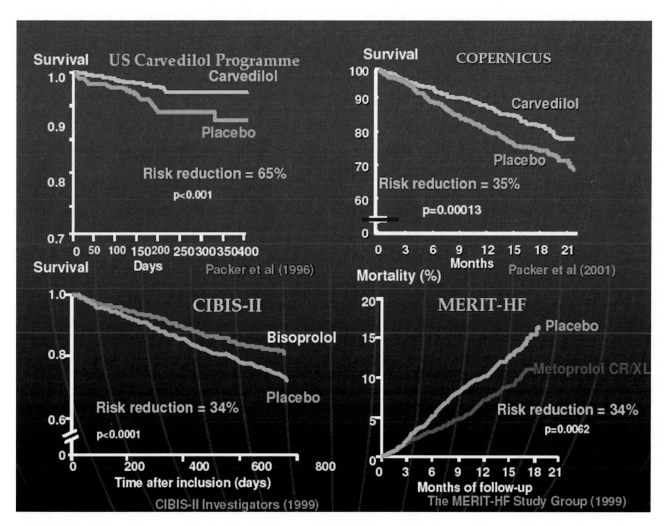

Fig. 20.1 Landmark trials of β-blockers in heart failure and systolic dysfunction

continue to have HF symptoms or hospitalizations, an ARB should be added [30, 31]. Aldosterone antagonists are effective in patients with post-MI HF or in chronic HF, especially if recently hospitalized for HF [32, 33]. Symptoms, blood pressure sitting and standing, heart rate, renal function, and electrolytes should be followed closely when combinations of drugs affecting the renin-angiotensin–aldosterone system are used.

A previous study compared an ACE inhibitors to isosorbide dinitrate (ISDN) and hydralazine combination and found the ACE inhibitor enalapril to reduce mortality at 2 years [22]. Therefore, in symptomatic patients with an LVEF ≤40%, the combination of hydralazine and ISDN may be used as an alternative if there is intolerance to both an ACE inhibitor and an ARB. The recent A-HeFT study [34] enrolled self-identified African American patients with systolic HF and demonstrated that adding a fixed dose combination of ISDN plus hydralazine to standard therapy reduced mortality as well as first hospitalization for HF and improved quality of life. Digoxin should not be used to treat patients with diastolic HF in sinus rhythm. By increasing contractility through increased intracellular calcium concentration, digoxin may increase LV stiffness in these patients, increasing LV filling pressure, and aggravating HF associated with normal LV ejection fraction [35]. At 37-month follow-up of 7,788 patients, mean age 64 years, with HF (6,800 with systolic HF and 988 with diastolic HF) in the Digitalis Investigator Group (DIG) study, the mortality was similar in patients treated with digoxin or placebo [36, 37]. HF hospitalization was significantly reduced (28%) in patients with systolic HF and insignificantly reduced (21%) in patients with diastolic HF [37]. All-cause hospitalization was significantly reduced in patients with systolic HF and insignificantly increased in patients with diastolic HF [37]. Hospitalization for suspected digoxin toxicity in patients treated with digoxin was 0.67% in patients aged 50–59 years, 1.91% in patients aged 60–69 years, 2.47% in patients aged 70–79 years, and 4.42% in patients aged ≥80 years [37]. A post-hoc subgroup analysis of data from women with systolic HF in the DIG study showed by multivariate analysis that digoxin significantly increased the risk of death among women (by 23%) [38]. A post-hoc subgroup analysis of data from men with systolic HF in the DIG study showed that digoxin significantly reduced mortality (by 6%) if the serum digoxin level was 0.5–0.8 ng/ml, insignificantly increased mortality (by 3%) if the serum digoxin level was 0.8–1.1 ng/ml, and significantly increased mortality (by 12%) if the serum digoxin level was ≥1.2 ng/ml [39]. Another post-hoc subgroup analysis of data from all 1,926 women with systolic or diastolic HF in the DIG study showed that digoxin significantly increased mortality (by 20%) in women [40].

Table 20.1 Evidence-based drugs and oral doses as demonstrated in large clinical trials

Drug	Start dose	Target dose
ACE inhibitor		
Captopril	6.25–12.5 mg TID	25–50 mg TID
Enalapril	1.25–2.5 mg BID	10 mg BID
Ramipril	1.25–2.5 mg BID	5 mg BID
Lisinopril	2.5–5 mg OD	20–35 mg OD
β-blockers		
Carvedilol	3.125 mg BID	25 mg BID
Bisoprolol	1.25 mg OD	10 mg OD
Metoprolol CR/XL	12.5–25 mg OD	200 mg OD
ARB		
Candesartan	4 mg OD	32 mg OD
Valsartan	40 mg BID	160 mg BID
Aldosterone antagonist		
Spironolactone	12.5 mg OD	50 mg OD
Eplerenone	25 mg OD	50 mg OD
Vasodilators		
Isosorbide dinitrate	20 mg TID	40 mg TID
Hydralazine	37.5 mg TID	75 mg TID

This retrospective analysis also showed that higher NYHA classes were associated with poorer outcomes in patients with diastolic HF [41]. On the basis of these data, women with systolic or diastolic HF and men with diastolic HF should probably not be treated with digoxin. Men with persistent symptoms due to systolic HF despite treatment with diuretics, ACE inhibitors and β- blockers may be treated with digoxin.

In practice, drugs that have been proven to be beneficial in large-scale clinical trials are recommended as the effective target doses are known (Table 20.1). The target drug dose should be either the dose used in large scale clinical trials or a lesser but maximum dose that is tolerated by the patient. If a drug with proven mortality or morbidity benefits does not appear to be tolerated by the patient (e.g., low blood pressure, slow heart rate, or renal dysfunction), other concomitant drugs with less proven benefit should be carefully reevaluated to determine if their dose can be reduced or the drug discontinued to allow better tolerance of the proven drug [42].

Cardiac Resynchronization Therapy

Up to one-third of patients with low EF and Class III to IV symptoms of HF have a QRS duration on their electrocardiograms that are greater than 0.12 s [43, 44]. This electrocardiographic manifestation of abnormal cardiac conduction has been used to identify subjects with dyssynchronous ventricular contraction. While not completely perfect, no other consensus definition of cardiac dyssynchrony exists as yet, although several echocardiographic measures have been employed. The mechanical consequences of dyssynchrony include suboptimal ventricular filling, a reduction in LV dP/dt (rate of rise of ventricular contractile force or pressure), prolonged duration (and therefore greater severity) of mitral regurgitation, and paradoxical septal wall motion [45, 46]. Ventricular dyssynchrony has also been associated with increased mortality in HF patients [47]. Dyssynchronous contraction can be reversed by electrically activating the right and left ventricles in a synchronized manner with a biventricular pacemaker device. This approach to HF therapy, commonly called cardiac resynchronization therapy (CRT), may enhance ventricular contraction and reduce the degree of secondary mitral regurgitation [48]. In addition, the short-term use of CRT has been associated with improvements in cardiac function and hemodynamics but without an accompanying increase in oxygen use [49] as well as adaptive changes in the biochemistry of the failing heart [48].

To date, more than 4,000 HF patients with LV dyssynchrony have been evaluated in randomized controlled trials comparing optimal medical therapy alone versus optimal medical therapy plus CRT, with or without an ICD. CRT, when added to optimal medical therapy in persistently symptomatic patients, has resulted in significant improvements in quality of life, functional class, exercise capacity and exercise distance during a 6-min walk test, and EF in patients randomized to CRT [50] or to combined CRT and ICD [51, 52]. In a meta-analysis of several CRT trials, HF hospitalizations were reduced by 32% and all-cause mortality by 25% [51]. The effect on mortality in this meta-analysis became apparent after approximately 3 months of therapy. In one study [53], subjects were randomized to optimal pharmacological therapy alone, optimal medical therapy plus CRT alone, or optimal medical therapy plus the combination of CRT and an ICD (Fig. 20.2).

Compared with optimal medical therapy alone, both device-treated arms significantly decreased the combined risk of all-cause hospitalization and all-cause mortality by approximately 20%, whereas the combination of a CRT and an ICD decreased all-cause mortality significantly by 36% [53]. More recently, in a randomized controlled trial comparing optimal medical therapy alone with optimal medical therapy plus CRT alone (without a defibrillator), CRT significantly reduced the combined risk of death of any cause or unplanned hospital admission for a major cardiovascular

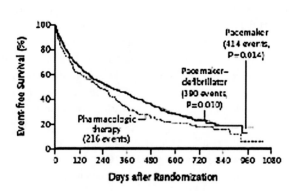

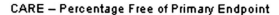

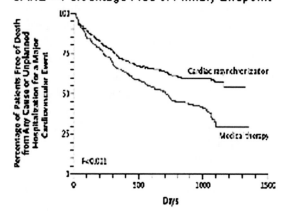

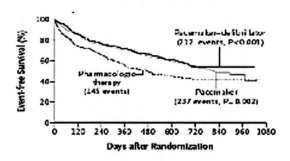

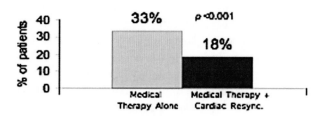

Fig. 20.2 Clinical outcomes in COMPANION and CARE

event (analyzed as time to first event) by 37% (see Fig. 20.2) [6]. In that trial, all-cause mortality was reduced by 36% and HF hospitalizations by 52% with the addition of CRT. Thus, there is strong evidence to support the use of CRT to improve symptoms, exercise capacity, quality of life, LVEF, and survival, and to decrease hospitalizations in patients with persistently symptomatic HF undergoing optimal medical therapy who have cardiac dyssynchrony (as evidenced by a prolonged QRS duration). The use of an ICD in combination with CRT should be on the basis of the indications for ICD therapy. With few exceptions, resynchronization trials have enrolled patients in normal sinus rhythm. Although the entry criteria required QRS duration only longer than 0.12 s, the average QRS duration in the large trials was longer than 0.15 s, with less information demonstrating benefit in patients with lesser prolongation of QRS. Two smaller studies, one randomized-controlled and the other observational [54, 55], have evaluated the potential benefit of CRT in HF patients with ventricular dyssynchrony in the presence of atrial fibrillation. Although both studies demonstrated the benefit of CRT in these patients, the total number of patients examined (<100) precludes a recommendation for CRT in otherwise eligible patients with atrial fibrillation. To date, only a small number of patients with "pure" right bundle-branch block have been enrolled in CRT trials. Similarly, the prolonged QRS duration associated with right ventricular pacing has also been associated with ventricular dyssynchrony that may be improved by CRT, but no published studies have addressed this clinical scenario as yet. Recommendations regarding CRT for patients with LVEF of less than or equal to 35%, NYHA functional class III, and ambulatory class IV symptoms or dependence on ventricular pacing have recently been updated to be consistent with the ACC/AHA/HRS 2008 Guidelines for Device-Based Therapy of Cardiac Rhythm Abnormalities [56]. A prospective, non-randomized multicenter study, the Predictors of Response to CRT (PROSPECT) trial [57] tested the performance of 12 echocardiographic parameters of dyssynchrony, based on both conventional and tissue Doppler-based methods to predict CRT response at 6 months. They enrolled 498 patients on a stable medical regimen with standard CRT indications (NYHA class III or IV symptoms, LV ejection fraction ≤35%, QRS≥130 ms). The sensitivity and specificity of these echocardiographic parameters to predict the clinical and remodeling composite outcomes varied widely, ranging from 6 to 74% for sensitivity and from 35 to 91% for specificity, with large variability in the analysis of the dyssynchrony parameters. Results of this study suggest that no single echocardiographic measurement of mechanical dyssynchrony may be recommended to improve patient selection for CRT beyond current guidelines. The benefit of CRT in patients with wide QRS is well established. However, some patients with narrow QRS complexes have echocardiographic evidence of LV mechanical dyssynchrony and may also benefit from CRT. The Cardiac Resynchronization Therapy in Patients with Heart Failure and Narrow QRS (RethinQ) trial enrolled 172 patients who had a standard indication for an ICD, LVEF<35%, moderate symptoms of HF (NYHA class III) caused by either ischemic or nonischemic cardiomyopathy, and a QRS interval <130 ms [58]. Patients received the CRT device and were randomly assigned to the CRT group or to a control group (no CRT) for 6 months. There was no change in the primary endpoint (peak oxygen consumption during cardiopulmonary exercise testing at 6 months), or change in quality-of-life scores, 6-min walking test, or ejection fraction.

To date, ten studies have reported on CRT implant morbidity and mortality. There were 13 deaths in 3,113 patients (0.4%). From a pooled assessment of 3,475 patients in 17 studies, the success rate of implantation was 90% [51]. Device-related problems during the first 6 months after implantation reported in 13 studies included lead malfunction or dislodgement in 8.5%, pacemaker problems in 6.7%, and infection in 1.4% of cases. These morbidity and mortality data are derived from trials that used expert centers. Results in individual clinical centers may vary considerably and are subject to a significant learning curve effects for each center; however, as implantation techniques evolve and equipment improves, complication rates may also decline [51].

Questions that remain to be answered include: exactly who benefits from CRT therapy? Why do all severely symptomatic patients with a wide QRS not benefit from this form of therapy? Does the QRS duration itself matter as much as the finding of cardiac dyssynchrony on echocardiography? What is the best way to evaluate cardiac dyssynchrony? What is the role of CRT in patients with chronic atrial fibrillation? Is there a better way to optimize CRT function by using certain echocardiographic parameters?. Should CRT be used in less symptomatic patients to prevent the progression of symptoms?. To address the last question, the recently published MADIT-CRT trial was designed to determine if CRT with biventricular pacing would reduce the risk of death or HF events in patients with mild cardiac symptoms, a reduced ejection fraction, and a wide QRS complex.[59] 1820 patients with ischemic or nonischemic cardiomyopathy, an ejection fraction ≤ 30%, QRS duration ≥ 130 msec, and NYHA class I or II symptoms were randomly assigned to receive CRT plus an ICD (1089 patients) or an ICD alone (731 patients). The primary end point of death or non-fatal HF event occurred in 187 of 1089 patients in the CRT–ICD group (17%) and 185 of 731 patients in the ICD-only group (25%) (hazard ratio in the CRT–ICD group, 0.66; 95% confidence interval [CI], 0.52 to 0.84; P = 0.001). Mortality, however, was not different. Another recent study, the REVERSE (REsynchronization reVErses Remodeling in

Systolic left vEntriculardysfunction) trial, [60] determined the effects of CRT in patients in NYHA I and II functional class with previous HF symptoms. Six hundred ten patients with NYHA functional class I or II HF with a QRS ≥ 120 ms and an ejection fraction 40% received a CRT device (±defibrillator) and were randomly assigned to active CRT (CRT-ON; n = 419) or control (CRT-OFF; n = 191) for 12 months. The primary end point was the HF clinical composite response, which scores patients as improved, unchanged, or worsened. The HF clinical composite response end point, which compared only the percent worsened, indicated 16% worsened in CRT-ON compared with 21% in CRT-OFF (p = 0.10). Patients assigned to CRT-ON experienced a greater improvement in LV end-systolic volume index. The current treatment guideline has not yet addressed the use of CRT in patients with milder symptoms of HF although the use of CRT in conjunction with defibrillator will likely increase in these patients in the near future.

Internal Cardiovertor Defibrillator Therapy

Patients with LV dilation and reduced LV ejection fraction frequently manifest ventricular tachydysrhythmias, both nonsustained ventricular tachycardia (VT) and sustained VT. The mortality of patients with all types of ventricular tachydysrhythmias is high. The high mortality results from progressive HF, as well as from sudden death. Sudden death is often equated with a primary dysrhythmic event, but multiple causes of sudden death have been documented and include ischemic events such as acute MI [61], electrolyte disturbances, pulmonary or systemic emboli, or other vascular events. Although ventricular tachydysrhythmias are the most common dysrhythmias associated with unexpected sudden death, bradycardia and other pulseless supraventricular rhythms are not uncommon in patients, particularly those with Stage D HF [62].

Patients with previous cardiac arrest or documented sustained ventricular dysrhythmias have a high risk of recurrent events. Implantation of an Internal Cardioverter Defibrillator (ICD) has been shown to reduce mortality in cardiac arrest survivors. An ICD is indicated for secondary prevention of death from ventricular tachydysrhythmias in patients with otherwise good clinical function and prognosis, for whom prolongation of survival is a goal. Patients with chronic HF and a low EF who experience syncope of unclear origin have a high rate of subsequent sudden death and should also be considered for placement of an ICD [63]. However, when ventricular tachydysrhythmias occur in a patient with a progressive and irreversible clinical HF decompensation, placement of an ICD is not indicated to prevent recurrence of sudden death, although an exception may exist for the minority of patients for whom definitive therapy such as cardiac transplantation is planned.

Patients with low EF but without prior history of cardiac arrest, spontaneous VT, or inducible VT have a risk of sudden death that is lower than for those who have experienced previous events, but the risk remains significant. Within this group, it has not yet been possible to identify those patients at highest risk, especially in the absence of prior MI. Approximately 50–70% of patients with low EF and symptomatic HF have episodes of nonsustained VT on ambulatory electrocardiographic monitoring; however, it is not clear whether the occurrence of complex ventricular dysrhythmias in these patients with HF contributes to the high frequency of sudden death or, alternatively, simply reflects the underlying disease process [64]. Antidysrhythmic drugs to suppress premature ventricular depolarizations and nonsustained ventricular dysrhythmias have not been shown improve survival [65], even though nonsustained VT may play a role in triggering ventricular tachydysrhythmias. Furthermore, most antidysrhythmic drugs have negative inotropic effects and can increase the risk of serious dysrhythmia; these adverse cardiovascular effects are particularly pronounced in patients with low EF [66]. This risk is especially high with the use of class IA agents (quinidine and procainamide) and class IC agents (flecainide and propafenone) [65, 67], which have increased mortality in post myocardial infarction trials [66]. Amiodarone is a class III antidysrhythmic agent but differs from other drugs in this class in having a sympatholytic effect [68]. Amiodarone has been associated with generally neutral effects on mortality when administered to patients with low EF and HF [69, 70]. Amiodarone therapy may also act through mechanisms other than antidysrhythmic effects because amiodarone has been shown in some trials to increase LVEF and reduce worsening HF [70]. Side effects of amiodarone have included thyroid abnormalities, pulmonary toxicity, hepatotoxicity, neuropathy, insomnia, and numerous other reactions. Therefore, amiodarone should not be considered as part of the routine treatment of patients with HF, with or without frequent premature ventricular beats or asymptomatic nonsustained VT; however, it remains the agent most likely to be safe and effective when antidysrhythmic therapy is necessary to prevent recurrent atrial fibrillation or symptomatic ventricular dysrhythmias. Indeed, other pharmacological antidysrhythmic therapies, apart from β-blockers, are rarely indicated in HF but may occasionally be used to suppress recurrent ICD shocks when amiodarone has been ineffective or discontinued owing to toxicity. The role of ICDs in the primary prevention of sudden death in patients without prior history of symptomatic dysrhythmias has been explored recently in a number of trials. If sustained ventricular tachydysrhythmias can be induced in the electrophysiology laboratory in patients with previous MI or chronic ischemic heart disease, the risk of sudden death in these patients is in the range of 5–6% per year and can be improved by ICD implantation [71]. The role of ICD for the primary prevention of sudden death in patients with HF and low EF and no history of spontaneous or inducible VT has been addressed by several large trials that used readily available clinical data as entry criteria [5, 72, 73]. The first of these trials, the Multicenter Automatic Defibrillator Implantation II (MADIT II) trial, demonstrated that ICDs, compared with standard medical therapy, decreased the occurrence of total mortality for patients with EF of 30% or less after remote MI [72]. Mortality was decreased in the ICD arm by an absolute of 5.6%, a relative decrease of 31% over 20 months. In a second trial, the Defibrillator in Acute Myocardial Infarction Trial (DYNAMIT), a survival benefit was not demonstrated with devices implanted within 6–40 days after an acute MI in patients who at that time had an EF less than 35% and abnormal heart rate variability. Although sudden deaths were decreased, there was an increase in other events, and ICD implantation did not confer any survival benefit in this setting [73]. A third trial, SCD-HeFT (Sudden Cardiac Death in Heart Failure Trial), examining the benefit of ICD implantation for patients with EF less than 35% and NYHA functional class II to III symptoms of HF included both ischemic and nonischemic causes of HF; absolute mortality was decreased by 7.2% over a 5-year period in the arm that received a simple ICD with backup pacing at a rate of 40 beats/min. This represented a relative mortality decrease of 23%, which was a survival increase of 11% [5]. There was no improvement in survival during the first year, with a 1.8% absolute survival benefit per year averaged over the next 4 years. The DEFINITE (Defibrillators in Non-Ischemic Cardiomyopathy Treatment Evaluation) trial compared medical therapy alone with medical therapy plus ICD in patients with nonischemic cardiomyopathy, NYHA class I to III HF, and an LV ejection fraction <36% [74]. ICD treatment was associated with a reduction in all-cause mortality that did not reach statistical significance but was consistent in terms of magnitude of effect (30%) with the findings of the MADIT II [72] and SCD-HeFT [5]. Results from systematic reviews of observational and randomized ICD trials confirm the favorable risk benefit ratio of this therapy [75].

In addition to cardiac status, consideration of other comorbid conditions, patient desires, and goals of therapy are essential components in the assessment for prescription of ICD therapy. In addition, close collaboration between the referring or HF physician and dysrhythmia specialist is essential not only in the initial assessment of these patients but also in their follow up. The inclusion of invasive hemodynamic monitoring as a component of the ICD implantation will mandate clear delineation of physician responsibilities in terms of responsibility and communication of monitoring results. A recent joint Heart Rhythm Society/ European society for Cardiology Task Force Statement has outlined important con-

siderations for these interactions [76]. There is an intrinsic variability in measurement of EF particularly shortly after recovery from an acute coronary syndrome event. Moreover, the pivotal primary prevention trials used a variable inclusion EF, ranging below 30 or 36%. Given the totality of the data demonstrating the efficacy of an ICD in reducing overall mortality in a population with dilated cardiomyopathy of either ischemic or nonischemic origins, the current recommendation is to include all patients with an LV ejection fraction ≤35%. ICDs are highly effective in preventing death due to ventricular tachydysrhythmias; however, frequent shocks from an ICD can lead to poor quality of life, whether triggered appropriately by life-threatening rhythms or inappropriately by sinus or other supraventricular tachycardia. For symptoms from recurrent discharges triggered by ventricular dysrhythmias or atrial fibrillation, antidysrhythmic therapy, most often amiodarone, may be added. For recurrent ICD discharges from VT despite antidysrhythmic therapy, catheter ablation may be effective [77]. ICDs have the potential to aggravate HF and have been associated with an increase in HF hospitalizations [72, 78]. This may result from right ventricular pacing that produces dyssynchronous cardiac contraction; however, the occurrence of excess events with ICDs placed early after MI suggests that other factors may also limit the overall benefit from ICDs. Careful attention to ICD implantation, programming, and pacing function is important for all patients with low EF who are treated with an ICD. The ACC/AHA/HRS 2008 Guidelines for Device-Based Therapy of Cardiac Rhythm Abnormalities [56] provides further discussion of the potential problem of worsening HF and LV function in all patients with right ventricular pacing. The decision regarding the balance of potential risks and benefits of ICD implantation for an individual patient thus remains a complex one. A decrease in incidence of sudden death does not necessarily translate into decreased total mortality, and decreased total mortality does not guarantee a prolongation of survival with meaningful quality of life. This concept is particularly important in patients with poor prognosis as a result of advanced HF or other serious comorbidities, because there had been no survival benefit observed from ICD implantation until after the first year in two of the major trials [5, 72]. Furthermore, the average age of patients with HF and low ejection fraction in the community is over 70 years, a population not well represented in any of the ICD trials. Comorbidities common in the elderly population, such as prior stroke, lung disease, and crippling arthritic conditions, as well as nursing home residence, should be factored into discussions regarding ICD. Atrial fibrillation, a common trigger for inappropriate shocks, is more prevalent in the elderly population. The gap between community and trial populations is particularly important for a device therapy that may prolong survival but has no real favorable impact on quality of life. Some patients may suffer a diminished quality of life because of device-site complications, such as bleeding, hematoma, or infections, or after ICD discharges, particularly those that are inappropriate. Consideration of ICD implantation is therefore recommended in patients with EF less than or equal to 35% and mild to moderate symptoms of HF and in whom survival with good functional capacity is otherwise anticipated to extend beyond 1 year. Because medical therapy may substantially improve EF, consideration of ICD implants should follow documentation of sustained reduction of EF despite a course of β-blockers and ACE inhibitors; however, ICDs are not warranted in patients with refractory symptoms of HF (Stage D disease) or in patients with concomitant diseases that would significantly shorten their life expectancy independent of HF. Before implantation, patients should be fully informed of their prognosis, including the risk of both sudden and non sudden mortality; the efficacy, safety, and risks of an ICD; and the morbidity associated with an ICD shock. Patients and families should clearly understand that the ICD does not improve clinical function or delay HF progression. Most importantly, the possible reasons and process for potential future deactivation of defibrillator features should be discussed long before functional capacity or outlook for survival is severely reduced.

Heart Transplantation

With a 1-year survival approaching 90%, a 5-year survival rate of approximately 70%, and a median survival in excess of 10 years, heart transplantation is now a valuable option for selected patients with end-stage HF despite optimal medical therapy [7]. The principal indications for heart transplantation remain to be advanced functional class, perception of poor 1-year survival, as exemplified by mixed $VO_2 < 15$ ml/kg/min, the absence of alternative or conventional surgical options, as well as the potential for cardiac rehabilitation. The absolute and relative contraindications include pulmonary hypertension after aggressive challenge with vasodilator or inotropic agents, primary systemic disease that may limit survival, persistent renal dysfunction despite adjustment of therapy, technical issues, psychosocial issues, morbid obesity, significant peripheral and cerebral vascular disease, and diabetes with end-organ damage [79]. The face of heart transplantation is constantly evolving. At the same time as older patients are being considered for heart transplantation, a greater proportion of younger patients being referred for evaluation have complex congenital heart disease (CHD) [7, 80]. There is also an increase in both the number of patients who require mechanical circulatory support (MCS) as a bridge to transplantation as well as the number of retransplant candidates [7]. This changing patient population brings new challenges to the transplant physicians. Among them, the risk of

having preformed antibodies directed against the donor heart (sensitized patients) is particularly challenging as it may increase the risk of rejection and allograft vasculopathy [7, 81]. Once considered an absolute contraindication to transplantation, older recipient age is now seen as a relative contraindication [82]. Older recipient age is usually considered a risk factor for reduced posttransplant survival, although many single-center studies report excellent survival in carefully selected older recipients [82]. The incidence of rejection is usually lower in older recipients while the incidence of infection and allograft vasculopathy is higher [7, 82].

An increasing number of patients with CHD are now surviving into adulthood. Many patients with CHD develop HF later in life, despite repair or palliation or as a result of uncorrected lesions [83, 84]. The most common congenital lesions in patients referred for transplantation include transposition of great arteries with a failing right ventricle and failed Fontan procedures. According to the International Society for Heart and Lung Transplantation (ISHLT) database, CHD is identified as one of the strongest risk factors for 1-year mortality after heart transplantation in adults [7, 83]. In contrast, in those who survive 3 years, CHD has a 10-year survival advantage independent of age. Similarly in the last decade, there has also been an increase in the number of patients requiring MCS as a bridge to transplantation [85]. The technology has allowed many severely ill adult and pediatric patients to survive until a suitable donor heart became available. Patients who require MCS are at increased risk for rejection, infection, stroke, and bleeding. The need for transfusions and possibly the mechanical devices themselves increase the risk of presensitization [7, 81]. Based on the International Society for Heart & Lung Transplantation (ISHLT) database, survival at 1 and 5 years is reduced in patients requiring MCS but still higher than 80 and 70%, respectively [7]. With the increasing number of patients transplanted at early ages, it is also expected that the need for retransplantation will become more common. For now, however, retransplantation comprises only a very small minority (<3%) of heart transplants [7]. Overall survival rates for transplant patients are significantly lower than for other transplant patients, possibly reflecting an increased risk of allosensitization as well as the consequence of years of immunosuppression [7, 86]. Risk factors for poor outcome include retransplantation early after primary transplantation (<6 months), retransplantation for acute rejection, or early allograft failure and retransplantation in an earlier era [86]. When selection criteria for retransplantation excluded retransplantation for primary allograft failure and intractable acute rejection occurring less than 6 months after transplantation, 1-, 2-, and 4-year survival rates after retransplantation were comparable to those after primary transplantation [86].

The surgical techniques for heart transplantation include two basically different surgical approaches, i.e., orthotopic (the donor heart implanted in the normal place of the native heart and heterotopic (donor heart implanted beside the native heart)) [87]. The biatrial technique for orthotopic heart transplantation, first introduced in a dog model by Lower and Shumway in 1960, has been the standard approach [88]. Preservation was provided by the use of topical hypothermia induced by immersion of the graft in iced saline [88]. In 1991, Sievers et al. [89] described a variation of the orthotopic procedure termed the bicaval technique where the donor right atrium is attached directly to the inferior and superior vena cava and the left atrial anastomosis is done as a cuff. Compared with the classical biatrial approach, the bicaval approach results in less disruption of the atrial geometry, better right ventricular function, less tricuspid and mitral valve regurgitation, and less sinus node dysfunction [90]. Despite increasing use of the bicaval technique, tricuspid regurgitation remains a difficult problem early and late after heart transplantation. Adding a tricuspid annuloplasty to the transplant operation has been recently shown to decrease the incidence of tricuspid regurgitation and may even improve survival [91]. Heterotopic heart transplantation was first performed by Barnard in 1974 as a left ventricular bypass and involves placing a donor heart in the right lower thorax where it is anastomosed to work in parallel to the recipient heart, which is left intact. The concept of having the donor and native heart side by side was more appealing in the early times of heart transplantation when the incidence of early

graft failure was high. Although rarely performed nowadays, there remain two potential indications for heterotopic heart transplantation: (1) patients with elevated pulmonary hypertension in whom the donor right ventricle is unable to tolerate the increased afterload; and (2) significant size mismatch (donor/recipient weight ratio <75%), especially seen in pediatric patients. Heart–lung transplantation may also represent an option for patients with irreversible elevation in pulmonary hypertension. Recent advances in organ preservation may also lead to further improvement in outcomes. One of the most promising new technologies is normothermic organ preservation, which provides warm blood perfusion of the donor organ, potentially decreasing reperfusion injury and graft dysfunction. If proven effective, this technology may decrease early graft failure and allow increased utilization of available organs. Its potential to decrease ischemic time may also give greater opportunity for prospective cross-matching in heart transplantation [92].

Conclusions

As with all diseases, prevention is the most important strategy. Once the diagnosis is established, the aim of treating HF is to relieve symptoms and to reduce mortality and mor-

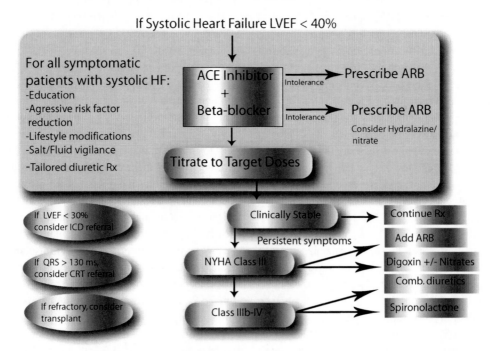

Fig. 20.3   Treatment algorithm of patients with chronic heart failure

bidity. General and nonpharmacologic measures are important components in the management. Cardiovascular risk factors should be aggressively managed with appropriate drugs and life style modifications to targets identified in other disease-specific national guidelines. Patients with symptoms should restrict their dietary salt intake and in patients with more advanced HF, fluid retention may be advised. Regular physical activity is recommended for all patients with stable HF symptoms and impaired LV systolic function. Exercise training should be considered for those with stable symptoms. All patients with HF and LVEF < 40% should be treated with an ACE inhibitor in combination with a β-blocker unless specific contraindications are present. CRT uses biventricular pacing to attempt to synchronize the activation of the septum and LV free wall and improve the overall LV function. Patients with class NYHA II–IV symptoms, despite optimal medical therapy, and who are in normal sinus rhythm with a QRS duration ≥120 ms and a LV ejection fraction ≤35%, should be considered for CRT. Consideration should be made for addition of ICD therapy to patients being referred for CRT who meet the requirements for ICD. Heart transplantation is now accepted therapy for end-stage HF and refractory symptoms despite optimal medical and surgical therapy. Apart from the shortage of donor hearts, the main challenge of heart transplantation is prevention of rejection of the allograft, which is responsible for a considerable percentage of deaths in the first postoperative year. Fortunately, refinement of donor and recipient selection methods, better donor heart management, and advances in immunosuppression have significantly improved survival. Future treatment options may include gene therapy or cell replacement therapy. An algorithm for the treatment of chronic HF using currently available strategies is summarized in Fig. 20.3.

Summary

- There have now been many landmark clinical trials and meta-analyses supporting the use of ACE inhibitors and β-blockers such that these agents have become standard therapy and should be considered in all patients diagnosed with HF with systolic dysfunction.
- Aldosterone receptor blockade should be considered in patients with LVEF < 30% and severe symptomatic chronic HF despite optimization of other recommended treatments, or acute heart failure with LVEF < 30% following acute myocardial infarction, if serum creatinine is <200 mmol/l and potassium is <5.2 mmol/l.
- The combination of isosorbide dinitrate and hydralazine should be considered in addition to standard therapy for African–Americans with systolic dysfunction and may be considered for other heart failure patients unable to tolerate other recommended standard therapy such as ACE inhibitors.
- Drugs that have been proven to be beneficial in large-scale clinical trials are recommended as the effective target doses. The target drug dose should be either the dose used in large-scale clinical trials or a lesser but maximum dose which is tolerated by the patient.
- Patients with symptomatic (NYHA III–IV) heart failure despite optimal medical therapy, and who are in normal sinus rhythm with a QRS duration ≥120 ms and a LV ejection fraction ≤35%, should be considered for cardiac resynchronization therapy (CRT).
- Consideration should be made for addition of ICD therapy to patients being referred for CRT who meet the requirements for ICD.
- Unanswered questions remain about exactly who benefits from CRT therapy. Based on available evidence, primary ICD therapy should be considered in patients with ischemic heart disease with or without mild to moderate HF symptoms and LV ejection fraction of less than or equal to 30%, measured at least 1 month post myocardial infarction and at least 3 months post coronary revascularization procedure. For example, why do not all severely symptomatic patients with a wide QRS benefit? Does the QRS duration itself matter as much as the finding of cardiac dyssynchrony on echocardiogram? What is the role of CRT in patients with chronic atrial fibrillation? An ICD should also be considered in patients with nonischemic cardiomyopathy present for at least 9 months, NYHA functional class II–III heart failure, and LVEF less than or equal to 30% or LV ejection fraction 31–35%.
- The decision to implant a device in a heart failure patient should be made with assessment and discussion between the heart failure and dysrhythmia specialist. An ICD should not be implanted in NYHA class IV heart failure in patients who are not expected to improve with any further therapy and who are not candidates for cardiac transplantation.
- Heart transplantation is the accepted therapy for selected patients with end-stage HF despite optimal medical and surgical therapy.
- As a result of advances in organ preservation, immunosuppressive therapy, improved surgical techniques, and optimal secondary prevention therapy, outcome continues to improve. In addition, a better understanding of the alloimmune response has led to improved monitoring of rejection and the development of better immunosuppressive regimens.
- In the future, advances in immunosuppression protocols, organ preservation, and the use of more specific immune monitoring tools are likely to lead to significant

improvements in outcomes. Until then, heart transplantation remains a treatment and not a cure.

References

1. (1991) Effect of enalapril on survival in patients with reduced left ventricular ejection fractions and congestive heart failure. The SOLVD Investigators. N Engl J Med 325:293–302
2. Packer M, Bristow MR, Cohn JN, Colucci WS, Fowler MB, Gilbert EM, Shusterman NH (1996) The effect of carvedilol on morbidity and mortality in patients with chronic heart failure. U.S. Carvedilol Heart Failure Study Group. N Engl J Med 334:1349–1355
3. Swedberg K, Kjekshus J (1988) Effects of enalapril on mortality in severe congestive heart failure: results of the Cooperative North Scandinavian Enalapril Survival Study (CONSENSUS). Am J Cardiol 62:60A–66A
4. (1999) The Cardiac Insufficiency Bisoprolol Study II (CIBIS-II): a randomised trial. Lancet 353:9–13
5. Bardy GH, Lee KL, Mark DB et al (2005) Amiodarone or an implantable cardioverter-defibrillator for congestive heart failure. N Engl J Med 352:225–237
6. Cleland JG, Daubert JC, Erdmann E, Freemantle N, Gras D, Kappenberger L, Tavazzi L (2005) The effect of cardiac resynchronization on morbidity and mortality in heart failure. N Engl J Med 352:1539–1549
7. Taylor DO, Edwards LB, Boucek MM et al (2007) Registry of the International Society for Heart and Lung Transplantation: twenty-fourth official adult heart transplant report – 2007. J Heart Lung Transplant 26:769–781
8. Butler J, Khadim G, Paul KM et al (2004) Selection of patients for heart transplantation in the current era of heart failure therapy. J Am Coll Cardiol 43:787–793
9. Zipes DP, Camm AJ, Borggrefe M et al (2006) ACC/AHA/ESC 2006 guidelines for management of patients with ventricular arrhythmias and the prevention of sudden cardiac death: a report of the American College of Cardiology/American Heart Association Task Force and the European Society of Cardiology Committee for Practice Guidelines (Writing Committee to Develop Guidelines for Management of Patients With Ventricular Arrhythmias and the Prevention of Sudden Cardiac Death. J Am Coll Cardiol 48:e247–e346
10. Jourdain P, Jondeau G, Funck F et al (2007) Plasma brain natriuretic peptide-guided therapy to improve outcome in heart failure: the STARS-BNP Multicenter Study. J Am Coll Cardiol 49:1733–1739
11. Pfisterer M, Buser P, Rickli H et al (2009) BNP-guided vs symptom-guided heart failure therapy: the Trial of Intensified vs Standard Medical Therapy in Elderly Patients With Congestive Heart Failure (TIME-CHF) randomized trial. JAMA 301:383–392
12. McKelvie RS, Teo KK, McCartney N, Humen D, Montague T, Yusuf S (1995) Effects of exercise training in patients with congestive heart failure: a critical review. J Am Coll Cardiol 25:789–796
13. Piepoli MF, Davos C, Francis DP, Coats AJ (2004) Exercise training meta-analysis of trials in patients with chronic heart failure (ExTraMATCH). BMJ 328:189
14. Pina IL, Apstein CS, Balady GJ et al (2003) Exercise and heart failure: a statement from the American Heart Association Committee on exercise, rehabilitation, and prevention. Circulation 107:1210–1225
15. Smart N, Marwick TH (2004) Exercise training for patients with heart failure: a systematic review of factors that improve mortality and morbidity. Am J Med 116:693–706
16. O'Connor CM, Whellan DJ, Lee KL et al (2009) Efficacy and safety of exercise training in patients with chronic heart failure: HF-ACTION randomized controlled trial. JAMA 301:1439–1450
17. (1987) Effects of enalapril on mortality in severe congestive heart failure. Results of the Cooperative North Scandinavian Enalapril Survival Study (CONSENSUS). The CONSENSUS Trial Study Group. N Engl J Med 316:1429–1435
18. (1992) Effect of enalapril on mortality and the development of heart failure in asymptomatic patients with reduced left ventricular ejection fractions. The SOLVD Investigattors. N Engl J Med 327:685–691
19. (1993) Effect of ramipril on mortality and morbidity of survivors of acute myocardial infarction with clinical evidence of heart failure. The Acute Infarction Ramipril Efficacy (AIRE) Study Investigators. Lancet 342:821–828
20. Kober L, Torp-Pedersen C, Carlsen JE et al (1995) A clinical trial of the angiotensin-converting-enzyme inhibitor trandolapril in patients with left ventricular dysfunction after myocardial infarction. Trandolapril Cardiac Evaluation (TRACE) Study Group. N Engl J Med 333:1670–1676
21. Pfeffer MA, Braunwald E, Moye LA et al (1992) Effect of captopril on mortality and morbidity in patients with left ventricular dysfunction after myocardial infarction. Results of the survival and ventricular enlargement trial. The SAVE Investigators. N Engl J Med 327:669–677
22. CIBIS-II Investigators and Committee (1999) The Cardiac Insufficiency Bisoprolol Study II (CIBIS-II): a randomised trial 37. Lancet 353:9–13
23. MERIT-HF Study Group (1999) Effect of metoprolol CR/XL in chronic heart failure: Metoprolol CR/XL Randomised Intervention Trial in Congestive Heart Failure (MERIT-HF). Lancet 353:2001–2007
24. Packer M, Coats AJ, Fowler MB et al (2001) Effect of carvedilol on survival in severe chronic heart failure. N Engl J Med 344:1651–1658
25. Flather MD, Yusuf S, Kober L et al (2000) Long-term ACE-inhibitor therapy in patients with heart failure or left-ventricular dysfunction: a systematic overview of data from individual patients. ACE-Inhibitor Myocardial Infarction Collaborative Group. Lancet 355:1575–1581
26. Shekelle PG, Rich MW, Morton SC et al (2003) Efficacy of angiotensin-converting enzyme inhibitors and beta-blockers in the management of left ventricular systolic dysfunction according to race, gender, and diabetic status: a meta-analysis of major clinical trials. J Am Coll Cardiol 41:1529–1538
27. Willenheimer R, van Veldhuisen DJ, Silke B et al (2005) Effect on survival and hospitalization of initiating treatment for chronic heart failure with bisoprolol followed by enalapril, as compared with the opposite sequence: results of the randomized Cardiac Insufficiency Bisoprolol Study (CIBIS) III. Circulation 112:2426–2435
28. Granger CB, McMurray JJ, Yusuf S et al (2003) Effects of candesartan in patients with chronic heart failure and reduced left-ventricular systolic function intolerant to angiotensin-converting-enzyme inhibitors: the CHARM-Alternative trial. Lancet 362:772–776
29. Pfeffer MA, McMurray JJ, Velazquez EJ et al (2003) Valsartan, captopril, or both in myocardial infarction complicated by heart failure, left ventricular dysfunction, or both. N Engl J Med 349:1893–1906
30. Cohn JN, Tognoni G (2001) A randomized trial of the angiotensin-receptor blocker valsartan in chronic heart failure 1. N Engl J Med 345:1667–1675
31. McMurray JJ, Ostergren J, Swedberg K et al (2003) Effects of candesartan in patients with chronic heart failure and reduced left-ventricular systolic function taking angiotensin-converting-enzyme inhibitors: the CHARM-Added trial 1. Lancet 362:767–771
32. Pitt B, Zannad F, Remme WJ et al (1999) The effect of spironolactone on morbidity and mortality in patients with severe heart failure. Randomized Aldactone Evaluation Study Investigators 19. N Engl J Med 341:709–717
33. Pitt B, Remme W, Zannad F et al (2003) Eplerenone, a selective aldosterone blocker, in patients with left ventricular dysfunction after myocardial infarction 20. N Engl J Med 348:1309–1321

34. Cohn JN, Johnson G, Ziesche S et al (1991) A comparison of enalapril with hydralazine-isosorbide dinitrate in the treatment of chronic congestive heart failure 3. N Engl J Med 325:303–310

35. Aronow WS (2005) Drug treatment of systolic and of diastolic heart failure in elderly persons. J Gerontol A Biol Sci Med Sci 60:1597–1605

36. (1997) The effect of digoxin on mortality and morbidity in patients with heart failure. The Digitalis Investigation Group. N Engl J Med 336:525–533

37. Rich MW, McSherry F, Williford WO, Yusuf S (2001) Effect of age on mortality, hospitalizations and response to digoxin in patients with heart failure: the DIG study. J Am Coll Cardiol 38:806–813

38. Rathore SS, Wang Y, Krumholz HM (2002) Sex-based differences in the effect of digoxin for the treatment of heart failure. N Engl J Med 347:1403–1411

39. Rathore SS, Curtis JP, Wang Y, Bristow MR, Krumholz HM (2003) Association of serum digoxin concentration and outcomes in patients with heart failure. JAMA 289:871–878

40. Ahmed A, Aronow WS, Fleg JL (2006) Predictors of mortality and hospitalization in women with heart failure in the Digitalis Investigation Group trial. Am J Ther 13:325–331

41. Ahmed A, Aronow WS, Fleg JL (2006) Higher New York Heart Association classes and increased mortality and hospitalization in patients with heart failure and preserved left ventricular function. Am Heart J 151:444–450

42. Arnold JM, Liu P, Demers C et al (2006) Canadian Cardiovascular Society consensus conference recommendations on heart failure 2006: diagnosis and management. Can J Cardiol 22:23–45

43. Silverman ME, Pressel MD, Brackett JC, Lauria SS, Gold MR, Gottlieb SS (1995) Prognostic value of the signal-averaged electro-cardiogram and a prolonged QRS in ischemic and nonischemic cardiomyopathy. Am J Cardiol 75:460–464

44. Fried AG, Parker AB, Newton GE, Parker JD (1999) Electrical and hemodynamic correlates of the maximal rate of pressure increase in the human left ventricle. J Card Fail 5:8–16

45. Xiao HB, Lee CH, Gibson DG (1991) Effect of left bundle branch block on diastolic function in dilated cardiomyopathy. Br Heart J 66:443–447

46. Grines CL, Bashore TM, Boudoulas H, Olson S, Shafer P, Wooley CF (1989) Functional abnormalities in isolated left bundle branch block. The effect of interventricular asynchrony. Circulation 79:845–853

47. Shamim W, Francis DP, Yousufuddin M, Varney S, Pieopli MF, Anker SD, Coats AJ (1999) Intraventricular conduction delay: a prognostic marker in chronic heart failure. Int J Cardiol 70:171–178

48. Kass DA, Chen CH, Curry C, Talbot M, Berger R, Fetics B, Nevo E (1999) Improved left ventricular mechanics from acute VDD pacing in patients with dilated cardiomyopathy and ventricular conduction delay. Circulation 99:1567–1573

49. Nelson GS, Berger RD, Fetics BJ, Talbot M, Spinelli JC, Hare JM, Kass DA (2000) Left ventricular or biventricular pacing improves cardiac function at diminished energy cost in patients with dilated cardiomyopathy and left bundle-branch block. Circulation 102:3053–3059

50. Abraham WT, Fisher WG, Smith AL et al (2002) Cardiac resynchronization in chronic heart failure. N Engl J Med 346:1845–1853

51. McAlister FA, Stewart S, Ferrua S, McMurray JJ (2004) Multidisciplinary strategies for the management of heart failure patients at high risk for admission: a systematic review of randomized trials. J Am Coll Cardiol 44:810–819

52. Young JB, Abraham WT, Smith AL et al (2003) Combined cardiac resynchronization and implantable cardioversion defibrillation in advanced chronic heart failure: the MIRACLE ICD Trial. JAMA 289:2685–2694

53. Bristow MR, Saxon LA, Boehmer J et al (2004) Cardiac-resynchronization therapy with or without an implantable defibrillator in advanced chronic heart failure. N Engl J Med 350: 2140–2150

54. Leclercq C, Walker S, Linde C et al (2002) Comparative effects of permanent biventricular and right-univentricular pacing in heart failure patients with chronic atrial fibrillation. Eur Heart J 23:1780–1787

55. Leon AR, Greenberg JM, Kanuru N et al (2002) Cardiac resynchronization in patients with congestive heart failure and chronic atrial fibrillation: effect of upgrading to biventricular pacing after chronic right ventricular pacing. J Am Coll Cardiol 39:1258–1263

56. Epstein AE, Dimarco JP, Ellenbogen KA et al (2008) ACC/AHA/HRS 2008 Guidelines for Device-Based Therapy of Cardiac Rhythm Abnormalities: a report of the American College of Cardiology/American Heart Association Task Force on Practice Guidelines (Writing Committee to Revise the ACC/AHA/NASPE 2002 Guideline Update for Implantation of Cardiac Pacemakers and Antiarrhythmia Devices) developed in collaboration with the American Association for Thoracic Surgery and Society of Thoracic Surgeons. J Am Coll Cardiol 51:e1–e62

57. Chung ES, Leon AR, Tavazzi L et al (2008) Results of the Predictors of Response to CRT (PROSPECT) trial. Circulation 117:2608–2616

58. Beshai JF, Grimm RA, Nagueh SF et al (2007) Cardiac-resynchronization therapy in heart failure with narrow QRS complexes. N Engl J Med 357:2461–2471

59. Moss AJ, Hall WJ, Cannom DS, Klein H, Brown MW, Daubert JP, Estes NA, III, Foster E, Greenberg H, Higgins SL, Pfeffer MA, Solomon SD, Wilber D, Zareba W (2009) Cardiac-resynchronization therapy for the prevention of heart-failure events. N Engl J Med 361:1329–1338

60. Linde C, Abraham WT, Gold MR, St John SM, Ghio S, Daubert C (2008) Randomized trial of cardiac resynchronization in mildly symptomatic heart failure patients and in asymptomatic patients with left ventricular dysfunction and previous heart failure symptoms. J Am Coll Cardiol 52:1834–1843

61. Uretsky BF, Thygesen K, Armstrong PW et al (2000) Acute coronary findings at autopsy in heart failure patients with sudden death: results from the assessment of treatment with lisinopril and survival (ATLAS) trial. Circulation 102:611–616

62. Luu M, Stevenson WG, Stevenson LW, Baron K, Walden J (1989) Diverse mechanisms of unexpected cardiac arrest in advanced heart failure. Circulation 80:1675–1680

63. Knight BP, Goyal R, Pelosi F, Flemming M, Horwood L, Morady F, Strickberger SA (1999) Outcome of patients with nonischemic dilated cardiomyopathy and unexplained syncope treated with an implantable defibrillator. J Am Coll Cardiol 33:1964–1970

64. Packer M (1992) Lack of relation between ventricular arrhythmias and sudden death in patients with chronic heart failure. Circulation 85:I50–I56

65. (1992) Effect of the antiarrhythmic agent moricizine on survival after myocardial infarction. The Cardiac Arrhythmia Suppression Trial II Investigators. N Engl J Med 327:227–233

66. Pratt CM, Eaton T, Francis M, Woolbert S, Mahmarian J, Roberts R, Young JB (1989) The inverse relationship between baseline left ventricular ejection fraction and outcome of antiarrhythmic therapy: a dangerous imbalance in the risk-benefit ratio. Am Heart J 118: 433–440

67. Coplen SE, Antman EM, Berlin JA, Hewitt P, Chalmers TC (1990) Efficacy and safety of quinidine therapy for maintenance of sinus rhythm after cardioversion. A meta-analysis of randomized control trials. Circulation 82:1106–1116

68. Du XJ, Esler MD, Dart AM (1995) Sympatholytic action of intravenous amiodarone in the rat heart. Circulation 91:462–470

69. Doval HC, Nul DR, Grancelli HO, Perrone SV, Bortman GR, Curiel R (1994) Randomised trial of low-dose amiodarone in severe congestive heart failure. Grupo de Estudio de la Sobrevida en la Insuficiencia Cardiaca en Argentina (GESICA). Lancet 344:493–498

70. Massie BM, Fisher SG, Radford M, Deedwania PC, Singh BN, Fletcher RD, Singh SN (1996) Effect of amiodarone on clinical status and left ventricular function in patients with congestive heart failure. CHF-STAT Investigators. Circulation 93:2128–2134

71. Klein HU, Reek S (2000) The MUSTT study: evaluating testing and treatment. J Interv Card Electrophysiol 4:45–50

72. Moss AJ, Zareba W, Hall WJ et al (2002) Prophylactic implantation of a defibrillator in patients with myocardial infarction and reduced ejection fraction. N Engl J Med 346:877–883

73. Hohnloser SH, Connolly SJ, Kuck KH et al (2000) The defibrillator in acute myocardial infarction trial (DINAMIT): study protocol. Am Heart J 140:735–739

74. Kadish A, Dyer A, Daubert JP et al (2004) Prophylactic defibrillator implantation in patients with nonischemic dilated cardiomyopathy. N Engl J Med 350:2151–2158

75. Ezekowitz JA, Rowe BH, Dryden DM, Hooton N, Vandermeer B, Spooner C, McAlister FA (2007) Systematic review: implantable cardioverter defibrillators for adults with left ventricular systolic dysfunction. Ann Intern Med 147:251–262

76. Wilkoff BL, Auricchio A, Brugada J et al (2008) HRS/EHRA expert consensus on the monitoring of cardiovascular implantable electronic devices (CIEDs): description of techniques, indications, personnel, frequency and ethical considerations. Heart Rhythm 5:907–925

77. Soejima K, Suzuki M, Maisel WH et al (2001) Catheter ablation in patients with multiple and unstable ventricular tachycardias after myocardial infarction: short ablation lines guided by reentry circuit isthmuses and sinus rhythm mapping. Circulation 104:664–669

78. Wilkoff BL, Cook JR, Epstein AE et al (2002) Dual-chamber pacing or ventricular backup pacing in patients with an implantable defibrillator: the Dual Chamber and VVI Implantable Defibrillator (DAVID) Trial. JAMA 288:3115–3123

79. Ross H, Hendry P, Dipchand A et al (2003) 2001 Canadian Cardiovascular Society Consensus Conference on cardiac transplantation. Can J Cardiol 19:620–654

80. Ventura HO, Muhammed K (2001) Historical perspectives on cardiac transplantation: the past as prologue to challenges for the 21st century. Curr Opin Cardiol 16:118–123

81. Kerman RH (2007) Understanding the sensitized patient. Heart Fail Clin 3:1–9

82. Aliabadi AZ, Zuckermann AO, Grimm M (2007) Immunosuppressive therapy in older cardiac transplant patients. Drugs Aging 24: 913–932

83. Hosseinpour AR, Cullen S, Tsang VT (2006) Transplantation for adults with congenital heart disease. Eur J Cardiothorac Surg 30: 508–514

84. Alkhaldi A, Chin C, Bernstein D (2006) Pediatric cardiac transplantation. Semin Pediatr Surg 15:188–198

85. Hunt SA (2007) Mechanical circulatory support: new data, old problems. Circulation 116:461–462

86. Johnson MR, Aaronson KD, Canter CE et al (2007) Heart retransplantation. Am J Transplant 7:2075–2081

87. Bernstein D, Naftel D, Chin C et al (2006) Outcome of listing for cardiac transplantation for failed Fontan: a multi-institutional study. Circulation 114:273–280

88. Lower RR, Shumway NE (1960) Studies on orthotopic homotransplantation of the canine heart. Surg Forum 11:18–19

89. Sievers HH, Weyand M, Kraatz EG, Bernhard A (1991) An alternative technique for orthotopic cardiac transplantation, with preservation of the normal anatomy of the right atrium. Thorac Cardiovasc Surg 39:70–72

90. Schnoor M, Schafer T, Luhmann D, Sievers HH (2007) Bicaval versus standard technique in orthotopic heart transplantation: a systematic review and meta-analysis. J Thorac Cardiovasc Surg 134:1322–1331

91. Jeevanandam V, Russell H, Mather P, Furukawa S, Anderson A, Raman J (2006) Donor tricuspid annuloplasty during orthotopic heart transplantation: long-term results of a prospective controlled study. Ann Thorac Surg 82:2089–2095

92. Jamieson RW, Friend PJ (2008) Organ reperfusion and preservation. Front Biosci 13:221–235

Chapter 21
Gene Therapy in Heart Failure: Forthcoming Therapies

Overview

After a decade of preclinical and early phase clinical investigations, gene therapy has emerged as a genuine therapeutic option with the potential to alter the way clinicians manage patients with coronary artery disease (CAD) and with HF. Initially conceived for the treatment of specific inherited monogenic disorders, gene therapy potential has been extended to also include acquired polygenic diseases, such as HF. True that some investigators believe that gene therapy may still be a long time away. Indeed, gene therapy had multiple "initial" successes followed by the realization that much of the enthusiasm for each success has been perhaps premature. Furthermore, much of the early excitement with regard to this approach has been dampened following the death of a young male in one clinical trial. However, as with all discoveries and new fields, problems will arise and they need to be and likely will be identified and overcome with time. In this chapter, we discuss the current state of gene therapy in cardiac disease, and particular HF, including vehicles for delivery and human clinical trials.

Introduction

Given the fact that patients with HF have an altered pattern of myocardial gene expression with a characteristic genetic fingerprint [1] using genes themselves as the vehicle for replacing or altering the expression of defective genes to treat patients at the molecular level is an attractive approach to therapy. In particular, muscular dystrophies constitute a good model to assess novel approaches of gene therapy in the setting of cardiomyopathy. These conditions are common and debilitating genetic diseases that frequently arise from single gene mutations. In humans and hamsters, mutations in the *SGCD* gene encoding δ-sarcoglycan (δ-SG) can cause limb girdle muscular dystrophy (LGMD) with accompanying DCM. A stable and safe gene delivery with minimal trauma is required for successful gene therapy. Recently, it has been reported that the therapeutic effect of systemic delivery of adeno-associated

virus (AAV) vectors carrying human *SGCD* gene in TO-2 hamsters, an HF and muscular dystrophy model with a δ-SG mutation [2]. A single injection of a double-stranded AAV vector carrying *SGCD* gene, without the need of physical or pharmaceutical interventions achieved near complete gene transfer and expression in the heart and skeletal muscles. Furthermore, sustained restoration of the missing δ-SG gene in the TO-2 hamsters corrected muscle cell membrane leakiness throughout the body and normalized serum creatine kinase levels. Echocardiography documented significant increase in the percent fractional shortening and decreased LV end-diastolic and end-systolic dimensions. The main objective of gene therapy in HF will be to achieve a reversal of the myocardial remodeling process with definitive improvement in cardiac function.

Why Gene Therapy for Cardiovascular Disease?

Gene therapy allows therapeutic concentrations of a gene product to be accumulated and maintained at optimally high levels at a localized target site of action. By avoiding high plasma levels of the gene product, it is possible to significantly reduce potential side effects.

Vectors and Targets

Both vascular and cardiac tissues have served as targets for gene therapy [3]. For myocardial gene therapy, the methods of gene delivery include: (a) direct injection into the epicardium, (b) catheter-mediated injection into the endocardium or into coronary arteries, (c) retroperfusion of coronary veins, and (d) intrapericardial delivery via catheter [4, 5]. The mechanics of delivery are continuously being up-dated and are dependent on the vector used; for instance, viral rather than nonviral vectors can be effectively delivered via coronary circulation approaches ((b) and (c) above). In addition, through ultrasound exposure, the uptake and expression of plasmid DNA in both

J. Marín-García, *Heart Failure*, Contemporary Cardiology,
DOI 10.1007/978-1-60761-147-9_21, © Springer Science+Business Media, LLC 2010

Table 21.1 Comparison of vectors for gene transfer and expression

Vector	Chromosomal integration	In vivo transfer efficiency	Target cells	Expression (level/ onset/duration)	Disadvantage of gene therapy
Liposome	No	+	Quiescent and dividing	+/rapid/transient	Low transduction efficiency and stability
Plasmid	No	+	Quiescent and dividing	+/moderate/transient	Low transduction efficiency
Adenovirus	No	++++	Quiescent and dividing	++++/rapid/transient	Immunogenic; viral mutation
Lentivirus	Yes	+++	Quiescent and dividing	+++/rapid/long term	Insertional mutagenesis
Retrovirus	Yes	++	Dividing	+++/rapid/long term	Oncogenic potential
AAV	Yes	+++	Quiescent and dividing	+++/slow/long term	Insertional mutagenesis

arteries and myocardium can be enhanced [6, 7]. Both viral vectors and naked plasmid DNAs have been employed in preclinical and clinical cardiovascular gene transfer studies. Naked plasmid DNA has been shown to have good entry and expression in normal and ischemic muscle [8]. However, the use of plasmid vectors pose limitations with lower efficiency of transfection.

It is important to keep in mind that the duration of transgene expression varies with the type of vector employed (Table 21.1), or the specific transgene. The requirements for sustained or long term gene expression will vary from case to case. For instance, certain cardiovascular disorders and/or clinical settings may require shorter-term gene expression, in which transgene expression is required only during a period of defined risk such as remodeling after myocardial infarct, or in preventing myocardial ischemia. In addition, short-term expression (e.g., 2–3 weeks) may be sufficient to promote neovascularization, or to inhibit restenosis [9].

Nature of Targeted Gene

A large assortment of genes has thus far been used in cardiovascular gene transfer and myocardial therapy; a representative list is presented in Table 21.2. Which genes to use in cardio-vascular gene therapy is markedly dependent on the specific disorder to be treated, as well as which cell type is being targeted. These genes range from SERCA, plasma membrane channel proteins, cytokines, and transcription factors to signaling pathway components. Early studies found the transfer of genes encoding extracellular secreted proteins such as VEGF rather than intracellular proteins was advantageous since a limited number of injections/transfections were needed to produce a large enough quantity of protein. This was particularly evident with vascular treatments involving therapeutic angiogenesis (e.g., VEGF, FGF). Active secretion can either be mediated by a native or ligated signal sequence. Features of the viral vector predetermine both the range of host cells that can be transduced as well as the efficiency, level and duration of transgene expression.

Adenoviral vectors, which are well manipulated and produced high titers [10] can transduce both dividing and nondividing cells and are particularly efficient in transfecting postmitotic cells including cardiomyocytes, and to a lesser extent vascular cells. A limitation of the adenoviral vectors is their provision of transient rather than prolonged transgene expression. Moreover, adenoviral vectors pose additional safety concerns; these vectors produce increased inflammation, and long term cell- and antibody-mediated immune responses have been reported [11, 12]. Nevertheless, to date no evidence of serious adverse effects have been reported in clinical trials of cardiovascular gene therapy using adenoviral vector involving over 150 subjects [11]. Other viral vectors such as adeno-associated virus (AAV) are being considered more promising, mainly in the context of gene therapy for chronic diseases such as HF [13], because its longer transgene expression and reduced immunogenicity. AAV is taken up more slowly into myocardial cells and transgene expression levels are lower when compared to adenovirus, but transgene expression can be longer term, being sustained in the rodent myocardium for 9–12 months. In addition, AAV vectors have a lower potential to induce unwanted immunocytotoxicity or inflammation [10, 14]. Liposomal carriers are also used, albeit less frequently.

Another alternative gene transfer approach uses oligonucleotides (e.g., antisense oligonucleotides) that regulate transcription of targeted endogenous genes and inhibit their expression. Moreover, double stranded oligonucleotides homologous to the *cis* regulatory sequences of the promoter of the gene of interest can be similarly employed. These function as decoys to bind transcription factors, and therefore block expression of genes requiring those transcription factors [15]. Transcription factors are attractive targets for gene therapy since they mediate the expression of a large number of genes involved in a coordinated cellular program. Competitively inhibiting the binding and activity of critical transcription factors such as NF-κB and E2f, involved in cell-cycle progression, cellular proliferation, and inflammatory responses, using the decoy approach has proved to be highly effective in treating myocarditis and intimal hyperplasia in preclinical studies, which will be discussed later. Which gene to use in gene therapy is highly

Table 21.2 Targeted gene expression in CVD

Function	Targeted gene	O or I
Antioxidant	Heme oxygenase (HO-1)	O
	Superoxide dismutase (SOD)	O
	Catalase (CAT)	O
	Glutathione peroxidase (GPx)	O
Pro-apoptotic proteins	p53	I
	Bad	I
	Fas ligand	I
Ca²⁺ regulation	β-adrenergic receptor kinase (β-ARK)	I
	β-adrenergic receptor (β-AR)	O
	Phospholamban (PLN)	I
	Sarcoplasmic reticulum Ca²⁺ ATPase (SERCA)	O
Channel proteins	Cardiac sodium channel (SCN5A)	O
	Hyperpolarization-activated cyclic nucleotide-gated channel (HCN2)	I
Coronary vessel tone	Endothelial nitric oxide synthase (eNOS)	O
	Adenosine receptor	O
Contractile proteins	Sarcomeric proteins	O
	Sarcoglycan (δ-SG)	O
Survival genes	Protein kinase B (Akt)	O
	Bcl-2	O
	Insulin-like growth factor (IGF-1)	O
Pro-angiogenic factors	Vascular endothelial growth factor (VEGF)	O
	Fibroblast growth factor (FGF)	O
	Hypoxia-inducing factor (HIF)-1α	O
Inflammatory cytokines	ICAM	I
	TNF-α	I
	NF-κB	I

O overexpression; *I* inhibition

dependent on the specific disorder to be treated as well as which cell-type is being targeted; a number of genes, thus far used (Fig. 21.1) will be discussed in the next section (Table 21.3).

Early experiments showed that the transfer of genes encoding extracellular (secreted proteins) rather than intracellular proteins (active secretion can either be mediated by a native or ligated signal sequence) was advantageous since a limited number of injections/transfections was needed to produce a large quantity of protein; this was particularly evident with vascular-treatments involving therapeutic angiogenesis (e.g., VEGF, FGF). Significantly, the regulation of transgene expression can be modulated by the addition of the appropriate regulatory sequences within the genetic construct to be introduced. These generally use constitutive promoters and enhancers. Promoter elements that are inducible in response to a variety of endogenous or exogenous molecular signals (e.g., steroid hormones, cytokines, and growth factors) are also available. Moreover, by the addition of specific peptide presequences to the transgene, targeting of the gene product to the appropriate cellular compartment can also be directed. In addition, prevention of unwanted transgene expression in nontarget cells can be

achieved by incorporation of tissue-specific regulatory elements, such as myocyte-specific promoter sequences of ventricle-specific myosin light chain-2 (MLC-2v) and cardiac troponin T (cTNT). Aiming gene therapies directly at the myocardium and at vascular tissues, transfection of cells with specific transgenes ex vivo followed by in vivo delivery of the transfected cells has broadened the possibilities associated with gene therapy, and potentially sidestepped a number of the safety concerns. Gene transfer of VEGF has been shown to augment the proliferative activity of bone marrow-derived endothelial progenitor cells, which increases neovascularization when administered to animals with limb or myocardial ischemia [41, 42]. New approaches are employing gene therapy to enhance the homing and engrafting of bone marrow derived progenitor cells to the heart and into areas damaged by ischemia promoting neovascularization for tissue repair.

Specific Examples of Cardiovascular Gene Therapy-Preclinical Studies

Specific examples of cardiovascular diseases in which gene therapy was initially employed will be discussed in this section. However, we must keep in mind that although the etiology of HF is diverse, the accompanied myocardial dysfunction may be elicited by similar mechanisms. These mechanisms include: (1) a defect in sarcoplasmic reticulum function, which is responsible for abnormal intracellular calcium handling, (2) activation of proapoptotic pathways, (3) dysregulation of β-adrenergic signaling, and (4) electrical remodeling [43, 44].

Coronary Artery Restenosis

One of the initial heart defect targeted for gene therapy was restenosis following coronary stenting and vein graft occlusion [16, 18–20, 45]. Vasculoproliferation, characteristic of these disorders, has been effectively inhibited in a variety of preclinical studies by the transfer and overexpression of genes, including isoforms of nitric oxide synthase [46] as well as by targeting gene expression of cell cycle progression, including the use of decoy and antisense genetic constructs to knock-out vasculoproliferative gene expression in vascular smooth muscle [47]. While advances in nongenetic treatments of these disorders, and concerns with their efficacy and safety have been raised, clinical trials for the use of gene therapy in restenosis are in place and will be discussed in a later section [14].

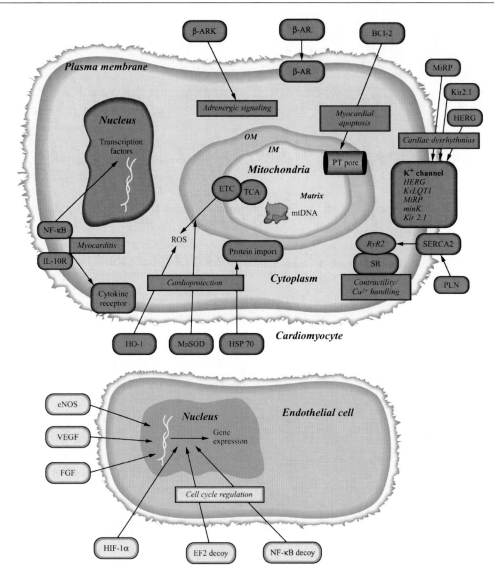

Fig. 21.1 Specific cellular targets of gene therapy in the cardiomyocyte and endothelial cell. A broad array of sub-cellular loci can be effective targets of cardiovascular gene therapy including (in cardiomyocyte as depicted in *Panel A*): Nuclear transcription factors, plasma membrane associated signaling pathways (cytokines, β-adrenergic signaling pathway and K⁺ channel), mitochondria (the primary site of energy and ROS generation by the electron transport chain (ETC)), and the sarcoplasmic reticulum (SR) (involved in Ca²⁺ cycling). Targets shown in the endothelial cell (*Panel B*) include the nucleus and signal transduction pathways which regulate cell cycle progression and endothelial cell proliferation. For each cell type, specific genes (*yellow boxes*) that have been effectively used in cardiovascular therapies are shown, and they are described in more detail in the text and in Table 21.3

Therapeutic Angiogenesis (Increasing Proliferation of Blood Vessels) to Limit Ischemia

The pioneering studies of the Isner laboratory [20, 48, 49] demonstrated that delivery of angiogenic peptides by gene transfer could enhance blood flow in ischemic tissue. In a number of animal models, vascular endothelial growth factor (VEGF), a secreted endothelial mitogen, markedly induced angiogenesis. Interestingly, gene transfer of hypoxia-inducible factor-1α (HIF-1α), a transcription factor known to regulate the transcription of hypoxia-inducible genes also induces

angiogenesis at ischemic sites [22]. Clinical trials using plasmid delivery of VEGF into ischemic limbs [50, 51] have initially proved to be promising and have been extended to include other angiogenic transgenes including other VEGF isoforms and fibroblast growth factor (FGF), which will be discussed later in this chapter.

Hypertension

Gene therapy has been effectively applied in preclinical studies with both systemic and pulmonary hypertension. Two

Table 21.3 Preclinical studies of gene therapy

Cardiovascular target	Gene used	Vector	Animal model	References
Restenosis	NOS	Adenovirus	Pig	[16]
	as-E2F decoy	Oligos	Rabbit	[17]
Therapeutic angiogenesis/ischemia	VEGF	Plasmid	Rabbit	[18–20]
	FGF	Plasmid	Rabbit	[21]
	HIF-1α	Plasmid	Rabbit	[22]
Hypertension	as-β-AR	Liposome	SH rat	[23]
	as-AT1R	AAV	SH rat	[24]
	Kallikrein	Adenovirus	Rat	[25]
	ANP	Adenovirus	Dahl rat	[26]
	Adrenomedullin	Adenovirus	SH rat	[27]
	eNOS	Plasmid	SH rat	[28]
Cardiac dysrhythmia	ShK	Adenovirus	Dog myocyte	[29]
	KIR2.5/SERCA	Adenovirus	Guinea pig	[30]
	MiRP	Plasmid	Pig	[31]
	Gα_{i2}	Adenovirus	Pig	[32]
Myocarditis	IL-10	Plasmid	Rat (EAM)	[33]
	NFκB/*cis* decoy	Oligos	Rat (EAM)	[34]
Myocardial protection	HO-1	AAV	Rat	[35]
	SOD	Adenovirus	Rat	[36]
	HSP 70	Liposome	Rat	[37]
	BCl-2	Adenovirus	Rabbit	[38]
Pulmonary hypertension	eNOS	Adenovirus	Mouse	[39]
	Kv1.5	Adenovirus	Rat	[40]

major approaches to gene therapy for treatment of systemic hypertension include the overexpression of vasodilator genes and reduction of vasoconstriction genes expression (usually accomplished by antisense inhibition). Preclinical studies in rat have demonstrated that the transfer and expression of genes, including an O_2-sensitive voltage-gated potassium channel (Kv1.5), endothelial nitric oxide synthase (eNOS), and prostaglandin I synthase, (PGIS) markedly improved pulmonary hypertension [40, 52].

Because antihypertensive treatments often are not aimed at a specific identifiable causes, traditional pharmacological therapy has focused on elements such as the renin–angiotensin system (RAS), which are known to be directly involved in the control of blood pressure [53]. The development of gene therapy directed at RAS represents a significant advance toward managing high blood pressure and reversing its associated pathophysiology. Delivery of antisense constructs to the angiotensin II type 1 receptor (AT1R) successfully prevented blood pressure elevation, alterations in calcium homeostasis, ion channel activity, and cardiovascular ultrastructure changes (for up to 18 months) in spontaneously hypertensive rats (SHRs), when compared to control rats. These results in animal models demonstrate that antisense gene delivery may be useful in the long-term treatment of hypertension. In addition to the angiotensin receptor, another genetic component of RAS targeted in the therapeutic treatment of hypertension by deploying antisense oligonucleotide therapies is angiotensinogen [24, 54, 55]. Antisense oligo-

nucleotides used in combination with an adeno-associated virus delivery system resulted in a significantly prolonged reduction of hypertension in adult rats and transgenic mice, with a single dose administration of AAV-antisense constructs [55]. Moreover, it has been shown that concomitant with the reduction of hypertension, the angiotensinogen and angiotensin receptor antisense therapies resulted in significant attenuation of cardiac hypertrophy [24, 56].

The adrenergic signaling system is another viable target for gene therapy, designed to stem hypertension by utilizing antisense technology. Transfer of antisense oligonucleotides against rat β1-adrenergic receptor (β1-AR) mRNA provided a significant and prolonged reduction in blood pressure in the SHR model [23].

Genes involved in the regulation of vasodilatation have also proved to be excellent targets for gene therapy of systemic hypertension. Several studies in adult rats demonstrated that systemic hypertension can be significantly reversed by transfer and overexpression of genes encoding atrial natriuretic peptide (ANP), kallikrein, adrenomedullin, and eNOS over a range of a 6–12 weeks [25–28]. Delivery of these genes employed either non-viral (naked DNA) or adenoviral vectors with several rat models of hypertension (including SHR and Dahl salt-sensitive rats). Interestingly, the decrease in blood pressure mediated by gene transfer and overexpression of kallikrein and adrenomedullin was also accompanied by an attenuation of both cardiac hypertrophy and myocardial apoptosis.

Cardiac Dysrhythmias

The treatment of cardiac dysrhythmias using gene therapy may be a desirable goal since current treatment options are limited. Several well defined genetic loci have been characterized, which can lead to ventricular dysrhythmias, including gene defects in the membrane transporters associated with potassium channels. Adenoviral-mediated transfection of a potassium channel gene has been performed with cardiomyocytes derived from failing dog hearts [29]. Interestingly, a moderate level of transgene expression increased the potassium current mimicked the nondisease phenotype. However, a robust level of transgene expression adversely impacted cardiomyocyte excitation–contraction coupling.

A dual gene therapy strategy was implemented to reverse K$^+$ channel deficiency or down-regulation without depressing contractility [30]. An adenoviral vector was constructed that enabled the coexpression of two genes driven by a single promoter. The genes encoding the potassium channel (Kir2.1) and SERCA1, to boost contractility, were directly injected into the myocardium. Both genes were amply expressed in myocytes from transfected hearts and exhibited significantly shorter action potentials and larger calcium transients, with unimpaired contractile function. In addition, plasmid-mediated gene transfer of specific mutant alleles of potassium channel genes has been used [31]. A mutant channel gene associated with the long QT syndrome (Q9E-hMiRP1) was introduced into human cell lines and implanted directly into the pig atria. Results from these in vitro and in vivo studies demonstrated significant levels of transgene expression and altered myocyte electrophysiological phenotype supporting the feasibility of site-specific gene transfer in the treatment of atrial dysrhythmias. Successful intracoronary adenoviral-mediated gene transfer of an inhibitory component (Gα_{i2}) of the β-adrenergic pathway, directed to the atrioventricular (AV) node to suppress AV node conduction, has also been reported [32].

Myocarditis

It is well established that the inflammatory cytokines play a critical role in the pathogenesis of viral myocarditis. In the rat model of experimental autoimmune myocarditis (EAM), introduction of plasmid DNA containing the gene encoding murine interleukin IL-10 into striated muscle (tibialis anterior) by electroporation significantly affected survival rates, attenuated myocardial damage, and improved hemodynamic parameters [33].

The transcription factor NFκB, by modulating the expression of TNF-α and inducible nitric oxide synthase (iNOS), as well as adhesion molecule (iCAM) genes, represents a potential target to control myocarditis using the same rat model of EAM. Decreasing the expression of NFκB, by introducing into the rat coronary artery a decoy sequence directed to the cis-regulatory sequence within the NFκB promoter, reduced the areas of myocarditis as well as myocardial gene expression of iNOS, iCAM, and TNF-α [34].

Myocardial Protection

Short-term protection of the heart from ischemia can be provided by gene transfer and overexpression of cardioprotective genes such as superoxide dismutase (SOD) or heme oxygenase (HO-1). Administration of a myocardial protective gene such as HO-1, employing a recombinant AAV vector, significantly reduced infarct size in a rat model of ischemia and reperfusion when introduced into myocardium prior to coronary ligation [35]. The resulting cardioprotective effect was maintained over 5 days, as gauged by echocardiography. In addition, gene-mediated cardioprotection against myocardial ischemia has been achieved by introducing and overexpressing genes for antioxidant enzyme SOD [36], the heat shock protein HSP70 [37], and the antiapoptotic protein BCl-2 [38]. It remains to be seen whether these vectors and genes can provide longer term cardioprotection against repeated, chronic forms of ischemic insult.

As a methodology for acute intervention in cardiac insults (e.g., myocardial ischemia), myocardial gene therapy may have limited efficacy. A period of time is clearly needed for transgene introduction, transcription, translation, and processing of the transgene product. Gene therapy in advance of specific insults, which prepares the cardiomyocyte to mount a protective response to an adverse event, may be more rewarding. Interestingly, a prototype cardioprotective vector has been developed called the "vigilant vector," designed to be expressed specifically in the heart and switch on therapeutic transgenes only during hypoxia [57]. It utilizes several elements including a cardiac-specific promoter (MLC-2v), a hypoxia response element (HRE), a therapeutic transgene (AT1R), and a reporter gene (green fluorescence protein) incorporated into an AAV vector. High levels of cardiac-specific expression of AT1R have been achieved with this vector in vitro with transfected cardiomyocytes (H9C2 cells), and in vivo with mice challenged with hypoxia.

Heart Failure

In preclinical studies of gene therapy in HF (Table 21.4), it has been shown that in both human and experimental animal models, sarcoplasmic reticulum Ca^{2+} ATPase (SERCA2)

Table 21.4 Preclinical studies of gene therapy in heart failure

Gene used	Vector	Animal model	References
β-ARK inhibitor	Adenovirus	Rabbit	[58]
SERCA2a	Adenovirus	Rat	[59]
SERCA2a, Parvalbumin	Adenovirus	Canine	[60]
SERCA2a	rAAV1	Swine	[61]

activity is decreased, resulting in abnormal calcium handling thought to contribute to severe reduction in cardiac contractility [58–61]. Myocardial SERCA2 Ca^{2+} pumping activity is inhibited by phospholamban. Adenovirus-mediated over-expression of SERCA2 by in vivo gene transfer in a pressure-overload rat model of HF restored cardiac function, including improved Ca^{2+} cycling and contractility [59]. Moreover, adenoviral-mediated transfer and overexpression of an antisense phospholamban construct or a dominant-negative mutant allele of phospholamban enhanced both SERCA2 activity and contractility in myocytes derived from failing rat and human hearts [62, 63]. Ablation of the phospholamban allele in some mouse models of HF reversed cardiac dysfunction, whereas in other models no beneficial effect was found [64, 65]. Furthermore, polymorphic null-alleles of phospholamban have been recently identified in individuals with lethal dilated cardiomyopathy (DCM) [66]. Caution must be used in applying these findings to human clinical trials since animal models of HF are different [64].

Hirsch et al. reported that genetic modification of intracellular calcium-handling proteins may reverse the diastolic dysfunction resulting from impaired ventricular relaxation, an important component of human HF [60]. They established a canine model of human-like diastolic dysfunction after 1 year of left ventricular (LV) pressure overload by coarctation of the descending thoracic aorta. Progressive increase in LV mass was documented by echocardiography, and diastolic dysfunction with preserved systolic function was evident at the whole organ and myocyte levels. Using gene transfer SERCA2a and parvalbumin (Parv), a fast-twitch skeletal muscle Ca^{2+} buffer, they were able to restore cardiac myocyte relaxation in a dose-dependent manner under baseline conditions. At high Parv concentrations, sarcomere shortening was depressed. On the other hand, during β-adrenergic stimulation, the expected enhancement of myocyte contraction (inotropy) was abrogated by SERCA2a, but not by Parv. These divergent effects of SERCA2a and Parv in a large animal model, with cardiac physiology closer to human than rodent models, appear to be of significant interest and may have potential toward the development of novel therapeutic strategies for human HF. Similarly, Kawase et al. [61] have recently evaluated the effects of SERCA2a gene transfer in a swine HF model. They found that long-term overexpression of SERCA2a by in vivo rAAV1-mediated intracoronary gene transfer preserved systolic function, potentially prevented diastolic dysfunction, and improved

ventricular remodeling. Interestingly, following on the above experiences with large animal models, designs for human clinical trials are in the making process. Haijar et al. [67] reported the design of a phase 1 clinical trial of intracoronary administration of AAV1/SERCA2a (MYDICAR) to subjects with HF divided into two stages: in Stage 1, subjects will be assigned open-label MYDICAR in one of up to four sequential dose escalation cohorts; in Stage 2, subjects will be randomized in parallel to two or three doses of MYDICAR or placebo in a double-blinded manner. Expectations are high to know the results of this trial.

It is well established that both experimental models and human HF exhibit marked abnormalities in β-adrenergic signaling, including the downregulation of β-adrenergic receptors (β-AR), their uncoupling with second messenger pathways, and modulation by upregulated β-AR kinase (β-ARK). Intracoronary transfer of an adenovirus encoding a peptide inhibitor of β-ARK, reversed cardiac dysfunction in both rabbit and mouse models of HF [58, 68]. Moreover, in vivo ventricular gene delivery to the failing heart of a β-adrenergic receptor kinase inhibitor reverses cardiac dysfunction [58]. However, with this approach, side-effects have been reported that may result in a sustained adrenergic stimulation, which can be both cardiotoxic and dysrhythmogenic [5].

Clinical Studies of Cardiovascular Gene Therapy Thus Far

Several small phase 1 and 2 clinical studies have been conducted with adenovirus- and plasmid-based VEGF and FGF gene constructs to provide therapeutic angiogenesis in coronary artery disease (CAD) and peripheral vascular disease (PVD) as shown in Table 21.5.

While recent studies have reported that new vessels are formed and functional, the potential efficacy has not yet been ascertained. Similarly, data are not yet available from large-scale randomized trials of VEGF treatment in patients with CAD and PVD; parenthetically, symptomatic relief in some patients with severe CAD has been reported. Obviously, prior to routine clinical use, additional data to develop the optimal dosage and delivery protocol are necessary. Moreover, concerns about the potential for retinal complications and tumor growth enhancement, due to increased vascularization will have to be further addressed reinforcing the need for critical subject selection and caution in VEGF use [78]. The Restenosis Gene Therapy (REGENT) trial, a phase 1 study, is still in progress and should provide information about dosage and safety. Inhibition of vasculoproliferation by targeting cell-cycle activation is also the rationale in clinical trials of antiproliferative gene therapy to prevent

Table 21.5 Clinical studies of gene therapy

Cardiovascular target	Gene used	Vector	Mode of Delivery	References
Restenosis	VEGF	Plasmid DNA	Balloon catheter	[69]
	E2F decoy	Oligonucleotide	Pressure-mediated transfection of vein grafts	[17]
CAD	VEGF-A	Naked DNA	Intramyocardial injection	[70]
	VEGF	Liposome/adenovirus	Infusion/perfusion	[71]
	VEGF	Adenovirus	Intramyocardial injection	[72]
	FGF-4	Adenovirus	Intracoronary injection	[73]
	VEGF-C	Naked DNA	Intramyocardial injection	[74]
	VEGF	Plasmid DNA	Intramyocardial injection	[49]
	FGF-4	Adenovirus	Intracoronary injection	[75]
	VEGF-A165	Plasmid DNA	Intramyocardial injection	[76]
	VEGF121	Adenovirus	Intramyocardial injection	[77]

bypass vein graft failure after coronary artery bypass surgery [17]. Data from the Project in Ex-Vivo Vein Graft Engineering via Transfection (PREVENT I and II), randomized, placebo-controlled studies have shown the safety and feasibility of using a synthetic DNA decoy to sequester the E2F family of transcription factors and arrest cells at the gap period (G1) checkpoint in the cell cycle. This mechanism can prevent intimal hyperplasia, associated with atherosclerosis and coronary graft failure; phase III trials are presently in progress [14].

In the Euroinject One phase II randomized double-blind trial, therapeutic angiogenesis of percutaneous intramyocardial plasmid gene transfer of vascular endothelial growth factor (phVEGF-A(165)) on myocardial perfusion, left ventricular function, and clinical symptoms has been assessed. Although the VEGF gene transfer did not significantly improve stress-induced myocardial perfusion abnormalities when compared with placebo, there was improved regional wall motion and confirmed that transient VEGF overexpression seems to be safe [76]. In the phase 2 of the REVASC study, cardiac gene transfer was optimized by direct intramyocardial delivery of a replication-deficient adenovirus-containing vascular endothelial growth factor (AdVEGF121), and the results showed objective improvement in exercise-induced ischemia in patients with refractory ischemic heart disease [77]. Taken the above observations together, gene therapy has shown potential usefulness for treating diseases, such as hypertension, myocardial ischemia, and HF, in various animal models. Some of these experimental therapies are now under evaluation in patients. However, further improvements in vector platforms and delivery together with critical documentation of clinical feasibility, safety, and efficacy are necessary through large multicenter randomized trials.

Gene-Targeting Approaches

In addition to transgene overexpression and activation, gene transfer approaches can be used to negatively modulate gene expression involving the use of antisense strategies (e.g., either ribozymes, antisense oligonucleotides, or RNA interference) as shown in Fig. 21.2. These approaches regulate the transcription of targeted endogenous genes, and selectively inhibit their expression, in both cultured cells and in specific animal and human tissues.

Ribozymes

Ribozymes are RNA molecules that catalyze the cleavage of RNA substrates, and the formation of covalent bonds in RNA strands at specific sites as shown in Fig. 21.3.

Ribozymes have been shown to be highly specific, efficient, and stable. They can be delivered to cells as preformed ribozymes using primarily lipofection or electroporation, or as ribozyme genes. Ribozyme genes can be packaged into viral vectors (e.g., adenovirus or AAV vectors) to enhance transfer into cells, and to achieve longer expression when compared with naked oligonucleotides. The choice of promoter (i.e., pol II, pol III, viral, etc.) can be critical for their expression. The "hammerhead" motif, approximately 30-nucleotide long, is a small endonucleolytic ribozyme. Hammerhead ribozymes can be directed against RNA sequences of interest, to selectively target their specific gene expression. Recently, a hammerhead ribozyme, directed against the mannose 6-phosphate/IGF-2 receptor (M6P/IGF2R), was used to probe the receptor's role in regulating cardiac myocyte growth and apoptosis. Downregulation of the expression of M6P/IGF2R in ribozyme-treated neonatal rat cardiac myocytes resulted in a marked increase in cell proliferation, and a reduced cell susceptibility to hypoxia- and TNF-induced apoptosis [79].

Antisense Oligonucleotides

The antisense oligonucleotide approach most commonly employs either single-strand RNA or DNA oligonucleotides

Gene Overexpression

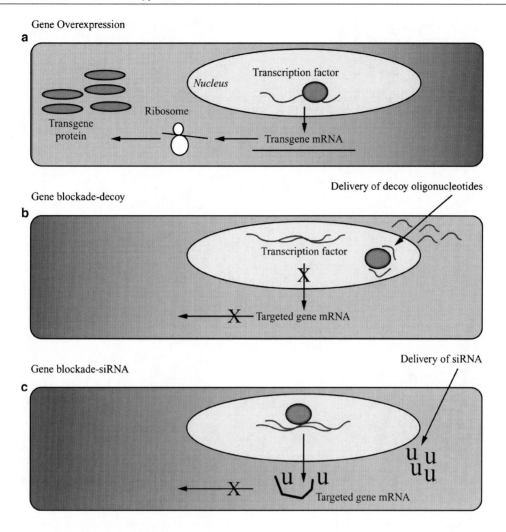

Fig. 21.2 Approaches to gene overexpression and targeting by decoy, and siRNA. (**a**) Gene transfer of a transgene by a vector allowing expression of a therapeutic protein in the host. The goal is gain-of-function, or enhanced function overcoming a deficiency in the host cell. (**b**) Gene blockade of a pathogenic pathway utilizing a transcriptional decoy (a double-stranded oligonucleotide containing the cis sequence bound by a transcription factor normally involved in the activation of pathogenic gene expression). Transfection of this decoy in molar excess prevents the binding and trans-activation of the host pathogenic genes. In this case neither the target gene mRNA nor protein product are expressed. (**c**) Gene blockade strategy is depicted using either an antisense oligonucleotide or small interfering RNA (siRNA). A small single-stranded antisense oligonucleotide or siRNA (around 21 nucleotides), complementary to the target mRNA, is transfected into the host cell, binds the target mRNA and prevents it from being translated

to target specific gene expression, and has been applied with success to modulating the progression of CVD in animal models [80–82]. These synthetic oligonucleotides are usually short ranging from 10 to 30 bp, and can be chemically modified to enhance stability; the substitution of sulfur for one of the oxygens in the phosphate backbone termed a phosphorothioate modification renders the oligonucleotide more stable to nuclease degradation.

Phosphorothiorate-modified antisense oligonucleotides have been shown to be more stable than natural oligomers to both serum and cellular nucleases. Another type of modified oligonucleotide is the phosphorodiamidate morpholino oligomers that comprise a novel class of nonionic antisense

agents that inhibit gene expression by binding to RNA and blocking its processing or translation (Fig. 21.4) [83, 84].

While morpholino oligonucleotides have shown improved sequence specificity, biostability, and low toxicity, compared to the phosphorothiorate-oligomers, making them effective antisense modulators of gene function in embryonic and adult tissues, their limited ability to cross cell membranes has restricted their use in cell culture. Morpholino oligonucleotides have proved to be a highly informative tool for "knocking-down" (inhibiting) specific transcripts in studies of early cardiac development in zebrafish, and other model organisms [85–90].

Another relevant modification of antisense oligonucleotides involves the addition of a conjugated peptide to the

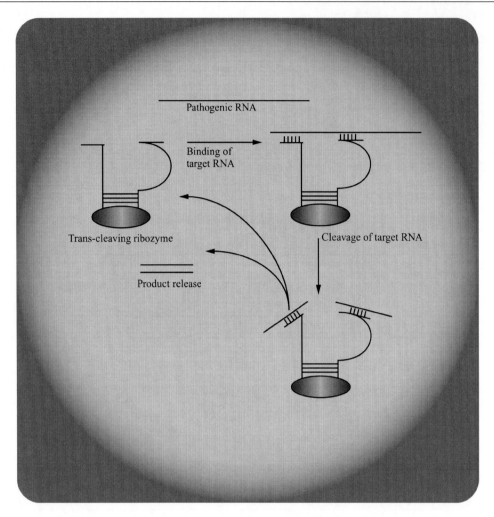

Fig. 21.3 Trans-cleaving ribozyme modulates level of specific RNA. Ribozymes can bind specific pathogenic targeted transcripts, cleave the target mRNA, release the cleaved products and repeat the process with other target mRNAs

oligonucleotide of interest. Peptide-conjugated nucleic acids (PNAs) has been applied in both cells and tissues [91, 92], and this approach can be used to better direct the oligonucleotide to the organelle of interest; for example, PNA-containing oligonucleotides fused with a mitochondrial targeting peptide can be specifically targeted to the mitochondrial organelle for mitochondrial gene repair.

RNA Interference

The RNA interference approach involves the use of a specific double-stranded RNA (dsRNA) construct to post-transcriptionally silence specific gene expression (RNAi). A dsRNA homologous in sequence to the silenced gene is processed into small interfering RNA (siRNA) by an RNAse III family member enzyme called Dicer, and the siRNAs are then incorporated into multicomponent RNA-induced silencing

ribonucleoprotein complexes (RISC), which find and cleave the target mRNA (see Fig. 21.4). The siRNA mediating this mRNA cleavage is usually 21–23 nucleotides, and can be expressed either as two separate strands or as a single short hairpin RNA (for further discussion see Chap. 3).

Expression cassettes encoding engineered siRNA (directed to specific mRNAs) can be efficiently introduced into the host cell utilizing viral vector systems (e.g., retroviral, adenoviral and lentiviral vectors) resulting in long-term silencing of target gene expression, both in cultured cells and in animal models [93–95]. Expression vectors for the induction of siRNA in mammalian cells frequently utilize polymerase III-dependent promoters (e.g., U6 or H1). They transcribe short hairpin RNAs (shRNA) that, after being directly processed into siRNAs, mediate target mRNA degradation. While preliminary data have shown that the use of siRNAs allows gene-specific knock-down without induction of the nonspecific interferon response in mammalian cells (which longer dsRNA species promote), new data have demonstrated

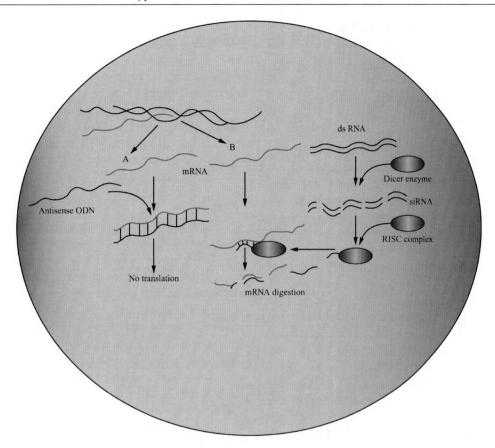

Fig. 21.4 Two post-transcriptional approaches to silence gene expression. After production of a specific mRNA, pathway A shows how a short single-strand antisense oligonucleotide, complementary to the mRNA can attenuate further specific protein translation. Pathway B, depicting the RNA interference (RNAi) approach, shows how a double-strand RNA (dsRNA) with sequence complementary to the mRNA of interest can be cleaved by the Dicer RNAse III enzyme to short dsRNA fragments (termed siRNA), which upon interaction with the RISC complex can present a short 20–21 bp single-strand RNA, homologous to and accessible for specific binding to the targeted mRNA, and enabling its endonucleolytic cleavage

an induction of interferon-activated gene expression in human cells transfected with siRNA. This interferon-mediated response to siRNA can be diminished by reducing the size (below 21 nucleotides), and changing the initiating nucleotide sequence of the siRNA. Exogenous delivery of synthetic siRNA to target cells can also be used to induce specific gene expression knock-down; however, the resulting gene silencing is transient, and tends to be less effective than with vectors. Specific RNA knock down by siRNA of the sarcoplasmic reticulum Ca^{2+} ATPase (SERCA) gene has been achieved in primary myocyte cultures from embryonic chickens, and neonatal rats [96].

While previous studies had displayed a low efficiency in the percentage of cells affected by cardiac myocyte siRNA transfection, the use of adenovirus vectors allowed effective introduction, and endogenous production of siRNA with marked reduction of SERCA2 gene expression. Interestingly, even with the pronounced reduction of SERCA2 protein and sarcoplasmic reticulum Ca^{2+} uptake and cycling, the cardiomyocytes retained the ability to increase cytosolic Ca^{2+} flux in response to stimulation. The intracellular store deficiency caused by reduced SERCA could be compensated for by Ca^{2+} fluxes through the plasma membrane, and this has been largely achieved by increased transcriptional activation of other Ca^{2+} proteins, including the up-regulation of transient receptor potential (TRP) channel proteins (TRPC4 and TRPC5), Na^+/Ca^{2+} exchanger, and related transcription factors such as stimulating protein 1 (Sp1), myocyte enhancer factor 2 (MEF-2) and nuclear factor of activated cells 4 (NFATc4), suggesting significant remodeling of the Ca^{2+} signaling pathway.

It is noteworthy, that RNA interference-mediated gene knock-down has shown a high level of specificity, and this approach seems particularly useful in assigning and differentiating the physiological actions of highly similar G-protein-coupled receptors (i.e., AT1a, AT1b and AT2) in response to angiotensin II. It was the development of specific siRNA to AT1a receptor (AT1aR) subtype, which had no significant effect on either AT1bR or AT2R subtypes that made it possible [97].

Conclusions and Future Directions

While the promise of effective gene therapy for a variety of cardiovascular disorders appears closer to be realized, with over 40 clinical trials in progress, more data concerning the safety, efficacy of delivery and long range consequences of cardiovascular gene therapy is critically needed. The utilization of epigenetic mechanisms of gene regulation to reversibly modulate the expression of cardiovascular transgenes in distinct fashion from endogenous gene expression, offers a potential added value for future therapeutic approaches.

Regarding the mode of delivery, it is worth noting the great expectations generated by adeno-associated vectors (AAV) as safe and effective vehicles for gene transfer because their small size allows to pass through vessel walls and to reach the myocardium. However, there are examples of dose-dependent generation of CD8+ T-cell responses to AAV capsid proteins in humans. In recent preclinical trial in a baboon model, McTiernan et al. [98] studied the comparative effects of gene transfer of type 2 AAV (AAV2) encoding TNFRII-Fc with empty AAV2 capsids in an effort to investigate the balance between induction of deleterious T-cell responses and operational immune tolerance to the AAV2, and payload gene proteins. Interestingly, these studies were carried out as preclinical safety studies of AAV2 TNFRII-Fc gene therapy for HF. However, the baboon developed myocarditis following the injection into the heart of AAV2 encoding TNFRII-Fc but not AAV2 empty capsids, which could be related to an immune response potentially directed toward the AAV capsids, or to an immune response directed toward the transgene TNFRII-Fc, and biological response induced by TNFRII-Fc. This response obviously has significantly limited the enthusiasm for use in human HF. Also, it is worth noting that Hajjar and Zsebo [99] in their analysis of McTiernan work suggested the possibility of an alternative explanation; that combination of anti-TNF coding transgenes and AAV results in cellular immune responses against AAV capsid proteins, which would not occur otherwise. Then, inhibition of TNF signaling may have resulted in myocarditis. Nevertheless, rather than giving up, we agree that McTiernan's findings may provide important information for further manipulation of the immune system with modalities that may enhance the potential success of AAV therapeutics.

A number of cardiovascular disorders have not yet been examined with regards to either preclinical or clinical studies of gene therapy. For example, there are cardiomyopathies with a mitochondrial-based cytopathy and bioenergetic dysfunction, a subset of which are due to defined mitochondrial DNA(mtDNA) or nuclear DNA mutations [100]. Potential gene therapy has been proposed for these mitochondrial cardiomyopathies utilizing ex vivo transfection of stem cells with their subsequent introduction to the diseased heart [101]. This approach would employ the introduction of mtDNA-repaired stem cells into a patient harboring an mtDNA mutation, thereby potentially transforming a bioenergetically dysfunctional heart into a healthy one. The mtDNA-repaired cell can be derived from the patient's own cells or from embryonic stem cells grown in vitro, whose endogenous defective mtDNA genome has been entirely eliminated by treatment with ethidium bromide, and replaced by entirely wild-type mtDNA genes. Similarly, a patient's nuclear DNA mutations might be replaced in ex vivo grown stem cells with wild-type alleles using site-specific homologous recombination or containing transplanted nuclei. While these scenarios have not yet been tested, they have become more feasible with the identification of cardiac-specific stem cells, which can be grown in vitro, and successfully transplanted into the heart [102].

To overcome acute and chronic rejection of cardiac allograft as well as ischemia/reperfusion injury associated with organ preservation, new approaches are being developed. Gene transfection of the donor organ during organ preservation is an attractive method, because the transfected genes would not affect recipients, and treatment could be delivered specifically to the site of inflammation. This method could be useful to prevent graft failure without systemic adverse effects [103].

While the pathophysiological relevance of small animal models (mouse, rat) to humans is in question, other alternatives such as viral gene delivery to larger mammals to sort out gene function are being developed. Still, no gene therapy compounds have been yet approved for clinical use in cardiovascular diseases in spite of the positive results obtained in therapeutic angiogenesis with vascular endothelial and fibroblasts growth factors. Nonetheless, the way is being cleared for clinical gene therapy trials using AAV8 and delta-sarcoglycan gene in human limb girdle muscular dystrophy [104], a disease that affect both skeletal and the heart. All together, it is obvious that we need to further develop safe and targeted gene transfer before this therapeutic modality can be used in the complex HF syndrome.

Summary

- Gene therapy has emerged as a genuine therapeutic option with the potential to alter the way clinicians manage patients with HF.
- Given the fact that patients with HF have an altered pattern of myocardial gene expression with a characteristic genetic fingerprint, using genes themselves as the vehicle for replacing or altering the expression of defective genes to treat patients at the molecular level is an attractive approach to therapy.

- The therapeutic effect of systemic delivery of adeno-associated virus (AAV) vectors carrying human SGCD gene in TO-2 hamsters, an HF and muscular dystrophy model with a δ-SG mutation, has been reported.

- Gene therapy allows therapeutic concentrations of a gene product to be accumulated and maintained at optimally high levels at a localized target site of action. By avoiding high plasma levels of the gene product, it is possible to significantly reduce potential side effects.

- Both viral vectors and naked plasmid DNAs have been employed in preclinical and clinical cardiovascular gene transfer studies.

- The duration of transgene expression varies with the type of vector employed, or the specific transgene.

- Which genes to use in cardio-vascular gene therapy is markedly dependent on the specific disorder to be treated, as well as which cell type is being targeted. These genes range from SERCA, plasma membrane channel proteins, cytokines, transcription factors to signaling pathway components.

- Adeno-associated virus (AAV) vectors are being considered more promising, mainly in the context of gene therapy for chronic diseases such as HF.

- AAV is taken up more slowly into myocardial cells and transgene expression levels are lower when compared to adenovirus, but transgene expression can be longer term, being sustained in the rodent myocardium for 9–12 months; in addition, AAV vectors have a lower potential to induce unwanted immunocytotoxicity or inflammation.

- Another alternative gene transfer approach uses oligonucleotides (e.g., antisense oligonucleotides) that regulate transcription of targeted endogenous genes and inhibit their expression.

- Aiming gene therapies directly at the myocardium and at vascular tissues, transfection of cells with specific transgenes ex vivo followed by in vivo delivery of the transfected cells has broadened the possibilities associated with gene therapy, and potentially sidestepped a number of the safety concerns.

- Gene transfer of hypoxia-inducible factor-1α, a transcription factor known to regulate the transcription of hypoxia-inducible genes also induces angiogenesis at ischemic sites.

- Gene therapy has been effectively applied in preclinical studies with both systemic and pulmonary hypertension.

- Preclinical studies in rat demonstrated that the transfer and expression of genes, including an O_2-sensitive voltage-gated potassium channel (Kv1.5), endothelial nitric oxide synthase (eNOS) and prostaglandin I synthase, (PGIS) markedly improved pulmonary hypertension.

- The development of gene therapy directed at renin–angiotensin system (RAS) represents a significant advance toward managing high blood pressure and reversing its associated pathophysiology.

- The β-adrenergic signaling system is another viable target for gene therapy, designed to stem hypertension by utilizing antisense technology.

- Genes involved in vasodilation regulation have also proved to be excellent targets for gene therapy of systemic hypertension.

- Successful intracoronary adenoviral-mediated gene transfer of an inhibitory component ($G\alpha_{i2}$) of the β-adrenergic pathway, directed to the atrioventricular (AV) node to suppress AV node conduction, has been reported.

- Decreasing the expression of NFκB in rats, by introducing into the rat coronary artery a decoy sequence directed to the cis-regulatory sequence within the NFkB promoter, reduced the areas of myocarditis as well as myocardial gene expression of iNOS, iCAM, and TNF-α.

- Short-term protection of the heart from ischemia can be provided by gene transfer and overexpression of cardioprotective genes such as superoxide dismutase (SOD) or heme oxygenase (HO-1).

- In preclinical studies of gene therapy in HF, it has been shown that in both human and experimental animal models, sarcoplasmic reticulum Ca^{2+} ATPase (SERCA2) activity is decreased, resulting in abnormal calcium handling thought to contribute to severe reduction in cardiac contractility.

- Intracoronary transfer of an adenovirus encoding a peptide inhibitor of β-ARK, reversed cardiac dysfunction in both rabbit and mouse models of HF.

- Several small phase 1 and 2 clinical studies have been conducted with adenovirus- and plasmid-based VEGF and FGF gene constructs to provide therapeutic angiogenesis in coronary artery disease and peripheral vascular disease.

- In the Euroinject One phase II randomized double-blind trial, therapeutic angiogenesis of percutaneous intramyocardial plasmid gene transfer of vascular endothelial growth factor (phVEGF-A(165)) on myocardial perfusion, left ventricular function, and clinical symptoms has been assessed.

- Although the VEGF gene transfer did not significantly improve stress-induced myocardial perfusion abnormalities when compared with placebo, there was improved regional wall motion and confirmed that transient VEGF overexpression seems to be safe.

- In the phase 2 of the REVASC study, cardiac gene transfer was optimized by direct intramyocardial delivery of a replication-deficient adenovirus-containing vascular endothelial growth factor (AdVEGF121), and the results showed objective improvement in exercise-induced ischemia in patients with refractory ischemic heart disease.

- Gene therapy has potential usefulness for treating diseases, such as hypertension, myocardial ischemia, and HF, in various animal models. Some of these experimental therapies are now under evaluation in patients.

- In addition to transgene overexpression and activation, gene transfer approaches can be used to negatively modulate gene expression involving the use of antisense strategies.
- Ribozyme genes can be packaged into viral vectors (e.g., adenovirus or AAV vectors) to enhance transfer into cells, and to achieve longer expression when compared with naked oligonucleotides.
- The antisense oligonucleotide approach most commonly employs either single-strand RNA or DNA oligonucleotides to target specific gene expression, and has been applied with success to modulating the progression of CVD in animal models.
- RNA interference-mediated gene knock-down has shown a high level of specificity, and this approach seems particularly useful in assigning and differentiating the physiological actions of highly similar G-protein-coupled receptors (i.e., AT1a, AT1b and AT2) in response to angiotensin II.
- While the promise of effective gene therapy for a variety of cardiovascular disorders appears closer to being realized, with over 40 clinical trials in progress, more data concerning the safety, efficacy of delivery and long range consequences of cardiovascular gene therapy is critically needed.
- While the pathophysiological relevance of small animal models (mouse, rat) to humans is in question, other alternatives such as viral gene delivery to larger mammals to sort out gene function are being developed.
- We need to further develop safe and targeted gene transfer to be used in the treatment of HF.

References

1. Tan FL, Moravec CS, Li J, Apperson-Hansen C, McCarthy PM, Young JB, Bond M (2002) The gene expression fingerprint of human heart failure. Proc Natl Acad Sci USA 99:11387–11392
2. Zhu T, Zhou L, Mori S et al (2005) Sustained whole-body functional rescue in congestive heart failure and muscular dystrophy hamsters by systemic gene transfer. Circulation 112:2650–2659
3. Nabel EG, Plautz G, Boyce FM, Stanley JC, Nabel GJ (1989) Recombinant gene expression in vivo within endothelial cells of the arterial wall. Science 244:1342–1344
4. Isner JM (2002) Myocardial gene therapy. Nature 415:234–239
5. Hajjar RJ, del Monte F, Matsui T, Rosenzweig A (2000) Prospects for gene therapy for heart failure. Circ Res 86:616–621
6. Lawrie A, Brisken AF, Francis SE, Cumberland DC, Crossman DC, Newman CM (2000) Microbubble-enhanced ultrasound for vascular gene delivery. Gene Ther 7:2023–2027
7. Chen S, Shohet RV, Bekeredjian R, Frenkel P, Grayburn PA (2003) Optimization of ultrasound parameters for cardiac gene delivery of adenoviral or plasmid deoxyribonucleic acid by ultrasound-targeted microbubble destruction. J Am Coll Cardiol 42:301–308
8. Baumgartner I, Isner JM (2001) Somatic gene therapy in the cardiovascular system. Annu Rev Physiol 63:427–450

9. Barbato JE, Kibbe MR, Tzeng E (2003) The emerging role of gene therapy in the treatment of cardiovascular diseases. Crit Rev Clin Lab Sci 40:499–545
10. Williams ML, Koch WJ (2004) Viral-based myocardial gene therapy approaches to alter cardiac function. Annu Rev Physiol 66:49–75
11. Isner JM, Vale PR, Symes JF, Losordo DW (2001) Assessment of risks associated with cardiovascular gene therapy in human subjects. Circ Res 89:389–400
12. Pislau S, Janssens SP, Gersh BJ, Simari RD (2002) Defining gene transfer before expecting gene therapy; putting the horse before the cart. Circulation 106:631–636
13. Vinge LE, Raake PW, Koch WJ (2008) Gene therapy in heart failure. Circ Res 102:1458–1700
14. Dzau VJ (2003) Predicting the future of human gene therapy for cardiovascular diseases: what will the management of coronary artery disease be like in 2005 and 2010? Am J Cardiol 92:32N–35N
15. Morishita R, Higaki J, Tomita N, Ogihara T (1998) Application of transcription factor "decoy" strategy as means of gene therapy and study of gene expression in cardiovascular disease. Circ Res 82:1023
16. Kibbe MR, Billiar TR, Tzeng E (2000) Gene therapy for restenosis. Circ Res 86:829–833
17. Mann MJ, Whittemore AD, Donaldson MC et al (1999) Ex-vivo gene therapy of human vascular bypass grafts with E2F decoy: the PREVENT single-centre, randomised, controlled trial. Lancet 354:1493–1498
18. Isner JM, Walsh K, Symes J et al (1996) Arterial gene transfer for therapeutic angiogenesis in patients with peripheral artery disease. Hum Gene Ther 7:959–988
19. Isner JM, Walsh K, Rosenfield K, Schainfeld R, Asahara T, Hogan K, Pieczek A (1996) Arterial gene therapy for restenosis. Hum Gene Ther 7:989–1011
20. Isner JM, Pieczek A, Schainfeld R et al (1996) Clinical evidence of angiogenesis after arterial gene transfer of phVEGF165 in patient with ischaemic limb. Lancet 348:370–374
21. Tabata H, Silver M, Isner JM (1997) Arterial gene transfer of acidic fibroblast growth factor for therapeutic angiogenesis in vivo: critical role of secretion signal in use of naked DNA. Cardiovasc Res 35:470–479
22. Vincent KA, Shyu KG, Luo Y et al (2000) Angiogenesis is induced in a rabbit model of hindlimb ischemia by naked DNA encoding an HIF-1a/VP16 hybrid transcription factor. Circulation 102:2255–2261
23. Zhang YC, Bui JD, Shen L, Phillips MI (2000) Antisense inhibition of b (1)-adrenergic receptor mRNA in a single dose produces a profound and prolonged reduction in high blood pressure in spontaneously hypertensive rats. Circulation 101:682–688
24. Kimura B, Mohuczy D, Tang X, Phillips MI (2001) Attenuation of hypertension and heart hypertrophy by adeno-associated virus delivering angiotensinogen antisense. Hypertension 37:376–380
25. Agata J, Chao L, Chao J (2002) Kallikrein gene delivery improves cardiac reserve and attenuates remodeling after myocardial infarction. Hypertension 40:653–659
26. Chao J, Jin L, Lin KF, Chao L (1998) Atrial natriuretic peptide gene delivery attenuates hypertension, cardiac hypertrophy and renal injury in salt-sensitive rats. Hum Gene Ther 9:1429–1438
27. Chao J, Kato K, Zhang JJ, Dobrzynski E, Wang C, Agata J, Chao L (2001) Human adrenomedullin gene delivery protects against cardiovascular remodeling and renal injury. Peptides 22:1731–1737
28. Lin KF, Chao L, Chao J (1997) Prolonged reduction of high blood pressure with human nitric oxide synthase gene delivery. Hypertension 30:307–313
29. Nuss HB, Johns DC, Kaab S, Tomaselli GF, Kass D, Lawrence JH, Marban E (1996) Reversal of potassium channel deficiency in cells from failing hearts by adenoviral gene transfer: a prototype for gene therapy for disorders of cardiac excitability and contractility. Gene Ther 3:900–912

30. Ennis IL, Li RA, Murphy AM, Marban E, Nuss HB (2002) Dual gene therapy with SERCA1 and Kir2.1 abbreviates excitation without suppressing contractility. J Clin Invest 109:393–400

31. Burton DY, Song C, Fishbein I et al (2003) The incorporation of an ion channel gene mutation associated with the long QT syndrome (Q9E-hMiRP1) in a plasmid vector for site-specific arrhythmia gene therapy: in vitro and in vivo feasibility studies. Hum Gene Ther 14:907–922

32. Donahue JK, Heldman AW, Fraser H et al (2000) Focal modification of electrical conduction in heart by viral gene transfer. Nat Med 6:1395–1398

33. Watanabe K, Nakazawa M, Fuse K et al (2001) Protection against autoimmune myocarditis by gene transfer of interleukin-10 by electroporation. Circulation 104:1098–1100

34. Yokoseki O, Suzuki J, Kitabayashi H et al (2001) Cis Element decoy against nuclear factor-k B attenuates development of experimental autoimmune myocarditis in rats. Circ Res 89:899–906

35. Melo LG, Agrawal R, Zhang L et al (2002) Gene therapy strategy for long-term myocardial protection using adeno-associated virus-mediated delivery of heme oxygenase gene. Circulation 105:602–607

36. Abunasra HJ, Smolenski RT, Morrison K et al (2001) Efficacy of adenoviral gene transfer with manganese superoxide dismutase and endothelial nitric oxide synthase in reducing ischemia and reperfusion injury. Eur J Cardiothorac Surg 20:153–158

37. Jayakumar J, Suzuki K, Sammut IA et al (2001) Heat shock protein 70 gene transfection protects mitochondrial and ventricular function against ischemia-reperfusion injury. Circulation 104:I303–I307

38. Chatterjee S, Stewart AS, Bish LT et al (2002) Viral gene transfer of the antiapoptotic factor Bcl-2 protects against chronic postischemic heart failure. Circulation 106:I212–I217

39. Champion HC, Bivalacqua TJ, D'Souza FM et al (1999) Gene transfer of endothelial nitric oxide synthase to the lung of the mouse in vivo. Effect on agonist-induced and flow-mediated vascular responses. Circ Res 84:1422–1432

40. Pozeg ZI, Michelakis ED, McMurtry MS et al (2003) In vivo gene transfer of the O2-sensitive potassium channel Kv1.5 reduces pulmonary hypertension and restores hypoxic pulmonary vasoconstriction in chronically hypoxic rats. Circulation 107:2037–2044

41. Kalka C, Tehrani H, Laudenberg B, Vale PR, Isner JM, Asahara T, Symes JF (2000) VEGF gene transfer mobilizes endothelial progenitor cells in patients with inoperable coronary disease. Ann Thorac Surg 70:829–834

42. Kawamoto A, Gwon HC, Iwaguro H et al (2001) Therapeutic potential of ex vivo expanded endothelial progenitor cells for myocardial ischemia. Circulation 103:634–637

43. Hajjar RJ, Samulski RJ (2006) Heart failure: a silver bullet to treat heart failure. Gene Ther 13:997

44. del Monte F, Hajjar RJ (2003) Targeting calcium cycling proteins in heart failure through gene transfer. J Physiol 546:49–61

45. Kullo I, Simari R, Schwartz R (1999) Vascular gene transfer: from bench to bedside. Arterioscler Thromb Vasc Biol 19:196–207

46. Kibbe MR, Tzeng E, Gleixner SL et al (2001) Adenovirus-mediated gene transfer of human inducible nitric oxide synthase in porcine vein grafts inhibits intimal hyperplasia. J Vasc Surg 34:156–165

47. Gascon-Irun M, Sanz-Gonzalez SM, Andres V (2003) Gene therapy antiproliferative strategies against cardiovascular disease. Gene Ther Mol Biol 7:75–89

48. Baumgartner I, Pieczek A, Manor O, Blair R, Kearney M, Walsh K, Isner JM (1998) Constitutive expression of phVEGF165 after intramuscular gene transfer promotes collateral vessel development in patients with critical limb ischemia. Circulation 97:1114–1123

49. Vale PR, Losordo DW, Milliken CE, Maysky M, Esakof DD, Symes JF, Isner JM (2000) Left ventricular electromechanical mapping to assess efficacy of phVEGF165 gene transfer for thera-peutic angiogenesis in chronic myocardial ischemia. Circulation 102:965–974

50. Fortuin FD, Vale P, Losordo DW et al (2003) One-year follow-up of direct myocardial gene transfer of vascular endothelial growth factor-2 using naked plasmid deoxyribonucleic acid by way of thoracotomy in no-option patients. Am J Cardiol 92:436–439

51. Grines C, Rubanyi GM, Kleiman NS, Marrott P, Watkins MW (2003) Angiogenic gene therapy with adenovirus 5 fibroblast growth factor-4 (Ad5FGF-4): a new option for the treatment of coronary artery disease. Am J Cardiol 92:24N–31N

52. Suhara H, Sawa Y, Fukushima N et al (2002) Gene transfer of human prostacyclin synthase into the liver is effective for the treatment of pulmonary hypertension in rats. J Thorac Cardiovasc Surg 123:855–861

53. Gelband CH, Katovich MJ, Raizada MK (2000) Current perspectives on the use of gene therapy for hypertension. Circ Res 87:1118–1122

54. Tomita N, Morishita R, Higaki J et al (1995) Transient decrease in high blood pressure by in vivo transfer of antisense oligodeoxynucleotides against rat angiotensinogen. Hypertension 26:131–136

55. Phillips MI (1997) Antisense inhibition and adeno-associated viral vector delivery for reducing hypertension. Hypertension 29:177–187

56. Reaves PY, Beck CR, Wang HW, Raizada MK, Katovich MJ (2003) Endothelial-independent prevention of high blood pressure in L-NAME-treated rats by angiotensin II type I receptor antisense gene therapy. Exp Physiol 88:467–473

57. Phillips MI, Tang Y, Schmidt-Ott K, Qian K, Kagiyama S (2002) Vigilant vector: heart-specific promoter in an adeno-associated virus vector for cardioprotection. Hypertension 39:651–655

58. Shah AS, White DC, Emani S et al (2001) In vivo ventricular gene delivery of a b -adrenergic receptor kinase inhibitor to the failing heart reverses cardiac dysfunction. Circulation 103:1311–1316

59. Miyamoto MI, del Monte F, Schmidt U et al (2000) Adenoviral gene transfer of SERCA2a improves left-ventricular function in aortic-banded rats in transition to heart failure. Proc Natl Acad Sci USA 97:793–798

60. Hirsch JC, Borton AR, Albayya FP, Russell MW, Ohye RG, Metzger JM (2004) Comparative analysis of parvalbumin and SERCA2a cardiac myocyte gene transfer in a large animal model of diastolic dysfunction. Am J Physiol Heart Circ Physiol 86:H2314–H2321

61. Ly KY, HQ PF et al (2008) Reversal of cardiac dysfunction after long-term expression of SERCA2a by gene transfer in a pre-clinical model of heart failure. J Am Coll Cardiol 51:1112–1119

62. He H, Meyer M, Martin JL et al (1999) Effects of mutant and antisense RNA of phospholamban on SR Ca(2+)-ATPase activity and cardiac myocyte contractility. Circulation 31:974–980

63. del Monte F, Harding SE, Dec GW, Gwathmey JK, Hajjar RJ (2002) Targeting phospholamban by gene transfer in human heart failure. Circulation 105:904–907

64. Dorn GW 2nd, Molkentin JD (2004) Manipulating cardiac contractility in heart failure: data from mice and men. Circulation 109:150–158

65. Minamisawa S, Hoshijima M, Chu G et al (1999) Chronic phospholamban-sarcoplasmic reticulum calcium ATPase interaction is the critical calcium cycling defect in dilated cardiomyopathy. Cell 99:313–322

66. Haghighi K, Kolokathis F, Pater L et al (2003) Human phospholamban null results in lethal dilated cardiomyopathy revealing a critical difference between mouse and human. J Clin Invest 111:869–876

67. Hajjar RJ, Zsebo K, Deckelbaum L et al (2008) Design of a phase 1/2 trial of intracoronary administration of AAV1/SERCA2a in patients with heart failure. J Card Fail 14:355–367

68. Rockman HA, Chien KR, Choi DJ et al (1998) Expression of a b -adrenergic receptor kinase 1 inhibitor prevents the development of myocardial failure in gene-targeted mice. Proc Natl Acad Sci USA 95:7000–7005

69. Vale PR, Losordo DW, Symes JF, Isner JM (1998) Gene therapy for myocardial angiogenesis. Circulation 98:I-322

70. Losordo DW, Vale PR, Symes JF (1998) Gene therapy for myocardial angiogenesis: initial clinical results with direct myocardial injection of phVEGF165 as sole therapy for myocardial ischaemia. Circulation 98:2800–2804

71. Laitinen M, Hartikainen J, Hiltunen MO et al (2000) Catheter-mediated vascular endothelial growth factor gene transfer to human coronary arteries after angioplasty. Hum Gene Ther 11:263–270

72. Rosengart TK, Lee LY, Patel SR, Kligfield PD, Okin PM, Hackett NR, Isom OW, Crystal RG (1999) Six-month assessment of a phase I trial of angiogenic gene therapy for the treatment of coronary artery disease using direct intramyocardial administration of an adenovirus vector expressing the VEGF121 cDNA. Ann Surg 230:466–470

73. Hammond KH, McKirnan DM (2001) Angiogenic gene therapy for heart disease: a review of animal studies and clinical trials. Cardiovasc Res 49:561–567

74. Yla-Herttuala S, Martin JF (2000) Cardiovascular gene therapy. Lancet 355:213–222

75. Grines CL, Watkins MW, Helmer G et al (2002) Angiogenic gene therapy (AGENT) trial in patients with stable angina pectoris. Circulation 105:1291–1297

76. Kastrup J, Jørgensen E, Rück A et al (2005) Direct intramyocardial plasmid vascular endothelial growth factor-A165 gene therapy in patients with stable severe angina pectoris A randomized double-blind placebo-controlled study: the Euroinject One trial. J Am Coll Cardiol 45:982–988

77. Stewart DJ, Hilton JD, Arnold JM et al (2006) Angiogenic gene therapy in patients with nonrevascularizable ischemic heart disease: a phase 2 randomized, controlled trial of AdVEGF(121) (AdVEGF121) versus maximum medical treatment. Gene Ther 13:1503–1511

78. Ratko TA, Cummings JP, Blebea J, Matuszewski KA (2003) Clinical gene therapy for nonmalignant disease. Am J Med 115:560–569

79. Chen Z, Ge Y, Kang JX (2004) Down-regulation of the M6P/IGF-II receptor increases cell proliferation and reduces apoptosis in neonatal rat cardiac myocytes. BMC Cell Biol 5:1

80. Tomita N, Morishita R (2004) Antisense oligonucleotides as a powerful molecular strategy for gene therapy in cardiovascular diseases. Curr Pharm Des 10:797–803

81. Morishita R, Aoki M, Kaneda Y (2001) Decoy oligodeoxynucleotides as novel cardiovascular drugs for cardiovascular disease. Ann N Y Acad Sci 947:294–301

82. Ehsan A, Mann MJ (2000) Antisense and gene therapy to prevent restenosis. Vasc Med 5:103–114

83. Arora V, Devi GR, Iversen PL (2004) Neutrally charged phosphorodiamidate morpholino antisense oligomers: uptake, efficacy and pharmacokinetics. Curr Pharm Biotechnol 5:431–439

84. Summerton J, Weller D (1997) Morpholino antisense oligomers: design, preparation, and properties. Antisense Nucleic Acid Drug Dev 7:187–195

85. Chen E, Ekker SC (2004) Zebrafish as a genomics research model. Curr Pharm Biotechnol 5:409–413

86. Heasman J (2002) Morpholino oligos: making sense of antisense? Dev Biol 243:209–214

87. Small EM, Warkman AS, Wang DZ, Sutherland LB, Olson EN, Krieg PA (2005) Myocardin is sufficient and necessary for cardiac gene expression in Xenopus. Development 132:987–997

88. Wood AW, Schlueter PJ, Duan C (2005) Targeted knockdown of insulin-like growth factor binding protein-2 disrupts cardiovascular development in zebrafish embryos. Mol Endocrinol 19:1024–1034

89. Shu X, Cheng K, Patel N, Chen F, Joseph E, Tsai HJ, Chen JN (2003) Na, K-ATPase is essential for embryonic heart development in the zebrafish. Development 130:6165–6173

90. Peterkin T, Gibson A, Patient R (2003) GATA-6 maintains BMP-4 and Nkx2 expression during cardiomyocyte precursor maturation. EMBO J 22:4260–4273

91. Chinnery PF, Taylor RW, Diekert K, Lill R, Turnbull DM, Lightowlers RN (1999) Peptide nucleic acid delivery to human mitochondria. Gene Ther 6:1919–1928

92. Tyler BM, Jansen K, McCormick DJ et al (1999) Peptide nucleic acids targeted to the neurotensin receptor and administered i.p. cross the blood-brain barrier and specifically reduce gene expression. Proc Natl Acad Sci USA 96:7053–7058

93. An DS, Xie Y, Mao SH, Morizono K, Kung SK, Chen IS (2003) Efficient lentiviral vectors for short hairpin RNA delivery into human cells. Hum Gene Ther 14:1207–1212

94. Arts GJ, Langemeijer E, Tissingh R et al (2003) Adenoviral vectors expressing siRNAs for discovery and validation of gene function. Genome Res 13:2325–2332

95. Hurtado C, Ander BP, Maddaford TG, Lukas A, Hryshko LV, Pierce GN (2005) Adenovirally delivered shRNA strongly inhibits Na(+)-Ca(2+) exchanger expression but does not prevent contraction of neonatal cardiomyocytes. J Mol Cell Cardiol 38:647–654

96. Seth M, Sumbilla C, Mullen SP et al (2004) Sarco(endo)plasmic reticulum Ca2+ ATPase (SERCA) gene silencing and remodeling of the Ca2+ signaling mechanism in cardiac myocytes. Proc Natl Acad Sci USA 101:16683–16688

97. Vazquez J, Correa de Adjounian MF, Sumners C, Gonzalez A, Diez-Freire C, Raizada MK (2005) Selective silencing of angiotensin receptor subtype 1a (AT1aR) by RNA interference. Hypertension 45:115–119

98. McTiernan CF, Mathier MA, Zhu X et al (2007) Myocarditis following adeno-associated viral expression of human soluble TNF receptor (TNFRII-Fc) in baboon hearts. Gene Therapy 14:1613–1622

99. Hajjar RJ, Zsebo K (2007) AAV vectors and cardiovascular disease: targeting TNF receptor in the heart: clue to way forward with AAV? Gene Ther 14:1611–1612

100. Marín-García J, Ananthakrishnan R, Goldenthal MJ, Pierpont ME (2000) Biochemical and molecular basis for mitochondrial cardiomyopathy in neonates and children. J Inherit Metab Dis 23: 625–633

101. Marín-García J, Goldenthal MJ (2002) Understanding the impact of mitochondrial defects in cardiovascular disease: a review. J Card Fail 8:347–361

102. Beltrami AP, Barlucchi L, Torella D et al (2003) Adult cardiac stem cells are multipotent and support myocardial regeneration. Cell 114:763–776

103. Isobe M, Kosuge H, Koga N, Futamatsu H, Suzuki J (2004) Gene therapy for heart transplantation-associated acute rejection, ischemia/reperfusion injury and coronary arteriosclerosis. Curr Gene Ther 4:145–152

104. Hajjar RJ, Samulski RJ (2006) Heart failure: a silver bullet to treat heart failure. Gene Ther 13:997

Chapter 22
Myocardial Cell-Based Regeneration in Heart Failure

Overview

Heart failure (HF) secondary to cardiomyopathy, myocardial infarction, and ischemia is associated with the irreversible loss of cardiomyocytes and vasculature, either via apoptosis or necrosis. However, the native capacity for the renewal and repair of myocardial tissue is inadequate as have been current therapeutic measures to prevent left ventricular remodeling. As an extraordinary example of translational medicine, cell transplantation has emerged as a potentially viable therapeutic approach to directly repopulate and repair the damaged myocardium. A detailed analysis and a vision for future progress in stem cell applications, both in research and clinical cardiology, are presented in this chapter, highlighting the use of a wide spectrum of stem or progenitor cell types including embryonic or fetal stem cells, myoblasts, and adult bone marrow stem cells. The roles that myocardial cell fusion and transdifferentiation play in stem cell transplantation, the specific shortcomings of available technologies, and recommendations for practical ways that these concerns can be overcome are also discussed.

Introduction

Recent progress in the field of stem cell research has confirmed the potential to be used in tissue regeneration since the cardiomyocyte native capacity for renewal and repair is inadequate, as have been the available therapeutic measures to prevent left ventricular remodeling. Cell transplantation represents a viable therapeutic approach for repairing the damaged myocardium. However, and in spite of remarkable progress in this field, significant problems remain, especially ethical problems and the tumorigenic and dysrhythmogenic potential that these techniques present for differentiation into somatic cells. Moreover, uncertainty remains about whether the cells formed new tissue or whether they released compounds that fortified existing cells. Because the limited potential of the myocardium for self-repair and renewal, a significant proportion of cardiac muscle loses its ability to perform work, and this loss may be the most important factor in the heart pump failure occurring in patients with coronary artery disease (CAD) and dilated cardiomyopathy (DCM).

Until recently, reperfusion of the ischemic myocardium was the only intervention available to restore the various cellular functions affected by myocardial ischemia, including preventing cell death by necrosis or apoptosis. Unfortunately, reperfusion may result in extensive myocardial damage, including myocardial stunning, and the functional recovery of the heart may appear only after a period of cardiac contractile dysfunction that may last for several hours or days. It is evident that the limited capacity of regeneration and proliferation of human cardiomyocytes can prevent neither the scar formation that follows myocardial infarction nor the loss of heart function occurring in patients with cardiomyopathy and HF. Replacement and regeneration of functional cardiac muscle is an important goal that could be achieved either by stimulation of autologous resident cardiomyocytes or by the transplantation of allogenic cells (e.g., embryonic stem cells, bone marrow mesenchymal cells, or skeletal myoblasts). However, a number of impediments to a successful implantation of these cells remain, and those will be addressed in this chapter.

Stem Cell Therapy

The most primitive of all stem cells are the embryonic stem (ES) cells that develop as the inner cell mass in the human blastocyst at day 5 after fertilization. At this early stage, ES cells have vast developmental potential since they can give rise to cells of the three embryonic germ layers. When isolated and grown in the appropriate culture media, the pluripotent mouse and human ES cells can undergo cell proliferation and form embryo-like aggregates (termed embryoid bodies) in vitro, some of which can spontaneously contract (Fig. 22.1). The beating embryoid bodies contain a mixed population of newly differentiated cell types including cardiomyocytes, based on the expression of cardiac-specific genes such as cardiac-myosin

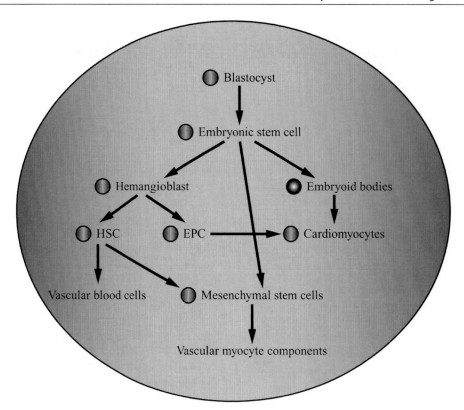

Fig. 22.1 Cell differentiation. Pluripotent embryonic stem cells spontaneously differentiate into endothelial progenitor cells (EPC), hemangioblasts, mesenchymal stem cells and embryoid bodies (embryo-like aggregates). Hemangioblasts further differentiate generating both hematopoietic stem cells (HSC) and EPC which give rise to both vascular blood and myocyte components. Under the appropriate conditions (most of which remain to be determined), cardiomyocytes can form from embryoid bodies as well as from EPC and mesenchymal stem cells

heavy chain, cardiac troponin I and T, atrial natriuretic factor, and cardiac transcription factors GATA-4, Nkx2.5, and MEF-2, cellular ultrastructure, and extracellular electrical activity [1–3]. These cardiomyocytes can be of the pacemaker-atrium and ventricle-like type, and they are distinguishable by their specific patterns of action potential [4–6].

While the precise cellular and molecular events comprising the pathway of ES cell cardiomyocyte-specific differentiation remain largely undetermined, significant progress has been made in identifying the regulatory factors which can enhance or inhibit the process (Fig. 22.2). Differentiation into a particular cell type is dependent on these factors. For instance, inhibition of bone morphogenetic protein (BMP) signaling by its antagonist Noggin induces cardiomyocyte differentiation from mouse ES cells [7], while retinoic acid specifically induces the formation of ventricular-specific cardiomyocytes [8].

Nitric oxide (NO) generated either by NO synthase activity or exogenous NO exposure has also been implicated in the promotion of cardiomyocyte-specific differentiation from mouse ES cells [9]. Cardiomyocyte differentiation of human ES cells could be enhanced by treatment with 5-aza-2′-deoxycytidine [10]. Also, IGF-1 promotes cardiomyocyte differentiation phenotype and the expression of the cardio-

myocyte phenotype in ES cells in vivo [11]. Interestingly, increased levels of oxidative stress appear to reduce the cardiotypic development of embryoid bodies [12].

Early experiments with both fetal cardiomyocyte and differentiating ES cell transplantation showed the successful formation of stable grafts and nascent intercalated discs between the grafted and the host myocardial cells [13, 14]. In addition, both fetal and embryonic stem cell-generated cardiomyocytes maintain myocardial electromechanical properties. Human ES cell-derived cardiomyocytes are able to effectively form structural and electromechanical connections with cultured rat cardiomyocytes [3]. Similarly, the transplanted human ES cell-derived cardiomyocytes were able to integrate and pace in vivo the swine heart with complete atrioventricular block, as demonstrated by detailed electrophysiological mapping and histopathological studies. The similarity in phenotype between the transplanted differentiating-ES cells and harder-to come-by (particularly in humans) fetal cardiomyocytes suggested that ES cells could be a useful surrogate for fetal cardiomyocytes in human cardiac engraftment procedures [14].

When fetal rat cardiomyocytes were transplanted into ischemic damaged hearts, a large percentage of cardiomyocytes died posttransplantation [15]. This, as well as the

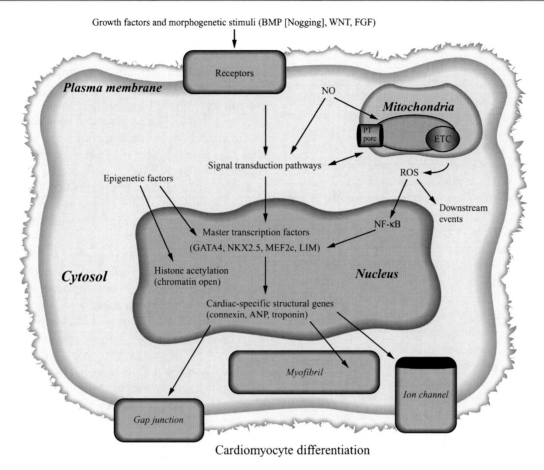

Growth factors and morphogenetic stimuli (BMP [Nogging], WNT, FGF)

Cardiomyocyte differentiation

Fig. 22.2 Signaling pathways potentially involved in cardiomyocyte differentiation. *BMP* bone morphogenetic protein; *Wnt* amalgam of wingless (Wg) and int (integration loci); *FGF* fibroblast growth factor; *ETC* electron transport chain; *NO* nitric oxide; permeability transition (PT) pore opening; *ANP* atrial natriuretic peptide

finding that no increase in graft size occurred while using increasing number of injected cardiomyocytes, has prompted a re-consideration of the clinical use of cardiomyocyte transplantation in the treatment of ischemic heart disease. It is apparent that more research is needed to develop a successful strategy that can maximize grafted cardiomyocyte cell survival and accelerate the differentiation process.

Advantages of ES Cell Transplantation

ES cells can be readily and reproducibly obtained from the inner layer of the blastocyst, and exhibit an excellent growth phenotype, both in vitro and in vivo. The development and application of ES-like cell lines (e.g., P19), which have been highly informative in the identification and characterization of regulatory factors, transcriptional activators and signal transduction events involved in cardiomyocyte differentiation, may also be useful in cell transplant therapy [16–18].

Preliminary data suggest that ES cells may be of a particular value in targeting and modifying congenital heart defect (CHD) phenotypes [19, 20]. Once their safety is confirmed, further clinical studies should address the use of targeted ES cell therapy in infants/children with severe cardiac diseases including cardiomyopathies, CHD and dysrhythmias. ES cells may also be more amenable to ex vivo engineering via DNA modifications (e.g., gene therapy, viral transfection, knockouts and over-expressed genes). In fact, the transformation of a normal cardiomyocyte into a pacemaker cell has been successfully achieved in animal models by the injection of plasmid or viral vectors carrying genes encoding specific therapeutic proteins [21–23]. In this manner, ES cells transfected with overexpressed β2-adrenergic receptors, or ion channel proteins could be transplanted to restore function in defective myocardial cells [23]. However, the safety and efficacy of these methodologies need to be absolutely proven prior to their use in humans with cardiac dysrhythmias.

Limitations and Concerns with ESC Transplantation

Considerable ethical and legal concerns about ES cells remain, and these concerns have significantly hampered further research efforts, which could provide needed cell lines as well as answers to many of the questions regarding the efficacy, long-term stability, function and even the extent of the negative effects of ES cell transplantation in cardiovascular disease (as well as in other human diseases).

A concern often raised regarding the use of ES cells relates to their source (i.e., whether they originate from a cell line or directly from embryo), primarily heterologous versus autologous, posing the potential problem of generating an allogenic response or immunorejection upon transplantation. In addition, pluripotent ES cells which have unlimited growth potential can have tumorigenic side-effects, making the screening for teratoma formation well-advised. In addition, there is evidence that differentiation of a heterogeneous ES cell population is rather inefficient, although several agents (e.g., retinoic acid) appear to be effective in activating a greater extent of ES cell-mediated cardiomyocyte specific differentiation. The long-term stability of ES cell-differentiated phenotype has also received mixed reviews since several studies have shown a loss of ES cell derived cardiomyocytes over time.

Transplanted ES cell progeny may not always have a normal function since ES cells may promote dysrhythmias in the transplanted hearts. On the other hand, the application of ES cells in repairing the damaged aging heart may also be limited; however, while this limitation has been proposed, currently there are no solid data to support it. Nevertheless, cell transplants (either ES or adult stem cells) in hearts of older individuals have frequently proved to be less effective. The inability of the damaged myocardium to provide the appropriate molecular signals for stem cells engraftment seems to limit their capacity for recruitment and integration into the aging myocardium [24].

Recently, major advances showing that stem cell therapy has great potential in the treatment of postmyocardial infarction HF have been reported. One report showed how bone marrow stem cells can regenerate myocardium in the infarct area of a mouse heart [25], whereas a second report showed the use of a subgroup of bone marrow stem cells to stimulate neovascularization and prevent remodeling in the infarct area of a rat heart [26]. In both studies, improved cardiac function was demonstrated.

Cardiomyogenic differentiation of marrow stem cells (MSCs) can occur in vivo [27]. Isogenic cultured MSCs were labeled with 4′, 6-diamidino-2-phenylindole (DAPI) and implanted into the LV wall of recipient rats. After 4 weeks, DAPI-labeled donor MSCs demonstrated myogenic differ-

entiation with the expression of sarcomeric myosin heavy chain in the cytoplasm. Orlic et al. have identified bone marrow stem cells that, when injected into MI mouse, migrate specifically into the infarct area, replenish it with cardiomyocytes, endothelial cells, and smooth muscle cells, and partially restore cardiac function [28]. In this study, the stem cells were isolated from donor mice and injected into recipients in viable myocardium bordering a 3–5 h old infarction. Nine days after injection, it was observed new myocardium complete with cardiomyocytes and vascular structures filling almost 70% of the infarcted region in 12 of the 30 mice. The treated mice showed significant improvement in LV function. At 9 days, the new myocardial cells were still proliferating and maturing.

An alternative approach to transplanting new myocardium to the infarcted heart is to help the heart in its own recovery by preventing remodeling. This approach was pursued by Kocher et al. [26] who identified a subpopulation of bone marrow stem cells with hemangioblast-like properties which, when injected into MI rats, migrate to the infarct zone, generate new blood vessels, and keep the hypertrophied cardiomyocytes viable as LV function restores. Left ventricular end-diastolic pressure declined by 36% and LV −dP/dt increased by 41%. At 2-week follow-up, significant increases in microvascularity and in the number of capillaries and feeding vessels, both within the infarct zone and at its perimeter, were observed. The revascularization of the infarct tissue resulted in a sixfold reduction in myocyte apoptosis and scar, and a significant restoration of cardiac function. The benefit was sustained up to 15 weeks, and LV ejection fraction increased by 34% [26, 29]. In the first human study, Strauer et al. transplanted the patient's bone marrow cells into his myocardium after an MI and found a significant improvement of the patient's heart function [30]. Ten weeks after stem cell implantation, there was a reduction of the infarct area and an increase of ejection fraction, cardiac index and stroke volume. The investigators assumed that the adult stem cells, which were transplanted into the necrotic areas of the myocardium, differentiated into cardiomyocytes, which regenerated the heart wall. Although at this point the hypothesis could not be proved, because tissue samples from the myocardium could not be extracted and analyzed, there is no other explanation for the improvement of the patient's heart function. After the first successful implantation six more patients have been treated with autologous bone marrow cells.

Clinical studies on stem cell therapy have so far been less compelling. A randomized, double blind, placebo-controlled study of stem cells in MI patients has failed to show an improvement in LV function, although there was a suggestion that such treatment could favorably affect infarct remodeling [31]. The randomized, open-label BOOST study has previously shown improvement of LV systolic function after transfer of stem cells, but this trial was not blinded. However, as bone-marrow aspiration and intracoronary injection can both induce cytokine release and therefore affect subsequent infarct healing and functional recovery, the control group must undergo exactly the same procedures as the active treatment group if the true benefit of cell transfer is to be fully appreciated. The investigators therefore followed up with a study of 67 patients, who all underwent bone-marrow aspiration 1 day after successful percutaneous coronary intervention for ST-elevation MI (STEMI). Patients were then assigned to intracoronary infusion of stem cells or placebo. The primary end point was the increase in LV ejection fraction, and secondary end points were change in infarct size and regional LV function at 4-month follow-up, all assessed by magnetic resonance imaging (MRI). The data showed no difference in LV function improvements between the two groups, although stem-cell infusion was associated with a significant reduction in myocardial infarct size and a better recovery of regional systolic function; no complications were associated with the treatment.

The first double blind, randomized, placebo-controlled trial of granulocyte colony stimulating factor (G-CSF) in patients with acute MI has been published and failed to show any benefit [32]. The Stem Cells in Myocardial Infarction (STEMI) clinical trial was assessed using G-CSF to mobilize stem cells in patients with STEMI after successful primary percutaneous coronary stent intervention. A total of 78 STEMI patients were evenly randomized to receive either a once-daily under-the-skin injection of G-CSF (10 μg/kg of body weight) or placebo for 6 days. Patients underwent angioplasty and stenting less than 12 h after the onset of symptoms, and 85% of patients were treated within 48 h. Although G-CSF proved safe, at 6-month follow-up there was no evidence of any significant benefit in the primary endpoint-change in systolic wall thickening in the infarct area from baseline, determined by cardiac MRI, which improved 17% in the G-CSF group and 17% in the placebo group. Comparable results were found in the infarct border, and noninfarcted myocardium. LVEF improved similarly in the two groups, as measured by both MRI and echocardiography. These findings differ from those observed in previous open-label trials of G-CSF, and underscore the importance of blinding and placebo controls in evaluating new, potentially antiangiogenic, stem-cell therapies.

Recommendations

1. The therapeutic use of ES cell transplantation in cardiac diseases primarily needs a rigorous demonstration that it can work in a stable fashion and with limited adverse effects.
2. Despite the limitations on federally-funded research presently imposed, new sources of ES cells and cell lines for ES cell transplantation studies need to be developed and likely will be, given the strong world-wide, corporate and state-funded interest in this technology and its purported benefits. Investigation into novel ways to isolate and culture autologous ES cells should also prove to be of significance.
3. Our overall understanding of the factors that may elicit the homing of ES cells to the heart and stimulate or direct the differentiation of ES cells to functional cardiomyocytes is presently rudimentary (a critique also applicable to adult stem cells). Identification of these factors as well as their mechanism of action will likely optimize both the homing and the differentiation processes, as well as contribute to defining the best-case scenarios in which ES cell transplantation will be beneficial.

Adult Skeletal Myoblast Cells

Transplanted satellite stem cells (myoblasts) from skeletal muscle can successfully home and engraft within a damaged myocardium, preventing progressive ventricular dilatation and improving cardiac function [33–36]. These myoblasts can be delivered into the myocardium by either intramural implantation or arterial delivery [36, 37], and recently effective deployment of a less invasive catheter approach has been reported [38]. Skeletal muscle satellite cells can proliferate abundantly in culture, and can be easily grown from the patient themselves (self-derived or autologous) thereby avoiding potential immune response.

Myoblasts are relatively ischemia-resistant (compared to cardiomyocytes, which become injured within 20 min) since they can withstand several hours of severe ischemia without becoming irreversibly injured [39]. The functional benefits of intramyocardially transplanted skeletal myoblasts in improving the damaged myocardium secondary to ischemia have been well documented [40]. Initial clinical trials have shown the efficacy of autologous skeletal myoblast transplantation in patients with left ventricular (LV) dysfunction [35]. The use of skeletal myoblasts, delivered by multiple intramyocardial injections, was effective in restoring left ventricular function in the genetically determined Syrian hamster model of DCM, demonstrating that the functional benefits of transplanted skeletal myoblast can be extended to non-ischemic cardiomyopathy [41].

Advantages to Myoblast Transplantation

Since myoblasts can be of autologous origin and can be robustly expanded in culture, a large number of cells can be obtained from only a small skeletal muscle biopsy sample (such as obtained from a patient) in a relatively short period of time. Compared to transplanted cardiomyocytes, myoblasts appear to be more resistant to ongoing apoptotic damage, which tends to be prevalent at ischemic sites.

Limitations and Concerns with Myoblast Transplantation

While several reports have suggested that a subpopulation of transplanted skeletal myoblasts were capable of transdifferentiation to a cardiomyocyte phenotype with increased expression of cardiac genes [42, 43], others have been unable to replicate the transdifferentiation of donor myoblasts to cardiomyocytes [44]. The present consensus of the majority of researchers in this field is that grafted myoblasts primarily remain non-cardiomyocytes. On the other hand, there is evidence that when myoblasts are implanted in the heart, their developmental program is influenced in such a way by the cardiac environment that it enables them to improve cardiac performance. Skeletal myoblasts engrafted to an injured myocardium differentiated to a fatigue-resistant, slow twitch phenotype adapted to cardiac workload [45]. Moreover, grafted myoblasts may display incompatible "wiring" or cell-to-cell connections with resident cardiomyocytes and do not respond in the same way to electrical signaling and stimuli [46].

While early preclinical studies did not detect the evidence of dysrhythmias, recent clinical studies have revealed that a subset of patients receiving skeletal myoblast transplant can experience severe and often life-threatening dysrhythmias [47]. The precise reason for these dysrhythmias remains unclear but may be related to the heterogeneous electrical properties and interactions between donor and recipient cells. On the other hand, the dysrhythmias may be promoted by the medium used to introduce the cells, rather than by the cells themselves [48]. Parenthetically, the functional benefits of myoblast transplantation may be related to the limitation of adverse post-infarction remodeling and/or the paracrine effects of transplanted myoblasts on recipient tissue, rather than to a grafted-myoblast contribution to enhance ventricular systolic function.

Further Recommendations

While preclinical studies with stem cell and myoblast transplantation have shown similar levels of efficacy [49, 50], there is a need for a detailed evaluation on the relative benefits, adverse effects and efficiency of skeletal myoblast and stem cell transplants in the clinical setting of HF vis a vis the

restoration of myocardial function. New methods to better assess and optimize post-transplanted myoblast recruitment and survival, particularly in the long-term, need to be developed and the repertoire of effective, less invasive cell delivery technologies needs to be expanded.

Trials with Autologous Skeletal Myoblast Transfer

Adult autologous skeletal myoblasts can be harvested from small peripheral muscle biopsy and if successfully isolated from the donor tissue, they will grow rapidly in culture. In a rat model of coronary artery ligation, evidence has been gathered that skeletal muscle myoblasts improve post-MI LV function to a similar degree as cardiomyocytes [51]. Ménasché first reported the transplantation of autologous skeletal myoblasts in a 72-year-old patient in HF secondary to multiple MIs [52]. About 800 million of skeletal myoblasts cultured from biopsies taken from the patient's leg, were injected into the infarcted tissue on the posterior wall of the heart during double-bypass surgery. Echocardiography and positron-emission tomography scanning prior to the transplant had shown that the area was metabolically non-viable. At 5 months follow-up, repeated studies reveal contraction in the area of the transplant, the magnitude of which increased when challenged with dobutamine. Later, further autologous skeletal myoblast transplantation was carried out in more patients with severe ischemic HF, and the technique was considered feasible, generally safe, and with signs of efficacy. Most patients have had symptomatic improvement, and echocardiographic studies revealed new systolic thickening in the implanted areas of the previous infarct, indicating contractility in implanted segments. Recently, Menasché et al. reported phase II of the randomized trial, the Myoblast Autologous Grafting in Ischemic Cardiomyopathy (MAGIC). This trial was carried out with a multicenter approach; this was the first randomized placebo-control study of myoblast transplantation in patients with LV dysfunction (ejection fraction $\leq 35\%$), myocardial infarction, and indication for coronary surgery [53]. Ninety-seven patients received myoblasts (400 or 800 million; $n = 33$ and $n = 34$, respectively) or placebo ($n = 30$). Interestingly, myoblast transfer did not improve regional or global LV function beyond what was seen in control patients. The absolute change in ejection fraction between 6 months and baseline was 4.4, 3.4, and 5.2% in the placebo, low-dose, and high-dose groups. Nonetheless, when compared with the placebo group the high-dose cell group showed significant decrease in LV volume. Although the dysrhythmic events were higher in the myoblast-treated patients, the 6-month rates of major cardiac adverse events and of ventricular dysrhythmias did not differ significantly between the treated and placebo groups. These data, revealed that myoblast injections in association with coronary surgery in patients with diminished LV function failed to improve heart function, as assessed by echocardiography. Moreover, there were increased early postoperative dysrhythmias after myoblast transplantation. However, an interesting finding was that the highest dose of myoblasts resulted in significant antiremodeling effect compared to placebo, and this merits further study in the future

Adult Bone Marrow Derived Stem Cells

Interest in bone marrow derived stem cells (BMCs) has been mainly motivated by their neovascularization and angiogenesis properties and these effects are enhanced by the presence of specific growth factors and cytokines (e.g., GCSF). The beneficial effects of these cells to a damaged vascular system were confirmed and subsequently extended to studies on myocardial damage in mice [54] in whom implanted BMCs can differentiate into myocytes and coronary vessels and thereby ameliorate the function of the injured heart. Since implantation of BMCs initially required surgical intervention and the procedure is often accompanied by a high mortality rate, with only a 40% rate of successful grafting, the development of noninvasive method became imperative. One such approach employed cytokine treatment, stem cell factor (SCF) and granulocyte-colony-stimulating factor (G-CSF), to mobilize endogenous BMCs and direct their integration or homing to the infarcted heart promoting repair. Mice injected with SCF (200 μg/kg/day) and G-CSF (50 μg/kg/day) exhibited a substantial increase in the number of circulating stem cells from 29 in nontreated controls to 7,200 in cytokine-treated mice. The endogenous BMCs were shown to give rise to new cardiac myocytes and coronary vasculature, and the BMC-derived myocardial regeneration resulted in improved cardiac function and survival. Similar findings of cell-mediated repair of myocardial infarction in the mouse were obtained using transplanted BMCs, which promoted proliferating myocytes and vascular structure [55].

It is important to remember that bone marrow contains several stem cell populations with overlapping phenotypes including, hematopoietic stem cells (HSCs), endothelial stem/precursor cells (EPCs), mesenchymal stem cells (MSCs), and multipotent adult progenitor cells (MAPCs). When EPCs, originating from a common hemangioblast precursor in bone marrow, are delivered to the myocardial target area they may implant, differentiate in situ and promote new vessel growth, an approach that has been applied to several animal models of myocardial ischemia [56]. These bone-marrow derived stem/precursor cells also can prevent the progression of cardiomyocyte apoptosis and stem cardiac remodeling [57].

Moreover, there is evidence showing that adult EPCs can transdifferentiate into active cardiomyocytes [58], although how extensively this occurs is presently not known. On the other hand, bone marrow-derived mesenchymal stem cells exhibit a high degree of plasticity allowing them to be employed as a self-renewing autologous source of progenitor cells (from adults), with the potential for differentiating into cardiomyocytes, and can be used in cellular cardiomyoplasty. Upon treatment with specific agents (e.g., 5-azacytidine), MSCs can differentiate into synchronously beating cardiomyocytes [59]. The injection of MSCs after their expansion in culture can also be used in the rescue of an abnormal mouse cardiac phenotype [60] and may prove effective in repairing a broader array of cardiac pathologies, including myocardial infarct and HF. In addition, bone marrow-derived HSCs and a subpopulation of HSCs termed SP cells have been reported following transplantation to repair infarcted myocardium, promoting new growth of cardiomyocytes, endothelial and smooth muscle cells [61]. While this cell-mediated myocardial repair was initially characterized as resulting from HSC's ability to transdifferentiate to cardiomyocytes, HSC plasticity has been difficult to reproduce and both its significance and basis remain undetermined.

Advantages of Adult BM Cells Transplantation

There is evidence that treatment with BMCs can ameliorate both myocardial and vascular damage with increasing angiogenesis. The effect of transplanted BMCs (which can include endothelial precursor cells) on vascular growth may significantly impact the recovery of the damaged heart, for example, by improving oxygen availability, although this may depend on the myocardial setting, whether acute myocardial infarction or established HF [57]. Moreover, autologously derived cells for transplantation are an attractive alternative, since bone marrow mesenchymal cells can be readily isolated in most cases. In addition, the expansion of BMC number by in vitro growth can be readily achieved by vigorous growth of mesenchymal cells in culture. It is significant that this method bypasses much of the ethical and legal maelstrom associated with the use of ESCs.

Limitations/Concerns with Adult BMC Transplant

The mechanism of BMC-mediated augmentation of cardiomyocyte number and function remains controversial. Some studies have suggested that the effects of adult stem cell transplantation on the recipient heart are not a consequence of transdifferentiation [62], but likely arise as a result of cell fusion with pre-existing cardiomyocytes or occur as a function of paracrine effects of transfected cells [63]; others maintain that there is evidence for a transdifferentiation event [56, 64–67].

Cell fusion has been demonstrated between cardiomyocytes and non-cardiomyocytes in vivo and in vitro [68, 69] and the data in support of transdifferentiation (particularly with HSCs) have not always been replicable. Further research is needed to clarify these issues and reconcile the contradictory claims, as well as to provide additional information about the extent of cell fusion and when it occurs. Similarly, a careful delineation of transdifferentiation from a well-defined adult stem cell type is warranted. Unfortunately, a critical problem in the replication of these experiments and in determining the effects of BMCs lies in the considerable heterogeneity of the populations of BMCs used. A limitation of the majority of the clinical studies with adult non-cardiac stem cell transplantation relates to the potential stability of the differentiated phenotype, since these studies have primarily examined the short-term benefits. However, it is important to underline the absence of adverse events in over 100 patients studied. This is in contrast with the dysrhythmia-prone myoblast transplantation [47].

Because of the paucity of successful techniques to effectively treat HF, there is mounting pressure (mainly from clinicians) to expedite the clinical application of cells transplant even before the mechanisms (as well as the long-term effects) are fully understood.

How Does the Preceding Information Translate to Human Clinical Studies?

Since most BMC research is presently performed in mice, a critical question is whether this model is truly applicable to humans. Preliminary studies in humans suggest that BMC transplantation and cytokines can home into areas of injury and promote neovascularization in those areas where they are needed. Whether enough BMCs can be transplanted to repair the damaged regions in the human heart, which tend to be larger in size than in the mouse heart, remains to be seen. Furthermore, it is questionable if adult human BM stem cell therapy works against any of the following: ischemic injury, cardiomyopathy/HF, the cardiomyopathy of aging, dysrhythmias and cardiac defects in infant/children.

Preliminary results of human clinical trials have shown a modest improvement in the cardiac function of patients with acute myocardial ischemia and infarct [70–73]. When cell transplantation was applied to patients with chronic myocardial disease the results were less definitive.

Cardiac Stem Cells

Cardiac stem cells (CSCs) are cells that can be isolated from the myocardium with a regenerative capacity higher than adult neonatal or fetal cardiomyocytes [73]. These cells can be isolated from mouse, rat and dog as well as human myocardium and are able to form all three major cardiovascular cell lineages: cardiomyocytes, endothelium and smooth muscle [74]. Interestingly, CSCs can be identified by different stem cell markers such as Sca-1 and c-kit. However, it is estimated that their number is very limited: about 1 CSC per 8,000–40,000 myocardial cells [75]; their potential for in vivo regeneration has been described in mouse, rat and dog studies after injected directly into the heart or via intracoronary administration after MI. Cells transdifferentiated in multiple cardiac lineages, regenerating the myocardium, preventing remodeling, and ameliorating left ventricular function [15]. However, despite their promising nature, especially the fact that they can be isolated from adult human hearts and thus form a source of autologous cells, many questions remain. The most important question is whether CSCs differentiate into true cardiomyocytes in vivo or just share some phenotypical characteristics.

Torella et al. [76] have reported that the adult heart has significant myocardial regenerative potential that stands against the accepted notion of terminal cardiomyocyte differentiation. The source of this regenerative potential is constituted by resident CSCs, and these CSCs through both cell transplantation and in situ activation have the capacity to regenerate significant segmental and diffuse myocyte losts, restoring anatomical integrity and ventricular function. It was suggested that CSC identification has started a brand new discipline of cardiac biology that could profoundly change the outlook of cardiac physiology and the potential for treatment of HF, and the potential of this new era should not be set back by premature attempts at clinical application before gathering the required scientifically reproducible data.

Adult Cardiac Stem Cells from Human and Animal Models

The findings that the adult heart contains stem cell niches that can regenerate myocytes and coronary vessels have raised the extraordinary possibility to regenerate dead myocardium after MI, to repopulate the failing heart with functioning cardiomyocytes and vessels, and probably to reverse ventricular dilation and wall thinning. Current information on various stem cell populations in the adult heart has emerged from research in several laboratories. However, many questions remain concerning the origin, structure, precise location, function, and regulation of these cells.

Beltrami et al. [77] reported the existence of Lin-c-kit⁺ cells in adult rat myocardium with the properties of stem cells. These cells are self-renewing and can be propagated for several months, expandable in culture, and multipotent, and can give rise to cardiomyocytes, smooth muscle, and endothelial cells. When injected into an ischemic heart, the Lin-c-kit⁺ cells contribute to the formation of endothelium and vascular smooth muscle and to the regeneration of myocardium in the region of necrosis, improving its pump function and ventricular chamber geometry [78].

The isolation and characterization of a small population of adult heart-derived cardiac progenitor cells (from postnatal mouse myocardium) expressing the surface marker stem cell antigen-1 (Sca-1⁺) and telomerase reverse transcriptase activity, associated with self-renewal potential, have been also reported [63, 79]. These adult cardiac stem (ACS) cells can be selectively isolated by a magnetic cell sorting system and express neither cardiac structural genes nor Nkx2.5. These cells can differentiate in vitro forming beating cardiomyocytes in response to the DNA demethylating agent 5'-azacytidine. Increased expression of other cardiogenic transcription factors (GATA-4, MEF-2C) has been shown by microarray profiling of differentiating ACS cells; previously found in bone marrow stromal cells with cardiogenic potential. Similarly, when treated with oxytocin, cardiac Sca-1⁺ stem cells expressed genes of cardiac transcription factors and contractile proteins and exhibited sarcomeric structure and spontaneous beating [73]. After intravenous delivery, the Sca-1⁺ cardiac stem cells can home to the myocardium injured by ischemia/reperfusion, and can functionally differentiate in situ.

Laugwitz et al. [82] have reported the presence of a population of cardioblasts in both embryonic and postnatal heart (from mouse, rat and human) numbering just a few hundred per heart. They were identified on the basis of their expression of a LIM-homeodomain transcription factor, Isl1. This group of cardiac stem cells was primarily localized in the atria, right ventricle, and outflow tract regions (where Isl1 is most prevalently expressed during cardiac organogenesis). These myocardial derived stem cells can be isolated, transplanted, survive and replicate in the damaged heart with evidence of functional improvement [83].

Advantages of ACS Cells

While the implantation of skeletal myoblasts and adult BMC transplantation appears promising, ACS cell transplantation might be more effective, since cardiac stem cells may be better programmed. The further identification, purification, and characterization of the ACS cells as well as a detailed knowledge of their interactions with the cardiac milieu or niche are essential if we are to achieve the major goal of regenerating/transplanting the tissue to treat myocardial damage.

Limitations of ACS Cells

Until recently, data on the presence of ACS cells have been scarce. This subset of stem cells appears to be extremely limited in number, difficult to identify and expand in culture thereby limiting their characterization and utilization, and likely contributing to difficulties in reproducing experiments concerning their isolation and transplantation. In addition, there is presently no consensus in the definition of selective markers specific for this cell type (see Table 22.1).

Table 22.1 Markers of stem cell-derived cardiomyocyte differentiation

Cell type	Differentiation agent	Markers of differentiated cardiomyocyte	Refs
ESC			
Embryonic stem cells	IGF-1, TGF-β	α-sarcomeric actin, connexin 43, major histocompatibility complex class I sarcomeric myosin, α-actin	[11, 84]
P19 embryonal carcinoma line	5'-azacytidine	Bone morphogenetic protein-2 (BMP-2), BMP-4, Bmpr 1a, Smad1, GATA-4, Nkx2.5, cardiac troponin I, desmin	[85]
BMC			
Bone marrow (MSC)	Insulin, ascorbic acid, dexamethasone	α-skeletal actin, β-myosin heavy chain (MHC), MLC-2v, CaV1.2, cardiac troponin I, sarcomeric tropomyosin, cardiac titin	[63, 86]
Cardiac stem cells			
Lin-c-kit⁺	Nd	c-kit⁺	[77]
isl1+	Nd	Csx/Nkx2.5, GATA-4	[82]
Sca-1+c-kit⁺	5'-azacytidine oxytocin	High telomerase activity, Sca-1+Csx/Nkx2.5, GATA-4, MEF-2C, α+ β-MHC, MLC-2, MLC-2v, Cardiac α-actin	[80–82, 87]
Cardiosphere	CKit+	Cardiac troponin I, myosin heavy chain, atrial natriuretic peptide	[83]
SP cells	Nd	ATP-binding cassette transporter (ABCG2)	[88, 89]

Nd not determined

Recommendations

Considerable work remains to fully delineate the relevant cardiac progenitor cell population and the optimization of conditions for their efficient transplantation, homing, differentiation, and integration into the myocardium. Understanding the factors that are responsible for growth, homing, and differentiation may allow specific ways to improve their production and functional benefits upon transplantation. Moreover, this information may also shed light on the activation of endogenous cardiac stem cells contributing to cardiac repair. Also, to be defined are the kinds of cardiac defects as well as type of injuries that can be best treated with these cells, including a clear knowledge of the best place in the heart to deliver or direct these cells. For instance, implanting cells within an area of necrosis and/or low oxygen availability may be unsuccessful, whereas implanting cells in regions of hibernating myocardium may be successful.

The long-term stability and functionality of transplanted ACS cells await definition. Whether ACS cells can be used as a platform for ex vivo gene modification, including the introduction of therapeutic genes, whether robust expression of specific genes can be directed in such cells, and if an increased proliferative response in the cardiac progenitor cells can be modulated by the introduction of cell-cycle progression genes remain to be seen.

Human Cardiac Stem Cells

The isolation and expansion in vitro of human cardiac stem cells (hCSCs) for autologous regeneration of dead myocardium in HF patients of ischemic and non ischemic etiology have been recently reported by Bearzi et al. [90]. These cells were identified in vitro as a class of human c-kit positive cardiac cells that possess the properties of stem cells: self-renewing, clonogenic and multipotent. Moreover, these cells can in vivo create cardiomyocytes and coronary vessels providing evidence that they play a role in cardiac homeostasis and myocardial regeneration. Again, these findings seem to contradict the previous concept that the heart is a post-mitotic organ unable to regenerate its own cells. Previously, Eberhard and Jockusch studied the pattern of clonal myocyte distribution during mammalian heart development, and found the presence of common progenitor cardiomyocytes prenatal and postnatally [91]. Embryo aggregation chimeras were employed, using as cellular markers enhanced jellyfish green fluorescent protein (eGFP) transgene and a desmin-promoter-driven, nuclear-localized β-galactosidase (nlacZ) knock-in. In neonatal, newly weaned mice, and adult chimeric atria and ventricles, irregularly formed patches of various sizes rather than highly dispersed cardiomyocytes were observed.

Most of the smaller patches and single cardiomyocytes were found in spatial neighborhood of large patches. This indicated a largely coordinated clonal growth during myocardial histogenesis combined with divergent displacement or active migration of myocytes. Interestingly, in the adult heart, large myocardial volumes devoid of eGFP-positive cardiomyocytes were found indicating a lack of secondary immigration of blood–borne stem cells into the myocardium. It is possible that similar patterns hold true for the human heart and that cell-lineage related pathological phenotypes may occur in patch patterns similar to those found in the mouse model. Recently, Anversa and Bolli et al. have further extended their work in this field. They have found that cardiac progenitor cells (CPCs) when implanted in the proximity of healed infarcts or resident CPCs, and stimulated locally by hepatocyte growth factor and IGF-1, invade the scarred myocardium and generate myocytes and coronary vessels improving the hemodynamics of the infarcted heart [92]. Injection of hCSCs regenerated the infarcted myocardium in the mouse heart 21 days after infarction, and human myocardium was present within the infarct area. Injection of CPCs led to the replacement of about 42% of the scar tissue with newly formed myocardium, decreased ventricular dilation and prevented the decline in function of the infarcted heart. Cardiac repair was probably mediated by the ability of CPCs to synthesize MMPs that degraded collagen proteins, forming tunnels within the fibrotic tissue during their migration across the scarred myocardium. Since the newly formed cardiomyocytes had a 2n karyotype and possessed 2 sex chromosomes cell fusion was excluded. They concluded that: (1) CPCs appear to be an ideal candidate cell for cardiac repair in HF patients; (2) CPCs isolated from myocardial biopsies and, following their expansion in vitro, can be administered back to the same patients avoiding the adverse effects associated with the use of nonautologous cells; (3) growth factors can be chosen instead and delivered locally to stimulate resident CPCs and promote myocardial regeneration, and (4) treatments could be repeated to reduce progressive tissue scarring and increase the working myocardium.

Using genetically engineered mice, the concept of the c-kit+ cells participating in the response to myocardial injury has been recently validated by Fransioli et al. [93]. The transgenic mouse expressing green fluorescent (GFP) protein driven by the c-kit promoter allows for unambiguous identification of this cell population; GFP driven by the c-kit promoter labeled a fraction of the c-kit+ cells recognized by antibody labeling for c-kit protein. Furthermore, the expression of GFP by the c-kit promoter and accumulation of GFP-positive cells in the myocardium appear relatively high at birth compared with adult and declines between postnatal weeks 1 and 2, which tracks in parallel with expression of c-kit protein and c-kit-positive cells. It was noted that acute cardiomyopathic injury by infarction prompts increased expression of both GFP protein and GFP-labeled cells in the region of infarction relative to remote myocardium, and that similar increases were observed for c-kit protein and cells with a slightly earlier onset and decline relative to the GFP signal. Cells coexpressing GFP, c-kit, and cardiogenic markers were apparent at 1–2 weeks postinfarction. Then, cardiac-resident c-kit$^+$ cell cultures derived from the transgenic line express GFP that is diminished in parallel with c-kit by induction of differentiation.

Finding Cell Identity

From the foregoing discussion, it should be evident that a critical element in the identification of the grafted cell in the heart and in a number of cases even prior to the transplant, is the unequivocal assignment of cell type identity. In Table 22.1, we provided a list of endogenous molecular markers that have been used to establish a differentiated cardiac phenotype resulting from transplanted different stem cell types, including BM cells, ES cells and CS cells. In addition to the endogenous markers available to establish cell identity, GFP has been extensively used as a reporter to define donor cells. Marking cells with the chromosome stain DAPI has been unsuccessful, since the DAPI stain from dead cells can be readily incorporated by non-marked cells [94]. Genotype marking is also a powerful tool in assessing cell identity. In several studies of cardiovascular self-repair in which female hearts were allografted into human male recipients, the presence of the Y chromosome was identified in the coronary vasculature and in cardiomyocytes [95–98], because the Y chromosome can be easily viewed by cytochemical staining or by fluorescence in situ hybridization. However, the assessment of the degree of cardiac chimerism reported in these studies reveals striking variation ranging from very low level of Y-chromosome containing cardiomyocytes (0.02–01%) [97, 98] to high levels (30%) [98], underscoring the critical need for establishing rigorous criteria by which chimerism is identified. The identification of a nucleus with a Y-chromosome is in itself not sufficient, but needs to be unequivocally associated with either myocardial vessels or cardiomyocyte structure (i.e., by confocal microscopy). Otherwise, it is possible to attribute the Y chromosome-positive nuclei to host cells involved in immune response and inflammatory infiltration, and not to cardiac regeneration. There is also some indication that the use of chromosomal analysis can result in the underestimation of the transfected cells due to the presence of nuclei that may not be counted in the histological section [58].

The detection of cell phenotype markers by real-time assays, confocal microscopy and non-invasive detection methodologies employing MRI has just begun to be applied in the assessment of cell transplant. Real-time visualization can provide identification of regions of myocardial infarction and precise MRI-guided delivery of therapeutic agents, with injection sites identified by contrast agents. Novel contrast agents permit MRI visualization of gene expression at a cellular resolution, and can be used as well to detect apoptotic cells [99, 100]. The appropriate labeling and detection of stem cells by MRI should enable the tracing of their in vivo distribution, and allow a glimpse of their destiny over time [101, 102].

Which Stem Cell Type to Use for HF

A brief comparison of the advantages and limitations of the cell types presently used in cardiac transplantation is shown in Table 22.2. While no clear-cut choice has yet emerged as to which cell type is best to transplant in myocardial repair, there are reasons to believe that the development of a multiplicity of approaches in the application of cell engineering will be required to develop novel therapies for the different cardiac disorders. HF may require the transplantation of cell types (e.g., skeletal myoblasts) that are different than those used in the targeted treatment of cardiac dysrhythmias, conduction disorders and congenital defects. It is also possible that the long-term repair of a fully functioning myocardium may require more than a single cell type – for instance, cardiomyocytes, fibroblasts, and endothelial cells – in the generation and integration of a stable and responsive cardiac graft.

Other Developing Technologies in Cell Engineering

The refinement of nuclear transfer, cybrid, and cell fusion techniques may allow further engineering of stem cells to provide cardioprotection, or stimulate antioxidant or antiapoptotic responses in the myocardium. These cell-engineering techniques might also allow the specific targeting of mitochondrial-based cytopathies [103]. Cardiomyopathies with a pronounced mitochondrial-based cytopathy and bioenergetic dysfunction have been reported and a subset of these has a genetic basis due to either defects in mtDNA or nuclear DNA [66]. Interestingly, introduction of mtDNA-repaired ES cells has been proposed in a patient harboring a mtDNA mutation, potentially transforming a diseased myocardium into a healthy one [103]. The mtDNA-repaired cells can be derived from the patient's own cells, whose endogenous defective mtDNA genome has been entirely eliminated by treatment with ethidium bromide, and replaced by entirely wild-type mtDNA genes. In a similar vein, treatment of a patient's nuclear DNA

Table 22.2 Myocardial transplants: advantages and limitations associated with cell-type

Cell-type	Source	Advantages	Limitations
Cardiac stem cells	Allogenic fetal, neonatal or adult heart	1. Recognition of myocardial growth factors and recruitment to myocardium are likely faster and more efficient than other cell types 2. In vivo electrical coupling of transplanted cells to existing myocardium has been demonstrated	1. Poor cell growth in vitro 2. Transplanted cells are very sensitive to ischemic insult and apoptotic cell death 3. Availability from either fetal (F), neonatal (N) or adult sources is low at present; likely immune rejection; F and N cells pose ethical difficulties
Skeletal myoblasts	Autologous skeletal muscle biopsy	1. Cells proliferate in vitro (allowing for autologous transplant) 2. Ischemia-resistant 3. Transplanted myoblasts can differentiate into slow-twitch myocytes (similar to cardiomyocytes) enabling cellular cardiomyoplasty 4. Reduces progressive ventricular dilatation and improves cardiac function 5. Can use adult cells	1. Likely do not develop new cardiomyocytes in vivo 2. Electrical coupling to surrounding myocardial cells is unclear (may cause dysrhythmias) 3. Long-term stability of differentiated phenotype unknown
Adult bone marrow stem cells	Autologous bone marrow stromal cells (mesenchymal) Bone marrow (endothelial progenitor cells)	1. Pluripotent stem cells can develop into cardiomyocytes 2. Stem cells are easy to isolate and grow well in culture 3. Neovascularization can occur at site of myocardial scar reducing ischemia 4. Transdifferentiation of cells into cardiomyocyte in vivo has been shown 5. Can be derived from autologous source; no immune-suppression treatment 6. Can improve myocardial contractile function	1. New program of cell differentiation is required 2. Efficiency of the differentiation into adult cardiomyocytes appears limited 3. Signaling, stability and regulation of differentiation unknown
Embryonic stem cells	Allogenic blastocyst (inner mass)	1. Easy propagation and well-defined cardiomyocyte differentiation process 2. In vivo electrical coupling of transplanted cells to existing myocardial cells 3. Pluripotent cells	1. Potential for tumor formation and immune rejection (allogenic) 2. Incomplete response to physiological stimuli 3. Legal and ethical issues 4. Donor availability

defects would involve either specific genetic replacement of the nuclear gene defect (site-specific homologous recombination can be readily undertaken in ES cells) or if the precise site of the nuclear defect is not known, by replacement of the entire nucleus of the patient with a wild-type nucleus. In the near future, ES cells therapy may be used in the treatment of mitochondrial-based cardiac diseases.

To identify aspects of the cardiac milieu that may contribute to the growth and development of transplanted myoblasts in vivo, three-dimensional matrices have been designed to serve as a novel in vitro system that mimic some aspects of the electrical and biochemical environment of the native myocardium. These structures may allow a finer resolution of electrical and biochemical signals that may be involved in myoblast proliferation and plasticity. Myoblasts have been grown on 3-D polyglycolic acid mesh scaffolds under control conditions in the presence of cardiac-like electrical current fluxes, and in the presence of culture medium that had been conditioned by mature cardiomyocytes [104]. Such scaffolds containing either fetal or neonatal aggregates of

contracting cardiac cells have been used to generate artificial cardiac grafts transplanted into injured myocardium with recuperation of ventricular function, and formation of functional gap junctions between the grafted cells and the myocardium [105, 106].

The combination of gene therapy and stem cell engineering is an attractive approach for treating cardiac disorders. Overexpression (and in some cases the inhibition of expression) of specific proteins can result in striking changes in cardiomyocyte and in cardiac phenotype. Specific cardiomyocyte functions, including ion channels, cardiac conduction, contractility and myocyte proliferation have been shown to be affected by gene transfer and expression of specific proteins [107–109]. Cell-based therapies for injured or dysfunctional hearts can be enhanced by using ex vivo genetically modified stem cells to deliver genes and proteins. For instance, transplanted mesenchymal stem cells appear to be effective devices to deliver channel proteins involved in pacemaking activity (e.g., channel protein HCN2) resulting in the modification of cardiac rhythm in vivo [23]. In an animal model of ischemic cardiomyopathy, the introduction of the vascular endothelial growth factor (VEGF) and its effect on both angiogenesis and left ventricular function was markedly enhanced in hearts with VEGF-transfected skeletal myoblasts in comparison to hearts directly injected with the adenoviral-VEGF construct [110].

Conclusions and Future Directions

The discovery of cardiogenesis in adult animals and human represents one of the most significant advances in cardiology in the last 25 years. Previously, most cardiologists believed that the birth of new cardiomyocytes was only confined to the fetal and neonatal heart. This dogma recently collapsed when researchers discovered that the heart of adult rat, mice and human undergo significant cardiac changes as a function of age. New cardiomyocytes were born/homing-in into myocardial areas relevant to cardiac pathways, and then could integrate structurally so that myocardial function could be restored and new tissue produced. These findings have set off a large number of parallel discoveries in rats, mice, and humans, with dramatic implications for how we think about cardiac plasticity and its potential role in rehabilitating individuals with acquired myocardial ischemia/infarct, HF and different types of cardiomyopathies, including the cardiomyopathy of aging.

Rigorous criteria are needed to evaluate the efficacy of cell transplantation, effects on stability and function of the transplanted cells and in the unequivocal identification of transplanted cells. To evaluate the most effective sources of transplanted cells, the following are necessary:

1. Collection of experimental data from large animals, whose anatomical and physiological characteristics are similar to human.
2. A careful analysis of isoforms of contractile protein genes, such as of myosin and α-actin comparing their phenotype with that of fetal ventricular cardiomyocytes.
3. Expression of cardiac transcription factors (e.g., Nkx2.5, eHAND, dHAND, GATA-4) and examination of both the timing and interaction of cardiac-specific transcription factors in the cascade pathway (see Fig. 22.2).
4. Immunocytological and ultrastructural analyses to examine whether the selected cardiomyocyte cultures are highly differentiated and evaluate the proportion of cells that are cardiomyocyte and fibroblast, as well as gauging their origin (double-labeling experiments are very effective).
5. Analysis of specific ion currents and action potentials characteristic of specific cardiomyocyte populations. Regenerated cardiomyocytes need to be capable of responding to appropriate adrenergic and muscarinic stimulation.

6. Identification of genes which control the power to produce efficient daughters cells from CSCs.

Moreover, the expression of specific transcription factors and structural markers of cardiac differentiation does not represent definitive proof of functionality. Establishing the best cell type for transplantation may require refinement of available imaging technology, as well as further studies to document efficiency in the production of cardiomyocytes and their stability and functioning in the myocardium.

An extraordinary prototype of translation from the bench to bedside, repair of a damaged heart is a formidable undertaken that soon will undergo clinical trials [111]. In their editorial to a review series, Benjamin and Schneider [112] posed several interesting and challenging questions: How might cell mobilization, homing, and migration best be enhanced?; to what extent do grafted cells function as replacements for cardiac muscle, and to what extent do their benefits depend on different mechanisms altogether, such as angiogenesis or the production of secreted cell-survival factors [113, 114]. Furthermore, what is the evidence for and against transdifferentiation? Parenthetically, in regard to the concept of transdifferentiation a note of caution is warranted since the use of this term, as proposed by David Tosh et al. [115] should be restricted *to irreversible switches of one differentiated cell type to another.*

The work of Anversa et al. has provided answer to questions on the presence of CPCs in the myocardium, and their properties and advantages over other types of cells. The discovery of CSCs [76], have opened a new field on cardiac regenerative biology that has changed the future of developmental and adult cardiac biology/physiology, as well as the potential treatment of HF. When transplanted into a damaged heart, CSCs have the capacity to generate significant new myocardial tissue and improve ventricular function. Furthermore, even more relevant for translational research and its application for future regeneration protocols, is that CSCs can also be activated by local injections of several growth factors or through the administration of systemic drugs, such as statins, to obtain beneficial results similar to those of CSC transplantation [116].

Finally, it would seem prudent to remember that the primary objective of the cell transplantation process in HF patients and in other cardiac diseases is to incorporate cells into myocardium that can perform cardiac work, respond appropriately to adjacent cardiomyocytes and be appropriately responsive to physiological stimuli. It is apparent that further procedures to establish proof-of-concept and others that have the potential for widespread clinical application are necessary. Whether the results obtained in animal models of HF secondary to ischemia or cardiomyopathy will be reproducible in human remains to be seen. Hopefully, with our increasing capacity to understand the function of different cardiomyocytes/cardiac differentiation pathways in detail, we will eventually be able to replace tissue, transplant others, and control imbalances in the molecular and biochemistry of the heart. However, without the required clinical trials, cell regeneration in the damaged human heart is a balancing act where in one side we have to place current proofs of safety and efficacy, and in the other the uncertainty of all tests available to measure results. It is our hope that with the beginning and eventually rapid progress in cell engineering, we may see the end of cardiac abnormalities that weaken human life and bankrupt the health care system.

Summary

- Cell transplantation represents a viable therapeutic approach for repairing the damaged myocardium.
- In spite of remarkable progress in this field, significant problems remain, especially ethical problems and the tumorigenic and dysrhythmogenic potential that these techniques present for differentiation into somatic cells.
- Because the limited potential of the myocardium for self-repair and renewal, a significant proportion of cardiac muscle loses its ability to perform work and this loss may be the most important factor in the heart pump failure occurring in patients with coronary artery disease and dilated cardiomyopathy.
- It is evident that the limited capacity of regeneration and proliferation of human cardiomyocytes can prevent neither the scar formation that follows myocardial infarction nor the loss of heart function occurring in patients with cardiomyopathy and HF.
- The most primitive of all stem cells are the embryonic stem (ES) cells that develop as the inner cell mass in the human blastocyst at day 5 after fertilization.
- While the precise cellular and molecular events comprising the pathway of ES cell cardiomyocyte-specific differentiation remain largely undetermined, significant progress has been made in identifying the regulatory factors which can enhance or inhibit the process.
- Nitric oxide (NO) generated either by NO synthase activity or exogenous NO exposure has also been implicated in the promotion of cardiomyocyte-specific differentiation from mouse ES cells.
- Also, IGF-1 promotes cardiomyocyte differentiation phenotype and the expression of the cardiomyocyte phenotype in ES cells in vivo.
- Early experiments with both fetal cardiomyocyte and differentiating ES cell transplantation showed successful formation of stable grafts and nascent intercalated discs between the grafted and the host myocardial cells.

- Human ES cell-derived cardiomyocytes are able to effectively form structural and electromechanical connections with cultured rat cardiomyocytes.
- The transplanted human ES cell-derived cardiomyocytes were able to integrate and pace in vivo the swine heart with complete atrioventricular block, as demonstrated by detailed electrophysiological mapping and histopathological studies.
- When fetal rat cardiomyocytes were transplanted into ischemic damaged hearts, a large percentage of cardiomyocytes die post-transplantation.
- ES cells can be readily and reproducibly obtained from the inner layer of the blastocyst, and exhibit an excellent growth phenotype, both in vitro and in vivo.
- The development and application of ES-like cell lines (e.g., P19), which have been highly informative in the identification and characterization of regulatory factors, transcriptional activators and signal transduction events involved in cardiomyocyte differentiation, may also be useful in cell transplant therapy.
- ES cells may also be more amenable to ex vivo engineering via DNA modifications (e.g., gene therapy, viral transfection, knockouts and over-expressed genes).
- ES cells transfected with overexpressed β_2-adrenergic receptors, or ion channel proteins could be transplanted to restore function in defective myocardial cells. However, the safety and efficacy of these methodologies need to be absolutely proven prior to their use in humans with cardiac dysrhythmias.
- Pluripotent ES cells which have unlimited growth potential can have tumorigenic side-effects, making the screening for teratoma formation well-advised.
- The inability of the damaged myocardium to provide the appropriate molecular signals for stem cells engraftment seems to limit their capacity for recruitment and integration into the aging myocardium.
- Major advances showing that stem cell therapy have great potentials in the treatment of post-myocardial infarction HF, have been reported.
- An alternative approach to transplanting new myocardium to the infarcted heart is to help the heart in its own recovery by preventing remodeling.
- The revascularization of the infarct tissue resulted in a sixfold reduction in myocyte apoptosis and scar, and a significant restoration of cardiac function.
- A randomized, double blind, placebo-controlled study of stem cells in MI patients has failed to show an improvement in LV function, although there was a suggestion that such treatment could favorably affect infarct remodeling.
- The first double blind, randomized, placebo-controlled trial of granulocyte colony stimulating factor (G-CSF) in patients with acute MI has been published and failed to show any benefit.

- Transplanted satellite stem cells (myoblasts) from skeletal muscle can successfully home and engraft within a damaged myocardium, preventing progressive ventricular dilatation and improving cardiac function.
- Skeletal muscle satellite cells can proliferate abundantly in culture, and can be easily grown from the patient themselves (self-derived or autologous) thereby avoiding potential immune response.
- The use of skeletal myoblasts, delivered by multiple intramyocardial injections, was effective in restoring left ventricular function in the genetically determined Syrian hamster model of dilated cardiomyopathy, demonstrating that the functional benefits of transplanted skeletal myoblast can be extended to non-ischemic cardiomyopathy.
- The present consensus of the majority of researchers in this field is that grafted myoblasts primarily remain noncardiomyocytes.
- There is evidence that when myoblasts are implanted in the heart, their developmental program is influenced in such a way by the cardiac environment that it enables them to improve cardiac performance.
- In a rat model of coronary artery ligation, evidence has been gathered that skeletal muscle myoblasts improve post-MI LV function to a similar degree as cardiomyocytes.
- Autologous skeletal myoblast transplantation has been carried out in patients with severe ischemic HF, and the technique has been considered feasible, generally safe, and with signs of efficacy.
- Myoblast injections in association with coronary surgery in patients with diminished LV function failed to improve heart function, as assessed by echocardiography.
- Interest in bone marrow derived stem cells has been mainly motivated by their neovascularization and angiogenesis properties and these effects are enhanced by the presence of specific growth factors and cytokines (e.g., GCSF).
- Endogenous BMCs have been shown to give rise to new cardiac myocytes and coronary vasculature, and the BMC-derived myocardial regeneration resulted in improved cardiac function and survival.
- When endothelial progenitor cells (EPCs), originating from a common hemangioblast precursor in bone marrow, are delivered to the myocardial target area, they may implant, differentiate in situ and promote new vessel growth, an approach that has been applied to several animal models of myocardial ischemia.
- The injection of MSCs after their expansion in culture can also be used in the rescue of an abnormal mouse cardiac phenotype and may prove effective in repairing a broader array of cardiac pathologies, including myocardial infarct and HF.
- The effect of transplanted BMCs (which can include endothelial precursor cells) on vascular growth may sig-

nificantly impact the recovery of the damaged heart, for example by improving oxygen availability, although this may depend on the myocardial setting, whether acute myocardial infarction or established HF.
- A limitation of the majority of the clinical studies with adult non-cardiac stem cell transplantation relates to the potential stability of the differentiated phenotype, since these studies have primarily examined the short-term benefits.
- Since most BMC research is presently performed in mice, a critical question is whether this model is truly applicable to humans.
- Preliminary studies in humans suggest that BMC transplantation and cytokines can home into areas of injury and promote neovascularization in those areas where they are needed.
- Whether enough BMCs can be transplanted to repair the damaged regions in the human heart, which tend to be larger in size than in the mouse heart, remains to be seen.
- Cardiac stem cells (CSCs) have been identified in vitro as a class of human c-kit positive cardiac cells that possess the properties of stem cells: self-renewing, clonogenic and multipotent.
- These cells can be isolated from mouse, rat and dog as well as human myocardium and are able to form all three major cardiovascular cell lineages: cardiomyocytes, endothelium and smooth muscle.
- The adult heart has significant myocardial regenerative potential that stands against the accepted notion of terminal cardiomyocyte differentiation.
- The source of this regenerative potential is constituted by resident CSCs, and these CSCs through both cell transplantation and in situ activation have the capacity to regenerate significant segmental and diffuse myocyte loss, restoring anatomical integrity and ventricular function.
- The findings that the adult heart contains stem cell niches that can regenerate myocytes and coronary vessels has raised the extraordinary possibility to regenerate dead myocardium after myocardial infarction, to repopulate the failing heart with functioning cardiomyocytes and vessels, and probably to reverse ventricular dilation and wall thinning.
- While the implantation of skeletal myoblasts and adult BMC transplantation appears promising, ACS cell transplantation might be more effective than adult BMC transplantation, since cardiac stem cells may be better programmed.
- Data on the presence of ACS cells have been scarce. This subset of stem cells appears to be extremely limited in number, difficult to identify and expand in culture thereby limiting their characterization and utilization, and likely contributing to difficulties in reproducing experiments concerning their isolation and transplantation.
- Considerable work remains to fully delineate the relevant cardiac progenitor cell population and the optimization of

conditions for their efficient transplantation, homing, differentiation and integration into the myocardium.

- The isolation and expansion in vitro of hCSCs for autologous regeneration of dead myocardium in HF patients of ischemic and non ischemic etiology have been recently reported.
- The detection of cell phenotype markers by real-time assays, confocal microscopy and non-invasive detection methodologies employing magnetic resonance imaging (MRI) has just begun to be applied in the assessment of cell transplant.
- While no clear-cut choice has yet emerged as to which cell type is best to transplant in myocardial repair, there are reasons to believe that the development of a multiplicity of approaches in the application of cell engineering will be required to develop novel therapies for the different cardiac disorders. HF may require the transplantation of cell types (e.g., skeletal myoblasts) that are different than those used in the targeted treatment of cardiac dysrhythmias, conduction disorders and congenital defects.
- The combination of gene therapy and stem cell engineering is an attractive approach for treating cardiac disorders.
- Rigorous criteria are needed to evaluate the efficacy of cell transplantation, effects on stability and function of the transplanted cells and in the unequivocal identification of transplanted cells.
- It is prudent to remember that the primary objective of the cell transplantation process in HF patients and in other cardiac diseases is to incorporate cells into myocardium that can perform cardiac work, respond appropriately to adjacent cardiomyocytes and be appropriately responsive to physiological stimuli.
- It is evident that further procedures to establish proof-of-concept and others that have the potential for widespread clinical application are necessary.

References

1. Doevendans PA, Kubalak SW, An RH, Becker DK, Chien KR, Kass RS (2000) Differentiation of cardiomyocytes in floating embryoid bodies is comparable to fetal cardiomyocytes. J Mol Cell Cardiol 32:839–851
2. Kehat I, Khimovich L, Caspi O et al (2004) Electromechanical integration of cardiomyocytes derived from human embryonic stem cells. Nat Biotechnol 22:1237–1238
3. Doetschman T, Shull M, Kier A, Coffin JD (1993) Embryonic stem cell model systems for vascular morphogenesis and cardiac disorders. Hypertension 22:618–629
4. He JQ, Ma Y, Lee Y, Thomson JA, Kamp TJ (2003) Human embryonic stem cells develop into multiple types of cardiac myocytes: action potential characterization. Circ Res 93:32–39
5. Muller M, Fleischmann BK, Selbert S et al (2000) Selection of ventricular-like cardiomyocytes from ES cells in vitro. FASEB J 14:2540–2548
6. Wobus AM, Boheler KR (2005) Embryonic stem cells: prospects for developmental biology and cell therapy. Physiol Rev 85:635–678
7. Yuasa S, Itabashi Y, Koshimizu U et al (2005) Transient inhibition of BMP signaling by Noggin induces cardiomyocyte differentiation of mouse embryonic stem cells. Nat Biotechnol 23:607–611
8. Wobus AM, Kaomei G, Shan J et al (1997) Retinoic acid accelerates embryonic stem cell-derived cardiac differentiation and enhances development of ventricular cardiomyocytes. J Mol Cell Cardiol 29:1525–1539
9. Kanno S, Kim PK, Sallam K, Lei J, Billiar TR, Shears LL 2nd (2004) Nitric oxide facilitates cardiomyogenesis in mouse embryonic stem cells. Proc Natl Acad Sci USA 101:12277–12281
10. Xu C, Police S, Rao N, Carpenter MK (2002) Characterization and enrichment of cardiomyocytes derived from human embryonic stem cells. Circ Res 91:501–508
11. Kofidis T, de Bruin JL, Yamane T et al (2004) Insulin-like growth factor promotes engraftment, differentiation, and functional improvement after transfer of embryonic stem cells for myocardial restoration. Stem Cells 22:1239–1245
12. Sauer H, Rahimi G, Hescheler J, Wartenberg M (2000) Role of reactive oxygen species and phosphatidylinositol 3-kinase in cardiomyocyte differentiation of embryonic stem cells. FEBS Lett 476:218–223
13. Koh GY, Soonpaa MH, Klug MG, Pride HP, Cooper BJ, Zipes DP, Field LJ (1995) Stable fetal cardiomyocyte grafts in the hearts of dystrophic mice and dogs. J Clin Invest 96:2034–2042
14. Klug MG, Soonpaa MH, Koh GY, Field LJ (1996) Genetically selected cardiomyocytes from differentiating embryonic stem cells form stable intracardiac grafts. J Clin Invest 98:216–224
15. Zhang M, Methot D, Poppa V, Fujio Y, Walsh K, Murry CE (2001) Cardiomyocyte grafting for cardiac repair: graft cell death and anti-death strategies. J Mol Cell Cardiol 33:907–921
16. Monge JC, Stewart DJ, Cernacek P (1995) Differentiation of embryonal carcinoma cells to a neural or cardiomyocyte lineage is associated with selective expression of endothelin receptors. J Biol Chem 270:15385–15390
17. Paquin J, Danalache BA, Jankowski M, McCann SM, Gutkowska J (2002) Oxytocin induces differentiation of P19 embryonic stem cells to cardiomyocytes. Proc Natl Acad Sci USA 99:9550–9555
18. Wobus AM, Kleppisch T, Maltsev V, Hescheler J (1994) Cardiomyocyte-like cells differentiated in vitro from embryonic carcinoma cells P19 are characterized by functional expression of adrenoceptors and Ca2+ channels. In Vitro Cell Dev Biol Anim 30A:425–434
19. Coburn B (2005) Beating congenital heart defects with embryonic stem cells. Clin Genet 67:224–225
20. Fraidenraich D, Stillwell E, Romero E, Wilkes D, Manova K, Basson CT, Benezra R (2004) Rescue of cardiac defects in id knockout embryos by injection of embryonic stem cells. Science 306:247–252
21. Qu J, Plotnikov AN, Danilo P Jr, Shlapakova I, Cohen IS, Robinson RB (2003) Rosen Expression and function of a biological pacemaker in canine heart. Circulation 107:1106–1109
22. Miake J, Marban E, Nuss HB (2002) Biological pacemaker created by gene transfer. Nature 419:132–133
23. Potapova I, Plotnikov A, Lu Z et al (2004) Human mesenchymal stem cells as a gene delivery system to create cardiac pacemakers. Circ Res 94:952–959
24. Dotson V, Horak K, Alwardt C, Larson DF (2004) Relationship of aging and cardiac IL-10. J Extra Corpor Technol 36:197–201
25. Orlic D, Kajstura J, Chimenti S, Jakoniuk I et al (2001) Bone marrow cells regenerate infarcted myocardium. Nature 410:701–705
26. Kocher AA, Schuster MD, Szabolcs MJ et al (2001) Neovascularization of ischemic myocardium by human bone-marrow-

derived angioblasts prevents cardiomyocyte apoptosis, reduces remodeling and improves cardiac function. Nat Med 7:430–436

27. Wang JS, Shum-Tim D, Galipeau J, Chedrawy E, Eliopoulos N, Chiu RC (2000) Marrow stromal cells for cellular cardiomyoplasty: feasibility and potential clinical advantages. J Thorac Cardiovasc Surg 120:999–1005

28. Orlic D, Hill JM, Arai AE (2002) Stem cells for myocardial regeneration. Circ Res 91:1092–1102

29. Rosenthal N, Tsao L (2001) Helping the heart to heal with stem cells. Nat Med 7:412–413

30. Strauer BE, Brehm M, Zeus T, Gattermann N, Hernandez A, Sorg RV, Kogler G, Wernet P (2001) Intracoronary, human autologous stem cell transplantation for myocardial regeneration following myocardial infarction. Dtsch Med Wochenschr 126:932–938

31. Janssens S, Dubois C, Bogaert J, Theunissen K (2006) Autologous bone marrow-derived stem-cell transfer in patients with ST-segment elevation myocardial infarction: double-blind, randomised controlled trial. Lancet 367:113–121

32. Ripa RS, Jorgensen E, Wang Y et al (2006) Stem cell mobilization induced by subcutaneous granulocyte-colony stimulating factor to improve cardiac regeneration after acute ST-elevation myocardial infarction. Result of the double-blind, randomized, placebo-controlled Stem Cells in Myocardial Infarction (STEMMI) trial. Circulation 113:1983–1992

33. Taylor DA, Atkins BZ, Hungspreugs P, Jones TR, Reedy MC, Hutcheson KA, Glower DD, Kraus W (1998) Regenerating functional myocardium: improved performance after skeletal myoblast transplantation. Nat Med 4:929–933

34. Kessler PD, Byrne BJ (1999) Myoblast cell grafting into heart muscle: cellular biology and potential applications. Annu Rev Physiol 61:219–242

35. Menasche P (2003) Skeletal muscle satellite cell transplantation. Cardiovasc Res 58:351–357

36. Robinson SW, Cho PW, Levitsky HI, Olson JL, Hruban RH, Acker MA, Kessler PD (1996) Arterial delivery of genetically labelled skeletal myoblasts to the murine heart: long-term survival and phenotypic modification of implanted myoblasts. Cell Transplant 5:77–91

37. Menasche P (2005) Skeletal myoblast for cell therapy. Coron Artery Dis 16:105–110

38. Brasselet C, Morichetti MC, Messas E et al (2005) Skeletal myoblast transplantation through a catheter-based coronary sinus approach: an effective means of improving function of infarcted myocardium. Eur Heart J 26:1551–1556

39. Jennings RB, Reimer KA (1981) Lethal myocardial ischemic injury. Am J Pathol 102:241–255

40. Van Den Bos EJ, Taylor DA (2003) Cardiac transplantation of skeletal myoblasts for heart failure. Minerva Cardioangiol 51: 227–243

41. Pouly J, Hagege AA, Vilquin JT et al (2004) Does the functional efficacy of skeletal myoblast transplantation extend to nonischemic cardiomyopathy? Circulation 110:1626–1631

42. Iijima Y, Nagai T, Mizukami M et al (2003) Beating is necessary for trans-differentiation of skeletal muscle-derived cells into cardiomyocytes. FASEB J 17:1361–1363

43. Winitsky SO, Gopal TV, Hassanzadeh S et al (2005) Adult murine skeletal muscle contains cells that can differentiate into beating cardiomyocytes in vitro. PLoS Biol 3:e87

44. Reinecke H, Poppa V, Murry CE (2002) Skeletal muscle stem cells do not transdifferentiate into cardiomyocytes after cardiac grafting. J Mol Cell Cardiol 34:241–249

45. Murry CE, Wiseman RW, Schwartz SM, Hauschka SD (1996) Skeletal myoblast transplantation for repair of myocardial necrosis. J Clin Invest 98:2512–2523

46. Leobon B, Garcin I, Menasche P, Vilquin JT, Audinat E, Charpak S (2003) Myoblasts transplanted into rat infarcted myocardium are functionally isolated from their host. Proc Natl Acad Sci USA 100:7808–7811

47. Menasche P, Hagege AA, Vilquin JT, Desnos M et al (2003) Autologous skeletal myoblast transplantation for severe postinfarction left ventricular dysfunction. J Am Coll Cardiol 41:1078–1083

48. Chachques JC, Herreros J, Trainini J, Juffe A, Rendal E, Prosper F, Genovese J (2004) Autologous human serum for cell culture avoids the implantation of cardioverter-defibrillators in cellular cardiomyoplasty. Int J Cardiol 95:S29–S33

49. Thompson RB, Emani SM, Davis BH, van den Bos EJ, Morimoto Y, Craig D, Glower D, Taylor DA (2003) Comparison of intracardiac cell transplantation: autologous skeletal myoblasts versus bone marrow cells. Circulation 108:II264–II271

50. Agbulut O, Vandervelde S, Al Attar N et al (2004) Comparison of human skeletal myoblasts and bone marrow-derived CD133+ progenitors for the repair of infarcted myocardium. J Am Coll Cardiol 44:458–463

51. Scorsin M, Hagege AA, Marotte F et al (1997) Does transplantation of cardiomyocytes improve function of infarcted myocardium? Circulation 96:II-93

52. Menasche P (2002) Cell transplantation for the treatment of heart failure. Semin Thorac Cardiovasc Surg 14:157–166

53. Menasché P, Alfieri O, Janssens S, McKenna W et al (2008) The Myoblast Autologous Grafting in Ischemic Cardiomyopathy (MAGIC) trial: first randomized placebo-controlled study of myoblast transplantation. Circulation 117:1189–1200

54. Orlic D, Kajstura J, Chimenti S et al (2001) Mobilized bone marrow cells repair the infarcted heart, improving function and survival. Proc Natl Acad Sci USA 98:10344–10349

55. Orlic D, Kajstura J, Chimenti S et al (2001) Bone marrow cells regenerate infarcted myocardium. Nature 410:701–705

56. Masuda H, Asahara T (2003) Post-natal endothelial progenitor cells for neovascularization in tissue regeneration. Cardiovasc Res 58:390–398

57. Itescu S, Kocher AA, Schuster MD (2003) Myocardial neovascularization by adult bone marrow-derived angioblasts: strategies for improvement of cardiomyocyte function. Heart Fail Rev 8: 253–258

58. Badorff C, Brandes RP, Popp R et al (2003) Transdifferentiation of blood-derived human adult endothelial progenitor cells into functionally active cardiomyocytes. Circulation 107:1024–1032

59. Tomita S, Li RK, Weisel RD, Mickle DA, Kim EJ, Sakai T, Jia ZQ (1999) Autologous transplantation of bone marrow cells improves damaged heart function. Circulation 100:II247–II256

60. Toma C, Pittenger MF, Cahill KS, Byrne BJ, Kessler PD (2002) Human mesenchymal stem cells differentiate to a cardiomyocyte phenotype in the adult murine heart. Circulation 105:93–98

61. Jackson KA, Majka SM, Wulf GG, Goodell MA (2002) Stem cells: a minireview. J Cell Biochem Suppl 38:1–6

62. Murry CE, Soonpaa MH, Reinecke H et al (2004) Haematopoietic stem cells do not transdifferentiate into cardiac myocytes in myocardial infarcts. Nature 428:664–668

63. Wollert KC, Drexler H (2005) Clinical applications of stem cells for the heart. Circ Res 96:151–163

64. Eisenberg LM, Burns L, Eisenberg CA (2003) Hematopoietic cells from bone marrow have the potential to differentiate into cardiomyocytes in vitro. Anat Rec A Discov Mol Cell Evol Biol 274: 870–882

65. Xu M, Wani M, Dai YS, Wang J, Yan M, Ayub A, Ashraf M (2004) Differentiation of bone marrow stromal cells into the cardiac phenotype requires intercellular communication with myocytes. Circulation 110:2658–2665

66. Zhang S, Wang D, Estrov Z, Raj S, Willerson JT, Yeh ET (2004) Both cell fusion and transdifferentiation account for the transformation of human peripheral blood CD34-positive cells into cardiomyocytes in vivo. Circulation 110:3803–3807

67. Kajstura J, Rota M, Whang B et al (2005) Bone marrow cells differentiate in cardiac cell lineages after infarction independently of cell fusion. Circ Res 96:127–137

68. Matsuura K, Wada H, Nagai T et al (2004) Cardiomyocytes fuse with surrounding noncardiomyocytes and reenter the cell cycle. J Cell Biol 167:351–363

69. Reinecke H, Minami E, Poppa V, Murry CE (2004) Evidence for fusion between cardiac and skeletal muscle cells. Circ Res 94:e56–e60

70. Galinanes M, Loubani M, Davies J, Chin D, Pasi J, Bell PR (2004) Autotransplantation of unmanipulated bone marrow into scarred myocardium is safe and enhances cardiac function in humans. Cell Transplant 13:7–13

71. Wollert KC, Meyer GP, Lotz J et al (2004) Intracoronary autologous bone-marrow cell transfer after myocardial infarction: the BOOST randomized controlled clinical trial. Lancet 364:141–148

72. Lee MS, Makkar RR (2004) Stem-cell transplantation in myocardial infarction: a status report. Ann Intern Med 140:729–737

73. van den Bos EJ, van der Giessen WJ, Duncker DJ (2008) Cell transplantation for cardiac regeneration: where do we stand? Neth Heart J 16:88–95

74. Beltrami AP, Barlucchi L, Torella D, Baker M, Limana F, Chimenti S et al (2003) Adult cardiac stem cells are multipotent and support myocardial regeneration. Cell 114:763–776

75. Anversa P, Kajstura J, Leri A, Bolli R (2006) Life and death of cardiac stem cells: a paradigm shift in cardiac biology. Circulation 113:1451–1463

76. Torella D, Ellison GM, Karakikes I, Nadal-Ginard B (2007) Resident cardiac stem cells. Cell Mol Life Sci 64:661–673

77. Beltrami AP, Barlucchi L, Torella D et al (2003) Adult cardiac stem cells are multipotent and support myocardial regeneration. Cell 114:763–776

78. Dawn B, Stein AB, Urbanek K et al (2005) Cardiac stem cells delivered intravascularly traverse the vessel barrier, regenerate infarcted myocardium, and improve cardiac function. Proc Natl Acad Sci USA 102:3766–3771

79. Oh H, Chi X, Bradfute SB, Mishina Y et al (2004) Cardiac muscle plasticity in adult and embryo by heart-derived progenitor cells. Ann N Y Acad Sci 1015:182–189

80. Oh H, Bradfute SB, Gallardo TD et al (2003) Cardiac progenitor cells from adult myocardium: homing, differentiation, and fusion after infarction. Proc Natl Acad Sci USA 100: 12313–12318

81. Matsuura K, Nagai T, Nishigaki N et al (2004) Adult cardiac Sca-1-positive cells differentiate into beating cardiomyocytes. J Biol Chem 279:11384–11391

82. Laugwitz KL, Moretti A, Lam J et al (2005) Postnatal isl1+ cardioblasts enter fully differentiated cardiomyocyte lineages. Nature 433:647–653

83. Messina E, De Angelis L, Frati G et al (2004) Isolation and expansion of adult cardiac stem cells from human and murine heart. Circ Res 95:911–921

84. Kumar D, Sun B (2005) Transforming growth factor-beta2 enhances differentiation of cardiac myocytes from embryonic stem cells. Biochem Biophys Res Commun 332:135–141

85. Choi SC, Yoon J, Shim WJ, Ro YM, Lim DS (2004) 5-azacytidine induces cardiac differentiation of P19 embryonic stem cells. Exp Mol Med 36:515–523

86. Hattan N, Kawaguchi H, Ando K et al (2005) Purified cardiomyocytes from bone marrow mesenchymal stem cells produce stable intracardiac grafts in mice. Cardiovasc Res 65:334–344

87. Oh H, Chi X, Bradfute SB et al (2004) Cardiac muscle plasticity in adult and embryo by heart-derived progenitor cells. Ann N Y Acad Sci 1015:182–189

88. Garry DJ, Martin CM (2004) Cardiac regeneration: self-service at the pump. Circ Res 95:852–854

89. Martin CM, Meeson AP, Robertson SM et al (2004) Persistent expression of the ATP-binding cassette transporter, Abcg2, identifies cardiac SP cells in the developing and adult heart. Dev Biol 265:262–275

90. Bearzi C, Rota M, Hosoda T et al (2007) Human cardiac stem cells. Proc Natl Acad Sci USA 104:14068–14073

91. Eberhard D, Jockusch H (2005) Patterns of myocardial histogenesis as revealed by mouse chimeras. Dev Biol 278: 336–346

92. Rota M, Padin-Iruegas ME, Misao Y, De Angelis A et al (2008) Local activation or implantation of cardiac progenitor cells rescues scarred infarcted myocardium improving cardiac function. Circ Res 103:107–116

93. Fransioli J, Bailey B, Gude NA et al (2008) Evolution of the c-kit-positive cell response to pathological challenge in the myocardium. Stem Cells 26:1315–1324

94. Borenstein N, Hekmati M, Bruneval P, Montarras D (2004) Unambiguous identification of implanted cells after cellular cardiomyoplasty: a critical issue. Circulation 109:e209–e210

95. Hruban RH, Long PP, Perlman EJ, Hutchins GM, Baumgartner WA, Baughman KL, Griffin CA (1993) Fluorescence in situ hybridization for the Y-chromosome can be used to detect cells of recipient origin in allografted hearts following cardiac transplantation. Am J Pathol 142:975–980

96. Taylor DA, Hruban R, Rodriguez ER, Goldschmidt-Clermont PJ (2002) Cardiac chimerism as a mechanism for self-repair: does it happen and if so to what degree? Circulation 106:2–4

97. Laflamme MA, Myerson D, Saffitz JE, Murry CE (2002) Evidence for cardiomyocyte repopulation by extracardiac progenitors in transplanted human hearts. Circ Res 90:634–640

98. Quaini F, Urbanek K, Beltrami AP et al (2002) Chimerism of the transplanted heart. N Engl J Med 346:5–15

99. Louie AY, Huber MM, Ahrens ET et al (2000) In vivo visualization of gene expression using magnetic resonance imaging. Nat Biotechnol 18:321–325

100. Zhao M, Beauregard DA, Loizou L, Davletov B, Brindle KM (2001) Non-invasive detection of apoptosis using magnetic resonance imaging and a targeted contrast agent. Nat Med 7:1241–1244

101. Taylor DA (2004) Cell-based myocardial repair: how should we proceed? Int J Cardiol 95:S8–S12

102. Thompson RB, van den Bos EJ, Davis BH et al (2005) Intracardiac transplantation of a mixed population of bone marrow cells improves both regional systolic contractility and diastolic relaxation. J Heart Lung Transplant 24:205–214

103. Zullo SJ (2001) Gene therapy of mitochondrial DNA mutations: a brief, biased history of allotopic expression in mammalian cells. Semin Neurol 21:327–335

104. Pedrotty DM, Koh J, Davis BH, Taylor DA, Wolf P, Niklason LE (2005) Engineering skeletal myoblasts: roles of three-dimensional culture and electrical stimulation. Am J Physiol Heart Circ Physiol 288:H1620–H1626

105. Leor J, Amsalem Y, Cohen S (2005) Cells, scaffolds, and molecules for myocardial tissue engineering. Pharmacol Ther 105: 151–163

106. Shimizu T, Yamato M, Isoi Y, Akutsu T, Setomaru T, Abe K, Kikuchi A, Umezu M, Okano T (2002) Fabrication of pulsatile cardiac tissue grafts using a novel 3-dimensional cell sheet manipulation technique and temperature-responsive cell culture surfaces. Circ Res 90:e40

107. Teng G, Zhao X, Cross JC, Li P, Lees-Miller JP, Guo J, Dyck JR, Duff HJ (2004) Prolonged repolarization and triggered activity induced by adenoviral expression of HERG N629D in cardiomyocytes derived from stem cells. Cardiovasc Res 61:268–277

108. Most P, Pleger ST, Volkers M et al (2004) Cardiac adenoviral S100A1 gene delivery rescues failing myocardium. J Clin Invest 114:1550–1563

109. Engel FB, Schebesta M, Duong MT, Lu G, Ren S, Madwed JB, Jiang H, Wang Y, Keating MT (2005) p38 MAP kinase inhibition enables proliferation of adult mammalian cardiomyocytes. Genes Dev 19:1175–1187

110. Askari A, Unzek S, Goldman CK, Ellis SG, Thomas JD, DiCorleto PE, Topol EJ, Penn MS (2004) Cellular, but not direct, adenoviral delivery of vascular endothelial growth factor results in improved left ventricular function and neovascularization in dilated ischemic cardiomyopathy. J Am Coll Cardiol 43:1908–1914

111. Dimmeler S, Zeiher AM, Schneider MD (2005) Unchain my heart: the scientific foundations of cardiac repair. J Clin Invest 115: 572–583

112. Benjamin IJ, Schneider MD (2005) Learning from failure: congestive heart failure in the postgenomic age. J Clin Invest 115:495–499

113. Bock-Marquette I et al (2004) Thymosin beta4 activates integrin-linked kinase and promotes cardiac cell migration, survival, and cardiac repair. Nature 432:466–472

114. Schneider MD (2004) Medicine: Prometheus unbound. Nature 432:451–453

115. Li WC, Yu WY, Quinlan JM, Burke ZD, Tosh D (2005) The molecular basis of transdifferentiation. J Cell Mol Med 9:569–582

116. Torella D, Indolfi C, Goldspink DF, Ellison GM (2008) Cardiac stem cell-based myocardial regeneration: towards a translational approach. Cardiovasc Hematol Agents Med Chem 6:53–59

Section XI
Looking to the Future

Chapter 23
Future Frontiers in Heart Failure

Overview

Heart failure (HF) is an pandemic health problem of great magnitude in the world. In spite of considerable clinical and research effort during the last decade and the development of new drugs and surgical modalities of therapy, the mortality and morbidity remain very high. Accordingly, breakthroughs in the treatment of HF are needed. Late-breaking molecular genetic technology has just begun to be applied in studies of HF with identification of a number of genes involved in its pathogenesis and may serve as prognosticators. Since the publication of the human genome, many changes in the field of genetic research have occurred providing investigators with a remarkable array of potential therapeutic genes to be tested in vivo in animal models. In this chapter, besides genetics we discuss current and future new technologies like proteomics, biomarkers, systems biology, bionics, and mitochondrial medicine. In addition, new approaches in developing methodologies that might advance HF diagnosis and therapy are analyzed.

Introduction

Current knowledge about the genetic and molecular changes that occur in HF has begun to find clinical applications in diagnosis, risk stratification and treatment. A number of cardiovascular pathological conditions that may culminate in HF are associated with defects in energy metabolism. Genetic modifications of key steps in the uptake and metabolism of glucose and fatty acids, by using transgenic technology, have enhanced our understanding of how these pathways may influence the pathogenesis of HF. In addition, metabolic shifts that accompany HF may contribute to the development of cardiac dysfunction.

In this chapter, we discuss the genetic and molecular changes that occur in HF that has begun to find clinical applications in diagnosis and management in conditions associated with the development of HF. Furthermore, the use of an integrative approach (i.e., method of integrating several approaches) that looks beyond the limits of a single approach, advances in technology for higher-throughput gene association studies, and other methodologies in the developmental phase are addressed.

Present and Emerging Concepts in the Integrative Approach to HF

In the development of LV dysfunction and HF, cardiac remodeling is a critical step. Its structural changes include hypertrophy and subsequent chamber dilatation with progressive impairment in function. This remodeling encompasses changes in both the myocytes and the extracellular matrix (ECM), the latter includes the activation of proteolytic enzymes that lead to the degradation and reorganization of collagens. In addition, neurohumoral signals acting through many interrelated signal transduction pathways lead to pathological cardiac hypertrophy and subsequently progression to HF. Many of such agonists act through cell surface receptors coupled with G-proteins to mobilize intracellular calcium, with consequent activation of downstream kinases and the calcium- and calmodulin-dependent phosphatase calcineurin; also, MAPK signaling pathways are interconnected at multiple levels with calcium-dependent kinases and calcineurin [1, 2].

Microarray technology has facilitated the way to simultaneously assess the expression of tens of thousands of gene transcripts in a single experiment, providing a resolution and precision of phenotypic characterization not previously possible. Within the heart, many examples of genetic and protein changes correlated with dysfunction have been noted both during normal growth and development and during the development of HF from diverse etiologies [3]. Furthermore, detailed gene profiling has been performed on structural and functional changes including energy metabolism and intracellular calcium handling.

Myocyte loss plays a critical role in the pathogenesis and pathophysiology of HF, mainly in HF following myocardial

J. Marín-García, *Heart Failure*, Contemporary Cardiology,
DOI 10.1007/978-1-60761-147-9_23, © Springer Science+Business Media, LLC 2010

infarction [4]. In animal models of HF, molecular and genetic studies have shown that cardiomyocyte apoptosis is a critical process, and if this paradigm is confirmed in humans, apoptosis regulation will be a logical target for novel HF therapies. On the other hand, it has been recently reported that although the failing human and monkey heart is characterized by significant myocyte apoptosis, in contrast to current concepts, the apoptosis in nonmyocyte cells was eight- to ninefold greater than in myocytes [5]. Notwithstanding, and despite successes in establishing the mechanistic link between apoptosis and HF, a clear understanding of the molecular mechanisms that regulate cell death, specifically in this complex HF syndrome remains incomplete. At present, fundamental questions still remain unanswered regarding the underlying molecular and biochemical mechanisms involved in HF, and how this information can be used to improve diagnosis and treatment. To address these questions, emerging technologies are being recruited, some tested so far in animal models and other are being investigated in clinical trials. These novel approaches include the integrated use of molecular genetics, microarrays, and proteomics under the so-called systems biology. This, together with an increasing number of novel cardiac biomarkers for cardiac diagnosis and the use of gene and cell transplantation therapies, represents some of the present and forthcoming advances in clinical cardiology.

Cardiac Biomarkers

Markers of HF and their effect on prognosis have been discussed to some extent in Chaps. 18 and 19. In this final chapter, we would like to emphasize that this is an area of research that needs continuous and intensive effort because of its importance in cardiovascular medicine. In this subsection, we comment on the identification and utilization of several markers from diverse tissues (e.g., endomyocardial biopsies, blood, and urine) and also on the physiological and genetic variants that are useful tools for diagnosis, and risk stratification of cardiovascular diseases (CVDs) in general, and HF in particular.

Clearly, cardiac biomarkers are of significant importance during the early stages of myocardial infarction (MI), acute coronary syndrome (ACS), and acute HF. In acute HF, the clinical signs and symptoms may not be completely informative; however, with biomarkers, early diagnosis can be rapidly established and early treatment can be started to reduce the extent of cardiac damage, and then enhancing patient survival. Several cardiac biomarkers have been shown to be excellent predictors of future cardiovascular events, morbidity and mortality, and they may be used not only in diagnosis, but also to develop strategies for prevention, treatment, and

risk stratification. A list of biomarkers, their association with an array of pathological processes, their use in diagnosis, as well as in risk stratification is presented in Table 23.1. These biomarkers range from markers of ischemia and resultant myocardial damage such as myocyte necrosis (e.g., cardiac troponins, myoglobin, creatine kinase-MB), markers of hemodynamic stress (e.g., brain natriuretic peptide (BNP) and N-terminal proBNP (NT-proBNP)), markers of neurohormonal imbalance secondary to genetic polymorphism of renin–angiotensin–aldosterone system and resultant congestive HF (genetic defects in some signaling components of the β-AR pathway are potential markers [6]), markers of systemic inflammatory processes (e.g., C-reactive protein, myeloperoxidase, matrix metalloproteinases, and interleukins), markers of platelet function (e.g., the soluble CD40 ligand, P-selectin), and markers of hemostasis, including fibrinogen and soluble fibrin, vWF [7]. These markers are all present in the blood allowing relatively low cost and noninvasive screening. In addition, the assays of these biomarkers are all relatively rapid, show high sensitivity and specificity, can be performed easily in a highly reproducible and accurate fashion, and display a low coefficient of variation. H-FABP, a cardiac-specific marker, behaves similarly to myoglobin, increasing within 3 h post-MI, and therefore is a useful gauge of cardiac injury in ACS and early MI [8]; it also allows the detection of minor myocardial injury in patients with HF and unstable angina, and can be used as a reliable marker of severe HF [9, 10]. Furthermore, H-FABP levels in early ACS are prognosticators of recurrent cardiac events [11]. Niizeki et al. have shown that serum H-FABP levels could be effectively used for risk stratification and prediction of cardiac events in elderly patients with severe HF [12]. Often, HF patients and patients with early coronary artery disease (CAD) may present a combination of genetic polymorphisms of the renin–angiotensin–aldosterone system (RAAS) that may result in the development of pathogenic neurohormonal mechanisms, likely independent of an association with diabetes, hypertension, obesity, and low ejection fraction [13, 14]. In patients with suspected HF, measurement of BNP and NT-proBNP has become a routine practice since their determination can facilitate the diagnosis and risk stratification, and also they can be used to guide the response to therapy. BNP is a marker of myocardial ischemia, and experimental studies have shown that BNP gene expression is markedly upregulated in the infarcted tissue and in surrounding ischemic tissue, but not in viable myocardium [15].

New biomarkers for HF are being evaluated. For example, galectin-3, a protein produced by active macrophages, may predict adverse outcomes in HF patients when its plasma levels are elevated. Van Kimmenade et al. have measured galectin-3 plasma levels in 599 patients who presented with dyspnea in the ER, of which 209 had acute HF [16]. Determination of NT-proBNP levels was superior to either

Table 23.1 Biomarkers function, and their use in diagnosis and risk stratification in myocardial ischemia/ACS/HF

Biomarker	Pathological process	Diagnostic indication	Prognostic indication
Troponin I (cTnI)	Ischemia/necrosis	Late MI/ACS	Death/MI
Troponin T (cTnT)	Ischemia/necrosis	Late MI/ACS	Death/MI/RI
Ischemia-modified albumin (IMA)	Early myocardial ischemia	ACS	a
Myoglobin	Myocardial ischemia/damage	Early-onset MI/RI	a
Creatine kinase MB (CK-MB)	Myocardial ischemia/damage	Late MI	Death
Myosin light chain	Myocardial ischemia/damage	Late MI	a
Brain natriuretic peptide (BNP)	Hemodynamic stress	Acute HF	Death/HF
N-terminal pro-brain natriuretic peptide (NT-proBNP)	Hemodynamic stress		Death/HF
High sensitivity C-reactive protein (hsCRP)	Inflammation		Death/MI/RI
Myeloperoxidase (MPO)	Inflammation	ACS	Death/MI
Interleukin-10 (IL-10)	Inflammation		a
Interleukin-6 (IL-6)	Inflammation		a
Monocyte chemoattractant protein (MCP-1)	Inflammation		Potential risk predictor in ACS
Matrix metalloproteinases (MMPs)	Inflammation		Death/MI
Soluble CD40 ligand (sCD40L)	Platelet function		Death/MI
P-selectin	Platelet function		a
von Willebrannd factor (vWF)	Hemostasis		Death
Fibrinogen	Hemostasis		ACS
Plasminogen activator inhibitor 1 (PAI-1)	Hemostasis		Death
Unbound free fatty acids (FFAU)	Myocardial ischemia	Early indicator of ischemia	Death/ventricular dysrhythmias
Heart fatty acid binding protein (H-FABP)	Myocardial ischemia/necrosis	AMI/stroke	Death/RI/HF
Fibrinopeptide A	Hemostasis		a
Soluble fiber	Hemostasis	Early marker of ischemia in unstable angina	a
Genetic polymorphism of renin–angiotensin–aldosterone system	Hemodynamic stress	ECAD/HF	Chronic HF
Chromogranin A	Hemodynamic stress Negative inotropic effect	MI/HF	Death/HF
Galectin-3	Inflammation	Acute HF	Death/HF
Osteoprotegerin	Inflammation (TNF family)	AMI/HF	MI/Death/HF

ACS acute coronary syndrome; *HF* heart failure; *AMI* acute myocardial infarct; *ECAD* early coronary artery disease; *RI* recurrent infarct
[a]Tests have not yet been in clinical use

apelin or galectin-3 in the diagnosis of acute HF; however, galectin-3 plasma levels were significantly higher in subjects with HF when compared with those without. Using a multivariate logistic regression analysis, an elevated level of galectin-3 was the best independent predictor of 60-day mortality or the combination of death/recurrent HF within 60 days. In addition, Kaplan–Meier analyses showed that the combination of an elevated galectin-3 and NT-proBNP was a better predictor of mortality than either one of the two markers alone. In contrast, measurement of apelin levels was not useful as a predictor of mortality or recurrence of HF.

Other markers being presently evaluated are osteoprotegerin, a member of the TNF receptor superfamily that has been implicated in the development of left ventricular dysfunction [17] and in predicting survival of HF patients after myocardial infarction [18]. Also, chromogranin A, a polypeptide hormone produced by the myocardium with potent negative inotropic properties, was found elevated in plasma of HF patients [19].

From the growing list of biomarkers, one can infer that there is no yet a perfect biomarker for all cardiac diseases/

events. For risk stratification and also to improve prognostication of HF patients, a combined, multimarkers analysis of biomarkers might help find the best, individualized strategy.

Proteomics in the Discovery of New Markers

Previously, in Chap. 19, we have extensively reviewed the use of proteomics in the development of new markers in cardiology diagnostics. In this chapter, it suffices to outline that two major approaches have been employed in proteomic research, the complete proteomic approach (large platforms) in which the entire proteome (all proteins) is characterized, and a more limited proteomic analysis which is either targeted to specific candidate proteins or limited to specific classes of proteins, or sub-proteomes [20]. A well-thought out argument has been presented regarding the limitation of current proteomic technology to carry out a complete proteomic analysis of plasma proteins [21]. This is mainly due to the high sensitivity required to evaluate in depth the plasma proteome, reflecting both the dynamic range of its constituent specific proteins, such as regulatory factors and cytokines, simply undetectable by present proteomic technology, as well as the surprisingly high levels of posttranslational modifications that most proteins undergo. Proteomic analysis can be used in the identification of novel markers of human cardiac allograft rejection. Besides cardiac allograft rejection, large platforms with hundreds of proteins will also be necessary for early detection of HF, for determining its pathogenesis, and for the assessment of HF patient's response to therapy.

Microarray and Genetic Biomarkers

Gene expression profiling may also be used to identify a pattern of genes (a molecular signature) that serves as biomarker of relevant clinical parameters of HF (e.g., disease presence, progression, or response to therapy) [22]. While not as easy or convenient to perform as the screening of circulating biomarkers, the deployment of gene/transcriptome profiling targeted to specific tissues or cell populations can often provide important information unavailable with other approaches, as well as augmenting the growing list of significant (and novel) biomarkers. For further discussion on microarray and biomarkers, see Chap. 19.

Role of Mitochondria

Abnormalities in mitochondrial function and structure have been increasingly recognized as a common feature in cardiomyopathy and HF, often presenting with heterogeneous patterns of changes in mitochondrial respiratory enzymatic function, as well as changes in organelle structure and mtDNA [23]. Animal studies have confirmed that changes in mitochondrial biogenesis because of targeted gene disruptions (e.g., mtTFA, ANT) can lead to DCM. Furthermore, mitochondria play a prominent role in the development of myocardial ischemia and in cardioprotection, partly through the generation of ROS and via its primary role in early apoptotic events, and through changes in mitochondrial metabolic function both in the utilization of fatty acids as substrate as well as in the efficiency of oxidative phosphorylation [24]. It is worth noting that mutations of mtDNA and mitochondrial respiratory changes, presumably resulting from oxidative damage may play an important role in HF and in the aging process. While there are several strong indications of mitochondrial involvement in cardiac dysfunction, the precise location of mitochondria in the subcellular pathways involved has not been clearly determined. Questions related to whether mitochondrial defects represent a primary event,

or are secondary to other myocardial changes contributing to the pathophysiology of cardiac dysfunction, have been largely unanswered [25]. Even in cases where mitochondrial-based cardiac disease is a certainty, there are indications that mitochondrial genetic abnormalities are markedly influenced by other genetic factors (modifiers), as well as by environmental factors leading to heterogeneity of phenotype. Whether situated upstream or downstream, the broad spectrum of mitochondrial defects evident in both clinical and experimental studies have spurred an increased interest in the potential application of mitochondrial medicine in both diagnosis and in the treatment of mitochondrial-associated cardiovascular pathologies.

Gene therapy to replace or repair defective mitochondrial genes could be an important adjunct in the treatment of mitochondrial-based CVD. However, mitochondria genes with their own genetic code as well as their multicopy status have proved to be rather refractory to genetic manipulation when compared to nuclear genes. Techniques of targeted mitochondrial gene transfection in animal studies have been rarely successful; electroporation and the use of the "gene gun" approach using biolistic transformation while successful in yeast and plants have not been extensively applied to incorporating genes into animal and human mitochondria [26, 27]. An alternative delivery system for nucleic acids into mitochondria involves the use of peptide nucleic acids (PNA) [28]. Early experiments employed PNA as a selective antisense inhibitor to target the replication of a pathogenic mtDNA allele in vitro, although this effect could not be demonstrated in cultured cells [29]. The difficulties associated with mitochondrial uptake of nucleic acids in living mammalian cells have been more recently surmounted by the addition of a mitochondrial-targeting leader peptide to the PNA-oligonucleotide molecule, and the introduction of the PNA-oligonucleotide construct in cationic liposomes [30, 31], and even more effectively, with cationic polyethylenimine [32]. The latter approach successfully allowed the import of PNA-oligonucleotides into the mitochondrial matrix of living cultured cells or isolated mitochondria, a critical step in potential mitochondrial gene-specific therapy. Similarly, a mitochondrial-specific delivery system has been recently developed using DQAsomes, liposome-like vesicles formed in aqueous medium from a dicationic amphiphile called *dequalinium* [33]. These DQAsomes can also bind and carry DNA (as well as drugs), are able to transfect cells with a high efficiency, and selectively accumulate in the mitochondrial organelle releasing their load [34]. Moreover, besides PNA-oligonucleotides, plasmid DNAs can be incorporated and condensed within the DQAsomes and exclusively delivered to the mitochondrial compartment [34]. In addition to modifying mtDNA genes, the selective delivery of a variety of compounds (e.g., antiapoptotic drugs, antioxidants, and proton uncouplers) to the mitochondria could be used as a potential alternative strategy in the treatment of a number of mitochondrial-based disorders with cardiac involvement. The previously mentioned DQAsome can also deliver drugs that trigger apoptosis to mitochondria and inhibit carcinoma growth in mice [35]. A synthetic ubiquinone analog (termed *mitoQ*) has been selectively targeted to mitochondria by the addition of a lipophilic triphenylphosphate cation [36]. These positively charged lipophilic molecules can rapidly permeate the lipid bilayers and accumulate at high levels within negatively charged energized mitochondria [37]. Significant doses of these bioactive compounds can be administered safely by mouth to mice over long periods of time and accumulate within most organs, including the heart and brain. The incorporation of mitoQ within mitochondria can prevent apoptotic cell death and caspase activation induced by H_2O_2 (in isolated Jurkat cells) and can function as a potent antioxidant, preventing lipid peroxidation and protecting the mitochondria from oxidative damage. Feeding mitoQ to rats significantly decreased heart dysfunction, cell death, and mitochondrial damage after ischemia–reperfusion [38].

Targeting bioactive molecules to mitochondria can be adapted to other neutral bioactive molecules, offering a potential vehicle for testing other mitochondrial-specific therapies. For instance, synthetic peptide antioxidants containing dimethyltyrosine, which are cell-permeable and concentrate 1,000-fold in the mitochondria, can reduce intracellular levels of ROS and cell death in a cell model. In ischemic hearts, these peptides potently improved contractile force in an ex vivo heart model [39]. In addition, the successful incorporation into the mitochondrial matrix of another modified antioxidant, a synthetic analog of vitamin E (MitoVitE), has been shown to significantly reduce mitochondrial lipid peroxidation and protein damage and can accumulate after oral administration at therapeutic concentrations within the cardiac tissue [37].

Besides direct modulation of mitochondria by introduction of "therapeutic" nucleic acids, proteins, and antioxidants, a variety of therapeutic agents have been used to indirectly affect the mitochondrial function either through bypassing specific steps leading to mitochondrial dysfunction (e.g., vitamins and metabolic cofactors such as riboflavin, thiamine, succinate, ascorbate) augmenting the "general" antioxidant balance in the cell (e.g., vitamin E, coenzyme Q_{10}), supplementing metabolites that might be reduced because of either defective synthesis or transport in patients with mitochondrial-based disease (e.g., carnitine) or by redirecting the metabolic pathways (e.g., drugs targeted to enhance glucose use and pyruvate oxidation energy, at the expense of FAO). While there have been multiple reports and case studies citing benefits with many of these compounds in treating cardiomyopathies, there have been no large-scale controlled studies supporting their efficacy in patients with mitochondrial cardiomyopathy. In some cases, these pharmacological treatments are being used,

in various combinations, as a therapeutic "cocktail." Knowledge of the precise site of the biochemical or molecular defect can be of critical importance regarding the choice of the therapeutic modality used.

In addition to a widening array of therapeutic strategies, advances are also been made in the area of diagnostic evaluation of mitochondrial defects, although many clinicians appear not to be aware either of the significance of mitochondrial defects in CVD or how to screen for them. While in some cases screening of different cell types (e.g., blood and biopsied skeletal muscle) can provide useful information about specific mtDNA mutations and bioenergetic defects (that often can exhibit a multisystemic phenotype), some defects (e.g., mtDNA deletions and some mtDNA point mutations) may not be present in active mitotic tissues such as blood. Unfortunately, direct examination of cardiac tissue although important can be limited by the invasive nature of a biopsy. Nevertheless, strong correlation between the mutation load (of a specific mtDNA mutation) present in postmitotic muscle and urinary epithelium, suggests that urinary epithelial cells may be the tissue of choice in a noninvasive diagnosis [40].

It is of critical significance to develop noninvasive methodologies that can evaluate both mtDNA and in vivo bioenergetic dysfunction. In this regard, techniques involving nuclear magnetic resonance spectrometry have been employed diagnostically (albeit in a limited fashion) as an in vivo diagnostic platform in animal models, and in healthy and diseased patients to assess mitochondrial energy reserves, OXPHOS rates, metabolite levels, pH, and energy coupling [41–46] (e.g., insulin-resistant patients with type 2 diabetes) [44]. Notwithstanding, the great majority of these studies have only evaluated skeletal muscle bioenergetics, not the heart. Of interest, positron emission tomography (PET) has been used as a noninvasive diagnostic method to evaluate myocardial mitochondrial Krebs cycle activity and dysfunction in children with cardiomyopathy [47].

Finally, the need for new treatments for HF is obvious, and currently a number of drugs are under development. Further research may bring in the near future a full understanding of the temporal order of changes in mitochondrial structure and function, as well as the organelle contribution to the pathophysiological events occurring in HF. These advances will facilitate a rational use of mitochondrial-targeted therapies.

Bionics Role in HF

Sophisticated CT, MRI, PET, and 3-D echo machines are representatives of the continual technological development in clinical cardiology, either for cardiovascular diagnoses and/or to be used as therapies. The latter are represented by the daily use of cardiac defibrillators, pacemakers, and circulatory assist devices (see Chap. 20) controlled by microprocessors that can deliver therapy, monitor disease, and rescue HF patients from sudden cardiac death. Clearly, a "bionics" era is developing, in which devices have the most significant impact in the treatment for HF. In 2005, Sunagawa [48] reported the development of a neurally regulated artificial pacemaker by unifying an artificial system with a native system allowing for bidirectional communication. Using the convolution integral of the impulse response with the instantaneous sympathetic activity, he could predict the precise sinus rate in real time. The clinical impact of direct manipulation of autonomic functions in CVDs may be of significance, and the case of central baroreflex failure (*failure of homeostatic mechanisms for maintaining blood pressure*) is the prototype of such application. In treating these diseases, an artificial bionic baroreflex system can be implemented as a kind of biological proxy capable of emulating the native central baroreflex function of the failing vasomotor center. The system operates as an intelligent negative feedback regulator, and in rats showed to be effective in restoring normal baroreflex functioning. Sunagawa also developed an artificial brain stem that takes over the native cardiac regulation [48]. This bionic brain stem consisted of an implantable pressure sensor with a radiotransmitter, an extra-corporeal microprocessor, and implantable radiocontrolled nerve stimulator, for the activation of vagal system. In a rat model of HF, the bionic brain stem performed better than the native brain stem, and the mortality rate at 140 days was reduced by 80%. Thus, bionic treatment of HF opens up an entirely new therapeutic paradigm for chronic HF patients. It is evident that the combination of microprocessors with nanomachine technology and quantitative systems physiology, will further expand the application of bionic medicine in the future.

Besides the aforementioned techniques (e.g., implantable cardioverter defibrillator, biventricular re-synchronization, and LVAD), other approaches have been developed that can affect the function of heart without developing a contraction, such as nonexcitatory cardiac contractility modulation (CCM) [49]. Recently, Butter et al. [50] have studied whether CCM-induced reverse molecular remodeling in myocardium of a group of HF patients. Endomyocardial biopsies were obtained at baseline and 3 and 6 months thereafter. The CCM signals were delivered in random order, on for 3 months and off for 3 months. Messenger ribonucleic acid expression was analyzed by investigators blinded to the treatment sequence. Expression of Atrial (ANP)-and B-type natriuretic peptides (BNP) and α-myosin heavy chain (MHC), the sarcoplasmic reticulum genes SERCA-2a, phospholamban and ryanodine receptors, and the stretch response genes p38 mitogen activated protein kinase and p21 Ras were measured using reverse transcription-polymerase chain reaction (RT-PCR) and bands quantified in densitometric units. The 3-month therapy off phase was associated with an increased expression of natriuretic peptides, p38 mitogen activated protein kinase, and p21 Ras and decreased expression of α-MHC, SERCA-2a, phospholamban, and ryanodine receptors. In contrast, the 3-month on therapy phase resulted in a decreased expression of ANP and BNP natriuretic peptides, p38 mitogen activated protein kinase, and p21 Ras and increased expression of α-MHC, SERCA-2a, phospholamban, and ryanodine receptors. Taken together, these findings showed that CCM signal treatment reverses the cardiac maladaptive fetal gene program and normalizes expression of key sarcoplasmic reticulum Ca^{2+} cycling and stretch response genes. These changes may contribute to the clinical effects of CCM.

It is safe to predict that further development of microengineering and sensor technologies will continue because the threshold of implanting a microprocessor that senses abnormal heart function and delivers therapy has already been crossed; with electrons now, and likely with drugs in the near future [51].

Modeling Systems Approaches

A major challenge facing cardiovascular medicine is how to translate the wealth of reductionist detail about molecules, cells and tissues into a real understanding of how these systems function in health and are perturbed in the disease processes. There is an increasing interest in integrating the large comprehensive and ever-growing databases containing genomic, proteomic, biochemical, anatomical, and physiological information that can be searched and retrieved via the Internet to further understand the functioning of the heart in health and disease. Eventually, a model of cardiac function at the genetic, molecular, and physiological levels will be available that may allow predictions about the potential interventions to be made. It is anticipated that such simulated modeling would also highlight the gaps in our knowledge and elicit new perspectives in how to fill them [52].

On a limited scale, early work on this type of integrative approach (prior to the acquisition of much of the proteomic/genomic/molecular data) has employed data on ion concentration and metabolite levels during cardiac ischemia to construct a simulated computer model that integrates cardiac energetics with electrophysiological changes (a novel approach to study myocardial ischemia). This model proved to be informative in predicting the effects of specific therapeutic interventions [53]. Furthermore, this model aided the identification of electrophysiological effects of therapeutic interventions such as Na^+–H^+ block, and suggested that it may be an effective strategy to control cardiac dysrhythmias during calcium overload, by regulating sodium–calcium exchange. In addition to myocardial ischemia, other types of cardiovascular disorders that so far have been "modeled" using this type of approach include cardiac contractile disorders [54–56].

The construction of these models, together with the array of data discussed earlier, requires an extensive and sophisticated mathematical and computer algorithmic treatment [57]. Its undertaking is clearly a multidisciplinary approach involving mathematics, computer skills, molecular and cell biology, genetics, physiology, and anatomy. A central premise of this recapitulates the maxim of the molecular biologist Sydney Brenner that genes can only specify the properties of the proteins they code for, and any integrative properties of the system must be "computed" by their interactions.

It is important to keep in mind that these models underscore that much more critical post-genomic data remain to be obtained, including the identification of gene–environmental factors and protein–protein interactions, which appear to underlie many phenotypic changes and signaling events in the cardiomyocyte. Biomolecular interactions revealed by proteomic information will be important for unraveling metabolic and signaling pathways operating in the cell, and in particular in response to disease and injury. The identification of functional interactions between signaling pathways and genetic networks will also be of key interest, as they will provide a window into regulation of the coordinate expression of functional groups of genes, with a few key pathways switching between alternative cell fates. Also, underlying these models is the important recognition that the heart and vascular system are dynamic and more than just electrical circuitry or mechanical pumps, and they have the ability to grow and remodel in response to changing environments, partly determined by genes and partly by their physical environment [58]. In the near future, a system approach may need to be applied to metabolic events occurring in the mitochondria of the failing heart, as well as to events occurring in both the aging heart and in early development.

Translation of Findings from the Bench into Clinical Application

In this section, we briefly discuss current and future methods involving the translation of the increasing myriad of physiological, genetic, molecular, biochemical, and cellular findings (mostly derived from preclinical studies), into an effective cardiovascular medicine for the twenty-first century.

Postgenomic biology has not only substantially increased our understanding of the mechanisms underlying CVD (as well as the events of aging), but has also provided an armamentarium of new approaches, which are gradually being adapted to clinical medicine and over the next decade should provide both improved diagnostic tools as well as gene and cell-based therapies. The biological information derived from increasing human-based studies may eventually be used in the context of an enhanced pharmacogenetic/genomic medicine, allowing a more individually tailored gauging of genetic susceptibility, environmental stresses, toxic insults, and even dietary requirements that might be required or avoided, and in addition delineating what could be the most effective treatment regimens for specific CVDs.

A primary step in the realization of this vision of postgenomic cardiovascular medicine is further acquisition of genetic data from human studies. The continued development of methodologies for increasingly powerful haplotype and SNP mapping throughout the human genome needs to be more widely examined throughout the general population. Data gathered from these genotyping techniques may be helpful in enhancing the identification of candidate genes (both known and novel loci), and in testing their association with HF and specific targeted CVD disorders. Pharmacogenetic analysis has recently allowed the identification of genetic factors that increase susceptibility to dysrhythmias and MI [59, 60]. Moreover, the underlying responsiveness to specific drug therapies targeting CVDs have been revealed by pharmacogenomic studies of statin responsiveness [61]. Critical factors that should also be stressed include the involvement and interest of the physician and a better educated lay public for understanding the significant ramifications of gathering as well as applying this information.

Unfortunately, despite the clear inroads made with respect to both identification of specific genes involvement in CVDs and cardioprotective treatments (both employing pharmacological and non-pharmacological approaches), as reported in numerous animal studies, few of these studies have been translated into human clinical practice. Some of the difficulties arise from the nature of the preclinical studies themselves; these are often conducted with models that do not approximate the human model (e.g., isolated cell/heart studies, variable levels of ischemia) and generally with young healthy animals and are primarily focused on illustrating/understanding the molecular and cellular mechanisms of injury and protection, rather than establishing the potential clinical efficacy of the interventions tested [62]. In addition, end-points in human studies are more difficult to precise measure and are often indirectly compared to animal studies, in which the duration of ischemia and size of infarct can be controlled, and appear to be subject to a myriad of confounding factors (e.g., concurrent use of medications, environmental stressors). For example, problems inherent in measuring patient infarct size may be alleviated by the use of novel imaging techniques including delayed contrast-enhanced MRI which provide higher resolution, highly quantitative, and noninvasive measures of infarct size in the clinical setting [63–65].

Awareness that large clinical trials need to be more targeted while inclusive of more perspectives in their design is increasing. A key suggestion that has been recently offered involves the increased use of patient subgroups. For instance, the rational selection of patient subgroups most likely to benefit from such cardioprotective therapies should enable the design of adequately powered studies with relatively small number of patients. However, there is an uncertainty as to which subgroups of patients will have postoperative complications. This is an important problem that may hinder further studies of cardioprotection.

The selection of drugs for specific subgroups of patients has also been proposed in other areas of medicine. Over half of withdrawn drugs (ranging from antihistamines, anticancer compounds, antiemetics, antibiotics, to antimigraine drugs) mandated by the FDA since 1998 has been attributable to cardiac side effects, most of them dysrhythmias [66]. This costly problem is largely attributable to the high degree of receptivity of one of the channel proteins, I_{Kr}, on which cardiac repolarization depends. A heart that is already prone to dysrhythmia, because of slowed conduction/and or failed repolarization, as a consequence of genetic or disease disturbance of sodium, or other channels and transporters, may therefore be tipped over into a fatal state by even a modest amount of I_{Kr} block. The advent of gene array technologies and proteomic analyses may be highly useful, not only in the identification of high-risk patients who are most likely to benefit by a specific treatment, but also in the identification of patients who are genetically prone to dysrhythmias. If these goals can be achieved, the benefits should be very significant.

Another relevant sub-group type analysis that may arise from a concerted pharmacogenetic analysis also includes the potential role of ethnicity, race, and gender. Evidence of racial/ethnic differences in CVD has been widely recognized for some time. For instance, the cause of HF is predominantly ischemic disease in nonblacks, but is related primarily to hypertension, which tends to be both more frequent and severe in blacks [67]; blacks appear to be stroke-prone, but relatively protected from coronary heart disease [68, 69]. In clinical trials, ethnic differences in the antihypertensive responses to β-blockers and ACE inhibitors, as therapeutic agents, have been reported; blacks exhibit somewhat reduced blood pressure responses to monotherapy with β-blockers and ACE inhibitors when compared to diuretics [70]. Recently, retrospective analyses of HF trials have suggested differences in the response to ACE inhibitors (e.g., enalapril) [68, 71]. Trials with the β-blocker carvedilol, when retrospectively reanalyzed by ethnicity, did not reveal differences in the benefit between blacks and whites [72]. However, in the BEST trial conducted with a diverse group of patients with NYHA class III and IV HF, treatment with the β-blocker bucindolol provided a significant increase in survival benefit in non-

black patients [73]. On the other hand, clinical studies have demonstrated that treatment with the NO donor isosorbide dinitrate, in combination with the antioxidant hydralazine when compared with placebo or prazosin conferred a survival advantage for black but not for white subjects [74]. The African-American Heart Failure Trial (A-HeFT), a randomized, placebo-controlled, double-blind trial involving 1,050 black patients with NYHA class III and IV HF confirmed the finding that a fixed dose of isosorbide dinitrate plus hydralazine, in addition to standard therapy for HF including neurohormonal blockers was efficacious and increased the survival of black patients with advanced HF [75, 76].

It remains to be seen whether a discrete DNA difference might underlie these different phenotypic responses to treatment. It also has been argued that the treatment of HF in blacks, which has a hypertensive component, might be more effective in targeting that pathology. Interestingly, the benefit of the combined isosorbide dinitrate and hydralazine in the treatment of HF has not been replicated by other antihypertensive medications. While the interpretation of these findings and their implications have been hotly debated, a majority of clinicians agree that the inclusion of diverse groups in significant numbers (for subgroup analysis) should be an intrinsic part of future clinical trials.

Diagnostic Challenges and Genetic Counseling

While the application of postgenomic technology in improving HF diagnosis and prognostication has been discussed previously, its use is of particular interest in prenatal diagnosis, and in preimplantation genetic diagnosis (PGD). The use of prenatal testing with DNA markers has been successful in identifying cases of X-linked cardiomyopathy (due to dystrophin mutations) [77], severe neonatal long QT syndrome (HERG mutations) [78], specific mutations associated with HCM [79, 80], and in Marfan syndrome (elastin mutations) [81]. It appears to be of a greater benefit when a specific mutation is suspected (due to family history), and can be directly screened. Specific mtDNA mutations leading to Leigh disease [82, 83], and respiratory deficiencies [84, 85] have been screened prenatally, in some cases using chorionic villi as the source of the genetic material, and in other cases with amniotic fluid [85, 86]. Analysis of mutant loads of the nt8993 mutations in fetal and adult tissues confirms that there is no substantial tissue variation, and suggested that the mutant load in a prenatal sample will represent the mutant load in other fetal tissues; the 8993 mutations show a strong correlation between mutant load and symptom severity, and between maternal blood mutant load and risk of a severe outcome [87].

As an adjunct to in vitro fertilization (IVF) technology, the application of PGD will be increasingly available to prevent the transmission of devastating diseases from affected parents to their children. Although this technique has not yet received widespread attention, the detection of mutant alleles of the TBX5 transcription factor resulting in Holt–Oram syndrome (HOS), which presents with multiple malformations, including congenital heart defect, has allowed the successful identification of fertilized eggs affected by HOS for potential embryo selection. Using molecular genotyping techniques, blastocysts containing wildtype genotypes were distinguishable from those containing mutant alleles, and their transfer to the mother resulted in the delivery of a normal child [88].

The use of transmitochondrial oocytes in human studies has a limited but controversial history. Ooplasmic transplantation has been reported in several studies in conjunction with IVF [89, 90]. The addition of a small amount of injected ooplasm, derived from fertile donor oocytes, into developmentally compromised oocytes from patients with recurrent preimplantation failure was reported to enhance embryo viability and led to the birth of 15 children. The mtDNA from the donor as well as the recipient cell mtDNA were found to be present in the blood of the child resulting from the transplanted oocyte at 1 year of age. Excluding the numerous ethical considerations provoked by this human germ-line genetic modification (going somewhat beyond screening for the wildtype genotype), several concerns have been raised by these studies, including the potential for long-term harm in chromosomal segregation and aberrant division (predicted by similar studies conducted in lower organisms), and negative epigenetic influences of foreign cytoplasm, as have been demonstrated in numerous studies of cytoplasmic transfer in mice [91]. In fact, two of the 15 pregnancies resulted in chromosomal abnormalities, including Turner syndrome. Moreover, the long-term deleterious influence of heteroplasmic mtDNA has also been considered an additional problem of this technique [92, 93]. If we are to fully appreciate the potential outcomes associated with embryo manipulation, extensive investigations with animal models that incorporate genetic, biochemical, and physiological analyses are mandated. Also, these investigations should be accompanied by careful clinical monitoring to demonstrate the suitability of these techniques for human use.

New and Future Therapeutic Options in Cardiovascular Medicine; Postgenomic Contributions

Advances in postgenomic cardiology may possibly make a brighter future for new HF therapies that offer greater specificity and breadth, some of which are already coming to frui-

tion. Molecular genetic analysis has substantially improved our understanding of the structure and functioning of the heart, both in early development and in aging, and has opened the door to further unraveling the order of molecular/cellular events and the principal molecules involved in both normal and malformed/dysfunctional hearts. Information derived from transgenic models has been instrumental in defining numerous therapeutic targets in the signaling pathways, how heart and cardiovascular system respond to stresses and insults, the elucidation of both apoptotic and survival/proliferative pathways affecting cardiomyocyte growth, oxidative stress, hypertrophy, aging and cell death, and in defining metabolic pathways essential for energy transduction, which is necessary for contractile function and electrical excitability. Animal models with specific gene dysfunction have been highly informative in defining the roles that specific contractile and ion channel proteins play in both, the normal and diseased heart. Some of this information has been very important in the design of pharmacological strategies to develop novel targets in the treatment of CVDs, ranging from HF to stroke, MI, and acute and chronic inflammatory diseases [94]. Therapies aimed at metabolic remodeling may be developed to effectively complement the treatment of myocardial ischemia, HF, the more obvious metabolic-based CVDs (i.e., metabolic syndrome), as well as underlying therapies such as calorie restriction aimed at modulating overall longevity and the aging processes [95–97].

The potential of combining genetic and cell engineering has been demonstrated in a number of animal models and in limited clinical studies, and this may be a useful adjunct in repairing the "broken" heart and damaged vessels, and in enhancing the heart's regenerative potential. Later in this chapter, we briefly review new developments in gene therapy, cell-based therapy, and in tissue re-engineering, and we discuss the possible future applications.

Bioengineering

The use of both embryonic and adult stem cells offers an exciting platform for repairing the damaged, failing heart. Direct transplantation of isolated myoblasts or bone marrow mononuclear cells, and recruitment of stem cells from bone marrow by cytokine administration (e.g., G-CSF) have already been clinically performed. Nevertheless, numerous and important unanswered questions have been raised concerning stem cell biology, including their differentiation process, the heterogeneity within stem cell populations, what effects are due to recruitment and activation of endogenous stem cell populations as compared to circulating stem cells originating in bone marrow (such as recently described in cardiac cells), what effects are due to cytokines and angiogenesis, and which factors impact in their differentiation and homing properties.

There is a considerable interest in combining the use and fabrication of biopolymers as a scaffolding matrix for rebuilding the damaged cardiac tissue with proliferating cells [98]. The importance of re-engineering the cardiac milieu so that stem cell can effectively adhere and be better functionally incorporated into the injured myocardium has been increasingly recognized. Cardiac tissue engineering research has also been centered on fabricating 3-D cardiac grafts and biodegradable scaffolds as alternatives of extracellular matrix [99]. Other alternatives include the use of beating myocardial tissue by layering cell sheets, which are harvested from cultured cells grafted with temperature-responsive polymer [100]. The transplantation of cardiomyocyte cell sheets in the treatment of HF, which eliminates the need for a donor, has reached the stage of preclinical testing. It is worth noting that skeletal myoblasts have been grown on polymer sheets in culture, and implanted into coronary artery-ligated rat hearts. This resulted in the repair of the damaged myocardium with markedly reduced fibrosis (compared with skeletal myoblast cell injection), and prevention of remodeling in association with a recruitment of hematopoietic stem cells through the release of stromal-derived factor 1, and other growth factors, suggesting their potential use in the treatment of patients with severe HF [101]. In addition, it is possible that the transplant-associated dysrhythmias, occurring with skeletal myoblasts in the heart (likely caused by the absence of gap junctions), might be eliminated by the ex vivo genetic modification of the myoblasts containing expression of the gap junction protein connexin 43 [102]. This antidysrhythmic engineering (achieved thus far only in cells in culture) may increase the safety (and perhaps the efficacy) of myoblast transplantation in patients.

Particular interest has been centered on the reengineering of heart valves [99]. Utilizing collagen scaffolds produced by a novel process termed rapid prototyping, valve interstitial cells isolated from three human aortic valves seeded on the scaffolds and cultured for up to 4 weeks remained viable and proliferating; an important step in the tissue engineering of an aortic valve. Repopulation of a scaffold of a decellularized valve matrix (usually porcine) in vitro with stem cells, in particular mesenchymal stem cells, has also been an area of intensive investigation [103–105]. While this approach has not yet been proved successful in neither animal models nor human clinical testing [105], conditions for the optimization of cell seeding and repopulation using either valve interstitial cells [106] or mesenchymal cells have recently been optimized. Creation of autologous semilunar heart valves in vitro with mesenchymal stem cells, and a biodegradable scaffold, has been reported following their implantation under cardiopulmo-nary bypass into the pulmonary valve position of the sheep. These valves underwent extensive remodeling in vivo, resembling the native heart valves, and functioned satisfactorily for periods of >4 months [107].

Targeting various regions of the heart associated with specific function has become another interesting approach. This has been focused on the possibility of grafting pacemaking cells, either derived from differentiating human embryonic stem cells, or engineered from mesenchymal stem cells into the myocardium [108]. Moreover, an initial proof that the use of gene therapy may create a biological pacemaker was provided by Miake et al. using an adenoviral gene transfer approach in guinea pig hearts [109]. By modifying the Kir2.1 gene encoding the inward rectifying potassium current I_{K1} (which pacemaker cells lack) and mutating it (i.e., obtaining a dominant-negative allele) to make a dysfunctional channel, a subset of transfected ventricular myocytes were converted to cells with pacemaker activity. A limitation of these studies was that the induced automaticity was threefold slower than normal, and genetic suppression of I_{K1} does not provide any direct mean to modulate the induced rhythm. In contrast, Xue et al. found that gene transfer of an engineered HCN1 construct to quiescent adult guinea pig ventricular cardiomyocytes can induce pacing with a normal firing rate [110]. Previous studies have reported that plasmids harboring the human β_2-adrenergic receptor injected into the right atria of Yorkshire pig hearts significantly enhanced porcine cardiac chronotropy upregulating the heart rate by 50% [111]. Other studies have found that transient overexpression of the channel protein HCN2 in the left atrium or bundle-branch system (in a canine model) could generate an ectopic biological pacemaker [112, 113]. This construct employed an adenoviral vector and vagal suppression was required to observe the effect. Moreover, transplanted stem cells (either MSCs or hESCs) can serve as platforms for the delivery of these pacemaker-conferring genes [110, 114]. In addition, it has been reported that hESC-derived cardiomyocytes (generated in vitro using the embryoid body differentiating system), when introduced into swine hearts with complete AV block, stably integrated, restored myocardial electromechanical properties acting as a rate-responsive biological pacemaker [115].

Vessel Engineering

It is well recognized that therapeutic angiogenesis/vasculogenesis can be achieved by supplementation of a variety of growth factors, or transplantation of vascular progenitor cells. This approach fosters the formation of arterial collaterals and promotes the regeneration of damaged tissues and therefore may be useful in treating ischemia [116, 117]. While angiogenic factors can be delivered in the form of recombinant proteins or by gene transfer using viral vectors, novel nonviral methods including liposomes, naked plasmid vectors, or cell-mediated gene transfer are promising alternatives with a safer profile [118–120]. Although growth factors offer distinct advantages in terms of efficacy, a number of approaches featuring the combination of several growth factors with cell transplantation are currently being explored both to initiate growth and stabilize vessels. Some angiogenic factors not only stimulate the growth of arterioles and capillaries, but also inhibit vascular destabilization triggered by metabolic and oxidative stress. Endothelial progenitor cells (EPCs) for the treatment of peripheral or myocardial ischemia can be transplanted either without any preliminary conditioning or after ex vivo genetic manipulation [121, 122]. Also, delivery of genetically modified autologous progenitor cells eliminates the drawback of immune response against viral vectors.

The formation of a microvascular network can be achieved by promoting vasculogenesis in situ, employing seeding vascular endothelial cells within a biopolymeric scaffolding construct; the inclusion of human smooth muscle cells seeded with EPC-derived endothelial cells can form capillary-like microvessel structures throughout the scaffold [123].

Genetic Engineering

A detailed discussion on gene therapy has been presented in Chap. 21. At this time, it is suffice to say that genetic engineering techniques besides its success in the development of new experimental mice models useful for research have begun to find some successes in diverse applications including the production of synthetic human insulin and erythropoietin in hamster ovary cells. In cardiovascular medicine, modification and introduction of specific genes could be successfully used to correct a number of specific myocardial defects resulting in cardiac dysfunction. Still, the limiting factor in clinical cardiology application of gene therapy is the timely development of safe and effective vectors/carriers for the transgene and their clinical testing.

Bioinformatics/Computational Biology in HF

To be useful, it is clear that the extensive amount of information coming from genomics, proteomics, and other molecular research technologies need to be integrated and standardized. This information will allow new interpretations and theories to be experimentally and clinically tested. The application of information technology, or *Bioinformatics*, to the field of

molecular cardiovascular biology will allow the creation and maintenance of database storing information coming from transcriptomics, miRNA, and protein level and sequences that will allow the profiling and identification of causal genes, and protein expression in HF. The actual process of analyzing and interpreting data is referred to as *computational biology*. Development of this type of database involved not only design issues, but the development of complex interfaces whereby researchers could both access the existing data as well as submit new or revised data. Bioinformatics has evolved in such a way that the most pressing task now involves the analysis and interpretation of various types of data, including nucleotide and amino acid sequences, protein domains, and protein structures.

What sets bioinformatics apart from other approaches is its focus on developing and applying computationally intensive techniques (e.g., data mining and machine learning algorithms). Major research in this field is being focused on sequence alignment, gene finding, genome assembly, protein structure alignment, protein structure prediction, prediction of gene expression and protein–protein interactions, and the modeling of evolution. It is evident that in order to understand how cardiomyocytes structure, function, and proliferation are altered in HF, the collected biological data must be combined to form a comprehensive picture. By doing so, new insights into the etiology, diagnostic and prognostication of HF, as well as new therapies for HF might be attained.

Conclusion

With the completion of the Human Genome Project, the likely identification of novel genes involved in HF will serve as an important foundation for our understanding of how specific gene defects generate the different HF phenotypes. Bioinformatic methods can be employed to search existing databases with the routine use of reverse genetics techniques, allowing subsequent cloning of novel genes/cDNAs of interest followed by the characterization of spatial-temporal patterns of specific gene expression. Moreover, both transcriptomic and proteomic methodologies can be used to further delineate the functions of the gene products, defining their precise role in pathogenesis, elucidating their interaction with other proteins in the subcellular pathways and potentially enabling their application as clinical markers of HF.

A critical area of research is the identification of molecular regulators that control cardiomyocyte proliferation in the human heart. Understanding the molecular basis of cardiomyocyte proliferation could greatly impact on our clinical attempts to repair the failing heart. Mechanism of cell growth regulation is being investigated by careful comparison of comprehensive gene expression profiles of adult, embryonic and post-natal myocytes, as well as by the generation of myocyte cell culture lines with the capacity to respond to proliferative inducers. Cellular transplantation is an alternative mechanism to augment myocyte number in the diseased, damaged heart. However, further research efforts will be necessary to define the optimal conditions necessary for cardiomyocyte differentiation and proliferation, and for the fully functional integration of stem cells in the myocardium, as well as to investigate the ability of transplanted stem cells to repair defects in the failing heart. It is of paramount significance to learn whether HF secondary to myocardial ischemia or DCM, myocardial infarct in adults, or children with Kawasaki disease and myocardial damage or with ARVD, can be treated with stem cell transplantation.

Research focusing on the basic science of stem cells, including isolation of factors involved in the acceleration of specific cell type differentiation, migration, homing and proliferation, in vitro as well as in vivo, and their responses to oxidative stress, apoptosis and injury may accelerate their potential use in clinical transplantation, and also as a new treatment modality of HF and other cardiovascular pathologies. Nonetheless, many of the methodologies discussed in this volume, such as gene profiling, proteomics, genetic analysis, development of relevant animal and cellular models, proteomics and pharmacogenomics, while promising at this times they all are relatively new approaches and still there is a good deal to be learned. This increasing armamentarium could contribute greatly to further understanding the role of basic cellular processes and their capacity for adaptation, including improving the understanding of organelle biology, metabolic modulation, DNA and protein damage and apoptosis, and their role as markers and causative factors in HF. In addition, findings from these basic studies and the use of integrative system biology methods will increase our knowledge of the critical interactions between multiple organ systems and their cross talk through hormonal and inflammatory/immune signaling, which have only recently been found to play a significant role in cardiovascular diseases. Furthermore, pharmacogenetics and pharmacogenomics may provide the necessary tools to realize the development of a more effective and individualized cardiovascular medicine.

Insights into the cardiovascular consequences of abnormal gene function and expression should ultimately impact on the development of targeted therapeutic strategies and disease management, and it will likely replace the less effective treatment modalities directed solely at rectifying structural cardiac defects and temporal improvement of function. With further progress in cell engineering, we will hopefully see the end of the complex HF syndrome, and other cardiovascular pathologies that so dramatically weaken human life and bankrupt the health care system all over the world. Finally, we are witnessing the transition from the Cardiology of the past to the study of systems biology, the constructive cycle of computational model building, and experimental verification capable to provide the necessary input to achieve new and exciting discoveries and also finding a renewing hope.

Summary

- Cardiac biomarkers widely used for diagnosis of MI include troponin I and T, CK-MB, and myoglobin. Combined use of biomarkers (i.e., multimarkers) increases the probability of correct diagnosis.
- While other markers appear to be better suited for detecting early myocardial ischemia and infarction, including unbound free fatty acids and ischemia-modified albumin, these are not widely tested or employed.
- Biomarkers of inflammation (e.g., CRP, cytokines, MCP) and hemodynamic function (BNP, N-T proBNP) are important prognostic indicators of future cardiovascular risk in both healthy individuals and in patients with acute coronary syndrome (ACS). BNP is also an excellent diagnostic marker of HF.
- Proteomic and gene profiling techniques are critical techniques that can be used in the identification of novel biomarkers. Also proteomic techniques such as mass spectroscopy and protein microarrays offer improved methods for rapid and highly accurate screening of multiple markers.
- Mitochondrial-based defects have been identified in a variety of CVDs because of the primary role of mitochondria in generating metabolic energy, as well as its role in oxidative stress signaling and ROS generation, and in the early events of apoptotic cell death.
- Mitochondria also play a pivotal role in myocardial ischemia, the development of cardioprotective responses, and cardiac aging.
- At present, therapies for mitochondrial-based diseases are limited, and they involve primarily metabolic bypasses of specific defects and antioxidant treatment (i.e., coenzyme Q_{10}).
- Direct genetic modulation of mitochondria involves novel gene therapeutic approaches since those previously used for nuclear gene therapy have not been successful.
- A variety of lipophilic carriers for bringing molecules into the mitochondria (modified nucleic acids, proteins, drugs, inhibitors and antioxidants) are being developed. Targeting mitochondria apoptotic function will likely involve new pharmacological development.
- Noninvasive diagnostic methods to detect mitochondrial defects in the cardiovascular system are presently being developed including magnetic resonance spectroscopy.
- Genetic screening has been employed to clinically detect prenatal defects in patients with congenital heart disease,

cardiac dysrhythmias, HCM, and Marfan syndrome. Similar tests will likely be used in preimplantation genetic diagnosis in association with IVF procedures.

- The use of gene therapy to target specific genetic defects or supplement deficiencies has an enormous potential with many possible useful applications; however, we are still awaiting the development of safe, effective, and easily testable vector systems.

- Cardiac targeted therapies may involve the direct modulation of myocardial cells with transfected genes or injected gene products, or the transplantation of cells or groups of cells (cell sheets).

- Cell-based therapies will likely play a critical role in the future since a number of cell types have shown the ability to be recruited into damaged myocardium with potentially beneficial results. These cells include several types of stem cells (either embryonic or adult), neonatal cardiomyocytes, and skeletal myocytes.

- Both stem cell biology and the cardiac milieu optimal for their homing, integration, and long-term survival need to be better characterized. In addition to cardiac transplantation, both stem cells and a combination of angiogenic factors can be utilized in therapeutic angiogenesis with its potential application in myocardial ischemia.

- A variety of biomaterials have been employed to simulate the cardiac environment, and they have been useful in tissue re-engineering of valves (e.g., aortic) and vessel remodeling.

- The application of information technology, or *Bioinformatics*, to the field of molecular cardiovascular biology will allow the creation and maintenance of database storing information coming from transcriptomics, miRNA and protein level and sequences that will allow the profiling and identification of causal genes, and protein expression in HF.

- What sets bioinformatics apart from other approaches is its focus on developing and applying computationally intensive techniques (e.g., data mining and machine learning algorithms).

- We are witnessing the transition from conventional cardiology practice to the study of systems biology, computational model building, and experimental verification capable to provide the necessary input to achieve new and exciting discoveries.

References

1. Sugden PH, Clerk A (1998) "Stress-responsive" mitogen-activated protein kinases (c-Jun N-terminal kinases and p38 mitogen-activated protein kinases) in the myocardium. Circ Res 83:345–352

2. McKinsey TA, Olson EN (2005) Toward transcriptional therapies for the failing heart: chemical screens to modulate genes. Clin Invest 115:538–546

3. Nanni L, Romualdi C, Maseri A, Lanfranchi G (2006) Differential gene expression profiling in genetic and multifactorial cardiovascular diseases. J Mol Cell Cardiol 41:934–948

4. Mani K, Kitsis RN (2003) Myocyte apoptosis: programming ventricular remodeling. J Am Coll Cardiol 41:761–764

5. Park M, Shen YT, Gaussin V, Heyndrickx GR, Bartunek J, Resuello RG, Natividad FF, Kitsis RN, Vatner DE, Vatner SF (2009) Apoptosis predominates in non-myocytes in heart failure. Am J Physiol Heart Circ Physiol 297:H785–H791

6. Dzimiri N (1999) Regulation of beta-adrenoceptor signaling in cardiac function and disease. Pharmacol Rev 51:465–501

7. Maisel AS, Bhalla V, Brunwald E (2005) Cardiac biomarkers; a contemporary status report. Nature 3:24–34

8. Azzazy HM, Pelsers MM, Christenson RH (2006) Unbound free fatty acids and heart-type fatty acid-binding protein: diagnostic assays and clinical applications. Clin Chem 52:19–29

9. Pelsers MM, Hermens WT, Glatz JF (2005) Fatty acid-binding proteins as plasma markers of tissue injury. Clin Chim Acta 352:15–35

10. Goto T, Takase H, Toriyama T, Sugiura T, Sato K, Ueda R, Dohi Y (2003) Circulating concentrations of cardiac proteins indicate the severity of congestive heart failure. Heart 89:1303–1307

11. Ishii J, Ozaki Y, Lu J et al (2005) Prognostic value of serum concentration of heart-type fatty acid-binding protein relative to cardiac troponin T on admission in the early hours of acute coronary syndrome. Clin Chem 51:1397–1404

12. Niizeki T, Takeishi Y, Arimoto T et al (2005) Serum heart-type fatty acid binding protein predicts cardiac events in elderly patients with chronic heart failure. J Cardiol 46:9–15

13. Pop D, Zdrenghea D, Procociuc LM, Popal A (2007) Gene polymorphism of angiotensin-converting enzyme and angiotensin II type 1 receptor in patients with congestive heart failure. Rom J Intern Med 45:349–354

14. Sekuri C, Cam FS, Ercan E, Tengiz I, Sagcan A, Eser E, Berdeli A, Akin M (2005) Renin-angiotensin system gene polymorphisms and premature coronary heart disease. J Renin Angiotensin Aldosterone Syst 6:38–42

15. Hama N, Itoh H, Shirakami G et al (1995) Rapid ventricular induction of brain natriuretic peptide gene expression in experimental acute myocardial infarction. Circulation 92:1558–1564

16. van Kimmenade RR, Januzzi JL Jr, Ellinor PT et al (2006) Utility of amino-terminal pro-brain natriuretic peptide, galectin-3, and apelin for the evaluation of patients with acute heart failure. J Am Coll Cardiol 48:1217–1224

17. Omland T, Drazner MH, Uehland T, Abedin M, Murphy SA, Aukrust P et al (2007) Plasma osteoprotegerin levels in the general population: relation to indices of left ventricular structure and function. Hypertension 49:1392–1398

18. Ueland T, Jemtland R, Godang K, Kjekshus J, Hognestad A, Omland T et al (2004) Prognostic value of osteoprotegerin in heart failure after acute myocardial infarction. J Am Coll Cardiol 44:1970–1976

19. Pieroni M, Corti A, Tota B, Curnis F, Angelone T, Colombo B et al (2007) Myocardial production of chromogranin A in human heart: a new regulatory peptide of cardiac function. Eur Heart J 28:1117–1127

20. Stanley BA, Gundry RL, Cotter RJ, Van Eyk JE (2004) Heart disease, clinical proteomics and mass spectrometry. Dis Markers 20:167–178

21. Anderson L (2005) Candidate-based proteomics in the search for biomarkers of cardiovascular disease. J Physiol 563:23–60

22. Kittleson MM, Hare JM (2005) Molecular signature analysis: using the myocardial transcriptome as a biomarker in cardiovascular disease. Trends Cardiovasc Med 15:130–138

23. Marin-Garcia J, Goldenthal MJ (2002) Understanding the impact of mitochondrial defects in cardiovascular disease: a review. J Card Fail 8:347–361

24. Marin-Garcia J, Goldenthal MJ (2004) Mitochondria play a critical role in cardioprotection. J Card Fail 10:55–66

25. Marin-Garcia J, Goldenthal MJ, Moe GW (2001) Mitochondrial pathology in cardiac failure. Cardiovasc Res 49:17–26

26. McGregor A, Temperley R, Chrzanowska-Lightowlers ZM, Lightowlers RN (2001) Absence of expression from RNA internalised into electroporated mammalian mitochondria. Mol Genet Genomics 265:721–729

27. Johnston SA, Anziano PQ, Shark K, Sanford JC, Butow RA (1988) Mitochondrial transformation in yeast by bombardment with microprojectiles. Science 240:1538–1541

28. Chinnery PF, Taylor RW, Diekert K, Lill R, Turnbull DM, Lightowlers RN (1999) Peptide nucleic acid delivery to human mitochondria. Gene Ther 6:1919–1928

29. Taylor RW, Chinnery PF, Turnbull DM, Lightowlers RN (1997) Selective inhibition of mutant human mitochondrial DNA replication in vitro by peptide nucleic acids. Nat Genet 15:212–215

30. Muratovska A, Lightowlers RN, Taylor RW, Turnbull DM, Smith RA, Wilce JA, Martin SW, Murphy MP (2001) Targeting peptide nucleic acid (PNA) oligomers to mitochondria within cells by conjugation to lipophilic cations: implications for mitochondrial DNA replication, expression and disease. Nucleic Acids Res 29:1852–1863

31. Geromel V, Cao A, Briane D, Vassy J, Rotig A, Rustin P, Coudert R, Rigaut JP, Munnich A, Taillandier E (2001) Mitochondria transfection by oligonucleotides containing a signal peptide and vectorized by cationic liposomes. Antisense Nucleic Acid Drug Dev 11:175–180

32. Flierl A, Jackson C, Cottrell B, Murdock D, Seibel P, Wallace DC (2003) Targeted delivery of DNA to the mitochondrial compartment via import sequence-conjugated peptide nucleic acid. Mol Ther 7:550–557

33. Weissig V, Lasch J, Erdos G, Meyer HW, Rowe TC, Hughes J (1998) DQAsomes: a novel potential drug and gene delivery system made from Dequalinium. Pharm Res 15:334–337

34. D'Souza GG, Rammohan R, Cheng SM, Torchilin VP, Weissig V (2003) DQAsome-mediated delivery of plasmid DNA toward mitochondria in living cells. J Control Release 92:189–197

35. Weissig V, Cheng SM, D'Souza GG (2004) Mitochondrial pharmaceutics. Mitochondrion 3:229–244

36. Kelso GF, Porteous CM, Coulter CV, Hughes G, Porteous WK, Ledgerwood EC, Smith RA, Murphy MP (2001) Selective targeting of a redox-active ubiquinone to mitochondria within cells: antioxidant and antiapoptotic properties. J Biol Chem 276:4588–4596

37. Smith RA, Porteous CM, Gane AM, Murphy MP (2003) Delivery of bioactive molecules to mitochondria in vivo. Proc Natl Acad Sci USA 100:5407–5412

38. Adlam VJ, Harrison JC, Porteous CM, James AM, Smith RA, Murphy MP, Sammut IA (2005) Targeting an antioxidant to mitochondria decreases cardiac ischemia-reperfusion injury. FASEB J 19:1088–1095

39. Zhao K, Zhao GM, Wu D, Soong Y, Birk AV, Schiller PW, Szeto HH (2004) Cell-permeable peptide antioxidants targeted to inner mitochondrial membrane inhibit mitochondrial swelling, oxidative cell death and reperfusion injury. J Biol Chem 279:34682–34690

40. McDonnell MT, Schaefer AM, Blakely EL, McFarland R, Chinnery PF, Turnbull DM, Taylor RW (2004) Noninvasive diagnosis of the 3243A > G mitochondrial DNA mutation using urinary epithelial cells. Eur J Hum Genet 12:778–781

41. Mattei JP, Bendahan D, Cozzone P (2004) P-31 magnetic resonance spectroscopy. A tool for diagnostic purposes and pathophysiological insights in muscle diseases. Reumatismo 56:9–14

42. Jucker BM, Dufour S, Ren J, Cao X, Previs SF, Underhill B, Cadman KS, Shulman GI (2000) Assessment of mitochondrial energy coupling in vivo by 13C/31P NMR. Proc Natl Acad Sci USA 97:6880–6884

43. Lebon V, Dufour S, Petersen KF, Ren J, Jucker BM, Slezak LA, Cline GW, Rothman DL, Shulman GI (2001) Effect of triiodothyronine on mitochondrial energy coupling in human skeletal muscle. J Clin Invest 108:733–737

44. Petersen KF, Dufour S, Befroy D, Garcia R, Shulman GI (2004) Impaired mitochondrial activity in the insulin-resistant offspring of patients with type 2 diabetes. N Engl J Med 350:664–671

45. Petersen KF, Befroy D, Dufour S, Dziura J, Ariyan C, Rothman DL, DiPietro L, Cline GW, Shulman GI (2003) Mitochondrial dysfunction in the elderly: possible role in insulin resistance. Science 300:1140–1142

46. Ingwall JS, Atkinson DE, Clarke K, Fetters JK (1990) Energetic correlates of cardiac failure: changes in the creatine kinase system in the failing myocardium. Eur Heart J 11:108–115

47. Leont'eva IV, Litvinova IS, Litvinov MM, Sebeleva IA, Sukhorukov VS, Tumanian MR, Koledinskii DG (2002) The use of positron emission tomography for noninva-sive diagnosis of mitochondrial dysfunction and assessment of myocardial compensatory reserve in children with cardiomyopathies. Kardiologiia 42:80

48. Sunagawa K (2005) Bionic cardiology: a new therapeutic modality for cardiology in the 21st century. Fukuoka Igaku Zasshi 96:63–66

49. Imai M, Rastogi S, Gupta RC et al (2007) Therapy with cardiac contractility modulation electrical signals improves left ventricular function and remodeling in dogs with chronic heart failure. J Am Coll Cardiol 49:2120

50. Butter C, Rastogi S, Minden HH, Meyhöfer J, Burkhoff D, Sabbah HN (2008) Cardiac contractility modulation electrical signals improve myocardial gene expression in patients with heart failure. J Am Coll Cardiol 51:1784–1789

51. Mudd JO, Kass DA (2008) Tackling heart failure in the twenty-first century. Nature 451:919–928

52. Bassingthwaighte JB, Qian H, Li Z (1999) The Cardiome Project. An integrated view of cardiac metabolism and regional mechanical function. Adv Exp Med Biol 471:541–553

53. Ch'en F, Clarke K, Vaughan-Jones R, Noble D (1997) Modeling of internal pH, ion concentration, and bioenergetic changes during myocardial ischemia. Adv Exp Med Biol 430:281–290

54. Noble D (2002) Modeling the heart from genes to cells to the whole organ. Science 295:1678–1682

55. Rudy Y (2000) From genome to physiome: integrative models of cardiac excitation. Ann Biomed Eng 28:945–950

56. Hunter P, Smith N, Fernandez J, Tawhai M (2005) Integration from proteins to organs: the IUPS Physiome Project. Mech Ageing Dev 126:187–192

57. Crampin EJ, Halstead M, Hunter P, Nielsen P, Noble D, Smith N, Tawhai M (2004) Computational physiology and the Physiome Project. Exp Physiol 89:1–26

58. Noble D (2002) Modelling the heart: insights, failures and progress. Bioessays 24:1155–1163

59. Roden DM (2005) Proarrhythmia as a pharmacogenomic entity: a critical review and formulation of a unifying hypothesis. Cardiovasc Res 67:419–425

60. Holloway JW, Yang IA, Ye S (2005) Variation in the toll-like receptor 4 gene and susceptibility to myocardial infarction. Pharmacogenet Genomics 15:15–21

61. Kajinami K, Akao H, Polisecki E, Schaefer EJ (2005) Pharmacogenomics of statin responsiveness. Am J Cardiol 96:65K–70K

62. Bolli R, Becker L, Gross G, Mentzer R Jr, Balshaw D, Lathrop DA (2004) NHLBI Working Group on the Translation of Therapies for Protecting the Heart from Ischemia. Myocardial protection at a crossroads: the need for translation into clinical therapy. Circ Res 95:125–134

63. Simonetti OP, Kim RJ, Fieno DS, Hillenbrand HB, Wu E, Bundy JM, Finn JP, Judd RM (2001) An improved MR imaging technique

for the visualization of myocardial infarction. Radiology 218:215–223

64. Klein C, Nekolla SG, Schwaiger M (2001) The role of magnetic resonance imaging in the diagnosis of coronary disease. Z Kardiol 90:208–217

65. Mahrholdt H, Wagner A, Holly TA, Elliott MD, Bonow RO, Kim RJ, Judd RM (2002) Reproducibility of chronic infarct size measurement by contrast-enhanced magnetic resonance imaging. Circulation 106:2322–2327

66. Noble D (2002) Unraveling the genetics and mechanisms of cardiac arrhythmia. Proc Natl Acad Sci USA 99:5755–5756

67. Gillum RF (1979) Pathophysiology of hypertension in blacks and whites: a review of the basis of racial blood pressure differences. Hypertension 1:468–475

68. Yancy CW (2000) Heart failure in African-Americans: a cardiovascular enigma. J Card Fail 6:183–186

69. Watkins LO (1984) Epidemiology of coronary heart disease in black populations. Am Heart J 108:635–640

70. Chobanian AV, Bakris GL, Black HR et al (2003) The Seventh Report of the Joint National Committee on Prevention, Detection, Evaluation, and Treatment of High Blood Pressure: the JNC 7 report. JAMA 289:2560–2572

71. Exner DV, Dries DL, Domanski MJ, Cohn JN (2001) Lesser response to angiotensin-converting-enzyme inhibitor therapy in black as compared with white patients with left ventricular dysfunction. N Engl J Med 344:1351–1357

72. Yancy CW, Fowler MB, Colucci WS, Gilbert EM, Bristow MR, Cohn JN et al (2001) US Carvedilol Heart Failure Study Group. Race and the response to adrenergic blockade with carvedilol in patients with chronic heart failure. N Engl J Med 344: 1358–1365

73. The Beta-Blocker Evaluation of Survival Trial Investigators (2001) A trial of the beta-blocker bucindolol in patients with advanced chronic heart failure. N Engl J Med 344:1659–1667

74. Carson P, Ziesche S, Johnson G, Cohn JN (1999) Racial differences in response to therapy for heart failure: analysis of the vasodilator-heart failure trials. J Card Fail 5:178–187

75. Taylor AL (2005) The African American Heart Failure Trial: a clinical trial update. Am J Cardiol 96:44–48

76. Taylor AL, Ziesche S, Yancy C, Carson P, D'Agostino R Jr, Ferdinand K et al (2004) African-American Heart Failure Trial Investigators. Combination of isosorbide dinitrate and hydralazine in blacks with heart failure. N Engl J Med 351:2049–2057

77. Rimessi P, Gualandi F, Duprez L, Spitali P, Neri M, Merlini L et al (2005) Genomic and transcription studies as diagnostic tools for a prenatal detection of X-linked dilated cardiomyopathy due to a dystrophin gene mutation. Am J Med Genet A 132:391–394

78. Johnson WH Jr, Yang P, Yang T, Lau YR, Mostella BA, Wolff DJ, Roden DM, Benson DW (2003) Clinical, genetic, and biophysical characterization of a homozygous HERG mutation causing severe neonatal long QT syndrome. Pediatr Res 53:744–748

79. Charron P, Heron D, Gargiulo M, Feingold J, Oury JF, Richard P, Komajda M (2004) Prenatal molecular diagnosis in hypertrophic cardiomyopathy: report of the first case. Prenat Diagn 24:701–703

80. Charron P, Heron D, Gargiulo M et al (2002) Genetic testing and genetic counselling in hypertrophic cardiomyopathy: the French experience. J Med Genet 39:741–746

81. Loeys B, Nuytinck L, Van Acker P et al (2002) Strategies for prenatal and preimplantation genetic diagnosis in Marfan syndrome (MFS). Prenat Diagn 22:22–28

82. Jacobs LJ, de Coo IF, Nijland JG et al (2005) Transmission and prenatal diagnosis of the T9176C mitochondrial DNA mutation. Mol Hum Reprod 11:223–228

83. Leshinsky-Silver E, Perach M, Basilevsky E, Hershkovitz E, Yanoov-Sharav M, Lerman-Sagie T, Lev D (2003) Prenatal exclusion of Leigh syndrome due to T8993C mutation in the mitochondrial DNA. Prenat Diagn 23:31–33

84. Amiel J, Gigarel N, Benacki A, Benit P et al (2001) Prenatal diagnosis of respiratory chain deficiency by direct mutation screening. Prenat Diagn 21:602–604

85. Niers L, van den Heuvel L, Trijbels F, Sengers R, Smeitink J; Nijmegen Centre for Mitochondrial Disorders, The Netherlands. Prerequisites and strategies for prenatal diagnosis of respiratory chain deficiency in chorionic villi. J Inherit Metab Dis 2003; 26:647–658

86. Thorburn DR, Dahl HH (2001) Mitochondrial disorders: genetics, counseling, prenatal diagnosis and reproductive options. Am J Med Genet 106:102–114

87. Dahl HH, Thorburn DR, White SL (2000) Towards reliable prenatal diagnosis of mtDNA point mutations: studies of nt8993 mutations in oocytes, fetal tissues, children and adults. Hum Reprod 15:246–255

88. He J, McDermott DA, Song Y, Gilbert F, Kligman I, Basson CT (2004) Preimplantation genetic diagnosis of human congenital heart malformation and Holt-Oram syndrome. Am J Med Genet A 126:93–98

89. Barritt JA, Brenner CA, Malter HE, Cohen J (2001) Mitochondria in human offspring derived from ooplasmic transplantation. Hum Reprod 16:513–516

90. Malter HE, Cohen J (2002) Ooplasmic transfer: animal models assist human studies. Reprod Biomed Online 5:26–35

91. Hawes SM, Sapienza C, Latham KE (2002) Ooplasmic donation in humans: the potential for epigenic modifications. Hum Reprod 17:850–852

92. St John JC (2002) Ooplasm donation in humans: the need to investigate the transmission of mitochondrial DNA following cytoplasmic transfer. Hum Reprod 17:1954–1958

93. Poulton J, Marchington DR (2002) Segregation of mitochondrial DNA (mtDNA) in human oocytes and in animal models of mtDNA disease: clinical implications. Reproduction 123:751–755

94. Kreuter M, Langer C, Kerkhoff C, Reddanna P, Kania AL, Maddika S, Chlichlia K, Bui TN, Los M (2004) Stroke, myocardial infarction, acute and chronic inflammatory diseases: caspases and other apoptotic molecules as targets for drug development. Arch Immunol Ther Exp 52:141–155

95. Roth GS, Lane MA, Ingram DK (2005) Caloric restriction mimetics: the next phase. Ann N Y Acad Sci 1057:365–371

96. Ingram DK, Anson RM, de Cabo R, Mamczarz J, Zhu M, Mattison J, Lane MA, Roth GS (2004) Development of calorie restriction mimetics as a prolongevity strategy. Ann N Y Acad Sci 1019:412–423

97. Dirks AJ, Leeuwenburgh C (2006) Caloric restriction in humans: potential pitfalls and health concerns. Mech Ageing Dev 127:1–7

98. Davis ME, Hsieh PC, Grodzinsky AJ, Lee RT (2005) Custom design of the cardiac microenvironment with biomaterials. Circ Res 97:8–15

99. Taylor PM, Sachlos E, Dreger SA, Chester AH, Czernuszka JT, Yacoub MH (2006) Interaction of human valve interstitial cells with collagen matrices manufactured using rapid prototyping. Biomaterials 27:2733–2737

100. Fukuda K (2005) Progress in myocardial regeneration and cell transplantation. Circ J 69:1431–1461

101. Memon IA, Sawa Y, Fukushima N et al (2005) Repair of impaired myocardium by means of implantation of engineered autologous myoblast sheets. J Thorac Cardiovasc Surg 130:1333–1341

102. Abraham MR, Henrikson CA, Tung L et al (2005) Antiarrhythmic engineering of skeletal myoblasts for cardiac transplantation. Circ Res 97:159–167

103. Knight RL, Booth C, Wilcox HE, Fisher J, Ingham E (2005) Tissue engineering of cardiac valves: re-seeding of acellular porcine aortic valve matrices with human mesenchymal progenitor cells. J Heart Valve Dis 14:806–813

104. Nagy RD, Tsai BM, Wang M, Markel TA, Brown JW, Meldrum DR (2005) Stem cell transplantation as a therapeutic approach to organ failure. J Surg Res 129:152–160

105. Vesely I (2005) Heart valve tissue engineering. Circ Res 97:743–755

106. Cushing MC, Jaeggli MP, Masters KS, Leinwand LA, Anseth KS (2005) Serum deprivation improves seeding and repopulation of acellular matrices with valvular interstitial cells. J Biomed Mater Res A 75:232–241

107. Sutherland FWH, Perry TE, Yu Y et al (2005) From stem cells to viable autologous semilunar heart valve. Circulation 111:2783–2791

108. Gepstein L (2005) cells as biological heart pacemakers. Expert Opin Biol Ther 5:1531–1537

109. Miake J, Marban E, Nuss HB (2002) Biological pacemaker created by gene transfer. Nature 419:132–133

110. Xue T, Cho HC, Akar FG, Tsang SY, Jones SP, Marban E, Tomaselli GF, Li RA (2005) Functional integration of electrically active cardiac derivatives from genetically engineered human embryonic stem cells with quiescent recipient ventricular cardiomyocytes: insights into the development of cell-based pacemakers. Circulation 111:11–20

111. Edelberg JM, Huang DT, Josephson ME, Rosenberg RD (2001) Molecular enhancement of porcine cardiac chronotropy. Heart 86:559–562

112. Qu J, Itskovitz-Eldor J, Shapiro SS, Waknitz MA, Cohen IS, Robinson RB, Rosen MR (2003) Expression and function of a biological pacemaker in canine heart. Circulation 107:1106–1109

113. Plotnikov AN, Sosunov EA, Qu J et al (2004) A biological pacemaker implanted in the canine left bundle branch provides ventricular escape rhythms having physiologically acceptable rates. Circulation 109:506–512

114. Potapova I, Plotnikov A, Lu Z et al (2004) Human mesenchymal stem cells as a gene delivery system to create cardiac pacemakers. Circ Res 94:952–959

115. Kehat I, Khimovich L, Caspi O et al (2004) Electromechanical integration of cardiomyocytes derived from human embryonic stem cells. Nat Biotechnol 22:1282–1289

116. Madeddu P (2005) Therapeutic angiogenesis and vasculogenesis for tissue regeneration. Exp Physiol 90:315–326

117. Hughes GC, Post MJ, Simons M, Annex BH (2003) Translational physiology: porcine models of human coronary artery disease: implications for preclinical trials of therapeutic angiogenesis. J Appl Physiol 94:1689–1701

118. Shimamura M, Sato N, Yoshimura S, Kaneda Y, Morishita R (2006) HVJ-based non-viral gene transfer method: successful gene therapy using HGF and VEGF genes in experimental ischemia. Front Biosci 11:753–759

119. Shah PB, Losordo DW (2005) Non-viral vectors for gene therapy: clinical trials in cardiovascular disease. Adv Genet 54:339–361

120. Lei Y, Haider HKh, Shujia J, Sim ES (2004) Therapeutic angiogenesis. Devising new strategies based on past experiences. Basic Res Cardiol 99:121–132

121. Riha GM, Lin PH, Lumsden AB, Yao Q, Chen C (2005) Review: application of stem cells for vascular tissue engineering. Tissue Eng 11:1535–1552

122. Sales KM, Salacinski HJ, Alobaid N, Mikhail M, Balakrishnan V, Seifalian AM (2005) Advancing vascular tissue engineering: the role of stem cell technology. Trends Biotechnol 23:461–467

123. Wu X, Rabkin-Aikawa E, Guleserian KJ et al (2004) Tissue-engineered microvessels on three-dimensional biodegradable scaffolds using human endothelial progenitor cells. Am J Physiol Heart Circ Physiol 287:H480–H487

Glossary

AC Adenylyl cyclase, a membrane-bound enzyme, which catalyzes the synthesis of the second messenger cyclic AMP from ATP in conjunction with specific signaling ligands (e.g., adrenergic), receptors, and G-proteins.

ACC Acetyl-CoA carboxylase, an enzyme that synthesizes malonyl-CoA from cytoplasmic and peroxisomal acetyl-CoA.

ACE Angiotensin converting enzyme, a central element of the renin–angiotensin system, converts the decapeptide angiotensin I to the potent pressor octapeptide angiotensin II (Ang II), mediating peripheral vascular tone, as well as glomerular filtration in the kidney.

Acetyl-CoA Small water-soluble molecule that carries acetyl groups linked to coenzyme A (CoA) by a thioester bond.

ACH Acetylcholine.

ACS cells Adult cardiac stem cells.

ADAM A disintegrin and metalloprotease; family of membrane-anchored metalloproteases.

ADE Adverse drug effect.

Adenovirus Common vector for gene transfer with high efficiency of transfection in vivo, but limited by transient transgene expression and host immunogenic response.

ADHERE Acute decompensated HF national registry.

ADHF Acute decompensated HF.

ADP Adenosine diphosphate.

Adrenoceptors Members of the G-protein-coupled receptor superfamily, linking adrenergic signaling from the sympathetic nervous system and the cardiovascular system, with integral roles in the rapid regulation of myocardial function.

AHFS Acute HF syndromes.

AIF Apoptosis-inducing factor. Released from mitochondrial intermembrane space in early apoptosis and subsequently involved in nuclear DNA fragmentation.

AKAP Specific PKA anchoring proteins; regulators of PKA function and signaling by directing and concentrating PKA at specific subcellular sites.

AKI Acute kidney injury.

Akt Protein kinase B (PKB). Myocardial Akt phosphorylates a number of downstream targets, including cardioprotective factors involved in glucose and mitochondrial metabolism, apoptosis and regulators of protein synthesis.

ALCAR Acetyl-L-carnitine, supplementation with lipoic acid (LA) appears to improve myocardial bioenergetics and decrease oxidative stress associated with aging.

Allele One of several alternate forms of a single gene occupying a given locus on a chromosome or mtDNA.

AMI Acute myocardial infarction.

AMP Adenosine monophosphate.

AMPK AMP-activated protein kinase.

ANG II Angiotensin II.

ANP Atrial natriuretic peptide.

ANT Adenine nucleotide translocator. A mitochondrial inner membrane carrier protein of ADP and ATP and part of the PT pore.

Apoptosis A form of programmed cell death.

Apoptosome Cytosolic complex involved in the activation of apoptotic caspases.

ARB Angiotensin receptor blocker.

ARIC Atherosclerosis risk in communities.

ARVD Arrhythmogenic right ventricular dysplasia; the most common symptoms are ventricular dysrhythmias, heart palpitations, fainting or loss of consciousness (syncope), and sudden death.

ASC Adult stem cell.

ATP Adenosine triphosphate.

ATPase Adenosine triphosphatase.

Bad Bcl-2/Bcl-X$_L$-associated death promotor. A death agonist.

β-AR Beta-adrenergic receptor, G-protein coupled receptors containing a seven transmembrane domain involved in signaling pathways of diverse cardiovascular functions including blood pressure control and cardiac contractility.

β-ARK Beta-adrenergic receptor kinase, a GRK, which mediates the desensitization of the β-adrenergic receptor by phosphorylation of agonist-occupied receptors.

Barth syndrome An X-linked recessive cardioskeletal myopathy with neutropenia and DCM with childhood onset caused by mutations in TAZ/G4.5 gene encoding the tafazzin protein.

Bcl-2 Family of apoptosis-related proteins. Also death antagonist.

BH domains Features of proapoptotic proteins, (BH1-4) are essential for homo- and heterocomplex formation, as well as to induce cell death. Proapoptotic homologues can be subdivided into 2 major subtypes, the multidomain Bax subfamily (e.g., Bax and Bak), which possesses BH1-3 domains, and the BH3-only subfamily (e.g., Bad and Bid).

Bid A proapoptotic Bcl-2 related protein, which links the extrinsic and intrinsic apoptotic pathways.

BMDC Bone-marrow-derived cells.

BMP Bone morphogenetic protein, a class of ligands, which bind specific membrane-bound receptors involved in signaling events in early cardiomyocyte differentiation.

BNP Brain natriuretic peptide, hemodynamic marker of neurohumoral and vascular stress.

BRDU Bromodeoxyuridine, a DNA synthesis inhibitor.

CAD Coronary artery disease.

Calcineurin Intracellular Ca^{2+}-regulated phosphatase implicated as a mediator of cardiac hypertrophy.

Calpains Calcium-dependent proteolytic enzymes expressed ubiquitously is regulated by the concentration of calcium ions.

Calsequestrin Major binding calcium protein present in the sarcoplasmic reticulum.

CaM Calmodulin, an intracellular Ca^{2+} sensor that selectively activates downstream signaling pathways in response to local changes in Ca^{2+}.

CaMK Ca^{2+}/CaM dependent protein kinase.

cAMP Cyclic AMP; second messenger used extensively in cell signaling. Product of adenylyl cyclase (AC).

Cardiac hypertrophy Growth of the heart in response to increased workload by enlarging myocyte size, rather than increasing myocyte number.

Cardiolipin Anionic phospholipid located primarily in the mitochondrial inner membrane.

Cardiomyocyte A single cell of a heart muscle.

Carnitine Carrier molecule involved in the transport of long-chain fatty acids into the mitochondria for β-FAO.

Caspases Intracellular cysteine proteases activated during apoptosis that cleave substrates at their aspartic acid residues.

Caveolae Flask-shaped specialized subdomains of the plasma membrane particularly abundant in cardiovascular cells that function both in protein trafficking and signal transduction.

Cell cycle The period between the release of a cell as one of the progeny of a division and its own subsequent division by *mitosis* into two daughter cells.

CETP Cholesteryl ester transfer protein plays role in reverse cholesterol transport with transfer of cholesteryl ester-rich HDL to triglyceride-rich lipoproteins (VLDL).

CHD Congenital heart defect.

Chromatin The complex of DNA and histone and nonhistone proteins found in the nucleus of a eukaryotic cell that constitutes the chromosomes.

Chromosome A very long, continuous piece of DNA, which hold together many genes, regulatory elements, and other intervening nucleotide sequences.

CHS Cardiovascular health study.

CI Confidence interval.

CIBIS Cardiac insufficiency bisoprolol study.

CK Creatine kinase. Both mitochondrial and cytosolic isoforms of this enzyme that catalyzes the reversible phosphorylation of creatine by ATP to form the high-energy compound phosphocreatine.

CL Cardiolipin, anionic phospholipid present in mitochondrial membranes. Deficiency in Barth syndrome. Involved in stabilization of ETC complexes and in apoptosis.

CNS Central nervous system.

Complex I NADH-ubiquinone oxidoreductase.

Complex II Succinate CoQ oxidoreductase.

Complex III CoQ-cytochrome *c* oxidoreductase.

Complex IV Cytochrome *c* oxidase.

Complex V Oligomycin-sensitive ATP synthase. Also termed F_0–F_1 ATPase.

COPD Chronic obstructive pulmonary disease.

CoQ Coenzyme Q (also ubiquinone). Electron carrier and antioxidant.

CPB Cardiopulmonary bypass.

CPT Carnitine palmitoyltransferase.

CPT-I Carnitine palmitoyltransferase I.

CPT-II Carnitine palmitoyltransferase II.

CR Caloric restriction, a restricted dietary regimen, which has been shown to increase lifespan in a number of organisms including mammals and may have anti-aging effects in the heart.

Cre-LoxP system A tool for tissue-specific deletion of genes that cannot be investigated in differentiated tissues because of their early embryonic lethality in mice with conventional knockouts. Conventional transgenic mice expressing Cre recombinase are mated to a strain with a gene flanked by LoxP sites ("a floxed gene"). The floxed gene is excised by recombination, and is thus inactivated, in whichever tissues Cre recombinase is expressed.

CR Chest roentgenogram.

CRP C-reactive protein; a significant marker of inflammation and atherosclerotic progression. Serum CRP levels are predictive of future cardiovascular events.

CRS Cardiorenal syndrome.

CRT Cardiac resynchronization therapy.

CRT-D CRT with or without implantable defibrillator.

cTnT Cardiac troponin T, widely used marker of myocardial ischemia and necrosis.

CTX Cholera toxin.

CVD Cardiovascular disease.

CPVT Catecholaminergic polymorphic ventricular tachycardia

CyP-D Cyclophilin D. CsA-binding mitochondrial matrix protein component of the PT pore.

Cytochrome A family of proteins that contain heme as a prosthetic group involved in electron transfer and identifiable by their absorption spectra.

Cytochrome c A mitochondrial protein involved in ETC at complex IV. Its release from the mitochondrial into the cytosol is a trigger of caspase activation and early myocardial apoptosis.

DAG Diacylglycerol.

DCM Dilated cardiomyopathy.

DHF 2′,7′-dichlorofluorescin, membrane-permeable fluorometric indicator of ROS levels (particularly in mitochondrial matrix).

Dicer An endonuclease that cleaves double-stranded RNA and that is required for microRNA biogenesis.

Differential display Technique used to identify genes that are differentially expressed; RNA from the samples being compared is reverse transcribed, and the cDNA is further amplified using random primers. Genes that are differentially expressed in the chosen samples can be identified by electrophoresis.

DIG Digitalis investigation group.

Double helix A molecular model of DNA made of two complementary strands of the bases guanine, adenine, thymine, and cytosine, covalently linked through phosphodiester bonds. Each strand forms a helix, and the two helices are held together through hydrogen bonds, ionic forces, hydrophobic interactions, and van der Waals forces.

Doxorubicin Also called *adriamycin*. Used to treat leukemia but also causes extensive mitochondrial defects, myocardial apoptosis and induces cardiomyopathy.

Dysrhythmia Any change in the regular rhythmic beating of the heart.

EB Embryoid bodies, aggregations of embryonic stem cells, which can differentiate spontaneously in vitro to a variety of cell types including cardiomyocytes.

ECLS Extracorporeal life support.

ECM Extracellular matrix.

ECMO Extracorporeal membrane oxygenation.

EF Ejection fraction.

EGF Epidermal growth factor.

EKG Electrocardiogram.

EMB Endomyocardial biopsy.

EPC Endothelial progenitor cell.

Epigenetic Acquired and reversible modification of genetic material (e.g., methylation).

Enhancer element A DNA sequence that, when bound by a specific transcription factor, can enhance the expression level of a nearby gene.

ER Endoplasmic reticulum. A membrane-bound cytosolic compartment where lipids and membrane-bound proteins are synthesized.

ErbB proteins Family of receptor tyrosine kinases, which mediate cell proliferation, migration, differentiation, adhesion, and apoptosis in numerous cell types, bind to a wide variety of ligands (e.g., EGF, neuregulins, TGF, and HB-EGF) and contribute to regulation of endocardial cushion remodeling and valve formation.

ERK Extracellular regulated kinase.

ES Embryonic stem cell.

ET Endothelin, signaling peptides (ET-1, ET-2, and ET-3) modulate contractile function and growth stimulation of cardiomyocytes by binding specific G-protein coupled receptors and triggering downstream signaling (e.g., DAG, IP3).

ETC Electron transport chain. A series of complexes in the mitochondrial inner membrane to conduct electrons from the oxidation of NADH and succinate to oxygen.

Expression vector A vector that contains elements necessary for high-level and accurate transcription and translation of an inserted cDNA in a particular host or tissue.

FA Friedreich ataxia. An autosomal-dominant neuromuscular disorder with frequent HCM.

FABP Fatty acid binding translocase.

FACS Fluorescence activated cell sorting, which can evaluate and isolate specific cell-types and cell-cycle stages.

FAD Flavin adenine dinucleotide. Common coenzyme of dehydrogenases. In the ETC, FAD is covalently linked to SDH.

FADD Fas-associated via death domain, adaptor protein recruiting procaspase into the apoptotic-promoting complex DISC.

FADH$_2$ Flavin adenine dinucleotide (reduced form).

FAO Fatty acid oxidation.

FasL Fas ligand, death ligand in extrinsic apoptotic pathway.

FAT Fatty acid translocase.

FCHL Familial combined hyperlipidemia, characterized by elevated levels of plasma triglycerides, LDL and VLDL-cholesterol or both is the most common discrete hyperlipidemia and a common cause of premature atherosclerosis.

FDA Fluorescein diacetate, a fluorochrome used to discriminate between necrosis and apoptosis in intact cardiomyocytes.

FGF Fibroblast growth factor.

FH Familial hypercholesterolemia is an autosomal dominant disorder characterized by elevated cholesterol, and premature CAD, is the result of mutations that affect the LDL receptor (LDLR).

FMN Flavin mononucleotide. A cofactor of complex I.

FoxO Forkhead box 0 transcription factors.

FRDA Friedreich's ataxia. An autosomal-dominant neuromuscular disorder with frequent HCM caused by mutations in gene for frataxin, a mitochondrial-localized protein.

Functional genomics A branch of molecular biology that makes use of the enormous amount of data produced by genome sequencing to delineate genome function.

GATA Family of zinc finger-containing transcription factors, which contribute to the activation of the cardiac-specific gene program involved in cardiac cell differentiation.

GC Guanylyl cyclase.

Gene product The protein, tRNA, or rRNA encoded by a gene.

Gene transfection Introduction of DNA into eukaryotic cells.

Genetic code Correspondence between nucleotide triplets (codon) and specific amino acids in proteins.

Genome Total genetic information carried by a cell or an organism.

Genomic library Collection of DNA fragments (each inserted into a vector molecule) representative of the entire genome.

Genotype Genetic constitution of a cell or an organism.

GFP Green fluorescent protein. Useful marker for imaging localized proteins.

GFR Glomerular filtration rate.

GH Growth hormone.

GIK Glucose, insulin, and potassium. Applied as a metabolic "cocktail" to provide beneficial preconditioning effects to injured myocardium.

GK rat Goto-Kakizaki rat, experimental model of type 2 diabetes.

GLP-1 Glucagon-like peptide 1, cardioprotective agent.

GLUT Glucose transporter.

Glycolysis Cytosolic-located metabolic pathway present in all cells catalyzing the anaerobic conversion of glucose to pyruvate.

Glycosylation An enzyme-directed site-specific process, resulting in the addition of carbohydrate residues to proteins and lipids.

GPCR G-protein coupled receptors.

G-protein A heterotrimeric membrane-associated GTP-binding protein involved in cell-signaling pathways; activated by specific hormone or ligand binding to a 7-helix transmembrane receptor protein.

GPx Glutathione peroxidase. An antioxidant enzyme with both mitochondrial and cytosolic isoforms.

GSH Glutathione.

GTP Guanosine triphosphate.

HA Hyaluronic acid, a glycosaminoglycan composed of alternating glucuronic acid and N-acetylglucosamine residues, present in the ECM, to expand the extracellular space, regulate ligand availability and direct remodeling events in the cardiac jelly.

HCM Hypertrophic cardiomyopathy.

HDL High-density lipoprotein.

Helicase Enzymes that separate the strands of DNA.

Heterochromatin Condensed regions of chromosomes containing less active genes.

Heteroplasmy Presence of more than 1 genotype in a cell.

H-FABP Heart-type fatty acid-binding protein, an intracellular binding protein, with potential clinical utility as an indicator of cardiac ischemia and necrosis.

5-HD 5-hydroxydecanoic acid, selective mitoK$_{ATP}$ channel blocker.

HF Heart failure.

HGP Human Genome Project.

HIF Hypoxia-inducible factor.

Histones Chief proteins of chromatin acting as spools around which DNA winds. They play a role in regulation of gene expression.

HLHS Hypoplastic left heart syndrome.

HNE 4-hydroxynonenal. A major product of endogenous lipid peroxidation.

H$_2$O$_2$ Hydrogen peroxide; a form of ROS and marker of oxidative stress.

HO-1 Heme oxygenase, antioxidant enzyme with cardioprotective function.

Homocysteine A reactive amino acid intermediate in methionine metabolism whose adverse effects include endothelial dysfunction with associated platelet activation and thrombus formation and accumulation of vascular atherosclerotic lesions.

Hop Homeodomain-only protein.

HPA Hypothalamic–pituitary–adrenal.

HR Hazard ratio.

HREs Hormone response elements.

HRT Hormone replacement therapy.

HSC Hematopoietic stem cells.

HSP Heat-shock protein. A family of chaperones involved in protein folding.

Hybridization Binding of nucleic acid sequences through complementary base pairing. The hybridization rate is influenced by temperature, G-C composition, extent of homology, and length of the sequences involved.

Hydrophobic Lipophilic. Insoluble in water.

ICA Ipsilateral carotid artery.

ICD Implantable cardioverter-defibrillator.

IFM Interfibrillar mitochondria.

IGF-1 Insulin-like growth factor, stimulates proliferative cardiomyocyte pathways and cell growth.

IMA Ischemia-modified albumin, indicator of early myocardial ischemia and acute coronary syndrome.

IMAC Anion channel of the inner mitochondrial membrane.

IMAGE Invasive monitoring attenuation through gene expression.

IML Intermediolateral cell column.

Infective endocarditis Microbial infection of the endocardial surface of the heart, which commonly involves the heart valves.

In situ hybridization Technique using DNA probes to localize specific transcripts within the cell in conjunction with microscopy.

Integrins Class of transmembrane, cell-surface receptor molecules that constitute part of the link between the extracellular matrix and the cardiomyocyte cytoskeleton and which act as signaling molecules and transducers of mechanical force.

Intermembrane space Space between inner and outer membranes.

Intron A segment of a nuclear gene that is transcribed into the primary RNA transcript but is excised during RNA splicing and not present in the mature transcript.

Ion channels Multisubunit transmembrane protein complexes that perform the task of mediating selective flow of millions of ions per second across cell membranes, and are the fundamental functional units of biological excitability.

Ionophore Small hydrophobic molecule that promotes the transfer of specific ions through the membrane bilayer.

IP3 Inositol trisphosphate, second messenger produced by phospholipase C.

IPC Ischemic preconditioning.

I/R Ischemia/reperfusion.

IRAK1 Interleukin-1 receptor-associated kinase 1.

Ischemic heart disease Also called coronary artery disease (CAD) and coronary heart disease (CHD), this condition is caused by narrowing of the coronary arteries, thereby causing decreased blood supply to the heart.

ISDN Isosorbide dinitrate.

ISHLT International Society for Heart & Lung Transplantation.

Isoforms Related forms of the same protein generated by alternative splicing, transcriptional starts or encoded by entirely different genes.

JC-1 Fluorometric dye used for measuring/imaging mitochondrial membrane potential.

Karyotype A snap-shot of the number of chromosomes in the normal diploid cell, as well as their size distribution.

KCOs Potassium channel openers (e.g., nicorandil, diazoxide, and pinacidil); can mediate cardioprotection.

KIR Potassium inward rectifier.

KLOTHO A single-pass transmembrane protein that functions in signaling pathways that suppress aging and which has β-glucuronidase activity.

Knock-out mutation A null mutation in a gene, abolishing its function (usually in transgenic mouse); allows evaluation of its phenotypic role.

Krebs cycle Central metabolic pathway of aerobic respiration occurring in the mitochondrial matrix; involves oxidation of acetyl groups derived from pyruvate to CO_2, NADH, and H_2O. The NADH from this cycle is a central substrate in the OXPHOS pathway. Also termed as TCA or citric acid cycle.

KSS Kearns–Sayre syndrome.

LA Lipoic acid, a potent thiol antioxidant and mitochondrial metabolite, appears to increase low molecular weight antioxidants, decreasing age-associated oxidative damage.

LAD Left anterior descending.

LBBB Left bundle branch block.

LBD Ligand binding domain.

LCAD Long-chain acyl-CoA dehydrogenase involved in FAO.

LCFA Long-chain fatty acid.

LCHAD Long-chain 3-hydroxylacyl-CoA dehydrogenase.

LDL Low-density lipoprotein, a cholesteryl ester-rich particle (containing only apoB100) whose plasma levels are elevated in several monogenic disorders of lipoprotein metabolism and lead to atherosclerosis.

LDLR Low-density lipoprotein receptor, cell-surface receptor in liver or peripheral tissues responsible for LDL removal from blood; defective LDLR results in FH.

Liddle's syndrome An autosomal dominant monogenic form of hypertension with both hypokalemia and increased sodium reabsorption due to specific defects in either the β or γ subunit of the epithelial sodium channel (*ENaC*) causing gain-of-function of channel activation.

Ligand Any molecule that binds to a specific site on a protein or a receptor molecule.

Ligase Enzyme that join together two molecules in an energy dependent process; involved in DNA replication and repair. Extensively used in manipulation with recombinant DNA.

Liposomes Lipid spheres with a fraction of aqueous fluid in the center used as vectors for gene transfection with plasmid DNA or oligonucleotides.

LQT Long QT syndrome; prolongation of the QT interval is a significant cause of syncope and SCD in children; delayed or prolonged repolarization of the cardiac myocyte can be acquired (e.g., drugs) or congenital (e.g., mutations in specific ion channels).

LTA Lymphotoxin-α, an inflammation-mediating cytokine implicated in coronary artery plaque formation; polymorphic gene variants associated with MI.

L-type Ca^{2+} channels Channels responsible for the activation of sarcoplasmic reticulum calcium release channels (RyR2). They are controllers of the force of muscle contraction generation in heart.

Luciferase ATP-dependent photoprotein luciferase used to fluorometrically assess the specific organelle ATP levels.

LV Left ventricle.

LVAD Left-ventricular assist devices.

LVEF Left ventricle ejection fraction.

LVH Left ventricular hypertrophy.

MAP Mean arterial pressure.

MAPCs Multipotent adult precursor cells.

MAPK Mitogen-activated protein kinases. A family of conserved serine/threonine protein kinases activated as a result of a wide range of signals involved in cell proliferation and differentiation; includes JNK and ERK.

Matrix Space surrounded by the mitochondrial inner membrane.

MBs Molecular beacons. Hairpin-forming oligonucleotides labeled at one end with a quencher, and at the other end with a fluorescent reporter dye.

MC Mineralocorticoid.

MCAD Medium-chain acyl-CoA dehydrogenase, FAO enzyme.

MCD Malonyl-CoA decarboxylase, an enzyme involved in regulation of malonyl-CoA turnover.

MCM Mitochondrial cardiomyopathy.

MCS Mechanical circulatory support.

MEF2 Myocyte enhancer factor-2.

MELAS Mitochondrial encephalomyopathy, lactic acidosis and stroke-like episodes.

Membrane potential Combination of proton and ion gradients across the mitochondrial inner membrane making the inside negative relative to the outside.

MERRF Mitochondrial cytopathy including myotonus, epilepsy, and ragged-red fibers.

MetSyn Metabolic syndrome.

MHC Myosin heavy chain.

MI Myocardial infarction.

Microarray A range of oligonucleotides immobilized onto a surface (chip) that can be hybridized to determine quantitative transcript expression or mutation detection.

MicroRNA Class of single-stranded RNA molecules of approximately 21–23 nucleotides in length that regulate gene expression post-transcriptionally.

Mineralocorticoid A monogenic autosomal dominant form of an early-onset hypertension, induced hypertension markedly exacerbated during pregnancy due to mutations in the *MR* hormone-binding domain.

Minisatellites Repetitive and variable DNA sequences, generally GC-rich, ranging in length from 10 to over 100 bp.

miRISC miRNA-induced silencing complexes.

Missense mutation Mutation that causes substitution of one amino acid for another.

MitoKATP channel ATP-sensitive K^+ channel in inner membrane of mitochondria. Activation of mitoKATP channel has been implicated as a central signaling event (both as trigger and end effector) in IPC and other cardioprotection pathways.

MitoQ Synthetic ubiquinone analog, which can be selectively targeted to mitochondria to provide antioxidant cardioprotection.

MLA Monophosphoryl lipid A, a nontoxic derivative of the endotoxin pharmacophore lipid A, cardioprotective agent.

MLC Myosin light chain.

MLP Muscle LIM protein, localized in the cardiomyocyte cytoskeleton, a positive regulator of myogenic differentiation.

MMPs Metalloproteinases, enzymes involved in extracellular matrix remodeling.

Mobile carrier Small molecule shuttling electrons between complexes in the ETC.

Modifier gene A gene that modifies a trait encoded by another gene.

MOMP Mitochondrial outer-membrane permeabilization, an apoptotic event in part mediated by binding of proapoptotic proteins (e.g., Bad, Bax, Bid) to mitochondria.

Motif homology searching Search for patterns between proteins, which can prove highly informative about the structural and functional properties of the encoded protein.

MPG N-2-mercaptopropionylglycine, a free radical scavenger.

MPI Myocardial performance index.

MPO Myeloperoxidase, indicator of pathological inflammation and for risk of ACS.

MR Mineralocorticoid receptor.

mRNA Messenger RNA. Specifies the amino acid sequence of a protein; translated into protein on ribosomes. Transcript of RNA polymerase II.

MSC Mesenchymal stem cells.

MT Metallothionein. An inducible antioxidant metal-binding protein with cardioprotective properties.

mtDNA Mitochondrial DNA.

mtTFA Mitochondrial transcription factor A (also called *TFAM*).

mTOR Mammalian target of rapamycin.

MTP Mitochondrial trifunctional protein, part of mitochondrial FAO.

Mutation Change occurring in the genetic material (usually DNA or RNA).

MVO$_2$ Myocardial oxygen consumption.

MVR Mitral valve regurgitation.

Na$^+$/Ca^{2+} exchanger The major plasma membrane transporting protein that can cause calcium to exit from the cardiac myocyte.

NADH Nicotinamide adenine dinucleotide (reduced form).

NEP Neutral endopeptidase.

NFAT Nuclear factor of activated T cells, a family of transcription factors controlled by the Ca^{2+}-regulated phosphatase, calcineurin.

NFATc A member of the NFAT family, exclusively expressed on the endocardium, which plays a prominent role in the morphogenesis of the semilunar valves and septa.

NF-κB Nuclear factor-κB. Family of transcription factors involved in the control of a number of normal cellular and organismal processes, including immune and inflammatory responses, developmental processes, cellular growth, and apoptosis.

NGF Nerve growth factor.

NHLBI National health lung and blood institute.

NHNES-1 National health and nutrition examination survey-1.

NO Nitric oxide; vasodilator.

Northern blot Molecular technique by which RNA separated by electrophoresis is transferred and immobilized for the detection of specific transcripts by hybridization with a labeled probe.

NOS Nitric oxide synthase.

NRF-1 and NRF-2 Nuclear respiratory factors.

Nt Nucleotide, the basic unit of DNA composed of a purine or pyrimidine base, a sugar (deoxyribose), and a phosphate group.

NTG Nitroglycerin.

NT-proBNP N-terminal pro-brain natriuretic peptide, indicator of hemodynamic stress and for risk of congestive HF.

Nucleases Enzymes that catalyze the degradation of DNA (DNAse) or RNA (RNAse); specific nucleases have been identified that target either the 5′ or 3′ ends of DNA (exonuclease) or that can digest nucleic acids from internal sites (endonucleases).

Null mutation Ablation or knock-out of a gene.

NYHA New York heart association.

OPTIMIZED-HF Organized program to initiate life-saving treatment in hospitalized patients with HF.

OS Oxidative stress.

OxLDL Oxidized LDL, a primary substrate for macrophage activation and involved in atherosclerosis progression.

OXPHOS Oxidative phosphorylation. A process in mitochondria in which ATP formation is driven by electron transfer from NADH and FADH$_2$ to molecular oxygen and by the generation of a pH gradient and chemiosmotic coupling.

PAI-1 Plasminogen activator inhibitor-1, a principal regulator of fibrinolysis.

PCMR Pediatric cardiomyopathy registry.

PCR Polymerase chain reaction. An amplification of DNA fragments using a thermostable DNA polymerase and paired oligonucleotide primers subjected to repeated reactions with thermal cycling.

PDGF Platelet-derived growth factor.

PDH Pyruvate dehydrogenase (also PDC).

PDK-1 Phosphoinositide dependent kinase 1, enzyme downstream of PIP3 production in the PI3K pathway, which becomes activated in part by its translocation to the plasma membrane, and proximity to its substrates which include Akt (PKB).

PEO Progressive external ophthalmoplegia.

Peroxisome Small organelle that uses oxygen to oxidize organic molecules, including fatty acids and contains enzymes that generate and degrade hydrogen peroxide (H_2O_2) (e.g., catalase).

PGC-1a Peroxisome proliferator-activated receptor gamma co-activator. Transcriptional regulator of mitochondrial bioenergetic and biogenesis operative during physiological transitions.

Pharmacogenetics Study of the role of inheritance in interindividual variation in drug response.

Phenotype Observable physical characteristics of a cell or organism resulting from the interaction of its genetic constitution (genotype) with its environment.

PI3K Phosphatidylinositol 3-kinase.

PIP3 Phosphatidylinositol 3,4,5-triphosphate, product of PI3K activity.

PKA Protein kinase A. Activated by cAMP.

PKB Protein kinase B; also called Akt.

PKC Protein kinase C.

Plasmid DNA capable of autonomous existence in an organism; can replicate and maintain itself without integrating into the genome; used as a vector.

PLC Phospholipase C, a potent effector enzyme catalyzing the hydrolysis of inositol phospholipids and production of second messengers such as IP3 and DAG in responce to activation by agonists (e.g., acetycholine) binding to membrane bound receptors in concert with G-proteins. This signaling promotes a downstream increase in intracellular Ca^{2+} levels, and PKC activation, which modulate myocardial contraction.

PLC1 Phospholipase C1.

PLE Protein-losing enteropathy.

Polycistronic A single RNA transcript encoding two or more gene products.

Porin Pore-forming protein in the outer mitochondrial membrane (see VDAC).

Posttranslational Postsynthetic modification of proteins by glycosylation, phosphorylation, etc.

Modification Proteolytic cleavage, or other covalent changes involving side chains or termini.

PPARs Peroxisome proliferator-activated receptors.

Primer Short nucleotide sequence that is paired with 1 strand of DNA and provides a free 3′ OH end at which a DNA polymerase starts the synthesis of a nascent chain.

Protein kinase Enzyme that transfers the terminal phosphate group of ATP to a specific amino acid of a target protein.

Proteome Entire complement of proteins contained within the eukaryotic cell.

PSF Preserved systolic function.

PRA Plasma renin activity.

PTLD Posttransplant lymphoproliferative disorder.

PT pore Permeability transition pore. A non-specific megachannel in the mitochondrial inner membrane.

PTPs Phosphoprotein tyrosine phosphatases.

PTX Pertussis toxin.

PUFA Polyunsaturated fatty acids.

PVN Paraventricular nucleus.

RA Retinoic acid; plays role in cardiomyocyte differentiation.

RAAS Renin–angiotensin–aldosterone system.

RACKs Receptors for activated C kinase.

Ras A small G protein (see small G proteins).

RCT Randomized controlled trial.

Real-time PCR Quantitative PCR technique employs simultaneous DNA amplification and quantification often using fluorescent dyes that intercalate with double-strand DNA, and modified DNA oligonucleotide probes which fluoresce when hybridized with a complementary DNA.

Recombinant DNA An artificial DNA sequence resulting from the combination of two DNA sequences in a plasmid.

Redox reactions Oxidation-reduction reactions in which there is a transfer of electrons from an electron donor (the reducing agent) to an electron acceptor (oxidizing agent).

Remote conditioning Preconditioning, which is not confined to one organ, but also limits infarct size in remote, non-preconditioned organs.

Reporter gene A gene that is attached to another gene or regulatory element to be identified in cell culture, animals, or plants.

Restenosis The re-closing or re-narrowing of an artery after an interventional procedure such as angioplasty or stent placement.

Restriction endonucleases Endonucleases that recognize a specific sequence in a DNA molecule (usually palindromic) and cleaves the DNA at or near that site.

RFLP Restriction fragment-length polymorphism. A variation in the length of restriction fragments due to presence or absence of a restriction site.

RGS proteins Regulators of G-protein signaling proteins, a family of proteins that accelerate intrinsic GTP hydrolysis on a subunits of trimeric G proteins and play crucial roles in the physiological regulation of G-protein-mediated cell signaling.

Rhod-2AM Fluorescent calcium indicator used to assess Ca^{2+} uptake, localization and levels in cardiomyocytes.

Rhodamine 123 A fluorescent dye used to stain mitochondria in living cells.

Ribosome A factory-like organelle that builds proteins from a set of genetic instructions. Composed of rRNA and ribosomal proteins, it translates mRNA into a polypeptide chain.

Ribozyme RNA molecule with endonucleolytic activity, which can be used to selectively target specific gene expression.

RNAi RNA interference, use of a specific double-stranded RNA (dsRNA) construct to posttranscriptionally silence specific gene expression.

RNA polymerase Enzyme responsible for transcribing DNA as template into RNA.

RNP Ribonucleic protein.

RNS Reactive nitrogen species.

ROC Receiver-operator curves.

ROS Reactive oxygen species, including superoxide, hydroxyl radicals, and hydrogen peroxide.

Rotenone Specific inhibitor of complex I activity.

RPF Renal plasma flow.

RRF Ragged red fiber.

rRNA Ribosomal RNA. A central component of the ribosome.

RSNA Renal sympathetic nerve activity.

RTK Receptor tyrosine kinase; this large family of proteins includes receptors for many growth factors and insulin; ligand binding results in dimerization and phosphorylation of downstream signaling targets as well as autophosphorylation.

RT-PCR Reverse transcription (RT) of RNA to DNA with the enzyme reverse transcriptase; can be combined with traditional PCR to allow the amplification and determination of the abundance of specific RNA.

RV Right ventricle.

RVLM Rostral ventrolateral medulla.

RXR Retinoid X receptor. On binding 9-cis retinoic acid, RXR acts as a heterodimer and as a repressor or activator of specific gene transcription, playing a key role in cardiac development and physiological gene expression.

Ryanodine receptor Major SR Ca^{2+} release channel in cardiac muscle; mutations in the cardiac isoform encoded by RyR2 result in ARVD and CVPT.

RyR2 A human gene that encodes a ryanodine receptor found in cardiac muscle sarcoplasmic reticulum. This ryanodine receptor is one of the components of a calcium channel.

SAGE Serial analysis of gene expression. Quantitative analysis of RNA transcripts by using short sequence tags to generate a characteristic expression profile.

SAH *S*-adenosylhomocysteine.

SCAD Short-chain acyl-CoA dehydrogenase involved in FAO.

SCD Sudden cardiac death.

SD Sudden death.

SDH Succinate dehydrogenase. A TCA cycle enzyme associated with complex II.

SERCA Sarcoplasmic reticulum Ca^{2+}-ATPase. There are 3 major isoforms, which are variably expressed in different muscle types.

SHR Spontaneously hypertensive rats.

Signalosome Multifunctional protein complex involved in many regulatory processes, including development and probably regulation of protein degradation.

siRISC siRNA-programmed RISC.

siRNA Small interfering RNA. Sometimes known as short interfering RNA. They are a class of 20–25 nucleotide-long RNA molecules that interfere with the expression of genes.

Small G proteins Superfamily of guanine nucleotide-binding proteins including Ras, Rho, Rab, Ran, and ADP ribosylation factor(s), which act as molecular switches to regulate cardiac myocyte hypertrophy and survival associated with cell growth and division, cytoskeletal events, vesicular transport, and myofibrillar apparatus. As with heterotrimeric G proteins, they are activated by exchange of GDP to GTP, and inactivated by return to a GDP-bound state but not mediated by agonist-occupied receptors rather primarily mediated by activation of guanine nucleotide exchange factors (GEFs).

SMC Smooth muscle cell.

SNGFR Single nephron filtration rate.

SNP Single nucleotide polymorphism.

SOD Superoxide dismutase. An antioxidant ROS-scavenging enzyme with both mitochondrial and cytosolic isoforms.

Southern blot Detection of separated DNA restriction fragments after size separation on agarose gels, transfer to membranes, and hybridization with labeled gene probes.

SPECT Single-photon emission computed tomography used to assess myocardial metabolism and screen for CAD.

SPI Serine protease inhibitors, termed as serpins are key regulators of numerous cardiovascular pathways that initiate inflammation, coagulation, angiogenesis, apoptosis, extracellular matrix composition and complement activation responses.

SR Sarcoplasmic reticulum. A network of internal membranes in muscle-cell cytosol that contain high Ca^{2+} concentration, which is released on excitation.

SRE Serum response element.

Statins HMG-CoA reductase inhibitors used to treat patients with elevated plasma LDL.

SUMO Small ubiquitin-like modifier.

SV Single ventricle.

SVR Systemic vascular resistance.

T3 Triiodothyronine.

TCA cycle Tricarboxylic acid cycle (see Krebs cycle).

TD Tangier disease, a rare monogenic autosomal co-dominant atherosclerotic disease characterized by the absence of HDL and very low plasma levels of apoA. It is caused by mutations in the ATP binding cassette transporter gene (*ABCA1*).

Telomerase An enzyme that recognizes the G-rich strand, and elongates it using an RNA template that is a component of the enzyme itself.

Telomere Special structure containing tandem repeats of a short G-rich sequence present at the end of a chromosome.

TERC Telomerase RNA component.

TERT Telomerase reverse transcriptase catalytic subunit.

TF Tissue factor.

TGF Transforming growth factor.

TH Thyroid hormone (also thyroxin), a stimulus of cardiac hypertrophic growth and myocardial mitochondrial biogenesis.

Thrombospondins Family of extracellular matrix glycoproteins with a role in platelet adhesion, modulation of vascular injury, coagulation, angiogenesis and MI.

TIM Protein complex in mitochondrial inner membrane required for protein import.

Titin Large polypeptide, anchored in the Z-disc spanning the sarcomere; contributes to sarcomere organization, myofibrillar elasticity, and myofibrillar cell signaling.

TLR Toll-like receptors involved in the innate-immunity signaling response of the macrophage, including pattern-recognition of pathogens and oxidized LDL, leukocyte recruitment and production of local inflammation and downstream signaling in atherosclerotic progression.

TNF-α Tumor necrosis factor α.

TOM Protein complex in mitochondrial outer membrane required for protein import.

Topoisomerases Enzymes that change the supercoiling of DNA.

tPA Tissue-type plasminogen activator, a primary regulator of fibrinolysis.

TR Thyroid hormone receptor, mediates both nuclear genomic effects of TH (largely as a transcription factor) as well as non-genomic effects of TH.

Transcript Specific RNA product of DNA transcription.

Transcription factor Protein required for the initiation of transcription by RNA polymerase at specific sites and functioning as a regulatory factor in gene expression.

Transcriptome Comprehensive transcript analysis for expression profiling.

Transgenesis Introduction an exogenous gene – called a transgene –into a living organism so that the organism will exhibit a new property, and transmit that property to its offspring.

Transgenic animal Animal that has stably incorporated one or more genes from another cell or organism.

Translation Synthesis of protein from the mRNA template at the ribosome.

Transposons Sequences of DNA that can move/transpose around to different locations within the genome of a cell.

TRF2 Telomere repeat-binding factor, telomere-associated protein critical for the control of telomere structure and function.

Triplet Repeat Syndromes Inherited neuromuscular disorders caused by expanded repeats of trinucleotide sequences within specific genes including Friedreich ataxia (FA) and myotonic muscular dystrophy (MMD).

tRNA Transfer RNA. A small RNA molecule used in protein synthesis as an adaptor between mRNA and amino acids.

Troponin C Part of a troponin complex that together with tropomyosin affects the interaction between actin and myosin leading to the development of myocardial contraction.

TTP Thrombotic thrombocytopenic purpura, an autosomal recessive relapsing form of severe thrombotic microangiopathy characterized by marked thrombocytopenia, systemic platelet aggregation, erythrocyte fragmentation, and organ ischemia and caused by mutations in the *ADAMTS13* gene.

TUNEL Terminal deoxynucleotidyl transferase dUTP nick end labeling.

Ubiquitylation Modification of a protein by the covalent attachment of one or more ubiquitin monomers.

UCP Uncoupling protein.

Uncoupler Protein or other molecule capable of uncoupling electron transport from oxidative phosphorylation.

UNOS United Network for Organ Sharing.

uPA Urokinase-type plasminogen activator.

UTR 3' untranslated region A section of mRNA following the coding region that contains several types of regulatory sequences that affect mRNA stability and translation, including microRNA-target sites.

Vasculogenesis The de novo formation of the first primitive vascular plexus and post-natal vascularization.

VCAM-1 Vascular cell adhesion molecule.

VDAC Voltage-dependent anion channel in mitochondrial outer membrane (see porin).

VDR Vitamin D receptor, involved in signaling cardiac morphogenesis.

VEGF Vascular endothelial growth factor.

Versican An ECM-localized chondroitin sulfate proteoglycan, which binds HA, is expressed in the pathways of neural crest cell migration and in prechondrogenic regions and has been associated with valvulogenesis in the developing heart.

VGCC Voltage-gated calcium channels.

VLCAD Very long-chain acyl-CoA dehydrogenase; enzyme involved in mitochondrial β-oxidation of fatty acids.

VLDL Very low density lipoprotein, a triglyceride-rich lipoprotein containing apoB100, which progressively becomes enriched in cholesteryl ester (CE) as a result of CE transfer from HDL and is converted by lipolysis to LDL and/or taken up as VLDL remnants by the liver.

von Willebrand disease Most common human congenital bleeding disorder, in which both quantitative and qualitative abnormalities of the vWF glycoprotein have been implicated.

VSD Ventricular septal defect.

vWF von Willebrand factor.

Western blot Immunochemical detection of proteins immobilized on a filter after size separation by PAGE.

Wild-type The common genotype or phenotype of a given organism occurring in nature.

WPW Wolff–Parkinson–White syndrome presents with hypertrophic cardiomyopathy, ventricular preexcitation, conduction defects, and accumulation of cardiac glycogen.

X-linked inheritance The presence of the gene of interest on the X-chromosome.

XO Xanthine oxidase, cytosolic enzyme involved in purine metabolism, involved in myocardial ROS production (e.g., superoxide radicals) particularly after I/R injury.

Z-discs Cardiomyocyte components positioned at the junction between the cytoskeleton and the myofilaments, providing a physical connection between the sarcomere, nucleus, membrane and sarcoplasmic reticulum (SR) with role in cardiac contraction and signaling.

Index

A

AAV. *See* Adeno-associated virus
AC. *See* Adenylyl cyclase
Acetyl-CoA carboxylase (ACC), 282
Acetyl-L-carnitine (ALCAR), 344–345
ACS. *See* Acute coronary syndrome; Adult cardiac stem cells
Acute coronary syndrome (ACS), 318, 432, 433
Acute heart failure syndrome (AHFS)
    categories, 10
    classification, 10
    definition, 10, 11
Adenine nucleotide translocator (ANT), 281
Adeno-associated virus (AAV), 393, 397
Adenomonophosphate activated protein kinase
    (AMPK), 282
Adenylyl cyclase (AC), 319
β-Adrenergic receptor kinase (β–ARK), 399
Adrenergic receptors (ARs), 177
α-Adrenergic receptor signaling
    changes, myocardial hypertrophy and failure, 166
    functional differences, 166
Adult cardiac stem (ACS) cells
    advantages and limitations, 417
    ex vivo gene modification, 418
Advanced glycation endproduct (AGE), 317
Adverse drug events (ADE), 345
AF. *See* Atrial fibrillation
Aging, cardiomyopathy and HF
    autophagy process
        coupled mitochondrial and lysosomal defects, 324
        macromolecules and organelles degradation, 325
        steps, 324
    biomarkers
        BNP and NT-proBNP, 359, 360
        BNP level, 343
        definition, 359
        interleukin-6 (IL-6), 343–344
        natriuretic peptide testing, 359, 360
    classification, 354
    clinical evaluation, patient
        CR and EKG, 356
        HIV screening, 357
        sensitivity and specificity, 355, 357
    clinical presentation and diagnostic challenges
        cardinal symptoms, 342
        cognitive impairment, 343
    CRT
        clinical and echocardiographic response, 346
        effects, elder *vs.* younger patients, 345–346
        survival rate, heart transplantation, 346–347
        usage, 345

DCM
    lamin A/C intracellular functions, 332–333
    LGMD, 332
    mutation, gene varieties, 330–332
    NICM and ICM specimens, 330
    subclasses detection, 329
definition, 353
description, 341, 353
diagnostic tests, 359
disease management programs, 345
echocardiography role
    preserved systolic function, 358–359
    systolic dysfunction, 357
    valvular regurgitation, 358
etiologies, 354
etiologies and precipitating factors, 342
evaluation, 353
HCM
    causing gene, 328–329
    mutations, 328
inflammatory signaling
    adrenergic and muscarinic receptors, 318–319
    cellular damage/cell loss, 322
    CRP level data, 318
    GH and IGF-I, 321–322
    GPCR, 319–320
    IL-6 and IL-1β markers, 318
    SERCA and thyroid hormone, 320–321
myocardial remodeling
    CPC and p66(Shc) longevity gene, 327
    DHF and SHF, 328
    fibroblasts activation, 327–328
    muscle mass loss, 325–326
    telomere length, 326
pathophysiology
    cardiomyocytes loss, 341
    cellular organelles interaction, 342
    mitochondrial stress response, 341
pharmacological therapy
    ADE, 345
    atypical clinical feature, frail elderly, 344–345
    HF-PEF, 344
    outcome trials, 344
RCM
    causes, 333
    hereditary hemochromatosis, 333
    HFE mutations, 333–334
    TTR mutation, 333
RHF
    causes, 355
    diagnosis, 355, 356

ROS
  FVB myocytes, 318
  generation and antioxidant enzymes, 316
  iNOS, 318
  mitochondrial OXPHOS, 317
  NADPH oxidase, 317
  role, 315
  somatic mtDNA damage, 316, 317
  telomeres
    and cell proliferation, 322, 323
    EPC, 323
    estrogen, 323
    in human and animal CVD, 324, 326
    length, 322
    mitochondrial dysfunction, 324, 325
  types, 354
AHFS. *See* Acute heart failure syndrome
Akt. *See* Protein kinase B (PKB)
ALCAR. *See* Acetyl-L-carnitine
AMP-dependent kinase A anchoring proteins (AKAPs)
  PKA function, 174
  targeting, 174
AMPK. *See* Adenomonophosphate activated protein kinase
Anemia
  definition, 263
  rHuEPO, 263
Animal models
  clinical phenotype, 110
  compensated cardiac hypertrophy, transition models
    cardiac remodeling and dysfunction, 113–114
    cardiomyopathic hamster, 112
    coronary artery ligation and
      microembolization, 112–113
    Dahl salt-sensitive rats, 111
    fluid retention and edema, 115
    neurohormonal and cytokine activation, 115–117
    pacing induced cardiomyopathy, 113
    SHR, 111–112
  mitochondria
    clinical studies, 94
    cytosolic proteins, defects, 93–94
    DNA integrity, transgenic mice, 89–91
    enzyme dysfunction, 82–87
    nuclear communication, 87–89
    PGC-1, 91–92
    PPARs, 92–93
    transcription, 89
    transgenic mice, 9
  pressure and volume overload
    aortic regurgitation, 109–110
    chronic mitral regurgitation, 111
    hypertrophy, 111
    Na^+/Ca^{2+}-exchanger, 110
  rat myocardium, 109
  transgenic
    antioxidants and ROS, 121
    genetic, 121–122
    metabolic defects, 120–121
    mutations, sarcomeric and intermediate filament
      proteins, 117–118
    signal transduction pathways, 118–120
ANP. *See* Atrial natriuretic peptide
ANT. *See* Adenine nucleotide translocator
Anteroventral third ventricle (AV3V), 237–238
Antioxidants therapy
  ACE inhibitors

    and carvedilol anti-oxidative properties, 205
    treatment, 205
  oxygen radical, 204
ARs. *See* Adrenergic receptors
Atrial fibrillation (AF)
  description, 265
  development, 265–266
  prediction, 365, 366
  rate control *vs.* rhythm control, 266
  risk, 265–266
  treatment, 266–267
  trial design, 266
Atrial natriuretic peptide (ANP), 359

B
Berlin Heart EXCOR device, 298–299
Best Pharmaceuticals for Children Act, 273
Bioenergetics and metabolic changes, failing heart
  abnormal fatty acid and glucose metabolism
    high-energy phosphates, 55
    LCFA transporters, 55
  animal and cellular models
    cardiac phenotypes, 57
    glucose utilization, 58
    isolated cardiomyocyte, 55
    lactate production, 58
    LCM, 58–59
    lipotoxicity, 59
    mRNA down-regulation, 56
    null mutations, 59
    PGC-1α overexpression, 58
    PPAR-α, 56–57
    RXR-α embryos, 59
  cardiomyocyte
    fatty acid transport, 48–49
    glucose transport, 49–51
  cellular location, FAO and glucose oxidation
    glycolytic enzymes, 51
    peroxisomal enzymes, 51
    PPAR regulation, 51
    transcriptional control mechanisms, 52
  diagnostics and metabolic therapies
    acylcarnitine analysis, 60
    β-blocker treatment, 59–60
    carnitine level determination, 60
    free fatty acids, 61
    polyunsaturated fatty acids, 61
    PPAR subtypes, 60
    ranolazine, 61
  down-regulation, 45
  fatty acid and glucose oxidation
    acetyl-CoA, 46
    AMPK, 48
    glycogen turnover, 47–48
    mitochondrial pathways, intersection, 46
    β-oxidation, 45–46
    PDC complex, 47
    phosphorylation, 47
  mitochondrial fatty acid β-oxidation
    cardiac remodeling and apoptosis, 53–54
    metabolism defects, 52–53
  molecular players and events
    CPT-II and MTP, 54
    MCAD and VLCAD, 54
    PGC-1, 55, 56
    PPAR, 45, 53–54

tissue-specific changes
    energy metabolism, alterations, 60
    skeletal muscle, 59
BMC. *See* Bone marrow cell
BNP. *See* Brain natriuretic peptide; B-type natriuretic peptide
Bone marrow cell (BMC) transplantation
    advantages, 415
    limitations/concerns, 415–416
Brain natriuretic peptide (BNP), 24, 25, 162, 274, 353, 359, 360, 365, 432, 433
B-type natriuretic peptide (BNP), 226, 247, 260, 267, 343, 353, 436

C

CABG. *See* Coronary artery bypass grafting
CAD. *See* Coronary artery disease
Calcium cycling, cardiac function
    changes, 16
    entry, plasma membrane
        cardiac myocytes, 16
        L-type Ca^{2+} channels, 15–16
        reduced expression, 16–17
    release, sarcoplasmic reticulum
        excitation–contraction coupling, 17
        ryanodine receptors, 17
    removal
        phospholamban, 18
        protein phosphorylation, 18
        SERCA2a, 18–19
    sarcoplasmic reticulum storage, 18
    sensitivity
        myocardial contraction, 17
        phosphorylation, 18
        troponin C, 17–18
    transients, 19
Calcium signaling
    Ca^{2+}-mediated
        calcineurin/calmodulin, 173–174
        sarcolemmal/stress-dependent pathways, 172–173
        transport and metabolism changes, 171–172
    effectors
        adenylyl cyclase, 185
        caveolae/caveolins, 186
        phospholipase C, 185
    extracellular signals and matrix, 188
    GPCRs
        β-ARK1, 176
        desensitization mechanism, 176
        GRKs pathophysiological role, 176
    MAP kinases, 176–177
    metabolic signals, 187–188
    PKA
        compartmentalization, 174
        leucine zipper motifs, 174
        structural organization, 174
    PKC
        anchoring proteins, 175
        cardiac phenotype, 174–175
    PKG
        cGMP, 175
        dependent pathways, 176
        intracellular mechanisms, 175–176
    receptors
        ARs, 177
        G-proteins, 183–184
        growth transcription factors, 179–178
        mAChR, 177

        neurohumoral, 177–179
        nuclear transcription factors, 184–185
        protease activated, 181
        TLR, 180–181
        tyrosine kinases, 181–183
    stress signals, 187
    transcription factors
        NF-κB, 186
        PPAR-α and cofactors, 187
Caloric restriction (CR)
    animal models, 140
    SIR2 activation, 140–141
Cardiac biomarkers, HF
    Kaplan–Meier analysis, 432
    multimarkers analysis, 433
    pathological process, 432
Cardiac contractility modulation (CCM), 436
Cardiac progenitor cells (CPCs), 327
Cardiac remodeling
    definition, 213
    ECM
        and cardiomyocyte cytoskeleton, 221–222
        metalloproteinases, 222–223
        perspectives, 222
    electrical, secondary and ventricular dysrhythmias
        T-wave memory, 223
        vs. ventricular tachycardia (VT), 223–224
    myocardial metabolism and neurohormonal signaling
        cell death and renewal, 219–221
        cellular hypertrophy, 218–219
        contractile elements, 218
        neurohormonal changes and cytokines, 217–218
        transgenic models, 216–217
    progression and transition, overt HF
        diacylglycerol, 214–215
        factors, 214
        mitochondrial UCP-2 gene expression, 215–216
        myocardial energy metabolism, 215
        neurohormonal/cytokine activation, 214
        pressure and volume, 215
    reversing
        LVADs, patients, 224–225
        remodeling and CRT, 225
        therapy approaches, 225–226
Cardiac resynchronization therapy (CRT)
    QRS duration, 382, 384
    REVERSE study, 384–385
    unplanned hospitalization, 383
    use, HF patients, 225
    ventricular dyssynchrony, 384
Cardiac stem cells (CSCs)
    ACS cells, 416–417
    description, 416
Cardiomyocytes
    fatty acid transport
        carnitine, 48–49
        import and oxidation, mitochondrial, 49
        metabolic utilization, 48
        metabolite malonyl CoA, 49
    glucose transport
        cardiac hypertrophy, 50–51
        diabetic cardiomyopathy, 50
        Goto-Kakizaki (GK) rat, 50
        insulin, 50
        metabolic flexibility, 51
        transmembrane glucose gradient, 49

Cardiorenal syndrome (CRS)
    classification, 245–246
    definition, 246
    type 1, 246
    type 3, 247
Cardiovascular diseases (CVDs), 432, 442
Cardiovascular profile score (CVPS), 278
Catalase (CA), 316
CCM. *See* Cardiac contractility modulation
Cell death and renewal
    apoptotic process, 219
    extrinsic and intrinsic pathways, 219–220
    homeostatic mechanism, 221
    protooncogenes expression, 220–221
Central and autonomic nervous system
    cytokine-CNS connection
        immune activation, 239
        PGE2, 239
    humoral heart–brain signaling
        AV3V, 237–238
        blood–borne neuroactive peptides, 236
        metabolic activity, 236–237
        mineralcorticoid receptors, 238–239
        renin–angiotensin–aldosterone system (RAAS), 238
    imbalance, 236
CHD. *See* Congenital heart defects; Coronary heart disease
Chemokine fractalkine (CX3CL1), 366
Chest roentgenogram (CR), 356
CHF. *See* Congestive HF
Chronic HF treatment
    algorithm, 388, 389
    CRT
        QRS duration, 382, 384
        REVERSE study, 384–385
        unplanned hospitalization, 383
        ventricular dyssynchrony, 384
    heart transplantation
        bicaval technique, 388
        MCS, 387
    ICD therapy
        ACC/AHA/HRS 2008 Guidelines, 386
        amiodarone, 385
        dysrhythmias, 385
        Stage D disease, 387
        trials, 386
    measures
        dietary instruction, 379
        exercise training programs, 380–381
        quality of life, 380
    pharmacologic therapy
        ACE inhibitors, 381–382
        β-blockers, 381
    prognostic model, 379
Chronic obstructive airway disease (COPD)
    β-blockers, 261
    diagnosis, 260–261
CK. *See* Creatine kinase
CK-MB. *See* Creatine kinase isoenzyme MB
Cognitive dysfunction, elderly
    delirium, 264–265
    depression, 264
    prevalence, 264
    screening instruments, 265
Comorbidities
    AF (*See* Atrial fibrillation)
    anemia, 263

cognitive dysfunction, elderly
    delirium, 264–265
    depression, 264
    prevalence, 264
    screening instruments, 265
definition, 257
diabetes mellitus
    cardiomyopathy, 259
    patient management, 259–260
    prevalence, 258–259
dysrhythmias, 265
prevalence
    data, 257–258
    risk, 258
pulmonary disorders, 260–261
renal dysfunction
    mechanism, 261
    patient management, 262–263
    risk, 262
Congenital heart defects (CHD), 273, 297
Congestive HF (CHF), 273–274
Coronary artery bypass grafting (CABG), 366
Coronary artery disease (CAD), 353
Coronary heart disease (CHD), 342
CPCs. *See* Cardiac progenitor cells
CR. *See* Caloric restriction; Chest roentgenogram
C-reactive protein (CRP), 318
Creatine kinase isoenzyme MB (CK-MB), 368
CRP. *See* C-reactive protein
CRS. *See* Cardiorenal syndrome
CRT. *See* Cardiac resynchronization therapy
CSCs. *See* Cardiac stem cells
CVDs. *See* Cardiovascular diseases
CVPS. *See* Cardiovascular profile score
CX3CL1. *See* Chemokine fractalkine
Cyclic nucleotides signaling
    α-adrenergic receptor
        functional differences, 166
        myocardial hypertrophy and failure, 166
    AMP and β-adrenergic receptors
        cardiac myocytes, 164
        cyclic AMP effectors, 165
        myocardial hypertrophy and failure, 165–166
        norepinephrine effect, 165
    and contractile function, 161
    GMP
        AMP level, 163
        degradation, 163
        effectors, 163
        production, guanylyl cyclase activation, 162–163
    myocardial hypertrophy and failure
        changes, GMP, 164
        GMPand natriuretic peptide levels, 163–164
        hypertrophy and HF, cyclic GMP, 164
        nitric oxide effects, 164
Cytomegalovirus (CMV), 308

D
DCD. *See* Donation after cardiac death
DCM. *See* Dilated cardiomyopathy
Defibrillator in acute myocardial infarction trial (DYNAMIT), 386
DHF. *See* Diastolic heart failure
Diabetes mellitus
    cardiomyopathy, 259
    patient management
        toxic effect mycardium, 259–260

treatment, 259
prevalence, 258–259
Diastolic heart failure (DHF), 328
Dicer expression, 29
Dilated cardiomyopathy (DCM)
    Dicer expression, 29
    estimated freedom, 275
    gene mutations, 37
    idiopathic, 24
    lamin A/C intracellular functions, 332–333
    LGMD, 332
    mutation, gene varieties, 330–332
    NICM and ICM specimens, 330
    subclasses detection, 329
Donation after cardiac death (DCD), 300, 302

E
ECM. *See* Extracellular matrix
ECMO. *See* Extracorporeal membrane oxygenation
EDMD. *See* Emery–Dreifuss muscular dystrophy
Effectors signaling
    adenylyl cyclase, 185
    caveolae/caveolins, 186
    phospholipase C, 185
Ejection fraction (EF), 354, 357, 358
Electrical remodeling secondary
    cardiac myocytes, 223
    ventricular dysrrhythmias *vs.* VT, 222–223
Electron transport chain (ETC), 52, 74, 143, 144, 201, 317, 396, 411
EMB. *See* Endomyocardial biopsy
Embryonic stem (ES) cell
    differentiation, 409–410
    nitric oxide (NO) generation, 410
    signaling pathways, 410–411
    transplantation
        advantages, 411
        limitations and concerns, 412–413
Emery–Dreifuss muscular dystrophy (EDMD), 332
Endomyocardial biopsy (EMB), 303
Endothelial progenitor cells (EPCs), 323
Enzyme dysfunction, mitochondria
    activities, 83
    cardiac metabolism, 82
    lipid peroxidation, 83
    myocardial apoptosis and oxidative stress levels, 83
    paced canine hearts, 82
    peptide levels, 84
    PKD phosphorylates, 87
    ROS, 82–83
    selected enzymes, mongrel dogs, 85, 86
    sub-populations, 84–85
    targeted therapies, 86
    thioredoxin, 87
    transcription, 84
    western immunoblot analysis, 83–84
EPCs. *See* Endothelial progenitor cells
ES cell. *See* Embryonic stem (ES) cell
Excitation contraction coupling (ECC), 17, 19, 96, 109, 172, 218, 398
Extracellular matrix (ECM)
    cardiac remodeling, 431
    and cardiomyocyte cytoskeleton, 221–222
    metalloproteinases, 222–223
    perspectives, 222
    production, 328
Extracorporeal membrane oxygenation (ECMO)
    Berlin Heart EXCOR device, 298–299

cardiopulmonary resuscitation, 298
mechanical circulatory support, 297–298
MEDOS-HIA VAD device, 299
MicroMed DeBakey VAD® device, 299
usage, 298

F
FAO. *See* Fatty acid oxidation
Fatty acid metabolism defects
    Barth syndrome, 52–53
    carnitine deficiency, 53
    and glucose, 53–54
    inherited, 52
Fatty acid oxidation (FAO)
    β-oxidation, 46
    cellular location, 51–52
    down-regulation, 45, 56
    gene transcription, 59
    inhibition, 61
    lamb heart increase, 282
    PPAR, 55
    ranolazine treatment, 61
    regulation, 45
Fetal heart failure
    arterial Doppler, 280
    combined cardiac ventricular output
        distribution, 277
    course, 277
    etiology, 277
    foramen ovale, 278
    heart size, 279–280
    hydrops, 279
    MHC profile, 278
    serum albumin level, 278
    treatment, 280
    umbilical venous Doppler, 279
Fibroblast growth factor (FGF), 395
Fontan procedure. *See* Single ventricle (SV) physiology

G
Gene profiling, failing heart
    DNA modification-methylation
        cardiac troponin gene, 34
        CpG methylation, 33
        epigenetic role model, 34
        hyperhomocysteinemia, 34
        hypomethylation, 35
    energy metabolism profiling
        LVAD treatment, 36
        metabolic switch, 35
        PPAR family, 35–36
    epigenetics
        chromatin remodeling regulators, 33
        heterochromatin assembly regulation, 33
        histone acetylation/chromatin remodeling, 32–33
        histone/chromatin modifications, 32
    expression
        molecular signature analysis, 24
        oligonucleotide microarrays, 24
        patient subgroups, 24
        post-translational and translational processes, 25
        transcriptomic biomarkers, 24–25
    global and specific analysis
        polymorphic variants, 26
        remodeling, 25
        susceptibility/modifier genes/RNAi, 25–27

Gene profiling, failing heart (*Con't*)
   human
      cardiac hypertrophy program, 37
      fetal gene activation, 37
      modifier genes, 38
      mutations, 37–38
      Ser49Gly polymorphism, 38
   intracellular calcium cycling profiling
      muscle contraction, 36
      phospholamban, 36
      protein dephosphorylation, 36–37
   microRNAs
      Alu transcription, 27
      biogenesis pathway, 28
      bioinformatic-prediction algorithms, 30
      cardiac, 29
      cardiomyocytes apoptosis, 30
      decipher gene expression regulation, 29
      definition, 27
      Dicer mutant muscles, 29
      dysregulated expression, 32
      guide molecules, 27
      mouse cardiovascular system, 29
      selective silencing, 28
      thyroid hormone nuclear receptor, 31
      transcription factor, 30
      validated heart/muscle-specific, 31
   myocardial function, 23
   transcriptional coactivator p300
      abnormal function, 35
      acetyltransferase activity, 35
Gene therapy, HF
   angiogenesis, 396
   antisense oligonucleotides, 400–402
   β-ARK, 399
   cardiac dysrhythmias, 398
   clinical studies, 399–400
   coronary artery restenosis, 395
   hypertension, 396–397
   myocardial protection, 398
   myocarditis, 398
   ribozymes, 400
   RNA interference, 402–403
   SERCA2, 398–399
   SGCD, 393
   vectors and targets
      AAV, 394
      approaches, 400
      cardiomyocyte and endothelial cell, 395, 396
      comparison, gene transfer and expression, 393, 394
      delivery methods, 393
      targeted gene expression, 394, 395
      transgene expression, 394
Genetic and molecular changes, HF
   bioengineering
      biological pacemaker, 440
      scaffolds, 440
      stem cell biology, 440
   bioinformatics/computational biology, 441
   bionic role, 435–436
   diagnostic challenges and counseling, 438–439
   integrative approach
      cardiac biomarkers, 432–433
      cardiac remodeling, 431
      microarray and biomarkers, 434
      myocyte loss, 431–432

      proteomics, 433–434
   mitochondria role
      biolistic transformation, 434
      mitoQ, 435
      PNA-oligonucleotides, 434
      therapeutic strategies, 435
   modeling systems approaches, 436–437
   therapeutic options
      animal models, 439
      transgenic models, 439
   translational findings
      β-blockers, 438
      CVD, 437
      patient subgroup analysis, 438
   vessel and genetic engineering, 440–441
GFP. *See* Green fuorescent protein
GH-releasing hormone (GHRH), 321
Glomerular filtration rate (GFR)
   diuretics, 287
   filtration fraction, 241
   hemodynamics, 242
   humoral mechanisms, 243
   microcirculatory, 244
   type 1 cardiorenal syndrome, 247
Glomerular hemodynamics
   adjustment, 242
   changes, 241–242
Glutathione peroxidase (GPx), 316
G-protein-coupled receptors (GPCRs). *See also* Calcium signaling
   ARs, 177
   calcium signaling, 171
   cardiomyocyte growth, 152
   cell growth and proliferation, 132
   hormones and neurotransmitters exertion, 183
   inflammatory mechanisms/signaling, 319–320
   phospholipase C (PLC) activation, 172–173
   signaling cascade activation, 132
G-protein regulated kinases (GRKs)
   β-ARK1, 176
   desensitization mechanism, 176
Green fuorescent protein (GFP), 418, 419

H
Half-width duration (HWD), 317
HCM. *See* Hypertrophic cardiomyopathy
Heart failure (HF)
   clinical phenotypes
      acute, 10
      systolic *vs.* diastolic, 9–10
   definition, 3
   economic burden, 6
   gender, age and ethnicity
      ADHF, 8
      age-adjusted incidence rate, 8
      elderly patients, 7
      men, 7
      multivariable analyses, 9
      racial differences, multiracial Singapore, 8–9
      women, 6–7
   mortality and morbidity
      discharges, 6
      etiologic factors, 5
      hospital admission, 5–6
      NHANES I, 5
   prevalence and incidence
      age groups, 3

definition, 11
diastolic and systolic dysfunction, 4
Framingham heart study, 4
incident hospitalizations, 4
LVEF, 3–4
risk factors
diabetes, 5
valvular heart diseases, 4
Heart fatty-acid-binding protein (H-FABP), 368
Heart transplantation, pediatrics
acute rejection
definition, 302
late, 302
noninvasive surveillance, 304
description, 299–300
donor organ availability, 301–302
ECMO
Berlin Heart EXCOR device, 298–299
cardiopulmonary resuscitation, 298
mechanical circulatory support, 297–298
MEDOS-HIA VAD device, 299
MicroMed DeBakey VAD® device, 299
usage, 298
EMB-based strategies, 303–304
immunosuppression, 307–308
indications
complex anatomy, 301
HLHS, 301
infection/malignancies, 308
late outcomes
CAV computation, Kaplan–Meier method, 307
conditional survival, recipient age, 304, 305
early rejection, impact, 304, 305
graft loss rate, 304
quality of life, 306
rehospitalization, 306
risk factors, 5 year mortality, 304, 306
pediatric donor and recipient variables
early mortality, 307
T-cells, 307–308
recipient age and indications
infant *vs.* older, 300
survival rate, under 1 year, 300
rejection surveillance, infant recipients
cardiac allograft rejection, 303
ECHO-A, 302
grade 3(2R) cellular rejection, 302
techniques, 297
HF. *See* Heart failure
H-FABP. *See* Heart fatty-acid-binding protein
HF-preserved ejection fraction (HF-PEF), 344
HLHS. *See* Hypoplastic left heart syndrome
Human Genome Project (HGP), 315
Humoral mechanisms, 243
Hypertrophic cardiomyopathy (HCM)
causal subgroups, 275
causing gene, 328–329
mutations, 328
Hypoplastic left heart syndrome (HLHS), 298, 301

I
ICD therapy. *See* Internal cardiovertor defibrillator
ICM. *See* Ischemic cardiomyopathy
IFM. *See* Interfibrillar mitochondria
IGF-1. *See* Insulin-like growth factor-1
Implantable cardioverter defibrillator (ICD), 345, 348

Inducible nitric oxide synthase (iNOS), 318
Infants and children, HF
β-blockers, 290–291
cardiac energy metabolism
ATP production rate, 281
CPT-I activity, 282
energy balance and FAO, newborn heart, 283
clinical signs and symptoms, 276
diuretics
furosemide, 287
renal blood flow and GFR, 287
etiology
CHD, 273, 274
CHF treatment, 273–274
Ross scoring system, 274
fetal
etiology, 277
heart size, 279–280
hydrops, 279
treatment, 280
umbilical venous Doppler, 279
growth retardation and nutrition
CHF treatment, 274–275
DCM and HCM, 275–276
estimated freedom, death/transplantation, 275
PCMR database, 275
survival rates by age, 275–276
vicious downward cycle, 276
inotropic agents
digoxin, 288
dopamine, 288
TH levels, 288
T$_3$ supplementation, 288–289
usage, 287
neonatal
diastolic filling abnormalities, 281
postnatal drop, PVR, 280
ventricular interdependence, 281
pharmacology, 286
phosphodiesterase inhibitors, 289
right ventricular dysfunction, CHD
vs. left ventricle, 282
percutaneous placement, 285
progressive dilation, 283
regurgitant fraction, 283–284
SV physiology
atrial dysrhythmias, 285
bidirectional cavopulmonary anastomosis, 285
PLE, 286
vasodilator therapy
ACE inhibitors, 289–290
nitroprusside, 289
Inferior vena cava (IVC), 279
Inflammatory mechanisms, aging
cellular damage/cell loss, 322
GH and IGF-I
Klotho protein, 32
risk, HF, 321
GPCR
β1-and β2-ARs, 319
GRK activity, 320
mAChR density, 319
SERCA and thyroid hormone
SERCA2a role, 320
TH signaling, 320–321
iNOS. *See* Inducible nitric oxide synthase

Insulin-like growth factor-1 (IGF-1)
  animal models, 137
  HF progression, 137–138
  HR-treated cardiomyocytes, 137
  and insulin receptor, 136–137
  I/R injury, 137
  mitochondrial DNA damage, 137
  mTOR and SIR2, 140
Interfibrillar mitochondria (IFM)
  aging-related defects, 317
  oxidative function, 84
  pacing-associated decline, 85
Internal cardiovertor defibrillator (ICD) therapy
  ACC/AHA/HRS 2008 guidelines, 386
  amiodarone, 385
  dysrhythmias, 385
  Stage D disease, 387
  trials, 386
Invasive Monitoring Attenuation Through Gene Expression (IMAGE)
    study, 304
Ischemia and reperfusion (I/R), 137, 316, 333
Ischemic cardiomyopathy (ICM), 330
Ischemic preconditioning (IPC) model, 198
IVC. *See* Inferior vena cava

K

Kaplan–Meier method, 300, 305, 307, 368, 432

L

LCFA. *See* Long-chain fatty acid
LCM. *See* Lipotoxic cardiomyopathy
Left ventricle assisting devices (LVADs), 226
Left ventricular ejection fraction (LVEF)
    African American patients, 8
    definition, 3
Length of hospital stay (LOS), 347
Limb girdle muscular dystrophy (LGMD), 332
Lipotoxic cardiomyopathy (LCM), 58–59
Long-chain fatty acid (LCFA)
    accumulation, 60
    transporters, 55
LOS. *See* Length of hospital stay
Loss-of-function model systems, 216
LVADs. *See* Left ventricle assisting devices
LVEF. *See* Left ventricular ejection fraction

M

mAChR. *See* Muscarinic acetylcholine receptor
MAPK. *See* Mitogen-activated protein kinases
Matrix metalloproteinases (MMPS), 328
Mechanical circulatory support (MCS), 387
Medium-chain acyl-CoA dehydrogenase (MCAD)
    deficiency, 53, 54
    expression, 54
MEDOS-HIA VAD device, 299
Metabolic signals
    metabolites, cardiomyocyte responds, 187–188
    UCP levels, mitochondria, 188
3-methyladenine (3MA), 325
MHC. *See* Myosin heavy chain
MI. *See* Myocardial infarction
MicroMed DeBakey VAD® device, 299
Mitochondria receptors
    K_{ATP} channel, 145–146
    ROS
      cell signaling, 145

      generation and signaling, 146
      negative effect, 143–145
Mitochondria role, HF
  animal models
    clinical studies, 94
    cytosolic proteins, defects, 93–94
    DNA integrity, transgenic mice, 89–91
    enzyme dysfunction, 82–87
    nuclear–mitochondrial communication, 87–89
    PGC-1, 91–92
    PPARs, 92–93
    transcription, 89
    transgenic mice, 89
  apoptosis and necrosis
    antiapoptotic proteins, 79–80
    autophagic cell death, 82
    Bcl-2 proteins, 81
    ETC function, 81
    intrinsic pathway, 79, 80
    morphological differences, 81
    outer membrane proteins, 79
    upstream death, 80
  cellular and molecular changes, 97
  centrality, cardiac bioenergetics
    animal models, 75
    Ant1 gene, 76
    ATP levels, 73
    creatine kinase reaction, 74
    energy metabolism, interactions, 74
    gene defects, 76
    OXPHOS, 73–74
    pathways, 75, 77
  gene profiling
    fatty acid and glucose oxidation, 94
    metabolic genes, 95
  metabolic damage
    calcium handing, homeostasis and contractility, 96–97
    Ca^{2+} levels, 96
    contractile dysfunction and cardiac remodeling, 95
  ROS generation and antioxidant response
    antioxidants, 78
    catalase overexpression, 78–79
    pathophysiologic role, 79
    superoxide and hydroxyl radicals, 77–78
  tissue specific events, 97–98
Mitogen-activated protein kinases (MAPK), 213
Mitral valve regurgitation (MVR), 358
MLCK. *See* Myosin light chain kinase
MMF. *See* Mycophenolate mofetil
MMPS. *See* Matrix metalloproteinases
Module Map algorithm, 371
MPI. *See* Myocardial performance index
Multicenter automatic defibrillator implantation II (MADIT II) trial,
    386
Muscarinic acetylcholine receptor (mAChR)
    GPCR signaling, 319, 320
    inotropic and chronotropic effects, 177
    stimulation, 177
MVR. *See* Mitral valve regurgitation
Mycophenolate mofetil (MMF), 308
Myoblast cells transplantation
    adult skeleton, 413
    advantages, 413–414
    autologous, trial, 414–415
    limitation, 414
Myocardial cell-based regeneration, HF

ACS
  advantages and limitations, 417
  ex vivo gene modification, 418
BMC
  advantages, 415
  limitations/concerns, 415–416
CSCs
  ACS cells, 416–417
  description, 416
ES cell
  differentiation, 409–410
  nitric oxide (NO) generation, 410
  signaling pathways, 410–411
  transplantation
    advantages, 411
    limitations and concerns, 412–413
finding cell identity, 419
myoblast cells transplantation
  adult skeleton, 413
  advantages, 413–414
  autologous, trial, 414–415
  limitation, 414
reperfusion, 409
stem cell-type, use, 419, 420
techniques, 419–421
Myocardial infarction (MI), 432, 433
Myocardial metabolism and neurohormonal signaling
  cellular hypertrophy
    mechanism and signal, 218
    miRNAs, 218–219
  changes and cytokines, 217–218
  contractile elements, 218
  transgenic models
    cardiac PPAR-α/PGC-1α, 217
    fatty acid defects, 217
    gain of function, 217
    loss-of-function, 216
    metabolopathies, 216
    MHC-ACS, 217
Myocardial performance index (MPI), 279
Myocarditis, 398
Myosin heavy chain (MHC), 278, 320, 328
Myosin light chain kinase (MLCK), 172

N
National Health and Nutrition Examination Survey (NHANES-1), 3
Natriuretic peptides (NP), 245, 353, 359, 360
Neurohumoral signaling
  angiotensin
    angiotensin II, 178
    AT1 and AT2, 179
    intracellular signals, 179
    renal dysfunction-associated HF, model, 178–179
  endothelin
    activation, 178
    kinase-phosphorylation effects, 178
    norepinephrine pathway, 178
NP. See Natriuretic peptides
Nuclear communication, animal models
  biogenesis and bioenergetic pathways, 88
  PPARγ, 89
  programmed changes, 87

O
Orthotopic heart transplantation (OHT), 347
OS. See Oxidative stress

Oxidative phosphorylation (OXPHOS)
  ATP synthesis, 74
  mitochondrial dysfunction, 82
  myocyte contractile activity, 73
Oxidative stress (OS)
  antioxidant
    defense, 203–204
    and metabolic treatment, 206
    therapy, 204–205
  and apoptosis, 202
  myocardial ischemia
    CAD, 200
    mitochondria, 199–200
  nitric oxide
    endothelial dysfunction, 202–203
    ETC, 202
  ROS
    aging failing heart, 200–202
    and cardiac pathology, 197–198
    and cell signaling, 196–197
    effects, 196
    production, 195–196

P
PCMR. See Pediatric Cardiomyopathy Registry
PDC. See Pyruvate dehydrogenase complex
Peak shortening (PS), 317
Pediatric Cardiomyopathy Registry (PCMR), 275
Peptide nucleic acids (PNA), 434
Peripheral changes, HF
  central and autonomic nervous system
    autonomic imbalance, 236
    cytokine-CNS connection, 239
    humoral heart–brain signaling, 236–239
  CRS (See Cardiorenal syndrome (CRS))
  endothelial dysfunction
    endothelial NO synthase (eNOS), 247–248
    shear dependent mechanisms, 248
  immune and cytokine activation
    biological effects, 249
    proinflammatory, 249
    TNF-α blood levels, 249–250
  renal adaptation and alterations
    effector mechanisms abnormalities, 241
    glomerular hemodynamics, 241–242
    humoral mechanisms, 243
    natriuretic peptides, 245
    physical factors, 242–243
    prostaglandins, 245
    renin–angiotensin–aldosterone system, 243–245
    sensing mechanisms, 240–241
    sympathetic nervous system, 243
Peroxisome proliferator-activated receptor (PPAR)
  cardiac metabolism, 35
  interacting coactivators, 55
  isoforms, 92
  ligand complex, 54
  loss-and gain-of-function models, 35–36
  α null mouse hearts, 58
  α protein levels, 56–57
  subtypes, 60
Phospholamban (PLB), 317
PKA. See Protein kinase A
PKB. See Protein kinase B
PKC. See Protein kinase C
PKG. See Protein kinase G

PLE. *See* Protein-losing enteropathy
PNA. *See* Peptide nucleic acids
Poly(ADP-ribose) polymerase (PARP), 204
PPAR. *See* Peroxisome proliferator-activated receptor
Prophylatic Intravenous Use of Milrinone After Cardiac Operation
    in Pediatrics (PRIMACORP) study, 289
Prostaglandins, 245
Protease activated receptors
    classes, 181
    vascular development, 181
Protein kinase A (PKA). *See also* Calcium signaling
    cyclic AMP-dependent, 165
    high F(passive), 328
    phosphorylation, 147
Protein kinase B (PKB)
    Akt signaling, 134
    description, 132
    and glycogen synthase kinase, 135
    oxidative stress and apoptosis
        antiapoptotic factor, 133
        phosphorylation activation, 133–134
    pacing-induced HF
        Akt phosphorylation, 132–133
        canine model, 132
    rapamycin, mammalian target, 134–135
Protein kinase C (PKC). *See also* Calcium signaling
    activation, 190
    cardiomyocytes, 146
    dependent and independent mechanisms, 214
    isoenzymes, 185
    ROS-activated, 136
Protein kinase G (PKG). *See also* Calcium signaling
    Ca^{2+} dependent signaling pathway, 176
    NO/PKGI signal transduction pathway, 175
Protein-losing enteropathy (PLE), 286
Protein-protein interaction (PPI) network, 371–372
Proteomics application, HF
    analysis
        cardiac biopsies, 368
        H-FABP, 368
        Kaplan–Meier analysis, 368
        Mass spectrometry (MS) technology, 367
        multivariate Cox proportional hazard, 368
        plasma proteins, 367
        protein biochip array technology, 367
    BNP, 365
    cardiac expression modules/integrative bioinformatics
        gene expression and PPI network, 371–372
        Module Map algorithm, 371
    drug targets and drug metabolism, genetic influences
        β-blockers, 370
        genetic variability, 370
    gene profiling
        AF, 365
        CABG, 366
        CX3CL1, 366
        microarray technology, 366
    integrative biology approach
        feature, 372
        top-down and bottom-up analysis, phenome, 372–373
    metabolic imaging
        CK, 369–370
        magnetic resonance spectroscopy (MRS), 370
    metabolome
        definiton, 368–369
        measurements, 369

pharmacogenetics/pharmacogenomics, 370–371
PS. *See* Peak shortening
Pulmonary disorders, 260–261
Pyruvate dehydrogenase complex (PDC)
    oxidative decarboxylation, 47
    phosphorylation, 47

R
RAAS. *See* Renin-angiotensin-aldosterone system
Randomized controlled trial (RCT), 359
RAS. *See* Renin–angiotensin system
RCM. *See* Restrictive cardiomyopathy
Reactive oxygen species (ROS)
    aging failing heart
        ANT, 200–201
        antioxidant mechanisms, 200
        Ca^{2+}, 202
        VDAC, 201–202
    antioxidant defense
        cell-damaging, 203
        iron and copper ions sequestering, 203
        mitochondrial isoform, 203
        PARP, 204
        respiration uncoupling, mitochondria, 203
    cardiac pathology
        canine model, 197–198
        mitochondrial functional plasticity, 199
        nonmitochondrial NADPH oxidase, 199
        source, 198
    cell signaling, 196–197
    effects
        lipids, 196
        mitochondrial respiration, 196
        protein modification, 196
    FVB myocytes, 318
    generation and antioxidant enzymes, 316
    iNOS, 318
    metabolism, 197
    mitochondrial OXPHOS, 317
    NADPH oxidase, 317
    production
        cellular sources, 196
        hydroxyl radical reactivity, 195–196
        physiological conditions, 196
    role, 315
    somatic mtDNA damage, 316, 317
Receptor tyrosine kinases (RTKs)
    cardiomyocyte signaling pathways, 182
    classes, 181
    erbB2 RTK, 182–183
    ligand binding, 181–182
    phosphorylation, 182
    vascular cells, 183
Recombinant human erythropoietin (rHuEPO), 263
Recombinant human growth hormone (rhGH), 321
Remodeling therapy
    carvedilol ACE inhibitor remodeling mild CHF (CARMEN), 225
    LVADs, 226
    RESOLVD, 225–226
Renal dysfunction
    mechanism, 261
    patient management
        function worsening, 262–263
        renal vasoconstriction, 262
    risk, 262
Renal sympathetic nerve activity (RSNA), 237

Renin-angiotensin-aldosterone system (RAAS)
    glomerular microcirculatory changes, 244
    renal sodium retention, 244
    systemic vasodilatation, 244–245
Renin–angiotensin system (RAS), 397
Restrictive cardiomyopathy (RCM)
    causes, 333
    hereditary hemochromatosis, 333
    HFE mutations, 333–334
    TTR mutation, 333
Retinoid X receptors (RXR), 320
Reversing cardiac remodeling
    CRT, 225
    LVADs, patients
        impact, 224–225
        paired test analysis, 224
RHF. *See* Right heart failure
rhGH. *See* Recombinant human growth hormone
rHuEPO. *See* Recombinant human erythropoietin
Right heart failure (RHF)
    causes, 355
    diagnosis, 355, 356
Right ventricular failure (RVF), 282
ROS. *See* Reactive oxygen species
RSNA. *See* Renal sympathetic nerve activity
RTKs. *See* Receptor tyrosine kinases
RVF. *See* Right ventricular failure
RXR. *See* Retinoid X receptors

S
Sarcolemmal K_{ATP} channel, 141–142
Sarcoplasmic reticulum Ca^{2+} ATPase (SERCA2), 398–399
Sarcoplasmic reticulum Ca-ATPase (SERCA)
    cardiac isoform, 18
    phospholamban, 18–19
Sensing mechanisms
    blood flow, arterial to venous circuit, 240
    cardiac output, 240
    fluid transudation, 241
    pressure–volume relationship, 240–241
    sodium retention, 241
SERCA. *See* Sarcoplasmic reticulum Ca-ATPase
SERCA2. *See* Sarcoplasmic reticulum Ca^{2+} ATPase
SHF. *See* Systolic heart failure
SHR. *See* Spontaneous hypertensive rats
Signaling cascades
    growth and pro-survival pathways
        SIR/sirtuins, 138–140
        TOR, 140
    mitochondria
        calcium, 148–149
        K_{ATP} channel, 145–146
        kinases, 147
        nuclear gene activation, 142
        protein kinases, 147
        receptors, 142–145
        retrograde, 148
        survival and stress impact heart, 149
        translocation, 148
    permeability transition (PT) pore, 146–147
    physiological cardiovascular growth
        cyclin D1, 131–132
        GPCRs, 132
        molecular mechanisms, 131
    plasma membrane, 141–142
    P53 pathways, 149–150

prosurvival pathways, Akt
    activator (*See* Insulin-like growth factor-1 (IGF-1))
    cardiac activation, 135–136
    expression and function, 132
    glycogen synthase kinase, 133
    mammalian target of rapamycin, 134–135
    oxidative stress and apoptosis, 133–134
    paced-induced HF, 132–133
    PI3K, 136
Silent information regulator 2 (SIR2)
    action, 139
    deacetylase activity, 140
    expression, 139
    identification, 138–139
Single nephron filtration rate (SNGFR)
    glomerular hemodynamics, 241
    humoral mechanism, 243
Single ventricle (SV) physiology
    atrial dysrhythmias, 285
    bidirectional cavopulmonary anastomosis, 285
    PLE, 286
SIR2. *See* Silent information regulator 2
SIRT1/SIRT2, 139
SNGFR. *See* Single nephron filtration rate
SOD. *See* Superoxide dismutase
Spontaneous hypertensive rats (SHR)
    calcium cycling, 111
    calcium influx, 112
Stress signals, 186
Subsarcolemmal mitochondrial (SSM), 317
Sudden cardiac death in heart failure (SCD-HeFT) trial, 386
Superoxide dismutase (SOD), 316
Sympathetic nervous system, 243
Systemic vascular resistance (SVR), 290
Systolic heart failure (SHF), 328

T
Target of rapamycin (TOR)
    action critical aspect, 141
    mammalian TOR (mTOR), 141
    PT pore modulation, 141
    signaling expression, 141
TDI. *See* Tissue Doppler imaging
Telomerase reverse transcriptase holoenzyme (TERT), 323
Telomere repeat-binding factor (TRF2), 323
TERT. *See* Telomerase reverse transcriptase holoenzyme
TH. *See* Thyroid hormone
TH-responsive elements (TREs), 320
Thyroid hormone (TH), 288
Tissue Doppler imaging (TDI), 358, 361
TLR. *See* Toll-like receptors
Toll-like receptors (TLR)
    activation, 180
    innate immune response proteins expression, 180
    signaling cascade, 180–181
TOR. *See* Target of rapamycin
Transcription factors
    NF-κB, 186
    PPAR-α and cofactors, 187
Transgenic models
    antioxidants and ROS
        age-mediated accumulation, 121
        catalase overexpression, 121
    genetic
        age-mediated cardiomyopathy, 121
        Ca^{2+} homeostasis, 122

Transgenic models (*Con't*)
    catecholamines, 122
    SHR strains, 122
    X-linked cardiac hypertrophy, 122
  metabolic defects
    energy status, 120
    FAO pathways, 120
    gain of function/overexpression, 120
    genes, 121
  mutations, sarcomeric and intermediate filament proteins
    age-specific phenotypic expression, 117
    cardiomyopathy, 117
    genes, 118
    LMNA mutant model, 118
  signal transduction pathways
    cytokine signaling and inflammation, 119–120
    Gαq levels, 119
    genes, 118–119
    intracellular Ca^{2+}, 118
Transition models
  cardiac remodeling and dysfunction
    atrial fibrillation, 114
    echocardiographic parameters comparison, 114
    hemodynamic and neurohormonal parameters, 113
    vulnerability and atrial fibrillation comparison, 114
  cardiomyopathic hamster, 112
  coronary artery ligation and microembolization
    hexokinase activity, 112
    LV dysfunction, 113
    myocardial infarction, 112
  Dahl salt-sensitive rats, 111
  fluid retention and edema, 115
  neurohormonal and cytokine activation
    β-adrenergic stimulation, 116
    cytokine blockade, 116
    disease progression, 115
    endothelin-1, 115
    NOS, 117
    proinflammatory cytokines, 116
  pacing induced cardiomyopathy, 113
  SHR
    calcium influx, 112
    cardiac pump function, 111
TREs. *See* TH-responsive elements
TRF2. *See* Telomere repeat-binding factor
Triiodothyronine for Infants and Children Undergoing
    Cardiopulmonary Bypass (TRICC) study, 289

V

Vascular endothelial growth factor (VEGF), 396
VEGF. *See* Vascular endothelial growth factor
Ventricular assist devices (VAD), 297
Ventricular septal defects (VSD), 273
Voltage dependent L-type Ca^{2+} channels
    (VDCC), 172

X

Xanthine oxidase (XO), 315, 316